City Hospital

WB00020263

D1454394

ur   at date

SWBH NHS TRUST

SITE – DRH

Queenan's Management of
High-Risk Pregnancy

Queenan's Management of High-Risk Pregnancy

An Evidence-Based Approach

EDITED BY

JOHN T. QUEENAN, MD
Professor and Chairman Emeritus
Department of Obstetrics and Gynecology
Georgetown University School of Medicine
Washington, DC, USA

CATHERINE Y. SPONG, MD
Bethesda, MD, USA

CHARLES J. LOCKWOOD, MD
Anita O'Keeffe Young Professor and Chair
Department of Obstetrics, Gynecology and Reproductive Sciences
Yale University School of Medicine
New Haven, CT, USA

SIXTH EDITION

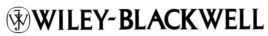
A John Wiley & Sons, Ltd., Publication

This edition first published 2012, © 2007, 1999 by Blackwell Publishing Ltd; 2012 by John Wiley and Sons, Ltd

Wiley-Blackwell is an imprint of John Wiley & Sons, Ltd, formed by the merger of Wiley's global Scientific, Technical and Medical business with Blackwell Publishing.

Registered office: John Wiley & Sons, Ltd, The Atrium, Southern Gate, Chichester, West Sussex, PO19 8SQ, UK

Editorial offices: 9600 Garsington Road, Oxford, OX4 2DQ, UK

The Atrium, Southern Gate, Chichester, West Sussex, PO19 8SQ, UK

350 Main Street, Malden, MA 02148-5020, USA

For details of our global editorial offices, for customer services and for information about how to apply for permission to reuse the copyright material in this book please see our website at www.wiley.com/wiley-blackwell.

Library of Congress Cataloging-in-Publication Data

Queenan's management of high-risk pregnancy : an evidence-based approach / edited by John T. Queenan, Catherine Y. Spong, Charles J. Lockwood. – 6th ed.
  p. ; cm.
Management of high-risk pregnancy
Rev. ed. of: Management of high-risk pregnancy / edited by John T. Queenan, Catherine Y. Spong, Charles J. Lockwood. 5th. 2007.
Includes bibliographical references and index.
ISBN-13: 978-0-470-65576-4 (hard cover : alk. paper)
ISBN-10: 0-470-65576-3 (hard cover : alk. paper)
1. Pregnancy–Complications.   I. Queenan, John T.   II. Spong, Catherine Y.
III. Lockwood, Charles J.   IV. Management of high-risk pregnancy.   V. Title:
Management of high-risk pregnancy.
[DNLM: 1. Pregnancy Complications.   2. Evidence-Based Medicine.   3. Pregnancy,
High-Risk.   WQ 240]
RG571.M24 2012
618.3–dc23
2011027303

A catalogue record for this book is available from the British Library.

Wiley also publishes its books in a variety of electronic formats. Some content that appears in print may not be available in electronic books.

Set in 9.25/12pt Palatino by Toppan Best-set Premedia Limited, Hong Kong
Printed and bound in Singapore by Markono Print Media Pte Ltd

1   2012

Contents

List of Contributors, vii

Foreword, xi

Preface, xii

Acknowledgments, xii

List of Abbreviations, xiii

Part 1 Factors of High-Risk Pregnancy

1 Overview of High-Risk Pregnancy, 1
John T. Queenan, Catherine Y. Spong,
and Charles J. Lockwood

2 Maternal Nutrition, 4
Edward R. Newton

3 Alcohol and Substance Abuse, 23
William F. Rayburn

4 Environmental Agents and Reproductive Risk, 32
Laura Goetzl

Part 2 Genetics

5 Genetic Screening for Mendelian Disorders, 41
Deborah A. Driscoll

6 Screening for Congenital Heart Disease, 47
Lynn L. Simpson

7 First- and Second-Trimester Screening for Fetal
Aneuploidy and Neural Tube Defects, 55
Julia Unterscheider and Fergal D. Malone

Part 3 Monitoring: Biochemical and Biophysical

8 Sonographic Dating and Standard Fetal Biometry, 63
Eliza Berkley and Alfred Abuhamad

9 Fetal Lung Maturity, 75
Alessandro Ghidini and Sarah H. Poggi

10 Antepartum Fetal Monitoring, 79
Brian L. Shaffer and Julian T. Parer

11 Interpreting Intrapartum Fetal Heart Tracings, 89
Michael Nageotte

Part 4 Maternal Disease

12 Sickle Cell Anemia, 93
Scott Roberts

13 Anemia, 98
Alessandro Ghidini

14 Thrombocytopenia, 102
Robert M. Silver

15 Inherited and Acquired Thrombophilias, 108
Michael J. Paidas

16 Thromboembolic Disorders, 121
Christian M. Pettker and Charles J. Lockwood

17 Cardiac Disease, 131
Stephanie R. Martin, Alexandria J. Hill,
and Michael R. Foley

18 Renal Disease, 151
David C. Jones

19 Pregnancy in Transplant Patients, 160
James R. Scott

20 Gestational Diabetes Mellitus, 168
Deborah L. Conway

21 Diabetes Mellitus, 174
George Saade

22 Hypothyroidism and Hyperthyroidism, 178
Brian Casey

23 Asthma, 183
Michael Schatz

24 Epilepsy, 193
Autumn M. Klein and Page B. Pennell

25 Chronic Hypertension, 204
Heather A. Bankowski and Dinesh M. Shah

26 Systemic Lupus Erythematosus, 209
Christina S. Han and Edmund F. Funai

27 Perinatal Infections, 218
    Jeanne S. Sheffield

28 Malaria, 231
    Richard M.K. Adanu

29 Group B Streptococcal Infection, 234
    Ronald S. Gibbs

30 Hepatitis, 238
    Patrick Duff

31 HIV Infection, 243
    Howard L. Minkoff

32 Pregnancy in Women with Physical
    Disabilities, 253
    Caroline C. Signore

Part 5 Obstetric Complications

33 Recurrent Spontaneous Abortion, 260
    Charles J. Lockwood

34 Cervical Insufficiency, 271
    John Owen

35 Gestational Hypertension, Preeclampsia, and
    Eclampsia, 280
    Labib M. Ghulmiyyah and Baha M. Sibai

36 Postpartum Hemorrhage, 289
    Michael A. Belfort

37 Emergency Care, 301
    Garrett K. Lam and Michael R. Foley

38 Rh and Other Blood Group Alloimmunizations, 307
    Kenneth J. Moise Jr

39 Multiple Gestations, 314
    Karin E. Fuchs and Mary E. D'Alton

40 Polyhydramnios and Oligohydramnios, 327
    Ron Beloosesky and Michael G. Ross

41 Prevention of Preterm Birth, 337
    Paul J. Meis

42 Pathogenesis and Prediction of Preterm Delivery, 346
    Catalin S. Buhimschi and Charles J. Lockwood

43 Preterm Premature Rupture of Membranes, 364
    Brian M. Mercer

44 Management of Preterm Labor, 374
    Vincenzo Berghella

45 Placenta Previa and Related Placental Disorders, 382
    Yinka Oyelese

Part 6 Complications of Labor and Delivery

46 Prolonged Pregnancy, 391
    Teresa Marino and Errol R. Norwitz

47 Induction of Labor, 399
    Nicole M. Petrossi and Deborah A. Wing

48 Cesarean Delivery, 406
    Michael W. Varner

49 Vaginal Birth After Cesarean Delivery, 414
    Mark B. Landon

50 Breech Delivery, 424
    Edward R. Yeomans and Larry C. Gilstrap

51 Operative Vaginal Delivery, 429
    Edward R. Yeomans

52 Obstetric Analgesia and Anesthesia, 434
    Gilbert J. Grant

53 Patient Safety, 439
    Christian M. Pettker

54 Neonatal Encephalopathy and Cerebral Palsy, 445
    *Maged M. Costantine, Mary E. D'Alton,
    and Gary D.V. Hankins*

Part 7 Procedures

55 Genetic Amniocentesis and Chorionic Villus
    Sampling, 453
    Ronald J. Wapner

56 Fetal Surgery, 464
    Robert H. Ball and Hanmin Lee

Index, 475

The color plate section can be found facing p. 192

List of Contributors

Alfred Abuhamad MD
Chairman, Department of Obstetrics and Gynecology
Director, Maternal-Fetal Medicine
Mason C. Andrews Professor of Obstetrics and Gynecology
Professor of Radiology
Eastern Virginia Medical School
Norfolk, VA, USA

Richard M.K Adanu MD, ChB, MPH, FWACS
Associate Professor of Obstetrics and Gynecology, Women's
Reproductive Health
University of Ghana Medical School
Accra, Ghana

Robert H. Ball MD
Associate Clinical Professor
Department of Obstetrics, Gynecology and Reproductive
Sciences
University of California
San Francisco, CA, USA

Heather A. Bankowski
Clinical Instructor, Maternal-Fetal Medicine
University of Wisconsin Medical School
Madison, WI, USA

Michael A. Belfort MBBCH, MD, PhD
Chairman and Professor
Department of Obstetrics and Gynecology
Baylor College of Medicine
Houston, TX, USA

Ron Beloosesky MD
Department of Obstetrics, Gynecology and Public Health
UCLA School of Medicine and Public Health;
Harbor-UCLA Medical Center
Torrance, CA, USA

Vincenzo Berghella MD
Professor
Department of Obstetrics and Gynecology
Thomas Jefferson University
Philadelphia, PA, USA

Eliza Berkley MD
Associate Professor
Department of Obstetrics and Gynecology
Eastern Virginia Medical School
Norfolk, VA, USA

Catalin S. Buhimschi MD
Associate Professor
Department of Obstetrics, Gynecology and Reproductive
Sciences
Yale University School of Medicine
New Haven, CT, USA

Brian Casey MD
Professor, Lead Doctor of Community Obstetrics
Department of Obstetrics and Gynecology
University of Texas Southwestern Medical Center
Dallas, TX, USA

Deborah L. Conway MD
Assistant Professor
Department of Obstetrics and Gynecology
University of Texas School of Medicine
San Antonio, TX, USA

Maged M. Costantine MD
Department of Obstetrics and Gynecology
University of Texas Medical Branch
Galveston, TX, USA

Mary E. D'Alton MD
Chair
Department of Obstetrics and Gynecology
Columbia University Medical Center;
Columbia Presbyterian Hospital
New York, NY, USA

Deborah A. Driscoll MD
Luigi Mastroianni Jr. Professor and Chair
Department of Obstetrics and Gynecology
Perelman School of Medicine at the University of Pennsylvania
Philadelphia, PA, USA

Patrick Duff MD
Professor of Obstetrics and Gynecology and Residency Program
Director
University of Florida College of Medicine
Gainesville, FL, USA

Michael R. Foley MD
Clinical Professor
Department of Obstetrics and Gynecology
University of Arizona
Tuscon, AZ, USA

Karin E. Fuchs MD
Assistant Clinical Professor
Department of Obstetrics and Gynecology
Columbia University Medical Center;
Columbia Presbyterian Hospital
New York, NY, USA

Edmund F. Funai MD
Professor
Department of Obstetrics and Gynecology
The Ohio State University College of Medicine
Columbus, OH, USA

Alessandro Ghidini MD
Professor of Obstetrics and Gynecology
Georgetown University Hospital
Washington, DC;
Perinatal Diagnostic Center
Inova Alexandria Hospital
Alexandria, VA, USA

Labib M. Ghulmiyyah
Department of Obstetrics and Gynecology
University of Cincinnati College of Medicine
Cincinnati, OH, USA

Ronald S. Gibbs MD
Professor and Chairman
Department of Obstetrics and Gynecology
University of Colorado School of Medicine
Denver, CO, USA

Larry C. Gilstrap III MD
Executive Director
American Board of Obstetrics and Gynecology
Dallas, TX, USA

Laura Goetzl MD, MPH
Associate Professor
Department of Obstetrics and Gynecology
Medical University of South Carolina
Charleston, SC, USA

Gilbert J. Grant MD
Associate Professor of Anesthesiology
New York University School of Medicine
New York, NY, USA

Christina S. Han MD
Assistant Professor
Department of Obstetrics and Gynecology
The Ohio State University College of Medicine
Columbus, OH, USA

Gary D. V. Hankins MD
Professor and Chairman
Department of Obstetrics and Gynecology
University of Texas Medical Branch
Galveston, TX, USA

Alexandria J. Hill MD
Department of Obstetrics and Gynecology
University of Arizona
Tucson, AZ, USA

David C. Jones MD
Associate Professor
Department of Obstetrics, Gynecology and Reproductive
Sciences
University of Vermont College of Medicine
Burlington, VT, USA

Autumn M. Klein MD, PhD
Department of Neurology
Brigham and Women's Hospital;
Harvard Medical School
Boston, MA, USA

Garrett K. Lam MD
Clinical Associate Professor
Dept of Obstetrics and Gynecology
University of Tennessee-Chattanooga
Chattanooga, TN

Mark B. Landon MD
Richard L. Meiling Professor and Chairman
Department of Obstetrics and Gynecology
Ohio State University
Columbus, OH, USA

Hanmin Lee MD
Associate Professor
Department of Surgery
Director, Fetal Treatment Center
University of California
San Francisco, CA, USA

Fergal D. Malone MD
Professor and Chairman
Department of Obstetrics and Gynaecology
Royal College of Surgeons in Ireland
Dublin, Ireland

Teresa Marino MD
Department of Obstetrics and Gynecology
Tufts Medical Center and
Tufts University School of Medicine
Boston, MA, USA

Stephanie R. Martin DO
Associate Professor
Department of Obstetrics and Gynecology
Baylor College of Medicine
Houston, TX, USA

Paul J. Meis MD
Professor Emeritus of Obstetrics and Gynecology
Department of Obstetrics and Gynecology
Wake Forest University School of Medicine
Winston-Salem, NC, USA

Brian M. Mercer BA, MD, FRCSC, FACOG
Director, Division of Maternal-Fetal Medicine
Metro Health Medical Center;
Professor, Reproductive Biology
Case Western Reserve University
Cleveland, OH, USA

Howard L. Minkoff MD
Chairman, Department of Obstetrics and Gynecology
Maimonides Medical Center;
Distinguished Professor of Obstetrics and Gynecology
SUNY Downstate Medical Center
New York, NY, USA

Kenneth J. Moise Jr MD
Professor, Obstetrics and Gynecology
Department of Obstetrics, Gynecology and Reproductive
Sciences
University of Texas School of Medicine at Houston and the
Texas Fetal Center of Memorial Hermann Children's Hospital
Houston, TX, USA

Michael Nageotte MD
Department of Obstetrics and Gynecology
University of California
Irvine, CA, USA

Edward R. Newton MD
Chair, Professor, Department of Obstetrics and Gynecology
East Carolina University
Brody School of Medicine
Greenville, NC, USA

Errol R. Norwitz MD, PhD
Louis E. Phaneuf Professor and Chair
Department of Obstetrics and Gynecology
Tufts Medical Center and
Tufts University School of Medicine
Boston, MA, USA

John Owen MD
Bruce A. Harris Jr. Endowed Professor
Department of Obstetrics and Gynecology
University of Alabama at Birmingham
Birmingham, AL, USA

Yinka Oyelese MD
Assistant Professor of Obstetrics and Gynecology
Department of Obstetrics and Gynecology
Jersey Shore University Medical Center;
UMDNJ-Robert Wood Johnson Medical School
New Brunswick, NJ, USA

Michael J. Paidas MD
Associate Professor
Department of Obstetrics, Gynecology and Reproductive
Sciences
Yale University School of Medicine
New Haven, CT, USA

Julian T. Parer MD, PhD
Professor
Department of Obstetrics, Gynecology and Reproductive
Sciences
University of California
San Fransisco, CA, USA

Page B. Pennell MD
Director of Research
Division of Epilepsy, EEG and Sleep Neurology
Department of Neurology
Brigham and Women's Hospital;
Harvard Medical School
Boston, MA, USA

Christian M. Pettker MD
Assistant Professor
Department of Obstetrics, Gynecology and Reproductive
Sciences
Yale University School of Medicine
New Haven, CT, USA

Nicole M. Petrossi
Department of Obstetrics and Gynecology
University of California
Irvine, CA, USA

Sarah H. Poggi MD
Associate Professor Obstetrics and Gynecology
Georgetown University Hospital
Washington, DC;
Perinatal Diagnostic Center
Inova Alexandria Hospital
Alexandria, VA, USA

William F. Rayburn MD
Seligman Professor and Chair of Obstetrics and Gynecology
University of New Mexico Health Sciences Center
Albuquerque, NM, USA

Scott Roberts MD
Professor and Lead Doctor in High Risk Obstetrics and
Gynecology
University of Texas Southwestern Medical Center
Dallas, TX, USA

Michael G. Ross MD
Professor of Obstetrics, Gynecology and Public Health
UCLA School of Medicine and Public Health;
Chairman, Department of Obstetrics and Gynecology
Harbor-UCLA Medical Center
Torrance, CA, USA

George Saade MD
Professor, Division Chief
Department of Obstetrics and Gynecology
University of Texas Medical Branch
Galveston, TX, USA

Michael Schatz MD
Chief, Department of Allergy
Kaiser Permanente Medical Center
San Diego, CA, USA

James R. Scott MD
Professor and Chair Emeritus
Department of Obstetrics and Gynecology
University of Utah
Salt Lake City, UT, USA

Brian L. Shaffer MD
Department of Obstetrics, Gynecology and Reproductive
Sciences
University of California
San Francisco, CA, USA

Dinesh M. Shah MD
Professor, Obstetrics and Gynecology
Director, Maternal-Fetal Medicine
University of Wisconsin Medical School
Madison, WI, USA

Jeanne S. Sheffield MD
Associate Professor, Obstetrics and Gynecology
University of Texas Southwestern Medical Center
Dallas, TX, USA

Baha M. Sibai MD
Professor of Clinical Obstetrics and Gynecology
Department of Obstetrics and Gynecology
University of Cincinnati College of Medicine
Cincinnati, OH, USA

Caroline C. Signore MD, MPH
Medical Officer, Obstetrics and Gynecology
Eunice Kennedy Shriver National Institute of Child Health and
Human Development
National Institutes of Health
United States Department of Health and Human Services
Bethesda, MD, USA

Robert M. Silver MD
Professor, Obstetrics and Gynecology
Division Chief, Maternal-Fetal Medicine
Medical Director, Labor and Delivery
Department of Obstetrics and Gynecology
University of Utah School of Medicine
Salt Lake City, UT, USA

Lynn L. Simpson MD
Associate Professor of Clinical Obstetrics and Gynecology
Columbia University Medical Center
New York, NY, USA

Julia Unterscheider MD
Clinical Lecturer and Research Registrar
Department of Obstetrics and Gynaecology
Royal College of Surgeons in Ireland
Dublin, Ireland

Michael W. Varner MD
Professor Obstetrics and Gynecology
University of Utah Health Sciences Center
Salt Lake City, UT, USA

Ronald J. Wapner MD
Director, Division of Maternal Fetal Medicine
Department of Obstetrics and Gynecology
Columbia University Medical Center
New York, NY, USA

Deborah A. Wing MD
Professor and Director
Department of Obstetrics and Gynecology
University of California
Irvine, CA, USA

Edward R. Yeomans MD
Professor, Chairman and Residency Program Director
Department of Obstetrics and Gynecology
Texas Tech University Health Sciences Center
Lubbock, TX, USA

Foreword

In 1980, the founding editor of *Contemporary OB/GYN*, Dr. John Queenan, assembled 67 chapters by 73 authors from the pages of *Contemporary OB/GYN* to create the first edition of the textbook, *Management of High-Risk Pregnancy*. This work became a classic. The fifth edition added two eminent co-editors, Dr. Catherine Y. Spong and Dr. Charles J. Lockwood, whose clinical and research experience further enhanced the publication's national reputation. The addition of Dr. Charles Lockwood, then and now the editor of *Contemporary OB/GYN*, cemented the close relationship between the evolution of this textbook and the journal. Credit for the success of this book most deservedly goes to Dr. John Queenan, whose vision and unique personal qualities make it difficult for most leaders in the field to say no to him!

As in past editions, this book focuses on factors affecting pregnancy, genetics, and fetal monitoring. These sections are followed by a review of maternal diseases in pregnancy, obstetric complications, intrapartum complications, a section on diagnostic and therapeutic procedures, perinatal asphyxia and neonatal considerations. The sixth edition includes important new chapters on maternal diseases – discussing iron deficiency anemia, malaria and placenta accreta. These additional chapters are timely and needed, as progress in maternal care in recent decades has lagged behind advances in fetal and neonatal care. In my opinion, we need to focus renewed resources and attention on coordinating care for mothers with complex medical and surgical complications, though focus should never be removed from enhancing fetal and neonatal care.

This edition also includes new chapters on induction of labor, operative vaginal delivery and patient safety on labor and delivery. These chapters are extremely valuable as the climate towards patient safety has changed: labor is more frequently induced in many hospitals; fewer obstetricians are being trained to perform operative vaginal deliveries; and the national attention on patient safety has led to higher expectations for successful outcomes on labor floors. Finally, this edition includes a new chapter on screening for congenital heart disease. As screening protocols for Down syndrome and neural tube defects have become standard, there is a need to focus on better national programs to screen for the most common, but perhaps the most difficult to diagnose condition, congenital heart disease.

The last 30 years have witnessed extraordinary advances in prenatal screening and diagnosis. Prenatal diagnosis of the majority of abnormalities is now possible. Severe Rh disease has been virtually eliminated and fetal surgery has been demonstrated to improve outcomes for some fetuses diagnosed with neural tube defects. The incidence of stillbirth and neonatal death has declined significantly, due to a combination of better antenatal and invasive care in our neonatal units. These advances have been beautifully and finely addressed in previous editions of this text. The sixth edition upholds the textbook's place as a classic, outlining a practical approach to management for physicians and trainees. I offer my congratulations to the editors for their ability to sustain excellence, and my humility for my small contribution.

Mary E. D'Alton, M.D.
Willard C. Rappleye Professor of Obstetrics
and Gynecology
Chair, Department of Obstetrics and Gynecology
Director, Obstetric and Gynecologic Services
Columbia University College of Physicians & Surgeons
New York, NY, USA

Preface

The sixth edition of *Queenan's Management of High-Risk Pregnancy*, like its predecessors, is directed to all health professionals involved in the care of women with high-risk pregnancies. A series of articles appearing in *Contemporary OB/GYN* was the inspiration for the first edition in 1980. The predominantly clinical articles provided a comprehensive perspective on diagnosis and treatment of complicated problems in pregnancy. The book contains clear, concise, practical material presented in an evidence-based manner. Each chapter is followed by an illustrative case report to help put the subject in perspective.

The major challenge has been to select the subjects most critical to providing good care, and then to invite the outstanding authorities on the subjects to write the articles. This dynamic process requires adding new chapters as the evidence dictates and eliminating others so that the reader is presented with clinically useful contemporary information. The addition of two editors for the fifth edition enhanced our ability to bring our readers the critical information: Catherine Y. Spong, MD, is Chief of the Pregnancy and Perinatology Branch at the National Institute of Child Health and Human Development. Charles J. Lockwood, MD, is Anita O'Keeffe Young Professor of Obstetrics, Gynecology, and Reproductive

Services, Yale University School of Medicine. They are outstanding experts in research and patient care.

We now present the sixth edition at a time when the setting for health care is rapidly changing. We have emphasized evidence-based information and clinical practicality and included chapters on timely topics such as safety, operative vaginal delivery, postpartum hemorrhage, and pregnancies in women with disabilities. In response to concern for health professionals in developing countries we have added chapters including maternal anemia, malaria, and HIV infection.

We are committed to bringing the reader the best possible clinical information. As a reader if you find an area that needs correction or modification, or have comments to improve this effort, please contact me at: JTQMD@aol.com.

John T. Queenan, MD
Professor and Chairman Emeritus
of Obstetrics and Gynecology
Georgetown University School of Medicine
Washington, DC
Deputy Editor *Obstetrics & Gynecology*

Acknowledgments

We are fortunate to work in cooperation with a superb editorial staff at Wiley Blackwell Publishing under the direction of our publisher Martin Sugden who has generously shared his wisdom and guidance. Lucinda Yeates, Rob Blundell, and Helen Harvey have also provided guidance and editorial skills which are evident in this edition.

We acknowledge with great appreciation and admiration the authors, experts all. Their contributions to this book are in the best traditions of academic medicine, and will be translated into a considerable decrease in morbidity and mortality for mothers and infants.

We wish to thank our editorial assistant Michele Prince who coordinated the assembly of the manuscripts in a professional and efficient manner. Her editorial and managerial skills are in large part responsible for the success of this book.

Use this book to improve the delivery of care for your patients. Your dedication to women's health has made it a joy to prepare this resource.

John T. Queenan, MD
Catherine Y. Spong, MD
Charles J. Lockwood, MD

List of Abbreviations

17P	17α-hydroxyprogesterone caproate
AAN	American Academy of Neurology
AAP	American Academy of Pediatrics
ABOG	American Board of Obstetrics and Gynecology
ABP	American Board of Pediatrics
AC	abdominal circumference
ACA	anticardiolipin antibody
ACE	angiotensin-converting enzyme
ACMG	American College of Medical Genetics
ACOG	American College of Obstetricians and Gynecologists
ACT	artemisin-based combination therapy
ACTH	adrenocorticotropin
adjOR	adjusted odds ratio
ADP	adenosine diphosphate
ADR	autonomic dysreflexia
AED	antiepileptic drugs
AES	American Epilepsy Society
AF	amniotic fluid
AFE	amniotic fluid embolism
AFI	Amniotic Fluid Index
AFP	α-fetoprotein
AIUM	American Institute of Ultrasound in Medicine
ALT	alanine aminotransferase
AMI	acute myocardial infarction
ANA	antinuclear antibodies
anti-β$_2$GPI	anti-β$_2$-glycoprotein-I
anti-dsDNA	anti-double-stranded DNA
anti-RNP	anti-ribonucleoprotein
anti-Sm	anti-Smith
AOI	Adverse Outcome Index
APA	antiphospholipid antibody
APAS	antiphospholipid antibody syndrome
APC	activated protein C
APE	acute pulmonary embolism
APO	adverse pregnancy outcome
APTT	activated partial thromboplastin time
AQP	aquaporin
ARB	angiotensin receptor blocker
ART	assisted reproductive technology
AS	aortic stenosis

ASCUS	atypical cells of undetermined significance
ASD	atrial septal defect
AST	aspartate aminotransferase
AT	antithrombin
AV	atrioventricular
BMI	Body Mass Index
BPA	bisphenol A
BPD	biparietal diameter
BPP	biophysical profile
BV	bacterial vaginosis
CBC	complete blood count
CBZ	carbamazepine
CCB	calcium channel blocker
CD	cesarean delivery
CDC	Centers for Disease Control
CDH	congenital diaphragmatic hernia
CHB	congenital heart block
CHD	congenital heart diseases
CI	confidence interval
CL	cervical length
CMV	cytomegalovirus
CNS	central nervous system
COX	cyclooxygenase
CP	cerebral palsy
CPAM	congenital pulmonary airway malformation
CRH	corticotropin-releasing hormone
CRL	crown–rump length
CSE	combined spinal–epidural
CST	contraction stress test
CT	computed tomography
CTPA	computed tomographic pulmonary angiography
CVS	chorionic villus sampling
CXR	chest x-ray
D&C	dilation and curettage
DAMP	damage-associated molecular pattern molecules
dDAVP	deamino arginine vasopressin
DES	diethylstilbestrol
DHEAS	dehydroepiandrosterone sulfate
DIC	disseminated intravascular coagulation
DM	diabetes mellitus

DVT	deep venous thrombosis	HIT	hemorrhage, infection, toxemia
ECG	electrocardiogram	HL	humeral length
ECM	extracellular matrix	HLA	human leukocyte antigen
ECMO	extracorporeal membrane oxygenation	HPA	human platelet antigen/
ECV	external cephalic version		hypothalamic–pituitary–adrenal
EDD	estimated date of delivery	HPV	human papillomavirus
EF	ejection fraction	HSV	herpes simplex virus
EFM	electronic fetal monitoring	IAI	intraamniotic infection
EFW	estimated fetal weight	ICD	implantable cardioverter-defibrillator
EI	erythema infectiosum	ICH	intracranial hemorrhage
EIA	enzyme immunoassay	IFA	immunofluorescent assay
ELISA	enzyme-linked immunosorbent assay	Ig	immunoglobulin
eNO	exhaled nitric oxide	IGFBP	insulin-like growth factor-binding
EP	erythropoietin		protein
EPCR	endothelial cell protein C receptor	IL	interleukin
ER-β	estrogen receptor-β	IM	intramuscular/intramembranous
FAS	fetal alcohol syndrome	INR	international normalized ratio
FDA	Food and Drug Administration	IOM	Institute of Medicine
FDP	fibrin degradation products	IT	intracranial translucency
FEV$_1$	forced expiratory volume in 1 sec	ITP	idiopathic thrombocytopenic purpura
fFN	fetal fibronectin	IU	international unit
FFP	fresh frozen plasma	IUD	intrauterine device
FHT	fetal heart rate tracing	IUFD	intrauterine fetal death
FIGS	fetal intervention guided by sonography	IUGR	intrauterine growth restriction
FiO$_2$	fraction of inspired oxygen	IUT	intrauterine transfusion
FL	femur length/fetal loss	IV	intravenous
FLM	fetal lung maturity	IVF	*in vitro* fertilization
FMF	frontomaxillary facial	IVH	intraventricular hemorrhage
FMH	fetomaternal hemorrhage	IVIG	intravenous immunoglobulin
FSI	Foam Stability Index	IVT	intravascular transfusion
fT$_4$	free thyroxine	KIR	killer cell immunoglobulin-like receptor
FVL	factor V Leiden	LAC	lupus anticoagulant
GBS	group B streptococci	LBC	lamellar body count
GCT	glucose challenge test	LBW	low birthweight
GDM	gestational diabetes mellitus	LDA	low-dose aspirin
GFR	glomerular filtration rate	LDH	lactate dehydrogenase
GP	glycoprotein	LEEP	loop electrosurgical excision procedure
GPL	anticardiolipin antibody of IgG isotype	LFT	liver function test
GTCS	generalized tonic-clonic seizures	LGA	large for gestational age
GTP	gestational thrombocytopenia	LMWH	low molecular weight heparin
GTT	glucose tolerance testing/gestational transient thyrotoxicosis	LPS	lipopolysaccharide
		LOS	length of stay
HAART	highly active antiretroviral therapy	LR	likelihood ratio
Hb	hemoglobin	LRD	limb reduction defect
HBV	hepatitis B	L:S	lecithin:sphingomyelin ratio
HBC	hepatitis C	LTG	lamotrigine
HC	head circumference/homocysteine	LUS	lower uterine segment
hCG	human chorionic gonadotropin	MCA	middle cerebral artery
Hct	hematocrit	MCD	minimal change disease
HDFN	hemolytic disease of the fetus and newborn	MCM	major congenital malformation
		MCV	mean corpuscular volume
HELLP	hemolysis, elevated liver enzymes, and low platelet count	MFMU	Maternal-Fetal Medicine Unit
		MMC	myelomeningocele
HFUPR	hourly fetal urine production rate	MMP	matrix metalloproteinase
HIE	hypoxic ischemic encephalopathy	MoM	multiples of the median

MOMS   Management of Myelomeningocele Study
MPL   anticardiolipin antibody of IgM isotype
MPR   multifetal pregnancy reduction
MR   magnetic resonance/mass restricted
MRI   magnetic resonance imaging
MS   multiple sclerosis
MSAFP   maternal serum α-fetoprotein
MSD   mean sac diameter
NAEPP   National Asthma Education and Prevention Program
NAIT   neonatal alloimmune thrombocytopenia
NCHS   National Center for Health Statistics
NEC   necrotizing enterocolitis
NICHD   National Institute of Child Health and Human Development
NICU   neonatal intensive care unit
NIH   National Institutes of Health
NK   natural killer
NLE   neonatal lupus erythematosus
NNRTI   nonnucleoside reverse transcriptase inhibitor
NOTSS   nontechnical surgical skills
NRTI   nucleoside analog reverse transcriptase inhibitor
NST   nonstress test
NT   nuchal translucency
NTD   neural tube defects
NYHA   New York Heart Association
OGTT   oral glucose tolerance test
OR   odds ratio
PAI   plasminogen activator inhibitor
PAMG   placental α-microglobulin
PAMP   pathogen-associated molecular pattern
PaPP-A   pregnancy-associated plasma protein A
PAR   protease-activated receptor
PB   phenobarbital
PC   protein C
PCA   patient-controlled analgesia
PCB   polychlorinated biphenyl
PCEA   patient-controlled epidural analgesia
PCOS   polycystic ovarian syndrome
PCR   polymerase chain reaction
PDA   patent ductus arteriosus
PE   pulmonary embolism
PEFR   peak expiratory flow rate
PG   phosphatidylglycerol/prostaglandin
PGDH   15-hydroxy-prostaglandin dehydrogenase
PGM   prothrombin G20210A gene mutation
PGS   preimplantation genetic screening
PHT   phenytoin
PI   protease inhibitor
PICC   peripherally inserted central catheter
PKA   protein kinase A

PKC   protein kinase C
PMC   placenta-mediated complications
PNV   prenatal vitamins
PPCM   peripartum cardiomyopathy
PPH   postpartum hemorrhage
PPROM   preterm premature rupture of membranes
PR   progesterone receptor
PRBC   packed red blood cell
PROM   premature rupture of membranes
PS   protein S
PT   prothrombin time
PTB   preterm birth
PTD   preterm delivery
PTH   parathyroid hormone
PTL   preterm labor
PTSD   posttraumatic stress disorder
PTT   partial thromboplastin time
PTU   propylthiouracil
PZ   protein Z
RA   rheumatoid arthritis
RAGE   receptor for advanced glycation end-products
RBC   red blood cell
RCA   root cause analysis
RDA   recommended dietary allowance
RDI   recommended daily intake
RDS   respiratory distress syndrome
RE   retinol equivalent
RFA   radiofrequency ablation
Rh   rhesus
RhIG   rhesus immunoglobulin
RIBA   recombinant immunoblot assay
RPF   renal plasma flow
RPR   rapid plasma reagin
RR   relative risk
SAB   spontaneous abortion
SAR   surfactant:albumin ratio
SB   spina bifida
SBE   systemic bacterial endocarditis
SCD   sickle cell disease
SCI   spinal cord injury
SCT   sacrococcygeal teratomas
S:D   systolic:diastolic
SDP   single deepest pocket
SELDI-TOF   surface-enhanced laser desorption ionization time-of-flight
SERPIN   serine protease inhibitor
SGA   small for gestational age
SLE   systemic lupus erythematosus
SMA   spinal muscular atrophy
SNP   single nucleotide polymorphism
ST   selective termination
SVT   supraventricular tachycardia

TAFI	thrombin-activatable fibrinolysis inhibitor		UFH	unfractionated heparin
TAT	thrombin–antithrombin		uPA	urokinase-type plasminogen activator
TEC	trauma, embolism, cardiac		UPD	uniparental disomy
TEE	transesophageal echocardiography		UTI	urinary tract infection
TF	tissue factor		VAS	vibroacoustic stimulation
TFPI	tissue factor pathway inhibitor		VBAC	vaginal birth after cesarean
TLR	Toll-like receptor		VDRL	Venereal Disease Research Laboratory
TNF	tumor necrosis factor		VOC	vasoocclusion
TOGV	transposition of the great vessels		VPA	valproic acid
TOL	trial of labor		V/Q	ventilation/perfusion
tPA	tissue-type plasminogen activator		VSD	ventricular septal defect
TRAP	twin reversed arterial perfusion		VTE	venous thromboembolism
TSH	thyroid-stimulating hormone		VUS	venous ultrasonography
TTTS	twin–twin transfusion syndrome		vWF	von Willebrand factor
TVU	transvaginal ultrasound		VZV	varicella zoster virus
TWR	tubular water reabsorption		WB	Western blot
TXA$_2$	thromboxane A$_2$		WHO	World Health Organization
UA	umbilical artery		WWE	women with epilepsy
UDS	urinary drug screen		ZDV	zidovudine
uE3	unconjugated estriol		ZPI	protein Z-related protease inhibitor

Chapter 1
Overview of High-Risk Pregnancy

John T. Queenan[1], Catherine Y. Spong[2] and Charles J. Lockwood[3]

[1]Department of Obstetrics and Gynecology, Georgetown University School Medicine, Washington, DC, USA

[2]Bethesda, MD, USA

[3]Department of Obstetrics, Gynecology and Reproductive Sciences, Yale University School of Medicine, New Haven, CT, USA

With the changing demographics of the United States population, including increasing maternal age and weight during pregnancy, higher rates of pregnancies conceived by artificial reproductive technologies and increasing numbers of cesarean deliveries, complicated pregnancies have risen. Although most pregnancies are low risk with favorable outcomes, high-risk pregnancies – the subject of this book – may have potentially serious occurrences. We classify any pregnancy in which there is a maternal or fetal factor that may adversely affect the outcome as high risk. In these cases, the likelihood of a positive outcome is significantly reduced. In order to improve the outcome of a high-risk pregnancy, we must identify risk factors and attempt to mitigate problems in pregnancy and labor.

Many conditions lend themselves to identification and intervention before or early in the perinatal period. When diagnosed through an appropriate work-up before pregnancy, conditions such as rhesus (Rh) immunization, diabetes, and epilepsy can be managed to minimize the risks of mortality and morbidity to both mother and baby. It is not possible, however, to predict other conditions, such as multiple pregnancies, preeclampsia, and premature rupture of membranes prior to pregnancy. To detect and manage these challenging situations, the obstetrician must maintain constant vigilance once pregnancy is established.

Although much progress has been made since the 1950s, there is still much to accomplish. Fifty years ago, the delivering physician and the nursing staff were responsible for newborn care. The incidence of perinatal mortality and morbidity was high. Pediatricians and pediatric nurses began appearing in the newborn nursery in the 1950s, taking responsibility for the infant at the moment of birth. This decade of neonatal awareness ushered in advances that greatly improved neonatal outcome.

Many scientific breakthroughs directed toward evaluation of fetal health and disease occurred in the 1960s, which is considered the decade of fetal medicine. Early in that decade, the identification of patients with the risk factor of Rh immunization led to the prototype for the high-risk pregnancy clinic. Rh-negative patients were screened for antibodies, and if none were detected, these women were managed as normal or "low-risk" cases. Those who developed antibodies were enrolled in a high-risk pregnancy clinic, where they could be carefully followed by specialists with expertise in Rh immunization. With the advent of scientific advances such as amniotic fluid bilirubin analysis, intrauterine transfusion, and, finally, Rh immune prophylaxis, these often perilous high-risk pregnancies generally became success stories.

A note of caution is in order. The creation of special Rh clinics for Rh-immunized mothers in the early 1960s was a logical strategy since the Rh-immunized mother with an Rh-positive fetus had a 50% chance of losing her baby either *in utero* or in the nursery. With increasing technologic and scientific advances physicians achieved markedly better outcomes. We are sensitive to the use of the term "high-risk pregnancy" and believe it should be avoided in patient counseling as it can cause unnecessary anxiety for the parents.

During the 1970s, the decade of perinatal medicine, pediatricians and obstetricians combined forces to continue improving perinatal survival. Some of the most significant perinatal advances are listed in Box 1.1. Also included are the approximate dates of these milestones and (where appropriate) the names of investigators who are associated with the advances.

Among the advances in perinatal medicine that occurred during the 1980s were the development of comprehensive evaluation of fetal condition with the biophysical profile, the introduction of cordocentesis for diagnosis and therapy, the development of neonatal surfactant

Queenan's Management of High-Risk Pregnancy: An Evidence-Based Approach, Sixth Edition. Edited by John T. Queenan, Catherine Y. Spong, Charles J. Lockwood.
© 2012 John Wiley & Sons, Ltd. Published 2012 by John Wiley & Sons, Ltd.

Box 1.1 Milestones in perinatology

Before 1950s

Neonatal care by obstetricians and nurses

1950s: decade of neonatal awareness

Pediatricians entered the nursery

1950	Allen and Diamond	Exchange transfusions
1953	du Vigneaud	Oxytocin synthesis
1954	Patz	Limitation of O_2 to prevent toxicity
1955	Mann	Neonatal hypothermia
1956	Tjio and Levan	Demonstration of 46 human chromosomes
1956	Bevis	Amniocentesis for bilirubin in Rh immunization
1958	Donald	Obstetric use of ultrasound
1958	Hon	Electronic fetal heart rate evaluation
1959	Burns, Hodgman, and Cass	Gray baby syndrome

1960s: decade of fetal medicine

Prototype of the high-risk pregnancy clinic

1960	Eisen and Hellman	Lumbar epidural anesthesia
1962	Saling	Fetal scalp blood sampling
1963	Liley	First intrauterine transfusion for Rh immunization
1964	Wallgren	Neonatal blood pressure
1965	Steele and Breg	Culture of amniotic fluid cells
1965	Mizrahi, Blanc, and Silverman	Necrotizing enterocolitis
1966	Parkman and Myer	Rubella immunization
1967		Neonatal blood gases
1967		Neonatal transport
1967	Jacobsen	Diagnosis of cytogenetic disorders *in utero*
1968	Dudrick	Hyperalimentation
1968	Nadler	Diagnosis of inborn errors of metabolism *in utero*
1968	Stern	NICU effectiveness
1968	Freda *et al*	Rh prophylaxis

1970s: decade of perinatal medicine

Refinement of NICU

Regionalization of high-risk perinatal care

1971	Gluck	L:S ratio and respiratory distress syndrome
1972	Brock and Sutcliffe	α-Fetoprotein and neural tube defects
	Liggins and Howie	Betamethasone for induction of fetal lung maturity
1972		
1972		Neonatal temperature control with radiant heat
1972	Quilligan	Fetal heart rate monitoring
1972	Dawes	Fetal breathing movements
1972	Ray and Freeman	Oxytocin challenge test

1972	ABOG	Maternal-Fetal Medicine Boards
1973	Sadovsky	Fetal movement
1973		Real-time ultrasound
1973	Hobbins and Rodeck	Clinical fetoscopy
1975	ABP	Neonatology Boards
1976	Schifrin	Nonstress test
1977	March of Dimes	Towards Improving the Outcome of Pregnancy I
1977	Kaback	Heterozygote identification (Tay–Sachs disease)
1978	Bowman	Antepartum Rh prophylaxis
1978	Steptoe and Edwards*	*In vitro* fertilization
1979	Boehm	Maternal transport

1980s: decade of progress

Technologic progress

1980	Bartlett	ECMO
1980	Manning and Platt	Biophysical profile
1981	Fujiwara, Morley, and Jobe	Neonatal surfactant therapy
1982	Harrison and Golbus	Vesicoamniotic shunt for fetal hydronephrosis
	Bang, Brock and Toll	First fetal transfusion under ultrasound guidance
1983	Kazy, Ward, and Brambati	Chorionic villus sampling
1985	Daffos, Hobbins	Cordocentesis
1986		DNA analysis
1986	NICHD	MFMU network established
1986	Michaels *et al*	Cervical ultrasound and preterm delivery

1990s: decade of managed care

Managed care alters practice patterns

1991	Lockwood *et al*	Fetal fibronectin and preterm delivery
1993	March of Dimes	Towards Improving the Outcome of Pregnancy II
		Fetal therapy
		Preimplantation genetics
		Stem cell research
1994	NIH Consensus Conference	Antenatal corticosteroids

2000s: decade of evidence-based perinatology

2000	Mari	Middle cerebral artery monitoring for Rh disease
2002	CDC	Group B streptococcus guidelines
	MFMU	Antibiotics for PPROM
2003	MFMU	Progesterone to prevent recurrent prematurity
2006	Merck	Immunization against human papillomavirus
2008	MFMU	Magnesium for prevention of cerebral palsy
2009	MFMU	Gestational diabetes trial

2010s: current decade

2010	NIH	Consensus conference on VBAC
2011	MOMS	Fetal surgery improves outcome for myelomeningocele

ABOG, American Board of Obstetrics and Gynecology; ABP, American Board of Pediatrics; CDC, Centers for Disease Control; ECMO, extracorporeal membrane oxygenation; L:S, lecithin:sphingomyelin ratio; MFMU, Maternal-Fetal Medicine Units; MOMS, Management of Myelomeningocele Study: NICU, neonatal intensive care unit; NICHD, National Institute of Child Health and Human Development; NIH, National Institutes of Health; PPROM, preterm premature rupture of membranes; VBAC, vaginal birth after cesarean.

*Recipient of the 2010 Nobel Prize in Medicine.

therapy, antenatal steroids and major advances in genetics and assisted reproduction. These technologic advances foreshadowed the "high-tech" developments of the 1990s. Clearly, the specialty has come to realize that "high tech" must be accompanied by "high touch" to ensure the emotional and developmental well-being of the baby and the parents. This decade was one of adjusting to the challenges of managed care under the control of "for profit" insurance companies.

The new millennium brought the decade of evidence-based perinatology. Clinicians became aware of the value of systematic reviews of the Cochrane Database. Major perinatal research projects by the Maternal-Fetal Medicine Units network of the Eunice Kennedy Shriver National Institute of Child Health and Human Development answered many clinical questions.

The future will bring better methods of determining fetal jeopardy and health. Continuous readout of fetal conditions will be possible during labor in high-risk pregnancies. Look for the new advances to be made in immunology and genetics. Immunization against group B streptococcus and eventually human immunodeficiency virus will become available. Preimplantation genetics will continue to provide new ways to prevent disease. Alas, prematurity and preeclampsia with their many multiple etiologies may be the last to be conquered.

New technology will increase the demand for trained workers in the healthcare industry. The perinatal professional team will expand to emphasize the importance of social workers, nutritionists, child development specialists, and psychologists. New developments will create special ethical issues. Finally, education and enlightened attitudes toward reproductive awareness and family planning will help to prevent unwanted pregnancies.

Chapter 2
Maternal Nutrition

Edward R. Newton

Department of Obstetrics and Gynecology, East Carolina University, Brody School of Medicine, Greenville, NC, USA

The medical profession and the lay public associate maternal nutrition with fetal development and subsequent pregnancy outcome. Classic studies from Holland and Leningrad during World War II [1] suggest that when maternal caloric intake fell acutely to below 800 kcal/day, birthweights were reduced 535 g in Leningrad and 250 g in Holland, the difference perhaps related to the better nutritional status of the Dutch women prior to the famine and the shorter duration of their famine. Exposure to famine conditions during the second half of pregnancy had the greatest adverse effect on birthweight and placental weight and to a lesser extent, birth length, head circumference, and maternal postpartum weight [2–5].

While these studies are used as *prima facie* evidence of a link between maternal nutrition and fetal development, a more discerning examination reveals many confounding variables that are common to the investigation of maternal nutrition and fetal development. While the onset of rationing was distinct and the birthweight and other anthropomorphic measurements were recorded reliably, other confounders were not identified. For example, menstrual data were notoriously unreliable, and the problem of poor determination of gestational dates was exacerbated by the disruption and stress of war.

In 2011, many of the most vulnerable mothers have little or no prenatal care (10–30%), often with unreliable menstrual data (15–35%). In Holland and Leningrad, the stress of war may have been associated with both preterm delivery and reduced birthweight. In a modern context, the urban war produces a similar stress through lack of social supports, domestic violence, and drugs. The content of the individual's diet in wartime Europe or the diet of underprivileged women in the United States in 2011 remains largely speculation; perhaps it is not the total number of kilocalories or protein content but an issue of overall quality that leads to decreased birthweights. In 2011, as in 1944–5, the link between maternal nutrition and pregnancy outcome relies on a relatively weak proxy for a woman's nutritional status: Body Mass Index (BMI). A prospective, longitudinal study that follows a sufficiently large cohort of women from preconception through each trimester and into the puerperium (with and without breastfeeding), measures the quality and quantity of women's diet, and correlates the diet with maternal and fetal and neonatal outcomes has not yet been performed.

The purpose of this chapter is to review the associations between maternal nutrition and perinatal outcome. It briefly summarizes the basic concepts of fetal growth, the multiple predictors of fetal growth, the use of maternal weight gain as a measure of maternal nutrition, adverse pregnancy outcomes as they relate to extremes in maternal weight gain, and the importance or controversy related to specific components of the diet (i.e. iron, calcium, sodium, and prenatal vitamins).

Fetal growth

Linear growth of the fetus is continuous, whereas the velocity of growth varies. Multiple researchers have studied linear fetal growth by examining birthweights or estimated fetal weights as determined by ultrasound, and found it to be nearly a straight line until approximately 35 weeks when the fetus grows 200–225 g/wk (Fig. 2.1). Thereafter, the curve falls such that by 40 weeks, the weight gain is 135 g/wk [6].

Twin pregnancies have a proportionately lower rate of growth, reaching a maximum at 34–35 weeks (monochorionic placentation, 140–160 g/wk; dichorionic placentation, 180–200 g/wk) [7]. Thereafter, the growth rate slows to 25–30 g/wk in both types of placentation. In 20–30% of term twin pregnancies, one or the other twin, or both, will have a birthweight less than the 10th percentile based on singleton growth charts. There is controversy as to whether singleton or separate twin charts should be the

Queenan's Management of High-Risk Pregnancy: An Evidence-Based Approach, Sixth Edition. Edited by John T. Queenan, Catherine Y. Spong, Charles J. Lockwood.
© 2012 John Wiley & Sons, Ltd. Published 2012 by John Wiley & Sons, Ltd.

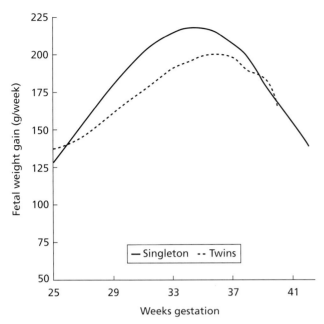

Figure 2.1 Fetal weight gain in grams among singleton and twin pregnancies.

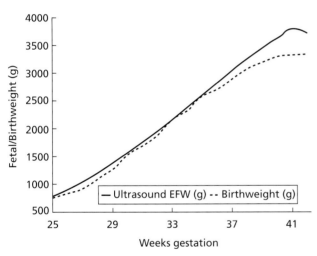

Figure 2.2 Fetal growth curves by method of estimation: ultrasound or birthweight. EFW, mean estimated fetal weight.

comparison resource in an individual pregnancy. Given the rapidly increasing incidence of twin and triplet pregnancies through assisted reproductive technologies, there is a need to resolve this controversy.

Fetal growth curves are based on two sources for fetal weight: birthweight [8] and estimated fetal weight based on ultrasound findings (Fig. 2.2). Birthweight sources encompass the pathophysiology that led to the preterm birth. Twenty to 25% of preterm births occur as the result of medical intervention in the setting of maternal pathology such as preeclampsia. In these cases, the effects of maternal nutrition (BMI) are muted significantly. Fetal growth curves derived by ultrasonographic estimation of

fetal weight reflect a more physiologic environment. Unfortunately, the comparison of coincidental estimated fetal weight and birthweight reveals a relatively large error; 20% of estimated fetal weights will differ from the actual weight by one standard deviation or more, 400–600 g at term.

The velocity of fetal growth is more instructive regarding the mechanisms of fetal growth restriction [9]. Length peaks earlier than weight, as the fetus stores fat and hepatic glycogen (increasing abdominal circumference) in the third trimester. When an insult occurs early, such as with alcohol exposure, severe starvation, smoking, perinatal infection (cytomegalovirus infection or toxoplasmosis), chromosomal or developmental disorders, or chronic vasculopathies (diabetes, autoimmune disease, chronic hypertension), the result is a symmetrically growth-restricted fetus with similarly reduced growth of its length, head circumference, and abdominal circumference. This pattern is often referred to as *dysgenic growth restriction* and these infants often have persistent handicaps (mental retardation, infectious retinopathy, i.e. toxoplasmosis infection) [10].

When the insult occurs after the peak in the velocity of length growth, the result is a disproportionately reduced body-length ratio (ponderal index), with a larger head circumference relative to abdominal circumference. This pattern is often referred to as *nutritional growth restriction* and usually is the result of developing vasculopathy (placental thrombosis/infarcts, preeclampsia) or a reduction of the absorptive capacity of the placenta (postdate pregnancy). The obstetrician uses the ultrasonographically defined ratio of head circumference to abdominal circumference as it compares to established nomograms. The pediatrician uses the ponderal index (birthweight [kg]/ height [cm³]) in a similar fashion. *Abnormality* is defined statistically (i.e. two standard deviations from the mean) rather than as it relates to adverse clinical outcomes. While the risk of adverse outcomes may be considerably higher, most small for gestational age babies (less than the 10th percentile) who are delivered at term have few significant problems. Likewise, the vast majority of term infants whose size is more than the 90th percentile at birth have few perinatal challenges.

Fetal growth requires the transfer of nutriments as building blocks and the transfer of enough oxygen to fuel the machinery to build the fetus. Maternal nutritional and cardiac physiology is changed through placental hormones (i.e. human placental lactogen) to accommodate the fetal-placental needs. The central role of the placenta in the production of pregnancy hormones, the transfer of nutriments, and fetal respiration is demonstrated by the fact that 20% of the oxygen supplied to the fetus is diverted to the metabolic activities of the placenta and placental oxygen consumption at term is about 25% higher than the amount consumed by the fetus as a whole.

Table 2.1 Weight gain in pregnancy

	Maternal gains		Fetal gains
Blood volume	2 kg (4.4 lb)	Fetus	3.5 kg (7.7 lb)
Uterine size	1 kg (2.2 lb)	Placenta	0.6 kg (0.7 lb)
Breast size	1 kg (2.2 lb)	Amniotic fluid	1.2 kg (2.6 lb)
Fat increase	3 kg (6.6 lb)		
Total weight gain	12.3 kg (27 lb)		

Table 2.2 Factors affecting fetal growth

Factors	Clinical examples
Genetics	Parental size
	Chromosomal disease
Uterine volume	Müllerian duct abnormalities
	Leiomyomata uteri
Maternal intake	Starvation
	Fad diets
	Iron deficiency anemia
	Neural tube defects (folic acid)
Maternal absorption	Inflammatory bowel disease
	Gastric bypass
Maternal hypermetabolic states	Hyperthyroidism
	Adolescent pregnancy
	Extreme exercise
Maternal cardiorespiratory function	Maternal cardiac disease
	Sarcoidosis
	Asthma
Uterine blood flow	Hypertension/preeclampsia
	β-Adrenergic blockers
	Diabetic vasculopathy
	Autoimmune vasculopathy
	Smoking (nicotine)
	Chronic environmental stress
Placental transfer	Infant of a diabetic mother
	Smoking (carbon monoxide)
Placental absorption	Placental infarcts or thrombosis
Fetal blood flow	Congenital heart disease
	Increased placental resistance
	Polycythemia
Fetal metabolic state	Drug effects (amphetamines)
	Genetic metabolic disease
Reduced fetal cell numbers	Alcohol abuse
	Chromosomal disease

The absorptive surface area of the placenta is strongly associated with fetal growth; the chorionic villus surface area grows from about 5 m² at 28–30 weeks to 10 m² by term.

The measured energy requirement of pregnancy totals 55,000 kcal for an 11,800 g weight gain [11] or 4.7 kcal/g of weight gain. This value is considerably less than the 8.0 kcal/g required for weight gain in the nonpregnant woman. This discrepancy is likely due to the poorly understood relationship between pregnancy hormones (i.e. human placental lactogen, corticosteroids, sex steroids) and the pattern of nutriment distribution. Table 2.1 describes the work as measured by weight that must occur to produce a well-grown fetus at term.

Weight gain is essentially linear throughout pregnancy [12]. The mean total weight gain (15th to 85th percentile) for white, non-Hispanic, married mothers delivering live infants was 13.8 (8.6–18.2) kg for small women (BMI below 19.8), 13.8 (7.7–18.6) kg for average women (BMI 19.8–26.0), 12.4 (6.4–17.3) kg for large women (BMI 26.1–29.0), and 8.7 (0.5–16.4) kg for obese women (BMI over 29) [11]. In general, average weight gains (15th to 85th percentile) per week are 0.15–0.69 kg for gestational ages 13–20 weeks, 0.31–0.65 kg for gestational ages 20–30 weeks, and 0.18–0.61 kg for gestational ages 30–36 weeks. The practical clinical rule of thumb is that a normal-weight woman with a normal pregnancy should gain about 4.5 kg (10 lb) in the first 20 weeks and 9.1 kg (20 lb) in the second 20 weeks of pregnancy. High-risk thresholds are weight gains less than 6.8 kg (15 lb) and more than 20.5 kg (45 lb) [12].

Many factors affect the transfer of nutriments and oxygen to the fetus. Table 2.2 lists factors and clinical examples where abnormalities change fetal growth.

Obstetric history reveals a strong tendency to repeat gestational age and birthweight as the result of shared genetic and environmental factors. Bakketeig *et al* analyzed almost 500,000 consecutive births in Norway over a 7-year period [13]. Table 2.3 depicts the results of their analysis.

In summary, fetal growth is affected by the quantity and quality of maternal diet, the ability of the mother to appropriately absorb and distribute digested micronutriments, maternal cardiorespiratory function, uterine blood flow, placental transfer, placental blood flow, and appropriate distribution and handling of nutriments and oxygen by the fetus. Additionally, genetics and uterine volume characteristics can greatly affect fetal size in the presence of normal physiology; birth size more closely reflects maternal rather than paternal morphometrics, and contractions of uterine volume (i.e. müllerian duct abnormalities or large uterine myomas) are associated with decreased birth size.

Ultimately, any evaluation of the effect of nutrition on fetal outcome must control for these confounders in the

Table 2.3 Obstetric history and birthweight

Incidence of adverse outcome in

First birth	Second birth	Subsequent birth (relative risk*)
Term AGA	–	1.4% (1.0)
Preterm low BW	–	13.1% (4.5)
Term SGA	–	8.2% (5.5)
BW > 4500 g	–	22.6% (9.0)
Post term	–	5.3% (2.2)
Term AGA	Term AGA	1.5% (0.5)
Preterm low BW	Preterm low BW	19.7% (6.8)
Term SGA	Term SGA	29% (19.3)
BW > 4500 g	BW > 4500 g	45.5% (18.2)
Post term	Post term	33.3% (13.9)

AGA, appropriate for gestational age; SGA, small for gestational age (2500 g); LGA, large for gestational age (4500 g); preterm, 36 weeks and 2500 g; post term, 44 weeks.
*The relative risk is the ratio of incidence of "poor" outcomes in the target cohort divided by the incidence of "poor" outcomes in the lowest risk cohort, women in whom all births were normal.
Source: Bakketeig [13].

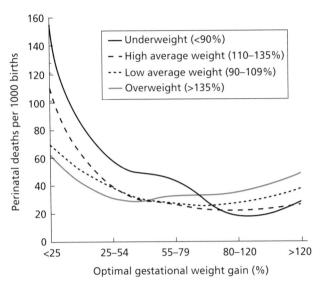

Figure 2.3 Perinatal mortality rates by prepregnancy weight and height (Metropolitan Life Insurance tables) and the percent of optimal weight gain. Reproduced from Naeye [14] with permission from Elsevier.

analysis. The presence of multiple variables requires large numbers of subjects to be included in the model for the study of main effects alone. As many variables (i.e. parity and preeclampsia) are interactive, the sample size necessarily increases geometrically by the analysis of secondary or higher interactive variables. The resultant complexity and difficulty in obtaining quality data on large numbers of pregnant women have led to purposeful exclusion of certain cohorts of women. Exclusions may include women with hypertension or diabetes, poorly dated gestations, late prenatal care, or middle- and upper-class white Anglo-Americans who seek care from private practitioners. The use of imprecise proxies to control for population differences in nutritional risk, such as educational and socio-economic level, age, parity or ethnicity adds to the variance. Likewise, determination of the quality and quantity of the maternal diet is severely limited by the time, personnel, and education required to obtain a valid measurement of that diet. As a consequence, most studies of maternal nutrition use the BMI (weight [kg]/(height in meters)^2) or maternal weight gain during pregnancy as a proxy for maternal nutrition; the quality and quantity of maternal diet are rarely measured. There is added imprecision with the measurement of weight gain. Most studies rely on reported prepregnancy weight, the accuracy of which is suspect. Additionally, the use of total weight gain in most studies does not account for the variance in the weight of the fetus, amniotic fluid or placenta. The use of net weight gain (total weight gain – birthweight) is used to reduce the resultant variance.

Body Mass Index, weight gain, and adverse pregnancy outcomes

Regardless of their imprecise measurement, weight gain and BMI have powerful associations with birthweight and pregnancy outcome. Naeye examined the association between weight gain and pregnancy outcome data obtained during the National Collaborative Perinatal Project (1959–65) [14]. In this project about 56,000 American women were followed from prenatal enrollment through birth. The infants were followed through the age of 7 years. The National Collaborative Perinatal Project demonstrated that progressive increases in prepregnancy weight or weight gain, or both, were significantly associated with increases in birthweight. Prepregnancy weight and weight gain appear to act independently of each other and their effects are additive. Increasing prepregnancy weight diminishes the influences of weight gain on birthweight. Among nonsmokers, the difference in birthweight across weight gains (less than 7.3 kg (16 lb) versus more than 15.9 kg (35 lb) in weight gain) was 556 g (19% difference) for underweight women, 509 g (16.4% difference) for normal-weight women, and 335 g (10% difference) for overweight women. Similarly, among smokers, the difference in birthweight was 683 g (27%) for underweight women, 480 g (16.4%) for normal-weight women, and 261 g (8%) for overweight women [14].

Perinatal mortality rates in underweight women (less than 90% of expected pregnancy weight in the Metropolitan weight-for-height charts) are strongly affected by weight gain (Fig. 2.3). Poor weight gain in underweight women is associated with a fivefold increase in perinatal mortality. Autopsies of fetuses and neonates in the same cohort demonstrated that body and organ size could be predicted by prepregnancy weight and weight gain [15]. Prior to 33 weeks, the relationship is less dramatic and is associated with a smaller liver and adrenals due to a reduction in cell numbers in underweight women with poor weight gain. After 33 weeks, when fetal weight gain is expected to be highest, the reduction in organ weights occurs in most organs with a reduction in cell size and numbers.

The Dutch famine during World War II [2–5], during which acute rationing was less than 800 kcal/day, resulted in different reductions in neonatal measurements depending on the gestational age when the rationing was instituted. The greatest adverse effects were seen when the rationing occurred in the last trimester, the parameters most affected being placental weight and birthweight and, to a lesser extent, birth length, head circumference, and maternal postpartum weight. With the progressive loss of calories, maternal weight absorbed the challenge until a critical threshold was met. Then maternal weight loss stabilized and the placental and then fetal weights were reduced. After the rationing was discontinued and intake was increased, maternal weight was the first to recover, followed by placental weight and finally birthweight.

The most representative data on total weight gain in the US population are from the 1980 National Natality Survey [16]. A probability sample of all livebirths to US women in 1980 was employed. BMI and weight gain were related to the incidence of term growth-restricted infants (less than 2500 g and more than 37 weeks' gestation) [16]. The analysis was adjusted for maternal age, parity, height, cigarette smoking, and education level. The relative risk (95% confidence interval [CI]) of delivering a term growth-restricted infant after a total weight gain of less than the 25th percentile was 2.4 (1.5–4.0) for small women (BMI below 19.8), 3.1 (2.2–4.5) for average women (BMI of 19.8 to 26.0), and 1.3 (0.6–2.8) for large women (BMI over 26). The effect of low weight gain in large women was not significant. Clinically, the expectation that an obese woman or large woman who is diagnosed with gestational diabetes should gain 11.4–13.6 kg (25–30 lb) is contrary to the later information. With documentation of a high-quality diet, these large women should gain 4.5–6.8 kg (10–15 lb). The Institute of Medicine has recently recommended guidelines on total weight gain during pregnancy (Table 2.4).

The interaction between weight gain, BMI, and the incidence of preterm delivery (weight less than 2500 g and before 37 weeks) is less clear; women who deliver prematurely have less opportunity to gain weight. The use of total weight gain or net weight gain is inappropriate. Net gain per week of gestation controls for the duration confounder. Subsequent analysis does not define a

Table 2.4 Recommended total weight gain during pregnancy [29]

Prepregnancy BMI (kg/m²)	Recommended total weight gain (kg/lb)
Underweight (BMI < 18.5)	12.7–18.2 kg (28–40 lb)
Normal (BMI 18.5–24.9)	11.4–15.4 kg (25–35 lb)
Overweight (BMI 25.0–29.9)	6.8–11.4 kg (15–25 lb)
Obese – all classes[a] (BMI ≥ 30)	5.0–9.1 kg (11–20 lb)

BMI, Body Mass Index.
[a]Class I: BMI 30–34.9, Class II: BMI 35–39.9, Class III: BMI ≥ 40

relationship between net weight gain per week, BMI, and preterm birth. More recently, a maternal prepregnancy weight less than 100 lb has been analyzed as a risk factor for preterm birth; low BMI appears to be a stronger predictor (primipara: odds ratio [OR] 2.31, 95% CI 1.37–3.92; multipara: OR 1.76, 95% CI 1.19–2.61) than race, social environment, or paying job during pregnancy, but less than prior preterm birth in multiparous women [17].

An important caveat for any analysis using gestational age as a co-variate is the inaccuracy of gestational age estimates. As many as 15–35% of women seeking prenatal care have poor documentation of the first day of their last menstrual period. If ultrasound dating is used (now in 90% or more of pregnancies), early growth restriction may be obscured; all fetuses are standardized to the size of fetus in the 50th percentile for that gestational age. The actual error in gestational age may be as high as 1 week by a first-trimester ultrasound scan, 2 weeks by a second-trimester ultrasound, and 3 weeks or more by a third-trimester ultrasound. At term, this systematic error may translate into an 800–1000 g (2–3 lb) discrepancy between estimated fetal weight and actual birthweight. Large epidemiologic studies have not had standard methods of defining gestational age. When patients with poor dates are eliminated, then the size of the group most vulnerable for nutritionally related fetal growth restriction is reduced significantly.

Many early studies that examined the relationship between prepregnancy BMI and preterm birth did not adequately control for the decreased exposure necessarily found in a pregnancy of shortened duration [18–21]. However, they found a consistent association in women whose total weight gain was lower and the incidence of preterm birth. The magnitude of the risk varied between a 50% and a 400% increase in preterm births. This variance might be explained by differences in study design. The lower threshold for weight gain varies considerably, by 11–20 lb of total weight gain. Some studies defined the preterm birth as any birthweight below 2500 g, which included many term, small-for-gestational-age (SGA) neonates.

The confounding nature of decreased exposure, preterm birth, is illustrated in the analysis of the data from the 1980 National Natality Study [16]. If total weight gain is used, the odds ratio (95% CI) for delivering a preterm infant according to prepregnancy BMI shows a significant relationship between preterm birth and poor weight gain (less than 11 kg): small women, 4.0 (2.7–6.0); average women, 2.8 (2.0–4.0); and large women, 1.6 (0.8–3.2) [16]. However, when the effect of pregnancy duration is controlled by measuring net weight gain per week, the relationship between prepregnancy BMI, poor weight gain, and preterm birth disappears: small women, 1.2 (0.8–1.9); average women, 1.0 (0.7–1.5); and large women, 1.0 (0.5–1.9) [16]. In contrast, two recent studies demonstrated a significant risk of preterm birth when weight gain per week was less than 0.23 kg (less than 0.5 lb/wk) or less than 0.27 kg (0.6 lb/wk) [22,23]. They demonstrated a 40–60% increase in preterm births.

Two recent epidemiologic studies detailed the association between prepregnancy BMI and net weight gain per week, and adverse pregnancy outcomes. Cnattingius *et al* [22] examined the municipal birth records of 204,555 infants born in Sweden, Denmark, Norway, Finland, and Iceland from 1992 to 1993. The final population included 167,750 women with singleton births for whom prepregnancy BMI data were available. The results were adjusted for maternal age, parity, maternal education, cigarette smoking, and whether the mother was living with the father. Prepregnancy BMI of 20 or greater was associated with a decrease in the incidence of SGA infants (adjusted OR 0.5–0.7; 95% CI 0.4–0.8). Weight gain of less than 0.25 kg/wk was associated with an adjusted OR of 3.0 (95% CI 2.5–3.5) for the incidence of SGA infants. Among low- and normal-weight women, there was no association with late fetal death or preterm delivery. Overweight (BMI above 24.9 and less than 30.0) and obese (BMI over 29.9) women were shown to have a risk of late fetal death (after 28 weeks' completed gestation). The adjusted ORs (95% CI) for fetal death were 1.7 (1.1–2.4) for overweight women and 2.7 (1.8–4.1) for obese women. In addition, large women have a 2–4-fold increase in diabetes (10–15%).

The failure of prepregnancy BMI to predict preterm birth was confirmed in a 1992–4 study supported by the NICHD-MFMU network [23]. A cohort of 2929 pregnancies from 11 centers was followed longitudinally through pregnancy. Subjects were examined at 22–24 weeks and biologic variables including cervical length, fetal fibronectin, bacterial vaginosis, contraction frequency, and the presence of vaginal bleeding were assessed. A positive fetal fibronectin finding and a cervical length below 2.5 cm were associated with spontaneous birth at less than 32, 35, and 37 weeks (adjusted OR 2.5–10.0). In multiparous women, a history of preterm birth was also associated with preterm birth (adjusted OR 2.6–5.0). Low prepregnancy BMI was associated with neither early nor late preterm birth. A cautionary note is warranted. The exclusion of net weight gain per week as an intercurrent variable fails to account for the effect of nutrition on outcome. Perhaps poor nutrition has an interactive effect by increasing the likelihood of a positive fetal fibronectin finding or a shortened cervix. The study only examined main effect variables and not interactive variables.

Examination of the effects of nutrition on other adverse pregnancy outcomes is complicated by a paucity of quality research. Nutrition in Western women does not seem to be associated with first- or second-trimester abortion, congenital abnormalities or lactational performance. Weight gain during pregnancy can be associated with preeclampsia or diabetes. Very high levels of total weight gain or late-occurring increases in net weight gain per week are quite common in primiparous pregnancies complicated by preeclampsia. If there were any effect from preeclampsia, one would expect a higher rate of fetal growth restriction and spontaneous preterm birth in women who gain excessive weight. The meager amount of existing data seems to support an association, but more research is needed.

Specific maternal conditions

Nutritional assessment

The strong associations between extremes in prepregnancy BMI, extremes in weight gain, and adverse pregnancy outcome dictate that a basic, patient-centered, individualized nutritional assessment and plan be incorporated in the primary care of women from preconception, throughout pregnancy, and during the postpartum period, with special attention for breastfeeding. The nutritional assessment relies on the patient's medical record, history, and physical examination. The main areas of focus are sociodemographic risk (age less than 2 years after menarche, high parity [>4], low socio-economic status, culture, previous nutritional challenge), obstetric history (SGA and large-for-gestational-age infants, preterm birth), medical history (bowel disease, diabetes, chronic hypertension, hyperthyroid, chronic infection such as tuberculosis or human immunodeficiency virus infection, allergies, autoimmune disease, renal failure), behavioral risks (substance abuse, excessive exercise), nutritional risks (eating disorders, pica, fad diets, strict vegetarian diet, medications), and current diet (deviations in quantity or quality).

In the 24-h recall method, the patient is asked to recall the type and amount of food and beverages she consumed during the previous day. This technique gives clues to eating behavior rather than providing a quantitative measurement. There is considerable day-to-day variation that relates to issues of memory, lack of knowledge concerning the content of food (i.e. what goes into a beef stew), and inability to estimate correct portion sizes [24–27]. Practical ways to improve reporting include 3 days

What you eat and some of the life-style choices you make can affect your nutrition and health now and in the future. Your nutrition can also have an important effect on your baby's health. Please answer these questions by circling the answers that apply to you.

Eating Behavior

1. Are you frequently bothered by any of the following? (circle all that apply)
    Nausea   Vomiting   Heartburn   Constipation

2. Do you skip meals at least 3 times a week?   No   Yes

3. Do you try to limit the amount or kind of food you eat to control your weight?   No   Yes

4. Are you on a special diet now?   No   Yes

5. Do you avoid any foods for health or religious reasons?   No   Yes

Food Sources

6. Do you have a working stove?   No   Yes
    Do you have a working refrigerator?   No   Yes

7. Do you sometimes run out of food before you are able to buy more?   No   Yes

8. Can you afford to eat the way you should?   No   Yes

9. Are you receiving any food assistance now? (circle all that apply)   No   Yes
    Food stamps   School breakfast   School lunch   WIC
    Donated food   Commodity Supplemental Food Program
    Food from a food pantry, soup kitchen, or food banks

10. Do you feel you need help in obtaining food?   No   Yes

Food and Drink

11. Which of these did you drink yesterday? (circle all that apply)
    Soft drinks   Coffee   Tea   Fruit drink
    Orange juice   Grapefruit juice Other juices   Milk
    Kool-Aid®   Beer   Wine   Alcoholic drinks
    Water   Other beverages (list) _____

12. Which of these foods did you eat yesterday (circle all that apply):
    Cheese   Pizza   Macaroni and cheese
    Yogurt   Cereal with milk
    Other foods made with cheese (such as tacos, enchiladas, lasagna, cheeseburgers)
    Corn   Potatoes   Sweet potatoes   Green salad
    Carrots   Collard greens   Spinach   Turnip greens
    Broccoli   Green beans   Green peas   Other vegetables
    Apples   Bananas   Berries   Grapefruit
    Melon   Oranges   Peaches   Other fruit
    Meat   Fish   Chicken   Eggs
    Peanut butter   Nuts   Seeds   Dried beans
    Cold cuts   Hot dog   Bacon   Sausage
    Cake   Cookies   Doughnut   Pastry
    Chips   French fries   Deep-fried foods, such
                                       as fried chicken or
                                       egg rolls
    Bread   Rolls   Rice   Cereal
    Noodles   Spaghetti   Tortillas
    Were any of these whole grain?   No   Yes

13. Is the way you ate yesterday the way you usually eat?   No   Yes

Life-style

14. Do you exercise for at least 30 minutes on a regular basis (3 times a week or more)? No   Yes

15. Do you ever smoke cigarettes or use smokeless tobacco?   No   Yes

16. Do you ever drink beer, wine, liquor, or any other alcoholic beverages?   No   Yes

17. Which of these do you take? (circle all that apply)
    Prescribed drugs or medications
    Any over-the-counter products (such as aspirin, acetaminophen, antacids, or vitamins)
    Street drugs (such as marijuana, speed, downers, crack, or heroin)

Figure 2.4 Sample of a standard nutrition survey from the Institute of Medicine [12].

or a week of written record on type and amount of food and drinks consumed, discussion with the individual who prepares the food in order to understand the content of mixed food (stew), and education of the patient about portion size. For example, a cup is roughly equal in volume to a clenched fist and a 3 oz piece of fish or meat is roughly the size and thickness of the palm of the hand.

Another method uses a standardized survey to identify the usual frequency or dietary history. The accuracy of the survey is improved when portion estimates are included. A major advantage of the survey is the speed with which an assessment can be performed. The precise nature of the data lends itself to population analysis using one of

many diet analysis computer programs available [28]. When personnel resources are limited, a standardized survey is useful as a screening tool for all pregnant women. The Institute of Medicine developed a standard nutritional survey and weight gain guidelines [29] (Fig. 2.4). If a high-risk individual is identified by the survey, a more detailed nutritional analysis and intervention are appropriate.

Obstetric care providers and nutritionists would appreciate a memory chip placed in the mouth which could automatically record the type and volume of the consumed food and drink: this will not happen any time soon! We have to rely on simultaneous written records or

Table 2.5 Dietary reference intakes[#], usual dietary intake, and prenatal vitamins in pregnant women

Nutriment	RDI	Usual intake	PNV	Intake plus PNV
Total carbohydrates (g/day)	2500	1900–2100[a]	None	2000[b]
Total protein (g/d)	60	68–91	None	80
Total fiber (g/d)	28			
Fat-soluble vitamins				
A (μg of RE)	770	1000–1400	450	1650
D (IU)	600*	40–60[a]	100	150
E (mg)	15	3.4–12.0[a]	22	30
K (μg)	90	300–500	None	465
Water-soluble vitamins				
Folate (μg)	600	168–245[a]	1000	1207
Thiamine (mg)	1.4	1.2–1.9[a]	3	8.5
Riboflavin (mg)	1.4	1.7–3.4	3.4	6.0
Pyridoxine (mg)	1.9	0.8–2.2[a]	10	26
Niacin (mg)	18	17–280	20	42
C (mg)	85	48–1440	100	298
B_{12} (μg)	2.6	2.6–5.70	12	16.5
Minerals				
Calcium (mg)	1000	668–1195[a]	250	1182
Magnesium (mg)	350	191–269[b]	25	255[b]
Iron (mg)	27	11.2–17.2[a]	60	74
Zinc (mg)	11	06.0–12.0[a]	25	34
Iodine (μg)	220	170[a]	150	320
Selenium (μg)	60	70	None	70

PNV, prenatal vitamins; RDI, recommended daily intake.
[a]Deficient without prenatal vitamins or supplement.
[b]Deficient after daily multivitamins.
#Institute of Medicine (2009): www.iom.edu.
*Institute of Medicine (2010): www.iom.edu.

patient recall. Unfortunately, the accuracy of both the 24-h recall and the nutritional survey depends on the accuracy of the patient's memory. In general, the accuracy is poor and may reflect what the provider wishes rather what was consumed [24–28]. The rather large variations in intake, yet the relative lack of demonstrable variation in adverse outcome, except in the extremes, raises concern about the practicality of obtaining a detailed dietary history from every pregnant woman. Because the extremes are important, more detailed nutritional assessment and counseling are needed for populations at high risk for poor dietary practices as defined by 24-h recall or the standardized survey. Table 2.4 describes the recommended weight gain, stratified by pregnancy BMI [29].

Tables 2.5 (pregnant) and 2.6 (nonsupplemented breastfeeding) compare the average daily intake of nutriments with and without prenatal multivitamins to the 2011 Dietary Reference Intakes [30,31]. The analysis reveals that the average American woman who is pregnant and taking one tablet daily of the prenatal multivitamins with 0.4–1.0 mg of folic acid requires only extra energy (500–600 kcal/day), magnesium (125 mg), and calcium

(300–600 mg). Likewise, lactating women who take one tablet daily of prenatal multivitamins and who are not supplementing the infant with formula and solids require the same micronutriments in similar amounts. The reader must keep in mind that the "usual" daily intake that the American medical environment emphasizes includes a higher intake of protein and dairy products during pregnancy and lactation. Recent focus on the fat content of dairy products will lead many women to reduce milk intake. If the liquid need is supplanted by beverages containing caffeine or phosphoric acid (carbonated sodas), the total intake of calcium or protein or both may be reduced.

Obesity

Obesity remains a major health issue for developed countries. United States data collected by the Centers for Disease Control (CDC) through 2009 suggests that the prevalence of obesity (BMI >30) rose from 19.8% in 2000 to 23.9% in 2005 and 26.7% in 2009 [32]. Obese women have many more adverse pregnancy outcomes. In addition to more gestational diabetes, hypertension, and

Table 2.6 Recommended dietary intakes[#], usual dietary intake, and prenatal vitamins in lactating women

Nutriment	RDI	Usual intake	PNV	Intake plus PNV
Total carbohydrates (g)	175	600	None	600
Total protein (g)	71	78–115	None	97
Total fiber (g)	29			
Fat-soluble vitamins				
A (µg of RE)	1300	1000–1200[a]	450	1550
D (IU)	600	136[a]	100	236[b]
E (mg)	19	4.5[a]	22	26.5
K (µg)	90	NR	None	NR
Water-soluble vitamins				
Folate (µg)	500	169–340[a]	1000	1255
Thiamine (mg)	1.4	1.39–2.1[a]	3	3.79
Riboflavin (mg)	1.6	1.87–2.8	3.4	5.7
Pyridoxine (mg)	2.8	1.11–1.69[a]	10	11
Niacin (mg)	17	16.3–70	20	63
C (mg)	120	108–199	100	253
B_{12} (µg)	2.8	2.88–7.96	12	17[b]
Minerals				
Calcium (mg)	1000	1004–1304[a]	250	1300
Magnesium (mg)	320	221[a]	25	227[b]
Iron (mg)	9	12.2–16.2[a]	60	74
Zinc (mg)	12	09.4–12.2[a]	25	36
Iodine (µg)	290	NR	150	150[b]
Selenium (µg)	70	84–870	None	85
Phosphorus (mg)	700	1350–20,050	None	1700

NR, not reported; PNV, prenatal vitamins; RDI, recommended daily intake.
[a]Deficient without prenatal vitamins or supplement.
[b]Deficient after daily multivitamins.
#Institute of Medicine (2009): www.iom.edu.
*Institute of Medicine (2010): www.iom.edu.

wound infections [33], overweight and obese women are more likely to have preterm birth or SGA neonates (relative risk [RR]1.24, 95% CI 1.18–1.37) [34] and more stillbirths (RR 2.07, 95% CI 1.59–2.74). A recent meta-analysis of the risks of obesity and birth defects revealed more neural tube defects (RR 1.87, 95% CI 1.62–2.15), more congenital heart defects (RR 1.30, 95% CI 1.12–1.51), more cleft lip and palate (RR 1.20, 95% CI 1.03–1.40), and more limb reduction defects (RR 1.34, 95% CI 1.03–0.73) among neonates of obese women. Interestingly, gastroschisis was less common (RR 0.17, 95% CI 0.1–0.3) among neonates of obese women [35,36].

The consequence of the concerns for obesity and adverse pregnancy outcomes were incorporated in the 1990 Institute of Medicine (IOM) guidelines for weight gain in pregnancy and their modification of the guidelines in 2009 (see Table 2.4). The guidelines and recommendations are in recent reviews [37,38]. An area ripe for outcomes study is to evaluate the impact of education and interventions to reduce the number of women entering

pregnancy obese, preconception counseling, and limiting excess gestational weight gain [38].

Early population-based outcome studies reveal interesting risks and benefits of the public health focus on obesity studies. For example, two papers came from Germany looking at about 820,000 births between 2000 and 2007. In the first [39], the prevalence of various adverse perinatal outcomes was measured among normal weight, overweight, and obese women who gained the recommended IOM amount of weight (Table 2.7). In a subset of the same population, the benefits and concerns for failure to gain weight in pregnancy are demonstrated. While hypertension and nonelective cesarean section were reduced in the overweight and class I obese women (30–34.9 kg/m²) (RR 0.65, 95% CI 0.51–0.83), the risk of SGA neonates was increased (RR 1.68, 95% CI 1.37–2.06) [40]. No differences were demonstrated when weight loss occurred in class II–III obesity (>35 kg/m²).

Retained weight postpartum plays a role in chronic morbidities. In general, while women with average

Table 2.7 The prevalence of adverse pregnancy outcomes associated with meeting Institute of Medicine targets

	Underweight	Normal weight	Overweight	Obese
Number	29,317	442,885	137,388	19,987
Preeclampsia	0.6%	0.88%	1.7%	4.9%
Gestational diabetes	0.6%	0.92%	2.3%	4.5%
Nonelective cesarean	9.3 %	10,6%	11.6%	14.3%
SGA	12.1%	8.4%	8.3%	7.3%
LGA	3.9%	7.1%	9.4%	13.9%
Preterm birth	5.2%	5.3%	8.1%	8.6%
Stillbirth	0.14%	0.16%	0.34%	0.51%
Early neonatal death	0.6%	0.04%	0.04%	0.21%

LGA, large for gestational age; SGA, small for gestational age.
Adapted from Beyerlein *et al* [39].

gestational weight gains retain about 1 kg (2.2 lb) postpartum, African-American women tend to retain more weight postpartum regardless of the prepregnancy BMI or prenatal weight gain [12,41,42]. African-American women with a normal prepregnancy BMI were twice as likely to retain more than 20 lb than were white women of the same build. Women with high weight gain tend to retain more weight. Researchers have reported that retention of more than 2.5 kg (5.5 lb) between the first and second pregnancy was associated with higher weight gain in the last half of pregnancy, 10–20 kg (22–26 lb) [12]. In the 1959 to 1965 Collaborative Perinatal Project, women who gained 16.4–18.2 kg (36–40 lb) or gained more than 18.2 kg (more than 40 lb) retained 5 kg (10.9 lb) and 8.0 kg (17.7 lb), respectively. The years when the latter two studies were performed suggest caution in the interpretation of the data. In 2011, more women gain high amounts of weight during pregnancy; the incidence of excessive weight retention must be higher.

Multifetal pregnancy

Multifetal pregnancy would be expected to increase the nutritional demand for the mother. Unfortunately, the confounders found in singleton pregnancies are more pronounced in multifetal pregnancy, and the nutritional component of adverse pregnancy outcomes is much harder to delineate. Multifetal pregnancies are associated with higher rates of preterm birth (40–50%), fetal growth restriction (20–40%), more perinatal deaths (fourfold to sixfold), more preeclampsia, more diabetes, and more frequent cesarean delivery. The analysis is complicated further by different fetal growth rates related to differences between like-sex and mixed-sex pregnancies or the differences between monozygotic and heterozygotic gestations. There has been limited study of the risks and concerns for weight gain in multifetal pregnancies. Goodnight *et al* diet recommendations include the following for twin pregnancies: 40–45 Kcal/kg (normal weight),

42–50 Kcal/kg (underweight), 30–35 Kcal/kg (overweight); 2500 gm calcium/day; Vitamin D 1000 IU/day; and Vitamin C 1000 mg/day. The nutritional recommendations for 3+ fetal pregnancies are speculation, perhaps an additional 10% per fetus [43].

Nutritional interventions

Nutritional intervention beyond prenatal multivitamins is not needed for most pregnant or lactating women who live in the United States. The critical issue is to identify the extremes in amounts: dietary restriction, nonfood competition (pica) or excess metabolic needs (see Table 2.2, Fig. 2.4). It must be remembered that nutritional supplementation most often uses mixed foods (nutritional drink supplying energy, protein, and micronutriments). Mixed food supplementation obscures the benefit of a specific nutriment. The following section provides a summary of the data concerning interventions related to nutriments.

Multivitamins

Prenatal multivitamins with at least 400 µg of folic acid are recommended for pregnant women in the United States. In developing countries, the use of multiple micronutriment supplements (prenatal vitamins) has been compared to supplements containing only folic acid and iron, with random assignment of treatment groups [44,45]. The results suggest an increase in birthweight of 50–100 g, less than the reduced birthweight with each pack of cigarettes smoked. Each pack of cigarettes smoked reduces birthweight by 100–150 g. The effect on other adverse outcomes, i.e. SGA neonates, prematurity, perinatal mortality, is less consistent and less clear. A more recent meta-analysis suggests benefits in undernourished populations: low birthweight (RR 0.83, 95% CI 0.71–0.91), SGA (RR 0.92, 95% CI 0.86–0.99), and anemia (RR 0.6, 95% CI 0.52–0.71) when used in populations of developing countries [45]. In developed countries there appears to be a reduction in birth defects (other than neural tube defects) with the use of multivitamins (RR 0.53–0.84) [46]. The use of prenatal vitamins in developed countries has not been shown to reduce adverse pregnancy outcomes or increase birthweight.

Energy and protein supplementation

Multiple comparative trials have addressed undernourished (less than 1500 kcal/day) populations in developing countries. When energy (200–800 kcal) and protein (40–60 g) are supplemented in undernourished women, there is a consistent increase in birthweight (100–400 g) and maternal weight gain (0.8–0.9 kg/month). Improvement in infant outcome is less clear; some studies showed a reduction in low birthweight and preterm birth, whereas others did not [12]. Among undernourished pregnant Gambian women, prenatal energy, protein, and micronutriment supplementation resulted in a decrease in the incidence of low birthweight from 23% in the control to 7.5% in the supplemented population [12].

In developing and industrialized countries where the nutrition is better (1600–2100 kcal/day), mixed food supplementation does not result in significant maternal weight gain or increases in birthweight. Few studies have demonstrated differences in perinatal outcomes between supplemented and unsupplemented pregnant women if their intake exceeds 2100–2300 kcal/day. These observations are supported by a systematic review of randomized trials [47,48].

Iron supplementation

Worldwide, iron deficiency anemia complicates the lives of nonpregnant (35%) and pregnant (51%) women. Among nonpregnant (2%) and pregnant (5–10%) women, industrialized countries have much lower incidences of iron deficiency anemia when defined by a low serum ferritin concentration (less than 12 µg/L) and a hemoglobin below 11.0, 10.5, and 11.0 g/dL in the first, second, and third trimesters, respectively (CDC definition). Adverse pregnancy outcomes, such as low birthweight, preterm birth, and increased perinatal mortality, are associated with a hemoglobin below 10.4 g/dL before 24 weeks of gestation [49–51]. Both the latter study and the National Collaborative Perinatal Project [12] demonstrated a U-shaped curve when adverse pregnancy outcomes are plotted against hemoglobin concentration. The incidence of poor outcome rises progressively when the hemoglobin falls below 10.4 g/dL or rises above 13.2 g/dL.

The pregnant woman has an additional need for absorbed, elemental iron (3.0 mg/day) above that of a nonpregnant reproductive-age woman (1.3 mg/day). Her extra needs arise from the 350 mg needed for fetal/placental growth, 250 mg for blood loss at delivery, 450 mg for increases in maternal red cell mass, and a baseline loss

of 250 mg. Blood loss at cesarean delivery is twofold to threefold higher than blood loss after a vaginal delivery without an episiotomy, an important consideration as 32% of American women have cesarean births. As a fully lactating woman less than 6 months after delivery is usually not menstruating, her needs are considerably lower, at 0.3 mg/day (men require 0.9 mg/day).

Luckily, 80% of American women receive daily prenatal multivitamins that contain 30–60 mg of iron, and iron absorption is doubled or tripled among pregnant women as opposed to nonpregnant women [52]. The absorption of iron is affected by many factors. The type of iron supplement is important; the absorption of iron sulfate is 20%, iron gluconate 12%, and iron fumarate 32%. Meat sources of iron absorb better than do plant sources (whole grains, legumes) by interaction with phytates, tannins, polyphenols, and plant calcium and phosphate moieties. Between-meal dosing will maximize the absorption of therapeutic iron because of the reduced number of binding compounds in the gastrointestinal tract. There appears to be a threshold for iron absorption; once the dose is increased to above 120 mg/day, the percentage absorption falls and the incidence of side-effects increases [53–55]. Orange juice or vitamin C (more than 200 mg) taken with the iron supplement will increase absorption twofold. On the other hand, excessive coffee or tea reduces iron absorption by one half.

The prevalence of iron deficiency anemia among nonpregnant women of child-bearing age was examined in the Second National Health and Nutrition Survey (1978–80) (NHANES2) [56]. The diagnosis of iron deficiency anemia was based on criteria defined by a mean corpuscular volume (MCV), iron/total iron binding capacity, and erythropoietin (EP) evaluation. The overall baseline incidence of iron deficiency anemia was 2% in middle- to upper-class non-Hispanic white women. The risk of iron deficiency anemia appears to be greater among the poor (7.8%), those with less than 12 years of education (13.2%), Mexican-Americans (11.2%), African-Americans (5.0%), and adolescents (4.9%), and in women who have given birth to three or four children (11.5%). Multiple pregnancy, maternal bowel disease, chronic infection (tuberculosis, human immunodeficiency virus), chronic aspirin use (0.2–2.0 mg iron loss/day), and persistent vaginal or rectal bleeding (second- and third-trimester bleeding, placenta previa, hemorrhoids) will increase the likelihood of anemia. In these populations prophylactic iron therapy (30 mg/day) is warranted.

Clinically, the diagnosis is based on the laboratory findings of anemia with hemoglobin below 10.5 g/dL, a low MCV, and a serum ferritin level below 12 µg/dL. Most studies using random assignment of subjects demonstrated that daily doses from 30–120 mg are equally effective in raising the hemoglobin 0.4–1.7 g/dL by 35–40 weeks' gestation [12]. The latest metaanalysis (2007) demonstrated that routine iron supplementation reduced anemia at delivery (RR 0.38, 95% CI 0.26–0.55) [57]. Unfortunately, the data on improvement in the incidence of adverse pregnancy outcomes are either not reported or obscured by small sample sizes [58].

Calcium

Approximately 99% of calcium and magnesium in pregnant women and their fetuses or infants is located in their bones and teeth. Pregnancy and lactation are associated with increased bone turnover in order to meet fetal or infant needs for calcium (50 mg/day at 20 weeks, 330 mg/day at 35 weeks, and 300 mg/day during lactation) and increased urinary excretion of calcium (200 mg/day). The fetus actively transports calcium, and fetal levels are higher than maternal calcium levels. The total fetal accretion of calcium is 30 g. The body maintains the serum ionized calcium level within a tight range (4.4–5.2 mg/dL) and if dietary deficiencies occur, maternal bone will supply its calcium to the fetus. While bone turnover is high in pregnant or lactating women, measures of net bone loss during pregnancy and lactation among women in developed countries are inconsistent (24% to 12%) [12]. One explanation for the varied results is increased absorption of dietary calcium related to pregnancy or lactation. Increased absorption is correlated with the highest fetal needs (nonpregnant, 27%; 5–6 months, 54%; and at term, 42%) [12]. Increased absorption is in part due to progressive increases in 1,25-dihydroxycholecalciferol (the active moiety of vitamin D). On the other hand, a diet high in plant phytates, phosphoric acid (carbonated sodas), aluminum-based antacids or over-the-counter medications containing bismuth reduces calcium absorption.

Increased calcium is associated with smooth muscle relaxation, and parathyroid hormone (PTH) has a stimulatory effect on angiotensin II-mediated secretion of aldosterone. Animal and human studies demonstrated a consistent reduction in blood pressure in nonpregnant animals or humans when their dietary calcium is increased. Hypocalciuria is a useful diagnostic tool in the differentiation of preeclampsia from other forms of hypertension in pregnancy [59]. These observations have led to controlled, clinical trials to test the hypothesis that calcium supplements during pregnancy reduce the incidence of pregnancy-induced hypertension (and perhaps preterm birth) [60–64]. In these studies, pregnant women were randomly assigned to receive 1500–2000 mg daily of calcium or no calcium. The effect on the incidence of pregnancy-induced hypertension has been mixed. The studies that reported a benefit demonstrated a dose–response effect and a reduction of vascular sensitivity to angiotensin II injection. There seemed to be a trend toward a reduction in the incidence of preterm birth. At least two other studies did not demonstrate a benefit from supplemental calcium. The discrepancy between the studies is likely to be related to patient selection and the handling of the analysis when compliance is an issue. A more recent metaanalysis has been more optimistic: calcium supplementation greater than 1 g/day resulted in a reduction in preeclampsia (RR 0.45, 95% CI 0.31–0.67), preterm birth (RR 0.76, 95% CI 0.6–0.9), and a composite of maternal death or serious morbidity (RR 0.8, 95% CI 0.65–0.97) [64].

Similarly, there does not seem to be a benefit from reduced salt diet in the prevention of preeclampsia [65,66].

At this point, there is no support for the routine supplementation of calcium (2000 mg/day) for all pregnant women. Pregnant women who have a diet deficient in calcium (less than 600 mg/day), prepregnancy hypertension, calcium-losing renal disease, a strong family or personal history of preeclampsia, or chronic use of certain medications (heparin, steroids) may benefit with little risk of toxicity from daily supplemental calcium (2000 mg of elemental calcium or 5000 mg of calcium carbonate). Young women (less than 25 years old) and those with mild dietary calcium deficiency (600–1200 mg/day) may be treated by extra servings of dairy products – 8 oz of milk or 1 oz of hard cheese, which supplies 300 mg of calcium per serving, or supplemental calcium, 600 mg (carbonate).

Calcium metabolism is more complex than the simple precepts outlined earlier indicated [67]. PTH is associated with increased calcium absorption from the intestine and increased bone absorption; a high level in late pregnancy would be expected. Unexpectedly, the biologically active form of PTH is associated with a 40% decrease during pregnancy. Calcitonin acts as a biologic balance to PTH, and as serum calcium levels are maintained within a tight range, higher levels of calcitonin would be expected. The studies that evaluated calcitonin levels during pregnancy had inconsistent results.

Magnesium

Magnesium is essential for the release of PTH from the parathyroid and the action of PTH on the intestines, bones, and kidneys. The fetus absorbs 6 mg of magnesium each day. Maternal magnesium levels remain constant during pregnancy despite inadequate intake (see Table 2.5). On the other hand, Spatling and Spatling performed a double-blind, placebo-controlled trial in which pregnant women (at less than 16 weeks) were assigned randomly to receive magnesium supplementation (360 mg/day) or placebo [68]. Of patients who reported compliance, the magnesium supplement group had 30% fewer hospitalizations, 50% fewer preterm births, and 25% more perinatal hemorrhages compared to the placebo supplement women. The outcomes were not analyzed on an intention-to-treat basis. A recent metaanalysis suggests that magnesium supplementation (350–450 mg/day) reduces preterm birth (RR 0.73, 95% CI 0.57–0.93), SGA (RR 0.70, 95% CI 0.53–0.93), and postpartum hemorrhage (RR 0.38, 95% CI 0.16–0.9) [69].

Vitamin D

Vitamin D is critical in the absorption, distribution, and storage of calcium. Sunlight is the major source of vitamin D, 1,25-hydroxycholecalciferol. Sunlight (ultraviolet light) converts 7-dehydroxycalciferol within the skin to vitamin D. Vitamin D is converted to 25-hydroxycholecalciferol (marker for adequate vitamin D) in the liver and subsequently to 1,25-hydroxycholecalciferol (active form) in the kidney. In latitudes higher than 40° North, especially where clouds obscure sunlight during the winter, the conversion of 7-dehydroxycholecalciferol to 1,25-hydroxycholecalciferol is insufficient to maintain adequate levels of vitamin D. For example, the serum levels of 25-hydroxycholecalciferol vary considerably between fall and spring: from 25 ng/dL in the fall to 17 ng/dL in the spring in England; from 18 ng/dL in the fall to 11 ng/dL in the spring in Finland. While few cases of vitamin D deficiency (less than 5 mg/dL) are encountered in England or the US, Finland records an incidence of 47% in the spring and 33% in the fall [12].

Relatively few foods are good sources of vitamin D. Vitamin D-fortified milk is the major dietary source in the United States. Eight ounces of fortified milk contains about 150 IU of vitamin D and 120 IU of vitamin A. Although vitamin D deficiency is very rare in the United States because of its latitude, propensity toward more exposure of bare skin, and the almost uniform vitamin D fortification of milk, selected populations may be at risk for low 25-hydroxycholecalciferol levels. These populations include culturally prescribed full clothing, the home-bound, or institutionalized patients who cannot (lactose intolerant) or will not drink milk. In these populations, intervention with vitamin D supplementation (600 IU/day) may be beneficial. No controlled trials have used vitamin D to correct a deficiency and subsequently demonstrate a change in its physiologic actions. In summary, uniform vitamin D supplementation is not recommended [70].

Folate

Folate participates in many bodily processes, especially rapidly growing tissue. It functions as a co-enzyme in the transfer of single carbon units from one compound to another. This step is essential to the synthesis of nucleic acids and the metabolism of amino acids. As the mother and fetus are rapidly developing new tissue, perturbation in folate intake might be expected to result in adverse pregnancy outcomes. In the last 10 years a clear and consistent relationship between low folate intake and fetal neural tube defects and, possibly, cleft lip and palate has been identified.

Folate deficiency works with multiple factors to cause birth defects [71]. Genetic factors appear to be a strong co-factor. The population rates of neural tube defects vary considerably: 1 per 1000 births in the United States, 6 per 1000 births in Ireland, and 10 per 1000 births in northern China. Women with a previous child with a neural tube defect have a 1.6–6.0% risk of recurrent neural tube defects. The level of risk is predicted by the frequency of occurrence of neural tube defects in the immediate family. Environmental exposures seem to be an additional co-factor. Preconceptual diabetes or first-trimester hyperglycemia is associated with a multiple-fold increase in the incidence of neural tube defects. Drugs such as valproic acid, carbamazepine, folate antagonists, and thalidomide are associated with a 1–4% risk of neural tube defects.

Folate is an essential nutriment for humans, as we cannot manufacture folates and must rely on dietary intake and absorption. Folates are present in leafy green vegetables, fruit, fortified breads and cereals, egg yolks, and yeast. Many multivitamins and fortified cereals contain 350–400 mg of folate. Prescription prenatal multivitamins contain 0.8–1.0 mg of folic acid. Eighty percent of folate intake in the United States is derived from polyglutamate forms of folate. The absorption of polyglutamate forms is about 60%; the absorption of monoglutamate forms is about 90%. Multivitamins contain the monoglutamate forms.

The recommended dietary allowance (RDA) of folate is 3 g per kilogram of bodyweight for nonpregnant and nonlactating women. Given a 60–70% absorption rate from their diet, pregnant women should acquire an extra 0.4 mg in their daily diet. Lactating women need an extra 0.2 mg/day. The average daily intake of folate in the United States is 0.20–0.25 mg despite the fact that 20% of American women consume multivitamins containing 0.36 mg or more of folic acid. Dietary deficiency of folic acid is a major public health issue. Public and individual interventions to increase folate intake raise awareness (62–72%), knowledge (21–45%), and consumption (14–23%) [72].

There is a progressive pattern of the pathophysiology of folate deficiency with increasing duration and intensity of folate deficiency. At 3 weeks, low serum folate levels (below 3 ng/mL) are manifest. At 5 weeks, neutrophils develop hypersegmentation (more than 3.5 lobes). At 7 weeks, the bone marrow demonstrates megaloblastic changes. At 17 weeks, the erythrocyte folate level is low (below 140 ng/mL). At 20 weeks, a generalized megaloblastic anemia (MCV above 105) is present.

Most interventions with folic acid have focused on the prevention of neural tube defects. In women with a previous history of a child with a neural tube defect, numerous studies involving randomized assignment demonstrated a 75% reduction in the frequency of recurrent neural tube defects when 4–5 mg of folic acid was taken daily for 1–2 months preconceptually and through the first trimester [12,73–75]. The most recent metaanalysis suggests that folate supplementation reduces neural tube and other birth defects by 72% (RR 0.28, 95% CI 0.15–0.52) [75]. The current standard of care requires documentation that the benefits of folic acid supplementation in preventing recurrent neural tube defects have been explained and that the supplement has been prescribed to the patient. The recommendation is to supplement with 4 mg of folic acid daily from 1 to 3 months preconceptually and through the first trimester.

More recently, daily multivitamins that contain 0.4–0.8 mg of folic acid have been shown to decrease the incidence of neural tube defects in low-risk women (no previous pregnancy or family history of neural tube defects). One study randomly assigned women to receive either a placebo plus trace elements or a multivitamin that contained 0.8 mg of folic acid [73,74]. Of 2104 women who received folic acid, no neural tube defects occurred and in 2065 women who received the placebo, six pregnancies were complicated by neural tube defects (P < 0.029). Women who are at mild risk (distant family history of neural tube defect, inadequate intake, multiple pregnancy [undergoing assisted reproductive technology]) and who are attempting pregnancy should have documentation of adequate dietary folate consumption or daily prescription multivitamins that contain at least 0.8 mg of folic acid from 1 to 3 months preconceptually through the first trimester.

Antioxidants and marine oils
Recently, antioxidant supplements, vitamin E, vitamin C and 3-N fatty acids (marine oils), have been suggested to decrease adverse pregnancy outcomes such as preeclampsia and preterm birth. However, a limited number of trials have not demonstrated a benefit from vitamin C or E in reducing preterm birth, preeclampsia, SGA neonates or perinatal mortality [76–78]. Supplemental marine oils and other prostaglandin precursors may have more benefit. One study suggested a reduction in preterm birth (RR 0.69, 95% CI 0.49–0.99) [79]. Other studies suggested better neurodevelopmental outcome in exposed children [80]. However, it is too early to recommend routine supplementation with marine oils for all pregnancies; much more study is required.

Other nutriments
The benefits of supplementing other specific nutriments in pregnant women have not been confirmed by blinded, placebo-controlled trials with random assignment of subjects, or the studies that do exist have major methodological weaknesses such as selection bias or inadequate sample size. An additional problem is outcome definition. Low maternal nutriment levels are very different from clinical deficiency states and many of the important outcomes (preterm birth, perinatal mortality, fetal growth restriction) have other predictors to obscure the relationship between nutrition and adverse pregnancy outcomes. Despite the latter observations, nutriments whose supplementation may benefit deficiency states include zinc, selenium, chromium (diabetes), fluoride, magnesium, vitamin A (less than 5000 retinol equivalent [RE]), vitamin B_6, and vitamin C.

Vitamin toxicity
The clinician is occasionally confronted with a woman who is taking unorthodox amounts of vitamins or minerals. Many of the data on toxic risk are based on animal studies and anecdotal cases, especially those concerning the ingestion of more obscure vitamins and minerals. The tragedy of thalidomide, fetal anomalies, and the lack of animal toxicity should caution interpretation of results of animal studies. Luckily, most water-soluble vitamins appear relatively safe for the mother and fetus; excess intake is readily excreted in the urine. Vitamin C taken in an amount greater than 6–8 g/day may cause loose stool. Vitamin B_6 intake greater than 500 mg/day is associated with a reversible peripheral neuropathy. Maternal or fetal toxicity has not been identified with the other water-soluble vitamins.

Toxicity is more of an issue with excess intake of fat-soluble vitamins. Vitamin A (retinol forms) is associated with a dose-dependent increase in fetal defects: hydrocephalus, microcephalus, and cardiac lesions. The risk of defects seems to be related to the retinol/retinyl ester forms of vitamin A. Carotenoid forms do not seem to have the same risks. The threshold intake where risk appears excessive has not been defined, but at doses lower than 10,000 RE of retinoid forms, the incidence of fetal abnormality is no greater than the baseline risk; with doses higher than 25,000 RE the risk of defects clearly exceeds the baseline risk. Huge doses (above 15 mg or 600,000 IU) of vitamin D have been associated with a variable degree of toxic symptoms (soft tissue calcification). Excess vitamin E or vitamin K use has not been associated consistently with adverse outcome for the mother or fetus.

Toxicity associated with excess mineral intake is associated with primarily maternal symptoms. Iron intake at more than 200 mg/day is associated with gastrointestinal symptoms (heartburn, nausea, abdominal pain, constipation) in a dose-dependent fashion (placebo 13%; 200 mg 25%; 400 mg 40%) [54]. Magnesium sulfate at more than 3 g/day is associated with catharsis and reduced iron absorption. Iodine excess is associated with goiter and hyperthyroidism. Selenium at more than 30 mg/day results in nausea, vomiting, fatigue, and nail changes. Molybdenum interferes with calcium absorption. Zinc intake at more than 45 mg/day has associated with preterm delivery and reduced iron and copper absorption. Fluoride at doses higher than 2 mg/L (fluoridated water plus supplemental fluoride) is associated with dental fluorosis of the primary teeth in the fetus.

Lactation

Breastfeeding and breast milk are unique gifts for the mother and newborn. Breast milk has nutritional qualities far superior to formula [81]. Formulas do not contain important enzymes and hormones to aid digestion, active or passive immunoglobulins, activated immune cells or antibacterial compounds (lactoferrin). Breast milk promotes growth of nonpathogenic bacterial flora in the infant's intestine, i.e. *Bifidobacterium* spp. Formula contains inappropriate fatty acid and lactose concentrations for optimal brain growth, and inconsistent amounts of essential vitamins and other micronutriments.

The unique qualities of breastfeeding and breast milk provide many benefits for the mother and infant. For the mother, the benefits include significant contraception and child spacing (lactational amenorrhea method), better mother–infant bonding, less cost for nutrition and equipment, fewer healthcare costs for the infant, less loss of work time and income to care for sick children, less postpartum retention of weight, and reduction in the risk of breast cancer. For the infant, the benefits include fewer deaths from infection, less morbidity from respiratory and gastrointestinal infections, appropriate growth patterns, less childhood obesity, less childhood cancer, better social interaction, higher intelligence, better orofacial development, and protection from allergies.

The documented benefits of breastfeeding and breast milk have prompted the World Health Organization (WHO), the US Surgeon General, and the American Academy of Pediatrics (AAP) [82] to recommend breastfeeding rather than formula feeding. The nutritional qualities of breast milk are sufficient for infant growth until 6 months, after which gradual introduction of food is appropriate. The AAP recommends breastfeeding for at least 12 months.

As breast milk is manufactured and secreted by the human breast, the nutritional quality and composition are remarkably constant regardless of the tremendous variation in maternal diet. The volume (700–1000 mL/day) of breast milk produced for the infant determines the mother's nutritional needs during lactation. If the fully lactating woman has an average diet and takes one prenatal multivitamin daily (see Table 2.6), her daily requirements for lactation are satisfied, except for magnesium and iodine. The deficiency in magnesium and iodine is not manifested by a variation in breast milk concentration. The infant is not at risk for deficiency.

In the fully breast-fed infant, the volume of breast milk consumed determines the amount of energy, protein, vitamins, and minerals obtained by the infant. Therefore, a review of the factors that can affect breast milk volume is appropriate. Less than 5% of women have anatomic limits for adequate volumes of breast milk. These include congenital hypoplasia (small, tubular shape), cosmetic breast surgery (reduction or augmentation), severe nipple inversion, and periareolar breast surgery. Pain (nipple trauma, injections), stress, and maternal insecurity inhibit the release of oxytocin and contraction of the myoepithelial cells surrounding the breast acini (interference with the letdown reflex). Some medications (bromocryptine, ergotrate/methergine, combination birth control pills, or testosterone analogs) can reduce milk volume.

Analysis of levels of maternal energy intake and the volume of breast milk reveals little risk for American women. Women who are below standards for BMI and who consume fewer than 1500 kcal/day preconceptually, during pregnancy, and during lactation (severely disadvantaged in developing countries) show little (less than 60 mL) difference in milk volume [83,84]. Nutritional supplementation studies in undernourished populations did not demonstrate an increase in milk volume. In developed countries, where the energy intake is at much higher levels, no reduction of milk volume is demonstrated. Short-term reduction in calorie intake (19–32%) in well-nourished lactating women did not reduce milk volume in those who restricted their intake to no less than 1500 kcal/day. In women who restricted their intake to less than 1500 kcal/day, the milk volume was reduced by 109 mL [84]. Gradual weight loss (2 kg/month) is associated with normal milk volumes. Regular postpartum exercise, which increases oxygen consumption by 25%, has no effect on breast milk volume [83,84].

Dietary recommendations for pregnancy and lactation

In 1990 the Institute of Medicine, after an exhaustive review of the literature, published its recommendations: *Nutrition During Pregnancy* [12] (revised in 2006 and 2009, see www.iom.edu) and *Nutrition During Lactation* [84]. The recommendations support accurate measurement of BMI at the preconceptual (preferred) or initial visit (see Table 2.4), subsequent measurement of weight at each prenatal and postpartum visit, standardized assessment of maternal diet (see Fig. 2.4), assessment of nutritional risk factors, patient education, and nutritional intervention.

One key component is different target levels of weight gain based on the mother's prepregnancy BMI. Table 2.4 describes the recommendations. Of equal importance, the amount and quality of the woman's diet should be assessed in a standardized fashion (see Fig. 2.4). A good daily diet will contain seven 1 oz servings of protein-rich foods (meat, poultry, fish, eggs, legumes, nuts), three 8 oz servings of milk or an equivalent amount of other dairy products, six or more servings of grain products (each serving one slice of bread, 1 oz of dry cereal, half a cup of cooked pasta, hot cereal or rice), and six or more servings of fruits and vegetables (each serving half a cup of cooked, one cup of raw, 6 oz of juice). Pregnant women younger than 24 years should consume one extra serving of dairy products daily [12,84]. This diet, when taken with one tablet of a prenatal multivitamin daily, will supply 2500–2700 kcal of energy per day and 1.3–1.5 g of protein per day as well as sufficient vitamins and minerals.

Once baseline information has been documented, the provider should counsel and educate the patient, continue accurate documentation of weight change, and intervene if necessary. Counseling and education involve setting a target goal (see Table 2.4) of weight gain for prepregnancy BMI. Intervention (except for routine prenatal vitamins) is based on the presence of nutritional risk factors or abnormal weight gain patterns.

The 1990 recommendations of the Institute of Medicine were evaluated using the Pregnancy Nutrition Surveillance System [85]. This analysis was limited to women who delivered live-born, singleton infants between 37 and 41 weeks' gestation. According to women, infant, children (WIC) clinic data, less than 32% of subjects had missing data concerning BMI, weight gain, birthweight or gestational age at delivery. The analysis included 220,170 women. Only 35% of non-Hispanic white women, 33.2% of non-Hispanic black women, and 36.4% of Hispanic-only women gained weight within the Institute's target range. Across the races, about 23% gained more than 10 lb above the Institute's recommendation. Overweight (38%) and obese (27.5%) women gained in excess of 10 lb above the recommendations; these are significant differences from the percentage deviation seen in underweight (11%) and normal-weight women (20%). Among underweight women across all races, failure to gain at least the Institute's recommended weight was associated with adjusted odds ratios of 1.5–3.2 for delivery of a term infant weighing less than 2500 g. Excessive weight gain was associated with a significant decrease in the incidence of term SGA infants. Weight gain in excess of 10 lb greater than the recommendations was associated with significant adjusted odds ratios (2.2–10.8) for a birthweight higher than 4500 g regardless of race. These data generally support the Institute's 1990 recommendations for weight gain based on prepregnancy BMI. The strong associations with adverse outcome, fetal growth restriction, and macrosomia, coupled with the frequency of excessive weight gain, predict the challenges of nutritional counseling in the 21st century.

Conclusion

Maternal nutrition plays an essential role in the health and well-being of the fetus and newborn. The single best evidence of adequate nutrition is appropriate weight gain for the woman's prepregnancy BMI: 28–40 lb for underweight, 25–35 lb for normal weight, 15–25 lb for overweight, and 11–20 lb for obese women. Dynamic weight gain charts and food intake surveys are clinically practical to allow intervention prior to term.

The average American woman who takes her prescribed prenatal vitamins consumes enough energy, protein, vitamins, and minerals (except for calcium) to prevent major adverse outcomes related to nutrition. Calcium deficiency is corrected easily by consuming an additional portion of dairy products each day. Unfortunately, many women gain much more than the recommended weight. Excessive nutrition can result in fetal macrosomia and postpartum weight retention. Postpartum weight retention plays a key role in the obesity of adult women. As a result, obese women are at greater risk for future obstetric complications, adult-onset diabetes, hypertension, atherosclerotic vascular disease, and early death.

Despite numerous dietary/nutritional interventions, relatively few have been shown to be helpful in adequately controlled and powered trials. The beneficial inventions include the following.
• Multiple micronutriments and protein/calorie supplements appear to be helpful in severely undernourished women who become pregnant, i.e. in developing countries.
• Folic acid supplementation of at least 0.4–0.8 mg daily reduces the incidence of neural tube defects in low-risk populations. Supplemental folic acid, 4–5 mg/daily, reduces the incidence of neural tube defects in high-risk populations.
• Modest iron supplementation (30 mg of elemental iron daily) reduces the incidence of anemia during pregnancy. The effect of iron supplementation on adverse pregnancy outcomes in the average American woman is less clear.
• Calcium > 1 g/d may reduce the incidence of hypertensive diseases in pregnancy.
• Marine fish oils may reduce adverse pregnancy outcomes but have not been "proven" by trials with randomized assignment to an intervention or placebo and sufficient numbers to assure true clinical relevance.
Many other individual nutriments have great theoretical benefit; however, the data are mixed as to their benefit in low-risk patients from industrialized countries.

The publications of the Institute of Medicine, *Nutrition During Pregnancy* [12] and *Nutrition During Lactation* [84], and the Institute of Medicine website, www.iom.edu, represent a unique resource and guide for the obstetric care provider. The assessment of maternal risk for nutritional risk factors, accurate measurement of weight and BMI, evaluation of current diet, establishment of target weight gain based on prepregnancy BMI, and ongoing assessment of weight gain during pregnancy are standards for preventative or therapeutic intervention.

CASE PRESENTATION

A 24-year-old gravida 1, para 1 is seen at a family planning office visit 2 years after the birth of her healthy child. She wants to stop her birth control pills and become pregnant again. Her second cousin has recently delivered a child with spina bifida. Your patient wishes to know what she can do to prevent the lesion in her fetus. Your evaluation is a good dietary history, especially for folic acid intake, and ascertainment of any additional environmental, genetic, familial or medical risk factors for developmental lesions, including neural tube defects. If her other risk factors are absent, her risk remains slightly increased for neural tube defect in her fetus. No example stands out more clearly than the recognition and intervention related to folic acid deficiency and neural tube defects. The preconceptual and first-trimester intake of more than 0.4 mg of folic acid prevents three-fourths of devastating neural tube defects. In counseling your patient about her slightly increased risk for neural tube defects, she needs to be educated about foods containing folic acid, start daily prenatal vitamins with 1 mg folic acid immediately, and wait at least 3 months off hormonal contraception before attempting pregnancy. If your patient has a first- or second-degree relative with a neural tube defect, 4 mg folic acid daily in addition to prenatal vitamins would be recommended.

References

1. Bergner L, Susser MW. Low birth weight and prenatal nutrition: an interpretative review. Pediatrics 1970;46:946–966.
2. Stein Z, Susser M, Saenger G, Marolla F. Famine and Human Development: The Dutch Hunger Winter of 1944–1945. New York: Oxford University Press, 1975.
3. Stein Z, Susser M. The Dutch famine, 1944–1945, and the reproductive process. I. Effects of six indices at birth. Pediatr Res 1975;9:70–76.
4. Stein Z, Susser M. The Dutch famine, 1944–1945, and the reproductive process. II. Interrelations of caloric rations and six indices at birth. Pediatr Res 1975;9:76–83.
5. Kyle UG, Pichard C. The Dutch famine of 1944–1945: a pathophysiological model of long-term consequences of wasting disease. Curr Opin Clin Nutr Metab Care 2006;9(4):388–394.
6. Luke B. Nutritional influences on fetal growth. Clin Obstet Gynecol 1994;37:538–549.
7. Ananth CV, Vintzileos AM, Shen-Schwarz S et al. Standards of birth weight in twin gestations stratified by placental chorionicity. Obstet Gynecol 1998;91:917–924.
8. Williams RL, Creasy RK, Cunningham GC et al. Fetal growth and perinatal viability in California. Obstet Gynecol 1982;59: 624–632.
9. Owen P, Donnet ML, Ogston SA et al. Standards for ultrasound fetal growth velocity. Br J Obstet Gynaecol 1996;103: 60–69.
10. Lubchenco LO. Assessment of gestational age and development of birth. Pediatr Clin North Am 1970;17:125–145.
11. Durnin JVGA. Energy requirements of pregnancy: an integration of the longitudinal data from the five-country study. Lancet 1987;2:1131–1133.
12. Institute of Medicine. Nutrition During Pregnancy. Washington, DC: National Academy, 1990, pp.97, 102, 107, 152–159, 262–263, 273, 320–321.
13. Bakketeig LS, Hoffman HJ, Harley EE. The tendency to repeat gestational age and birth weight in successive births. Am J Obstet Gynecol 1979;135:1086–1103.
14. Naeye RL. Weight gain and the outcome of pregnancy. Am J Obstet Gynecol 1979;135:3–9.
15. Kleiman JC. Maternal Weight Gain During Pregnancy: Determinants and Consequences. NCHS Working Paper Series No. 33. Hyattsville, MD: National Center for Health Statistics, Public Health Service, US Department of Health and Human Services, 1990.
16. Taffel SM. Maternal Weight Gain and the Outcome of Pregnancy: United States. Vital Health Statistics, Series 21, No. 44. DHHS Publication No. (PHS) 86–1922. Hyattsville, MD: National Center for Health Statistics, Public Health Service, US Department of Health and Human Services, 1986, p.25.
17. Mercer BM, Goldenberg RL, Das A et al. The preterm prediction study: a clinical risk assessment system. Am J Obstet Gynecol 1996;174(6):1885–1893.
18. Naeye RL, Blanc W, Paul C. Effects of maternal nutrition on the human fetus. Pediatrics 1973;52:494–503.
19. Papiernik E, Kaminski M. Multifactorial study of the risk of prematurity at 32 weeks of gestation. A study of the frequency of 30 predictive characteristics. J Perinat Med 1974;2:30–36.
20. Berkowitz GS. An epidemiologic study of preterm delivery. Am J Epidemiol 1981;113:81–92.
21. Picone TA, Allen L, Olsen P, Ferris M. Pregnancy outcome in North American women. II. Effects of diet, cigarette smoking, stress, and weight gain on placentas, and on neonatal physical and behavioral characteristics. Am J Clin Nutr 1982;36: 1214–1244.
22. Cnattingius S, Bergstrom R, Lipworth L, Kramer M. Prepregnancy weight and the risk of adverse pregnancy outcomes. N Engl J Med 1998;338:147–152.
23. Goldenberg RL, Iams JD, Mercer BM et al. The preterm prediction study: the value of new vs. standard risk factors in

predicting early and all spontaneous preterm births. Am J Public Health 1998;88:233–238.

24. Beaton GH, Milner J, Corey P et al. Sources of variance in 24-hour dietary recall data: implications for nutrition study design and interpretation. Am J Clin Nutr 1979;32:2546–2559.

25. Beaton GH, Milner J, McGuire V et al. Source of variance in 24-hour dietary recall data: implications for nutrition study design and interpretation. Am J Clin Nutr 1983;37:986–995.

26. Block G, Hartman AM. Issues in reproducibility and validity of dietary studies. Am J Clin Nutr 1989;50:1133–1138.

27. Magkos F, Yannakoulia M. Methodology of dietary assessment in athletes: concepts and pitfalls. Curr Opin Clin Nutr Metab Care 2003;6(5):539–549.

28. Frank GC, Pelican S. Guidelines for selecting a dietary analysis system. J Am Diet Assoc 1986;86:72–75.

29. Institute of Medicine. Weight Gain During Pregnancy: Reexamining the Guidelines. Washington, DC: National Academic Press, 2009. www.iom.edu.

30. www.nap.edu: dietary reference intakes for energy, carbohydrate, fiber, fatty acids, cholesterol, protein and amnio acids.

31. www.nao.edu. Dietary reference intakes for calcium, phosphorus, magnesium, vitamin D, and fluoride (1997), thiamin, riboflavin, vitamin B_6, folate, vitamin B_{12}, pantothenic acid, biotin, and choline (1998), vitamin C, vitamin E, selenium, and carotenoids (2000), vitamin A, vitamin K, arsenic, boron, chromium, copper, iodine, iron, manganese, molybdenum, nickel, silicon, vanadium, and zinc (2001), water, potassium, sodium, chloride, and sulfate (2005), calcium and vitamin D (2011).

32. Center for Disease Controls. State specific obesity among adults. United States. MMWR 2010. http://www.cdc.gov/obesity/data/trend.html.

33. Catalano PM. Management of obesity in pregnancy. Obstet Gynecol 2007;109:419–433.

34. McDonald SD, Han Z, Mulla S, Beyene J. Overweight and obesity in mothers and risk of preterm birth and low birth weight infants: systematic review and meta-analyses. Knowledge Synthesis Group. BMJ 2010;341:c3428.

35. Rasmussen SA, Chu SY, Kim SY, Schmid CH, Lau J. Maternal obesity and risk of neural tube defects: a metaanalysis. Am J Obstet Gynecol 2008;198(6):611–619.

36. Stothard KJ, Tennant PW, Bell R, Rankin J. Maternal overweight and obesity and the risk of congenital anomalies: a systematic review and meta-analysis. JAMA 2009;301(6):636–650.

37. Rasmussen KM, Catalano PM, Yaktine AL. New guidelines for weight gain during pregnancy: what obstetrician/gynecologists should know. Curr Opin Obstet Gynecol 2009;21(6):521–526.

38. Rasmussen KM, Abrams B, Bodnar LM, Butte NF, Catalano PM, Maria Siega-Riz A. Recommendations for weight gain during pregnancy in the context of the obesity epidemic. Obstet Gynecol 2010;116(5):1191–1195.

39. Beyerlein A, Lack N, von Kries R. Within-population average ranges compared with Institute of Medicine recommendations for gestational weight gain. Obstet Gynecol 2010;116(5):1111–1118.

40. Beyerlein A, Schiessl B, Lack N, von Kries R. Associations of gestational weight loss with birth-related outcome: a retrospective cohort study. Br J Obstet Gynecol 2011;118(1):55–61.

41. Parker JD. Postpartum weight change. Clin Obstet Gynecol 1994;37:528–537.

42. Greene GW, Smicikla-Wright H, School TO, Karp RJ. Postpartum weight change: how much of the weight gain in pregnancy will be lost after delivery? Obstet Gynecol 1988;71:701–707.

43. Goodnight W, Newman R. Optimal nutrition for improved twin pregnancy outcome. Society of Maternal-Fetal Medicine. Obstet Gynecol 2009;114(5):1121–1134.

44. Osrin D, Vaidya A, Shrestha Y et al. Effects of antenatal multiple micronutrient supplementation on birthweight and gestational duration in Nepal: double-blind, randomised controlled trial. Lancet 2005;365:955–962.

45. Haider BA, Bhutta ZA. Multiple-micronutrient supplementation for women during pregnancy. Cochrane Database Syst Rev 2006;4:CD004905.

46. Botto LD, Olney RS, Erickson JD. Vitamin supplements and the risk for congenital anomalies other than neural tube defects. Am J Med Genet Part C Semin Med Genet 2004;125C(1):12–21.

47. Kramer MS, Kakuma R. Energy and protein intake in pregnancy. Update of Cochrane Database Syst Rev 2000;2:CD000032. Cochrane Database Syst Rev 2003;4:CD000032.

48. Kramer MS. Isocaloric balanced protein supplementation in pregnancy. Cochrane Database Syst Rev 2000;2:CD000118.

49. Murphy JF, O'Riordan J, Newcombe RG et al. Relation of haemoglobin levels in first and second trimesters to outcome of pregnancy. Lancet 1986;1:992–995.

50. Garn SM, Ridella SA, Petzold AS, Falkner F. Maternal hematologic level and pregnancy outcomes. Semin Perinatol 1981;5:155–162.

51. Chanarin I, Rothman D. Further observations on the relation between iron and folate status in pregnancy. BMJ 1971;2:81–84.

52. Hallberg L, Bjorn-Rasmussen E, Ekenved G et al. Absorption from iron tablets given with different types of meals. Scand J Haematol 1978;21:215–224.

53. Hallberg L, Brune M, Rossander L. Iron absorption in man: ascorbic acid and dose-dependent inhibition by phytate. Am J Clin Nutr 1989;49:140–144.

54. Hallberg L. Bioavailability of dietary iron in man. Annu Rev Nutr 1981;1:123–147.

55. Hallberg L, Ryttinger L, Solvell L. Side effects of oral iron therapy: a double-blind study of different iron compounds in tablet form. Acta Med Scand 1967;459(Suppl):3–10.

56. Life Sciences Research Office. Assessment of the Iron Nutritional Status of the U.S. Population Based on Data Collected in the Second National Health and Nutrition Examination Survey, 1976–1980. Bethesda, MD: Federation of American Societies for Experimental Biology, 1984.

57. Reveiz L, Gyte GM, Cuervo LG. Treatments for iron-deficiency anaemia in pregnancy. Update of Cochrane Database Syst Rev 2001;2:CD003094. Cochrane Database Syst Rev 2007;2:CD003094.

58. Mahomed K. Iron supplementation in pregnancy. Cochrane Database Syst Rev 2006;3:CD000117.

59. Grunewald C. Biochemical prediction of pre-eclampsia. Acta Obstet Gynecol Scand 1997;164(Suppl):104–107.

60. Belizan JM, Villar J, Gonzales L et al. Calcium supplementation to prevent hypertensive disorders of pregnancy. N Engl J Med 1991;325:1399.

61. Sanchez-Ramos L, Briones DK, Kaunitz AM et al. Prevention of pregnancy-induced hypertension by calcium supplementation in angiotensin II-sensitive patients. Obstet Gynecol 1994;84:349–353.

62. Bucher HC, Guyatt GH, Cook RJ et al. Effect of calcium supplementation on pregnancy-induced hypertension and preeclampsia: a meta-analysis of randomized control trials. JAMA 1996;275:1113–1117.

63. Levine RJ, Hauth JC, Curet LB et al. Trial of calcium to prevent preeclampsia. N Engl J Med 1997;337:69–76.

64. Hofmeyr GJ, Lawrie TA, Atallah AN, Duley L. Calcium supplementation during pregnancy for preventing hypertensive disorders and related problems. Update of Cochrane Database Syst Rev 2006;3:CD001059. Cochrane Database Syst Rev 2010;8:CD0001059.

65. Duley L, Henderson-Smart D. Reduced salt intake compared to normal dietary salt, or high intake, in pregnancy. Cochrane Database Syst Rev 2000;2:CD001687.

66. Duley L, Henderson-Smart D, Meher S. Altered dietary salt for preventing pre-eclampsia, and its complications. Cochrane Database Syst Rev 2005;4:CD005548.

67. Pitkin RM, Reynolds WA, Williams GA, Hargis GK. Calcium metabolism in normal pregnancy: a longitudinal study. Am J Obstet Gynecol 1979;133:781–790.

68. Spatling L, Spatling G. Magnesium supplementation in pregnancy. A double blind study. Br J Obstet Gynaecol 1988;95:120–125.

69. Makrides M, Crowther CA. Magnesium supplementation in pregnancy. Update of Cochrane Database Syst Rev 2000;2:CD000937. Cochrane Database Syst Rev 2001;4: CD000937.

70. Mahomed K, Gulmezoglu AM. Vitamin D supplementation in pregnancy. Cochrane Database Syst Rev 2000;2:CD000228.

71. Rose NC, Mennuti MT. Periconceptional folate supplementation and neural tube defects. Clin Obstet Gynecol 1994;37: 605–620..

72. Chivu CM, Tulchinsky TH, Soares-Weiser K, Braunstein R, Brezis M.A systematic review of interventions to increase awareness, knowledge, and folic acid consumption before and during pregnancy. Am J Health Promot 2008;22(4):237–245.

73. Czeizel AE, Dudas I. Prevention of the first occurrence of neural-tube defects by peri-conceptional vitamin supplementation. N Engl J Med 1992;327:1832–1835.

74. Lumley J, Watson L, Watson M, Bower C. Periconceptional supplementation with folate and/or multivitamins for preventing neural tube defects. Cochrane Database Syst Rev 2001;3:CD001056.

75. De-Regil LM, Fernandez-Gaxiola AC, Dowswell T, Pena-Rosas JP. Effects and safety of periconceptional folate supplementation for preventing birth defects. Cochrane Database Syst Rev 2010;10:CD007950.

76. Polyzos NP, Mauri D, Tsappi M et al. Combined vitamin C and E supplementation during pregnancy for preeclampsia prevention: a systematic review. Obstet Gynecol Surv 2007; 62(3):202–206.

77. Rumbold A, Crowther CA. Vitamin E supplementation in pregnancy. Cochrane Database Syst Rev 2005;2:CD004069.

78. Rumbold A, Crowther CA. Vitamin C supplementation in pregnancy. Cochrane Database Syst Rev 2005;2:CD004072.

79. Makrides M, Duley L, Olsen SF. Marine oil, and other prostaglandin precursor, supplementation for pregnancy uncomplicated by pre-eclampsia or intrauterine growth restriction. Cochrane Database Syst Rev 2006;3:CD003402.

80. Mendez MA, Torrent M, Julvez J et al. Maternal fish and other seafood intakes during pregnancy and child neurodevelopment at age 4 years. Public Health Nutr 2009;12(10): 1702–1710.

81. Newton ER. Breastmilk: the gold standard. Clin Obstet Gynecol 2004;47(3):632–642.

82. American Academy of Pediatrics Work Group on Breastfeeding. Breastfeeding and the use of human milk. Pediatrics 1997;100:1035–1039.

83. Strode MA, Dewey KG, Lonnerdal B. Effects of short-term caloric restriction on lactational performance of well-nourished women. Acta Paediatr Scand 1986;75:222–229.

84. Institute of Medicine. Nutrition During Lactation. Washington, DC: National Academy Press, 1991, pp.68–70.

85. Schieve LA, Cogswell ME, Scanlon KS. An empiric evaluation of the Institute of Medicine's pregnancy weight gain guidelines by race. Obstet Gynecol 1998;91:878–884.

Chapter 3
Alcohol and Substance Abuse

William F. Rayburn

Department of Obstetrics and Gynecology, University of New Mexico Health Sciences Center, Albuquerque, NM, USA

Alcohol and substance abuse are most prevalent in reproductive age adults. Among women aged 15–44, almost 90% have used alcohol, approximately 44% have used marijuana, and at least 14% have used cocaine [1]. Combined 2002–2007 national survey data show that past-month alcohol use among women aged 18–44 was highest for those who were not pregnant and did not have children living in the household (63%) but comparatively low for women in the first trimester of pregnancy (19%), and even lower for those in the second (7.8%) or third trimester (6.2%); similar patterns were seen with marijuana, cigarette, and binge alcohol use [2]. Even though cessation in alcohol, illicit drug use or cigarette smoking usually occurs during pregnancy, some women may not reduce or alter their patterns until pregnancy is confirmed or well under way.

Care of alcohol- or substance-using pregnant women is complex, difficult, and often demanding. Healthcare providers must be aware of their patient's unique psychological and social needs and the related legal and ethical ramifications surrounding pregnancy.

Screening for substance use

Screening for alcohol or other substances should be undertaken on all women known to be or suspected of being pregnant. The goal of screening should be for public health purposes, not for criminal prosecution. Identification of substance use most often depends on a history given voluntarily by the patient. Pregnant and postpartum women who use and abuse alcohol or other drugs are more stigmatized than nonpregnant women. They may therefore deny their drug habit and its potential harmful effects and not seek help. Young, poor women can be especially fearful of the medical and social welfare system because of their naivety or desire to hide their pregnancy.

Questions about alcohol, illicit substances, and cigarette smoking should be routine at the initial prenatal visit. A history of past and present substance use should be taken in a nonjudgmental manner and by questioning about the frequency, amount, and time during gestation of a specific substance(s) [3]. If alcohol is reported, you may then ask the following using the CAGE questionnaire: "Have you ever felt that you should cut down on your drinking? Have people annoyed you by criticizing your drinking? Have you ever felt guilty about your drinking? Have you ever needed an "eye-opener" drink when you get up in the morning?" [4].

Testing for drugs or metabolites after obtaining informed consent is recommended among those pregnant women with multiple medical, obstetric, and behavior characteristics (Table 3.1). A positive screen can facilitate referral to a comprehensive care program or compliance requirements for treatment continuation. About half of women with positive urine drug screens deny any drug use [3]. Random testing of all gravidas raises several legal issues, including the right to privacy, lack of probable cause, and admissibility of test results [5].

Urine is the preferred source for drug testing, because it is easily obtainable in large quantities. There are no national guidelines for urine screening, however. Except for chronic marijuana use, most substances or their metabolites are measurable in urine for less than 72 h and alcohol for less than 12 h. Therefore, substances may not be identified unless urine specimens are tested frequently [6]. In the evaluations for cocaine and opiate exposure, hair analysis of the mother or newborn infant is also effective [5,7].

Effects on the fetus

Virtually all chemicals cross the placenta easily because of their lipid solubility, low molecular weight, pKa not

Table 3.1 Examples of obstetric, behavior, and medical patterns in pregnant women suggestive of alcohol and substance use disorders

Obstetric	Behavioral and personal	Medical
Abruptio placentae	Alcohol- or drug-abusing partner	Anemia
Birth outside hospital	Bizarre or inappropriate behavior	Arrhythmias
Congenital anomalies	Child abuse or neglect	Bacterial endocarditis
Fetal alcohol spectrum disorder	Chronic unemployment	Cellulitis or phlebitis
Fetal distress	Difficulty concentrating	Cerebrovascular accident
Fetal growth restriction	Domestic violence	Drug overdose or endocarditis
Neonatal abstinence syndrome	Family history of substance abuse	Hepatitis B and C
Prenatal care – none, sporadic, or late prenatal care	Frequent emergency department visits	HIV seropositivity
Preterm labor and delivery	Incarceration	Lymphedema
Preterm rupture of the membranes	Noncompliance with appointments	Myocardial ischemia or infarction
Spontaneous abortion	Poor historian	Pancreatitis
Stillbirth	Prostitution	Poor dental hygiene
Sudden infant death syndrome	Psychiatric history (depression, anxiety, posttraumatic stress)	Poor nutritional status
	Restless, agitation, demanding	Septicemia
	Slurred speech or staggering gait	Sexually transmitted infections
		Tuberculosis

being high, and not being too protein bound. Unlike prescription or nonprescription drugs, alcohol and substances of abuse may be intentionally or inadvertently taken at toxic doses. Consuming many drinks per occasion (i.e. binge drinking, ≥5 drinks) may be more harmful to the developing fetus than the same amount spread over several days, because of higher peak blood alcohol content [8]. Moreover, the impurity of most illicit drugs and the common practice of using multiple substances (including smoking) make it difficult to ascribe specific fetal effects and perinatal outcomes to a certain drug. Accurate evaluation of dosage and timing of exposure are encouraged but usually inaccurate.

Teratogenic effects on the fetus depend on the developmental stage: from fertilization to implantation (abortion), from second through eighth weeks (anomalies), and from ninth week to birth (shortened gestation, restricted growth, neurobehavior impairment). Maternal alcohol and substance use places the fetus at risk for spontaneous abortion, low birthweight, small head circumference, prematurity, and a variety of developmental complications. Furthermore, alcohol consumption is the most widely recognized cause of severe mental and developmental delay in the baby. Table 3.2 lists effects in the human fetus/infant from *in utero* exposure to specific substances. This list was compiled using data from two or more reports in humans [9]. Although the table serves as a guideline, counseling about absolute risk is unreasonable. The risk of structural anomalies is not increased in most cases of substance exposure, although the background risk of major structural malformations at birth is 3% and another 3% by age 5, with 8–10% of persons having one or more functional abnormalities by age 18 [10]. For this reason, a

screening scan at midgestation should include a search for common sites for anomalies such as the face, intracranium, heart, abdominal wall, and urine collecting system.

Prenatal counseling about fetal effects from alcohol and substance abuse is often limited to case reports or small series and retrospective cohort studies [11]. These reports are limited by the frequent use of multiple substances, predominant experience with first-trimester exposure only, animal studies not reliably predicting human response, retrospective and uncontrolled methodology, patient recall often later during gestation, and selective acceptance by editors of only reports with positive findings. Large populations are required to determine the relative teratogenic risks. A fetal ultrasound is important to confirm gestation dating and, if possible, to screen for any structured abnormalities. Maternal serum screening, chorionic villous sampling, amniocentesis, and fetal blood sampling have no role in determining direct fetal effects from alcohol or any other substance.

Ascribing a fetal disorder to alcohol or a specific substance is extremely difficult. Regular high alcohol intake during pregnancy (5 drinks/day) increases the risk of congenital anomalies. Lower intake levels and binge patterns of drinking have been implicated in some studies with fetal death, congenital malformations, and abnormalities of development. Fetal alcohol syndrome (FAS), the only clearly defined syndrome of defects, may be as infrequent as 4% among heavy daily users [11]. Subtle craniofacial anomalies cannot be reliably viewed on fetal ultrasound. In the case of illicit drugs, evidence is neither sufficient nor consistent to identify with reasonable certainty which substance produced which effect and at what level. Furthermore, evidence to untangle the

Table 3.2 Impact of *in utero* exposure of specific substances on the fetus and newborn infant and on obstetric complications*

Complications	Fetal/neonatal effects	Obstetric complications
Alcohol	Microcephaly; growth deficiency; CNS dysfunction including mental retardation and behavioral abnormalities; craniofacial abnormalities (i.e. short palpebral fissures, hypoplastic philtrum, flattened maxilla); behavioral abnormalities	Spontaneous abortion
Cigarettes	No anomalies; reduced birthweight (200 g lighter); facial clefting (?); attention deficit hyperactivity disorder (?)	Spontaneous abortion Preterm birth Placenta previa Placental abruption Reduced risk of preeclampsia

Cannabis
  Marijuana
  THC
  Hashish
	No anomalies; corresponding decrease in birthweight; subtle behavioral alterations (reduced executive functioning)	Reduction of gestation 0.8 weeks

CNS sedatives
  Barbiturates
  Diazepam
  Flurazepam
  Meprobamate
  Methaqualone
	No pattern of anomalies; depression of interactive behavior; impaired "executive function" behavioral (?)	

CNS stimulants
  Antiobesity drugs
  Cocaine
  Methylphenidate
  Methamphetamines
  Phenmetrazine
	No clear association with malformations; excess activity *in utero*; congenital anomalies (heart?, biliary atresia?); depression of interactive behavior; urinary tract defects; symmetric growth restriction; placental abruption; cerebral infarction; brain lesions; fetal death; neonatal necrotizing enterocolitis	Spontaneous abortion
		Premature birth
		Placental abruption

Hallucinogens
  LSD
  Ketamine
  Mescaline
  Dimethyltryptamine
  Phencyclidine (PCP)
	No anomalies; chromosomal breakage (?) (LSD); dysmorphic face; behavioral problems	Spontaneous abortions

Opiates
  Codeine
  Heroin
  Hydromorphone
  Hydrocodone
  Meperidine
  Methadone
  Morphine
  Opium
  Pentazocine (& tripelennamine)
	No anomalies; intrauterine withdrawal with increased fetal activity; depressed breathing movements; fetal growth restriction; perinatal mortality; neonatal withdrawal	Preterm delivery
		Preterm rupture of the membranes
		Meconium-stained amniotic fluid

Inhalants
  Gasoline
  Glue
  Hairspray
  Paint
	Similar to the fetal alcohol and fetal hydantoin syndromes (?); growth restriction; increased risk of leukemia in children (?); impaired heme synthesis	Preterm labor

*≥Two investigations in humans as reported in reference [9].
CNS, central nervous system; THC, tetrahydrocannabinol.

environmental factors (such as poverty and the corresponding poor nutrition and lack of easy access to prenatal care) from alcohol- and substance abuse-related factors is limited, conflicting, or nonexistent.

The long-term impact of prenatal alcohol and other substances on infant and child development presents other challenges. Although animal studies have shown that alcohol and drugs reduce the density of cortical neurons and change dendritic connections, the significance to human development is unclear [12]. Studies of behaviors in animals have shown long-term changes, and abnormal neurobehavioral findings in the newborn raise concerns about how those conditions may affect subsequent development. It has been suggested that consumption of less than one alcoholic drink per day early in the pregnancy does not impair cognitive abilities when measured in offspring at age 14 years [13]. Another consideration about effects on the human fetus is the number of drinks consumed per occasion by the mother, not just the number of drinks per day or week. Maternal binge drinking may lead to the eventual childhood finding of more social disinhibition and defects in numerical and language skills [14].

Specific therapy for pregnancy

Psychological and pharmacological treatments are intertwined in managing pregnant patients with a chemical dependency. Support includes individual counseling, group therapy, exercise, lifestyle change training, and self-help groups such as Alcoholics Anonymous and Cocaine Anonymous. Relapse prevention methods, which utilize peer support and learning principles, are directed toward avoiding situations that elicit conditioned cravings for alcohol or other substances and toward developing better coping skills. Under supervision, mothers can become drug free, learn effective parenting skills, and experience improved relationships with their children. This reunification model with the family also unburdens foster care systems by assuring the safety of the child(ren) in a therapeutic milieu.

Psychosocial intervention

Our ability to determine the best psychosocial intervention for reducing alcohol consumption before and during pregnancy is limited by the paucity of studies, number of participants, high risk of bias, and complexity of interventions [15,16]. Nevertheless, forms of behavioral therapy include self-management procedures, motivational interviewing, relaxation training, contingency contracting, and skills training. Contingency contracting involves rearranging the individual's environment so that positive consequences follow desired behavior, while either negative or neutral consequences follow undesired behaviors.

These techniques require reinforcement from others, such as spouses or boyfriends, other family members, employers, or healthcare providers. Individuals admitting to a relapse of substance use or having positive urine drug screening are subject to negative consequences. A systematic review by Terplan and Liu found that contingency management is effective in improving retention of pregnant women in illicit drug treatment programs but with minimal effects on their abstaining from illicit drugs [17]. They found that motivational interviewing over 3–6 sessions may, if anything, lead to poorer retention in treatment.

Women with alcohol or other substance abuse present with higher prevalence rates of psychiatric co-morbidities than do men, making psychiatric assessment and treatment crucial to women to overcome barriers [18]. Psychiatric disorders such as depression or anxiety among substance users are so common that it is difficult to ascertain whether they contributed to or resulted from the substance use. In many instances, abstinence from substance use results in an amelioration of those conditions. Specific psychosocial interventions or pharmacotherapy may result in resolution of both the psychiatric disorder and the substance use among women whose psychiatric disorder either antedated the substance use or co-existed with the addiction process [14,15].

Pharmacotherapy

There is a need for high-quality research to determine the effectiveness of pharmacologic intervention in pregnant women enrolled in illicit drug or alcohol treatment programs, since select drug therapy with extensive counseling is an important modality [15]. Unfortunately, drug therapy is often metabolized and eliminated more rapidly during pregnancy, so a higher daily dose is often required.

A prime example of pharmacotherapy during pregnancy is methadone, which has been prescribed for years in treating opiate dependence during pregnancy. Methadone maintenance (usually 60–120 mg daily) reduces the risk of relapse, enhances retention in treatment and prenatal programs, and improves perinatal outcomes [18,19]. We do permit breastfeeding during methadone maintenance therapy.

Buprenorphine is another medication prescribed for opiate addiction, especially for those with no access to methadone treatment programs. Its effectiveness during pregnancy has not been proven, although preliminary reports suggest that it may lead to less neonatal withdrawal [20]. Subutex, rather than suboxone (buprenorphine with naloxone), may be prescribed by physicians who have taken special coursework for those who decline methadone for mild-to-moderate withdrawal.

Minozzi and colleagues searched for randomized controlled trials enrolling opiate-dependent pregnant women [21]. They found three trials with 96 pregnant women:

two compared methadone with buprenorphine and one methadone with oral slow morphine. No significant differences were observed between the drugs compared both for mother and for child outcomes. However, the trials were too few and the sample size too small to make firm conclusions about the superiority of one treatment over another.

Cocaine dependence remains a major public health problem because of the high relapse rates and poor treatment responses. Drug trials for cocaine addiction (tricyclic antidepressants, dopamine agonists, lithium, amino acids, and vitamins) have not been conducted during gestation and are not universally effective. Cocaine blocks the uptake of neurotransmitters, leading to their depletion. Further research is needed to determine whether dopamine agonists (bromocriptine, amantadine), used to replenish neurotransmitters from cocaine exposure, are effective and safe.

Other forms of maintenance therapy for alcohol or other substance use are not customarily prescribed during pregnancy [16]. Benzodiazepines and phenobarbital are used to withdraw pregnant women who abuse alcohol, with antidepressants after withdrawal. Disulfiram, naltrexone, and acamprosate are used in more severe pregnancy cases to decrease cravings and maintain abstinence [16].There is no conclusive evidence about the effects of long-term consequences of these drugs during pregnancy [16].

Alcohol and smoking education

While alcohol and cigarette smoking are the most commonly used substances before and shortly after conception, a paucity of women report heavy use after pregnancy recognition [22]. The obstetrician can approach the pregnant woman who smokes in a stepwise manner. A patient who smokes should be advised to stop by providing clear, strong advice to quit with personalized messages about the benefits of quitting and about the harmful impact of continued smoking on the fetus and newborn and on herself. Her willingness to attempt to quit smoking should be assessed within the next 30 days [23].

Smoking interventions have demonstrated a greater likelihood of smoking cessation by late pregnancy and less low birthweight and preterm delivery [23]. Patients interested in quitting should be assisted by providing pregnancy-specific, self-help smoking cessation materials. Regular follow-up visits are encouraged to track the progress of the patients who attempt to quit smoking. Daytime delivery of nicotine through gum or transdermal patches should be considered for use during pregnancy only when nonpharmacologic treatments (e.g. counseling) have failed, and if the increased likelihood of smoking cessation, with its potential benefits, outweighs the unknown risk of nicotine replacement and potential concomitant smoking [23].

Comprehensive prenatal care

Care should be taken by professionals with training and expertise in the area of substance use. The most common complaint by healthcare professionals is the feeling of ineffectiveness, because their patients are generally unmotivated, noncompliant, and difficult to retain in treatment programs [3,24]. Professionals willing to work with this population must tackle the many issues associated with alcoholism or substance use: poverty, lack of education and job training, poor parenting skills, domestic violence in the form of physical and sexual abuse, child abuse, family and other personal relations, communicable disease, child development, and such psychiatric disorders as depression, anxiety, bipolar disorders, posttraumatic stress disorder, and psychosis [24,25].

The most important aspect of this comprehensive preventive care is to encourage a woman to take an active role in reaching her ultimate goal: a drug-free environment for herself and especially the fetus. This aspect is important, especially when realizing that prenatal care is occasionally sought late [25]. Engaging patients with treatment of their substance use is not a guarantee that they will seek prenatal care. Some women have either "kicked the habit" or feel that their habit is too infrequent for time-consuming multidisciplinary care using other drug therapy that may not benefit them.

Several reports of substance use treatment in multidisciplinary prenatal settings suggest that even minimal drug interventions (such as methadone maintenance) and counseling, combined with prenatal care, can lead to better pregnancy and infant outcomes [23,26]. Although comprehensive interventions such as this show promise for reducing substance use and harm to the fetus, few clinics are dedicated to assessing and treating pregnant addicts [24,27].

Favorable outcomes relate directly to the time dedicated by an experienced multidisciplinary team [24,25]. Providers need to be sensitive to the feelings and cultural background of pregnant alcoholic or substance-using women and offer care in an environment that is supportive, nurturing, and nonjudgmental [28]. As the patient becomes more involved, a strong and more positive relationship often develops with the staff. The ability of providers to be flexible and to provide an environment that is safe and fosters self-esteem and interpersonal growth is essential.

By way of example, organization of primary/preventive care, laboratory, and behavioral services at our specialized prenatal clinic is shown in Table 3.3 [29]. This comprehensive program serves not only pregnant and postpartum women who are chemically dependent, but also their infants. Our goal is not only to promote cessation of alcohol, tobacco, and other substance use, but also to effect lifestyle changes since addiction disorders in a

Table 3.3 Guidelines for organization of preventive/prenatal care, laboratory, and behavioral counseling services in a comprehensive prenatal care program

Visit	Preventive/prenatal care	Labs/studies	Behavioral counseling
New OB	Discuss proper nutrition and supplements Focus on any poor obstetric history (IUFD, repeated losses, anomalies, preterm deliveries, LBW) Smoke cessation, alcohol avoidance	Thorough drug use history (past and present) Thorough physical exam (signs of current/recent use) New OB labs, HIV (need consent); UDM; urine C&S Place Tbc skin test and order hepatitis panel, LFTs Dating ultrasound and first-trimester screen	Assess patient's willingness/attempt to quit Encourage attendance at Milagro counseling sessions/methadone group Identify barriers to quitting and help identify solutions Counsel patient regarding potential anomalies, fetal effects, and high-risk problems (preterm labor, abruption, preeclampsia) that could occur with the particular drug being abused Discuss/treat co-morbid disorders (depression, anxiety)
15–19 wks	Examine oral cavity; review oral hygiene Discuss elements of prenatal care; avoid frequent emergency visits Review STD labs	Maternal serum quadruple screen (need consent) Check UDM Consider 20–22 week ultrasound to r/o anomalies	Motivational counseling for successes/failures Encourage continued attendance at counseling sessions/groups Educate and answer questions regarding effects of particular drug on fetus at this stage
20–24 wks	Encourage compliance with appointments Fitness counseling; smoke cessation Discuss asthma and URIs		Observe for signs of withdrawal/overdose Inquire about job satisfaction Discuss any issues relating to prostitution or incarceration
25–28 wks	Examine skin (cellulitis, abscesses, phlebitis, acne, lymphedema, dermatitis) Discuss signs and symptoms of hepatitis, pancreatitis Explain about preterm labor/PPROM precautions	1 h glucola and Hct Check UDM Rhogam (if Rh neg)	Encourage continued attendance at counseling sessions/groups Educate regarding effects of particular drug on fetus at this stage and on neonatal withdrawal symptoms and complications
29–30 wks	Use of safety belts; firearms Discuss about urinary tract infections Postpartum contraception counseling	Consent for any tubal	Observe for signs of overdose/withdrawal Focus on any psychiatric history
31–32 wks	Discuss headaches Encourage childbirth classes Discuss safe sex	Begin daily fetal movement charting	Encourage attendance of counseling sessions Ask about current drug use Discuss domestic violence
33–34 wks	Review vaccination history (rubella, tetanus, travel immunizations, influenza, pneumococcal) Encourage childbirth classes Discuss asthma and upper airway problems	Repeat hepatitis panel, LFTs (if Hep C+) Repeat RPR and HIV Check UDM	Motivational counseling for successes/failures Observe for signs of overdose/withdrawal Discuss/make plans for ongoing counseling/drug treatment PP
35–36 wks	Discuss breastfeeding issues related to particular drug being abused Discuss breast conditioning and disorders	Consider ultrasound for fetal growth GC/chlamydia/GBS cultures Maternal viral load (if Hep C+)	Inquire about support at home Educate about potential neonatal withdrawal symptoms and complications Discuss future employment

Table 3.3 (*Continued*)

Visit	Preventive/prenatal care	Labs/studies	Behavioral counseling
37 wks	Rediscuss labor precautions Confirm pediatrician/family physician Review plans for postpartum contraception	Check UDM	Motivational counseling for successes/failures Encourage continued attendance at counseling sessions/groups Ask about current drug use Review social work support (Los Pasos) and ongoing counseling/drug treatment
≥38 wks	Explain about postpartum "blues" and anatomic changes		Educate about analgesic options during labor Educate about potential neonatal withdrawal symptoms and complications
6 wk PP	Provide birth control counseling and prescriptions Review written information about general health care/annual exam	Pap; GC/C	Ask about current drug use Screen for depression Encourage continued attendance at counseling sessions/groups Discuss employment plans

C&S, culture and sensitivity; GBS, group B streptococcus; GC/C, gonorrhea/chlamydia; Hct, hematocrit; IUFD, intrauterine fetal death; LBW, low birthweight; LFT, liver function test; maternal serum α-fetoprotein; OB, obstetric; Pap, Papanicolaou test; PP, postpartum; PPROM, preterm rupture of the membranes; Rh, Rhesus; r/o, risk of/rule out; RPR, rapid plasma reagin test; STD, sexually transmitted disease; Tbc, tuberculosis; UDM, urine drug and metabolites; URI, upper respiratory infection.

holistic sense also involve the family and whole community.

Each patient receives prenatal care using a protocol established for chemically dependent women. This protocol includes more frequent prenatal visits (bimonthly until 32 weeks, then weekly), ultrasound to monitor fetal growth and to promote maternal bonding, proper dating of the pregnancy, and a 24-h on-call staff. Patients are often screened twice during pregnancy for hepatitis B and C, HIV, chlamydia, gonorrhea, and syphilis. Tuberculosis skin testing is performed at the initial visit. Routine counseling about healthy pregnancies includes nutrition counseling, childbirth classes, tours of the inpatient obstetrics and newborn facilities, analgesia/anesthesia classes (including regional, IV, and local anesthesia), and breastfeeding. We check constantly for signs of substance overdose and withdrawal. We observe for unusual behavior, agitation, dilated or constricted pupils, elevated or decreased blood pressure, rapid or slow heart rate or respiratory rate, and altered reflexes. These can be confused with the physiologic adaptive changes of pregnancy but are essential to document as a means of assessing the adequacy of therapy.

Hospital and postpartum care

Ideally, the same physicians or midwives providing prenatal care will follow the patient in the hospital. Notification of anesthesia staff about any substance use is recommended during early labor. In this manner, continuity of care is better maintained, and patients feel more secure during the transition from pregnancy to care of the infant.

Many states require hospitals to report women presenting for delivery who are suspected of heavy alcohol and other drug use to local public health authorities or the criminal justice system [5,24]. This reporting may cause women to be even more wary of acknowledging their problem and seeking prenatal care and hospital delivery, particularly if they have other children who are in the custody of Child Protective Services (CPS) or who are living with relatives. In many states, protective services, foster care placements, and review boards base their decisions on the length of time for which the child is away from the mother. These decisions also serve as deterrents to women seeking effective long-term substance abuse treatment if childcare is unavailable.

A low pain threshold is often observed during labor. Relief is better provided with epidural analgesia, with spinal blocks being preferred during a cesarean. Higher doses of oral narcotics or postoperative patient-controlled analgesia are often required after delivery. Neonatal signs of substance use withdrawal during the first 72h may present as irritability, tremors, seizure-like action, a high-pitched cry, abnormal muscle tone, poor feeding, vomiting or diarrhea, and impaired temperature maintenance.

These signs, as well as unexplained fetal growth restriction and placental abruption, are valid reasons for newborn urine screening or meconium testing (more sensitive but not timely results).

In general, breastfeeding should be encouraged unless the new mother is either HIV positive or hepatitis C positive with bleeding from her nipples [29]. Alcohol and illicit substances are excreted in small amounts of breast milk. Contradictions to breastfeeding are either theoretical or focused on case reports. Offering a consultation with a lactation consultant is a reasonable option.

National survey data suggest that substance use increases following childbirth. For example, marijuana use was higher for recent mothers with children under 3 months old in the household (3.8%) than for women in the third trimester of pregnancy (1.4%), suggesting resumption of use among mothers in the first 3 months after childbirth [2]. Many chemically dependent women lose interest in the clinics once the baby has been born. If the neonate is healthy, the new mother may feel that her drug use is not that dangerous.

Contraception is the primary prevention of pregnancy-related problems resulting from alcohol or other substance abuse. Screening for sexually transmitted disease is especially important with intrauterine devices, while assessing liver function is important when offering hormonal contraception to those with alcohol abuse or hepatitis.

It is the moral responsibility of a substance use program not to let these patients become lost to follow-up. Once this happens, the patient is set up for failure and often reverts back to substance use. Health professionals need to continue monitoring pregnant women after delivery for signs and symptoms of substance use. These nonpunitive monitoring efforts are intended to motivate behaviors in adults to enhance attention to their children and to identify early developmental delays in children in order to begin early intervention services. Home visits after birth increase the engagement of these women in drug treatment programs, but data are insufficient to say whether such visits improve the health of the babies and mother [27].

CASE PRESENTATION

A 26-year-old G3P1021 was seen for a postpartum exam after scant prenatal care. Four weeks ago, she delivered vaginally a 34w 2d fetus weighing 4 lb 5 oz after preterm ruptured membranes and labor. The nonanomalous infant was discharged from the intensive care nursery 2 weeks later and is now being cared for by the grandmother. The patient declined to breastfeed.

She admitted to using methamphetamines and crack cocaine occasionally during the pregnancy but has not been using for 3 months. She has a history of poor family relationships, sexual and physical abuse, depression, housing and transportation difficulties, and limited prostitution. She was charged with drug possession once and with parole violations three times. Her prenatal laboratory tests were positive for hepatitis C, ASCUS (atypical cells of undetermined significance) on Pap test, and hematocrit 34% (microcytic hypochromic anemia).

Her pelvic examination today revealed normal reparative changes. A Pap test and cultures were obtained. She

states that she is not currently sexually active, and the baby's father remains in jail. Our plan was to arrange for an intrauterine device (IUD) insertion following discussion about various methods of contraception. If an ASCUS result persists on cervical cytology, then human papillomavirus (HPV) testing will be useful to detect high-risk (16 or 18) serotypes and, if positive, immediate colposcopy.

The patient is currently living at a shelter. Our social work staff continues to assist on housing, possible employment, and legal issues. Counseling has already helped her in overcoming her drug-seeking behavior and in developing a more stable family relationships. Precautions were explained about hepatitis C transmission. She is aware that there is effective long-term antiviral treatment for hepatitis C which could be considered after her childcare support is certain and continued drug rehabilitation shows signs of improvement.

References

1. American College of Obstetricians and Gynecologists. Substance abuse in pregnancy. ACOG Tech Bull 1994;195:825–831.
2. Substance Abuse and Mental Health Services Administration, Office of Applied Studies. The NSDUH Report: Substance Use Among Women During Pregnancy and Following Childbirth.

Rockville, MD: Substance Abuse and Mental Health Services Administration, 2009.
3. Chasnoff I, Neuman K, Thornton C, Callaghan M. Screening for substance use in pregnancy: a practical approach for the primary care physician. Am J Obstet Gynecol 2001;184(4):112–119.
4. Ewing J A. Detecting alcoholism: the CAGE questionnaire. JAMA 1984;252:1905–1907.

5. Foley E. Drug screening and criminal prosecution of pregnant women. J Obstet Gynecol Neonatal Nursing 2002;31:133–137.

6. Wolff K, Farrell M, Marsden J et al. A review of biological indication of illicit drug use, practical considerations and clinical usefulness. Addiction 1999;94:1279–1298.

7. Macgregor S, Keith L, Bachicha J, Chasnoff I. Cocaine abuse during pregnancy: correlation between prenatal care and perinatal outcome. Obstet Gynecol 1989;74:882–885.

8. Bailey B, Delaney-Black V, Covington C et al. Prenatal exposure to binge drinking and cognitive and behavioral outcomes at age 7 years. Am J Obstet Gynecol 2004;191:1037–1043.

9. Reprotox® database, Reproductive Toxicology Center, Bethesda MD, 2010. http://reprotox.org/Members/AgentDetail.aspx?a=1290.

10. Cunningham F, Leveno K, Bloom S, Hauth J, Rouse D, Spong C. Teratology and medications that affect the fetus. In: Williams Obstetrics, 23rd edn. New York: McGraw-Hill, 2010, p.312.

11. Abel EL. An update on the incidence of FAS: FAS is not an equal opportunity birth defect. Neurotoxicol Teratol 1995;17:437–443.

12. Sampson PD, Streissguth AP, Bookstein FL. Incidence of fetal alcohol syndrome and prevalence of alcohol-related neurodevelopmental disorder. Teratology 1997;56:317–326.

13. O'Callaghan FV, O'Callaghan M, Najman JM, Williams GM, Bor W. Prenatal alcohol exposure and attention, learning and intellectual ability at 14 years: a prospective longitudinal study. Early Hum Dev 2007;83:115–123.

14. Lui S, Terplan M, Smith EJ. Psychosocial interventions for women enrolled in alcohol treatment during pregnancy. Cochrane Database Syst Rev 2008;3:CD006753.

15. Smith EJ, Lui S, Terplan M. Pharmacologic interventions for pregnant women enrolled in alcohol Treatment. Cochrane Database Syst Rev 2009;3:CD007361.

16. Zilberman ML, Tavares H, Blume SB, el-Guebaly N. Substance use disorders: sex differences and psychiatric comorbidities. Can J Psychiatry 2003;48:5–15.

17. Terplan M, Lui S. Psychosocial interventions for pregnant women in outpatient illicit drug treatment programs compared to other interventions. Cochrane Database Syst Rev 2007;4:CD006037.

18. Kranzler H, Amin H, Lowe V, Oncken C. Pharmacologic treatments for drug and alcohol dependence. Psych Clin North Am 1999;22(2):212–239.

19. Rayburn WF, Bogenschutz MP. Pharmacotherapy for pregnant women with addictions. Am J Obstet Gynecol 2004;191:1885–1897.

20. Kakko J, Heilig M, Sarman I. Buprenorphine and methadone treatment of opiate dependence during pregnancy: comparison of fetal growth and neonatal outcomes in two consecutive case series. Drug Alcohol Depend 2008;96:69–78.

21. Minozzi S, Amato L, Vecchi S, Davoli M. Maintenance agonist treatments for opiate dependent pregnant women. Cochrane Database Syst Rev 2008;2:CD006318.

22. Bauer C, Shankaran S, Bada H et al. The maternal lifestyle study: drug exposure during pregnancy and short-term maternal outcomes. Am J Obstet Gynecol 2002;186(3):487–495.

23. American College of Obstetricians and Gynecologists. Smoking Cessation During Pregnancy. ACOG Committee Opinion 316. Washington, DC: American College of Obstetricians and Gynecologists, 2005.

24. American College of Obstetricians and Gynecologists. At-risk Drinking and Illicit Drug Use: Ethical Issues in Obstetric and Gynecologic Practice. ACOG Committee Opinion 422. Washington, DC: American College of Obstetricians and Gynecologists, 2008.

25. American College of Obstetricians and Gynecologists. Psychosocial Risk Factors: Perinatal Screening and Intervention. ACOG Committee Opinion 343. Washington, DC: American College of Obstetricians and Gynecologists, 2006.

26. Dashe J, Sheffield J, Jackson G et al. Relationship between maternal methadone dosage and neonatal withdrawal. Am J Obstet Gynecol 2002;100(6):1244–1249.

27. US Dept Health and Human Services. Outreach To and Identification of Women: Practical Approaches in the Treatment of Women Who Abuse Alcohol and Other Drugs. Rockville, MD: US Department of Health and Human Services, Public Health Service, 1994, pp.124–126.

28. Ramirez W, Strickland L, Meng C, Beraun C, Rayburn W. Medical students' comfort levels toward pregnant women with substance use disorders. Birth Defects Res 2005;73:346.

29. Rayburn W. Maternal and fetal effects from substance use. Clin Perinatol 2007;34:559–571.

Chapter 4
Environmental Agents and Reproductive Risk

Laura Goetzl

Department of Obstetrics and Gynecology, Medical University of South Carolina, Charleston, SC, USA

Obstetricians are frequently asked about the reproductive risks of specific environmental, work-related, or dietary exposures. While few exposures have been associated with a measurable increase in risk of congenital anomaly, fetal death, or growth impairment, ongoing research continues to identify new areas of concern. Research linking low levels of environmental exposures is hampered by the cost and difficulty of prospective cohort studies with accurate ascertainment of exposure to specific agents at various gestational periods. In this chapter, we discuss the principles concerning the evaluation of the developmental toxicity of occupational and environmental exposures in general, and review selected agents that have been associated with reproductive toxicity.

Background incidence of adverse outcome

Increased attributable risk of an individual environmental agent must be placed in the context of the background incidence of adverse pregnancy outcome in the general population. Approximately 30% of recognized pregnancies result in miscarriage and 3% result in children with major malformations, defined as a malformation requiring medical or surgical attention, or resulting in functional or cosmetic impairment. This high background risk introduces statistical problems in the identification of toxicity. If the increase in adverse outcome is relatively small, it is likely to go undetected unless the study sample size is quite large.

Biologic evidence of toxicity

Two types of evidence are generally employed when evaluating agents for evidence of reproductive toxicity: animal studies and epidemiologic studies in human populations.

Studies with experimental animals offer the advantage of studying varying levels of exposure (from minimal to substantial) at specific key developmental time periods. In addition, outcomes are standardized and typically include measures of fertility, fetal weight, viability, and presence and patterns of malformations. If low doses of a compound produce an increase in malformations, a role for the agent in disrupting embryo development is possible. Limitations of animal testing include species variations in toxicity (i.e. compounds may be toxic to human embryos but not to various animal embryos, and vice versa). Further, evaluation of functional attributes such as behavior or immunocompetence is not a part of standard testing schemes. Therefore, absence of toxicity in animal protocols provides only limited information on possible adverse effects on human development.

Human epidemiologic studies can be subdivided, in increasing order of scientific merit, into case reports, case–control studies, retrospective cohort studies, and well-designed prospective cohort studies. Often, case reports of malformations or pregnancy loss will emerge first, raising hypotheses that lead to further study. However, case reports alone are insufficient evidence on which to establish the presence or degree of risk. The evaluation of toxicity requires comprehensive assessment of both exposures and outcomes. Accurate occupational and environmental exposures are difficult to measure in humans and it is even more difficult to pinpoint precise exposure at a specific gestational age. Outcome assessment can also be difficult because the identification of abnormalities in children is affected by the age of the child and the thoroughness with which abnormalities are sought. Relying on birth certificates or obstetrician reports, for example, will yield a lower rate of identification of abnormalities than will examination by a trained dysmorphologist using a standardized assessment protocol.

Queenan's Management of High-Risk Pregnancy: An Evidence-Based Approach, Sixth Edition. Edited by John T. Queenan, Catherine Y. Spong, Charles J. Lockwood.

Table 4.1 Reproductive toxicology sources

Individual source	Web address	Practitioner cost 2010
Reprotox	www.reprotox.org	$199/year
Teris	http://depts.washington.edu/terisweb/teris/	$150/year
Reprorisk	www.micromedex.com/products/reprorisk/	$765/year
OTIS	www.otispregnancy.org/	Free
	Limited number of fact sheets for download	
Toxnet	http://toxnet.nlm.nih.gov/	Free
DART (Developmental and Reproductive Toxicology) database	http://toxnet.nlm.nih.gov/cgi-bin/sis/htmlgen?DARTETIC	Free

General principles

Principles of reproductive toxicity apply to environmental agents just as they do to pharmaceuticals and these principles are summarized here. These ideas were popularized by Wilson [1] in the 1950s based on his work with experimental animals, but they remain applicable decades later in a discussion of human risk.

• A large proportion of adverse outcomes are unrelated to exposures. Only 5% of congenital malformations are estimated to be attributable to exposure to a chemical agent or pharmaceutical [2].

• A specific agent may be nontoxic at low doses but toxic at higher doses. For example, x-ray exposures of >50 rad during pregnancy have been associated with microcephaly and mental retardation, but x-ray exposures in the range of most diagnostic procedures (<1 rad) are not associated with an increase in adverse pregnancy outcome.

• Each fetus will respond differently to a given exposure based on their genetic susceptibility and other factors. For a given toxic exposure, responses can range from unaffected to significantly affected.

• The timing of exposure during pregnancy will influence the response. Target tissues will have different sensitivities to toxicity at different times during gestation. Although the first trimester is typically the most sensitive time period for many congenital malformations (e.g. limb and heart defects), there are a number of examples of severe toxicity from exposures at other times in pregnancy. For example, agents that affect fetal growth and neurologic development, such as mercury and ethanol, will continue to be toxic throughout the second and third trimesters.

• Toxicity must occur via a biologically plausible mechanism. Therefore, chemicals that cannot cross the placenta or agents such as microwaves that cannot penetrate into the uterus are unlikely causes of reproductive toxicity.

Specific agents

Research demonstrating adverse reproductive effects of various chemical and environmental agents is continuously evolving. In this section we present a snapshot of the current knowledge. Computerized databases are available and can provide access to regularly updated summaries of chemical exposures (Table 4.1).

Lead

Lead can cross the placenta readily [3,4]. In women with significant occupational lead exposure (pottery glazes, batteries), rates of stillbirth and miscarriage are increased [5] as well as rates of premature rupture of membranes and premature birth [6–8]. Over time, with the reduction in lead alkyl additives in gasoline and the use of lead-based paints, lead levels in women of reproductive age have declined. Surveillance from the 1980s suggested that 9% of white women and 20% of African-American women exceeded blood lead levels of $10\,\mu g/dL$ [9]. More recently, overall percentages have declined to 0.5% [10].

While significant occupational exposures are rare in the USA, lower levels of perinatal lead exposure have been linked to adverse reproductive outcomes. Even mild elevations in maternal lead levels have been associated with an increased risk of miscarriage (5–9 $\mu g/dL$, odds ratio [OR] 2.8; 10–14 $\mu g/dL$, OR 5.4; >15 $\mu g/dL$, OR 12.2) [11]. Increased maternal bone and blood lead levels have also been associated with a minor-to-moderate increased risk of pregnancy-induced hypertension [12,13]. Cord blood concentrations less than $30\,\mu g/dL$, and perhaps as low as $10\,\mu g/dL$ [14,15], have been linked to measurable deficits in early cognitive development. Although the results are not consistent, elevated maternal lead levels during pregnancy have been associated with lower IQ scores at age 8 [16] and tests of attention and visuoconstruction at ages 15–17 [17]. There is some suggestion that male fetuses may be more susceptible to adverse *in utero* effects of lead exposure on subsequent neurodevelopment [18]. Although isolated studies have linked maternal lead exposure to an increased fetal risk of neural tube defects [19] and total anomalous pulmonary venous return [20], these findings have not been consistent. One potential mechanism through which lead may result in adverse developmental effects is the inverse relationship between maternal lead levels and fetal DNA methylation [21].

Sources of lead exposure include lead solders, pipes, storage batteries, construction materials (e.g. lead-based paints), dyes, and wood preservatives. A validated questionnaire for screening pregnant women is not available. Risk factors for maternal lead levels that exceed $10\,\mu g/mL$ include occupational exposures and house remodeling; however, screening high-risk women still fails to identify approximately 30% of cases [22]. Women at risk of lead exposure should be evaluated prior to pregnancy. If the blood level is higher than $30\,\mu g/dL$, chelation therapy should be considered prior to conception. There is no agreement on how to manage women with lower levels of blood lead, although our preference at the time of writing would be to use chelation therapy to reduce blood lead concentrations to $10\,\mu g/dL$ or less. Pregnancy itself may lead to a mobilization of bone stores of lead, with increased exposure [23–25]. Calcium treatment (1000–1200 mg/day) decreases bone mobilization during pregnancy and may provide modest reduction of maternal blood lead levels during pregnancy $(-1\,\mu g/dL)$ [23,26,27]. Current pregnancy is a relative contraindication to chelation therapy as ethylenediaminetetra-acetic acid (EDTA) may chelate other key minerals necessary for development and has been linked to malformations in animal models [28]. Chelation therapy during pregnancy should be individualized based on the maternal serum lead level and the gestational age.

Mercury

Methyl mercury, a byproduct of such industries as incineration of solid waste and fossil fuel combustion facilities, pollutes our oceans and waterways. Methyl mercury crosses the placenta freely and accumulates in fetal tissues at concentrations exceeding maternal levels [29,30]. At high levels, methyl mercury can result in fetal neurotoxicity with microcephaly, cerebral palsy, deafness, and blindness (Minimata Bay, Japan [31,32]), but is not reproducibly associated with congenital malformations. However, most exposure to mercury occurs at low levels from fish consumption (methyl mercury), dental amalgams (mercury vapor), or the vaccine preservative thimerosal (ethyl mercury). Thimerosal has been removed from most vaccines in the USA and is therefore an unlikely potential source of exposure.

Fish consumption remains a modifiable source of fetal and childhood mercury exposure. Several large cohort

---

Box 4.1 Commercial fish and levels of mercury

High levels: avoid in pregnancy

- Swordfish
- Shark
- King mackerel
- Tile fish

Moderate levels: limit consumption to 6 oz/week

- Canned albacore tuna
- Fresh tuna
- Orange roughy
- Halibut
- Grouper
- Sea bass
- Local fish if no specific information is available

Low levels: current recommendation is to limit consumption to 12 oz/week but higher consumption may be beneficial if risks and benefits considered

- Shrimp
- Canned light tuna
- Salmon
- Pollack
- Catfish
- Haddock
- Scallops
- Tilapia

www.cfsan.fda.gov/~frf/sea-mehg.html provides mercury levels in commercially bought fish

---

studies have addressed the effects of low levels of *in utero* mercury exposure from maternal fish consumption on neuropsychologic development. Studies from the Faroe Islands (>1000 mother–infant pairs) and New Zealand (237 pairs) [33,34] found subtle deficits in language, attention, intelligence, and memory in school-aged children. Another, more recent study from the Seychelles (779 mother–infant pairs) did not find an association between *in utero* mercury exposure and outcome at 9 years; however, the final power to detect these outcomes was only 50% [35]. In 2001, based on these findings and a 2000 report from the National Research Council (NRC) [36], the Environmental Protection Agency (EPA) issued advice urging pregnant women to limit consumption of fish high in mercury (Box 4.1). A benchmark blood level of $<5.8\,\mu g/L$ was recommended by the NRC; exposure above this level was associated with a doubling in the risk of adverse neurologic outcomes. Among women of child-bearing age in the United States between 1999 and 2002, 4–8% exceeded this benchmark level [37]. More recent iterations of this advice balance concerns over mercury exposure with the known benefits of fish consumption (www.epa.gov/ost/fishadvice/factsheet.html). Moderate intake of relatively safer fish should not be discouraged, as increasing fish consumption has been linked with higher measures of infant cognition [38,39]. The 2004 EPA and FDA recommendations are as follows.

- Do not eat shark, swordfish, king mackerel, or tilefish because they contain high levels of mercury.
- Eat up to 12 ounces (two average meals) a week of a variety of fish and shellfish that are lower in mercury.
- Five of the most commonly eaten fish that are low in mercury are shrimp, canned light tuna, salmon, pollock, and catfish.
- Another commonly eaten fish, albacore ("white") tuna, has more mercury than canned light tuna. So, when choosing your two meals of fish and shellfish, you may eat up to 6 ounces (one average meal) of albacore tuna per week.
- Check local advisories about the safety of fish caught by family and friends in your local lakes, rivers, and coastal areas. If no advice is available, eat up to 6 ounces (one average meal) per week of fish you catch from local waters, but don't consume any other fish during that week.

In 2009, the FDA released a draft of a summary of its updated position which weighed the risks and benefits of fish consumption during pregnancy on fetal neurodevelopmental outcome [40]. The overall conclusion of its risk/benefit assessment was that consumption of fish with low mercury levels has a significantly greater probability of resulting in net benefit as measured by verbal development, although the maximum benefit was modest. The FDA solicited commentary prior to moving forward with a final draft. The EPA responded with an extensive commentary expressing concerns about various aspects of the scientific method used but supporting a comprehensive analysis of risks and benefits of fish consumption and urging consideration of agents in addition to mercury [41]. Updated joint recommendations have not yet been updated.

Mercury exposure from dental amalgams is usually at low level and is not easily modified. Both placement and removal of dental amalgams are associated with transient increased levels of mercury exposure and should be avoided during pregnancy [42,43]. Dental personnel may also be exposed to inorganic mercury in vapors released from dental amalgams. Although evidence of documented harm in dental personnel is limited, current studies lack the power to detect subtle neurodevelopmental deficits. Safe levels of mercury during pregnancy have not been established although suggested guidelines are that environments have a mercury vapor concentration less than $0.01 \, mg/m^3$ (one-fifth of Occupational Safety and Health Administration [OSHA] limits of $0.05 \, mg/m^3$).

Pesticides and herbicides

A diverse group of agents is used to control pests such as insects and unwanted plants. While most exposures are agricultural, significant household exposure can occur, especially in the inner city [44]. The majority of pesticides cross the placenta readily [44]. Methodologically, it is difficult to isolate a single agent in epidemiologic studies; exposure to pesticides has been estimated by maternal recall, proximity to agricultural pesticide use, or maternal pesticide levels. Of concern, several pesticides act as endocrine disruptors; serum levels of hexachlorobenzene, a fungicide used to treat seed, have been associated with an increased risk of hypospadias in male offspring [45]. Several studies have linked occupational exposure to pesticides with an increased risk of miscarriage [46,47] and birth defects such as musculoskeletal [48,49] and limb reduction abnormalities [50]. No association or weak associations have been found between parental pesticide exposure and adverse pregnancy outcomes including low birthweight [51], preterm delivery, or early neurodevelopmental outcomes [52]. While several maternal recall case–control studies have linked household pesticide use with an increased risk of childhood cancer [53,54], no association was found when exposure was estimated by proximity to agricultural pesticide use [55].

Minimizing occupational pesticide exposure through the use of protective clothing, adequate ventilation, respiratory masks, and hand washing is recommended. Limiting everyday exposure by minimizing household pesticide use (especially aerosolized pesticides), washing fruits and vegetables or buying organic produce is of uncertain benefit, but is easily accomplished.

Polychlorinated biphenyls

Polychlorinated biphenyls (PCBs) are a heterogeneous group of more than 200 lipid-soluble chemicals that were used extensively in industry until 1979, particularly in the manufacture of electrical transformers. Low-level maternal exposure is largely related to meat, dairy, and fish consumption, particularly fish from contaminated areas such as the Great Lakes. PCBs cross the placenta easily (fetal to maternal serum ratios of 0.6:1.1) and also accumulate in human breastmilk (breastmilk to maternal ratios of 0.6:1.8), contributing to postnatal exposure [56]. The overall effect on birthweight appears to be modest (290 g difference between <10th and >90th percentile exposure) [57] in some studies and insignificant in others [58].

Studies of *in utero* exposure to low levels of PCBs and subsequent neurodevelopment have produced various results. Several studies have shown no relationship between maternal serum levels of PCBs and mental and motor development in infancy/early childhood [59] and at school age [60,61]. Other studies have suggested minor deficits in attention, memory, and motor skills in vulnerable populations of children; deficits were not observed in children in more advantageous circumstances or in those who were breastfed [62,63]. PCBs can also act as endocrine disruptors.

While levels of individual PCB compounds are not significant, total PCB load >2.0μg/L has been linked to increased risks of hypospadias [64]. Local fish advisories should be consulted to determine which fish should not be eaten during pregnancy (http://water.epa.gov/scitech/swguidance/fishshellfish/fishadvisories/states.cfm).

Organic solvents

Many women work in industries where they may be exposed to organic solvents, including dry cleaning and manufacturing using solvent-based adhesives, paints, or lacquers. Common organic solvents include toluene, benzene, and xylene. Significant occupational exposure has been associated with small (160 g) reductions in birthweight and an increased risk of major malformations (relative risk [RR] 13.0, 95% confidence interval [CI] 1.8–99.5) [65]. The risk of any major malformation was 10% and the overwhelming majority of malformations occurred in women with symptomatic exposure. Maternal occupational exposure to solvents is also associated with an increase in major malformations (oral clefts, urinary malformations, and male genital malformations) [66], increased rates of hyperactivity [67] and subtle decreases in visual acuity and abnormalities in red/green color vision [68]. An increase in childhood acute lymphoblastic leukemia has also been associated with self-reported occupational exposure to solvents and petroleum in the UK [69]. Purposeful maternal solvent abuse (sniffing) has been associated with a fetal syndrome similar to fetal alcohol syndrome in 12.5% of cases, as well as major malformations (16.1%) and neonatal hearing loss (10.7%) [70].

Occupational exposure to solvents should be identified and minimized; similarly, women should avoid exposure to solvents at home, especially in poorly ventilated areas. Regarding non-occupational exposures to paint fumes, the Danish National Birth Cohort Study found an inverse relationship between exposure to paint fumes and low birthweight in a cohort of 19,000 mothers [71].

Video display terminals

Initial concerns regarding the reproductive risks of video display terminals (VDTs) centered on early reports linking occupational exposure with an increased risk of spontaneous pregnancy loss [72]. However, subsequent well-designed studies suggested no increased risk [73,74]. Therefore patients can be reassured that there are no known fetal risks associated with working at VDTs.

Bisphenol A

There has been recent attention focused on the possible adverse affects of bisphenol A (BPA) on pregnancy and childhood development. BPA is a hormone disrupter with estrogenic effects that is commonly found in hard plastic items such as food storage containers, bottled water, in the lining of some canned goods, in thermal coatings of cash register receipts, and some dental sealants. In general, plastics that are marked with recycle codes 1, 2, 4, 5, and 6 are very unlikely to contain BPA. Some, but not all, plastics that are marked with recycle codes 3 or 7 may contain BPA.

In 2008 the National Toxicology Program released an expert report and a monograph on the potential adverse effects of BPA on humans and outlined the critical missing data [75,76]. The potential adverse effects of BPA on the fetus, largely identified in animal models, include effects on the brain, especially related to sex-related differences, developing endocrine and reproductive organs such as the prostate and breast tissue, and detrimental neurobehavioral effects. There is scant human data regarding maternal blood levels of BPA in the US. In one study of 40 Michigan mothers, blood levels of BPA ranged from 0.5 to 23ng/mL [77]. In *ex vivo* placental perfusion models, BPA has been found to cross the human placenta in its active form even when present in low levels [78]. In one study, third-trimester maternal urine BPA levels were not correlated with birthweight [79]. In a prospective study of 249 mother–infant pairs, maternal urine BPA levels at ≤16 weeks were associated with increased aggressive (externalizing) behaviour in 2-year-old girls [80].

In January of 2010, the FDA stated that while standardized toxicity tests support the safety of current low levels of human exposure to BPA, subtle human effects were possible [81]. Therefore, at this time, it is reasonable for pregnant women to avoid the use of products that contain BPA where possible. Fact sheets for pregnant women (www.niehs.nih.gov/health/docs/bisphenol-a-factsheet.pdf) and new parents (www.hhs.gov/safety/bpa/) are available.

CASE PRESENTATION

A 38-year-old G1 presents at 8 weeks' gestation for her first prenatal visit. She reports that her husband is an avid fisherman and she is concerned about the risks of mercury and other toxins to her pregnancy from eating fish that he has caught. On the other hand, she does not want to offend him by spurning his fish if the risks are low.

Adequately counseling this patient requires knowledge both of the amount of fish that she is consuming and local fish advisories. Local fish advisories are common (Fig. 4.1). Possible fish contaminants triggering a local advisory include mercury, PCBs, chlordane, dioxins, and DDT. Patients should be advised not to consume any locally caught fish covered by a fish advisory during pregnancy. If no advisory is found, the patient may be counseled that she can eat up to 6 oz (one average meal) per week of fish her husband catches from local waters. However, she should not consume any other fish during that week. At the same time, the potential health benefits to her fetus of fish consumption during pregnancy should be reviewed. Ideally, fish consumption should continue during pregnancy, but should be limited to fish and shellfish with relatively low levels of contaminants, especially mercury. Locally caught fish may not be ideal for this purpose, especially in the Great Lakes area. More recently, there are unknown health effects of the Gulf oil spill. Links to the latest local fish advisories can be found at http://water.epa.gov/scitech/swguidance/fishshellfish /fishadvisories/states.cfm.

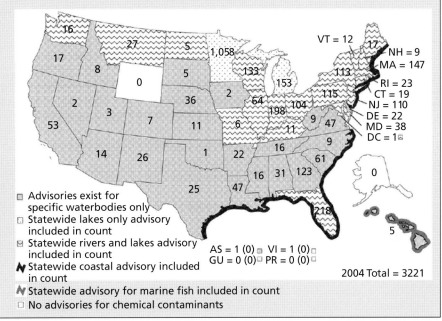

Figure 4.1 Fish consumption advisories by state (2006 data, from the Environmental Protection Agency). Please note that states may have a different counting method for fish advisories from the national method, so advisory in the figure may be slightly different from those reported by individual states.

□ Advisories exist for specific waterbodies only
▣ Statewide lakes only advisory included in count
☒ Statewide rivers and lakes advisory included in count
Ν Statewide coastal advisory included in count
Ν Statewide advisory for marine fish included in count
□ No advisories for chemical contaminants

AS = 1 (0)   VI = 1 (0)
GU = 0 (0)   PR = 0 (0)

2004 Total = 3221

References

1. Wilson JG. Current status of teratology: general principles and mechanisms derived from animal studies. In: Wilson JG, Fraser FC, eds. Handbook of Teratology. New York: Plenum, 1977, pp.47–74.
2. Czeizel A, Rácz J. Evaluation of drug intake during pregnancy in the Hungarian case–control surveillance of congenital anomalies. Teratology 1990;42:505–512.
3. McClain RM, Becker BA. Teratogenicity, fetal toxicity, and placental transfer of lead nitrate in rats. Toxicol Appl Pharmacol 1975;31:72–82.
4. Barltrop D. Transfer of lead to the human foetus. In: Barltrop D, Burland WL, eds. Mineral Metabolism in Pediatrics. Oxford: Blackwell Science, 1969, pp.135–151.
5. Scanlon JW. Dangers to the human fetus from certain heavy metals in the environment. Rev Environ Health 1975;2: 39–64.
6. Nogaki K. On action of lead on body of lead refinery workers: particularly conception, pregnancy and parturition in case of females and on vitality of their newborn. Igaku Kenkyu 1957;27:1314–1338.
7. Fahim MS, Fahim Z, Hall DG. Effects of subtoxic lead levels on pregnant women in the state of Missouri. Res Commun Chem Pathol Pharmacol 1976;13:309–331.
8. Wilson AT. Effects of abnormal lead content of water supplies on maternity patients. Scott Med J 1966;11:73–82.
9. Crocetti AF, Mushak P, Schwartz J. Determination of numbers of lead-exposed women of childbearing age and pregnant women: an integrated summary of a report to the US Congress

on childhood lead poisoning. Environ Health Perspect 1990;89:121–124.

10. Brody DJ, Pirkle JL, Kramer RA et al. Blood lead levels in the US population. Phase I of the Third National Health and Nutrition Examination Survey (NHANES III). JAMA 1994; 272:277–283.

11. Borja-Aburto VH, Hertz-Picciotto I, Lopez MR et al. Blood lead levels measured prospectively and risk of spontaneous abortion. Am J Epidemiol 1999;150:590–597.

12. Rothenburg SJ, Kondrashov V, Manalo M et al. Increases in hypertension and blood pressure during pregnancy with increased bone lead levels. Am J Epidemiol 2002;156; 1079–1087.

13. Yazbeck C, Thiebaugeorges O, Moreau T et al. Maternal blood lead levels and the risk of pregnancy-induced hypertension: the EDEN cohort study. Environ Health Perspect 2009;117: 1526–1530.

14. Bellinger D, Leviton A, Waternaux C et al. Longitudinal analyses of prenatal and postnatal lead exposure and early cognitive development. N Engl J Med 1987;316:1037–1043.

15. Dietrich KN, Krafft KM, Bornschein RL et al. Low-level fetal lead exposure effect on neurobehavioral development in early infancy. Pediatrics 1987;80:721–730.

16. Wasserman GA, Liu X, Popovac D et al. The Yugoslavia Prospective Lead Study: contributions of prenatal and postnatal lead exposure to early intelligence. Neurotoxicol Teratol 2000;22:811–818.

17. Ris MD, Dietrich KN, Succop PA et al. Early exposure to lead and neurophyschological outcome in adolescence. J Int Neuropsychol Soc 2004;10; 261–270.

18. Jedrychowski W, Perera F, Jankowski J et al. Gender specific differences in neurodevelopmental effects of prenatal exposure to very low lead levels: the prospective cohort study in three-year olds. Early Human Dev 2009;85:503–510.

19. Bound JP, Harvey PW, Francis BJ et al. Involvement of deprivation and environmental lead in neural tube defects: a matched case–control study. Arch Dis Child 1997;76:107–112.

20. Jackson LW, Correa-Villasenor A, Lees PS et al. Parental lead exposures and total anomalous pulmonary venous return. Birth Defects Res Part A Clin Mol Teratol 2004;70: 185–193.

21. Pilsner JR, Hu H, Ettinger A et al. Influence of prenatal lead exposure on genomic methylation of cord blood DNA. Environ Health Perspect 2009;117:1466–1471.

22. Fletcher AM, Gelberg KH, Marshall EG. Reasons for testing and exposure sources among women of childbearing age with moderate blood lead levels. J Commun Health 1999;24: 215–227.

23. Gulson BL, Mizon KJ, Korsch MR et al. Mobilization of lead from human bone tissue during pregnancy and lactation: a summary of long term research. Sci Total Environ 2003;303: 79–104.

24. Gulson BL, Mizon KJ, Palmer JM et al. Blood lead changes during pregnancy and postpartum with calcium supplementation. Environ Health Perspect 2004;112:499–507.

25. Manton WI, Angle CR, Stanek KL et al. Release of lead from bone in pregnancy and lactation. Environ Res 2003;92: 139–151.

26. Hernandez-Avila M, Gonzalez-Cossio T, Hernandez-Avila JE et al. Dietary calcium supplements to lower blood lead levels in lactating women: a randomized placebo-controlled trial. Epidemiology 2003;14:206–212.

27. Ettinger AS, Lamadrid-Figueroa H, Tellez-Rojo MM et al. Effect of calcium supplementation on blood lead levels in pregnancy; a randomized placebo-controlled trial. Environ Health Perspect 2009;117:26–31.

28. Brownie CF, Brownie C, Noden D, Krook L, Haluska M, Aronson AL. Teratogenic effect of calcium edetate (CaEDTA) in rats and the protective effect of zinc. Toxicol Appl Pharmacol 1986;82:426–443.

29. Tsuchiya H, Mitani K, Kodama K et al. Placental transfer of heavy metals in normal pregnant Japanese women. Arch Environ Health 1984;39:11.

30. Bjornberg KA, Vahter M, Berglund B, Niklasson B, Blennow M, Sandborgh-Englund G. Transport of methylmercury and inorganic mercury to the fetus and breast-fed infant. Environ Health Perspect 2005;113:1381–1385.

31. Matsumoto H, Koya G, Takeucki T. Fetal Minimata disease: a neuropathological study of two cases of intrauterine intoxication by a methyl mercury compound. J Neuropathol Exp Neurol 1965;24:563–574.

32. Muramaki U. The effect of organic mercury on intrauterine life. Acta Exp Biol Med Biol 1972;27;301–336.

33. Grandjean P, Weihe P, White RF et al. Cognitive deficit in 7-year old children with prenatal exposure to methylmercury. Neurotoxicol Teratol 1997;19:417–428.

34. Crump KS, Kjellstrom T, Shipp AM, Silvers A, Stewart A. Influence of prenatal mercury exposure upon scholastic and psychological test performance: benchmark analysis of a New Zealand cohort. Risk Anal 1998;18:701–713.

35. Myers GJ, Davidson PW, Cox C et al. Prenatal methylmercury exposure from ocean fish consumption in the Seychelles child development study. Lancet 2003;361:1686–1692.

36. National Research Council. Toxicological effects of methylmercury. Washington, DC: National Academy Press, 2000.

37. Blood mercury levels in young children and childbearing-aged women, United States, 1999–2002. MMWR 2004;53:1018–1020.

38. Oken E, Wright RO, Kleinman KP et al. Maternal fish consumption, hair mercury, and infant cognition in an US cohort. Environ Health Perspect 2005;113:1376–1380.

39. Daniels JL, Longnecker MP, Rowland AS, Golding J and the ALSPAC Study Team. Fish intake during pregnancy and early cognitive development of offspring. Epidemiology 2004;15: 394–402.

40. Docket No. FDA-2009-N-0018. Report of Quantitative Risk and Benefit Assessment of Commercial Fish Consumption, Focusing on Fetal Neurodevelopmental Effects (Measured by Verbal Development in Children) and on Coronary Heart Disease and Stroke in the General Population, and Summary of Published Research on the Beneficial Effects of Fish Consumption and Omega-3 Fatty Acids for Certain Neurodevelopmental and Cardiovascular Endpoints. Federal Register 2009;74:3615–3617.

41. Environmental Protection Agency. Comments on the draft FDA report assessing risks and benefits from fish. 2009. http://water.epa.gov/scitech/swguidance/fishshellfish/ fishadvisories/upload/2009_04_20_fish_epa-comments-fda.pdf.

42. Molim M, Bergman B, Marklund SI, Schutz A, Skerfving S. Mercury, selenium and glutathione peroxidase before and after amalgam removal in man. Acta Odontol Scand 1990;48:189–202.

43. Razagui IB, Haswell SJ. Mercury and selenium concentrations in maternal and neonatal scalp hair: relationship to amalgam-based dental treatment received during pregnancy. Biol Trace Elem Res 2001;81:1–19.

44. Whyatt RM, Barr DB, Camann DE et al. Contemporary-use pesticides in personal air samples during pregnancy and blood samples at delivery among urban minority mothers and newborns. Environ Health Perspect 2003;111:749–756.

45. Giordano F, Abballe A, de Felip E et al. Maternal exposures to endocrine disrupting chemicals and hypospadias in offspring. Birth Defects Res 2010;88:241–250.

46. Arbuckle TE, Lin Z, Mery LS, Curtis KM. An exploratory analysis of the effect of pesticide exposure on the risk of spontaneous abortion in an Ontario farm population. Environ Health Perspect 2001;109:851–857.

47. Garry VF, Harkins M, Lybuvimov A, Erickson L, Long L. Reproductive outcomes in the women of the Red River Valley of the North. The spouses of pesticide applicators: pregnancy loss, age at menarche and exposures to pesticides. J Toxicol Environ Health 2002;65:769–786.

48. Hemminki K, Mutanen P, Luoma K, Saloniemi I. Congenital malformations by the parental occupation in Finland. Int Arch Occup Environ Health 1980;46:93–98.

49. Garry VF, Schreinemachers D, Harkins ME, Griffith J. Pesticide appliers, biocides and birth defects in rural Minnesota. Environ Health Perspect 1996;104:394–399.

50. Engel LS, O'Meara ES, Schwartz SM. Maternal occupation in agriculture and risk of adverse birth outcomes in Washington state, 1980–1991. Am J Epidemiol 2000;26:193–198.

51. Kristensen P, Ingens LM, Andersen A, Bye A, Sundheim L. Gestational age, birth weight, and perinatal death among births to Norwegian farmers, 1967–1991. Am J Epidemiol 1997;146:329–338.

52. Young JG, Eskenazi B, Gladstone EA et al. Association between in utero organophosphate pesticide exposure and abnormal reflexes in neonates. Neurotoxicology 2005;26:199–209.

53. Daniels JL, Olshan AF, Savitz DA. Pesticides and childhood cancers. Environ Health Perspect 1997;105:1068–1077.

54. Zahm SH, Ward MH. Pesticides and childhood cancer. Environ Health Perspect 1998;106:893–908.

55. Reynolds P, von Behren J, Gunier RB, Goldberg DE, Harnly M, Hertz A. Agricultural pesticide use and childhood cancer in California. Epidemiology 2005;16:93–100.

56. DeKoning EP, Karmaus W. PCB exposure in utero and via breastmilk: a review. J Expo Anal Environ Epidemiol 2000;10:285–293.

57. Hertz-Picciotto I, Charles MJ, James RA, Keller JA, Willman E, Teplin S. In utero polychlorinated biphenyl exposure in relation to fetal and early childhood growth. Epidemiology 2005;16:648–656.

58. Longnecker MP, Klebanoff MA, Brock JW, Guo X. Maternal levels of polychlorinated biphenyls in relation to preterm and small for gestational age birth. Epidemiology 2005;16:641–647.

59. Daniels JL, Longnecker MP, Klebanoff MA et al. Prenatal exposure to low level polychlorinated biphenyls in relation to mental and motor development at 8 months. Am J Epidemiol 2003;157:485–492.

60. Gray KA, Klebanoff MA, Brock JW et al. In utero exposure to background levels of polychlorinated biphenyls and cognitive functioning among school age children. Am J Epidemiol 2005;162:17–26.

61. Gladen BC, Rogan WJ. Effects of perinatal polychlorinated biphenyls and dichlorodiphenyl dichloroethene on later development. J Pediatr 1991;119:58–63.

62. Vreugdenhil HJI, Lanting CI, Mulder PGH, Boersma ER, Weisglas-Kuperus N. Effects of prenatal PCB and dioxin background exposure on cognitive and motor abilities in Dutch children at school age. J Pediatr 2002;140:48–56.

63. Jacobsen JL, Jacobsen SW. Perinatal exposure to polychlorinated biphenyls and attention at school age. J Pediatr 2003;143:780–788.

64. McGlynn KA, Guo X, Graubard BI et al. Maternal pregnancy levels of polychlorinated biphenyls and risk of hypospadias and cryptorchidism in male offspring. Environ Health Perspect 2009;117:1472–1476.

65. Katthak S, K-Moghtader G, McMartin K, Barrera M, Kennedy D, Koren G. Pregnancy outcome following gestational exposure to organic solvents. JAMA 1999;281:1106–1109.

66. Gariantezec R, Monfort C, Rouget F et al. Maternal occupational exposure to solvents and congenital malformations: a prospective study in the general population. Occupat Environ Med 2009;66:456–463.

67. Laslo-Baker D, Barrera M, Knittel-Keren D et al. Child neurodevelopment outcome and maternal occupational exposure to solvents. Arch Pediatr Adolesc Med 2004;158:956–961.

68. Till C, Westall CA, Koren G, Nulman I, Rovet JF. Vision abnormalities in young children exposed prenatally to organic solvents. Neurotoxicology 2005;26:599–613.

69. McKinney PA, Raji OY, van Tongeren M et al. The UK Childhood Cancer Study: maternal occupational exposures and childhood leukaemia and lymphoma. Rad Protect Dosimetry 2008;132:232–240.

70. Scheeres JJ, Chudley AE. Solvent abuse in pregnancy: a perinatal perspective. J Obstet Gynaecol Can 2002;24:22–26.

71. Sorensen M, Andersen AM, Raaschou-Nielsen O. Non-occupational exposure to paint fumes during pregnancy and fetal growth in a general population. Environ Research 2010;110:383–387.

72. Gold EB, Tomich E. Occupational hazards to fertility and pregnancy outcome. Occup Med (Lond) 1994;9:435–469.

73. Blackwell R, Chang A. Video display terminals and pregnancy: a review. Br J Obstet Gynaecol 1988;95:446–453.

74. Rothenberg SJ, Manalo M, Jiang J et al. Maternal blood lead level during pregnancy in South Central Los Angeles. Arch Environ Health 1999;54:151–157.

75. NIH Publication No. 08 – 5994. NTP-CERHR Monograph on the Potential Human Reproductive and Developmental Effects of Bisphenol A. 2008 http://cerhr.niehs.nih.gov/evals/bisphenol/bisphenol.pdf.

76. Chapin RE, Adams J, Boekelheide K et al. NTP-CERHR Expert Panel Report on the Reproductive and Developmental Toxicity of Bisphenol A. Birth Defects Research Part B 2008;83:157–395.

77. Padmanabhan V, Siefert K, Ransom S et al. Maternal bisphenol-A levels at delivery: a looming problem? J Perinatol 2008;28:258–263.

78. Balakrishnan B, Henare K, Thorstensen EB et al. Transfer of bisphenol A across the human placenta. Am J Obstet Gynecol 2010;202:e1–7.

79. Wolff MS, Engel SM, Berkowitz GS et al. Prenatal phenol and phthalate exposures and birth outcomes. Environ Health Perspect 2008; 116:1092–1097.

80. Braun JM, Yolton K, Dietrich KN et al. Prenatal bisphenol A exposure and early childhood behavior. Environ Health Perspect 2009;117:1945–1952

81. US Food and Drug Administration. Update on Bisphenol A for Use in Food Contact Applications. 2010. www.fda.gov/downloads/NewsEvents/PublicHealthFocus/UCM197778.pdf.

Chapter 5
Genetic Screening for Mendelian Disorders

Deborah A. Driscoll

Department of Obstetrics and Gynecology, Perelman School of Medicine at the University of Pennsylvania, Philadelphia, PA, USA

Genetic screening to identify couples at risk for having offspring with inherited conditions such as Tay–Sachs disease, sickle cell disease, and cystic fibrosis has been integrated into obstetric practice. The number of genetic conditions for which carrier screening and genetic testing is available has increased as a result of the Human Genome Project and advances in technology. Further, the demand for genetic screening and testing has increased. The decision to offer population-based genetic screening is complex. Factors to consider include disease prevalence and carrier frequency; nature and severity of the disorder; options for treatment; intervention and prevention; availability of a sensitive and specific screening and diagnostic test; positive predictive value of the test; and cost [1]. Care must be taken to avoid the potential for psychological harm to the patient and the misuse of genetic information and possible discrimination. Successful implementation of genetic screening programs requires adequate educational materials for providers and patients and genetic counseling services. This chapter reviews mendelian inheritance, indications for genetic screening, and the current carrier screening guidelines for common genetic disorders.

Family history

Genetic screening begins with an accurate family history, which should be a routine part of a patient's complete evaluation. It is useful to summarize this information in a pedigree to demonstrate the family relationships and which relatives are affected. The family history should include three generations; the sex and state of health should be noted. Stillbirths and miscarriage should be recorded. A history of the more common genetic diseases, chromosomal abnormalities, and congenital malformations such as cardiac defects, cleft lip and palate, and neural tube defects should be routinely sought. The

history should also include cognitive and behavioral disorders such as mental retardation, autism, developmental delay, and psychiatric disorders. Cancer and age at diagnosis should be noted. Genetic diagnoses should be confirmed by review of the medical records whenever possible. Pedigree analysis is important in determining the type of inheritance of a given mendelian disorder, and is important in providing accurate risk estimate.

Mendelian inheritance

Mendelian inheritance refers to genetic disorders that arise as a result of transmission of a mutation in a single gene. Most single-gene disorders are uncommon, usually occurring in 1 in 10,000–50,000 births. Over 11,000 single-gene disorders or traits have been described and can be found in the Online Mendelian Inheritance in Man (OMIM) (www3.ncbi.nlm.nih.gov/omim/) [2]. Obstetricians should be familiar with the inheritance patterns and some of the common disorders for which carrier screening is available.

There are three basic patterns of mendelian inheritance:
- autosomal dominant
- autosomal recessive
- X-linked.

Genes occur in pairs; one copy is present on each one of a pair of chromosomes. If the effects of an abnormal gene are evident when the gene is present in a single dose, then the gene is said to be dominant. A carrier of an autosomal dominant disorder has a 50% chance of transmitting the disorder to his or her offspring. In general, pedigree analysis shows the disease in every generation with some exceptions. In some families, the disorder may not be expressed in every individual who inherits the gene. This is referred to as incomplete or reduced penetrance. Affected relatives may have a variable phenotype as a

Queenan's Management of High-Risk Pregnancy: An Evidence-Based Approach, Sixth Edition. Edited by John T. Queenan, Catherine Y. Spong, Charles J. Lockwood.

result of differences in expression. Modifying genes and/or the environment can influence the phenotype and hence it may be difficult to predict the outcome accurately. Autosomal dominant disorders may also arise as a result of a sporadic or *de novo* mutation. If this occurs then a couple does not have a 50% risk of having a subsequent affected child unless germline mosaicism exists. Germline mosaicism refers to the existence of a population of cells with the mutation in the testes or ovary.

For an autosomal recessive disorder to be expressed, both copies of the gene must be abnormal. Carriers of autosomal recessive disorders are detected either through carrier screening or after the birth of an affected child or relative. Pedigree analysis typically shows only siblings to be affected. In general, carriers are healthy although at the cellular level they may demonstrate reduced enzyme levels; this is not sufficient to cause disease. For example, Tay–Sachs carriers have a reduced level of hexosaminidase A. When both parents are carriers there is a 25% chance of having an affected child in each pregnancy. There is a two-thirds likelihood that their offspring is a carrier.

X-linked diseases such as Duchenne muscular dystrophy or hemophilia primarily affect males because they have a single X chromosome. In contrast, female carriers are less likely to be affected because of the presence of two X chromosomes. A female carrier may show manifestations of the disease because of unfavorable lyonization or inactivation of the X chromosome with the normal copy of the gene. A female who carries a gene causing an X-linked recessive condition has a 50% chance of transmitting the gene in each pregnancy; 50% of the male fetuses will be affected and 50% of the females will be carriers. X-linked disorders can also occur as a result of a *de novo* mutation. The mother of a child with an X-linked condition is not necessarily a carrier. Similar to autosomal dominant disorders, germline mosaicism must also be considered. A male with an X-linked disorder will pass the abnormal gene on his X chromosome to all of his daughters who will be carriers; his sons receive his Y chromosome and hence will be unaffected. X-linked dominant disorders such as incontinentia pigmenti are rare and affect females; they tend to be lethal in males.

It is now recognized that some genetic conditions do not follow simple mendelian inheritance. Some genes contain a region of trinucleotide repeats (i.e. $(CCG)_n$) that are unstable and may expand during transmission from parent to offspring. When the number of repeats reaches a critical level, the gene becomes methylated and is no longer expressed (e.g. fragile X syndrome). Testing is available to determine if an individual with a positive family history of mental retardation carries a premutation, which may expand to a full mutation in their offspring [3]. Trinucleotide repeats are also implicated in several neurologic disorders such as Huntington disease and myotonic dystrophy [4].

Carrier screening

Carrier screening refers to the identification of an individual who is heterozygous or has a mutation in one of two copies of the gene. The screening test may identify an individual with two mutations who is so mildly affected it has escaped medical attention. Ideally, carrier screening should be offered to patients and their partners prior to conception to provide them with an accurate assessment of their risk of having an affected child and a full range of reproductive options. Most screening takes place during pregnancy and should be performed as early as possible to allow couples an opportunity to have prenatal diagnostic testing. When both parents are carriers, genetic counseling is recommended and they are informed of the availability of prenatal diagnostic testing, preimplantation genetic diagnosis, donor gametes (eggs or sperm), and adoption to avoid the risk for having an affected child. It is helpful to explore their attitudes towards prenatal testing and termination of pregnancy. In addition, they may consider contacting their relatives at risk and informing them of the availability of carrier screening.

In the USA, preconception or prenatal genetic screening tests are available for many inherited conditions. The decision to offer testing is based on family history, or ethnic or racial heritage associated with an increased risk for a specific condition. Information about specific genetic disorders and testing can be found at www.genetests.org. Screening should be voluntary and informed consent is desirable. Patients should be provided with information about the disorder, the prevalence, severity, and treatment options. Test information including detection rates and limitations should be reviewed with the patient. When the detection rate is less than 100%, it is important for the patient to understand that a negative screening test reduces the likelihood that an individual is a carrier and at risk for having an affected offspring but does not eliminate the possibility. For some patients, genetic counseling may assist with the decision-making process. Patients should also be assured that their test results are confidential.

Guidelines for carrier screening for the hemoglobinopathies [5], cystic fibrosis [6], and genetic diseases more commonly found among individuals of Eastern European Jewish heritage [7] have been developed by the American College of Obstetricians and Gynecologists (ACOG). These disorders are briefly described below and in Table 5.1. DNA-based tests to assess an individual's carrier status for other inherited conditions such as spinal muscular atrophy, fragile X mental retardation or Huntington

Table 5.1 Mendelian disorders frequent among individuals of Eastern European Jewish ancestry

Disorder	Carrier rate	Clinical features
Tay–Sachs disease	1 in 30	Hypotonia, developmental delay, loss of developmental milestones, mental retardation beginning at 5–6 months, loss of sight at 12–18 months, usually fatal by age 6
Canavan disease	1 in 40	Hypotonia, developmental delay, seizures, blindness, large head, gastrointestinal reflux
Familial dysautonomia	1 in 32	Abnormal suck, feeding difficulties, episodic vomiting, abnormal sweating, pain and temperature instability, labile blood pressure, absent tearing, scoliosis
Cystic fibrosis	1 in 24	Chronic pulmonary infections, malabsorption, failure to thrive, pancreatitis, male infertility because of congenital absence of the vas deferens
Fanconi anemia type C	1 in 89	Limb, cardiac, and genitourinary anomalies, microcephaly, mental retardation, developmental delay, anemia, pancytopenia, and increased risk for leukemia
Niemann–Pick type A	1 in 90	Jaundice and ascites caused by liver disease, pulmonary disease, developmental delay and psychomotor retardation, progressive decline in cognitive ability and speech, dysphagia, seizures, hypotonia, abnormal gait
Bloom syndrome	1 in 100	Prenatal and postnatal growth deficiency, predisposition to malignancies, facial telangiectasias, abnormal skin pigmentation, learning difficulties, mental retardation
Mucolipidosis IV	1 in 127	Growth and severe psychomotor retardation, corneal clouding, progressive retinal degeneration, strabismus
Gaucher disease	1 in 15	Chronic fatigue, anemia, easy bruising, nosebleeds, bleeding gums, menorrhagia, hepatosplenomegaly, osteoporosis, bone and joint pain

Note: carrier rates apply to individuals of Eastern European Jewish ancestry; clinical features may vary in presentation, severity, and age of onset.

disease are available but in general are only offered if an individual is at an increased risk to be a carrier based on family history, or at the patient's request.

When a family history suggests that a patient or her partner may be at increased risk to be a carrier or to have a child with an inherited condition, the first step is to determine if the gene for that disorder has been identified. If the gene is known, the optimal strategy is to test the affected relative. Many disorders are caused by mutations unique to a family, and DNA sequencing is required to identify the disease-causing mutation. Once a mutation is confirmed in the affected individual, testing relatives at risk to be carriers is possible. In some cases, DNA sequencing can be used as a carrier screening test but it is expensive and less reliable than testing the affected person. Testing for disorders that are the result of one or more common mutations can be utilized for carrier testing provided that the diagnosis in the affected relative is correct. For example, a carrier test has been developed for spinal muscular atrophy (SMA), a common autosomal recessive disorder caused by a deletion in exon 7 of the SMN1 gene [8]. This is a highly accurate carrier test because the vast majority of cases are caused by this deletion and carrier screening is recommended for individuals with a family history of SMA or SMA-like disease. The ACOG has been cautious about recommending population-based screening in the absence of appropriate genetic counseling since the severity and life expectancy are highly variable and difficult to predict based on the genetic test results [9].

Carrier screening tests may be helpful when a particular diagnosis is suspected based on ultrasound findings in the pregnancy. The antenatal evaluation of a fetus with a congenital malformation typically includes a thorough ultrasound examination and fetal echocardiogram to look for associated anomalies, as well as a fetal karyotype. Single-gene disorders are often considered in the differential diagnosis but until recently were not amenable to prenatal testing. Now that the molecular basis of many of these disorders has been elucidated, either carrier screening of the parents or diagnostic testing of the pregnancy is possible when a particular diagnosis is suspected. For example, carrier screening for Fanconi anemia type C may be considered as part of the evaluation of a fetus with absent radius [10], particularly if the couple are of Eastern European Jewish ancestry, because the carrier frequency is 1 in 90 in this population and a single mutation accounts for 99% of the disease-causing mutations. Testing the parents to determine their carrier status can help establish or exclude a diagnosis in the fetus with an anomaly.

Carrier testing may be carried out on request because of heightened anxiety and concern. It is not uncommon for patients to request a test based on a personal experience, recent newspaper article, or television show. In these instances, it is important for them to understand their individual risk of being a carrier and having an affected child, as well as the risks, benefits, and limitations of testing. Pre- and posttest counseling is very important. For most rare disorders, this is not a very cost-conscious approach but with the availability of high-throughput molecular technology, testing is becoming more affordable. Direct to consumer marketing, advocacy organizations and laboratories offer genetic screening regardless of family or medical history, and although it has become feasible to perform these tests, our ability to predict outcome and future risks associated with carrier status is sometimes limited. In many cases, longitudinal studies of carriers will be needed to better define the risks and benefits of testing.

Hemoglobinopathies

The hemoglobinopathies include structural hemoglobin variants and the thalassemias. Sickle cell disease, a severe form of anemia, is an autosomal recessive disorder common among individuals of African origin but also found in Mediterranean, Arab, southern Iranian, and Asian Indian populations. Approximately 1 in 12 African-Americans is a carrier or has sickle cell trait (Hb AS). The underlying abnormality is a single nucleotide substitution (GAG to GTG) in the sixth codon of the β-globin gene. This mutation leads to the substitution of the amino acid valine for glutamic acid. Sickle cell disorders also include other structural variants of β-hemoglobin. Screening is best accomplished by complete blood count (CBC) with red blood cell (RBC) indices and a hemoglobin electrophoresis.

The thalassemias are a heterogeneous group of hereditary anemias brought about by reduced synthesis of globin chains. α-Thalassemia results from the deletion of 2–4 copies of the α-globin gene. The disorder is most common among individuals of South East Asian descent. If one or two of the genes are deleted, the individual will have α-thalassemia minor, which is usually asymptomatic. Deletion of three genes results in hemoglobin H disease, which is a more severe anemia, and a fetus with deletions of all four α-chain genes can only make an unstable hemoglobin (Bart hemoglobin) that causes lethal hydrops fetalis and is associated with preeclampsia. α-Thalassemia is also common among individuals of African descent but typically does not result in hydrops.

The β-thalassemias are caused by mutations in the β-globin gene that result in defective or absent β-chain synthesis. β-Thalassemia is more common in Mediterranean countries, the Middle East, South East Asia, and parts of India and Pakistan. The heterozygous carrier (β-thalassemia minor) is not usually associated with clinical disability, except in periods of stress. Individuals who are homozygous (β-thalassemia major or Cooley anemia) have severe anemia, failure to thrive, hepatosplenomegaly, growth retardation, and bony changes secondary to marrow hypertrophy. The mean corpuscular volume (MCV) is performed as an initial screening test for patients

at risk. Individuals with low MCV (<80 μL^3) should undergo hemoglobin electrophoresis; β-thalassemia carriers have an elevated HbA_2 ($>3.5\%$). Diagnosis of α-thalassemia trait is by exclusion of iron deficiency and molecular detection of α-globin gene deletions.

Cystic fibrosis

In 2001, the ACOG and the American College of Medical Genetics (ACMG) recommended that carrier screening for cystic fibrosis, an autosomal recessive disorder that primarily affects the pulmonary and gastrointestinal system, be offered to non-Hispanic Caucasian patients planning a pregnancy or currently pregnant [6]. Cystic fibrosis screening is available to any patient; however, the prevalence and carrier rates are lower in other populations and the detection rates are also reduced, resulting in a less effective screening test. The ACMG recommends that a panel of 23 panethnic mutations be used for screening the general population [11]. For individuals with a family history of cystic fibrosis, screening with an expanded panel of mutations or complete analysis of the CFTR gene by sequencing may be indicated, if the mutation has not been previously identified in the affected relative. Patients with a reproductive partner with cystic fibrosis or congenital absence of the vas deferens may benefit from this approach to screening. Genetic counseling in these situations is usually beneficial. Cystic fibrosis carrier screening may also identify individuals with two mutations who have not been previously diagnosed as having cystic fibrosis. These individuals may have a milder form of the disease and should be referred to a specialist for further evaluation.

Jewish genetic diseases

There are a number of autosomal recessive conditions that are more common in individuals of Eastern European Jewish (Ashkenazi) descent. Several of these conditions are lethal or associated with significant morbidity. Tay–Sachs was the first disorder amenable to carrier screening based on the measurement of serum or leukocyte hexosaminidase A levels [12]. Today, similar detection rates can be achieved with mutation testing [13]. With the identification of the genes and disease-causing mutations for other disorders, carrier screening became feasible. The ACOG recommends that in addition to Tay–Sachs, carrier testing for Canavan disease, familial dysautonomia, and cystic fibrosis be offered when one or both parents are of Eastern European Jewish descent [7]. These disorders share similar prevalence and carrier rates (see Table 5.1). The sensitivity of these tests is also very high (95% or higher) and thus, a negative result indicates that the risk of having a child with the disorder is very low. Carrier testing is also available for less common conditions such as Fanconi anemia, Bloom syndrome, mucolipidosis type IV, Niemann–Pick type A and Gaucher disease, which is a less severe and treatable condition. However, it is important to recognize that, with the exception of Tay–Sachs and cystic fibrosis, the prevalence and the nature of the gene mutations in the non-Jewish population are unknown and hence carrier screening of a non-Jewish individual is of limited value.

Table 5.1 lists the disorders for which carrier testing is available and provides a brief list of the clinical features. Many of these disorders are less frequent and therefore the decision to pursue screening is left to the patient.

Prenatal diagnosis

Invasive prenatal diagnostic testing is available for patients identified through carrier screening to be at increased risk for having an affected offspring (see Chapter 54). Molecular testing for the specific gene mutations can be performed on cells obtained through chorionic villus sampling (CVS) at 10–12 weeks' gestation or amniocentesis after 15 weeks' gestation. It is critical that the laboratory perform maternal cell contamination studies to ensure the accuracy of the test results.

Newborn screening

Carriers of mendelian disorders may also be identified through state newborn screening programs. Newborn screening was designed to identify newborns with inherited metabolic disorders who would benefit from early detection and treatment. However, advances in genetics and technology have led to expanded screening programs which include testing for hemoglobinopathies, endocrine disorders, hearing loss, and infectious diseases. Newborn screening for most mendelian disorders is performed by collecting capillary blood from a heel puncture onto a filter paper. Specimens are then sent to a reference laboratory where they are assayed for the specified diseases. Confirmatory testing is necessary because of the high false-positive rate on the initial screen. In addition to the appropriate referral of the infant for treatment, genetic counseling of the couple is recommended to review the recurrence risk and reproductive options.

CASE PRESENTATION

A 26-year-old healthy primigravida presents for prenatal care at 8 weeks' gestation. There is no family history of congenital malformations, genetic disorders, mental retardation, neurologic or psychiatric conditions. The patient's ancestors are Eastern European Jewish. Her partner is Caucasian and his ancestors are Northern European. She denies any medication use and has been taking multivitamins.

Based on the patient's Eastern European Jewish ancestry, the obstetrician discusses the availability of carrier screening tests to determine if she is a carrier of Tay–Sachs disease, Canavan disease, familial dysautonomia, and cystic fibrosis as well as less common or less severe conditions such as Fanconi anemia, Bloom syndrome, mucolipidosis type IV, Niemann–Pick type A and Gaucher disease. The patient is provided with a pamphlet containing information about the disorders, the prevalence and carrier rate, risk of an affected child, test sensitivity, limitations, and possible outcomes. If the test is negative then her risk of being a carrier is markedly reduced and it is highly improbable that she will have a child with one of these disorders. If the test indicates that she is a carrier then her partner should be counseled and offered screening. The obstetrician informs the patient that the decision to proceed with carrier screening is hers and testing is voluntary.

The patient is informed of the following risks to be a carrier: about 1 in 30 for Tay–Sachs and familial dysautonomia, 1 in 24 for cystic fibrosis, and 1 in 40 for Canavan disease. The screening tests, performed on a sample of blood from the patient, analyze her DNA for the common mutations that cause each of these disorders. The detection rates are greater than 95%. Because the patient is pregnant, serum hexosaminidase A levels are unreliable; in lieu of DNA testing, leukocyte testing can be performed and has a high detection rate (98%). The patient inquires if there are other disorders she should be worried about. Her obstetrician informs her that carrier testing is available for a number of other inherited conditions that are common among individuals of Eastern European Jewish ancestry (see Table 5.1). With the exception of Gaucher disease, which can be mild and is treatable, the other disorders occur less frequently and the chance that she is a carrier is approximately 1 in 90 or higher.

The patient asks if her partner should be tested. The obstetrician informs the patient that most of these disorders are less common among non-Jewish individuals and the detection rate is unknown. Therefore, carrier screening is not recommended for her partner unless the test indicates that she is a carrier. Cystic fibrosis is an exception; the carrier rate among Caucasians of Northern European ancestry is similar and the test detection rates

Continued

are high. She may ask her partner to have cystic fibrosis carrier screening so that if they are both carriers she would learn early in the pregnancy and have the option of CVS if she desires prenatal diagnostic testing.

The patient elects to have the carrier screening performed for Tay–Sachs, Canavan, familial dysautonomia, and cystic fibrosis. Her obstetrician calls to inform her that the test results indicate that she is not a carrier of one of the common mutations that cause Tay–Sachs, Canavan, or familial dysautonomia and therefore she is unlikely to have an affected child. However, she is a carrier of ΔF508, the most common cystic fibrosis mutation found in approximately 70% of cystic fibrosis patients. The obstetrician recommends screening for cystic fibrosis in her partner and offers genetic counseling to obtain additional information. The partner agrees and the screening test demonstrates that he does not have any of the 23 common mutations that cause cystic fibrosis. Therefore, based on the partner's ethnicity and the test sensitivity, his risk of being a carrier has been reduced to approximately 1 in 208 and the risk that this couple will have an affected child is 1 in 832 ($1 \times 1/208 \times 1/4$). Prenatal testing is not recommended. The obstetrician informs the patient that she inherited the mutation from one of her parents so her siblings may also be carriers, and recommends that she share this information with them.

References

1. Holtzman NA. Newborn screening for Genetic-Metabolic Diseases: Progress, Principles and Recommendations. Publication No. (HSA) 78–5207. Washington, DC: Department of Health, Education, and Welfare, 1977.

2. Mendelian Inheritance in Man, OMIM™. Center for Medical Genetics, Johns Hopkins University, Baltimore, MD, and National Center for Biotechnology Information, National Library of Medicine, Bethesda, MD, 1998. www.ncbi.nlm.nih.gov/omim/.

3. Sherman S, Pletcher BA, Driscoll DA. Fragile X syndrome: diagnostic and carrier testing. Genet Med 2005;7:584–587.

4. Wenstrom KD. Fragile X and other trinucleotide repeat diseases. Obstet Gynecol Clin North Am 2002;29:367–388.

5. American College of Obstetricians and Gynecologists. Clinical Management Guidelines for Obstetrician-Gynecologists. Hemoglobinopathies in Pregnancy. Practice Bulletin No. 64. Obstet Gynecol 2005;106:203–210.

6. American College of Obstetricians and Gynecologists, American College of Medical Genetics. Preconception and Prenatal Carrier Screening for Cystic Fibrosis. Washington, DC: American College of Obstetricians and Gynecologists, 2001.

7. American College of Obstetricians and Gynecologists Committee on Genetics. Prenatal and preconceptional carrier screening for genetic diseases in individuals of Eastern European Jewish descent. Obstet Gynecol 2009;114:950–953.

8. Ogino S, Wilson RB. Genetic testing and risk assessment for spinal muscular atrophy (SMA). Hum Genet 2002;111:477–500.

9. American College of Obstetricians and Gynecologists Committee on Genetics. Spinal muscular atrophy. Obstet Gynecol 2009;113:1194–1196.

10. Merrill A, Rosenblum-Vos L, Driscoll DA, Daley K, Treat K. Prenatal diagnosis of Fanconi anemia (Group C) subsequent to abnormal sonographic findings. Prenat Diagn 2005;25:20–22.

11. Watson MS, Cutting GR, Desnick RJ et al. Cystic fibrosis population carrier screening: 2004 revision of American College of Medical Genetics mutation panel. Genet Med 2004;6:387–391.

12. American College of Obstetricians and Gynecologists Committee on Genetics. Screening for Tay–Sachs disease. Obstet Gynecol 2005;106:893–894.

13. Eng CM, Desnick RJ. Experiences in molecular-based screening for Ashkenzi Jewish genetic disease. Adv Genet 2001;44:275–296.

Chapter 6
Screening for Congenital Heart Disease

Lynn L. Simpson
Department of Obstetrics and Gynecology, Columbia University Medical Center, New York, NY, USA

Obstetric ultrasound completed after the first trimester requires an assessment of fetal anatomy and both the American Institute of Ultrasound in Medicine (AIUM) and the American College of Obstetricians and Gynecologists (ACOG) recommend that the four-chamber view of the fetal heart and the ventricular outflow tracts be routinely evaluated on all patients [1,2]. As outlined in a joint guideline from the AIUM, the ACOG, the Society for Maternal-Fetal Medicine, and the American College of Radiology, fetal echocardiography with multiple cardiac views and specialized assessments is indicated for patients at high risk for congenital heart disease [3].

Screening low-risk populations

Congenital heart disease is a common condition that warrants prenatal screening of all pregnancies. With a prevalence of 6 per 1000 livebirths, it is estimated that 10 of every 1000 fetuses scanned in the second trimester will have a heart anomaly and half of these will be major with serious consequences [4,5]. Intrauterine fetal death occurs in 20–30% of cases, neonatal death in 40–60%, and long-term survival rates are low, ranging from 15% to 40% [6]. The presence of extracardiac anomalies and chromosomal abnormalities contributes to the poor outlook. Overall, 25–45% of fetuses with congenital heart disease have other malformations and 15–50% have abnormal karyotypes [7–9]. Other poor prognostic signs include associated fetal arrhythmias, hemodynamic abnormalities, and the presence of hydrops.

Benefits of cardiac screening

Early prenatal diagnosis of major heart defects is important for counseling patients about pregnancy options, therapeutic interventions, changes in obstetric care, and alternative plans for delivery. Studies have shown that when major congenital heart disease is diagnosed in the second trimester of pregnancy, many patients opt for termination [10]. In one survey of 65 women who previously had borne a child with congenital heart disease, 58% said they would elect to terminate a subsequent affected pregnancy [11].

Without universal screening, the prenatal diagnosis of congenital heart disease is often made late in gestation when options are limited. With early screening and detection of congenital heart disease, patients and their families have time to consider the implications of the condition and to make choices that are best for them. Therapeutic interventions and improved neonatal survival are possible when particular heart malformations are detected prenatally and the timing, mode, and location of delivery can be planned [12]. Referral to a tertiary care center where immediate therapeutic and palliative interventions are available can be life saving. Prompt infusion of prostaglandin E_1 or balloon atrial septostomy can significantly improve prognosis for newborns with certain cardiac defects that require postnatal maintenance of fetal flow pathways. Immediate institution of extracorporeal membrane oxygenation can make the difference between life and death in complex cardiac anomalies, particularly when associated with other structural defects such as congenital diaphragmatic hernia. Experienced neonatologists, pediatric cardiologists, and cardiac surgeons may have a significant impact of an infant's condition and ultimate outcome.

Universal screening for major cardiac anomalies in the general population is essential to reduce the long-term morbidity and mortality of this disease. In experienced centers, routine screening can reassure patients that the fetal heart is normal or identify those patients in need of fetal echocardiography.

Queenan's Management of High-Risk Pregnancy: An Evidence-Based Approach, Sixth Edition. Edited by John T. Queenan, Catherine Y. Spong, Charles J. Lockwood.
© 2012 John Wiley & Sons, Ltd. Published 2012 by John Wiley & Sons, Ltd.

High-risk populations for fetal echocardiography

The conventional strategy for the prenatal detection of congenital heart disease has been to refer patients identified to be at risk for fetal echocardiography [3]. Unfortunately, it is estimated that over half of prenatal detected heart anomalies are found in patients with no preexisting risk factors and that most cardiac malformations would be missed if fetal echocardiography were done based on these factors alone [13,14]. Despite the initial enthusiasm for nuchal translucency as a screening tool for congenital heart disease, its performance in large studies of unselected and low-risk populations has been disappointing [15,16]. However, it is a reasonable marker or risk factor for major heart anomalies and warrants referral for fetal echocardiography.

Interestingly, the factor most predictive of congenital heart disease is an abnormal cardiac examination at the time of prenatal ultrasonography. In one study of fetal echocardiography, only 4% of patients were referred because of an abnormal cardiac screen, yet defects were detected at a rate of 68% in this group, far in excess of the rate for all other risk factors combined [13]. In many centers, an abnormal cardiac screen during routine obstetric ultrasonography has become the most common reason for referral for fetal echocardiography with a high yield for heart defects [14,17].

See Box 6.1.

Normal fetal heart anatomy

Normal fetal heart anatomy can be visualized with confidence as early as 13–14 weeks gestation by the transvaginal approach in highly specialized centers [6]. While patients at risk may benefit from early echocardiography, screening for normal fetal heart anatomy at 20 weeks' gestation seems ideal for the low-risk patient [1,2]. For low-risk populations, the four-chamber view and views of the ventricular outflow tracts comprise a reasonable cardiac screen. Fetal echocardiography is an extended examination with multiple views using additional imaging modalities for patients identified as being at increased risk for congenital heart disease, including those with an abnormal cardiac screen at the time of routine ultrasound [3].

Technique

Two-dimensional cross-sectional imaging

The transabdominal approach is most often used for fetal cardiac screening performed beyond the first trimester of pregnancy. The determination of fetal lie and presentation in the uterus is critical for the evaluation of cardiac and

---

Box 6.1 Reasons to refer for fetal echocardiography [3]

Maternal indications

- Autoimmune antibodies (e.g. SSA/SSB)
- Familial inherited disorders (e.g. Marfan syndrome)
- First-degree relative with congenital heart disease
- *In vitro* fertilization
- Metabolic diseases (e.g. diabetes mellitus)
- Teratogen exposure (e.g. retinoids)

Fetal indications

- Abnormal cardiac screen
- Abnormal fetal heart rate or rhythm
- Fetal chromosomal abnormality
- Extracardiac anomalies
- Hydrops
- Increased nuchal translucency
- Monochorionic twins
- Unexplained polyhydramnios

---

abdominal situs. A transverse sweep through the fetus can quickly confirm normal situs with the stomach and apex of the heart on the left side of the fetus (Fig. 6.1). During this sweep, the cardiac position in the fetal chest, cardiac axis, and size of the heart can be subjectively evaluated. On transverse imaging of the fetal abdomen, the inferior vena cava can be seen to the right of the fetal spine and the descending aorta to the left and anterior to the fetal spine.

Four-chamber view

The most important image of the fetal heart is obtained on a cross-sectional transverse view

through the fetal chest and heart. The horizontal position of the heart in the chest during fetal life makes this plane easy to obtain in most instances. While the appearance of the four-chamber view will vary depending on fetal lie and presentation, the landmarks remain the same. A transverse view of the fetal chest will be circular with the bony vertebral body posteriorly, the sternum anteriorly, and complete ribs laterally. A simple approach to the four-chamber view includes an evaluation of size, position, anatomy, and function of the fetal heart.

The four-chamber view is obtained on a transverse image of the fetal thorax just above the diaphragm (Fig. 6.2). In this transverse plane, the fetal heart occupies about one-third of the area of the fetal chest with an axis about 45 to the left. The atrial and ventricular chambers, interventricular septum, foramen ovale, and atrioventricular valves can all be assessed on the four-chamber view. The two atria and two ventricles should be similar in size, with the left atrium closest to the spine and the right ventricle closest to the sternum. In this transverse cross-sectional plane, the pulmonary veins may be seen entering the left atrium and the aorta descending between the left atrium and the spine (Fig. 6.3). The flap of the

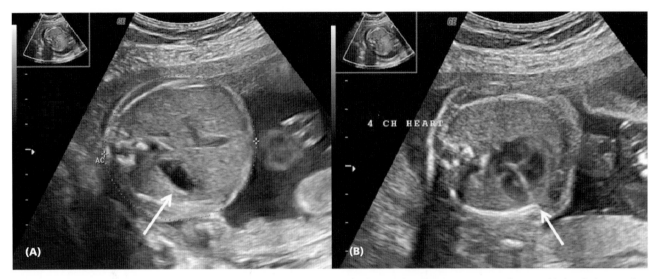

Figure 6.1 (A) Transverse two-dimensional ultrasound of the abdomen of a fetus in breech presentation with normal left-sided stomach (*arrow*). (B) Transverse view of the chest of the same fetus demonstrating normal left axis of fetal heart (*arrow*).

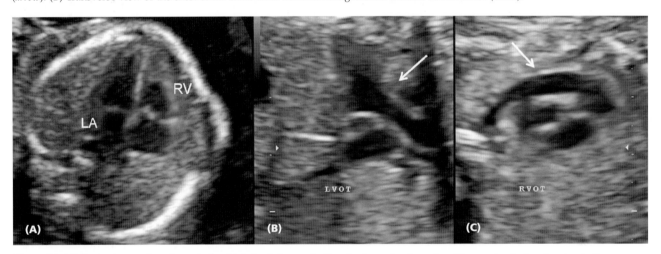

Figure 6.2 (A) A transverse view through the fetal chest demonstrating the four-chamber view. The most anterior chamber is the trabeculated right ventricle (RV) and the most posterior chamber adjacent to the spine is the left atrium (LA). The interventricular septum appears intact and the patent foramen ovale can be seen between the two atria. The atrioventricular valves are closed. (B) Long-axis view of the left ventricular outflow tract (LVOT) (*arrow*). Note the continuity between the interventricular septum and the aorta. (C) Short-axis view of the right ventricular outflow tract (RVOT) (*arrow*) wrapping around the aorta as it exits the heart.

foramen ovale should project into the left atrium through a patent foramen ovale. The internal surface of the left ventricle is smooth compared with the trabeculated right ventricle containing the moderator band. The two atrioventricular valves meet at the junction of the interatrial and interventricular septa to form the crux of the heart. The mitral and tricuspid valves should move freely, with the tricuspid valve attached slightly more towards the apex than the mitral valve on the interventricular septum. Ventricular systolic function can be assessed subjectively by observing the ventricular wall movement during systole. The presence of a pericardial effusion also can be identified on the four-chamber view. Systematic evaluation of the four-chamber view can easily be incorporated into a routine 30-min screening midtrimester ultrasound with adequate visualization in over 95% of fetuses [18]

Ventricular outflow tracts

A major limitation of cardiac screening with the four-chamber view alone is that conotruncal anomalies can easily be missed. Normal four-chamber screening can occur with transposition of the great arteries, tetralogy of Fallot, double-outlet right ventricle, pulmonary and aortic stenosis, and coarctation of the aorta [10]. It is estimated that defects of the great vessels are only associated with an abnormal four-chamber view in about 30% of cases [19]. Consequently, both the AIUM and ACOG now recommend that views of the aortic and pulmonary outflow tracts be included with an evaluation of the four-chamber view when screening for congenital heart disease [1,2].

With adequate training and experience, it is possible to visualize the four-chamber view and outflow tracts in

90% of pregnant women [20]. The long-axis view of the left ventricular outflow tract and the short-axis view of the right ventricular outflow tract are common images used to evaluate the proximal ventriculoarterial

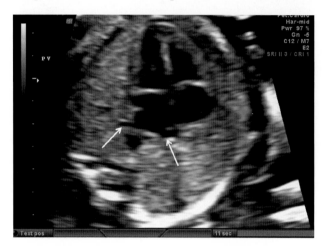

Figure 6.3 Pulmonary veins (PV) entering the posterior left atrium (*arrows*). At least one pulmonary artery from each lung should be identified during a screening fetal echocardiogram.

connections (see Fig. 6.2). The aortic and pulmonary outflow tracts are approximately equal in size in the midtrimester and should be seen to cross as they arise from their respective ventricles during real-time imaging. The aorta arises from the posterior ventricle and has branches originating from its arch that supply the head and upper extremities. The pulmonary artery arises from the anterior ventricle and branches into the ductus arteriosus and pulmonary arteries. The two semilunar valves should be seen to open and close with the pulmonary valve anterior and cranial to the aortic valve.

Experts in fetal echocardiography extend the examination of the fetal heart beyond the four-chamber view and proximal ventricular outflow tracts. A simple stepwise approach to the fetal heart may help to standardize two-dimensional fetal echocardiography [21]. This approach begins with a complete assessment of the four-chamber view followed by serial cephalad transverse planes to assess the great arteries and their connections, the three-vessel view, and the aortic arch (Fig. 6.4). Sweeping cephalad from the four-chamber view displays the five-chamber view, demonstrating the aorta arising from the

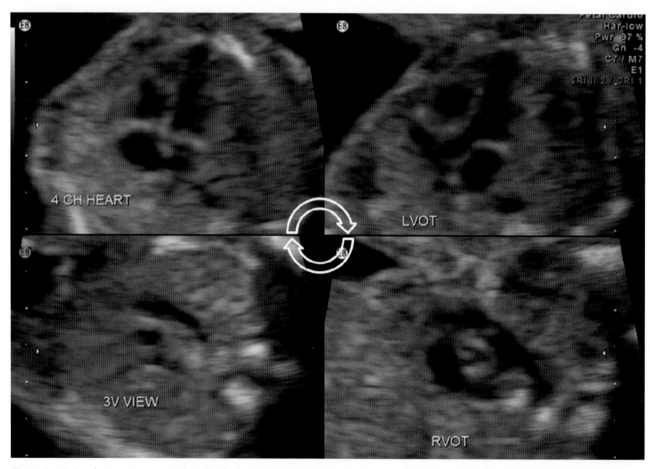

Figure 6.4 A simple stepwise approach to the fetal heart can help to standardize two-dimensional imaging of the fetal heart during routine obstetric ultrasound. This approach begins with a complete assessment of the four-chamber view followed by serial cephalad transverse planes to assess the left ventricular outflow tract (LVOT), right ventricular outflow tract (RVOT), their connections, and the three-vessel view.

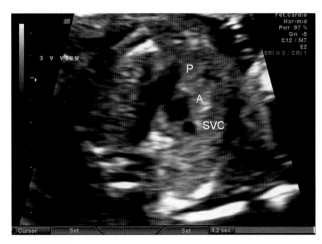

Figure 6.5 Transverse three-vessel view of the fetal heart demonstrating the anterior pulmonary artery (P), aorta (A), and posterior superior vena cava (SVC). The diameter of the aorta and pulmonary artery should be similar in size in this view.

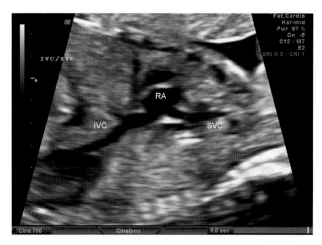

Figure 6.6 The superior vena cava (SVC) and inferior vena cava (IVC) seen entering the right atrium (RA).

left ventricle towards the right shoulder of the fetus. Cross-sectional transverse imaging just cephalad to this view shows the pulmonary artery arising from the anterior right ventricle directed posteriorly to the fetal spine. During this sweep towards the fetal head, the left and right ventricular outflow tracts can be observed to cross at their origins with the aortic root located posterior to the main pulmonary trunk. The traditional three-vessel view of the superior vena cava, aorta, and pulmonary artery lies in a transverse plane just above the origins of the great arteries and the transverse aortic arch lies just superior to the three-vessel view (Fig. 6.5).

While the transverse views of the fetal heart are often sufficient to evaluate the normal cardiac anatomy and screen for major anomalies, long-axis and oblique views of the heart may be useful when transverse views are difficult to obtain or when a cardiac defect is suspected. These images may include the short-axis view of the right ventricle and its outflow tract, the long-axis view of the left ventricle and its outflow tract, views of the ductal arch and aortic arch, and the inferior vena cava and superior vena cava entering the right atrium (Plate 6.1, Fig. 6.6). These additional two-dimensional views complete the cross-sectional assessment of the major anatomic structures of the fetal heart and can be used to confirm normal venoatrial inflows, atrioventricular connections, and ventriculoarterial outflows.

Color Doppler imaging

Color flow mapping of the fetal heart is utilized by those trained to perform basic cardiac screening as well as those experienced in advanced fetal echocardiography. In general, the cardiac examination is repeated briefly using color Doppler to demonstrate normal directional blood flow through the fetal heart (Plate 6.2). In addition to confirming normal blood flow patterns, it can identify structures that can be difficult to visualize by two-dimensional ultrasound alone. For example, the small pulmonary veins are often best demonstrated with the use of color flow mapping. Color Doppler can also be used to identify defects that might be missed on two-dimensional imaging (Plate 6.3). Some ventricular septal defects may only be visible when color Doppler is applied with the ultrasound beam perpendicular to the interventricuular septum. Color flow mapping can also identify abnormal flow patterns associated with complex heart defects, valvular stenosis, coarctation, and hemodynamic compromise such as regurgitation and poor contractility. For example, the retrograde aortic flow in hypoplastic left heart syndrome and the reversed ductal flow with pulmonary atresia are easily identified with the use of color Doppler. Turbulent flow or aliasing on color Doppler may be indicative of valvular stenosis or coarctation. In general, color Doppler should be obtained when the ultrasound beam is parallel to the interrogated vessel with less than 20 angle correction.

The addition of color Doppler is now considered an important component of a cardiac screening exam in many centers. Normal flow patterns determined by color flow mapping provide further reassurance to patients and their families that their offspring has no evidence of major structural or functional heart disease.

Expectations from cardiac screening

See Table 6.1.

Four-chamber view

The four-chamber view was introduced as a screening tool for the prenatal detection of heart anomalies in the 1980s [22,23]. Initial reports suggested that the

Table 6.1 Detection of major congenital heart disease

Screening tool	Prenatal detection rate
Preexisting risk factors	<10%
Nuchal translucency	15–50%
Four-chamber view	40–50%
Four-chamber view and ventricular outflow tracts	60–80%
Fetal echocardiography	>85%

four-chamber view could detect 80–90% of fetuses with congenital heart disease [23,24]. However, the sensitivity of the four-chamber view in detecting cardiac anomalies varied widely in subsequent studies. For example, only 16% of fetuses with heart defects were detected using the four-chamber view in the highly publicized Routine Antenatal Diagnostic Imaging with Ultrasound (RADIUS) trial of prenatal ultrasonographic screening, and no cardiac malformations were detected before 24 weeks' gestation in facilities other than tertiary-level referral centers [25].

There are many possible explanations for the inconsistent performance of the four-chamber view in screening for congenital heart disease. Different ultrasonographers with varying levels of skill use the four-chamber view under a variety of conditions in clinical practice. Performance is also significantly influenced by factors such as a community setting versus a tertiary care center, high-risk versus low-risk patients, level of ascertainment, and availability of outcome information. Screening by skilled sonographers, experienced perinatologists, and expert pediatric cardiologists at teaching hospitals and tertiary reference centers is expected to be superior to that performed in the community. This is reflected in the poor detection rate reported in nontertiary care centers in the RADIUS study [25]. The sensitivity of any screening test also depends on the prevalence of disease in the population being studied. Tertiary care hospitals will see more affected fetuses because they are the facilities to which women with abnormal serum screening, advanced maternal age, and high-risk factors for congenital heart disease are referred for evaluation. The prevalence of congenital heart disease in many tertiary care centers is twice that expected in the general population [26].

The ability to image the fetal heart is also influenced by gestational age, fetal position, amniotic fluid volume, previous abdominal surgery, and maternal body habitus. Even when the four-chamber view is achieved, it is unreasonable to expect that it will identify all cases of congenital heart disease. Certain defects are easily missed on the four-chamber view, such as ventricular septal defects, atrial septal defects, coarctation, tetralogy of Fallot, transposition of the great arteries, double-outlet right ventricle, truncus arteriosus, and total anomalous pulmonary venous return [27]. Prenatal diagnosis of patent foramen

ovale and patent ductus arteriosus is precluded by their normal patency *in utero*. The superior aspect of the interventricular septum tends to be thin, particularly in the apical view, and can be incorrectly diagnosed as a subaortic ventricular septal defect. Small muscular ventricular septal defects are the defects most commonly missed on prenatal ultrasonography. Certain cardiac malformations, such as transposition of the great vessels, double-outlet right ventricle, and tetralogy of Fallot, can be associated with a normal four-chamber view.

Although most congenital heart defects occur during the period of organogenesis, some defects are known to evolve over the course of gestation and may be missed at the time of midtrimester screening. Flow abnormalities such as valvular pulmonic stenosis, aortic stenosis, and coarctation of the aorta are not easy to detect on the four-chamber view. Ventricular hypoplasia has been observed to develop as pregnancy advances and may not be evident on cardiac imaging in the second trimester [28]. Abnormalities of the distal pulmonary arteries and pulmonary veins are not commonly appreciated prenatally due to limited flow and filling of these vessels *in utero*. Even under optimal conditions, some defects will not be detected at a midtrimester scan by the four-chamber view.

When used as a screening tool in the general population, the four-chamber view can be expected to detect 40–50% of cases of congenital heart disease [23,29]. The four-chamber view should be considered abnormal if there is ventricular or atrial disproportion, myocardial hypertrophy, dilation or hypoplasia of the chambers, septal defects apart from the foramen ovale, or abnormalities of the atrioventricular valves. Congenital heart disease may also be associated with abnormal positioning of the heart in the fetal chest and with axis deviation. Defects expected to be associated with an abnormal four-chamber view include hypoplasia of the right or left ventricle, atrioventricular septal defect, double-inlet ventricle, Ebstein anomaly, single ventricle, and large ventricle septal defect. Screening with the four-chamber view may also identify dextrocardia, situs inversus, ectopia cordis, cardiomyopathies, pericardial effusion, cardiac tumors, valvular atresia, stenosis, and insufficiency. Hypoplastic ventricles and atrioventricular septal defects are the defects most often detected prenatally by the four-chamber view [10,27,29].

Addition of outflow tract views

Overall, the prenatal detection of cardiac anomalies can be increased from 40–50% with the four-chamber view alone to 60–80% when the ventricular outflow tracts are also assessed [7,30,31]. Although the best detection rates of congenital heart disease have been reported in high-risk populations screened at referral centers, a sensitivity of 66% was observed in a study of primarily low-risk patients screened with views of the four-chamber and outflow tracts [29]. It is clear that multiple cardiac views are crucial for midtrimester screening for many serious congenital heart defects and that the 20–30% increase in detection rate that results from including the outflow tracts along with the four-chamber view can be of clinical importance. Inclusion of the three-vessel view, which includes the pulmonary artery, aorta, and superior vena cava, along with color flow mapping has been reported to increase the detection rate of outflow tract abnormalities in low-risk populations [32,33]. Universal screening with the four-chamber and ventricular outflow tract views, utilizing two-dimensional ultrasound with color flow mapping, may be optimal for midtrimester cardiac assessment of low-risk populations.

Conclusion

Despite the widespread use of obstetric ultrasound, only a third of infants with congenital heart disease born in the United States since the turn of the century have been detected prenatally [12,34]. One explanation is that most infants with heart anomalies are born to low-risk women. Universal routine screening of all patients utilizing a standard approach has the potential to significantly improve the prenatal diagnosis of congenital heart disease [21]. Another explanation for the low antenatal detection rate is that the performance of cardiac screening falls well below expectations. The four-chamber view should detect 40–50% of defects and the addition of ventricular outflow views should increase detection to 60–80%. Recent studies have shown that an abnormal cardiac screen at the time of routine obstetric ultrasound has become the most common indication for fetal echocardiography. With detection rates consistently over 85% in experienced centers, it might be optimal for all patients to undergo screening fetal echocardiography [35]. However, with limited resources, a major goal for providers of obstetric ultrasound must be to improve the quality of cardiac screening so that abnormal fetal hearts are promptly recognized and referred to those skilled in fetal echocardiography.

CASE PRESENTATION

A 26-year-old gravid 3 para 2 presents at 18 weeks' gestation for an ultrasound examination. During the fetal survey, the four-chamber view of the fetal heart appears to be normal but the outflow tracts are not well seen. She reports that there was some concern at the time of the first-trimester risk assessment about fluid at the back of the fetal neck but that she was told the likelihood of Down syndrome was low based on the final results. She has no other known risk factors for congenital heart disease. She returns 4 weeks later for a follow-up ultrasound examination and again the outflow tracts are difficult to image but they appear to arise in a parallel fashion from the heart. Upon further evaluation, transposition of the great arteries is diagnosed with the pulmonary artery arising from the posterior left ventricle and the aorta arising from the anterior right ventricle. She is distraught at this news and asks why this was not detected earlier and what should be done now.

The majority of infants with cardiac malformations are born to women with normal pregnancies and no identifiable risk factors for congenital heart disease. However, fetal echocardiography is now recommended when the nuchal translucency is increased at the time of first-trimester screening for aneuploidy. Different cut-off values are used in different centers but an absolute nuchal translucency measurement of ≥3–3.5 mm between 11–13 weeks' gestation is a reasonable threshold to flag patients for referral for fetal echocardiography.

Transposition of the great arteries is often associated with a normal four-chamber view and can easily be missed if views of the outflow tracts are not routinely evaluated and seen at the time of the second-trimester anatomic survey of the fetus. One of the clues to this diagnosis is the fact that the outflow tracts do not cross normally as they exit their respective ventricles. A repeat ultrasound or referral for fetal echocardiography is indicated if the fetal heart cannot be adequately visualized as congenital heart disease is the most common of the major anomalies adversely affecting survival. Fortunately, simple transposition of the great vessels has a favorable prognosis but certain steps should be taken when this diagnosis is made. First, a careful examination for additional cardiac and extracardiac anomalies should be performed. The interventricular septum should be carefully examined as those cases with an intact septum should have a timed delivery in a center capable of performing an emergency atrial septostomy. Genetic counseling should be offered and fetal karyotyping considered, particularly if extracardiac anomalies are identified. However, the risk for aneuploidy is low in cases of isolated transposition of the great arteries.

A multidisciplinary team including the obstetrician, maternal-fetal medicine specialist, geneticist, pediatric cardiologist, pediatric cardiothoracic surgeon, and neonatologist should be involved in the counseling of the patient and her family about this condition and its implications. It is only then that the patient can fully understand the diagnosis, her options, and the plan for management, delivery, and neonatal care.

References

1. American Institute of Ultrasound in Medicine. AIUM practice guideline for the performance of obstetric ultrasound examinations. J Ultrasound Med 2010;29:157–166.

2. American College of Obstetricians and Gynecologists. Ultrasonography in pregnancy. ACOG Practice Bulletin No. 101. Obstet Gynecol 2009;113:451–461.

3. American Institute of Ultrasound in Medicine. AIUM practice guideline for the performance of fetal echocardiography. J Ultrasound Med 2011;(in press).

4. Hoffman JIE, Kaplan S. The incidence of congenital heart disease. J Am Coll Cardiol 2002;39:1890–1900.

5. Buskens E, Steyerberg EW, Hess J, Wladimiroff JW, Grobbee DE. Routine prenatal screening for congenital heart disease: what can be expected? A decision-analytic approach. Am J Public Health 1997;87:962–967.

6. Johnson B, Simpson LL. Screening for congenital heart disease: a move towards earlier echocardiography. Am J Perinatol 2007;24:449–456.

7. Bromley B, Estroff JA, Sanders SP, Parad R, Roberts D, Frigoletto FD, Benacerraf BR. Fetal echocardiography: accuracy and limitations in a population at high and low risk for heart defects. Am J Obstet Gynecol 1992;166:1473–1481.

8. Copel JA, Pilu G, Kleinman CS. Congenital heart disease and extracardiac anomalies: associations and indications for fetal echocardiography. Am J Obstet Gynecol 1986;154:1121–1132.

9. Paladini D, Calabro R, Palmieri S, d'Andrea T. Prenatal diagnosis of congenital heart disease and fetal karyotyping. Obstet Gynecol 1993;81:679–682.

10. Sharland GK, Allan LD. Screening for congenital heart disease prenatally. Results of a 2½-year study in the South East Thames Region. Br J Obstet Gynaecol 1992;9:220–225.

11. Bjorkhem G, Jorgensen C, Hanseus K. Parental reactions of fetal echocardiography. J Matern Fetal Med 1997;6:87–92.

12. Friedberg MK, Silverman NH, Moon-Grady AJ et al. Prenatal detection of congenital heart disease. J Pediatr 2009;155: 26–31.

13. Cooper MJ, Enderlein MA, Dyson DC, Roge CL, Tarnoff H. Fetal echocardiography: retrospective review of clinical experience and an evaluation of indications. Obstet Gynecol 1995; 86:577–582.

14. Simpson LL. Indications for fetal echocardiography from a tertiary care obstetric sonography practice J Clin Ultrasound 2004;32:123–128.

15. Simpson LL, Malone FD, Bianchi DW et al. Nuchal translucency and the risk of congenital heart disease. Obstet Gynecol 2007;109:376–383.

16. Sananes N, Guigue V, Kohler M et al. Nuchal translucency and cystic hygroma in screening for fetal major congenital heart defects in a series of 12,910 euploid pregnancies. Ultrasound Obstet Gynecol 2010;35:273–279.

17. Friedberg MK, Silverman NH. Changing indications for fetal echocardiography in a university center population. Prenat Diagn 2004;24:781–786.

18. Tegnander E, Eik-Nes SH, Linker DT. Incorporating the four-chamber view of the fetal heart into the second-trimester routine fetal examination. Ultrasound Obstet Gynecol 1994;4: 24–28.

19. Paladini D, Rustico M, Todros T et al. Conotruncal anomalies in prenatal life. Ultrasound Obstet Gynecol 1996;8:241–246.

20. Devore GR. The aortic and pulmonary outflow tract screening examination in the human fetus. J Ultrasound Med 1992;11: 345–348.

21. Allan L. Technique of fetal echocardiography. Pediatr Cardiol 2004;25:223–233.

22. Devore GR. The prenatal diagnosis of congenital heart disease: a practical approach for the fetal sonographer. J Clin Ultrasound 1985;13:229–245.

23. Allan LD, Crawford DC, Chita SK, Tynan MJ. Prenatal screening for congenital heart disease. BMJ 1986;292:1717–1719.

24. Copel JA, Pilu G, Green J, Hobbins JG, Kleinman CS. Fetal echocardiographic screening for congenital heart disease: the importance of the four-chamber view. Am J Obstet Gynecol 1987;157:648–655.

25. Crane JP, Lefevre ML, Winborn RC et al. A randomized trial of prenatal ultrasonographic screening: impact on the detection, management, and outcome of anomalous fetuses. Am J Obstet Gynecol 1994;171:392–399.

26. Buskens E, Stewart PA, Hess J, Grobbee DE. Efficacy of fetal echocardiography and yield by risk category. Obstet Gynecol 1996;87:423–428.

27. Allan LD, Sharland GK, Milburn A et al. Prospective diagnosis of 1,006 consecutive cases of congenital heart disease in the fetus. J Am Coll Cardiol 1994;23:1452–1458.

28. Hornberger LK, Need L, Benacerraf BR. Development of significant left and right ventricular hypoplasia in the second and third trimester fetus. J Ultrasound Med 1996;15:655–659.

29. Kirk JS, Comstock CH, Lee W, Smith RS, Riggs TW, Weinhouse E. Sonographic screening to detect fetal cardiac anomalies: a 5-year experience with 111 abnormal cases. Obstet Gynecol 1997;89:227–232.

30. Bronshtein M, Zimmer EZ, Gerlis LM, Lorber A, Drugan A. Early ultrasound diagnosis of fetal congenital heart defects in high-risk and low-risk pregnancies. Obstet Gynecol 1993;82:225–229.

31. Carvalho JS, Mavrides E, Shinebourne EA, Campbell S, Thilaganathan B. Improving the effectiveness of routine prenatal screening for major congenital heart defects. Heart 2002;88:387–391.

32. Wong SF, Ward C, Lee-Tannock A, Le S, Chan FY. Pulmonary artery/aorta ratio in simple screening for fetal outflow tract abnormalities during the second trimester. Ultrasound Obstet Gynecol 2007;30:275–280.

33. Del Bianco A, Russo S, Lacerenza N et al. Four chamber view plus three-vessel and trachea view for a complete evaluation of the fetal heart during the second trimester. J Perinat Med 2006;34:309–312.

34. Acherman RJ, Evans WN, Luna CF et al. Prenatal detection of congenital heart disease in southern Nevada. J Ultrasound Med 2007;26:1715–1719.

35. Randall P, Brealey S, Hahn S, Khan KS, Parsons JM. Accuracy of fetal echocardiography in the routine detection of congenital heart disease among unselected and low risk populations: a systematic review. Br J Obstet Gynaecol 2005; 112:22–30.

Chapter 7
First- and Second-Trimester Screening for Fetal Aneuploidy and Neural Tube Defects

Julia Unterscheider and Fergal D. Malone
Department of Obstetrics and Gynaecology, Royal College of Surgeons in Ireland, Dublin, Ireland

Prenatal screening for Down syndrome and other aneuploidies, such as trisomies 13 and 18, has advanced significantly since its advent in the 1980s. Historically, women 35 years or older were offered prenatal genetic counseling and the option of a diagnostic test such as chorionic villus sampling or amniocentesis. With this screening approach, only 20% of the fetal Down syndrome population are detected antenatally. Sonographic and biochemical markers are now employed to screen for aneuploidies and neural tube defects in the first and second trimester. Maternal serum screening for Down syndrome in the second trimester started in the mid-1980s, with low levels of the analyte α-fetoprotein (AFP) associated with an increased risk of fetal Down syndrome. Today, an increased nuchal translucency in the first trimester and/or a thickened nuchal fold in the second trimester are highly specific sonographic markers in trisomy 21 fetuses. Prenatal diagnosis should be made available, if requested, after appropriate counseling, including risks and benefits, to all pregnant women, regardless of maternal age.

First-trimester sonographic screening

The single most powerful discriminator of Down syndrome from euploid fetuses is first-trimester sonographic measurement of the nuchal translucency space, generally performed between 11 0/7 and 13 6/7 weeks' gestation, corresponding with a fetal crown–rump length between 45 and 84 mm [1]. Nuchal translucency (NT) refers to a clearly demarcated fluid-filled or sonolucent space behind the fetal neck. It is present in all fetuses (Fig. 7.1). An increased NT measurement is significantly associated with fetal aneuploidy, structural malformations, and adverse pregnancy outcome.

Because the average NT measurement is only 0.5–1.5 mm in thickness, it is absolutely essential that sonographic technique be meticulous, follows an agreed protocol, and is performed only by those with adequate training and experience. An error of only a millimeter can have a significant impact on the Down syndrome risk quoted to an individual patient. Critical components of good NT sonographic technique are demonstrated in Figure 7.1, and include imaging the fetus in a neutral position in the midsagittal plane, including visualization of the palate, mesencephalon and nasal bone, adequate magnification to focus only on the fetal head and upper thorax, discrimination between the nuchal skin and amniotic membrane, and caliper placement on the inner borders of the echolucent space. NT sonography is a more powerful discriminator of Down syndrome fetuses from euploid fetuses at 11 weeks, rather than 13 weeks, and therefore this form of screening should be performed as close to 11 weeks as possible [1].

Several large prospective population screening studies have now been completed in the US and Europe, and each has confirmed that NT sonography, when performed by trained and experienced sonographers, is an effective screening tool for fetal aneuploidy [1–5]. At a 5% false-positive rate, NT sonography (combined with maternal age) detects 70% of cases of Down syndrome at 11 weeks, but decreases to 64% detection at 13 weeks' gestation [1]. In general, NT measurement has limited usefulness as a stand-alone test because of the increased sensitivity and improved positive predictive value achieved with incorporation of other sonographic and maternal serum markers.

Credentialing programs, provided by the US Nuchal Translucency Quality Review Program or the UK Fetal Medicine Foundation, ensure that clinicians are adequately trained and certified in obtaining reproducible

Queenan's Management of High-Risk Pregnancy: An Evidence-Based Approach, Sixth Edition. Edited by John T. Queenan, Catherine Y. Spong, Charles J. Lockwood.

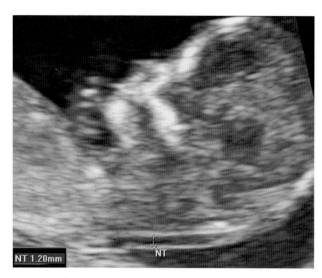

Figure 7.1 Sonographic examination at 12 weeks and 4 days' gestation demonstrating measurement of the fetal nuchal translucency (NT).

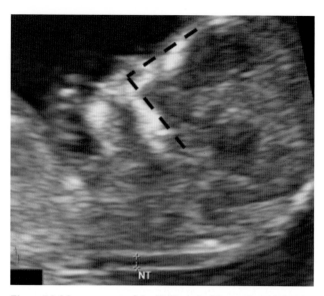

Figure 7.2 Measurement of the FMF angle. The angle is defined by a line along the upper surface of the palate and a line from the upper corner of the anterior aspect of the maxilla extending to the external surface of the frontal bone.

NT measurements. These programs are highly important for ongoing quality review and evaluation of provider proficiency.

Other sonographic tools that are available for first-trimester screening for fetal aneuploidy include nasal bone sonography and facial angle, ductus venosus Doppler waveform analysis, and tricuspid regurgitation.

The use of nasal bone sonography in the first trimester for general population screening is controversial. A large prospective observational study in a high-risk population [6] described the absence of nasal bone ossification in 73% of fetuses affected by trisomy 21 versus 0.5% in euploid fetuses. It was estimated that 85% and 93% of trisomy 21 cases would be detected at false-positive rates of 1% and 4%, respectively. The authors concluded that the visualization of the fetal nasal bone would result in a major reduction in the need for invasive testing and a substantial increase in sensitivity. The same investigators suggested a 97% detection rate for Down syndrome with a 5% false-positive rate when combining nasal bone measurements with nuchal translucency and serum markers [7]. In contrast, the FASTER trial [8] did not find that nasal bone assessment is useful in general population screening for Down syndrome as nine of 11 fetuses with trisomy 21 had nasal bones present. Significant variability has been observed in nasal bone assessment, posing some limitations to its usefulness. Until such time as nasal bone evaluation is subjected to the same rigorous standardization process as nuchal translucency, its application as a screening tool will be likely confined to a second-line assessment once a pregnancy has already been deemed to be at high risk.

The ductus venosus is a fetal blood vessel that carries oxygenated blood from the umbilical vein to the inferior vena cava. A normal first-trimester ductus venosus Doppler waveform is triphasic in appearance, with constant forward flow (Plate 7.1). Reversed flow in the ductus venosus (Plate 7.2) has been associated with both fetal aneupoidy and congenital heart disease [9]. However, the reproducibility of this measurement has been questioned and, like nasal bone sonography, it is likely that this form of first-trimester sonography will remain a second-line screening tool at select expert centers [10].

The presence of significant tricuspid regurgitation at the time of NT sonography is also a useful marker for fetal Down syndrome [11]. A study by Falcon *et al* [12] identified tricuspid regurgitation as an independent risk factor for fetal aneupoidy. However, further population screening studies are still needed to validate the role of first-trimester tricuspid regurgitation for this indication.

Finally, measurement of the facial angle has been suggested to improve first-trimester screening for Down syndrome. The frontomaxillary facial (FMF) angle describes the relative position of the maxilla to the forehead between the upper surface of the palate and the frontal bone in a midsagittal view of the fetal face (Fig. 7.2). A prospective study of 782 euploid and 108 trisomy 21 fetuses found that 69% of those affected by trisomy 21 had a FMF angle over 85° and suggested that this novel sign was an independent marker for trisomy 21 [13]. Accurate assessment and reproducibility, however, are highly dependent on a sonographer's skills and experience in first-trimester ultrasound scanning; therefore, it is unlikely that this measurement will be incorporated into routine first-trimester screening in all cases at this time.

When considering newer forms of ultrasound evaluation for fetal Down syndrome, a balance needs to be struck between exciting new modalities and robust sonographic techniques that can be easily implemented at a general population level. Just because a new technique may perform well in select expert hands when evaluating high-risk patients does not imply that it will be a useful addition to general population screening.

Combined first-trimester serum and sonographic screening

In Down syndrome pregnancies, first-trimester serum levels of pregnancy-associated plasma protein A (PAPP-A) are decreased compared with euploid pregnancies, and human chorionic gonadotropin (hCG) levels are increased. Because these two serum markers are relatively independent of each other, and of both maternal age and NT measurements, improvements in Down syndrome risk assessment can be achieved by a combined serum and sonographic screening approach. Several large population studies have now confirmed that such combined first-trimester screening is significantly better than screening for Down syndrome based on NT sonography alone [1,3]. At a 5% false-positive rate, such combined first-trimester screening detects 87% of cases of Down syndrome at 11 weeks, decreasing to 82% at 13 weeks' gestation (compared with 70% and 64% detection rates, respectively, for NT alone) [1]. Looked at differently, to achieve an 85% Down syndrome detection rate at 11 weeks' gestation, screening using NT sonography alone would yield a false-positive rate of 20%, while combined first-trimester screening would have a false-positive rate of only 3.8% [1].

It is now clear that first-trimester screening for fetal Down syndrome should be provided using the combination of NT sonography with appropriate serum markers. The only exception to this may be the presence of a multiple gestation where it can be very difficult to interpret the relative contributions of different placentas to maternal serum marker levels. In this latter situation, it is reasonable to provide a Down syndrome risk assessment based on NT sonography alone.

Another practical problem for the implementation of first-trimester combined screening in the US is limited access to assays for the free β-subunit of hCG (fβhCG). Both total hCG and fβhCG are very effective discriminators of Down syndrome and euploid pregnancies, but when evaluated as univariate markers, fβhCG is more powerful (15% versus 28% detection rates, respectively, for a 5% false-positive rate at 11 weeks) [3]. However, in actual clinical practice fβhCG is never used on its own to screen for fetal Down syndrome, but instead will always be used in combination with other serum markers, such

as PAPP-A and NT sonography. When the combination of first-trimester NT, PAPP-A, and fβhCG is compared with the combination of NT, PAPP-A, and total hCG, their performance is actually very similar, with Down syndrome detection rates of 83% and 80%, respectively, for a 5% false-positive rate [3]. Therefore, for clinicians in practice, if fβhCG is not available at their local laboratory it would still be possible to achieve similar Down syndrome screening performance using the more widely available total hCG.

Cross-trimester repeated measures testing [14] evaluated maternal serum samples from the same patient in the first and second trimester (fβhCG, unconjugated estriol [uE3], PAPP-A). Maternal blood samples were obtained at 11–13 and 15–18 weeks' gestation. The most promising marker for repeated measures was PAPP-A, with increased detection rates and reduced false-positive rates for Down syndrome, but only when the first-trimester sample was collected before 13 weeks' gestation. This benefit decreased with increased gestational age at the time of the first sample. There was no evidence of improvement in screening performance for uE3 or hCG. Until the potential benefits of repeated measurements of PAPP-A with samples from early in the first trimester are confirmed in a prospective study, these promising results should be interpreted with caution.

First-trimester cystic hygroma

It has now become clear that there is a subgroup of fetuses with enlarged NT measurements which are at sufficiently high risk for aneuploidy and other adverse outcomes that delaying invasive diagnostic testing until serum markers are available is not necessary. The finding of an increased NT space, extending along the entire length of the fetus, and in which septations are clearly visible, is referred to as septated cystic hygroma, and is an easily identifiable feature during first-trimester sonography (see Plate 7.1). Septated cystic hygroma will be encountered in approximately 1 in every 300 first-trimester sonographic evaluations [15]. Once this diagnosis is made, patients should be counseled regarding a 50% incidence of fetal aneuploidy, with the most common abnormalities being Down syndrome, followed by Turner syndrome and trisomy 18 [15]. Of the remaining euploid fetuses, half will have major structural malformations such as congenital heart defects, diaphragmatic hernias, skeletal dysplasias, and a variety of genetic syndromes. Less than 20% of such pregnancies will result in a healthy liveborn infant at term.

The American College of Medical Genetics states that women carrying a fetus with an NT over 4 mm or where a septated cystic hygroma is present should be offered immediate invasive diagnosis using chorionic villus sampling (CVS) as the addition of serum markers would not significantly alter the risk for Down syndrome [16]. Results from the FASTER trial showed that a NT measurement of 3 mm or greater yields a minimum risk of aneuploidy of 1 in 6, so invasive testing should be offered at this cut-off. Given the association with congenital malformations, fetuses with increased NT or first-trimester cystic hygroma should undergo targeted sonography and/or echocardiogram at 18–20 weeks' gestation.

Second-trimester sonographic screening

The mainstay for antenatal Down syndrome screening for over 20 years has been second-trimester sonographic evaluation of fetal anatomy, also frequently referred to as the genetic sonogram. Two general approaches have been used in the second trimester: sonographic detection of major structural fetal malformations, and sonographic detection of minor markers for Down syndrome.

The detection of certain major structural malformations that are known to be associated with aneuploidy should prompt an immediate consideration of genetic amniocentesis. The major structural malformations that are associated with Down syndrome include cardiac malformations (atrioventricular [AV] canal defect, ventricular septal defect, tetralogy of Fallot), duodenal atresia, cystic hygroma, and hydrops fetalis. The major malformations associated with trisomy 18 include cardiac malformations (AV canal defect, ventricular septal defect, double-outlet right ventricle), meningomyelocele, omphalocele, esophageal atresia, rocker-bottom feet, cleft lip or palate, cystic hygroma, and hydrops fetalis. While the genetic sonogram can be performed at any time during the second and third trimesters, the optimal time is likely to be at 17–18 weeks' gestation, which is late enough to maximize fetal anatomic evaluation yet early enough to allow for amniocentesis results to be obtained. When a major structural malformation is found, such as an AV canal defect or a double-bubble suggestive of duodenal atresia, the risk of Down syndrome in that pregnancy can be increased by approximately 20–30-fold [17]. For almost all patients, such an increase in their background risk for aneuploidy will be sufficiently high to justify immediate genetic amniocentesis.

Second-trimester sonography can also detect a range of minor markers for aneuploidy. The latter are not considered structural abnormalities of the fetus *per se* but, when noted, may be associated with an increased probability that the fetus is aneuploid. The minor markers that have been commonly linked to Down syndrome include nuchal fold thickening (Fig. 7.3), nasal bone absence or hypoplasia, mild ventriculomegaly, short femur or humerus, echogenic bowel, renal pyelectasis,

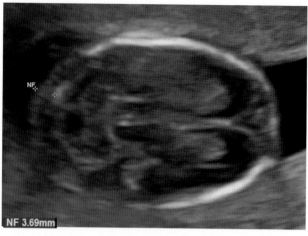

Figure 7.3 Second-trimester sonographic measurement of the fetal nuchal fold (NF) at 15 5/7 weeks' gestation. The measurement is taken in the axial plane at the level of the posterior fossa, with calipers placed from the outer skull edge to the outer skin edge.

echogenic intracardiac focus, clinodactyly, sandal gap toe, and widened iliac angle [18]. The minor markers that are associated with trisomy 18 include nuchal fold thickening, mild ventriculomegaly, short femur or humerus, echogenic bowel, enlarged cisterna magna, choroid plexus cysts, micrognathia, single umbilical artery, clenched hands, and fetal growth restriction. It should be noted that almost all data supporting the role of second-trimester sonography for minor markers for aneuploidy are derived from high-risk populations, such as patients of advanced maternal age or with abnormal maternal serum screening results. It is still unclear what the relative contribution of screening for such minor markers will be in lower risk patients from the general population.

To objectively counsel patients following the prenatal diagnosis of a minor sonographic marker, likelihood ratios can be used to create a more precise risk assessment for the patient that her fetus might be affected with Down syndrome. Their use in clinical practice is simply to multiply the relevant likelihood ratio by the *a priori* risk. Table 7.1 summarizes the likelihood ratios that can be used to modify a patient's risk for Down syndrome, depending on which minor marker is detected. If no markers are present, the patient's *a priori* risk can be multiplied by 0.4, effectively reducing her chances of carrying a fetus with Down syndrome by 60% [18]. The likelihood ratio values listed for each marker assume that the marker is an isolated finding. By contrast, when more than one minor marker is noted in the same fetus, different likelihood ratios must be used, with the risk for Down syndrome being increased by a factor of 10 when two minor markers are detected and by a factor of 115 when three or more minor markers are found [18]. It should also be noted that the 95% confidence interval (CI) values for each marker's

Table 7.1 Likelihood ratios for Down syndrome when an isolated minor sonographic marker is detected*

Table 7.1 Likelihood ratios for Down syndrome when an isolated minor sonographic marker is detected*

Minor marker	Likelihood ratio	95% Confidence interval
Nuchal fold >5mm	11	6–22
Echogenic bowel	6.7	3–17
Short humerus	5.1	2–17
Short femur	1.5	0.8–3
Echogenic intracardiac focus	1.8	1–3
Pyelectasis	1.5	0.6–4
Any two minor markers	10	6.6–14
Any three or more minor markers	115	58–229
No markers	0.4	0.3–0.5

*The patient's *a priori* risk is multiplied by the appropriate positive likelihood ratio to yield an individualized posttest risk for fetal Down syndrome.

Reproduced from Nyberg *et al* [18] with permission from the American Institute of Ultrasound in Medicine.

likelihood ratios are rather wide. These values should therefore be used only as a general guide for counseling patients, and care should be exercised to avoid implying too much precision in the final risk estimates. Accuracy of risk estimates, however, can be maximized by using the best available *a priori* risk value for a particular patient, such as the results of maternal serum marker screening or first-trimester combined screening, rather than maternal age, when available.

The role of second-trimester genetic sonography after Down syndrome screening has been evaluated in a study of 7842 pregnancies, including 59 with trisomy 21 [19]. For a 5% false-positive rate, genetic sonography increased detection rates substantially for combined and quadruple tests, from 81% to 90%, respectively and for the integrated test from 93% to 98%. Detection rates for sequential protocols were only modestly improved with the genetic sonogram: from 97% to 98% with the stepwise test and from 95% to 97% with the contingent test.

Second-trimester serum screening

Maternal serum levels of AFP and uE3 are both approximately 25% lower in pregnancies complicated by Down syndrome compared with euploid pregnancies [20]. By contrast, levels of hCG and inhibin-A are approximately twice as high in pregnancies complicated by Down syndrome [20]. Maternal serum levels of AFP, uE3, and hCG all tend to be decreased in pregnancies complicated by trisomy 18. The combination of AFP, uE3, and hCG, commonly known as the triple screen, can detect 69% of cases of Down syndrome, for a 5% false-positive rate [1]. When

inhibin-A is added to this test, commonly known as the quad screen, the Down syndrome detection rate increases to 81%, for a 5% false-positive rate [1,3].

Performance of serum screening tests can be maximized by accurate ascertainment of gestational age and, wherever possible, sonographic dating should be used instead of menstrual dating. It is optimal to provide serum screening between 15 and 16 weeks' gestation, thereby allowing the results to be available at the time of second-trimester sonographic evaluation. Subsequently, if the genetic sonogram reveals any minor markers, the Down syndrome risk quoted from serum screening should be used with the appropriate likelihood ratio (as summarized in Table 7.1) to determine the final Down syndrome risk.

Combined first- and second-trimester screening

It is now clear that both first- and second-trimester approaches to screening for Down syndrome are highly effective, with first-trimester combined screening being superior to second-trimester serum quad screening only when performed as early as 11 weeks' gestation [1]. However, rather than restricting patients to one or another screening option, it is now possible to improve screening performance even further by combining screening tests across both trimesters. There are currently three approaches to this: integrated screening, sequential screening, and contingent screening.

Integrated screening

Integrated screening is a two-step screening protocol, with results not being released until all screening steps are completed. Sonographic measurement of NT, together with serum assay for PAPP-A, are obtained between 10 and 13 weeks' gestation, followed by a second serum assay for AFP, hCG, uE3, and inhibin-A obtained between 15 and 16 weeks' gestation. A single risk assessment is then calculated at 16 weeks' gestation. This "fully integrated" test has a Down syndrome detection rate of 95%, for a 5% false-positive rate [1,3]. A variant of this approach, referred to as the "serum integrated" test, involves blood tests only, including PAPP-A in the first trimester, followed by AFP, hCG, uE3, and inhibin-A in the second trimester. This latter test, which does not require an NT ultrasound assessment, has a Down syndrome detection rate of 86%, for a 5% false-positive rate [1,3].

For some patients who are anxious to receive rapid screening results, or for those who might wish to have a first-trimester CVS, it is possible that such integrated screening tests might not be acceptable, as a delay inevitably exists between the time of first-trimester screening measurements and release of results in the second trimester. However, for patients who may not be interested in, or have access to, first-trimester CVS, the efficiency of being provided with a single Down syndrome risk assessment result, which maximizes detection and minimizes false positives, may make such integrated screening tests appear attractive.

Sequential screening

In contrast to integrated screening, stepwise sequential screening refers to multiple different Down syndrome screening tests being performed, with risk estimates being provided to patients upon completion of each step. A key concept in performing stepwise screening is to ensure that each subsequent screening test that is performed uses the Down syndrome risk from the preceding test as the new *a priori* risk for later screening, or includes all previous marker results in risk calculation. If sequential screening tests are performed independently for Down syndrome without any modification being made for earlier screening results, the positive predictive value of the later tests will inevitably deteriorate, and it is likely that the overall false-positive rate will increase [21].

A potential advantage of stepwise screening over integrated screening is that it allows patients in the first trimester to avail themselves of an immediate CVS, should their risk estimate justify this test, without having to wait until 16–18 weeks when the integrated screening results are provided. Patients could therefore achieve the benefit of early diagnosis associated with first-trimester screening, as well as the higher detection rate for Down syndrome associated with integration of both first- and second-trimester screening tests.

Contingent screening

Finally, one of the major disadvantages of providing all possible first- and second-trimester screening tests for patients is the cost involved and the patient anxiety inherent with prolongation of the screening process over several months. A possible solution to this is to utilize contingent screening, in which patients have first-trimester screening with NT, PAPP-A, and fβhCG, and only those patients with extremely high-risk results (e.g. greater than 1 in 30) are offered CVS. Patients with extremely low-risk results that are unlikely to be significantly changed by additional later tests (e.g. less than 1 in 1500) are reassured and are not offered additional Down syndrome screening tests. Finally, borderline risk patients (e.g. with risks between 1 in 30 and 1 in 1500) return at 15 weeks for quad serum markers and these are combined with the earlier first-trimester markers to provide a final Down syndrome risk. The advantage of this approach is that it may focus the benefits of CVS with the highest risk patients, while significantly reducing the number of second-trimester screening tests performed.

The FASTER trial evaluated 32,269 unaffected and 86 Down syndrome pregnancies and found a 91% detection rate for contingent screening, coupled with a 4.5% false-positive rate. Therefore, contingent screening is comparable with stepwise and integrated screening and substantially reduces the number of patients needing to return for second-trimester testing [22]. While this appears to be an exciting approach that may be quite cost-effective, it still requires validation by actual population trials before it can be endorsed for clinical application.

Screening in multiple gestations

Combined first-trimester serum screening for multifetal gestations is less sensitive than in singleton pregnancies. Nuchal translucency measurement in dichorionic twin gestations has comparable detection rates to those in singleton pregnancies [23]. NT measurement in monochorionic gestations is less reliable, however, given the recognition of increased or discordant NT as an early sign for twin-to-twin transfusion syndrome. Maternal serum screening has not been widely utilized in the setting of multiple gestations because of the potential for discordancy between twins and the impact of different placentas on the various analytes. Options for first-trimester screening for Down syndrome therefore include a fetus-specific risk based on NT alone, or providing an overall pregnancy risk based on combined serum and sonographic markers. In a series of 448 twin pregnancies, NT alone yielded an 88% detection rate for a 7% false-positive rate [24]. Another series of 206 twin pregnancies included maternal serum markers and reported a 75% detection rate for a 5% false-positive rate [25].

Currently, the method of choice for screening in multiple gestations is debatable but avoiding serum markers and providing a fetus-specific risk based on NT alone is a reasonable strategy. Sonographic evaluation of each individual fetus in the second trimester for major structural malformations or minor markers will allow for the calculation of fetus-specific risks for aneuploidy.

Screening for neural tube defects

Screening tests to identify patients at risk for fetal open neural tube defects (NTD) utilize both maternal biochemical markers and ultrasonography to achieve highest detection rates. While second-trimester serum screening has been available over the past two decades, first-trimester tests are now available to allow for earlier diagnosis and optimized management options to be offered to the patient, including pregnancy termination. Between 75% and 90% of open NTDs and over 95% of anencephaly can be detected by elevated maternal serum AFP (MSAFP).

MSAFP also detects 85% of abdominal wall defects. Screening for NTD can be performed between 15 and 22 weeks' and optimally between 16 and 18 weeks' gestation. Factors influencing MSAFP are multiple gestations, maternal ethnicity, insulin-dependent diabetes mellitus, and a positive family history of open NTD. Cut-off levels for NTD screening are 2.0–2.5 multiples of the median (MoM) in singleton pregnancies and 4.0–5.0 MoM in twin gestations. These cut-off levels may be laboratory specific [16].

In pregnancies with elevated MSAFP, a targeted ultrasound examination is recommended. If optimal views of spine, abdominal wall, and intracranial anatomy are not obtained at a targeted ultrasound, consideration may be given to amniocentesis to evaluate for amniotic fluid AFP and acetylcholinesterase levels. Given the association of NTDs with trisomy 18, amniotic fluid should also be sent for genetic evaluation. Sonographic markers observed in most fetuses with NTDs in the second trimester include scalloping of the frontal bones ("lemon" sign) and caudal displacement of the cerebellum ("banana" sign) due to Chiari malformation [26]. Often those fetuses have a small biparietal diameter (BPD) early in the second trimester [27]. Spina bifida can be indicated in the first trimester, between 11 and 13 weeks' gestation, by the absence of the intracranial translucency (IT) [28]. The IT represents the fourth cerebral ventricle which can be visualized on the same midsagittal plane of the fetal face as for measurement of NT and assessment of the nasal bone. The two lines that define the IT are the posterior border of the brainstem anteriorly and the choroid plexus of the fourth ventricle posteriorly. It is unclear, however, what the precise sensitivity and specificity for this marker will be, if used in clinical practice.

CASE PRESENTATION 1

A healthy 35-year-old primigravida presents at 11 weeks' gestation requesting reassurance regarding the possibility of fetal Down syndrome. After appropriate pretest counseling, in which the various screening tests and the relative advantages and disadvantages of screening versus invasive diagnostic tests are discussed, the patient agrees to proceed with combined first-trimester screening. NT sonography is performed by a sonographer experienced in this technique, and the fetal crown–rump length (CRL) is measured at 45 mm, while the NT space is measured at 1.6 mm. A maternal blood sample is obtained and sent to a prenatal screening laboratory for assay of PAPP-A and fβhCG, together with the sonographer's credentialing ID number (to facilitate an NT quality assurance scheme) and the fetal CRL and NT data. Four days later, a laboratory report confirms that the patient's *a priori* age-related risk for Down syndrome is 1 in 270, and that this has been reduced to 1 in 1500 by combined first-trimester screening. The patient is informed of this result, feels reassured, and declines CVS.

Subsequently, the patient has a detailed sonographic fetal anatomic survey performed at 18 weeks' gestation and no major malformations are found. The fetus is noted to have a single echogenic intracardiac focus in the left ventricle, but no other minor markers are seen. The patient is informed of this finding and its possible association with Down syndrome. The physician knows that this marker has a likelihood ratio of 1.8 for Down syndrome and calculates that the final risk of Down syndrome in this patient's case is 1 in 830 ([1/1500] × 1.8). The patient is again reassured and declines genetic amniocentesis. Approximately 5 months later, she delivers a healthy female infant at term.

CASE PRESENTATION 2

A 32-year-old para 1 is referred from the early pregnancy assessment unit with an increased NT. She attends the prenatal diagnosis clinic at 11 0/7 weeks' gestation and a septated cystic hygroma is identified (see Plate 7.1). Following careful counseling regarding the associated risks of aneuploidy and congenital structural abnormalities, the patient agrees to proceed with a transabdominal CVS. Genetic evaluation reveals a normal male karyotype. She attends again at 18 0/7 and 23 4/7 weeks' gestation. The first-trimester cystic hygroma has entirely resolved and genetic sonography and echocardiogram reveal no abnormalities. Her pregnancy progresses without complications and she delivers a healthy male infant by vacuum delivery at 40 5/7 weeks' gestation, weighing 4500 g.

References

1. Malone FD, Canick JA, Ball RH et al. A comparison of first trimester screening, second trimester screening, and the combination of both for evaluation of risk for Down syndrome. N Engl J Med 2005;353:2001–2011.

2. Snijders RL, Noble P, Sebire N, Souka A, Nicolaides KH. UK multicenter project on assessment of risk of trisomy 21 by maternal age and fetal nuchal-translucency thickness at 10–14 weeks of gestation. Lancet 1998;351:343–346.

3. Wald NJ, Rodeck C, Hackshaw AK, Walters J, Chitty L, Mackinson AM. First and second trimester antenatal screening for Down's syndrome: the results of the Serum, Urine and Ultrasound Screening Study (SURUSS). Health Technol Assess 2003;7:1–77.

4. Wapner R, Thom E, Simpson JL et al. First-trimester screening for trisomies 21 and 18. N Engl J Med 2003;349:1405–1413.

5. Malone FD, d'Alton MD, for the Society for Maternal-Fetal Medicine. First trimester sonographic screening for Down syndrome. Obstet Gynecol 2003;102:1066–1079.

6. Cicero S, Curcio P, Papageorghiou A, Sonek J, Nicolaides KH. Absence of nasal bone in fetuses with trisomy 21 at 11–14 weeks of gestation: an observational study. Lancet 2001;358: 1665–1667.

7. Cicero S, Rembouskos G, Vandecruys H, Hogg M, Nicolaides KH. Likelihood ratio for trisomy 21 in fetuses with absent nasal bone at the 11–14-week scan. Ultrasound Obstet Gynecol 2004;23:218–223.

8. Malone FD, Ball RH, Nyberg DA et al. First trimester nasal bone evaluation for aneuploidy in the general population: results from the FASTER Trial. Obstet Gynecol 2004;104: 1222–1228.

9. Matias A, Gomes C, Flack N, Montenegro N, Nicolaides KH. Screening for chromosomal abnormalities at 10–14 weeks: the role of ductus venosus blood flow. Ultrasound Obstet Gynecol 1998;12:380–384.

10. Hecher K. Assessment of ductus venosus flow during the first and early second trimesters: what can we expect? Ultrasound Obstet Gynecol 2001;17:285–287.

11. Faiola S, Tsoi E, Huggon IC, Allan LD, Nicolaides KH. Likelihood ratio for trisomy 21 in fetuses with tricuspid regurgitation at the 11 to 136 week scan. Ultrasound Obstet Gynecol 2005;26:22–27.

12. Falcon O, Auer M, Gerovassili A et al. Screening for trisomy 21 by fetal tricuspid regurgitation, nuchal translucency and maternal serum free beta-hCG and PAPP-A at 11+0 to 13+6 weeks. Ultrasound Obstet Gynecol 2006;27:151–155.

13. Borenstein M, Persico N, Kagan KO, Gazzoni A, Nicolaides KH. Frontomaxillary facial angle in screening for trisomy 21 at 11+0 to 13+6 weeks. Ultrasound Obstet Gynecol 2008; 32:5–11.

14. Wright D, Bradbury I, Malone F et al. Cross-trimester repeated measures testing for Down's syndrome screening: an assessment. Health Technol Assess 2010;14(33):iii–iv.

15. Malone FD, Ball RH, Nyberg DA et al. First trimester septated cystic hygroma: prevalence, natural history, and pediatric outcome. Obstet Gynecol 2005;106:288–294.

16. Driscoll DA, Gross SJ for the Professional Practice Guidelines Committee. Screening for fetal aneuploidy and neural tube defects. Genet Med 2009;11(11):818–821.

17. Nyberg DA, Luthy DA, Resta RG, Nyberg BC, Williams MA. Age-adjusted ultrasound risk assessment for fetal Down's syndrome during the second trimester: description of the method and analysis of 142 cases. Ultrasound Obstet Gynecol 1998;12:8–14.

18. Nyberg DA, Souter VL, El-Bastawissi A, Young S, Luthhardt F, Luthy DA. Isolated sonographic markers for detection of fetal Down syndrome in the second trimester of pregnancy. J Ultrasound Med 2001;20:1053–1063.

19. Aagaard-Tillery KM, Malone FD, Nyberg DA et al. Role of second-trimester genetic sonography after Down syndrome screening. Obstet Gynecol 2009;114(6):1189–1196.

20. Wald NJ, Kennard A, Hackshaw A, McGuire A. Antenatal screening for Down's syndrome. J Med Screening 1994;4: 181–246.

21. Platt LD, Greene N, Johnson A et al. Sequential pathways of testing after first-trimester screening for trisomy 21. Obstet Gynecol 2004;104:661–666.

22. Cuckle HS, Malone FD, Wright D et al. Contingent screening for Down syndrome – results from the FASTER trial. Prenat Diagn 2008;28:89–94.

23. Sebire NJ, Snijders RJM, Hughes K et al. Screening for trisomy 21 in twin pregnancies by maternal age and fetal nuchal translucency thickness at 10–14 weeks of gestation. Br J Obstet Gynaecol 1996;103:999–1003.

24. Sebire NJ, Souka A, Skentou H et al. Early prediation of severe twin-to-twin transfusion syndrome. Hum Reprod 2000;15: 2008–2010.

25. Spencer K, Nicolaides KH. Screening fo trisomy 21 in twins using first trimester ultrasound and maternal serum biochemistry in a one stop clinic: a review of three years experience. Br J Obstet Gynaecol 2003;110:276–280.

26. Nicolaides KH, Campbell S, Gabbe SG, Guidetti R. Ultrasound screening for spina bifida: cranial and cerebellar signs. Lancet 1986;8498:72–74.

27. Wald NJ. Prenatal screening for open neural tube defects and Down syndrome: three decades of progress. Prenat Diag 2010;30:619–621.

28. Chaoui R, Nicolaides KH. From nuchal translucency to intracranial translucency: towards the early detection of spina bifida. Ultrasound Obstet Gynecol 2010;35:133–138.

Chapter 8
Sonographic Dating and Standard Fetal Biometry

Eliza Berkley and Alfred Abuhamad
Department of Obstetrics and Gynecology, Eastern Virginia Medical School, Norfolk, VA, USA

Pregnancy dating

Accurate pregnancy dating is a critical component of prenatal management. Precise knowledge of gestational age is essential for the management of high-risk pregnancies and in particular fetal growth restriction. Although uterine size, as measured by the fundal height, provides a subjective assessment of the fetal size, ultrasound has a far more precise role in confirming gestational age [1].

Overestimation of gestational age based on menstrual dates is responsible for a preponderance of misdated pregnancies and results from delayed ovulation in the conception cycle. Overestimation of true gestational age by the menstrual history results in an underestimate of the rate of preterm delivery [2] and an overestimate of the postdates pregnancies. In a retrospective review of a routinely scan-dated population, Gardosi *et al* [3] found that 72% of inductions carried out for postterm pregnancy (>294 days) according to menstrual dates were not actually post term according to ultrasound dating.

Ultrasound has an integral role in confirming gestational age, with a high accuracy when performed in the first or second trimesters. A study involving *in vitro* fertilization (IVF) pregnancy has shown that ultrasound has an accuracy in pregnancy dating of 3–4 days when performed between 14 and 22 weeks' gestation [1]. Dating during the third trimester is less predictive because of heterogeneity in individual fetal growth rates, and should be avoided.

First trimester

Dating by ultrasound in the first half of pregnancy has become a routine part of antenatal care in many institutions around the world. Before 6 weeks' gestation, dating can be carried out by measurement and observation of the gestational sac [4]. The gestational sac is visible as early as 4 weeks, and should always be visible by 5 weeks. The size of the gestational sac can be correlated with gestational age [5]. Because the mean sac diameter (MSD) grows at a rate of 1 mm/day, gestational age can be estimated by the formula:

$$\text{Gestational age (days)} = 30 + \text{MSD (mm)} \, [6]$$

Among all fetal biometry measurements, determination of the maximum embryonic length (crown–rump length [CRL]) up to 14 weeks' gestation is the most accurate for determining gestational age. The random error is in the range of 4–8 days at the 95th percentile [7–12].

Second and third trimesters

When the CRL is above 60 mm, other biometric parameters are more useful for dating the pregnancy [13]. Standardized measurements include the biparietal diameter (BPD), head circumference (HC), femur length (FL), humeral length (HL), and abdominal circumference (AC). These grow in a predictable way and so can be correlated with gestational age. Virtually any other bone or organ can be measured and compared with gestational age.

In a study that involved pregnancies conceived with IVF, the HC was the most predictive parameter of gestational age between 14 and 22 weeks' gestation as it predicts gestational age within 3.4 days [1]. Other parameters such as the BPD, AC, and FL also have good accuracy. Combining various biometric parameters improves the prediction of gestational age slightly over the use of HC alone [1].

The AC is a measure of fetal girth. It includes soft tissues of the abdominal wall as well as a measure of internal organs, primarily the liver. Unlike other commonly used fetal measurements, it is not influenced by bone growth or morphology. At term, 95% of newborns are found to be within 20% of an expected length of 20 cm, whereas infant weight may vary by 100% or more. Therefore, differences in weight must be explained

Queenan's Management of High-Risk Pregnancy: An Evidence-Based Approach, Sixth Edition. Edited by John T. Queenan, Catherine Y. Spong, Charles J. Lockwood.
© 2012 John Wiley & Sons, Ltd. Published 2012 by John Wiley & Sons, Ltd.

primarily by variations in girth and, not surprisingly, the AC is among the least predictive measures of fetal age but the most predictive of fetal growth [14–16].

Estimation of fetal weight

The best overall measure of fetal size is obtained by estimating fetal weight. Numerous formulas for estimating fetal weight have been described and utilized [17–19]. Using standard biometry, some formulas use head measurements and AC, others use long bone measurements and AC, and others use all these measurements. The AC is included in all commonly used formulas of estimated fetal weight, and it also strongly influences fetal weight estimates [20]. Weight estimates based on AC alone have also been reported [21,22].

Hadlock [17], Dudley [18], Coombs *et al* [19], Rose and McCallum [23], and Medchill *et al* [24] estimations of weight formulas, which include BPD, HC, AC, and FL, result in a mean absolute error of approximately 10% [25,26]. Some formulas for estimating fetal weight are volume based and would be expected to be more accurate in predicting fetal weight; however, these volume-based equations have not been shown to be consistently more accurate and some studies have resulted in large systematic errors [27].

In experienced hands, nearly 80% of estimated weights are within 10% of the actual birthweights and most of the remaining are within 20% of birthweights. However, accuracy decreases when less experienced sonographers perform exams [28]. A number of studies have documented that prediction of fetal weight by ultrasound is limited. In one study, Baum *et al* [28] found that sonographic estimation of fetal weight was no better than clinical or patient estimates at term.

Intrauterine growth restriction

Definition

The term "small for gestational age" (SGA) is commonly used to describe all fetuses that are small. SGA fetuses represent a heterogeneous group of both constitutionally small but "normal" and pathologically growth-restricted fetuses.

It should be clear that estimated weights and weight percentiles only evaluate fetal size. This approach cannot distinguish growth-restricted potentially compromised fetuses from otherwise healthy fetuses that are simply constitutionally small for gestational age. Therefore, it is important to correlate estimates of fetal size with other correlates of fetal health, including amniotic fluid, Doppler flow studies, and fetal activity. For this reason, use of the term "intrauterine growth restriction" (IUGR) should be limited to fetuses who are SGA and who show other evidence of reduced uteroplacental blood flow, chronic

hypoxemia or malnutrition. Nevertheless, in actual day-to-day practice, the terms SGA and IUGR are frequently used interchangeably.

Dynamic evaluation of fetal growth with serial ultrasound examinations is more important than a single examination when fetal measurements are below the 10th percentile. This is true independent of methods used, including cross-sectional or longitudinal growth charts, customized growth charts, or predicted fetal growth. The optimal measurement interval in small fetuses that combines acceptable technical variability with useful clinical data while minimizing intra- and interobserver variabilities appears to be approximately 10 days [29]. However, longer time intervals will reflect fetal growth in low-risk patients more accurately [30].

Several definitions exist in the literature for the diagnosis of IUGR. The definition that is most commonly used in clinical practice is an estimated fetal weight at less than the 10th percentile for gestational age. At this diagnostic threshold, approximately 70% of "affected" fetuses will be constitutionally small and have no increase in perinatal morbidity or mortality [31]. Using the 5th percentile as a cut-off for the diagnosis of IUGR may be more clinically applicable, given that perinatal morbidity and mortality have been shown to increase beyond this threshold [32].

Of all the ultrasound-derived biometric parameters, the AC is the most sensitive indicator for growth restriction in the fetus. An AC of less than the 2.5th percentile for gestational age carries a sensitivity of greater than 95% for the diagnosis of IUGR [33,34]. The growth profile of the AC should therefore be monitored closely in fetuses at risk for growth abnormalities. Furthermore, when estimating fetal weights by ultrasound, the appropriate growth curves should be used. Curves generated at high altitudes will underestimate IUGR by approximately 50% for sea-level population [35].

Customized growth curves, which take into account genetic factors which affect fetal growth such as maternal height, maternal weight, parity, ethnic origin, and fetal gender, have been developed. Studies suggest that such customized curves are better than population-derived curves at correlating growth restriction with low Apgar scores, stillbirth, and neonatal death and at differentiating between physiologically and pathologically small newborns [36]. In addition, some studies have shown an ability to decrease antenatal testing and improve the correlation of SGA with adverse outcome when customized growth curves are used for the diagnosis of IUGR [36–38]. However, customized growth curves have not attained wide application in clinical practice primarily due to the complexity of this approach. Furthermore, customized growth curves that are currently available do not reference the Hispanic population, which accounts for about 24% of deliveries in the United States [36,39].

Symmetric versus asymmetric

"Symmetric" IUGR has been used to describe the growth pattern when all biometric measurements appear affected to the same degree, whereas "asymmetric" IUGR has been used to characterize a smaller AC compared with other growth parameters. Asymmetric IUGR would then show abnormal ratios such as the HC:AC or FL:AC ratio [40].

When first introduced, symmetric IUGR was suggested as more likely to reflect underlying fetal condition including aneuploidy, whereas asymmetric IUGR supposedly reflected underlying uterine–placental vascular dysfunction. However, these assumptions have proved to be largely false. Asymmetric IUGR was more likely to be associated with a major fetal anomaly in one study [41], may also be seen with aneuploidy (e.g. triploidy), and severe uteroplacental vascular insufficiency can initially present as symmetric IUGR [42]. Fetuses with symmetric and asymmetric IUGR also show a similar degree of acid–base impairment [43]. The FL:AC ratio has also been found to be useful for prediction of IUGR [44].

Risk factors

Causes of and associations with IUGR are shown in Box 8.1. The most common associations are with maternal hypertension and/or a history of IUGR in previous pregnancies. Conversely, a history of a prior SGA fetus is a risk factor for preeclampsia [45].

Underlying uterine–placental dysfunction is a commonly cited cause for otherwise unexplained IUGR. Uterine–placental dysfunction has been correlated with a range of pathologic findings including failure of physiologic transformation of uterine spiral arteries by endovascular trophoblast, smaller placentas, increase in the thickness of tertiary stem villi vessel wall, and decrease in lumen circumference of spiral arterioles. Also, confined placental mosaicism has been found to carry a higher risk of IUGR and adverse outcome, including fetal death [46]. Uterine–placental dysfunction produces fetal hypoxemia which results in subnormal growth, oligohydramnios, and alterations in blood flow [47].

Various chromosome abnormalities including those confined to the placenta (confined placental mosaicism) may exhibit delayed growth as a prominent feature. Abnormal growth and development have also been associated with disturbed genomic imprinting (expression of genes depending on whether they are located on the maternal or the paternal chromosome). This has led to the suggestion that genomic imprinting has evolved as a mechanism to regulate embryonic and fetal growth [48].

Many fetuses with chromosomal anomalies or other genetic syndromes may exhibit growth delay as a dominant feature (Box 8.2). It may be the primary or in some cases the only sonographic evidence of underlying fetal anomalies. Early-onset IUGR is a common manifestation

---

Box 8.1 Causes of and associations with intrauterine growth restriction

Maternal

- Pregnancy-induced hypertension/preeclampsia
- Severe chronic hypertension
- Severe maternal diabetes mellitus
- Collagen vascular disease
- Heart disease
- Smoking
- Poor nutrition
- Renal disease
- Lung disease/hypoxia
- Environmental agents
- Endocrine disorders
- Previous history of IUGR

Uterine–placental

- Uterine–placental dysfunction
- Placental infarct
- Chronic abruption
- Multiple gestation/twin transfusion syndrome
- Confined placental mosaicism

Fetal

- Chromosome abnormalities
- Anomalies
- Skeletal dysplasias
- Multiple anomaly syndromes (see Box 8.2)
- Infection
- Teratogens

---

of major chromosome abnormalities, particularly trisomies 18 and 13, and triploidy [49,50].

Among other variables, smaller fetal size tends to reflect both maternal and paternal birth weights. Magnus *et al* [51] found the mean maternal birthweight was significantly less among those who had experienced two SGA births compared with those with no SGA births (3127 ± 54 g versus 3424 ± 22 g). Interestingly, the mean paternal birthweight was also lower (3497 ± 88 g versus 3665 ± 24 g) from affected pregnancies with two previous SGA births.

Outcome

Failure to recognize fetal growth restriction may result in a 50% rate of unexplained term stillbirths [52]. In addition to an increased risk of perinatal mortality, when compared with appropriately grown fetuses matched for gestational age, IUGR fetuses have an increased risk of perinatal morbidity [53]. Long-term follow-up studies have shown an increased incidence of physical handicap and neurodevelopmental delay in growth-restricted fetuses [54,55]. The presence of chronic metabolic acidemia

Box 8.2 Genetic syndromes that include intrauterine growth restriction

- **Aarskog syndrome**. X-linked. Associated with brachydactyly, shawl scrotum, hypertelorism, vertebral anomalies, and moderate short stature. DNA testing is available
- **Ataxia-telangiectasia syndrome**. Autosomal recessive. Associated with growth deficiency sometimes evident prenatally, ataxia, telangiectasias, and immunodeficiency. DNA testing is available
- **Bloom syndrome**. Autosomal recessive. More common in Ashkenazi Jewish population. Associated with prenatal growth deficiency, butterfly telangiectasia of the face, microcephaly, mild mental retardation in some cases, and occasional syndactyly and/or polydactyly. DNA analysis is available
- **Cornelia de Lange/Brachman syndrome**. Autosomal dominant, often *de novo*. Associated with prenatal growth deficiency, micromelia, mental retardation, and synophrys. DNA testing is available
- **CHARGE syndrome**, characterized by coloboma, heart disease, choanal atresia, retarded growth (typically postnatal onset) or development, CNS abnormalities, genital anomalies, and ear anomalies and/or deafness. DNA testing is available
- **Coffin–Siris syndrome**. Autosomal recessive. Characterized by prenatal growth deficiency, mental retardation, coarse facies, absence of terminal phalanges, and hypoplastic to absent fingernails and toenails. DNA testing is not currently available
- **Dubowitz syndrome**. Autosomal recessive. Characterized by microcephaly, prenatal growth deficiency, mental retardation, dysmorphic facies, 2,3 toe syndactyly, and eczema. DNA testing is not currently available
- **Fanconi anemia**. Autosomal recessive. Characterized by radial ray defects including aplasia of the thumbs or supernumerary thumbs, short stature often of prenatal onset, pancytopenia, renal or other urinary tract abnormalities, cardiac defects, and gastrointestinal abnormalities. DNA testing is available
- **Johanson–Blizzard syndrome**. Autosomal recessive. Rare syndrome associated with prenatal growth deficiency, hypoplastic alae nasi, mental retardation, microcephaly, hydronephrosis, and pancreatic insufficiency. DNA testing is not currently available
- **Neu–Laxova syndrome**. Autosomal recessive. Rare syndrome associated with severe prenatal growth deficiency, microcephaly, exophthalmos, subcutaneous edema, micrognathia, sloping forehead, syndactyly, contractures, often with pterygia, polyhydramnios, small placenta, and short umbilical cord. Majority of patients are stillborn. DNA testing is not available
- **Noonan syndrome**. Autosomal dominant. Associated with pulmonic stenosis, other congenital heart defects, webbed neck/increased nuchal translucency, short stature typically of postnatal onset, dysmorphic facies, pectus excavatum, and vertebral anomalies. DNA analysis is available
- **Pena–Shokier phenotype**. Autosomal recessive in some families. Characterized by prenatal growth deficiency, arthrogryposis, clubfoot, rocker-bottom feet, micrognathia, pulmonary hypoplasia, polyhydramnios, abnormal placenta, and short umbilical cord. DNA testing is not available
- **Roberts syndrome/Roberts phocomelia**. Autosomal recessive with variable expression. Characterized by thalidomide-type limb reduction defects often more severe in the upper limbs, microcephaly, severe prenatal growth deficiency, mental retardation, cleft lip and/or palate. DNA testing is not available
- **Seckel syndrome**. Autosomal recessive. Characterized by severe prenatal growth deficiency, mental retardation, microcephaly, prominent nose, micrognathia, and missing ribs. DNA analysis is not available
- **Silver–Russell syndrome**. Typically sporadic but has been associated with maternal uniparental disomy of chromosome 7 in about 10% of cases. Characterized by prenatal growth deficiency, asymmetry of the limbs, triangular facies, relative microcephaly, and small and/or curved fifth finger. Uniparental disomy testing is available
- **Smith–Lemli–Opitz syndrome**. Autosomal recessive. Characterized by failure to thrive, microcephaly, 2,3 toe syndactyly, genital abnormalities, polydactyly, and congenital heart defects. Affected fetuses may have low unconjugated estriol MoM on maternal serum screening. Diagnostic testing available
- **Williams syndrome**. Autosomal dominant microdeletion syndrome caused by a deletion of 7p11.23. Characterized by mild prenatal growth deficiency, congenital heart defect particularly supravalvular aortic stenosis, mental retardation, dysmorphic features, contractures, abnormal curvature of the spine, and renal anomalies. Diagnostic testing available by fluorescence *in situ* hybridization analysis

in utero, rather than actual birthweight, appears to be the best predictor of long-term neurodevelopmental delay [56]. Progression of fetal hypoxemia to acidemia is an important antecedent to adverse short- and long-term outcomes. Therefore, antenatal surveillance aims to detect fetal responses that accompany such deterioration [57]. In contrast, early delivery can result in significant neonatal complications secondary to prematurity [58].

Results of both randomized and observational studies suggest that gestational age remains the major contributor to adverse perinatal outcome in fetuses delivered prior to 32–34 weeks' gestation [58,59]. While there is evidence of increased morbidity with late preterm birth, it should be noted that these findings may not be applicable to fetuses with suboptimal growth and abnormal

fetal surveillance [60–62]. Therefore, in pregnancies with growth-restricted fetuses, timing of the delivery is the most critical step in clinical management. Balancing the risk of prematurity with the risk of long-term neurodevelopmental delay is a serious challenge facing physicians involved in the care of these pregnancies. In addition, IUGR fetuses may face long-term adverse adult health outcomes including accelerated atherosclerotic vascular disease, hypertension, and diabetes.

Management

Traditionally, the management of pregnancies with fetal growth restriction relied on cardiotocography for fetal surveillance. During cardiotocography, the physician looks for heart rate variability as a sign of fetal well-being.

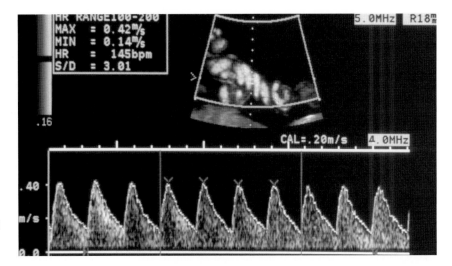

Figure 8.1 Normal Doppler waveforms obtained from the umbilical artery in the third trimester. In the third trimester of pregnancy, the umbilical circulation is a low-impedance circulation. Note the increased amount of flow at end diastole (*white arrow*). Reproduced from Abuhamad [104] with permission from Thieme Medical Publishing.

Heart rate variability is the final result of the rhythmic integrated activity of autonomic neurons generated by organized cardiorespiratory reflexes [63]. In growth-restricted fetuses, higher baseline rates, decreased long- and short-term variability, and delayed maturation of reactivity are seen in heart rate tracings [64,65]. These studies have relied on computer-generated analyses of fetal heart rate tracings in their evaluation. Unaided visual analyses of fetal heart rate records have been shown to have limited reliability and reproducibility [66,67]. Furthermore, overtly abnormal patterns of fetal heart rate tracings represent late signs of fetal deterioration [68,69].

Doppler ultrasound has been shown to improve outcome in high-risk pregnancies [70]. The use of Doppler ultrasound in the management of pregnancies with fetal growth restriction has received significant attention in the literature. Several cross-sectional and longitudinal studies have highlighted the fetal cardiovascular adaptation to hypoxemia and the progressive stages of such adaptation [71–76]. Findings from these studies and the use of Doppler ultrasound in the management of the growth-restricted fetus are discussed in the following section.

Fetal arterial Doppler

Umbilical circulation

The umbilical arterial circulation is normally a low-impedance circulation, with an increase in the amount of end-diastolic flow with advancing gestation (Fig. 8.1) [77]. Umbilical arterial Doppler waveforms reflect the status of the placental circulation, and the increase in end-diastolic flow that is seen with advancing gestation is a direct result of an increase in the number of tertiary stem villi with placental maturation [78]. Diseases that obliterate small muscular arteries in placental tertiary stem villi result in a progressive decrease in end-diastolic flow in

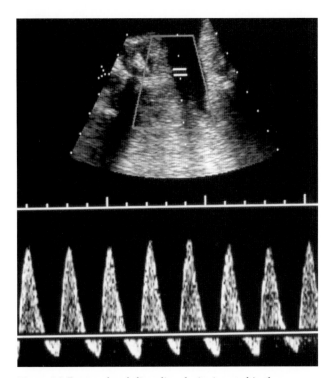

Figure 8.2 Reversed end-diastolic velocity is noted in the umbilical circulation when downstream impedance is increased. These Doppler waveforms are associated with significant fetal compromise. Reproduced from Abuhamad [104] with permission from Thieme Medical Publishing.

the umbilical arterial Doppler waveforms until absent and then reverse flow during diastole is noted (Fig. 8.2) [79]. Reversed diastolic flow in the umbilical arterial circulation represents an advanced stage of placental compromise and is associated with obliteration of more than 70% of placental tertiary villi arteries [80,81]. The presence of absent or reversed end-diastolic flow in the umbilical artery is commonly associated with severe IUGR and oligohydramnios [82].

Doppler waveforms of the umbilical arteries can be obtained from any segment along the umbilical cord. Waveforms obtained from the placental end of the cord show more end-diastolic flow than those obtained from the abdominal cord insertion [83]. Differences in Doppler indices of arterial waveforms obtained from different anatomic locations of the same umbilical cord are generally minor and have no significance in clinical practice [77].

Middle cerebral circulation

The cerebral circulation is normally a high-impedance circulation with continuous forward flow throughout the cardiac cycle [84]. The middle cerebral artery is the cerebral vessel most accessible to ultrasound imaging in the fetus and it carries more than 80% of cerebral blood flow [85]. In the presence of fetal hypoxemia, central redistribution of blood flow occurs, resulting in an increased blood flow to the brain, heart, and adrenals, and a reduction in flow to the peripheral and placental circulations. This blood flow redistribution is known as the brain-sparing reflex and has a major role in fetal adaptation to oxygen deprivation [84,86].

The right and left middle cerebral arteries represent major branches of the circle of Willis in the fetal brain. The circle of Willis, which is supplied by the internal carotids and vertebral arteries, can be imaged with color flow Doppler ultrasound in a transverse plane of the fetal head obtained at the base of the skull. In this transverse plane, the proximal and distal middle cerebral arteries are seen in their longitudinal view, with their course almost parallel to the ultrasound beam (Fig. 8.3). Middle cerebral artery Doppler waveforms, obtained from the proximal

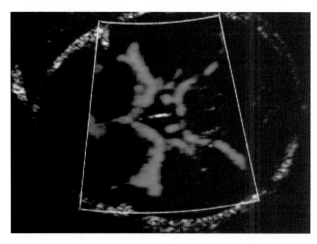

Figure 8.3 Axial view of the fetal head in the second trimester with color Doppler showing the circulation at the level of the circle of Willis. Note the course of the middle cerebral arteries, almost parallel to the ultrasound beam. Reproduced from Abuhamad [104] with permission from Thieme Medical Publishing.

portion of the vessel, immediately after its origin from the circle of Willis, have shown the best reproducibility [87].

Arterial Doppler and fetal growth restriction

Central redistribution of blood flow to the brain, known as the brain-sparing reflex, represents an early stage in fetal adaptation to hypoxemia [73–76], and follows the lag in fetal growth [88]. At this early stage, the brain-sparing reflex is clinically evident by increased end-diastolic flow in the middle cerebral artery (lower middle cerebral artery pulsatility or resistance index) and decreased end-diastolic flow in the umbilical artery (higher umbilical artery resistance index or S:D ratio). The cerebroplacental ratio, derived by dividing the cerebral resistance index by the umbilical resistance index, defines the brain-sparing reflex and has been shown to predict outcome in IUGR fetuses at less than 34 weeks' gestation. This ratio is a better predictor of a constitutionally small fetus than the umbilical artery or middle cerebral artery pulsatility index alone [71,89–91].

In the presence of IUGR, Doppler changes in the umbilical artery precede the decrease in cerebroplacental ratio and middle cerebral artery pulsatility or resistance index [73,88]. However, middle cerebral artery Doppler waveforms are of clinical value in differentiating a growth-restricted/hypoxemic fetus from a constitutionally small/normoxemic fetus. In the clinical setting of a constitutionally small fetus, the presence of normal middle cerebral artery Doppler waveforms, obtained at less than 32 weeks' gestation, has a 97% negative predictive value for major adverse perinatal outcomes [92].

Several studies have shown that this early stage of arterial redistribution is not associated with the presence of fetal metabolic acidemia [73–76]. It is therefore inferred that infants delivered at this early stage of fetal adaptation are expected to have no adverse long-term neurodevelopmental complications. However, several recent studies challenge these inferences. Controversy now exists as to whether cerebral vasodilation, brain sparing, is merely protective or on the contrary may be an indicator of future poor neurological development. In fact, the ability to diagnose the SGA fetus, defined by IUGR and normal umbilical artery Doppler studies, from the truly growth-restricted fetus has been called into question. Full-term SGA fetuses, as previously defined, have been shown to have poorer neonatal-behavioral-assessment scores in all areas, a higher incidence of suboptimal neurodevelopmental outcome with lower communication and problem-solving skills [93,94]. Larger studies with longer neonatal and infant follow-up will be required to solve this controversy.

Venous Doppler and fetal growth restriction

Chronic fetal hypoxemia results in decreased preload, decreased cardiac compliance, and elevated end-diastolic

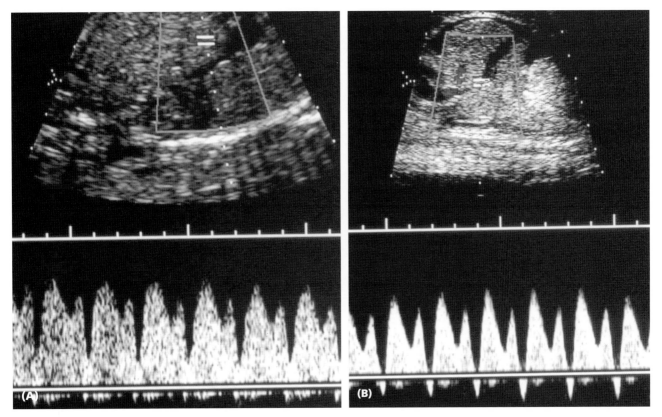

Figure 8.4 Doppler velocity waveforms of the ductus venosus in a normal fetus (A) and a severely compromised fetus (B) in the third trimester of pregnancy. Note the presence of reverse flow during late diastole in the severely compromised fetus (B). Reproduced from Abuhamad [104] with permission from Thieme Medical Publishing.

pressure in the right ventricle [72,95–98]. These changes are evident by an elevated central venous pressure in the chronically hypoxemic fetus, which is manifested by an increased reverse flow in Doppler waveforms of the ductus venosus (Fig. 8.4) and the inferior vena cava (Fig. 8.5) during late diastole. Changes in the fetal central venous circulation are associated with an advanced stage of fetal hypoxemia. At this late stage of fetal adaptation to hypoxemia, cardiac decompensation is often noted with myocardial dysfunction [97]. Furthermore, fetal metabolic acidemia is often present in association with Doppler waveform abnormalities of the inferior vena cava and ductus venosus [68,72,73].

Clinical application

In clinical practice, Doppler ultrasound provides important information on the extent of fetal compromise and thus may aid in the timing of delivery for IUGR fetuses. Arterial Doppler abnormalities, at the level of the umbilical and middle cerebral arteries (brain-sparing reflex), confirm the presence of hypoxemia in the growth-restricted fetus and present early warning signs. Once arterial centralization occurs, however, no clear trend is noted in the observational period and thus arterial

redistribution may not be helpful for the timing of delivery [99–101]. On the other hand, the presence of reversed diastolic flow in the umbilical arteries is a sign of advanced fetal compromise, and strong consideration should be given to delivery except in cases of extreme prematurity. Cesarean delivery following a course of corticosteroids, when appropriate, should be given preference in this setting as labor may cause further fetal compromise.

The current literature suggests that venous Doppler abnormalities in the inferior vena cava and ductus venosus and abnormal fetal heart rate monitoring follow arterial Doppler abnormalities and are thus associated with a more advanced stage of fetal compromise [73–76,102]. Furthermore, in the majority of severely growth-restricted fetuses, sequential deterioration of arterial and venous Doppler precedes biophysical profile score deterioration [74]. At least one-third of fetuses will show early signs of circulatory decompensation 1 week before biophysical profile deterioration and, in most cases, Doppler deterioration precedes deterioration of biophysical profile scores by 1 day [74].

The occurrence of such abnormal late-stage changes of vascular adaptation in the IUGR fetus appears to

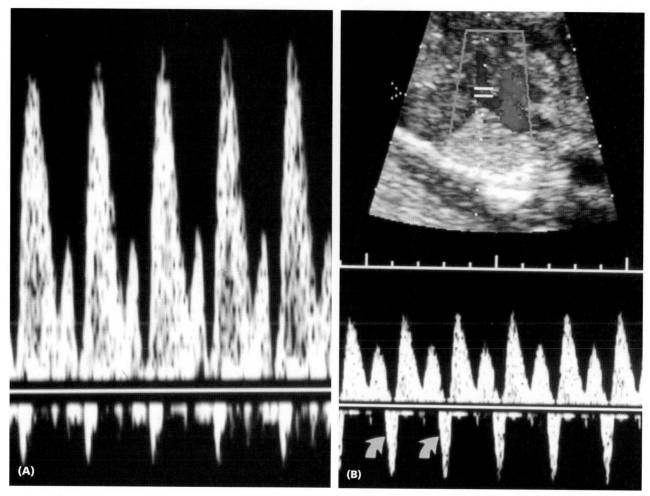

Figure 8.5 Doppler velocity waveforms of the inferior vena cava (IVC) in a normal fetus (A) and a severely compromised fetus (B) in the third trimester of pregnancy. The IVC Doppler waveforms have reverse flow during late diastole (atrial kick) in the normal fetus. Note the increase in reverse flow during late diastole in the severely compromised fetus (B) (*white arrowhead*). (A) Reproduced from Abuhamad [105] with permission from Elsevier; (B) Reproduced from Abuhamad [104] with permission from Thieme Medical Publishing.

be the best predictor of perinatal death, independent of gestational age and weight [76]. In a longitudinal study on Doppler and IUGR fetuses, all intrauterine deaths and all neonatal deaths, with the exception of one case, had late Doppler changes at the time of delivery, whereas only a few of the surviving fetuses showed such changes [76].

This sequential deterioration of the hypoxemic, growth-restricted fetus is rarely seen at gestations beyond 34 weeks [88,37]. Indeed, normal umbilical artery Doppler is common in growth-restricted fetuses in late gestation and cerebroplacental ratios have poor correlation with outcome of IUGR fetuses at more than 34 weeks' gestation [71]. Caution should therefore be exercised when umbilical artery Doppler is used in the clinical management of IUGR fetuses beyond 34 weeks' gestation.

The natural history and pathophysiology of fetal growth restriction have not been fully elucidated as recent studies have highlighted the presence of significant variation in fetal adaptation to hypoxemia. The pattern of incremental deterioration of arterial Doppler abnormalities, followed by venous Doppler abnormalities, then followed by fetal heart tracings and biophysical profile abnormalities is not seen in approximately 20% of preterm IUGR fetuses [73]. Furthermore, only 70% of IUGR fetuses showed significant deterioration of all vascular beds by the time they were delivered and approximately 10% showed no significant circulatory change by delivery time [74]. In a prospective observational study, more than 50% of IUGR fetuses delivered because of abnormal fetal heart rate tracings did not have venous Doppler abnormalities [76]. In view of these findings, the universal introduction of venous Doppler in the clinical management of the growth-restricted fetus should await the results of randomized trials on this subject.

It is currently evident that fetal growth restriction is a complex disorder involving multiple fetal organs and systems [103]. While fetal biometry and arterial Doppler provide information on the early compensatory phase of this disorder, venous Doppler, fetal heart rate analysis, and the biophysical profile provide information on the later stages, commonly associated with fetal cardiovascular collapse. It is hoped that future studies will shed more light on the pathophysiology of this disease and on the various interactions of diagnostic tools in fetal surveillance.

CASE PRESENTATION

The patient is a 40-year-old G3 P2002 with a pregnancy resulting from assisted reproduction with IVF. She presented to her obstetrician at 29 weeks' gestation for a routine prenatal visit. Prenatal care thus far had been uneventful except for abnormal quad screen with elevated maternal serum AFP and hCG. Detailed ultrasound examination at 19 weeks showed normal fetal anatomy.

Fundal height measured 26 cm and the patient was referred for an obstetric ultrasound examination. The patient reported good fetal movements, and vital signs were within normal limits with no proteinuria. Ultrasound examination revealed the following.

- Cephalic presentation.
- Normal amniotic fluid volume.
- BPD and HC at the 26th percentile for gestational age.
- AC at the 5th percentile for gestational age.
- Estimated fetal weight at the 7th percentile for gestational age.

When the biometric data were reported to the obstetrician, Doppler studies were ordered. Doppler studies revealed the following.

- Umbilical artery S:D = 8.0 (abnormal for 29 weeks).
- Middle cerebral artery pulsatility index = 1.50 (abnormal for gestational age).
- Forward flow in the ductus venosus during the entire cardiac cycle (normal).

In view of the presence of IUGR with abnormal arterial Doppler waveforms, the patient was sent to Labor and Delivery where a course of steroids was initiated and a nonstress test (NST) showed reactive fetal heart rate. The patient was discharged home with the following plan.

- Modified bedrest.
- Home nurse visitation in 24 h to complete the steroid course.
- Twice-weekly NSTs, including amniotic fluid assessment.
- Weekly Doppler studies to include the umbilical artery, the middle cerebral artery, and the ductus venosus.
- Follow-up fetal growth in 3 weeks.

At 31 weeks' gestation, 3 weeks from diagnosis, absent end-diastolic velocity in the umbilical artery was noted. The patient was admitted to the hospital for daily testing, a second course of steroids, and twice-weekly Doppler studies. Fetal biometry showed estimated fetal weight at the 4th percentile with decreased amniotic fluid volume. The patient reported normal fetal activity. Fetal surveillance studies on admission showed the following.

- Absent end-diastolic velocity with intermittent reversed end-diastolic velocity noted in the umbilical artery.
- Middle cerebral artery pulsatility index = 1.35.
- Absent flow in late diastole in the ductus venosus.
- NST with normal reactivity.

On the second day of hospitalization, the patient reported decreased fetal movements, NST showed spontaneous decelerations, and Doppler studies showed persistent reversed end-diastolic velocity in the umbilical artery with persistent reversed flow during late diastole (atrial kick) in the ductus venosus. Biophysical profile scored 4/8. The patient had a cesarean delivery of a male infant, weighing 1150 g with Apgar scores of 4 and 7 at 1 and 5 min, respectively. Arterial pH was 7.10 with base excess of −11. Both infant and mother did well with no major complications.

References

1. Chervenak FA, Skupski DW, Romero R et al. How accurate is fetal biometry in the assessment of fetal age? Am J Obstet Gynecol 1998;178:228–237.
2. Goldenberg RL, Davis RO, Cutter GR et al. Prematurity, postdates, and growth retardation: the influence of use of ultrasonography on reported gestational age. Am J Obstet Gynecol 1989;160:462–470.
3. Gardosi J, Vanner T, Francis A. Gestational age and induction of labour for prolonged pregnancy. Br J Obstet Gynaecol 1997;104:792–797.
4. Warren WB, Peisner DB, Raju S, Rosen MG. Dating the early pregnancy by sequential appearance of embryonic structures. Am J Obstet Gynecol 1989;161:747.
5. Daya S. Accuracy of gestational age estimation by means of fetal crown–rump length measurement. Am J Obstet Gynecol 1987;168:903–908.
6. Nyberg DA, Mack LA, Laing FC, Patten RM. Distinguishing normal from abnormal gestational sac growth in early pregnancy. J Ultrasound Med 1987;6:23–27.
7. Robinson HP, Fleming JE. A critical evaluation of sonar "crown–rump length" measurement. Br J Obstet Gynaecol 1975;82:702–710.

8. Drumm JE, Clinch J, McKenzie G. The ultrasonic measurement of fetal crown rump length as a method of assessing gestational age. Br J Obstet Gynaecol 1976;83:417–421.

9. Daya S, Woods S, Ward S, Lappainen R, Caco C. Early pregnancy assessment with transvaginal ultrasound scanning. Can Med Assoc J 1991;144:441–446.

10. Lasser DM, Peisner DB, Wollenbergh J, Timor-Trisch I. First trimester fetal biometry using transvaginal sonography. Ultrasound Obstet Gynecol 1993;3:104–108.

11. McGregor SN, Tamura RK, Sabbagha RE, Minogue JP, Gibson ME, Hoffman DI. Underestimation of gestational age by conventional crown rump length dating curves. Am J Obstet Gynecol 1987;70:344–348.

12. Wisser J, Dirscheld P. Estimation of gestational age by transvaginal sonographic measurement of greatest embryonic length in dated human embryos. Ultrasound Obstet Gynecol 1994;4:457–462.

13. Hadlock FP. Sonographic estimation of fetal age and weight. Radiol Clin North Am 1990;28:39–50.

14. Kurjak A, Kirkinen P, Latin V. Biometric and dynamic ultrasound assessment of small-for-dates infants: report of 260 cases. Obstet Gynecol 1980;56:281–284.

15. Landon MB, Mintz MC, Gabbe SG. Sonographic evaluation of fetal abdominal growth: predictor of the large for gestational age infant in pregnancies complicated by diabetes mellitus. Am J Obstet Gynecol 1989;160:115–121.

16. Basel D, Lederer R, Diamant YZ. Longitudinal ultrasonic biometry of various parameters in fetuses with abnormal growth rate. Acta Obstet Gynecol Scand 1987;66:143–149.

17. Hadlock FP. Ultrasound evaluation of fetal growth. In: Callen PW, ed. Ultrasonography in Obstetrics and Gynecology. Philadelphia: WB Saunders, 1994, pp.129–143.

18. Dudley NJ. Selection of appropriate ultrasound methods for estimation of fetal weight. Br J Radiol 1995;68:385–388.

19. Coombs CA, Jaekle RK, Rosenn B, Pope M, Miodovnik M, Siddiqi TA. Sonographic estimation of fetal weight based on a model of fetal volume. Obstet Gynecol 1993;82:365–370.

20. Hadlock FP, Harrist RB, Carpenter RJ, Deter RL, Park SK. Sonographic estimation of fetal weight. Radiology 1984;150:535–540.

21. Smith GCS, Smith MFS, McNay MB, Flemming JEE. The relation between fetal abdominal circumference and birthweight: findings in 3512 pregnancies. Br J Obstet Gynaecol 1997;104:186–190.

22. Gore D, Williams M, O'Brien W, Gilby J. Fetal abdominal circumference for prediction of intrauterine growth restriction. Obstet Gynecol 2000;95(Suppl 1):S78–79.

23. Rose BI, McCallum WD. A simplified method for estimating fetal weight using ultrasound measurements. Obstet Gynecol 1987;69:671–675.

24. Medchill MT, Peterson CM, Garbaciak J. Prediction of estimated fetal weight in extremely low birth weight neonates (500–1000 g). Obstet Gynecol 1991;78:286–290.

25. Robson SC, Gallivan S, Walkinshaw SA, Vaughan J, Rodeck CH. Ultrasonic estimation of fetal weight: use of targeted formulas in small for gestational age fetuses. Obstet Gynecol 1993;82:359–364.

26. Sabbagha RE, Minogue J, Tamura RK, Hungerford SA. Estimation of birth weight by use of ultrasonographic formulas targeted to large-, appropriate-, and small-for-gestational-age fetuses. Am J Obstet Gynecol 1989;160:854–862.

27. Edwards A, Goff J, Baker L. Accuracy and modifying factors of the sonographic estimation of fetal weight 26: Aust N Z J Obstet Gynaecol 2001;41:187–190.

28. Baum JD, Gussman D, Wirth JC 3rd. Clinical and patient estimation of fetal weight vs. ultrasound estimation. J Reprod Med 2002;47:194–198.

29. Divon M, Chamberlain P, Sipos L, Manning F, Platt L. Identification of the small for gestational age independent indices of fetal growth. Am J Obstet Gynecol 1986;155:1197–2003.

30. Owen P, Maharaj S, Khan KS, Howie PW. Interval between fetal measurements in predicting growth restriction. Obstet Gynecol 2001;97:499–504.

31. Ott WJ. The diagnosis of altered fetal growth. Obstet Gynecol Clin North Am 1988;15; 237–263.

32. Manning FA. Intrauterine growth restriction. Diagnosis, prognostication, and management based on ultrasound methods. In: Manning FA, ed. Fetal Medicine: Principles and Practice. Norwalk, CT: Appleton and Lange, 1995.

33. Hadlock FP, Deter RL, Harrist RB, Roecker E, Park SK. A date-independent predictor of intrauterine growth retardation: femur length/abdominal circumference ration. Am J Roentgenol 1993;141:979–984.

34. Brown HL, Miller JM Jr, Gabert HA, Kissling G. Ultrasonic recognition of the small-for-gestational-age fetus. Obstet Gynecol 1987;69:631–635.

35. Creasy RK, Resnick R. Intrauterine growth retardation. In: Creasy RK, Resnick R, eds. Maternal Fetal Medicine: Principles and Practice. Philadelphia: Saunders, 1984.

36. Powell K, Sanderson M, Chauhan SP. Inadequate identification of small for gestational age: experience at urban teaching hospital. Int J Obstet Gynecol 2010;109:140–143.

37. Hecher K, Campbell S, Doyle P, Harrington K, Nicolaides K. Assessment of fetal compromise by Doppler ultrasound investigation of the fetal circulation. Arterial, intracardiac, and venous blood flow velocity studies. Circulation 1995;91:129–138.

38. Gardosi J, Francis A. Adverse pregnancy outcome and association with small for gestational age birthweight by customized and population-based percentiles. Am J Obstet Gynecol 2009;201(1):28.

39. American College of Obstetricians and Gynecologists. Intrauterine Growth Restriction. ACOG Practice Bulletin No. 12. Washington, DC: American College of Obstetricians and Gynecologists, 2000.

40. David C, Gabrielli S, Pilu G, Bovicelli L. The head-to-abdomen circumference ratio: a reappraisal. Ultrasound Obstet Gynecol 1995;5:256–259.

41. Dashe JS, McIntire DD, Lucas MJ, Leveno KJ. Effects of symmetric and asymmetric fetal growth on pregnancy outcomes. Obstet Gynecol 2000;96:321–327.

42. Vik T, Vatten L, Jacobsen G, Bakketeig LS. Prenatal growth in symmetric and asymmetric small-for-gestational-age infants. Early Hum Dev 1997;48:167–176.

43. Blackwell SC, Moldenhauer J, Redman M, Hassan SS, Wolfe HM, Berry SM. Relationship between the sonographic pattern of intrauterine growth restriction and acid–base status at the

time of cordocentensis. Arch Gynecol Obstet 2001;264: 191–193.

44. Benson CB, Doubilet PM, Saltzman DH, Jones TB. FL/AC ratio: poor predictor of intrauterine growth retardation. Invest Radiol 1985;20:727–730.

45. Rasmussen S, Irgens LM, Albrechtsen S, Dalaker K. Predicting preeclampsia in the second pregnancy from low birth weight in the first pregnancy. Obstet Gynecol 2000;96:696–700.

46. Stipoljev F, Latin V, Kos M, Miskovic B, Kurjak A. Correlation of confined placental mosaicism with fetal intrauterine growth retardation: a case–control study of placentas at delivery. Fetal Diagn Ther 2001;16:4–9.

47. Mitra SC, Seshan SV, Riachi LE. Placental vessel morphometry in growth retardation and increased resistance of the umbilical artery Doppler flow. J Matern Fetal Med 2000;9: 282–286.

48. Devriendt K. Genetic control of intra-uterine growth. Eur J Obstet Gynecol Reprod Biol 2000;92:29–34.

49. Snijders RJ, Sherrod C, Gosden CM, Nicolaides KH. Fetal growth retardation: associated malformations and chromosomal abnormalities. Am J Obstet Gynecol 1993; 168:547–555.

50. Dicke JM, Crane JP. Sonographic recognition of major malformations and aberrant fetal growth in trisomic fetuses. J Ultrasound Med 1991;10:433–438.

51. Magnus P, Bakketeig LS, Hoffman H. Birth weight of relatives by maternal tendency to repeat small-for-gestational-age (SGA) births in successive pregnancies. Acta Obstet Gynecol Scand 1997;165(Suppl):35–38.

52. Pedersen NG, Figueras F, Wojdemann KR, Tabor A, Gardosi J. Early fetal size and growth as predictors of adverse outcome. Obstet Gynecol 2008;112(4):765–771.

53. Bernstein IM, Horbar JD, Badger GJ, Ohlsson A, Golan A. Morbidity and mortality among very-low-birth weight neonates with intrauterine growth restriction. Am J Obstet Gynecol 2000;182:198–202.

54. Kok JH, den Ouden AL, Verloove-Vanhorick SP, Brand R. Outcome of very preterm small for gestational age infants: the first nine years of life. Br J Obstet Gynaecol 1998;105: 162–168.

55. Fattal-Valevski A, Leitner Y, Kutai M et al. Neurodevelopmental outcome in children with intrauterine growth retardation: a 3-year follow-up [Abstract]. J Child Neurol 1999;14:724–727.

56. Soothill PW, Ajayi RA, Campbell S et al. Relationship between fetal academia at cordocentesis and subsequent neurodevelopment. Ultrasound Obstet Gynecol 1992;2:80–83.

57. Froen JF, Gardosi JO, Thurmann A, Francis A, Stray-Pedersen B. Restricted fetal growth in sudden intrauterine unexplained death. Acta Obstet Gynecol Scand 2004;83(9):801–807.

58. Turan S, Miller J, Baschat AA. Integrated testing and management in fetal growth restriction. Semin Perinatol 2008; 32(3):194–200.

59. GRIT Study Group. A randomised trial of timed delivery for the compromised preterm fetus: short term outcomes and Bayesian interpretation. Br J Obstet Gynaecol 2003;110(1): 27–32.

60. Baschat AA, Cosmi E, Bilardo CM et al Predictors of neonatal outcome in early-onset placental dysfunction. Obstet Gynecol 2007;109:253–261.

61. Lubow JM, How HY, Habli M, Maxwell R, Sibai BM. Indications for delivery and short-term neonatal outcomes in late preterm as compared with term births. Am J Obstet Gynecol 2009;200(5):e30–33.

62. Cheng YW, Nicholson JM, Nakagawa S, Bruckner TA, Washington AE, Caughey AB. Perinatal outcomes in low-risk term pregnancies: do they differ by week of gestation? Am J Obstet Gynecol 2008;199(4):370.

63. Hanna BD, Nelson MN, White-Traut RC et al. Heart rate variability in preterm brain-injured and very-low-birth-weight infants. Biol Neonate 2000;77:147–155.

64. Nijhuis IJ, ten Hof J, Mulder EJ et al. Fetal heart rate in relation to its variation in normal and growth retarded fetuses. Eur J Obstet Gynecol Reprod Biol 2000;89:27–33.

65. Vindla S, James D, Sahota D. Computerised analysis of unstimulated and stimulated behaviour in fetuses with intrauterine growth restriction. Eur J Obstet Gynecol Reprod Biol 199;83:37–45.

66. Devoe L, Golde S, Kilman Y, Morton D, Shea K, Waller J. A comparison of visual analyses of intrapartum fetal heart rate tracings according to the new National Institute of Child Health and Human Development guidelines with computer analyses by an automated fetal heart rate monitoring system. Am J Obstet Gynecol 2000;183:361–366.

67. Bracero LA, Roshanfekr D, Byrne DW. Analysis of antepartum fetal heart rate tracing by physician and computer. J Matern Fetal Med 2000;9:181–185.

68. Hecher K, Hackeler B. Cardiotocogram compared to Doppler investigation of the fetal circulation in the premature growth-retarded fetus: longitudinal observations. Ultrasound Obstet Gynecol 1997;9:152–160.

69. Ribbert LS, Visser GH, Mulder EJ, Zonneveld MF, Morssink LP. Changes with time in fetal heart rate variation, movement incidences and haemodynamics in intrauterine growth retarded fetuses: a longitudinal approach to the assessment of fetal well being. Early Hum Dev 1993;31:195–208.

70. Zarko A, Neilson JP. Doppler ultrasonography in high-risk pregnancies: systematic review with meta-analysis. Am J Obstet Gynecol 1995;172:1379–1387.

71. Bahado-Singh RO, Kovanci E, Jeffres A et al. The Doppler cerebroplacental ratio and perinatal outcome in intrauterine growth restriction. Am J Obstet Gynecol 1999;180:750–756.

72. Rizzo G, Capponi A, Talone PE, Arduini D, Romanini C. Doppler indices from inferior vena cava and ductus venosus in predicting pH and oxygen tension in umbilical blood at cordocentesis in growth-retarded fetuses. Ultrasound Obstet Gynecol 1996;7:401–410.

73. Baschat AA, Gembruch U, Reiss I, Gortner L, Weiner CP, Harman CR. Relationship between arterial and venous Doppler and perinatal outcome in fetal growth restriction. Ultrasound Obstet Gynecol 2000;16:407–413.

74. Baschat AA, Gembruch U, Harman CR. The sequence of changes in Doppler and biophysical parameters as severe fetal growth restriction worsens. Ultrasound Obstet Gynecol 2001;18:571–577.

75. Hecher K, Bilardo CM, Stigter RH et al. Monitoring of fetuses with intrauterine growth restriction: a longitudinal study. Ultrasound Obstet Gynecol 2001;18:564–570.

76. Ferrazzi E, Bozzo M, Rigano S et al. Temporal sequence of abnormal Doppler changes in the peripheral and central

circulatory systems of the severely growth-restricted fetus. Ultrasound Obstet Gynecol 2002;19:140–146.

77. Fleischer A, Schulman H, Farmakides G, Bracero L, Blattner P, Randolph G. Umbilical artery waveforms and intrauterine growth retardation. Am J Obstet Gynecol 1985;151: 502–505.

78. Giles WB, Trudinger BJ, Baird PJ. Fetal umbilical artery flow velocity waveforms and placental resistance: pathological correlation. Br J Obstet Gynaecol 1987;157:900–902.

79. Trudinger BJ, Stevens D, Connelly A et al. Umbilical artery flow velocity waveforms and placental resistance: the effect of embolizations of the umbilical circulation. Am J Obstet Gynecol 1987;157:1443–1448.

80. Kingdom JC, Burrell SJ, Kaufmann P. Pathology and clinical implications of abnormal umbilical artery Doppler waveforms. Ultrasound Obstet Gynecol 1997;9:271–286.

81. Morrow RJ, Adamson SL, Bull SB, Ritchie JW. Effect of placental embolization on the umbilical arterial velocity waveform in fetal sheep. Am J Obstet Gynecol 1989;161: 1055–1060.

82. Copel JA, Reed KL. Doppler Ultrasound in Obstetrics and Gynecology. New York: Raven Press, 1995, pp.187–198.

83. Trudinger BJ. Doppler ultrasonography and fetal well being. In: Reece EA, Hobbins JC, Mahoney M, Petrie RH, eds. Medicine of the Fetus and Mother. Philadelphia: JB Lippincott, 1992.

84. Mari G, Deter RL. Middle cerebral artery flow velocity waveforms in normal and small-for-gestational age fetuses. Am J Obstet Gynecol 1992;166:1262–1270.

85. Veille JC, Hanson R, Tatum K. Longitudinal quantitation of middle cerebral artery blood flow in normal human fetuses. Am J Obstet Gynecol 1993;169:1393–1398.

86. Berman RE, Less MH, Peterson EN, Delannoy CW. Distribution of the circulation in the normal and asphyxiated fetal primate. Am J Obstet Gynecol 1970;108:956–969.

87. Mari G, Abuhamad AZ, Brumfield J, Ferguson JE III. Doppler ultrasonography of the middle cerebral artery peak systolic velocity in the fetus: reproducibility of measurement. Am J Obstet Gynecol 2001;185:Abstract 669.

88. Harrington K, Thompson MO, Carpenter RG et al. Doppler fetal circulation in pregnancies complicated by pre-eclampsia or delivery of a small for gestational age baby: 2. Longitudinal analysis. Br J Obstet Gynaecol 1999;106:453–466.

89. Wladimoroff JW, van den Wijingaard JAGN, Degani S, Noordam MJ, van Eyck J, Tonge HM. Cerebral and umbilical arterial blood flow velocity waveforms in normal and growth retarded pregnancies: a comparative study. Obstet Gynecol 1987;69:705–709.

90. Gramellini D, Folli MC, Raboni S, Vadora E, Marialdi A. Cerebral–umbilical Doppler ratio as a predictor of adverse perinatal outcome. Obstet Gynecol 1992;74:416–420.

91. Arduini D, Rizzo G. Prediction of fetal outcome in small for gestational age fetuses: comparison of Doppler measurements obtained from different fetal vessels. J Perinat Med 1992;20:29–38.

92. Fong KW, Ohlsson A, Hannah ME et al. Prediction of perinatal outcomes in fetuses suspected to have intrauterine growth restriction: Doppler US study of fetal cerebral, renal and umbilical arteries. Radiology 1999;213:681–689.

93. Cruz-Martinez R, Figueras F, Oros D et al. Cerebral blood perfusion and neurobehavioral performance in full-term small-for-gestational-age fetuses. Am J Obstet Gynecol 2009;201:474.

94. Eixarch E, Meler E, Iraola A et al. Neurodevelopmental outcome in 2-year-old infants who were small-for-gestatioinal-age term fetuses with cerebral blood flow redistribution. Ultrasound Obstet Gynecol 2008;32:894–899.

95. Rizzo G, Arduini D. Fetal cardiac function in intrauterine growth retardation. Am J Obstet Gynecol 1991;165:876–882.

96. Chang CH, Chang FM, Yu CH, Liang RI, Ko HC, Chen HY. Systemic assessment of fetal hemodynamics by Doppler ultrasound. Ultrasound Med Biol 2000;26:777–785.

97. Mäkikallio K, Vuolteenaho O, Jouppila P, Räsänen J. Ultrasonographic and biochemical markers of human fetal cardiac dysfunction in placental insufficiency. Circulation 2002;105:2058–2062.

98. Tsyvian P, Malkin K, Wladimiroff JY. Assessment of mitral a-wave transit time to cardiac outflow tract and isovolumic relaxation time of left ventricle in the appropriate and small-for-gestational-age human fetus. Ultrasound Med Biol 1997;23:187–190.

99. Baschat AA, Gembruch U, Gortner L et al. Coronary artery blood flow visualization signifies hemodynamic deterioration in growth restricted fetuses. Ultrasound Obstet Gynecol 2000;16:425–431.

100. Senat MV, Schwarzler P, Alcais A et al. Longitudinal changes in the ductus venosus, cerebral transverse sinus and cardiotocogram in fetal growth restriction. Ultrasound Obstet Gynecol 2000;16:19–24.

101. Baschat AA, Gembruch U, Weiner CP et al. Longitudinal changes of arterial and venous Doppler in fetuses with intrauterine growth restriction [Abstract]. Am J Obstet Gynecol 2001;184:103.

102. Pardi G, Cetin I, Marconi AM et al. Diagnostic value of blood sampling in fetuses with growth retardation. N Engl J Med 1993;328:692–696.

103. Romero R, Kalache KD, Kadar N. Timing the delivery of the preterm severely growth-restricted fetus: venous Doppler, cardiotocography or the biophysical profile? Ultrasound Obstet Gynecol 2002;19:118–121.

104. Abuhamad A. Uterine size less than dates: a clinical dilemma. In: Bluth EI, Benson CB, Ralls PW, Siegel MJ, eds. Ultrasound: Practical Approach to Clinical Problems, 2nd edn. New York: Thieme Medical Publishing, 2006, pp.56–60.

105. Abuhamad A. Doppler ultrasound in obstetrics. Ultrasound Clin 2006;6:293–301.

Chapter 9
Fetal Lung Maturity

Alessandro Ghidini and Sarah H. Poggi

Department of Obstetrics and Gynecology, Georgetown University Hospital, Washington, DC, and Perinatal Diagnostic Center, Inova Alexandria Hospital, Alexandria, VA, USA

Fetal lung maturity tests are performed on amniotic fluid and they evaluate fetal lung maturation either by quantifying components of pulmonary surfactant (e.g. lecithin, phosphatidylglycerol, or lamellar bodies) or by measuring the surface active effects of the phospholipids in the surfactant.

Indications for assessment of fetal pulmonary maturity

Fetal pulmonic maturity should be documented before scheduled delivery at less than 39 weeks' gestation [1]. Examples of clinical scenarios that may suggest the need to assess for fetal lung maturity include preterm labor (as tocolysis is generally contraindicated in the presence of mature fetal lungs), iatrogenic preterm delivery (although fetal lung maturity test is contraindicated when delivery is required for fetal or maternal indications), or presence of unsure dates. Testing is not recommended before 32 weeks given the high likelihood of respiratory distress syndrome even in the presence of results suggestive of mature fetal lungs [2].

Techniques for obtaining amniotic fluid

Amniocentesis
Amniocentesis performed under ultrasonographic guidance in experienced hands is associated with low rates of failure or of bloody fluid collection, and a lower than 1% risk of complications, such as emergency delivery [3].

Vaginal pool collection
Tests for fetal pulmonary maturity can be performed on fluid obtained from vaginal pool specimens in the presence of premature rupture of membranes. Vaginally free-flowing collected fluid can be evaluated for determination of lecithin:sphingomyelin (L:S) ratio, surfactant:albumin ratio (SAR), phosphatidylglycerol (PG), and lamellar body counts (LBC), yielding results similar to those observed with samples obtained with amniocentesis.

Specific tests for lung maturity

Lecithin:sphingomyelin ratio
The concentrations of these two substances are approximately equal until about 32 weeks, when the concentration of pulmonary lecithin increases significantly while the nonpulmonary sphingomyelin concentration remains unchanged. Determination of the ratio involves thin-layer chromatography after centrifugation to remove the cellular component and organic solvent extraction. The technique is expensive, time consuming and requires highly trained personnel.

An L:S ratio of 2.0 or greater predicts absence of respiratory distress syndrome (RDS) in 98% of neonates. With a ratio of 1.5–1.9, approximately 50% of infants will develop RDS [4]. Maternal serum has a L:S ratio ranging from 1.3 to 1.9; thus, blood-tinged samples can falsely lower a result (but a mature test can reliably predict pulmonary maturity). The presence of meconium can interfere with test interpretation, increasing the L:S ratio by 0.1–0.5, thus leading to an increase in falsely mature results.

Phosphatidylglycerol
Phosphatidylglycerol (PG) is a minor constituent of surfactant that becomes evident in amniotic fluid several weeks after the rise in lecithin [5]. Its presence indicates a more advanced state of fetal lung development and function, as PG enhances the spread of phospholipids on the alveoli.

Phosphatidylglycerol testing can be performed by thin-layer chromatography (which requires time and

Queenan's Management of High-Risk Pregnancy: An Evidence-Based Approach, Sixth Edition. Edited by John T. Queenan, Catherine Y. Spong, Charles J. Lockwood.

expertise) or slide agglutination (AmnioStat FLM), which is quicker and cheaper. PG determination is not generally affected by blood, meconium or vaginal secretion. The results are typically reported qualitatively as positive or negative, where positive represents an exceedingly low risk of RDS. Due to its late appearance in pregnancy, there is a high falsely immature rate (i.e. negative PG results in neonates without RDS).

Surfactant:albumin ratio (TDx test)

The fluorescence polarization assay uses polarized light to evaluate the competitive binding of a probe to both albumin and surfactant in amniotic fluid. The SAR is determined, with amniotic fluid albumin used as an internal reference. The TDx test requires 1 mL amniotic fluid and can be run in less than 1 h.

A recent commercial modification of the assay (TDx-FlxFLM II) allows simple, automated, and rapid results. A SAR of 55 mg/g has been proposed as the optimal threshold to indicate maturity [6]. Values of 35–55 are considered "borderline." The test is affected by blood contamination, as red blood cell phospholipids may falsely lower the TDx-FLM result, but a mature test can reliably predict pulmonary maturity.

Lamellar body counts

Lamellar bodies, the storage form of surfactant, are released into the amniotic fluid by fetal type II pneumocytes. Because they are the same size as platelets, the amniotic fluid concentration of lamellar bodies may be determined using a commercial cell counter. The test requires less than 1 mL amniotic fluid and takes only 15 min to perform. Although initial studies employed centrifugation, it is now agreed that the sample should be processed without spinning as centrifugation reduces the number of lamellar bodies.

Values of 40,000–50,000/μL generally indicate pulmonary maturity, while a count below 15,000/μL suggests a significant risk for RDS [7]. However, ideally, laboratories should develop their own reference standards [8]. The test compares favorably with L:S for diagnostic ability (sensitivity and false mature test results) in predicting RDS [9,10]. Meconium does not affect LBC results, whereas bloody fluid can increase the count because the platelets are counted as lamellar bodies.

Foam Stability Index

The Foam Stability Index (FSI) is derived from the shake test, an assay of surfactant function that evaluates the ability of pulmonary surfactant to generate stable foam in the presence of ethanol. The commercially prepared test kit contains wells with a predispensed volume of ethanol. Adding amniotic fluid to each test well produces final ethanol concentrations ranging from 44% to 50%. After shaking the amniotic fluid–ethanol mixture, one reads the FSI as the highest well in which a rim of stable foam persists at meniscus. RDS has been reported to be unlikely with an FSI of 47% or higher; however, a negative test often occurs in the presence of a mature lung. The FSI cannot be derived from an amniotic fluid specimen contaminated by blood or meconium [11].

Multiple tests or cascade?

Faced with different assays for fetal lung maturity, some laboratories perform multiple tests simultaneously, leaving the clinician with the possibility of results both indicative and not of pulmonary maturity from the same amniotic fluid specimen. In general, any "mature" test result is indicative of fetal pulmonic maturity given the high predictive value of any single test (5% or less of false mature rates). Conversely, the use of a "cascade" approach has been proposed to minimize the costs. In this approach, a rapid and inexpensive test is performed first, with follow-up tests performed only in the face of immaturity of the initial test (e.g. LBC or TDx-FLM as the initial test and L:S ratio as the final test).

Clinical conditions affecting risk of respiratory distress syndrome and predictive value of pulmonary maturity tests

Although optimal cut-offs for prediction of fetal lung maturity are available for each test, several variables affect the risk of RDS and modify the predictive value of pulmonary maturity tests, including gestational age, ethnicity, maternal conditions (e.g. poorly controlled diabetes or red blood cell isoimmunization), fetal gender, and mode of delivery [12–16]. In African-Americans, lung maturity is achieved at lower gestational ages and at lower L:S ratios (1.2 or greater) than in white people. Female gender is associated with acceleration of lung maturation. In contrast, poorly controlled maternal diabetes and red blood cell isoimmunization are associated with a delay in fetal lung maturation. Some authors have recommended the use of higher thresholds of L:S ratio (e.g. a cut-off ratio of 3) to establish pulmonic maturity in these conditions [17]. Presence of PG is commonly considered as the gold standard for documentation of fetal lung maturity with diabetes or red blood cell isoimmunization.

In twin gestations with discordant gender or discordant weight, it is commonly recommended that the sac of the male twin or the larger twin be sampled at amniocentesis [18]. The reasoning is that if the sampled twin has mature pulmonic results, the other twin is even more likely to be mature.

Less need for testing?

Recent changes in clinical practice have, in many cases, reduced the need for determining fetal lung maturity. More obstetricians are scheduling ultrasound examinations early in pregnancy, thereby establishing gestational age more accurately. The result is that elective deliveries at term can be scheduled without determining fetal lung maturation. Similarly, in pregnancies complicated by diabetes mellitus, excellent maternal glucose control through self-monitoring of blood glucose levels and therapy, combined with intensive antepartum fetal surveillance, has reduced the need for induction of labor at 39 weeks or less, making amniocentesis to establish fetal lung maturity unnecessary.

CASE PRESENTATION

A 32-year-old white, G3P2002 patient has a known complete previa in the setting of poorly controlled gestational diabetes and is carrying a male fetus. She is at 35–37 weeks, with the uncertainty a result of her late entry to prenatal care and the possibility of a large for gestational age (LGA) baby because of her diabetes. An amniocentesis for lung maturity is recommended to aid with delivery planning.

The lamellar count comes back within the hour at 42,000. Because of concern that this is not over the threshold value of 50,000 recommended for diabetic mothers and because results may be falsely increased, at least initially, by blood contamination, the decision is made to wait for L:S and PG results before delivery (a cascade approach).

Later that day, the L:S ratio is noted to be 1.9 and the PG is negative. The decision is made to defer delivery and continue antepartum testing. Assuming no bleeding from the previa or fetal issues that would prompt delivery regardless of fetal lung maturity status, the amniocentesis will be repeated in 1 week.

References

1. American College of Obstetricians and Gynecologists. Fetal lung maturity. ACOG Educational Bulletin No. 97. Washington, DC: American College of Obstetricians and Gynecologists, 2008.
2. Ghidini A, Hicks C, Lapinski R, Lockwood CJ. Morbidity in the preterm infant with mature lung indices. Am J Perinatol 1997;14:75–78.
3. Hodor JG, Poggi SH, Spong CY et al. Risk of third-trimester amniocentesis: a case-control study. Am J Perinatol 2006; 23:177–180.
4. Harper MA, Lorenz WB. Immature lecithin/sphingomyelin ratios and respirator course. Am J Obstet Gynecol 1993;168: 495.
5. Towers CV, Garite TJ. Evaluation of the new Amniostat-FLM test for the detection of phosphatidylglycerol in contaminated fluids. Am J Obstet Gynecol 1989;160:298.
6. Kesselman EJ, Figueroa R, Garry D, Maulik D. The usefulness of the TDx/TDxFLx fetal lung maturity II assay in the initial evaluation of fetal lung maturity. Am J Obstet Gynecol 2003;188:1220–1222.
7. Neerhof MG, Dohnal JC, Ashwood ER, Lee IS, Anceschi MM. Lamellar body counts: a consensus on protocol. Obstet Gynecol 2001;97:318–320.
8. Janicki MB, Dries LM, Egan JF, Zelop CM. Determining a cutoff for fetal lung maturity with lamellar body count testing. J Matern Fetal Neonatal Med 2009;22:419–422.
9. Ghidini A, Poggi SH, Spong CY, Goodwin KM, Vink J, Pezzullo JC. Role of lamellar body count for the prediction of neonatal respiratory distress syndrome in non-diabetic pregnant women. Arch Gynecol Obstet 2005;271:325–328.
10. Wijnberger LD, Huisjes AJ, Voorbij HA, Franx A, Bruinse HW, Moll BV. The accuracy of lamellar body count and lecithin/sphingomyelin ratio in the prediction of neonatal respiratory distress syndrome: a meta-analysis. Br J Obstet Gynaecol 2001;108:585–588.
11. Lipshitz J, Whybrew W, Anderson G. Comparison of the Lumadex-foam stability test, lectithin:sphingomyelin ratio, and simple shake test for fetal lung maturity. Obstet Gynecol 1984;63:349.
12. Karcher R, Sykes E, Batton D et al. Gestational age-specific predicted risk of neonatal respiratory distress syndrome using lamellar body count and surfactant-to-albumin ratio in amniotic fluid. Am J Obstet Gynecol 2005;193:1680–1684.
13. Parvin CA, Kaplan LA, Chapman JF, McManamon TG, Gronowski AM. Predicting respiratory distress syndrome using gestational age and fetal lung maturity by fluorescent polarization. Am J Obstet Gynecol 2005;192:199–207.
14. Wijnberger LDE, de Kleine M, Voorbij HAM et al. Comparison of vaginal and transabdominal collection of amniotic fluid for fetal lung maturity tests. J Matern Fetal Neonatal Med 2010;23:613–616.
15. De Luca AK, Nakazawa CY, Azevedo BC etal. Influence of glycemic control on fetal lung maturity in gestations affected by diabetes or mild hyperglycemia. Acta Obstet Gynecol Scand 2009;88:1036–1040.

16. Bennasar M, Figueras F, Palacio M et al. Gestational age-specific cutoff levels of TDx-FLM II for the prediction of neonatal respiratory distress syndrome. Fetal Diagn Ther 2009;25:392–396.

17. Ghidini A, Spong CY, Goodwin K, Pezzullo JC. Optimal thresholds of lecithin/sphingomyelin ratio and lamellar body count for the prediction of the presence of phosphatidyl-glycerol in diabetic women. J Matern Fetal Neonatal Med 2002;12:95–98.

18. Mackenzie MW. Predicting concordance of biochemical lung maturity in the preterm twin gestation. J Matern Fetal Neonatal Med 2002;12:50–58.

Chapter 10
Antepartum Fetal Monitoring

Brian L. Shaffer and Julian T. Parer
Department of Obstetrics, Gynecology and Reproductive Sciences, University of California, San Francisco, CA, USA

The goal of antenatal surveillance is to prevent fetal injury and death. Antenatal testing should improve long-term neurologic outcome through optimal timing of delivery while avoiding unnecessary intervention, such as cesarean or preterm delivery.

The US National Center for Health Statistics (NCHS) defines intrauterine fetal death (IUFD) as death prior to birth, 20 or more weeks in gestation, without evidence of life such as neonatal breathing, pulsation of the umbilical cord, a heartbeat, and without voluntary movements. However, gasping, fleeting movements, transient cardiac contractions, and respiratory gasps are not considered signs of life [1].

To assist in reaching the Healthy People 2010 goal of an IUFD incidence of 4.1/1000 [2], the etiology of IUFD must be clarified. Several approaches based on the timing of the event, gestational age, and specifying the abnormal "compartment" (i.e. maternal, fetal, or placental) have been proposed [3].

The most common etiologies in those less than 27 weeks include infection, abruption, and lethal congenital anomalies. In comparison, the most frequent causes of stillbirth at more than 28 weeks are growth restriction and abruption. However, unexplained deaths account for 27–50% of cases of IUFD after 20 weeks [3–5].

Those mothers who are at increased risk for IUFD are often referred for some type of antenatal surveillance. Despite performing antepartum testing for several decades, unequivocal evidence does not clearly illustrate for whom, at what gestational age, how frequently, and which specific test should be employed to improve perinatal outcomes. The standard should be determined by the performance of each specific test— in this case the sensitivity and specificity, compared with the rate of stillbirth and the week-specific mortality rate.

There are several antepartum testing modalities from which to choose, including fetal movement or "kick counts," the nonstress test (NST), the Amniotic Fluid Index (AFI) combined with the NST (modified biophysical profile), the contraction stress test (CST), the biophysical profile (BPP), and use of Doppler velocimetry. Our aim is to present a reasonable guide to answer the "who, what, when, where and why" of antepartum fetal monitoring.

Fetal movement or "kick counts"

Decreased fetal movement may precede fetal death by several days [6]. Because up to 50% of those with IUFD have no risk factors and thus undergo no formal antepartum surveillance, some have recommended kick counts for all patients [6,7]. One study of intervention after decreased movements

has been associated with decreasing the IUFD rate [7]. Defining what constitutes "decreased movement" varies, and regardless of the method, once decreased fetal movement has been diagnosed, a back-up test is employed. One evaluation of maternal perception of kick counts used 10 movements in 2h. After implementing formal fetal movement counts, the authors found a decreased stillbirth rate from 8.7/1000 to 2.1/1000 [7]. However, Grant *et al* [8] found no difference in mortality in those who presented after decreased fetal movement. The authors reported that women with decreased movement presented earlier with stillborns, whereas those in routine care were diagnosed at the next visit. The authors asserted that fetal death was predictable but not preventable and large amounts of provider and maternal time were necessary to prevent a single IUFD. Specifically, 1250 women would have to perform movement counts to prevent a single stillbirth [8]. In contrast, Froen [9], in a meta-analysis, highlights the shortcomings of the Grant *et al* study and asserts that vigilance toward maternal perception of fetal movements significantly reduces avoidable stillbirth rates in those with risk factors and is nearly

Queenan's Management of High-Risk Pregnancy: An Evidence-Based Approach, Sixth Edition. Edited by John T. Queenan, Catherine Y. Spong, Charles J. Lockwood.

statistically lower in women without risk factors while "costing" only an additional antenatal visit in 2–3% of pregnancies. With few patients returning for unscheduled visits, this low "false alarm" rate seems acceptable as fetal movement monitoring may reduce fetal deaths in women with and without risk factors for fetal death.

Nonstress test

The NST is a recording of fetal heart rate and uterine activity and is performed with the patient in the semi-Fowler position with left lateral tilt. The fetal heart rate transducer and tocodynamometer are placed on the maternal abdomen. A "reactive" or normal test is one in which there is a normal fetal heart rate tracing (FHT) baseline (110–160 beats per minute [beats/min]), with moderate variability (6–25 beats/min), and two accelerations (FHT peaks 15 beats/min above the baseline for ≥15 sec). A reactive NST is associated with survival for 7 days in 99% of cases [10]. The duration of an NST is normally 20 min but an additional 20 min may be added if needed.

The variability and baseline of the FHT are governed by a functioning cortex, brainstem, and cardiac conduction system. However, a reactive NST does not necessarily reflect an entirely normal central nervous system, as a fetus affected by holoprosencephaly may still have a reactive NST [11].

The value of the NST relies on several assumptions, which can be made after a few characteristics are observed. In the presence of a normal baseline rate, variability, and accelerations, the fetus is presumed to be nonacidemic and nonhypoxic. The acceleration is a response to fetal movement. Adequate accelerations have been associated with sonographically detected fetal movement in 99% of cases [12]. Several factors have been identified as modulators of accelerations, including sympathetic discharge, fetal circadian rhythm, gestational age, and maternal medication or illicit drug exposure. Maternal smoking has been associated with decreased FHT reactivity [13,14]. Similarly, assumptions can be made about the fetal status when accelerations are absent during an NST. Fetal sleep cycles usually last 20–40 min but may be longer. Fetal movement and accelerations are less likely to occur during sleep. Also, non-REM sleep is associated with reduced FHT variability [15]. Thus, extending the NST duration to 40 min allows for variation in sleep–wake cycle. Lack of accelerations, however, may indicate a fetal state of hypoxemia or acidemia, central nervous system (CNS) depression, or congenital anomalies.

Variable decelerations during an NST are not infrequent and may occur in up to 50% of those undergoing testing. If variable decelerations are nonrepetitive, lasting less than 30 sec, and occur in the setting of an otherwise reactive NST, there is no need for intervention [16]. However, three or more variable decelerations in 20 min have been associated with increased cesarean rates for nonreassuring FHT [17,18]. Decelerations lasting more than 60 sec have been associated with IUFD and cesarean for nonreassuring FHT [19–21].

A nonreactive NST over a 40-min testing period may indicate fetal compromise, but there is a considerable false-positive rate and gestational age must be considered because in one study 50% of healthy fetuses between 24 and 28 weeks had a nonreactive NST [22]. At 28–32 weeks, only 15% of normal fetuses were not reactive [23].

Vibroacoustic stimulation (VAS) can be used without compromising the detection of the impaired fetus while shortening the time to produce a reactive test [24–27]. Often, VAS is used after a period of nonreactive FHT. The provider gives a 1-sec stimulation and may repeat after 60 sec if no fetal acceleration occurs. A third stimulation may be administered for up to 3 sec in duration if no acceleration occurs after previous attempts. Using VAS may not actually decrease the duration of testing, producing prolonged accelerations in approximately one-third of cases [28]. Despite common assumptions, manual stimulation and maternal administration of a glucose-containing drink do not improve the reactivity of the NST [29].

The nonreactive NST has a false-positive rate (fetal survival >1 week after a nonreactive NST) of up to 50%, requiring back-up testing (e.g. CST/BPP). Adverse outcome (e.g. perinatal death, low 5-min Apgar score, late decelerations during labor) occurs only in 20% of cases with a nonreactive NST. In the largest series of patients (n = 5861) undergoing antepartum surveillance with the NST, the false-negative (i.e. fetal death <1 week after a reactive NST) rate was 3.1/1000, while others have found similar results (1.9–5/1000) (Table 10.1) [30–34]. However, the use of the NST is "widely integrated into clinical practice" [35] and despite the lack of definitive evidence of a beneficial effect on fetal mortality, it will probably continue to be utilized liberally in modern obstetric practice [36] (see Table 10.1).

Table 10.1 False-negative and false-positive rates for antenatal testing modalities

Test	False negative*	False positive†
Nonstress test	1.9–5 [30–34]	50% [31]
Modified biophysical profile	0–0.8 [24,25,38,39]	60% [25]
Contraction stress test	0.4 [31,45,46]	40% [48]
Biophysical profile	0.6 [43]	40% [43]

*Risk of fetal mortality (per 1000 livebirths) <1 week after a negative test result.

†Fetal survival >1 week after a positive test result.

Modified biophysical profile (nonstress test/ Amniotic Fluid Index)

The risk of short-term hypoxemia is addressed with the NST. Measuring the AFI is a surrogate for fetal renal perfusion and reflects long-term placental function via the amniotic fluid status. The AFI acts as a measure of redistribution of fetal blood flow as hypoxemia can lead to decreased renal perfusion, urine output, and oligohydramnios [24,37]. The modified BPP has a lower false-negative rate than the NST alone, 0–0.8/1000, but the false-positive rate (i.e. a normal fetus despite a positive test result) remains 60% [24,25,38,39]. When utilizing the modified BPP, a back-up test must be performed for any of the following: nonreactive NST, significant variable or late decelerations, or AFI <5.

Intervention based on surveillance with the modified BPP may not be without consequence as its use in one study was associated with a higher rate of cesarean (relative risk [RR] 2.09; 95% confidence interval [CI], 1.69–2.57). Further, intervention in those with a false-positive test led to iatrogenic premature delivery in 1.5% of women tested [25]. However, it appears that the modified BPP is similar in its incidence of adverse outcomes following a negative result (risk of fetal mortality after a negative test result) compared with the CST, with a risk of IUFD of approximately 1 in 1000 in both tests. The modified BPP is probably currently the primary means of antenatal surveillance [39,40].

Biophysical profile

The BPP consists of an NST with ultrasound observation of the fetus for up to 30 min, and reflects acute and chronic fetal hypoxia. The BPP has five separate variables: the NST, fetal breathing, movement, tone, and the AFI (Table 10.2). The AFI is the chronic marker while the other four components reflect potential acute hypoxia. Each component scores either 0 or 2 points. Each component score is tallied and a composite score is given, yet not all measures are equal. Indeed, low AFI is independently associated with increased risk of acidemia [41]. The BPP can be employed for primary antepartum surveillance, follow-up of nonreactive NST, or for further information after positive or suspicious CST.

The management of the BPP is as shown in Table 10.3. Eight and 10 out of 10 are normal and repeat testing should be performed as typically scheduled. However, if points are lost for oligohydramnios, this may confer fetal jeopardy and delivery should be considered if the gestational age permits. Alternatively, more frequent surveillance, including assessment of fetal growth, should be performed.

A score of 6/10 is equivocal and should be repeated within 12–24 h if less than 34 weeks. However, if the fetus is 34 or more weeks, delivery should be considered. If oligohydramnios is noted, delivery should be considered, as the test is likely a true positive if the fetus loses points for nonreactive NST or breathing movements. In contrast, the test is more likely a false positive if the fetus has normal fluid and loses points for nonreactive NST and another parameter [42].

A score of 4/10 requires immediate evaluation and intervention and may warrant delivery unless the fetus is very premature (i.e. <28 weeks). If delivery is not carried out, repeat assessments are needed every 12–24 h.

On the other hand, a score of 2/10 generally requires delivery, particularly if the score persists after extending

Table 10.2 Scoring for biophysical profile

Variable	Normal (score = 2 for 1–5)	Abnormal (score = 0 for 1–5)
1 Fetal breathing movement (FBM)	≥1 episode of FBMs of ≥30 sec in duration	<30 sec of sustained FBMs
2 Fetal movement	≥3 discrete body/limb movements (simultaneous limb and trunk movements are counted as a single movement)	≤2 movements
3 Fetal tone	≥1 episode of active extension with rapid return	Either slow extension with return to partial flexion or movement of limb in full trunk, or hand extension, or absent fetal movement
4 Fetal heart rate tracing (FHT) over 20 min	≥2 accelerations of ≥15 beats/min, peak amplitude lasting ≥15 sec from the baseline with moderate variability in 20 min	<2 accelerations or accelerations <15 beats/min peak amplitude or accelerations <15 sec duration in 20 min. Variability less than moderate
5 Amniotic Fluid Index (AFI) For twins, deepest vertical pocket (DVP) in each sac	≥5.0 cm ≥2.0 cm	<5.0 cm <2.0 cm

Table 10.3 Biophysical profile scoring and management

Score	Risk of hypoxia	Management	Perinatal mortality*
10/10 8/10 (AFI nl)	Nearly zero	Follow as clinical course dictates	<1/1000
8/10 (Oligo)	Chronic hypoxia likely	If normal urinary tract, no ROM; consider delivery after corticosteroids	20–30/1000
6/10 (AFI nl) 6/10 (Oligo)	Hypoxia not excluded Chronic hypoxia likely	Repeat testing. If persistent 6/10, deliver at >37 weeks; if immature repeat within 24h; if less than 6/10 delivery	50/1000 >50/1000
4/10	Acute likely, if oligohydramnios, risk of acute and chronic increases	Delivery, continuous FHT	115/1000 >115/1000 (if oligo)
2/10	Acute with chronic hypoxia likely	Delivery, typically via cesarean	220/1000
0/10	Nearly certain	Deliver immediately	550/1000

AFI, Amniotic Fluid Index; FHT fetal heart rate tracing; ROM, rupture of membranes.
*Risk of fetal mortality per 1000 livebirths within 1 week without any fetal intervention [64].

testing for 120 min [43]. As with the above, the final decision depends on the actual fetal diagnosis, gestational age, and possibly betamethasone window for acceleration of fetal lung maturity.

Contraction stress test

The CST is a measure of fetal response to stress. The uterus contracts and the spiral arteries are occluded, decreasing flow to the intervillous space and resulting in decreased oxygenation of the fetus. In the suboptimally oxygenated fetus, the baseline oxygen deficit will be worsened and late decelerations on FHT may be apparent. The advantage of the CST is that subtle hypoxia prior to acidosis is more easily detected when compared with the BPP/NST, and the CST is helpful in predicting tolerance of labor.

The CST is performed with the patient in the lateral recumbent position. An adequate test is assessment of the FHT and uterine contractions with three contractions in 10 min, each lasting at least 40 sec in duration. Oxytocin can be employed for uterine contractions (0.5 mU/min, increased every 20 min to a maximum of 10 mU/min) or manual stimulation of the maternal nipple may be used. This is done by rubbing one nipple through clothing for 2 min or until a contraction begins. If no contractions are observed after 2 min, a second stimulation is performed after 5 min. An alternative technique is to apply warm packs to the breasts for a maximum of 2 min followed by a 5-min break prior to restimulation.

Nipple stimulation was approximately 50% faster than intravenous oxytocin in one evaluation of the time to an adequate CST [44]. Contraindications to the CST include preterm labor, preterm premature rupture of the membranes (PPROM), abnormal vaginal bleeding and contraindications for vaginal delivery (e.g. placenta previa, prior classic cesarean, extensive uterine surgery).

The CST test result is "negative" if there are no late decelerations or significant variable decelerations in the setting of a normal baseline fetal heart rate. If three adequate contractions occur in 10 min, a negative and reactive CST has a false-negative rate of 0.4–1/1000 and more than 99% survival over a week [45–47]. A CST is deemed positive if more than 50% of uterine contractions have associated late decelerations. A positive CST is associated with a 50% rate of poor perinatal outcome, including perinatal death, increased cesarean for nonreassuring fetal status and low 5-min Apgar score.

While a positive CST is associated with adverse outcomes, the fetus may tolerate labor and therefore a trial of labor induction is recommended, unless there is an obstetric contraindication to vaginal delivery [48]. A reactive, positive CST is one with normal FHT variability and baseline but late decelerations after more than 50% of contractions. This generally calls for delivery, continuous or close follow-up surveillance at a very early gestational age. A test deemed equivocal or suspicious is one in which there are 50% or fewer late decelerations, variable decelerations (i.e. possibly indicating IUGR, oligohydramnios), or an abnormal fetal heart rate baseline. These can be managed by delivery or more frequent testing, depending on gestational age.

If there are five or more uterine contractions in 10 min or contractions lasting more than 90 sec in the setting of

Table 10.4 Follow-up for contraction stress test

CST result	Follow-up
Reactive –negative	Repeat, 7 days
Nonreactive – negative	Repeat, 24 h Evaluation for nonreactivity Fetus <28 weeks, normal variability, repeat in 7 days
Reactive – equivocal	Repeat, 24 h
Nonreactive – equivocal	Repeat, 24 h
Reactive – positive	Gestational age >37 weeks, trial of induction Preterm: further evaluation
Nonreactive – positive	Term: delivery via cesarean Preterm: further evaluation

fetal heart rate decelerations then the CST is equivocal – tachysystole. Finally, a tracing is considered unsatisfactory if there are fewer than three contractions or the FHT is of poor quality (see Table 10.4 for management of CST results).

Doppler velocimetry

Doppler velocimetry is used as an adjunct to other testing modalities and is particularly useful in the growth-restricted fetus [49]. It is not generally used as a primary means of surveillance, nor for screening in a low-risk population. The fetal umbilical artery is used to assess the hemodynamic components of placental vascular impedance. In some fetuses with IUGR, there is increased systolic:diastolic (S:D) ratio (above 3) blood flow velocity in the umbilical artery signifying increased umbilical vascular impedance. In severe IUGR, with high placental impedance, there may be absent or reversed diastolic flow in the umbilical artery [50–52]. Fetal mortality is increased with reversed or absent end-diastolic flow [53] and asphyxia in SGA fetuses is associated with absent end-diastolic flow in the umbilical artery [54]. The use of Doppler velocimetry in high-risk pregnancies was associated with decreases in induction of labor, and antepartum admission, and may result in decreased perinatal mortality (adjusted odds ratio [OR] 0.71, 95% CI 0.50–1.01) [55].

An increased S:D ratio in pregnancies at risk was more likely to have "abnormal" perinatal outcome than those with values of less than 3.0 (2.3–2.9); however, gestational age-specific tables exist. The S:D ratio was a better predictor of poor outcome than suboptimal fetal growth [56]. The best predictor of poor long-term outcomes may be in those with IUGR and associated with umbilical cord S:D ratio abnormalities [57].

Poorer neurodevelopmental outcome in children aged 5–12 years was associated with reversed end-diastolic flow compared with normal and absent flow [57]. Other adverse outcomes have been associated with absent and reversed end-diastolic flow in the umbilical artery: mortality (28–45%), neonatal intensive care unit (ICU) admission (84–98%), and cesarean section (73%) for fetal distress [53,58].

Abnormal Doppler indices alone should not dictate intervention, but rather indicate the level of antenatal surveillance needed. For instance, a growth-restricted fetus less than 32 weeks' gestation, with absent end-diastolic flow in the umbilical artery, continuous FHT and a reassuring BPP, may allow for maternal and fetal evaluation, corticosteroid administration, magnesium for neuroprophylaxis, and preparation for delivery. In the setting of IUGR, absent end-diastolic flow should trigger continuous fetal surveillance with prolongation of the pregnancy dictated only by a reassuring BPP score, NST, and early gestational age.

In normal fetuses, impedance of the vessels in the brain is relatively higher than in the umbilical artery (UA) and S:D ratios average above 5; however, gestational age-specific tables exist. In the fetus with IUGR, and especially in those with asymmetric IUGR, the impedance decreases, further reflecting an increased perfusion and presumably oxygen delivery. This increase in the UA S:D ratio, and decrease in the middle cerebral artery (MCA) S:D ratio, can be used as an index of the fetal compensatory mechanisms, and indicates a more severe response to IUGR [59–61].

Venous Doppler, specifically the ductus venosus waveform, may be helpful when cardiac dysfunction is suspected (e.g. in the setting of IUGR due to increased placental resistance). The ductus venosus has the most rapidly moving blood in the fetus and thus is easy to identify. Abnormal flow in the ductus venosus has been shown to be one of the final markers of fetal decline; its utility lies in strong specificity and positive predictive values for stillbirth. Absence or reversal of the a-wave (absence or reversal of forward blood flow during atrial systole) is ominous and most commonly indicates growth restriction due to placental insufficiency, metabolic disturbance leading to poor cardiac contractility, or redistribution of hepatic flow and injury. Regardless of the etiology, this finding is considered worrisome, and in the setting of abnormal UA waveforms, the greatest risk of fetal death. Prompt intervention, as suggested above, is warranted. [62,63].

Specific indications and onset of testing

The appropriate initiation and frequency of testing are determined by the indication for the test as well as gestational age. Typically, testing is begun at 32 weeks and is performed on a weekly to twice-weekly basis. However, maternal or fetal situations may dictate daily testing (e.g. unstable hypertension, poorly controlled diabetes) [41]. The specifics of many recommendations are often based on sparse evidence while others are opinion based and quite controversial. Table 10.5 shows the antenatal testing guidelines for the University of California, San Francisco.

Table 10.5 Fetal surveillance: diagnostic conditions and frequency. The basic formal testing scheme is NST/AFI (modified BPP)

Indications	GA of initiation	Frequency
Post dates	40½ wks (earlier if EDD unsure)	Twice weekly
Hypertensive diseases:	At Dx	Twice weekly (or more frequently depending on severity)
Preeclampsia (including r/o preeclampsia)	32 wks	
Chronic hypertension	See IUGR	Weekly
Chronic hypertension with IUGR		See IUGR
Diabetes mellitus	Kick counts only	Twice weekly
GDM	32 wks	Twice weekly
On diet & exercise (A1) – good control (FBG <95 mg/dL, PPBG <140 mg/dL)	32 wks	Twice weekly
On insulin or oral agent (A2) – good or poor control	28 wks	Twice weekly
Pregestational (type I, type II)	28 wks or when complications arise	
W/out complications – good control		
W/out complications – poor control		
W/complications (e.g. poor growth, vascular disease)		
Advanced maternal age	32 wks	Weekly
>40 years	36 wks	Weekly
35–39 years		
Severe maternal conditions (e.g. cardiac, pulmonary, severe asthma, sickle cell)	32 wks	Weekly or more frequently
Active drug/ETOH abuse or methadone use	32 wks	Weekly
SLE or antiphospholipid syndrome	32 wks (earlier if microvascular disease)	Weekly or more frequently
Thyroid disease	32 wks	Twice weekly
Uncontrolled	36 wks	Weekly
Maternal Graves disease		
w/TSI >130%		
Cholestasis	At Dx (begin before bile acid results)	Twice weekly
Herpes gestationis	At Dx	Weekly
HIV (on combination therapy)	32 wks	Weekly
Seizure disorder (poorly controlled)	28 wks	Weekly
IVF	36 wks	Weekly
	40 wks	Twice weekly

Table 10.5 (*Continued*)

Indications	GA of initiation	Frequency	
History abruption previous pregnancy	2 wks prior to GA of previous abruption	Weekly	
Abnormal maternal serum screening: AFP >2.5 MoM, 2nd trimester hCG >2 MoM, estriol <0.15 MoM, inhibin >2 MoM, PAPP-A <1st % (<0.23 MoM)	32 wks	Weekly	
Decreased fetal movement	When occurs	May only require single test	
Oligohydramnios	At Dx	As indicated	
Polyhydramnios	At Dx	Weekly	
IUGR (<10th percentile) or r/o IUGR (sono pending)	At Dx	Twice weekly	
Twins:	32 wks	Weekly	
di/di w/normal growth	36 wks	Twice weekly	
and normal AFV	28 wks	Weekly	NST/Deepest pocket in each sac
mono/di w/normal growth and concordant/ normal AFV	32 wks	Twice weekly	
di/di w/IUGR and/or discordant growth (>20%) and/or abnormal AFV	At Dx	Twice weekly	
mono/di w/IUGR and/or discordant growth (>20%) and/or discordant AFV	At Dx	Twice weekly	
mono/mono	At GA of intervention	Daily	
Triplets	Same as mono/di twins	Same as mono/di twins	
Hx previous IUFD	32 wks or if previous demise <32 wks, then begin 2 wks prior to date of previous demise	Weekly	
Fetuses with certain abnormalities (e.g. CDH, persistent echogenic bowel, increased NT [>3.0 mm])	32 wks	Weekly	
Fetal gastroschisis	28 wks	Twice weekly	
Fetal arrhythmia (i.e. SVT, PACs, etc.)	At Dx	Weekly (BPP if unable to obtain FHR strip)	
Fetal heart block	At Dx (>28 wks)	Weekly BPP	
Fetal blood disorders (e.g. Rh alloimmunization, parvovirus, NAIT)	>28 wks or at onset of disease	Weekly or more frequently	

AFI, Amiotic Fluid Index; BPP, biophysical profile; CDH, congenital diaphragmatic hernia; di, dichorionic; Dx, diagnosis; EDD, estimated date of delivery; ETOH, alcohol abuse; FBG, fasting blood glucose; FHR, fetal heart rate; GA, gestational age; GDM, gestational diabetes mellitus; Hx, history; IUGR, intrauterine growth restriction; IVF, *in vitro* fertilization; mono, monochorionic, monoamniotic; MSAFP, maternal serum α-fetoprotein; MSHCG, maternal serum human chorionic gonadotropin; NAIT, neonatal alloimmune thrombocytopenia; NST, nonstress test; NT, nuchal translucency; PAC, premature atrial contractions; PAPP-A, pregnancy-associated plasma protein A; PPBG, postprandial blood glucose; r/o, rule out; Rh, rhesus; SLE, systemic lupus erythematosus; SVT, supraventricular tachycardia; TSI, thyroid stimulating immunoglobin.

CASE PRESENTATION

A 36-year-old white gravida 1, para 0 had chronic hypertension. She initiated prenatal care at 8 weeks and was maintained on labetalol, 400 mg twice daily. Baseline urine analysis revealed 213 mg protein and a serum creatinine of 0.9 mg/dL. At 16 weeks an amniocentesis was performed for increased risk of Down syndrome on integrated screening, revealing a chromosomally normal male fetus.

Serial sonograms were performed for fetal growth, beginning at 26 weeks. At 28 weeks, antenatal testing was initiated with twice-weekly modified BPP. The initial NST result was nonreactive despite acoustic stimulation after 20 min. The AFI was 11.0.

Although the NST result may have been nonreactive as a result of the prematurity of the fetus, other etiologic factors were explored. The patient was questioned about her eating and drug habits; she had a normal breakfast prior to the test and denied any illicit drug use. A BPP was performed to follow up the nonreactive NST, with a score of 8/10 (loss of 2 points for NST result). With a reassuring BPP, the nonreactive tracing was attributed to the fetal prematurity.

At 29 weeks, there was a reactive NST result and an AFI of 9.7. However, blood pressure was 167/105 mmHg and the fundal height was 26 cm. She was hospitalized, and biometry revealed that the fetus was 820 g (<5%), and a presumptive diagnosis of IUGR was made. Umbilical artery Doppler velocimetry was performed which revealed an increased S:D ratio of 5.3–6.0, with forward end-diastolic flow present. In addition, the MCA S:D ratio measured 3.0–3.8.

During her hospitalization, she experienced a severe exacerbation of hypertension, the labetalol was increased and a second agent, nifedipine, was begun. On admission, the complete blood cell count (CBC), liver function test (LFT), and urine protein values were normal. An NST on the day of admission was reactive; the AFI was 5.0. Owing to the severity of the hypertension and abnormal cord Doppler indices, twice-daily NST testing was initiated and a course of betamethasone was given for acceleration of fetal pulmonary maturity.

A plan for weekly Doppler velocimetry was devised. Three days later, the NST result was nonreactive and the AFI was 4.0. A BPP was performed, with an equivocal score of 6/10 (loss of 2 points for nonreactive NST and oligohydramnios). Repeat testing was scheduled for the next morning (12 h later). On hospital day 5, she complained of midepigastric pain. Laboratory tests revealed a hematocrit of 42%, platelet count of $102,000 \times 10^9/L$, and serum aspartate transaminase and alanine transaminase levels of 960 U/L and 1020 U/L, respectively.

The repeat BPP score was 4/10 with the additional loss of fetal breathing. Preparations for induction of labor were made because of the deteriorating fetal and maternal conditions, and a male infant weighing 875 g was delivered vaginally. Apgar scores were 5 at 1 min and 8 at 5 min. Cord umbilical artery (CUA) and vein (CUV) blood gas values were obtained: CUA pH 7.27, PCO_2 48 mmHg, PO_2 33 mmHg, base excess −4.4 and CUV pH 7.30, PCO_2 42 mmHg, PO_2 39 mmHg, base excess −3.4.

The newborn required intubation for 48 h, was weaned from all oxygen support by day 12 of life, and discharged on day 46 of life. The mother was treated with magnesium sulfate for 48 h postpartum, her abnormal laboratory values were normal by day 5 postpartum, and she was discharged.

References

1. MacDorman MF, Kirmeyer S. Fetal and perinatal mortality, United States, 2005. National vital statistics reports; vol 57, no 8. Hyattsville, MD: National Center for Health Statistics, 2009. www.cdc.gov/nchs/data/nvsr/nvsr57/nvsr57_08.pdf.

2. MacDorman M, Kirmeyer S. The challenge of fetal mortality. NCHS Data Brief No. 16. Hyattsville, MD: National Center for Health Statistics, 2009.

3. Fretts RC. Etiology and prevention of stillbirth. Am J Obstet Gynecol 2005;193:1923–1935.

4. Huang DY, Usher RH, Kramer MS et al. Determinants of unexplained antepartum fetal deaths. Obstet Gynecol 2000;95:215–221.

5. Incerpi MH, Miller DA, Samadi R, Settlage RH, Goodwin TM. Stillbirth evaluation: what tests are needed? Am J Obstet Gynecol 1998;178:1121–1125.

6. Pearson JF, Weaver JB. Fetal activity and fetal wellbeing: an evaluation. BMJ 1976;1:1305–1307.

7. Moore TR, Piacquadio K. A prospective evaluation of fetal movement screening to reduce the incidence of antepartum fetal death. Am J Obstet Gynecol 1989;160:1075–1080.

8. Grant A, Elbourne D, Valentin L, Alexander S. Routine formal fetal movement counting and risk of antepartum late death in normally formed singletons. Lancet 1989; 8659:345–349.

9. Froen JF. A kick from within: fetal movement counting and the canceled progress in antenatal care. J Perinat Med 2004;32:13–24.

10. Schifrin BS. The rationale for antepartum fetal heart rate monitoring. J Reprod Med 1979;23:213–221.

11. Cardosi RJ, Heffron JA, Spellacy WN. Reactive nonstress test despite severe congenital brain damage. What does the test measure? J Reprod Med 1997;42:251–252.

12. Rabinowitz R, Persitz E, Sadovsky E. The relation between fetal heart rate accelerations and fetal movements. Obstet Gynecol 1983;61:16–18.

13. Graca LM, Cardoso CG, Clode N, Calhaz-Jorge C. Acute effects of maternal cigarette smoking on fetal heart rate and fetal body movements felt by the mother. J Perinat Med 1991;19:385–390.

14. Oncken C, Kranzler H, O'Malley P, Gendreau P, Campbell WA. The effect of cigarette smoking on fetal heart rate characteristics. Obstet Gynecol 2002;99:751–755.

15. Nijhuis JG, Prechtl HF, Martin CB Jr, Bots RS. Are there behavioural states in the human fetus? Early Hum Dev 1982;6:177–195.

16. Meis PJ, Ureda JR, Swain M, Kelly RT, Penry M, Sharp P. Variable decelerations during nonstress test are not a sign of fetal compromise. Am J Obstet Gynecol 1986;154:586–590.

17. Anyaegbunam A, Brustman L, Divon M, Langer O. The significance of antepartum variable decelerations. Am J Obstet Gynecol 1986;155:707–710.

18. O'Leary JA, Andrinopoulos GC, Giordano PC. Variable decelerations and the nonstress test: an indication of cord compromise. Am J Obstet Gynecol 980;137:704–706.

19. Druzin ML, Gratacos J, Keegan KA, Paul RH. Antepartum fetal heart rate testing. VII. The significance of fetal bradycardia. Am J Obstet Gynecol 1981;139:194–198.

20. Bourgeois FJ, Thiagarajah S, Harbert GM Jr. The significance of fetal heart rate decelerations during nonstress testing. Am J Obstet Gynecol 1984;150:213–216.

21. Pazos R, Vuolo K, Aladjem S, Lueck J, Anderson C. Association of spontaneous fetal heart rate decelerations during antepartum nonstress testing and intrauterine growth retardation. Am J Obstet Gynecol 1982;144:574–577.

22. Bishop EH. Fetal acceleration test. Am J Obstet Gynecol 1981;141:905–909.

23. Druzin ML, Fox A, Kogut E, Carlson C. The relationship of the nonstress test to gestational age. Am J Obstet Gynecol 1985;153:386–389.

24. Clark SL, Sabey P, Jolley K. Nonstress testing with acoustic stimulation and amniotic fluid volume assessment: 5973 tests without unexpected fetal death. Am J Obstet Gynecol 1989;160:694–697.

25. Miller DA, Rabello YA, Paul RH. The modified biophysical profile: antepartum testing in the 1990s. Am J Obstet Gynecol 1996;174:812–817.

26. Smith CV, Phelan JP, Platt LD, Broussard P, Paul RH. Fetal acoustic stimulation testing. II. A randomized clinical comparison with the nonstress test. Am J Obstet Gynecol 1986;155:131–134.

27. Zimmer EZ, Divon MY. Fetal vibroacoustic stimulation. Obstet Gynecol 1993;81:451–457.

28. Newnham JP, Burns SE, Roberman BD. Effect of vibratory acoustic stimulation on the duration of fetal heart rate monitoring tests. Am J Perinatol 1990;7:232–234.

29. Tan KH, Sabapathy A. Maternal glucose administration for facilitating tests of fetal wellbeing. Cochrane Database Syst Rev 2001;4:CD003397.

30. Boehm FH, Salyer S, Shah DM, Vaughn WK. Improved outcome of twice weekly nonstress testing. Obstet Gynecol 1986;67:566–568.

31. Freeman RK, Anderson G, Dorchester W. A prospective multi-institutional study of antepartum fetal heart rate monitoring. I. Risk of perinatal mortality and morbidity according to antepartum fetal heart rate results. Am J Obstet Gynecol 1982;143:771–777.

32. Druzin ML, Gratacos J, Paul RH. Antepartum fetal heart rate testing. VI. Predictive reliability of "normal" tests in the prevention of antepartum deaths. Am J Obstet Gynecol 1980;137:745–747.

33. Devoe LD. The non stress test. In: Eden RD, Boehm FH, eds. Assessment and Care of the Fetus: Physiological, Clinical, and Medicolegal Principles. Norwalk, CT: Appleton and Lange, 1990.

34. Phelan JP, Lewis PE Jr. Fetal heart rate decelerations during a nonstress test. Obstet Gynecol 1981;57:228–232.

35. American College of Obstetricians and Gynecologists Practice Bulletin. Antepartum fetal surveillance. ACOG Educational Bulletin No. 238. Washington, DC: American College of Obstetricians and Gynecologists, 1999.

36. Grivell RM, Alfirevic Z, Gyte GML, Devane D. Antenatal cardiotocography for fetal assessment. Cochrane Database Syst Rev 2010;1:CD007863.

37. Seeds AE. Current concepts of amniotic fluid dynamics. Am J Obstet Gynecol 1980;138:575–586.

38. Vintzileos AM, Knuppel RA. Multiple parameter biophysical testing in the prediction of fetal acid–base status. Clin Perinatol 1994;21:823–848.

39. Nageotte MP, Towers CV, Asrat T, Freeman RK, Dorchester W. The value of a negative antepartum test: CST and modified BPP. Obstet Gynecol 1994;84:231–234.

40. Nageotte MP, Towers CV, Asrat T, Freeman RK, Dorchester W. The value of a negative antepartum test: CST and modified BPP. Obstet Gynecol 1994;84:231–234.

41. Devoe LD, Gardner P, Dear C, Castillo RA. The diagnostic values of concurrent nonstress testing, amniotic fluid measurement, and Doppler velocimetry in screening a general high-risk population. Am J Obstet Gynecol 1990;163:1040–1047.

42. Hanley ML, Vintzileos AM. Biophysical testing in premature rupture of the membranes. Semin Perinatol 1996;20:418–425.

43. Manning FA, Morrison I, Lange IR, Harman CR, Chamberlain PF. Fetal assessment based on fetal biophysical profile scoring: experience in 12,620 referred high-risk pregnancies. I. Perinatal mortality by frequency and etiology. Am J Obstet Gynecol 1985;151:343–350.

44. Huddleston JF, Sutliff G, Robinson D. Contraction stress test by intermittent nipple stimulation. Obstet Gynecol 1984;63:669–673.

45. Evertson LR, Gauthier RJ, Collea JV. Fetal demise following negative contraction stress tests. Obstet Gynecol 1978;51:671–673.

46. Lagrew DC. The contraction stress test. Clin Obstet Gynecol 1995;38:11–25.

47. Schrifrin BS. The rationale for antepartum fetal heart rate monitoring. J Reprod Med 1979;23:213–221.

48. Thacker SB, Berkelman RL. Assessing the diagnostic accuracy and efficacy of selected antepartum fetal surveillance techniques. Obstet Gynecol Surv 1986;41:121–141.

49. Hayley J, Tuffnell DJ, Johnson N. Randomised controlled trial of cardiotocography versus umbilical artery Doppler in the

management of small for gestational age fetuses. Br J Obstet Gynaecol 1997;104:431–435.

50. Erskine RL, Ritchie JW. Umbilical artery blood flow characteristics in normal and growth retarded fetuses. Br J Obstet Gynaecol 1985;92:605–610.

51. Gudmundsson S, Marsal K. Umbilical and uteroplacental blood flow velocity waveforms in pregnancies with fetal growth retardation. Eur J Obstet Gynecol Reprod Biol 1988;27:187–196.

52. Reuwer PJ, Bruinse HW, Stoutenbeek P, Haspels AA. Doppler assessment of the fetoplacental circulation in normal and growth-retarded fetuses. Eur J Obstet Gynecol Reprod Biol 1984; 18:199–205.

53. Karsdorp VH, van Vugt JM, van Geijn HP et al. Clinical significance of absent or reversed end diastolic velocity waveforms in umbilical artery. Lancet 1994;344:1664–1668.

54. Nicolaides KH, Bilardo CM, Soothill PW, Campbell S. Absence of end diastolic frequencies in umbilical artery: a sign of fetal hypoxia and acidosis. BMJ 1988;297:1026–1027.

55. Neilson JP, Alfirevic Z. Doppler ultrasound for fetal assessment in high risk pregnancies. Cochrane Database Syst Rev 1996;4:CD000073.

56. Maulik D, Yarlagadda P, Youngblood JP, Ciston P. The diagnostic efficacy of the umbilical arterial systolic/diastolic ratio as a screening tool: a prospective blinded study. Am J Obstet Gynecol 1990;162:1518–1523.

57. Schreuder AM, McDonnell M, Gaffney G, Johnson A, Hope PL. Outcome at school age following antenatal detection of absent or reversed end diastolic flow velocity in the umbilical artery. Arch Dis Child Fetal Neonatal Ed 2002;86:108–114.

58. Maulik D, ed. Doppler Ultrasound in Obstetrics and Gynecology. New York: Springer-Verlag, 1997.

59. Strigini FA, de Luca G, Lencioni G, Scida P, Giusti G, Genazzani AR. Middle cerebral artery velocimetry: different clinical relevance depending on umbilical velocimetry. Obstet Gynecol 1997;90:953–957.

60. Fong KW, Ohlsson A, Hannah ME et al. Prediction of perinatal outcome in fetuses suspected to have intrauterine growth restriction: Doppler US study of fetal cerebral, renal, and umbilical arteries. Radiology 1999;213:681–689.

61. Bahado-Singh RO, Kovanci E, Jeffres A et al. The Doppler cerebroplacental ratio and perinatal outcome in intrauterine growth restriction. Am J Obstet Gynecol 1999;180: 750–756.

62. Baschat AA, Gembruch U, Weiner CP, Harman CR. Qualitative venous Doppler waveform analysis improves prediction of critical perinatal outcomes in premature growth-restricted fetuses. Ultrasound Obstet Gynecol 2003;22:240–245.

63. Mari G, Hanif F. Fetal Doppler: umbilical artery, middle cerebral artery, and venous system. Semin Perinatol 2008;32: 253–257.

64. Manning FA. Fetal biophysical profile. Obstet Gynecol Clin 1999;26:557–578.

Chapter 11
Interpreting Intrapartum Fetal Heart Tracings

Michael Nageotte

Department of Obstetrics and Gynecology, University of California, Irvine, CA, USA

Over the past 30 years, electronic fetal heart rate monitoring (EFM) has become an accepted means of assessing fetal status during labor. More than 85% of livebirths in the USA are so monitored despite a frequent lack of agreement on strip interpretation and management decisions [1]. This has resulted in an increased rate of cesarean delivery in patients monitored with EFM accompanied by a lack of clear evidence of efficacy. EFM is unquestionably a labor-saving device for nurses and is unlikely to be displaced from what is an accepted standard obstetric practice. Further, monitoring of the fetal heart rate (FHR) is a highly reliable modality in identifying the well-oxgenated fetus. This is because the brain controls the heart rate and changes in both cerebral blood flow and blood oxygenation in turn affect the FHR. Certain patterns in the heart rate of the fetus can be used to determine oxygen status with excellent concordance between normal fetal oxygenation and the presence of normal baseline FHR accompanied by FHR accelerations. While the concordance between normal oxygenation and the presence of FHR accelerations provides clinical reassurance, the absence of accelerations does not necessarily predict abnormality in fetal oxygenation. In fact, the correlation between abnormalities of the FHR (e.g. late or variable decelerations, elevated baseline) and adverse neonatal outcomes is at best tenuous [2]. That is to say, the positive predictive value of an abnormal FHR pattern to predict adverse outcome is very poor. Consequently, EFM should be understood and employed cautiously and used only as a diagnostic tool in the management of a woman's labor. It is only with the correct interpretation of the information provided from such a modality that appropriate management decisions can be made.

Interpretation guidelines for electronic fetal heart rate monitoring

In order to understand the FHR and communicate interpretation accurately among healthcare providers, there needs to be an appreciation of certain aspects of the FHR. These include baseline rate, variability, accelerations, and decelerations. The overall pattern appearance, changes over time, and response to certain clinical interventions must also be considered. In 2008, the National Institute of Child Health and Human Development, the American College of Obstetricians and Gynecologists (ACOG) and the Society for Maternal-Fetal Medicine collaborated on updating both definitions and interpretations of electronic fetal monitoring [3]. In 2009, a new ACOG Practice Bulletin was published in support of this collaboration [4]. Agreement was reached that efforts at classification of fetal heart rate tracings should fall into three categories. Category I tracings are normal, category II tracings are indeterminate, and category III tracings are abnormal.

Evaluation frequency

Assessment of FHR should occur frequently during active labor. For women with complicated pregnancies, such evaluations using auscultation should be every 15 min in the first stage of labor and every 5 min in the second stage [5]. The recommended evaluation frequency for laboring women without complications is auscultation every 30 min in the first stage of labor and every 15 min in the second stage. Similarly, when using EFM, the frequency of tracing review would apply. Unfortunately, at times there is lack of concordance in the FHR strip interpretation among physicians and nurses. While there is generally excellent agreement when a strip is category I, for those FHR patterns in category II there is poor agreement regarding interpretation and management. Such interpretation is further challenged by clinically important confounders including gestational age, parity, maternal vital signs, medications, and progress in labor. Category III patterns are expected to be consistently interpreted correctly.

Queenan's Management of High-Risk Pregnancy: An Evidence-Based Approach, Sixth Edition. Edited by John T. Queenan, Catherine Y. Spong, Charles J. Lockwood.

Fetal heart rate pattern definitions

Baseline

The baseline FHR is the mean rate rounded in increments of 5 beats per min (bpm) over a minimum of 10-min segments, excluding periodic or episodic changes, periods of marked variability or when segments of tracing reveal difference of baseline of more than 23 bpm. Normal is 110–160 bpm. Bradycardia is when the baseline is less than 110 bpm and tachycardia is when the baseline is greater than 160 bpm.

Variability

Irregular fluctuations in the baseline FHR of two or more cycles per minute that are irregular in amplitude and frequency describe variability. FHR variability is either absent, minimal (amplitude range ≤5 bpm), moderate (amplitude range >5–25 bpm), or marked (amplitude range >25 bpm). Of note, the sinusoidal heart rate has a smooth sine wave-like pattern of regular amplitude and frequency with a cycle frequency of 3–5 per min and persists for at least 20 min. The sinusoidal pattern is excluded from the FHR variability definition.

Accelerations

An abrupt increase from baseline FHR to peak within 30 sec of at least 15 bpm lasting at least 15 sec but less than 2 min from onset to return is termed an acceleration. Gestational age has a role in this definition, with fetuses less than 32 weeks having accelerations defined as increases at least 10 bpm above baseline lasting at least 10 sec.

Decelerations

• *Late deceleration:* a gradual and visually apparent decrease of baseline FHR lasting at least 30 sec with return to baseline associated with a uterine contraction. Late decelerations are delayed in onset with the nadir of deceleration occurring after the contraction peak. Early deceleration is defined as a gradual and visually apparent decrease and return to baseline of the FHR coincident with a contraction.

• *Early deceleration:* a gradual and visually apparent decrease and return to baseline of the FHR associated with contraction. An early deceleration has its nadir occurring with the peak of the uterine contraction and mirrors the onset, peak, and ending of the contraction.

• *Variable deceleration:* a sudden, rapid decrease of the FHR to its nadir in less than 30 sec. The decrease must be at least 15 bpm lasting at least 15 sec with return to baseline in less than 2 min.

• *Prolonged deceleration:* a decrease in the FHR of at least 15 bpm lasting for longer than 2 min but less than 10 min before return to baseline. If a deceleration lasts 10 min or longer, it is a baseline change.

Category I fetal heart rate

Category I FHR tracings have a normal baseline, moderate variability, no early, variable or late decelerations, and accelerations may be present or absent. The most reliable marker of adequate fetal oxygenation and normal acid–base status is the presence of FHR accelerations. An additional marker of reassurance is the presence of normal FHR variability. Caution must be employed in the interpretation of EFM when variability is present when accompanied by concerning characteristics of the FHR such as persistent decelerations [6]. It is very rare for an entire FHR to remain category I throughout labor and delivery.

Category II and III fetal heart rate

Category II FHR tracings include all FHR tracings not categorized as category I or category III. Category III FHR tracings include absent baseline variability and recurrent late decelerations, recurrent variable decelerations, and/or bradycardia. A sinusoidal FHR pattern is considered category III. The absence of accelerations in the FHR, particularly when accompanied by persistent decelerations, may be a concerning finding in the EFM. The presence of recurrent late, variable, or prolonged decelerations with absent FHR variability is a pattern which requires close attention by the healthcare providers. Possible causes of such decelerations and their remedies should be considered. Treatment options include cervical examination to determine dilation and assess for umbilical cord prolapse. Repositioning the patient to the left or right lateral recumbent position is recommended. Discontinuation or diminishing of Pitocin or other uterine stimulants and consideration of treatment with a tocolytic agent are additionally recommended. Employing one or more of these treatments will often result in rapid improvement of the concerning FHR.

Further assessment of such FHR patterns should include ancillary tests of the fetal status. The most commonly used modalities are scalp stimulation or vibroacoustic stimulation of the fetus with observation for the occurrence of an immediate acceleration of the FHR. This modality does not have any value in a prolonged deceleration. However, appropriate fetal response indicates the presence of a normal fetal pH. Specifically, if there is an acceleration of the FHR accompanying either direct digital scalp or vibroacoustic stimulation, fetal acidosis (pH ≥7.21) is excluded at that point in time [7]. This allows for the continuation of labor in a patient with nonreassuring FHR changes. In the absence of accelerations of the FHR with such stimulation, there is the possibility of an abnormal fetal pH. Traditionally, obtaining a sample of fetal blood from the scalp has been utilized as a means to determine the fetal pH. However, this technique is currently rarely employed and for most practitioners is not even available. Further, there is poor sensitivity and specificity of a scalp pH less than 7.21 predicting umbilical artery acidosis (pH < 7.0) or adverse neonatal neurologic outcome. Consequently, direct assessment of fetal blood pH levels no longer occurs in most centers.

Fetal resuscitation

Management of category III FHR patterns is often limited to immediate delivery, commonly by cesarean section. However, use of various ancillary techniques should be considered and frequently result in improved FHR tracing. The association of maternal hypotension and concerning changes in the FHR is commonly seen. Correction of such hypotension with maternal position change or ephedrine infusion (following epidural) is encouraged. Perhaps the most common technique is the administration of oxygen to the laboring patient along with rapid intravenous infusion of fluids. Not surprisingly, such interventions have not been shown to be efficacious but nonetheless are widely employed. What has been shown to have efficacy is the use of various forms of tocolytic therapy [8]. These most commonly include β-agonists such as terbutaline and ritodrine although other agents such as magnesium sulfate or calcium channel blockers can be considered. However, while improvement of the FHR commonly occurs following such therapy, there is no evidence to suggest overall improvement in newborn or neonatal outcome. Additionally, use of amnio-infusion in patients experiencing recurrent variable decelerations of the FHR has been shown to reduce the frequency and severity of variable decelerations as well as the need for cesarean delivery for fetal intolerance to labor [9]. This is a simple technique which is readily available in most labor and delivery units.

CASE PRESENTATION

The patient is a 32-year-old gravida 3, para 2002, at 39 weeks' gestation in active labor. Cervical examination reveals 5cm dilation with vertex well applied to the cervix. Artificial rupture of the membranes is performed with return of clear amniotic fluid. Within minutes, the FHR changes from a normal pattern without deceleration to one of persistent variable decelerations, a category II pattern (Fig. 11.1, panel 1). Through the previously placed intrauterine pressure catheter, amnio-infusion of normal saline is begun at 10mL/min for 1h. The subsequent FHR reveals marked change in the FHR to a category I pattern (Fig. 11.1, panels 2, 3). The patient subsequently has a vaginal delivery of a healthy newborn with Apgars of 8 and 9 at 1 and 5min, respectively.

This case demonstrates the potential value of amnio-infusion in patients experiencing recurrent variable decelerations. Although the exact mechanism of action is unknown, it is thought that the infused fluid relieves compression of the umbilical cord which is the etiology of the FHR decelerations.

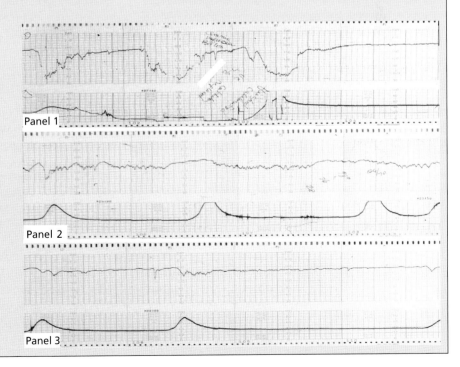

Figure 11.1 Fetal heart rate measurements.

References

1. Martin JA, Hamilton BE, Venture SJ, Menacker F, Park MM, Sutton PD. Births: final data for 2002. Natl Vital Stat Rep 2003;52:1–113.

2. Nelson KB, Dambrosia JM, Ting TY, Grether JK. Uncertain value of electronic fetal monitoring in predicting cerebral palsy. N Engl J Med 1996;324:613–618.

3. Macones GA, Hankins GDV, Spong CY, Hauth J, Moore T. The 2008 National Institute of Child Health and Human Development Workshop Report on Electronic Fetal Monitoring. Obstet Gynecol 2008;112:661–616.

4. American College of Obstetricians and Gynecologists. Intrapartum fetal heart rate monitoring: nomenclature, interpretation, and general management principles. ACOG Practice Bulletin No. 106. Washington, DC: American College of Obstetricians and Gynecologists, 2009.

5. Vitzileos AM, Nochimson DJ, Antsakis A, Vavarigos I, Guzman EF, Knuppel RA. Comparison of intrapartum electronic fetal heart rate monitoring versus intermittently auscultation in detecting fetal academia at birth. Am J Obstet Gynecol 1995; 173:1021–1024.

6. Samueloff A, Langer O, Berkus M, Field N, Xenakis E, Ridgway L. Is fetal heart rate variability a good predictor of fetal outcome? Acta Obstet Gynecol Scand 1994;73:39–44.

7. Skupzki DW, Rosenberg CR, Egllinton GS. Intrapartum fetal stimulation tests: a meta-analysis. Obstet Gynecol 2001;99: 129–134.

8. Kulier R, Hofmeyr GJ. Tocolytics for suspected intrapartum fetal distress. Cochrane Database Sys Rev 1998;1:CD00035.

9. Hofmeyr GJ. Amnioinfusion for umbilical cord compression in labor. Cochrane Database Syst Rev 1998;1:CD00013.

Chapter 12
Sickle Cell Anemia

Scott Roberts
Department of Obstetrics and Gynecology, University of Texas Southwestern Medical Center, Dallas, TX, USA

Sickle cell disease is a member of a family of genetic disorders involving abnormal hemoglobin. Each hemoglobin molecule is made up of two α-globin (141 amino acids) and two β-globin chains (146 amino acids). These chains conform to facilitate solubility, oxygen affinity and transport, and a stable biconcave structure in the red blood cell (RBC). Solubility and reversible oxygen binding are the key properties which are deranged in hemoglobinopathies. Sickle hemoglobin (S) results from the substitution of glutamic acid by valine in the β-globin chain at position 6, and hemoglobin C from substitution of the same amino acid but by lysine. The β-globin genes are expressed codominantly so that homozygous SS or the compound heterozygote SC must be expressed for clinical morbidity to be significant. In contrast, the β-thalassemia variant of the β-globin gene causes the production of normal hemoglobin A to be absent or reduced.

The most prevalent hemoglobinopathy is sickle cell anemia resulting from the homozygous SS genotype. One of every 12 African-Americans is a carrier for the hemoglobin S gene and hence $(1/12 \times 1/12 \times 1/4 = 1/576)$ approximately 1 in 600 African-American newborns has sickle cell anemia [1]. The overall rate of sickle cell disorders at birth for African-Americans is 1 in 300 [2]. The prevalence of the hemoglobin C allele is approximately 1 in 40 and the β-thalassemia gene approximately 1 in 40 to 1 in 50 in this population. These disorders are associated with increased maternal and perinatal morbidity and mortality.

Red blood cells with hemoglobin S undergo sickling under conditions of decreased oxygen tension. This results in hemolysis, increased viscosity, and vasoocclusion (VOC), and leads to further decreased oxygenation. This VOC leads to local infarction in all major organ systems, and all surviving adults with sickle cell anemia have undergone autosplenectomy after multiple episodes of VOC and infarction. The bone pain, so typical of sickle cell crises, represents VOC in the bone marrow.

Other chronic and acute changes from sickling include bony abnormalities such as osteonecrosis of the femoral and humeral heads, renal medullary damage, hepatomegaly, ventricular hypertrophy, pulmonary infarctions, pulmonary hypertension, cerebrovascular accidents, leg ulcers, and a susceptibility to infection and sepsis [3–5].

Because of hemolysis of defective RBCs, most patients with sickle cell anemia have hemoglobin values of approximately 7–8 g/dL. Iron therapy will not treat their anemia and may worsen their condition due to iron overload. Folic acid requirements, however, are considerable as there is intense hematopoiesis occurring to compensate for the markedly shortened RBC lifespan. Patients with SC disease are usually less anemic, with hemoglobin levels near 10 g/dL, and painful crises occur less frequently. Manifestations of S/β-thalassemia disease are quite variable, but can present similarly to severe SS disease. In either SC disease or S/ β-thalassemia, iron studies should be performed and iron supplemented if indicated.

Pregnancy is a serious burden to women with sickle hemoglobinopathies, especially those with hemoglobin SS disease. Pregnancy usually results in an increased frequency of sickle cell crises. Infections and pulmonary complications are common. Maternal mortality has decreased dramatically over the years because of improvements in medical care, but remains high. According to the Nationwide Inpatient Sample from the Healthcare Cost and Utilization Project of the Agency for Healthcare Research and Quality, for the years 2000–2003, the maternal mortality rate was 72.4 deaths per 100,000 deliveries in women with sickle cell disease (SCD), compared with a mortality rate of 12.7 deaths per 100,000 deliveries for women without SCD [6–8]. Significant maternal risks are faced by women with SCD during pregnancy (Table 12.1). Although women with SCD comprise 0.1% of the delivering population, they account for 1% of maternal deaths

Queenan's Management of High-Risk Pregnancy: An Evidence-Based Approach, Sixth Edition. Edited by John T. Queenan, Catherine Y. Spong, Charles J. Lockwood.
© 2012 John Wiley & Sons, Ltd. Published 2012 by John Wiley & Sons, Ltd.

[6]. Some overall statistical demographics from the National Inpatient Sample are listed in Table 12.2 [9].

Hemoglobin SC disease

In nonpregnant women, morbidity and mortality from sickle cell/hemoglobin C disease are much lower than those seen with SS homozygous disease. Fewer than half of the women with SC disease have ever been symptomatic prior to pregnancy. However, during pregnancy and the puerperium, attacks of severe bone pain and episodes of pulmonary infarction and embolization become more common [10]. A particularly worrisome complication is acute chest syndrome seen in both SS and SC disease related to embolization of necrotic fat and cellular bone marrow, and VOC sickling, with resultant respiratory insufficiency. This syndrome is characterized by a noninfectious pulmonary infiltrate with fever, leading to hypoxemia and acidosis, and, infrequently, death. Acute chest syndrome is the leading cause of death among patients with sickle cell disease [11].

Table 12.1 Increased rates for maternal complications in pregnancies complicated by sickle cell syndromes [6]

Complications	OR	P-value
Preexisting medical disorders		
Cardiomyopathy	3.7	<0.001
Pulmonary hypertension	6.3	<0.001
Renal failure	3.5	0.9
Pregnancy complications		
Cerebral vein thrombosis	4.9	<0.001
Pneumonia	9.8	<0.001
Pyelonephritis	1.3	0.5
Deep venous thrombosis	2.5	<0.001
Pulmonary embolism	1.7	0.08
Sepsis syndrome	6.8	<0.001
Delivery complications		
Gestational hypertension/preeclampsia	1.2	0.01
Eclampsia	3.2	<0.001
Placental abruption	1.6	<0.001
Preterm delivery	1.4	<0.001
Fetal growth restriction	2.2	<0.001

OR, odds ratio.

Perinatal mortality is higher in SC disease (75 in 1000) than in the general population, but not as high as with SS disease (175 in 1000) (Table 12.3).

Hemoglobin S/β-thalassemia disease

This heterozygous condition usually is much milder than either SS or SC disease. Variable amounts of hemoglobin A are produced depending on the variant of the β-thalassemia allele inherited. Hemoglobin F is made in abundance with extramedullary hematopoiesis to make up for abnormally low hemoglobin A. In its most usual form, a level of A2 above 3.5% on hemoglobin electrophoresis is diagnostic. In the most severe form of S/β-thalassemia disease, no hemoglobin F is made and the resulting phenotypic expression is of severe SS disease.

Either of the above sickle cell variants can have symptoms as bad as or worse than any particular SS patient. Particularly unnerving and dangerous is the previously asymptomatic SC or S/β-thalassemia patient who presents with acute chest syndrome in pregnancy.

Management during pregnancy

Close observation of these patients is mandatory during pregnancy. They are at increased risk for infection, which in turn can aggravate sickling crises. With the increased RBC mass typically required during pregnancy, folate supplementation is important. Any strain that impairs erythropoiesis or increases RBC destruction aggravates the anemia. Clinical presentations that cause anemia and pain may be overlooked (e.g. placental abruption, ectopic pregnancy, appendicitis, and pyelonephritis). The diagnosis of sickle cell crisis should be reserved until other possible causes are ruled out.

Covert bacteriuria and acute pyelonephritis are increased in these patients. Frequent (monthly or every trimester) screening urine cultures should be employed to discover asymptomatic bacteriuria and treat before it becomes symptomatic. Acute pyelonephritis can result in the release of endotoxin which lyses sickle cells and suppresses hematopoiesis, resulting in severe anemia and sickle crises. Pneumonia is common, caused by *Streptococcus pneumoniae*, and the polyvalent

Table 12.2 Demographic and obstetric outcomes in SCD 2002–2004 [9]

Number	SCD	Age	%AA	Renal failure	PROM	LOS	OR Hosp	No. Hosp	Cesarean delivery
14,000,000	4352	25.3	89.4	0.5%	4.4%	5.3 days	5.56	11,928	1936

AA, African American; LOS, length of stay; OR, odds ratio; PROM, premature rupture of membranes; SCD, sickle cell disease.

Table 12.3 Pregnancy outcomes reported since 1956 for women with sickle cell anemia and hemoglobin SC disease [6,7,22–29]

	Sickle cell disease (SS)	Hemoglobin SC disease
Women	1213	351
Pregnancies	2214	798
Maternal deaths (per 100,000)	~2500	~2300
Perinatal mortality (per 1000)	~175	~75

pneumococcal vaccine is recommended. Annual inactivated influenza vaccine should be administered. Hepatitis B vaccination is recommended. For patients who have undergone autosplenectomy, vaccination against *Haemophilus influenzae* type B is recommended.

Crises are hallmarked by intense pain, usually from involved bone marrow. As many as 40% of sickle cell patients have acute chest syndrome [9]. Episodes can develop acutely and do so more often late in pregnancy. Intravenous hydration along with opioid analgesics should be given. Oxygen by nasal cannula will decrease the sickling at the capillary level and improve symptoms. Any focus of infection should be discovered and treated as it may be responsible for the crisis. The risks of low birthweight, fetal growth restriction, preterm delivery, and preeclampsia are increased. Cardiac dysfunction is prevalent in sickle cell disease. After years of pulmonary infarction, restrictive airway disease can lead to ventricular hypertrophy and pulmonary hypertension [12]. There is increased preload and decreased afterload with a normal ejection fraction. This condition is augmented by the increasing volume of pregnancy. Chronic hypertension can aggravate the preexisting cardiac dysfunction. Severe preeclampsia, sepsis or secondary pulmonary hypertension can lead to heart failure. A multidisciplinary approach should be used involving obstetricians, hematologists, and anesthesiologists [13].

Prophylactic red blood cell transfusions

Some institutions utilize prophylactic RBC transfusions. Managed correctly, sickle crises can be held to a minimum. Hematocrit and hemoglobin electrophoresis are monitored monthly and transfusion effected to keep the hematocrit between 25% and 30% and the S fraction of hemoglobin no greater than 60%. Prophylactic transfusions will not modify an existing sickle crisis. However, exchange transfusion in the face of crisis, acute chest syndrome, stroke, and infection can be valuable.

Transfusion is not without its complications. Transfusion-related lung injury occurs in approximately 1 in 5000 units of blood products transfused [14]. Delayed hemolytic transfusion reactions are reported in as many as 10% of patients [15]. The rate of viral infection from transfusion is exceedingly low with modern pretransfusion blood screening techniques. The highest rate is from hepatitis B at 1 in 100,000 and that from hepatitis C and HIV at approximately 1 in 2,000,000 [16]. The rate of alloimmunization has been reported at 3% per unit in the sickle disease population [17]. Because of the concern for the aforementioned and the usual need for repeated transfusions in this population, all blood should be typed and crossed and leukocyte reduced. There is no reported benefit in maternal or perinatal mortality from the use of prophylactic transfusions [18].

Much of the decrease in perinatal and maternal morbidity and mortality is ascribed to improved perinatal care in the sickle disease population. Managing without prophylactic transfusions, however, can involve multiple long and painful hospitalizations [10,18].

In our institution, SCD patients are managed conservatively, reserving prophylactic blood transfusions, if at all, for unique situations in which perinatal morbidity seems to be the highest: low hemoglobin F concentration, frequent pain crises, history of acute chest syndrome or severe anemia. Worsening anemia, painful crisis or chest syndrome may benefit from exchange transfusion [19].

Fetal assessment

Pregnancies in women with sickle cell disease are at increased risk for spontaneous abortion, preterm labor, fetal growth restriction, and stillbirth [20]. Frequent assessment for the detection of fetal growth restriction, oligohydramnios, and assurance of fetal activity is important. Formal antepartum surveillance may be used to augment fetal assessment (e.g. biophysical profile, umbilical artery Doppler in the presence of fetal growth restriction). Published data concerning antepartum surveillance in pregnancies complicated by sickle cell disease are limited.

Labor and delivery

Management should take into account the degree of underlying cardiac dysfunction. Preparatory consultation with an anesthesiologist is helpful. Route of delivery otherwise should be based solely on obstetric indications. Epidural anesthesia is ideal and will keep the patient comfortable during a long labor process. If a difficult vaginal or cesarean delivery is foreseen, and the patient's hematocrit is less than 20%, packed RBCs should be administered. Blood should be typed and crossed and readily available. Fluid administration should be conservative to avoid circulatory overload and pulmonary edema.

Genetic evaluation

Prenatal genetic evaluation is possible for the sickle hemoglobinopathies. Maternal and paternal electrophoresis will elucidate the potential genotypes. When there is reasonable suspicion and probability, amniocentesis or chorionic villus sampling should be offered and polymerase chain reaction (PCR) utilized to detect abnormal fetal genotypes. Most couples with foreknowledge of an SS fetus will opt to carry the pregnancy forward [21], but some will not.

CASE PRESENTATION

The patient is a 28-year-old, gravida 1, para 0, Nigerian woman with SS disease. She was first seen at 15–16 weeks with painful sickle crisis involving her extremities, and pleuritic chest pain. She was found to have a hematocrit of 28.5% and was transfused previously during the pregnancy; electrophoresis now had S 60% and A 40%. She was alloimmunized with anti-c and anti-E antibodies, titers too low to report. Ultrasound showed diamnionic/dichorionic twins. Baseline renal function showed 24-h urine protein of 122 mg and urine culture was negative. Chest x-ray revealed left retrocardiac opacity which was stable in appearance from a previous chest x-ray 1 year previously and probably represented old pulmonary infarction. Cardiomegaly and a small calcified spleen were noted on computed tomography (CT) scan from 1 year before. Influenza vaccination was given. Pneumococcal vaccine had been given previously. Significant pathology (e.g. appendicitis, acute chest syndrome) was ruled out. Her crisis was managed with intravenous hydration, opioid analgesics, and oxygen by nasal cannula. She remained hospitalized for the next 2 weeks and was discharged on 4 mg/day folate.

She was seen in the clinic thereafter every 2 weeks. At 20, 26, and 30 weeks, ultrasound evaluation revealed size less than dates with 4%, 8%, and 14% discordance, respectively, between twins. The father of the babies was unavailable for zygosity testing concerning maternal antibodies, and fortunately anti-c and anti-E titers were never significantly elevated. From 18 weeks onward the patient was transfused approximately every month to achieve a hematocrit of at least 25% with hemoglobin S percentages less than 60%. She presented to the hospital three more times during gestation for painful VOC, one of which was complicated by a hemoglobin S fraction of 78% with a hematocrit of 23.6%. However, because of subsequent and continued adequate hematocrit and hemoglobin A versus S fractions and absence of objective morbidity, exchange transfusion was not performed.

Her last admission occurred at 32–33 weeks. At this time she had mildly elevated blood pressures and a hematocrit of 22.7%. With limited intravenous (IV) access, the patient had a peripherally inserted central catheter (PICC) line placed and received transfusion to a hematocrit of 30%. Her 24-h urine protein was 3.8 g. She was managed with ward rest and maternal fetal surveillance. At 33–34 weeks, her hypertension increased and the decision was made to deliver for severe preeclampsia. A low transverse cesarean was performed per hospital protocol and seizure prophylaxis was instituted until 24 h postpartum. She recovered unremarkably, without further crises or transfusions during the puerperal period. Both babies did well in the special care nursery and went home within 2 weeks.

We note the lack of apparent benefit in this patient with prophylactic transfusions on significantly decreasing the number of painful crises she endured. We believe that this patient's management was complicated by opioid tolerance and/or dependence. She was never pain free beginning with her first admission at 15–16 weeks, and was managed as an outpatient with oral hydromorphone between admissions. Difficulties were also encountered in achieving IV access in this patient who had received multiple transfusions in her lifetime. Although premature and complicated by preeclampsia, both maternal and perinatal outcome were good.

We believe this case highlights some of the significant and not atypical problems with SS disease in pregnancy. It should be emphasized that some of the worst morbidity occurs in SC and S/β-thalassemia disease, and that evaluation and management should be similar to those of the SS patient.

References

1. Angastiniotis M, Modell B. Global epidemiology of hemoglobin disorders. Ann N Y Acad Sci 1998;850:251–269.
2. Motulsky AG. Frequency of sickling disorders in US Blacks. N Engl J Med 1973;288:31–33.
3. Driscoll MC, Hurlet A, Styles L et al. Stroke risk in siblings with sickle cell anemia. Blood 2003;101:2401–2404.
4. Gladwin MT, Sachdev V, Jison ML et al. Pulmonary hypertension as a risk factor for death in patients with sickle cell disease. N Engl J Med 2004;350:886–895.
5. Weatherall DJ, Provan AB. Red cell I: inherited anaemias. Lancet 2000;355:1169–1175.
6. Villers MS, Jamison MG, DeCastro LM, James AH. Morbidity associated with sickle cell disease in pregnancy. Am J Obstet Gynecol 2008;199:125.
7. Powars DR, Sandhu M, Niland-Weiss J et al. Pregnancy in sickle cell disease. Obstet Gynecol 1986;67:217–228.
8. Poddar D, Maude GH, Plant MJ, Scorer H, Serjeant GR. Pregnancy in Jamaican women with homozygous sickle cell disease: fetal and maternal outcome. Br J Obstet Gynaecol 1986;93:927–932.

9. Chakravarty EF, Khanna D, Chung L. Pregnancy outcomes in systemic sclerosis, pulmonary hypertension, and sickle cell disease. Obstet Gynecol 2008;111:927–934.

10. Cunningham FG, Pritchard JA, Mason R. Pregnancy and sickle hemoglobinopathy: results with and without prophylactic transfusions. Obstet Gynecol 1983;62:419–424.

11. Vichinsky EP, Neumayr LD, Earles AN et al. Causes and outcomes of the acute chest syndrome in sickle cell disease. N Engl J Med 2000;342:1855–1865.

12. Powars D, Weidman JA, Odom-Maryon T, Niland JC, Johnson C. Sickle cell chronic lung disease: prior morbidity and the risk of pulmonary failure. Medicine (Baltimore) 1988;67:66–76.

13. Rees DC, Olujohungbe AD, Parker NE, Stephens AD, Telfer P, Wright J. Guidelines for the management of the acute painful crisis in sickle cell disease. British Committee for Standards in Haematology General Haematology Task Force by the Sickle Cell Working Party. Br J Haematol 2003;120:744–752.

14. Silliman CC, Boshkov LK, Mehdizadehkashi Z et al. Transfusion-related acute lung injury: epidemiology and a prospective analysis of etiologic factors. Blood 2003;101: 454–462.

15. Garratty G. Severe reactions associated with transfusion of patients with sickle cell disease. Transfusion 1997;37:357–361.

16. Jackson BR, Busch MP, Stramer SL, AuBuchon JP. The cost-effectiveness of NAT for HIV, HCV, and HBV in whole-blood donations. Transfusion 2003;43:721–729.

17. Cox JV, Steane E, Cunningham G, Frenkel EP. Risk of alloimmunization and delayed hemolytic transfusion reactions in patients with sickle cell disease. Arch Intern Med 1988; 148:2485–2489.

18. Koshy M, Burd L, Wallace D, Moawad A, Baron J. Prophylactic red-cell transfusions in pregnant patients with sickle cell disease: a randomized cooperative study. N Engl J Med 1988;319:1447–1452.

19. National Institutes of Health, National Heart, Lung, and Blood Institute, and Division of Blood Diseases and Resources. The Management of Sickle Cell Disease. NIH Publication No. 02–2117. Bethesda, MD: National Institutes of Health, 2002.

20. Serjeant GR, Loy LL, Crowther M, Hambleton IR, Thame M. Outcome of pregnancy in homozygous sickle cell disease. Obstet Gynecol 2004;103:1278–1285.

21. Alter BP. Prenatal diagnosis of hematologic diseases: 1986 update. Acta Haematol 1987;78:137–141.

22. Morris JS, Dunn DT, Poddar D, Sergeant GR. Haematological risk factors in pregnancy outcome in Jamaican women with homozygous sickle cell disease. Br J Obstet Gynaecol 1994 Sep;101(9):770–3.

23. Smith JA, Espeland M, Bellevue R, Bonds D, Brown AK, Koshy M. Pregnancy in sickle cell disease: experience of the cooperative study of sickle cell disease. Obstet Gynecol 1996;87:199–204.

24. Charache S, Scott J, Niebyl J, Bonds D. Management of sickle cell disease in pregnant patients. Obstet Gynecol 1980;55:407–410.

25. El-Shafei AM, Dhaliwal JK, Sandhu AK. Pregnancy in sickle cell disease in Bahrain. Br J Obstet Gynaecol 1992;99:101–104.

26. Howard RJ, Tuck SM, Pearson TC. Pregnancy in sickle cell disease in the UK: results of a multi-centre survey of the effect of prophylactic blood transfusion on maternal and fetal outcome. Br J Obstet Gynaecol 1995;102:947–951.

27. Milner PF, Jones BR, Dobler J. Outcome of pregnancy in sickle cell anemia and sickle cell-hemoglobin C disease. Am J Obstet Gynecol 1980;138:239–245.

28. Seoud MA, Cantwell C, Nobles G, Levy DL. Outcome of pregnancies complicated by sickle cell and sickle-C hemoglobinopathies. Am J Perinatol 1994;11:187–191.

29. Sun PM, Wilburn W, Raynor BD, Jamieson D. Sickle cell disease in pregnancy: twenty years of experience at Grady Memorial Hospital, Atlanta, Georgia. Am J Obstet Gynecol 2001;184:1127–1130.

Chapter 13
Anemia

Alessandro Ghidini

Department of Obstetrics and Gynecology, Georgetown University Hospital, Washington, DC, and Perinatal Diagnostic Center Inova Alexandria Hospital, Alexandria, VA, USA

A comprehensive review of all causes of anemia is often intimidating for the general obstetrician. Moreover, most algorithms are not targeted to conditions highly prevalent in obstetric populations consisting mainly of healthy young women. The current chapter proposes an initial evaluation of anemia, which will allow the identification and appropriate therapy of the majority of cases encountered in a pregnant population. The few cases which defy the initial evaluation are probably better managed in consultation with a hematologist.

Definition

The fall in hemoglobin (Hb) level seen in healthy normal pregnant women, also known as physiologic or dilutional anemia of pregnancy, is caused by a relatively greater expansion of plasma volume (50%) compared with the red blood cell (RBC) volume (25%). The fall in hematocrit (Hct) reaches a nadir during the late second to early third trimester, when normal values in pregnancy range from 33% to 44%. The Centers for Disease Control and Prevention (CDC) define anemia as a Hb or Hct level below the 5th centile for a healthy, iron-supplemented population, i.e. a Hb <11 g/dL or a Hct <33% in the first trimester, and Hb <10.5 or Hct <32% afterwards [1]. Severe anemia is usually defined as Hb level at or below 8.5 mg/dL. The two most common causes of anemia during pregnancy and the puerperium are iron deficiency and acute blood loss.

Consequences

According to the World Health Organization (WHO), severe anemia contributes to 40% of maternal deaths in underdeveloped countries [2]. In developed countries, severe anemia has been associated with increased risk of preterm birth, preterm premature rupture of membranes, infections, and fetal growth restriction [3–6]. The symptoms of mild anemia are often indistinguishable from those related to pregnancy, and include fatigue, breathlessness, palpitations, difficulty in concentration, and lower intellectual and productive capacity.

Diagnostic work-up and treatment

Traditionally, evaluation of anemia starts with mean corpuscular volume (MCV), based on which anemias are defined as microcytic (<80 fL), normocytic (80–100 fL) or macrocytic (>100 fL). However, mixed nutritional deficiencies (folate and iron) often lead to normocytic anemia, and most anemias at the beginning are normocytic. The red cell distribution width (RDW) is a useful indicator of anemias due to nutritional deficiencies (i.e. it increases above 15% in the presence of iron, folate or vitamin B_{12} deficiencies).

Macrocytic anemia

Appropriate work-up of macrocytic anemia (MCV >100 fL) should begin with assessment of serum folate and vitamin B_{12} levels.

Vitamin B_{12} deficiency is rare, as most healthy individuals have 2–3 years' storage available in the liver. However, vitamin B_{12} deficiency can be encountered in individuals who have undergone bariatric surgery and are not compliant with the recommended vitamin B_{12} supplementation (350 μg/day sublingually plus 1000 μg intramuscularly (IM) every 3 months if needed). It also occurs in individuals with pernicious anemia, an extremely uncommon autoimmune disease in women of reproductive age which is diagnosed by the presence of serum intrinsic factor antibodies, and in those with malabsorption (e.g. Crohn disease or ileal resection).

Queenan's Management of High-Risk Pregnancy: An Evidence-Based Approach, Sixth Edition. Edited by John T. Queenan, Catherine Y. Spong, Charles J. Lockwood.

Folate deficiency is less common nowadays given US fortification of grains with folate. In addition to macrocytic anemia, folate deficiency often also causes thrombocytopenia. Recommended folate requirements are 400 μg/day during the pregnant state and 500 μg/day for lactating women [7]. However, higher dosages are recommended in the presence of multiple gestations, hemolytic disorders (such as sickle cell anemia or thalassemia), and in patients taking antiepileptic therapies or sulfa-containing drugs (e.g. sulfasalazine). If a diagnosis of folate deficiency is made or the woman previously had an infant with a neural tube defect, the recommended dose of folic acid is 4 mg/day. By 4–7 days after beginning treatment, the reticulocyte count should be increased. In the case of macrocytic anemia with normal folate and vitamin B_{12} levels, a consultation with a hematologist is indicated for bone marrow biopsy.

Normocytic anemia

The pertinent laboratory work-up of normocytic anemia (MCV between 80 and 100 fL) should start with a reticulocyte count. A high reticulocyte count suggests recent blood loss due to hemolysis (e.g. drug induced or immune based, as witnessed by a positive direct Coombs test) or hemorrhage.

Low reticulocyte count is usually seen in the early stage of iron deficiency, and it should prompt assessment of a serum ferritin level. Serum ferritin is the most sensitive screening test for iron deficiency, with a level <16 ng/mL indicating depleted iron stores. Normal or high serum ferritin levels can be seen in the presence of hypothyroidism or chronic disorders (such as inflammatory bowel disease, systemic lupus erythematosus or rheumatoid arthritis). Hematology consultation for further assessment is indicated in these circumstances.

Microcytic anemia

Because most cases of microcytic anemia (MCV <80 fL) in pregnancy are due to iron deficiency and because serum ferritin is an excellent indicator of body iron stores, the initial step should be assessment of serum ferritin levels. Low serum ferritin would diagnose iron deficiency. A high or normal serum ferritin level should indicate a hemoglobin electrophoresis, which would allow identification of heterozygous thalassemia (characterized by high percentage levels of Hb A_2 and F). Normal hemoglobin A_2 and F should prompt DNA probes for α-thalassemia and a request for hematology consultation.

Prophylaxis of iron deficiency

In a typical singleton gestation, maternal iron requirements, related to the expansion of the maternal RBC mass, fetal and placental requirements, average 1 g over the course of pregnancy. In a landmark study of healthy, non-anemic, menstruating young women who agreed to bone marrow biopsy, 66% had inadequate iron stores [8]. For the above reasons, and because gastrointestinal side-effects of oral iron supplementation, which include constipation, nausea and diarrhea, are negligible with doses less than 45–60 mg, in the US supplementation with elemental iron (30 mg/day) is recommended for all pregnant nonanemic women [7]. This prophylaxis should be continued until 3 months postpartum in areas with high prevalence of anemia. Despite such recommendations, a large study has shown that 50% of women develop iron deficiency anemia by 26 weeks' gestation [9].

A review of randomized clinical trials generally performed in Western countries shows that routine supplementation in nonanemic women results in higher maternal Hb levels at term and 1 month postpartum, higher serum ferritin levels, lower rates of anemia at term (relative risk [RR] 0.27, 95% confidence interval [CI] 0.17–0.42) and of iron deficiency anemia in particular (RR 0.33, 95% CI 0.16–0.69), and higher serum ferritin levels in the infants [10]. However no differences are noted in most clinical outcomes, such as preterm delivery, preeclampsia, or need for transfusion, birthweight, small for gestational age, perinatal mortality or need for neonatal intensive care unit (NICU) admissions [10].

Treatment of iron deficiency anemia

Higher doses of iron are required for therapy of anemia than for prophylaxis (up to 120–150 mg/day).

Oral iron: Table 13.1 lists the most commonly available formulations of oral iron. Enteric-coated forms should be avoided because they are poorly absorbed; absorption is increased by intake of iron on an empty stomach and with concomitant ingestion of vitamin C or orange juice. Although several trials have been conducted to compare types of iron, it is not possible to assess the efficacy of the treatments due to the use of different drugs, doses, and routes [11]. Gut absorption of iron decreases with increasing doses of iron: divide the total daily dose into 2–3 doses. A relationship is present between dose of oral iron and gastrointestinal side-effects. Occurrence of such side-effects leads to discontinuation of therapy in 50% of women [12]. To ensure patient compliance, it is thus important to minimize the side-effects. Suggested strategies include:

• prescribe ferric iron, which seems to have fewer side-effects than ferrous fumarate or ferrous sulfate [12]
• increase doses of iron gradually
• instruct the patient to take the large doses at bedtime. Stool softeners may be needed to prevent constipation. Serum reticulocyte count can be checked after 7–10 days of therapy to document appropriate response. The rate of increase of Hct is typically 1% per week. To replenish iron stores, oral therapy should be continued for 3 months after the anemia has been corrected.

Type of iron	Elemental iron (mg)	Brand
Ferrous fumarate	64–200	Femiron, Feostat, Ferrets, Fumasorb, Hemocyte, Ircon, Nephro-Fer, Vitron-C
Ferrous sulfate	40–65	Chem-Sol, Fe50, Feosol, Fergensol, Ferinsol, Ferogradumet, Ferosul, Ferratab, FerraTD, Ferrobob, Ferrospace, Ferrotime, Moliron, Slowfe, Yieronia
Ferrous gluconate	38	Fergon, Ferralet, Simron
Ferrous fumarate and ferrous asparto-glycinate	81	Replica 21/7
Ferric 5	0–150	Ferrimin, Fe-Tinic, Hytinic, Niferex, Nu-iron

Table 13.1 Oral preparations for therapy of iron deficiency anemia

Intravenous iron is more effective than oral therapy at improving hematological indices, with higher maternal Hb levels at 4 weeks of therapy and lower rates of gastrointestinal side-effects [11]. However, randomized trials have not shown significant differences in need for maternal blood transfusion, neonatal birthweight, or neonatal anemia. Therefore, intravenous (IV) therapy is indicated only in cases of severe anemia with intolerance to oral therapy or malabsorption [13]. Different formulations of IV iron are available: dextran iron (INFeD®) should not be used because it is associated with side-effects in 8.7% of cases, including delayed serum sickness reactions, fever, urticaria, and anaphylactic reactions leading to maternal death. Ferric gluconate (Ferrlecit®) is safer, with only a 2% rate of side-effects and no recorded cases of anaphylaxis. Iron sucrose (Venofer®) has also been recently introduced onto the market.

The required dose of IV iron can be calculated according to the formula:

$$\text{IV iron dose (mg)} = \text{blood volume (dL)} \times$$
$$\text{Hb deficit (g/dL)} \times 3.3$$

in which the blood volume can be estimated as $65\,\text{mL} \times \text{weight}/100$, the Hb deficit is the difference between the observed and desired Hb level (usually $12\,\text{g/dL}$), and 3.3 reflects the amount of iron in each gram of Hb.

Erythropoietin is not indicated in the treatment of iron deficiency anemia unless the anemia is caused by chronic renal failure or other chronic conditions, such as those outlined above among causes of normocytic anemias with low reticulocyte count and normal or high serum ferritin levels. Erythropoietin is an expensive medication with risk of side-effects, ranging from flu-like illness to pure red cell aplasia.

Blood transfusion is indicated only for anemia associated with hypovolemia from blood loss or in preparation for a cesarean delivery in the presence of severe anemia.

CASE PRESENTATION

A 28-year-old woman, gravida 6, para 3023, presented at 35 weeks with a long history of severe anemia and poor attendance to prenatal visits. She had been prescribed iron prophylaxis during pregnancy, but she had been noncompliant with it. Initial laboratory evaluation revealed Hb 7.9 g/dL, Hct 23.9%, and MCV 85, suggesting a diagnosis of normocytic anemia. Reticulocyte count was low, at 1.9%, thus prompting assessment of serum ferritin, which was <15, thus establishing a diagnosis of iron deficiency anemia. There was no co-existent deficiency of folate (RBC folate 16.6, normal values 3–18) or vitamin B_{12} (342, normal values 248–894). Given the documented lack of compliance, it was decided to implement replacement therapy with IV iron. It was calculated that the iron deficit was 400 mg. IV ferric gluconate (Ferrlecit®) 125 mg elemental iron was administered daily for 3 days. After 3 days, the reticulocyte count had increased appropriately to 2.6%, and at delivery 4 weeks later the Hct had appropriately increased to 28%.

References

1. Centers for Disease Control and Prevention. CDC criteria for anemia in children and childbearing-aged women. MMWR 1989;38:400.

2. Viteri FE. The consequences of iron deficiency and anemia in pregnancy. Adv Exp Med Biol 1994;352:127.

3. Kadyrov M, Kosanke G, Kingdom J et al. Increased fetoplacental angiogenesis during first trimester in anaemic women. Lancet 1998;352:1747.

4. Klebanoff MA, Shiono PH, Selby JV et al. Anemia and spontaneous preterm birth. Am J Obstet Gynecol 1991;164:59.

5. Lieberman E, Ryan KJ, Monson RR et al. Risk factors accounting for racial differences in the rate of premature birth. N Engl J Med 1987;317:743.

6. Scanlon KS, Yip R, Schieve LA et al. High and low hemoglobin levels during pregnancy: differential risk for preterm birth and small for gestational age. Obstet Gynecol 2000;96:741.

7. American College of Obstetricians and Gynecologists. Clinical Management Guidelines for Obstetrician-Gynecologists. Practice Bulletin No. 44, July 2003. Obstet Gynecol 2003;102:203.

8. Scott DE, Pritchard JA. Iron deficiency in healthy young college women. JAMA 1967;199:147.

9. Goldenberg RL, Tamura T, DuBard M et al. Plasma ferritin and pregnancy outcome. Am J Obstet Gynecol 1996;175:1356.

10. Pena-Rosas JP, Viteri FE. Effects of routine oral iron supplementation with or without folic acid for women during pregnancy. Cochrane Pregnancy and Childbirth Group. Cochrane Database Syst Rev 2009;3:CD004736.

11. Reveiz L, Gyte GML, Cuervo LG. Treatments for iron-deficiency anaemia in pregnancy. Cochrane Pregnancy and Childbirth Group. Cochrane Database Syst Rev 2007;2:CD003094.

12. Melamed N, Ben-Haroush A, Kaplan B, Yogev Y. Iron supplementation in pregnancy – does the preparation matter? Arch Gynecol Obstet 2007;276:601–604.

13. Faich G, Strobos J. Sodium ferric gluconate complex in sucrose: safer intravenous iron therapy than iron dextrans. Am J Kidney Dis 1999;33:464–470.

Chapter 14
Thrombocytopenia

Robert M. Silver

Department of Obstetrics and Gynecology, University of Utah School of Medicine, Salt Lake City, UT, USA

The antepartum diagnosis of maternal thrombocytopenia has become more common because platelet counts are now routinely obtained as part of prenatal screening. Although thrombocytopenia is classically defined as a platelet count of less than 150,000/μL, there is a physiologic drop in platelet count during pregnancy of 10–30% secondary to hemodilution and increased consumption. The most common causes of maternal thrombocytopenia include gestational thrombocytopenia, preeclampsia/ HELLP (hemolysis, elevated liver enzymes, and low platelet count) syndrome, and autoimmune thrombocytopenia. These conditions have implications for both mother and fetus. Thus, it is important to consider both maternal and fetal thrombocytopenia.

Maternal thrombocytopenia

Gestational thrombocytopenia (GTP), also termed incidental thrombocytopenia of pregnancy, describes a mild (usually more than 70,000/μL platelet count), common (up to 5%), asymptomatic thrombocytopenia that occurs during pregnancy [1,2]. This accounts for more than 70% of thrombocytopenias in pregnant women [2,3]. The cause of thrombocytopenia in these women is unclear, but may be an acceleration of the physiologic pattern of increased platelet destruction [1]. Women with this diagnosis are healthy, not at risk for fetal thrombocytopenia or bleeding complications, and have no history of autoimmune thrombocytopenia. Platelet counts return to normal after delivery. It can be difficult to distinguish GTP from autoimmune thrombocytopenia. If thrombocytopenia is found late in pregnancy and counts are more than 70,000/μL, GTP is the most likely diagnosis. However, other causes of thrombocytopenia, including preeclampsia, should be excluded. Women with GTP do not require additional testing or specialized care.

Autoimmune thrombocytopenia, also termed idiopathic thrombocytopenic purpura (ITP), is a syndrome characterized by immunologically mediated thrombocytopenia. The disorder is caused primarily by autoantibodies to platelet membrane glycoproteins, leading to increased platelet destruction. In adults, ITP is typically a chronic disorder. It can be difficult to distinguish from other causes of thrombocytopenia and is a diagnosis of exclusion. The most common signs and symptoms include petechiae, ecchymoses, easy bruising, epistaxis, gingival bleeding, and menorrhagia. Serious spontaneous bleeding complications are rare, even in severely thrombocytic individuals with platelet counts of less than 10,000/μL [4]. When thrombocytopenia is profound and detected early in pregnancy, suspicion is high that the diagnosis is ITP. It often co-exists with pregnancy because the disease usually presents in the second to third decades of life and has a female preponderance of 3:1 in the mid-adult years (30–60 years) [5].

Few diagnostic tests are useful in the evaluation of ITP. A complete blood count (CBC) and peripheral blood smear are helpful to exclude other causes of thrombocytopenia (e.g. pancytopenia, leukemias). The peripheral smear may show an increased proportion of slightly enlarged platelets. Bone marrow biopsy is sometimes helpful to clarify the diagnosis as increased numbers of immature megakaryocytes may be seen and inadequate platelet production may be excluded. Although antiplatelet antibodies are present in most individuals with ITP, they are very nonspecific and testing is not recommended for the routine evaluation of maternal thrombocytopenia [6].

The focus of maternal therapy is to avoid bleeding complications associated with severe thrombocytopenia. Because labor and delivery pose a substantial risk for bleeding, most authorities recommend more aggressive medical therapy for women in the late second or third trimesters. Current recommendations about maternal

Queenan's Management of High-Risk Pregnancy: An Evidence-Based Approach, Sixth Edition. Edited by John T. Queenan, Catherine Y. Spong, Charles J. Lockwood.

therapy for ITP are derived largely from expert opinion. Pregnant women who are asymptomatic and who have platelet counts of over 50,000/µL do not require treatment. In the first and second trimesters, asymptomatic women with platelet counts of 30,000–50,000/µL also do not require treatment. Treatment is considered appropriate [7]:

- for women with platelet counts of less than 20,000/µL at any gestational age
- for women with mucocutaneous bleeding and thrombocytopenia at any gestational age
- to produce an increase in platelet count to a level considered safe for procedures. This is controversial but is considered to be 50,000/µL for cesarean delivery and 75,000/µL for regional anesthesia. Thus, more aggressive treatment is often considered during the third trimester in anticipation of delivery.

Glucocorticoids are standard first-line treatment in both pregnant and nonpregnant adults. Prednisone is initiated at a dosage of 1–2 mg/kg/day and is typically continued for 2–3 weeks. If platelet counts reach acceptable levels, the drug is tapered by 10–20% per week until the lowest dosage required to maintain the platelet count at an acceptable level is achieved. Some increase in platelet count occurs in approximately 70% of patients, and complete remission has been reported in up to 25% of cases [8]. A response to glucocorticoids is usually apparent in 3–7 days and will reach a maximum in 2–3 weeks [5]. The benefits of steroids appear to outweigh the risks in women requiring treatment for ITP.

Intravenous immunoglobulin (IVIG) is an appropriate initial treatment for pregnant women with platelet counts of:

- less than 10,000/µL in the third trimester
- 10,000–30,000/µL who are bleeding.

Intravenous immunoglobulin is also used in cases refractory to treatment with glucocorticoids. The optimal dose for treatment is uncertain. IVIG 400 mg/kg/day given for 2–5 consecutive days is the most widely used regimen, although similar results have been obtained using higher doses for a shorter duration. This dose of IVIG will substantially increase the platelet count in 75% of patients and will restore normal platelet counts in 50% of patients [6,9]. However, in 70% of cases, the platelet count will return to pretreatment levels within 1 month after treatment [6,9]. Mild side-effects of IVIG are common, but serious side-effects are rare. The most substantial drawback of IVIG therapy may be expense. It should therefore be used in cases of severe thrombocytopenia, hemorrhage or nonresponse to steroids.

Intravenous anti-D immunoglobulin has been used to successfully and safely treat ITP in rhesus (Rh)-positive individuals [10–13]. There is a theoretical risk of causing fetal anemia by administering high doses to pregnant women with Rh-positive fetuses. Acute hemolysis and disseminated intravascular coagulation (DIC) may be rare but potentially severe complications of anti-D administration [14]. In general, anti-D antibodies appear to be safe for both mother and fetus [11,13]. The use of anti-D is attractive because it is less expensive and has a shorter infusion time than IVIG.

Splenectomy was the first therapy recognized to be effective for ITP and induces complete remission in approximately 80% of patients. The postsplenectomy platelet counts increase rapidly and are often normal within 1–2 weeks. The procedure is usually avoided during pregnancy but can be safely accomplished, although preferably in the second trimester. Splenectomy during pregnancy is reserved for women with platelet counts of less than 10,000/µL who are bleeding and who fail to respond to steroids and IVIG [6]. The procedure is not recommended for asymptomatic women with platelet counts of more than 10,000/µL.

There are few data regarding the use of other medical therapies for ITP during pregnancy. One approach in refractory cases is to combine treatment with IVIG and steroids. Azathioprine and cyclosporine may be reasonable choices in extremely refractory cases [7].

Platelet transfusions should be used only as a temporary measure to prepare a patient for splenectomy or surgery, or for life-threatening hemorrhage. However, the usual elevation in platelet counts of approximately 10,000/µL per unit of platelet concentrate transfused is not achieved in patients with ITP because antiplatelet antibodies also bind to donor platelets. Thus, 6–10 units of platelet concentrate should be transfused. The ITP practice guideline panel recommends platelet transfusions before delivery in women with platelet counts of less than 10,000/µL undergoing planned cesarean delivery or with mucous membrane bleeding and anticipated vaginal delivery [6].

Mothers with ITP require little specialized care beyond attention to platelet count. These patients should be instructed to avoid salicylates, nonsteroidal antiinflammatory agents, and trauma. Regardless of route of delivery, platelets, fresh frozen plasma (FFP), and IVIG should be readily available.

Other causes

Other causes of thrombocytopenia during pregnancy include preeclampsia/HELLP syndrome, systemic lupus erythematosus, antiphospholipid syndrome, human immunodeficiency virus (HIV) infection, hepatitis C virus (HCV) infection, DIC, drug-induced thrombocytopenia, thrombotic thrombocytopenic purpura, hemolytic uremic syndrome, and pseudothrombocytopenia as a result of laboratory artefact. These disorders can be excluded with an appropriate history, physical examination, assessment of blood pressure, HIV and HCV serology, and laboratory studies (e.g. liver function tests).

Fetal thrombocytopenia

Autoimmune thrombocytopenia

Fetal thrombocytopenia and, rarely, bleeding complications may occur with ITP because maternal immunoglobulin-G (IgG) antiplatelet antibodies are actively transported across the placenta. Avoidance of fetal hemorrhagic complications is the central issue in the obstetric management of these women. Occasionally, minor clinical bleeding such as purpura, ecchymoses, hematuria, or melena is observed. Rarely, fetal thrombocytopenia can lead to intracranial hemorrhage (ICH) which can result in severe neurologic impairment or even death. It is important to emphasize that the risk of serious fetal bleeding with maternal ITP is very low [3].

Strategies intended to minimize or avoid fetal bleeding complications include corticosteroids, IVIG, and splenectomy. Currently, no maternal treatment has been found to be consistently effective in the prevention of fetal/neonatal thrombocytopenia or to improve fetal outcome [15–18]. The risk of neonatal bleeding is inversely proportional to the platelet count and bleeding complications are rare with platelet counts over 50,000/μL [3,17]. Attempts have been made to determine which fetuses are severely thrombocytopenic and at higher risk for ICH. Unfortunately, no maternal factor has been identified that can predict fetal thrombocytopenia in all cases and current evidence does not support the routine use of fetal scalp sampling and cordocentesis in women with ITP [19,20].

Route of delivery was once considered critical to neonatal outcome in women with ITP. Passage through the birth canal was proposed as the reason for bleeding in thrombocytopenic fetuses and this together with anecdotal reports and case series led to recommendations for delivery by cesarean section [21]. However, vaginal delivery has never been proven to cause ICH and several studies have shown no association between route of delivery and neonatal bleeding complications [3,17,22]. At this time, it seems prudent to deliver by cesarean section for the usual obstetric indications without determination of the fetal platelet count in most women. However, the matter remains controversial.

In all cases of possible fetal thrombocytopenia, whether secondary to ITP or alloimmune thrombocytopenia, a neonatologist or other clinician familiar with the condition should be present to care for potential bleeding complications and the anticipated decrease in neonatal platelet count during the first several days after birth. The use of scalp electrodes, forceps, and vacuum extractors should be avoided in these patients. Although there is a theoretical risk of neonatal thrombocytopenia, women with ITP should not be discouraged from breast-feeding [23].

Alloimmune thrombocytopenia

Fetal and neonatal alloimmune thrombocytopenia (NAIT) is a serious and potentially life-threatening disorder that affects 1 in 1000–2000 live infants [24–27]. The condition is analogous to Rh isoimmunization, except that maternal IgG alloantibodies are directed against fetal platelet antigens. Several polymorphic, diallelic platelet antigen systems are responsible for this condition. Uniform nomenclature has been adopted describing these antigen systems as human platelet antigens (e.g. HPA-1, HPA-2), with alleles designated as "a" or "b." The most frequent cause of severe NAIT in white people is the HPA-1a antigen. Although approximately 1 in 42 pregnancies are incompatible for HPA-1a, NAIT develops in only about 10% of these cases [28]. This may be because the disorder is subclinical in some cases, and it may also be because, in addition to antigen exposure, an immunologic susceptibility (possibly related to HLA type DRB3*0101) is necessary.

In contrast to Rh isoimmunization, NAIT can occur during a first pregnancy without prior exposure to the offending antigen. It is usually diagnosed after birth when an infant is found to have thrombocytopenia, petechiae, or ecchymoses. Affected infants are often severely thrombocytopenic, and 10–20% have ICH [29,30]. The rate of ICH is considerably lower in cases detected by routine screening rather than based on thrombocytopenic infants [28]. Fetal ICH can occur *in utero* and a significant number of cases can be diagnosed by antenatal ultrasound. The recurrence risk is substantial and has been estimated to be up to 100% in cases of HPA-1a incompatibility, depending upon paternal zygosity for HPA-1a [25,31]. Thrombocytopenia tends to worsen as pregnancy progresses in untreated fetuses.

The goal of the obstetric management of pregnancies at risk of NAIT is to prevent ICH and its associated complications. In contrast to ITP, the dramatically higher frequency of ICH associated with NAIT justifies more aggressive interventions. Also, therapy must be initiated antenatally because of the risk of *in utero* ICH. Possible NAIT should be suspected in cases of otherwise unexplained fetal or neonatal thrombocytopenia, ICH, or porencephaly. In most cases, the diagnosis of NAIT can be determined by testing the parents; testing fetal or neonatal blood is confirmatory and occasionally helpful. Appropriate assays include serologic confirmation of maternal antiplatelet antibodies that are specific for paternal or fetal/neonatal platelets. In addition, individuals should undergo platelet typing with paternal zygosity testing. This can be determined serologically or with DNA-based tests. It is unnecessary to repeat testing in a family with a previously confirmed case of NAIT. Antibody titers are poorly predictive of risk to the current pregnancy and need not be obtained once the diagnosis is made. If the father is heterozygous for the offending antigen, fetal HPA typing can be accomplished with chorionic villi or amniocytes, or using free fetal DNA in maternal blood. Fetal genotyping avoids additional expensive and risky interventions in approximately 50% of such cases.

If the fetus is determined to be at risk, cordocentesis may be considered to determine the fetal platelet count. This strategy avoids treatment of fetuses that have normal platelet counts and provides feedback about treatment response in cases of thrombocytopenia. However, the risk of hemorrhagic complications with cordocentesis is increased in pregnancies affected by NAIT [32]. The overall perinatal loss rate for cordocentesis has been reported to be 2.7% [33] and is likely higher in the setting of severe fetal thrombocytopenia. Even with prophylactic transfusion of maternal platelets at the time of cordocentesis, the percentage of bleeding complications may be unchanged [34]. The risk of bleeding at the site of cordocentesis has prompted some clinicians to empirically treat pregnancies at risk for NAIT without determining the fetal platelet count. This strategy is usually reserved for cases of HPA-1a sensitization with a known antigen-positive fetus and is strongly recommended in cases with severely affected siblings [35]. Disadvantages include the potential for unnecessary and expensive treatment and the inability to assess treatment efficacy or to institute salvage therapy in cases of treatment failure. The benefits of cordocentesis may outweigh the risks in some cases, but the matter remains controversial. The number of cordocenteses should be minimized, especially in early gestation when the consequence of hemorrhage is greatest.

The optimal timing of the initial cordocentesis also is uncertain. ICH can occur early in gestation, but such cases are rare [36,37]. Active transport of IgG is limited until the late second and third trimesters. It is therefore likely that in most instances fetal blood sampling and treatment can be delayed until viability or even until the third trimester [38]. It seems prudent to individualize management of these cases depending on the antigen involved and the severity of NAIT during previously affected pregnancies.

Proposed therapies to increase fetal platelet counts and prevent ICH include maternal treatment with steroids and IVIG, fetal treatment with IVIG, and fetal platelet transfusions. No therapy is effective in all cases. Low-dose maternal steroids do not appear to improve fetal platelet counts. The efficacy of high-dose steroids is uncertain. IVIG administered directly to the fetus has had inconsistent results. Platelet transfusions are effective but the short half-life of transfused platelets requires weekly procedures. The potential risks involved with multiple transfusions as well as the potential for increased sensitization limit the attractiveness of this treatment. Platelet transfusions are likely best reserved for severe cases refractory to other therapies. Administration of IVIG to the mother appears to be the most consistently effective antenatal therapy for NAIT. Weekly infusions of 1 g/kg maternal weight of IVIG will often stabilize or increase the fetal platelet count [30,39,40]. ICH is extremely rare in pregnancies treated with IVIG [30].

Berkowitz *et al* and Bussel *et al* further refined the optimal therapy for NAIT during pregnancy (HPA-1a sensitization and antigen-positive fetus) in several recent clinical trials [38,41–43]. They advise the following.

- Initiate treatment with IVIG at 12 weeks' gestation in women with prior infants with ICH. The dose should be 1 or 2 g/kg/week of IVIG unless the previous ICH occurred prior to 28 weeks' gestation. In that case 2 g/kg/wk is advised.
- If there was no ICH in a prior pregnancy, treat with IVIG at 1 g/kg/week and prednisone 0.5 mg/kg/day starting at 20–26 weeks' gestation.
- Cordocentesis can be done at 32 weeks' gestation with an increase in the dose of IVIG if the fetus has a platelet count <30,000/µL. Alternatively, the dose can be empirically increased without doing a cordocentesis.
- Another option (in patients whose prior infant did not have ICH) is to start treatment with 2 g/kg/week of IVIG and use prednisone as salvage therapy.

Most authorities recommend cesarean delivery for fetuses with platelet counts less than 50,000/µL. As discussed in the section on ITP, vaginal delivery has never been shown to cause ICH and cesarean delivery has never been shown to prevent it. Nonetheless, the substantial rate of ICH probably justifies cesarean delivery in pregnancies with severe NAIT. Cordocentesis at about 37 weeks' gestation is used to document a safe platelet count for vaginal delivery. It is reasonable to consider a platelet count >100,000/µL at 32 weeks to be an adequate threshold for allowing a trial of labor.

There are no compelling data to support population-wide screening for HPA incompatibility. Studies are ongoing to address the efficacy and cost-effectiveness of such programs and the issue remains controversial [44]. Screening relatives of affected women also remains of unproven benefit.

CASE PRESENTATION 1

A healthy 34-year-old gravida 3, para 2002, at 36 weeks' gestation, presents for evaluation of regular contractions. The cervix is 3 cm dilated and 50% effaced. Routine CBC is notable for a platelet count of 94,000/µL. Her blood pressure is 116/72 mmHg. She denies headache, visual changes, abdominal pain, or bleeding of any type. Prenatal HIV serology is negative, and hematocrit, liver enzymes, and creatinine are normal. A platelet antibody test is positive. The clinician is concerned about possible ITP and wonders about the need for treatment.

When a clinician evaluates a mother with thrombocytopenia, a careful history should be obtained with emphasis on discovering a history of underlying bleeding diathesis, medication use, and medical conditions associated with thrombocytopenia. A physical examination

should be performed to look for petechiae or ecchymoses. A peripheral smear should be considered to evaluate platelet morphology and to exclude platelet clumping. Although antiplatelet antibodies are present in most individuals with ITP, tests for these antibodies are nonspecific, poorly standardized, and subject to a large degree of interlaboratory variation. Antiplatelet antibody tests cannot distinguish between GTP and ITP and are not recommended for the routine evaluation of maternal thrombocytopenia.

In this case, there is no evidence of preeclampsia or other medical conditions associated with thrombocytopenia. Gestational thrombocytopenia is the most likely diagnosis and no additional testing or treatment is warranted.

CASE PRESENTATION 2

A 26-year-old gravida 2, para 1001 presents for prenatal care at 8 weeks' gestation. Her prior pregnancy was uncomplicated, resulting in vaginal birth of a healthy infant at 39 weeks' gestation. However, her infant had petechiae and neonatal platelet count was determined to be 22,000/µL. There was no evidence of sepsis, preeclampsia, or other explanation for the thrombocytopenia. The platelet count increased after platelet transfusion and the child has had no medical problems or persistent thrombocytopenia. The couple asks whether the current fetus is at risk for thrombocytopenia and if anything can be done to prevent it.

The clinician should consider a diagnosis of NAIT in any case of current or prior unexplained fetal or neonatal thrombocytopenia. Both parents should be tested for platelet antigen type and zygosity, and the mother should be tested for specific antiplatelet antibodies against paternal platelet antigens. Testing is best accomplished in a specialized laboratory with expertise in NAIT; testing for

generic antiplatelet antibodies in the mother is not clinically useful.

In this case, the mother is HPA-1b homozygous and the father is HPA-1a/HPA-1b heterozygous. The mother has specific antibodies against HPA-1a. The couple should be advised that there is a 50% chance that the fetus carries the HPA-1a gene and is at risk for NAIT. Amniocentesis for fetal platelet antigen genotyping should be offered. If the fetus is HPA-1b, no further evaluation is required. If the fetus is HPA-1a, consideration should be given to treatment with IVIG and possible assessment of the fetal platelet count. The couple should be referred for consultation with a maternal-fetal medicine specialist to discuss the risks and benefits of specific management options. Trial of labor should only be allowed in cases wherein fetal platelet count is documented to be more than 50,000/µL and delivery should occur in a setting with neonatal expertise in NAIT.

References

1. Burrows RF, Kelton JG. Incidentally detected thrombocytopenia in healthy mothers and their infants. N Engl J Med 1988;319:142–145.

2. Burrows RF, Kelton JG. Thrombocytopenia at delivery: a prospective survey of 6715 deliveries. Am J Obstet Gynecol 1990;162:731–734.

3. Burrows RF, Kelton JG. Fetal thrombocytopenia and its relation to maternal thrombocytopenia. N Engl J Med 1993;329:1463–1466.

4. Lacey JV, Penner JA. Management of idiopathic thrombocytopenic purpura in the adult. Semin Thromb Hemost 1977;3:160–174.

5. George JN, El-Harake MA, Raskob GE. Chronic idiopathic thrombocytopenic purpura. N Engl J Med 1994;331:1207–1211.

6. George JN, Woolf SH, Raskob GE et al. Idiopathic thrombocytopenic purpura: a practice guideline developed by explicit methods for the American Society of Hematology. Blood 1996;88:3–40.

7. Provan D, Stasi R, Newland AC et al. International report on the investigation and management of primary immune thrombocytopenia. Blood 2010:115:168–207.

8. Karpatkin S. Autoimmune thrombocytopenic purpura. Am J Med Sci 1971;261:127.

9. Bussel JB, Pham LC. Intravenous treatment with gamma globulin in adults with immune thrombocytopenia purpura: review of the literature. Vox Sang 1987;52:206.

10. Boughton BJ, Chakraverty R, Baglin TP et al. The treatment of chronic idiopathic thrombocytopenia with anti-D (Rho) immunoglobulin: its effectiveness, safety, and mechanism of action. Clin Lab Haematol 1988;10:275–284.

11. Newman GC, Novoa MV, Fodero EE et al. A dose of 75 mg/kg/d of i.v. anti-D increased the platelet count more rapidly than 50 mg/kg/d in adults with immune thrombocytopenic purpura. Br J Haematol 2001;112:1076–1078.

12. Michel M, Novoa MV, Bussel JB. Intravenous anti-D as a treatment for immune thrombocytopenic purpura (ITP) during pregnancy. Br J Haematol 2003;123:142–146.

13. Sieunarine K, Shapiro S, Al Obaidi MJ, Girling J. Intravenous anti-D immunoglobulin in the treatment of resistant immune thrombocytopenic purpura in pregnancy. Br J Obstet Gynaecol 2007;114:505–507.

14. Gaines AR. Disseminated intravascular coagulation associated with acute hemoglobinemia or hemoglobinuria following Rh(0)(D) immune globulin intravenous administration for immune thrombocytopenic purpura. Blood 2005;106:1532–1537.

15. Kaplan C, Daffos F, Forestier F et al. Fetal platelet counts in thrombocytopenic pregnancy. Lancet 1990;336:979–982.

16. Christiaens GCML, Nieuwenhuis HK, von dem Borne AEGK et al. Idiopathic thrombocytopenic purpura in pregnancy: a randomized trial on the effect of antenatal low dose corticosteroids on neonatal platelet count. Br J Obstet Gynaecol 1990;97:893–898.

17. Cook RL, Miller RC, Katz VL, Cefalo RC. Immune thrombocytopenic purpura in pregnancy: a reappraisal of management. Obstet Gynecol 1991;78:578–583.

18. Scott JR, Rote NS, Cruikshank DP. Antiplatelet antibodies and platelet counts in pregnancies complicated by autoimmune thrombocytopenic purpura. Am J Obstet Gynecol 1983;145:932–939.

19. Silver RM. Management of idiopathic thrombocytopenic purpura in pregnancy. Am J Obstet Gynecol 1998;41:436–448.

20. Silver RM, Branch DW, Scott JR. Maternal thrombocytopenia in pregnancy: time for a reassessment. Am J Obstet Gynecol 1995;173:479–482.

21. Carlos HW, McMillan R, Crosby WH. Management of pregnancy in women with immune thrombocytopenic purpura. JAMA 1980;224:2756–2758.

22. Laros RK, Kagan R. Route of delivery for patients with immune thrombocytopenia. Am J Obstet Gynecol 1984;148:901–908.

23. American Society of Hematology ITP Practice Guideline Panel. Diagnosis and treatment of idiopathic thrombocytopenic purpura: recommendation of the American Society of Hematology. Ann Intern Med 1997;126:319–326.

24. Blanchette VS, Chen L, Defreideberg A et al. Alloimmunization to the PLA1 platelet antigen: results of a prospective study. Br J Haematol 1990;74:209–215.

25. Bussel JB, Zabusky MR, Berkowitz RL, McFarland JG. Fetal alloimmune thrombocytopenia. N Engl J Med 1997;337:22–26.

26. Dreyfus M, Kaplan C, Verdy E et al. Frequency of immune thrombocytopenia in newborns: a prospective study: Immune Thrombocytopenia Working Group. Blood 1997;89:4402–4406.

27. Williamson LM, Hackett G, Rennie J et al. The natural history of fetomaternal alloimmunization to the platelet-specific antigen HPA-1a (PL^{A1}, Zw^a) as determined by antenatal screening. Blood 1998;92:2280–2287.

28. Kjeldsen-Kragh J, Killie MK, Tomter G et al. A screening and intervention program aimed to reduce mortality and serious morbidity associated with severe neonatal alloimmune thrombocytopenia. Blood 2007;110:833–839.

29. Mueller-Eckhardt C, Kiefel V, Grubert A et al. 347 cases of fetal alloimmune thrombocytopenia. Lancet 1989;1:363–366.

30. Bussel JB, Skupski DW, McFarland JG. Fetal alloimmune thrombocytopenia: consensus and controversy. J Matern Fetal Med 1996;5:281–292.

31. Kaplan C, Murphy MF, Kroll H, Waters AH. Feto-maternal alloimmune thrombocytopenia: antenatal therapy with IvIgG and steroids: more questions and answers. European Working Group on Feto-maternal Alloimmune Thrombocytopenia. Br J Haematol 1998;100:62–65.

32. Paidas MJ, Berkowitz RL, Lynch L et al. Alloimmune thrombocytopenia: fetal and neonatal losses related to cordocentesis. Am J Obstet Gynecol 1995;172:475–479.

33. Ghidini A, Sepulveda W, Lockwood CJ, Romero R. Complications of fetal blood sampling. Am J Obstet Gynecol 1993;168:1339–1344.

34. Silver RM, Porter TF, Branch DW et al. Neonatal alloimmune thrombocytopenia: antenatal management. Am J Obstet Gynecol 1999;182:1233–1238.

35. Murphy MF, Bussel JB. Advances in the management of alloimmune thrombocytopenia. Br J Haematol 2007;136:366–378.

36. Giovangrandi Y, Daffos E, Kaplan C et al. Very early intracranial hemorrhage in alloimmune thrombocytopenia. Lancet 1990;2:310.

37. Reznikoff-Etievant MF. Management of alloimmune neonatal and antenatal thrombocytopenia. Vox Sang 1988;5:193–201.

38. Berkowitz RL, Lesser ML, McFarland JG et al. Antepartum treatment without early cordocentesis for standard risk alloimmune thrombocytopenia: a randomized controlled trial. Obstet Gynecol 2007;110:249–255.

39. Bussel JB, Berkowitz RL, McFarland JG et al. Antenatal treatment of neonatal alloimmune thrombocytopenia. N Engl J Med 1988;319:1374–1378.

40. Lynch L, Bussel JB, McFarland JG et al. Antenatal treatment of alloimmune thrombocytopenia. Obstet Gynecol 1992;80:67–71.

41. Berkowitz RL, Kolb EA, McFarland JG et al. Parallel randomized trials of risk-based therapy for fetal alloimmune thrombocytopenia. Obstet Gynecol 2006;107:91–96.

42. Berkowitz RL, Bussel JB, McFarland JG. Alloimmune thrombocytopenia: state of the art 2006. Am J Obstet Gynecol 2006;195:907–913.

43. Bussel JB, Berkowitz RL, Hung C et al. Intracranial hemorrhage in alloimmune thrombocytopenia: stratified management to prevent recurrence in the subsequent affected fetus. Am J Obstet Gynecol 2010;203:135.

44. Husebekk A, Killie MK, Kjeldsen-Kragh J, Skogen B. Is it time to implement HPA-1 screening in pregnancy? Curr Opin Hematol 2009;16:497–502.

Chapter 15
Inherited and Acquired Thrombophilias

Michael J. Paidas

Department of Obstetrics, Gynecology and Reproductive Sciences, Yale University School of Medicine, New Haven, CT, USA

Thrombophilias present an evolving, controversial story. Predominant thrombophilic mutations include the factor V Leiden (FVL) mutation, prothrombin G20210A gene mutation (PGM), and deficiencies of the natural anticoagulants proteins C (PC) and S (PS), and antithrombin (AT). Prospective cohort studies have provided an accurate assessment of the risk for placenta-mediated complications (PMC) posed by common inherited thrombophilic conditions. Acquired thrombophilic conditions consist of the antiphospholipid antibody syndrome (APAS) and hyperhomocysteinemia. Well-conducted, placebo-controlled, randomized trials have demonstrated no benefit of anticoagulation in women with recurrent pregnancy loss and inherited thrombophilia. The routine use of anticoagulation to prevent other PMC in the setting of inherited thrombophilia should be considered experimental until the results of adequate clinical trials are available. Heparin and antiplatelet therapy are the cornerstones of treatment of APAS in pregnancy.

Hemostatic changes in pregnancy

Pregnancy is associated with significant elevations of a number of clotting factors. Fibrinogen concentration is doubled, factors VII, VIII, IX, X, and XII increase 20–1000%, and von Willebrand factor (vWF) increases 20–1000%, with maximum levels reached at term [1]. Prothrombin and factor V levels remain unchanged while levels of factors XIII and XI decline modestly. The overall effect of these changes is to increase thrombin generating potential. Coagulation activation markers are elevated in uncomplicated pregnancy, as evidenced by increased thrombin activity, increased soluble fibrin levels (9.2–13.4 nmol/L), increased thrombin–antithrombin (TAT) complexes (3.1–7.1 µg/L), and increased levels of fibrin D-dimer (91–198 µg/L) [2]. Fifty percent of women had elevated TAT levels (11/22) and 36% of women had elevated levels of D-dimers (9/25) in the first trimester.

During pregnancy there are significant changes in the natural anticoagulant and fibrinolytic systems. Protein S levels significantly decrease. Mean free PS antigen levels have been reported to be $38.9 \pm 10.3\%$ and $31.2 \pm 7.4\%$ in the second and third trimesters, respectively [3]. The PS carrier molecule, complement 4B-binding protein, is increased in pregnancy, and is one explanation for the diminished PS levels in pregnancy. Levels of plasminogen activator inhibitor-1 (PAI-1) increase three- to four-fold during pregnancy; plasma PAI-2 values are low prior to pregnancy and reach concentrations of 160 µg/L at term. Table 15.1 summarizes the relevant pregnancy-associated changes in the hemostatic system. These prothrombotic hemostatic changes are exacerbated by pregnancy-associated venous stasis in the lower extremities resulting from compression of the inferior vena cava and pelvic veins (left greater than right) by the enlarging uterus, as well as a hormone-mediated increase in deep vein capacitance secondary to increased circulating levels of estrogen and local production of prostacyclin and nitric oxide.

Substantial changes must occur in local decidual and systemic coagulation, anticoagulant, and fibrinolytic systems to meet the hemostatic challenges of pregnancy, including avoidance of hemorrhage at implantation, placentation, and third stage of labor. In addition to the systemic prothrombotic, anticoagulant, and fibrinolytic changes, there are potent local hemostatic effectors in the decidua [4,5]. Progesterone augments perivascular decidual cell tissue factor (TF) and PAI-1 expression. Decidual TF is critical in maintaining hemostasis, as evidenced by experiments with transgenic TF knockout mice which have a significant risk of fatal postpartum hemorrhage [6].

Queenan's Management of High-Risk Pregnancy: An Evidence-Based Approach, Sixth Edition. Edited by John T. Queenan, Catherine Y. Spong, Charles J. Lockwood.

Table 15.1 Hemostatic changes in pregnancy

Variables (mean ± SD)	1st trimester*	2nd trimester*	3rd trimester*	Normal range
Platelet (×10⁹/L)	275 ± 64	256 ± 49	244 ± 52	150–400
Fibrinogen (g/L)	3.7 ± 0.6	4.4 ± 1.2	5.4 ± 0.8	2.1–4.2
Prothrombin complex (%)	120 ± 27	140 ± 27	130 ± 27	70–30
Antithrombin (U/mL)	1.02 ± 0.10	1.07 ± 0.14	1.07 ± 0.11	0.85–1.25
Protein C (U/mL)	0.92 ± 0.13	1.06 ± 0.17	0.94 ± 0.2	0.68–1.25
Protein S, total (U/mL)	0.83 ± 0.11	0.73 ± 0.11	0.77 ± 0.10	0.70–1.70
Protein S, free (U/mL)	0.26 ± 0.07	0.17 ± 0.04	0.14 ± 0.04	0.20–0.50
Soluble fibrin (nmol/L)	9.2 ± 8.6	11.8 ± 7.7	13.4 ± 5.2	<15
Thrombin-antithrombin (μg/L)	3.1 ± 1.4	5.9 ± 2.6	7.1 ± 2.4	<2.7
D-dimers (μg/L)	91 ± 24	128 ± 49	198 ± 59	<80
Plasminogen activator inhibitor-1 (AU/mL)	7.4 ± 4.9	14.9 ± 5.2	37.8 ± 19.4	<15
Plasminogen activator inhibitor-2 (μg/L)	31 ± 14	84 ± 16	160 ± 31	<5
Cardiolipin antibodies positive	2/25	2/25	3/23	0
Protein Z (μg/mL)†	2.01 ± 0.76	1.47 ± 0.45	1.55 ± 0.48	
Protein S (%)†	34.4 ± 11.8	27.5 ± 8.4		

*1st trimester, weeks 12–15; 2nd trimester, week 24; 3rd trimester, week 35.
†First trimester, 0–14 weeks; second trimester, 14–27 weeks; third trimester ≥27 weeks.
Source: Bremme [1], Paidas *et al* [3].

Table 15.2 Inherited thrombophilias and their association with venous thromboembolism

Ratio thrombophilia life-time	Inheritance	Prevalence in European pop. (from large cohort studies)	Prevalence in patients with VTE (range)	Relative risk or odds VTE (95% CI)
FVL (homozy.)	AD	0.07%*	<1%*	80 (22–289)
FVL (heterozy.)	AD	5.3%	6.6–50%	2.7 (1.3–5.6)
PGM (homozy.)	AD	0.02%*	<1%	>80-fold*
PGM (heterozy.)	AD	2.9%	7.5%	3.8 (3.0–4.9)
FVL/PGM (compound heterozy.)	AD	0.17%*	2.0%	20.0 (11.1–36.1)
Hyperhomocysteinemia	AR	5%	<5%	3.3 (1.1–10.0)†
Antithrombin def (<60% activity)	AD	0.2%	1–8%	17.5 (9.1–33.8)
Protein S def Heerlen S460P mutation or free S antigen <55%	AD	0.2%	3.1%	2.4 (0.8–7.9)
Protein C (<60% activity)	AD	0.2%	3–5%	11.3 (5.7–22.3)

AD, autosomal dominant; AR, autosomal recessive; CI, confidence interval; FVL, factor V Leiden; PGM, prothrombin gene mutation G20210A; VTE, venous thromboembolism.
*Calculated based on a Hardy–Weinberg equilibrium.
†Odds ratio (OR) adjusted for renal disease, folate and vitamin B_{12} deficiency, while OR are adjusted for these confounders.
Source: American College of Obstetricians and Gynecologists [10].

Inherited thrombophilias

In 1965, Egberg, a Norwegian physician, reported a family with a partial AT deficiency, and in his classic article suggested the term thrombophilia, referring to hereditary or acquired conditions that predispose individuals to thromboembolic events [7]. After the description of AT deficiency, deficiencies of proteins C and S were described in the 1980s [8,9]. Table 15.2 describes the association between inherited thrombophilias and venous thromboembolism (VTE) [10].

Factor V Leiden mutation

Interest in thrombophilia grew following the discovery of this relatively common genetic predisposition to clotting. In 1994, Dahlback [11] reported an association between a mutation in the factor V gene and increased thrombotic risk, termed the FVL mutation. It results from a substitution of adenine for guanine at the 1691 position of the 10th exon of the factor V gene, causing an amino switch of glutamine for arginine at position 506 in the factor V polypeptide (FV Q506). Factor V then is rendered resistant to cleavage by activated protein C. The frequency of

FVL varies among different ethnic groups: 5.2% of US Caucasians, 1.2% of African-Americans [12], and 5–9% of Europeans, while it is rare in Asian and African populations [13]. FVL is primarily inherited in an autosomal dominant fashion [14].

Heterozygosity of FVL confers a 5–10-fold increased risk of VTE, while homozygosity confers a greater than 25-fold increased risk of VTE [15]. Although FVL is present in 40% of pregnant patients with VTE, given the low incidence of thrombosis in pregnancy (1 in 1400) and the high incidence of the mutation in European-derived populations, the estimated risk of VTE among heterozygous pregnant patients without personal or family history of thrombosis is only 1.5%. However, retrospective studies suggest the risk may be up to 17% among pregnant women with a personal or strong family VTE history [16]. In contrast, a multicenter prospective observational National Institute of Child Health and Human Development (NICHD)-sponsored study identified 134 FVL carriers among 4885 gravidas (2.7%) [17]. In this study, no thromboembolic events occurred among the FVL carriers (0%, 95% confidence interval [CI] 0–2.7%), while three pulmonary emboli (PE) and one deep venous thrombosis occurred (0.08%, 95% CI 0.02–0.21%) among noncarriers. In this study, maternal FVL carriage was not associated with increased fetal loss (FL), preeclampsia, placental abruption, or small for gestational age (SGA) births.

Prothrombin gene mutation 20210A

A mutation in the prothrombin gene discovered in 1996 was associated with a significantly increased risk of thrombosis [18]. The prothrombin G20210 A polymorphism (PGM) is a point mutation causing a guanine to adenine switch at nucleotide position 20210 in the 3'-untranslated region of the gene [19]. This nucleotide switch results in increased translation and increased circulating levels of prothrombin. The prevalence of PGM heterozygosity ranges from 2% to 3% of Europeans and increases circulating levels of prothrombin 150–200% [13]. It accounted for 17% of thromboembolism in pregnancy in one large case–control study [20]. The actual risk of clotting in an asymptomatic pregnant carrier is approximately 1 in 200 or 0.5%. Rare, PGM homozygosity likewise confers a high risk of thrombosis, equal to that of homozygosity for FVL [13].

Protein S deficiency

Protein S is a vitamin K-dependent 69 kDa molecular weight glycoprotein which has several anticoagulant functions including its activity as a nonenzymatic cofactor to the anticoagulant serine protease activated protein C (APC) [21]. Protein S has a plasma half-life of 42 h, longer than protein C whose half-life is approximately 6–8 h. Circulating PS exists in both free (40%) and bound (60%) forms. Plasma PS is reversibly bound (60%) to C4b-binding protein (C4BP), which serves as a carrier protein for protein S. Protein S also has an APC-independent anticoagulant function in the direct inhibition of the prothrombinase complex. Protein S also inhibits the antifibrinolytic protein, thrombin activatable fibrinolysis inhibitor (TAFI) [22]. Protein S deficiency occurs in 0.03–1.3% of the population, and inheritance is autosomal dominant [23]. Protein S deficiency presents with one of three phenotypes: type I, marked by reduced total and free forms; type II, characterized by normal free PS levels but reduced APC co-factor activity; and type III, in which there are normal total but reduced free PS levels. Of note, different mutations have highly variable procoagulant sequelae, making it extremely difficult to predict which patients with PS deficiencies will develop thrombotic sequelae.

Pregnancy is associated with decreased levels of PS activity and free PS antigen in most patients [24]. Most normal pregnancies acquire some degree of resistance to APC when measured by the first-generation global assays and tests that measure endogenous thrombin potential [25,26]. Factor X's activation to factor Xa and its involvement in the activation of prothrombin is a central element in the generation of thrombin.

Paidas *et al* [3] compared second and third trimester PS levels in 51 healthy women with a normal pregnancy outcome with 51 healthy women with a poor pregnancy outcome. Protein S levels were significantly lower in the second and third trimesters among patients with adverse pregnancy outcome (APO). A small case–control study performed in subjects from a larger, multicenter, prospective study also found lower levels of PS activity and free antigen in the second and third trimesters [17].

Protein C deficiency

Protein C is a vitamin K-dependent 62 kDa molecular weight glycoprotein substrate that is a precursor to a serine protease, APC [27]. Protein C is activated to APC by thrombin in the presence of thrombomodulin (TM) on the surface of endothelial cells. APC, with PS and factor V as co-factors, inactivates factors Va and VIIIa, which decreases the generation of thrombin. Deficiencies of PC result from numerous mutations, although two primary types are recognized: type I, in which both immunoreactive and functionally active PC levels are reduced; and type II, where immunoreactive levels are normal but activity is reduced [28]. The prevalence of PC deficiency is 0.2–0.5%, and its inheritance is autosomal dominant.

The reported pregnancy and puerperal risk of VTE with PC and PS deficiencies appears modest, ranging from 5–20%, and may be overstated because of ascertainment biases [28]. Preston *et al* [29] have reported that the risk of stillbirth is modestly increased with an adjusted odds ratio (OR) of 2.3 (95% CI 0.6–8.3). The risk of miscarriage appears to be minimal with PC deficiencies (OR 1.4, 95% CI 0.9–2.2)] or not increased [28,30].

Antithrombin deficiency

Antithrombin, a vitamin K-independent glycoprotein, is a pivotal component of the natural anticoagulant system, acting as a major inhibitor of thrombin and other serine proteases. The anticoagulant effect of heparin occurs via an increase in AT's thrombin inhibitory activity. Deficiency of AT is the most thrombogenic of the inherited thrombophilia, with a 70–90% lifetime risk of VTE [28]. In addition to its thrombin inhibitory properties, AT can also inactivate factors Xa, IXa, VIIa, and plasmin. The anticoagulant activity of AT is increased 5000–40,000-fold by heparin binding. Deficiencies in AT result from numerous point mutations, deletions, and insertions, and are usually inherited in an autosomal dominant fashion [26]. The two classes of AT deficiency are: type I, the most common deficiency, characterized by concomitant reductions in both antigenic protein levels and activity; and type II, which is characterized by normal antigenic AT levels but decreased activity. Type II deficiency is further classified by the site of the mutation (e.g. RS, reactive site; HBS, heparin binding site; PE, pleiotropic functional defects). The type II-HBS variant appears to have the least clinical significance.

Because the prevalence of AT deficiency is low, at 1 in 1000 to 1 in 5000, it is only present in 1% of patients with VTE. The risk of thrombosis among affected patients is as high as 60% during pregnancy and 33% during the puerperium [28]. With no previous history of VTE, 31% of patients with hereditary AT will develop thrombosis during pregnancy, and if there is a history of previous VTE, the recurrence rate is 49% [32]. Preston *et al* [29] reported adjusted ORs of 1.7 (95% CI 1.0–2.8) and 5.2 (95% CI 1.5–18.1) for miscarriage and stillbirth, respectively. However, because of its low prevalence compared with that of fetal loss, preeclampsia, SGA, and abruption, AT deficiency is rarely the cause of these disorders [31].

Polymorphisms of the thrombomodulin gene are associated with an increased risk of thrombosis, but the pregnancy implications are unclear at this time [33]. Interestingly, pregnant patients with thrombophilia and subsequent APO have been demonstrated to exhibit a decreased first-trimester response to thrombomodulin in an activated partial thromboplastin time (APTT) system [34].

Protein Z deficiency

Protein Z (PZ) is a 62 kDa vitamin K-dependent plasma protein that serves as a co-factor for a protein Z-dependent protease inhibitor (ZPI) of factor Xa [35,36]. Protein Z is critical for regulation of factor Xa activity in addition to TF pathway inhibitor [37–39]. It increases rapidly during the first months of life followed by slow increases during childhood, with adult levels reached during puberty [40,41]. Protein Z deficiency influences the prothrombotic phenotype in FVL patients, and low plasma PZ levels have been reported in patients with antiphospholipid antibodies (APA) [42,43]. There is a high prevalence of PZ deficiency in patients with unexplained early fetal loss (10th–19th weeks) [44]. Gris *et al* [45] found an increased risk of fetal loss associated with PZ deficiency (OR 6.7, 95% CI 3.1–14.8, P < 0.001), and noted that the patients with late fetal loss and recurrent miscarriages had lower PZ levels.

Paidas *et al* [3] found that there was a significant decrease in the PZ levels in patients (n = 51) with a variety of APO, including SGA, preeclampsia, preterm delivery, and bleeding in pregnancy, compared with women (n = 51) with normal pregnancy outcomes (second trimester 1.5 ± 0.4 versus 2.0 ± 0.5 μg/mL, P < 0.0001; third trimester 1.6 ± 0.5 versus 1.9 ± 0.5 μg/mL, P < 0.0002) [3].

Protein Z levels at the 20th percentile (1.30 μg/mL) were associated with an increased risk of APO (OR 4.25, 95% CI 1.5–11.8), with a sensitivity of 93% and specificity of 32%. Mean first-trimester PZ level was significantly lower among patients with APO compared with pregnant controls (1.81 ± 0.7 versus 2.21 ± 0.8 μg/mL, respectively; P < 0.001). Gris *et al* [45] carried out a prospective, randomized trial comparing the low molecular weight heparin (LMWH) enoxaparin (40 mg/day) with low-dose aspirin (LDA) (100 mg/day), in 160 women with one unexplained fetal loss (≥10th week of gestation) and FVL, PGM, or PS deficiency. The livebirth rate was 86% in the enoxaparin-treated women versus 29% in the aspirin-treated group (OR for livebirth with LMWH 15.5, 95% CI 7–34). Birthweights were higher and there were fewer SGA infants in the enoxaparin group. Gris *et al* [45] found that PZ deficiency or PZ antibodies was more frequently present in cases of treatment failures (P = 0.20 and 0.019, respectively) as was the complex of PZ deficiency positive anti-PZ antibodies (P = 0.004); 15 of the 20 cases led to pregnancy failure, nine being treated with aspirin and six with enoxaparin. Both groups of patients received 5 mg/day folic acid, in addition to LDA or heparin therapy.

Elevated levels of type 1 plasminogen activator inhibitor

Plasminogen activator inhibitors are serine protease inhibitors, often referred to as serpins (serine protease inhibitors), with diverse functions, including blood coagulation, fibrinolysis, and cell migration [46,47]. The PAI-1 and PAI-2 molecules inhibit tissue-type and urokinase-type plasminogen activators (tPA and uPA, respectively). The tPA and uPA molecules promote fibrin degradation by converting plasminogen to plasmin, and are also involved in the remodeling of extracellular matrix [48]. PAI-1 and PAI-2 are found in the blood of women with normal pregnancies, and their levels tend to rise with advancing gestation [49]. In preeclamptic patients, the vascular endothelium is responsible for the majority of the elevated PAI-1 plasma levels, with platelets accounting for a smaller proportion [50]. Unlike PAI-1, which is found in a variety of nonpregnant disease states, PAI-2 expression has been identified in a limited number of cells, principally placental trophoblasts, macrophages, and various malignant cell lines [50,51].

Higher levels of PAI-1 are noted in cases of preeclampsia and SGA (either during manifestations of the disease process or shortly prior to their manifestation). Homozygosity for the 4G/4G mutation in the PAI-1 gene leads to a three- to fivefold increased level of circulating PAI-1. The significance of the 4G/4G PAI-1 mutation is uncertain. Its contribution to VTE events has been called into question, as evidenced by the review by Francis [52].

Hyperhomocysteinemia and MTHFR C677T and MTHFR A1298C

Homocysteine (HC) is generated from the metabolism of the amino acid methionine. It normally circulates in the plasma at concentrations of 5–16 μmol/L. Deficiencies in vitamins B_6, B_{12}, and folic acid can result in elevated levels of HC in the setting of inherited hyperhomocysteinemia. Homocysteine levels can vary with diet, however, and normal levels in pregnancy are slightly lower than nonpregnant values. Hyperhomocysteinemia can be diagnosed by measuring fasting HC levels by gas chromatography mass spectrometry or other sensitive biochemical means. The disorder is classified into three categories according to the extent of the fasting HC elevation: severe (>100 μmol/L), moderate (25–100 μmol/L), or mild (16–24 μmol/L). Methionine loading can improve diagnostic sensitivity. Severe hyperhomocysteinemia results from an autosomal recessive homozygous deficiency in cystathionine β-synthase (CBS) (prevalence of 1 in 200,000). Clinical manifestations of hyperhomocysteinemia include neurologic abnormalities, premature atherosclerosis, and recurrent thromboembolism.

The mild and moderate forms can result from autosomal dominant (heterozygote) deficiencies in CBS (0.3–1.4% of population) or from homozygosity for the 667C-T MTHFR thermolabile mutant, present in 11% of white European populations [28]. Hyperhomocysteinemia can also result from the presence of combined heterozygousity for the MTHFR C677T and another common missense mutation at base pair 1298, which converts a glutamate to an alanine residue, and is termed MTHFR A1298C [53]. Patients with mild or moderate hyperhomocysteinemia are at risk for atherosclerosis, thromboembolism, fetal neural tube defects, and possibly recurrent abortion.

There are conflicting data on the link between hyperhomocysteinemia and recurrent spontaneous abortion [54–56]. An older metaanalysis of the association between hyperhomocysteinemia and fetal loss prior to 16 weeks suggested a weak association with an OR of 1.4 (95% CI 1.0–2.0) [57]. The natural history of the MTHFR mutation in pregnancy has not been well documented. The metaanalysis by Rey [30] concluded that MTHFR was not associated with an increased risk of fetal loss. A subsequent metaanalysis concluded that MTHFR C677T mutation was not associated with early fetal loss [58].

Inherited thrombophilia and pregnancy complications

Inherited thrombophilic conditions have been evaluated in a variety of obstetric complications, including preeclampsia and related conditions, early and late fetal loss, intrauterine growth restriction (IUGR), and abruption.

Preeclampsia

A systematic review and metaanalysis, encompassing 10 prospective cohort studies [17,56,59–66] and evaluating the association of FVL, PGM and PMC in prospective cohort studies, demonstrated no significant association between FVL and preeclampsia (OR 1.23, 95% CI 0.89–1.70) or between PGM and preeclampsia (OR 1.25, 95% CI 0.79–1.99) [67].

Intrauterine growth restriction

Infante-Rivard *et al* [68] found rates of 4.5% and 2.5% for FVL and PGM, respectively, when IUGR was defined as <10th percentile. In a systematic review, FVL and PGM were associated with an increased risk of IUGR (OR 2.7, 95% CI 1.3–5.5, and OR 2.5, 95% CI 1.3–5.0), respectively, in 10 case–control studies [69]. However, in five cohort studies (three prospective, two retrospective), the relative risk (RR) was 0.99 (95% CI 0.5–1.9) [56,59,70–72]. Howley *et al* concluded that both FVL and PG confer an increased risk of giving birth to an IUGR infant, although this may be driven by small, poor-quality studies that demonstrated extreme associations. Rodger *et al* demonstrated no significant association between FVL and SGA (OR 1.0, 95% CI 0.80–1.25) or PGM and SGA (OR 1.25, 95% CI 0.92–1.70) [67]. Prevalence rates of 11–23% have been reported for PS deficiency [73–75].

Abruptio placentae

The determination of the relationship between thrombophilia and abruption has been challenging because of the limited number of studies and confounding variables, including chronic hypertension, and cigarette and cocaine use [76,77]. De Vries [74] found that 9/31 (29%) patients with abruption had a PS deficiency, compared with their general population prevalence of 0.2–2%. The prevalence of FVL, PGM, and PS deficiency was in the ranges 22–30%, 18–20%, and 0–29%, respectively [1,78].

In the multicenter prospective observational Maternal-Fetal Medicine Units Network report from 2005, nested carrier–control analysis revealed no difference between FVL carriers and noncarriers in development of abruption [17]. Rodger *et al* demonstrated no significant association between FVL and abruption (OR 1.85, 95% CI 0.92–3.70) or PGM and abruption (OR 2.02, 95% CI 0.81–5.02) [67]. Regarding MTHFR and hyperhomocysteinemia, in a case–control study from the New Jersey Placental Abruption Group, homozygosity for neither the C677CT (OR 0.60, 95% CI 0.33–1.18) nor the A1298C (OR 2.28, 95% CI 0.82–6.35) variants in MTHFR was associated with abruption [79].

Fetal loss

Several studies have found strong associations between FVL and second/third-trimester fetal loss, but not with early first-trimester fetal loss. The gaseous milieu of the uteroplacental circulation during early pregnancy is one containing low oxygen levels, with intervillous oxygen pressures at 8–10 weeks of 17 ± 6.9 mmHg, and rising to 60.7 ± 8.5 mmHg by 13 weeks [80]. The hypoxic environment may result from trophoblast plugging of the spiral arteries and low Doppler flow in the uterine vasculature, and allows for undetectable levels of the damaging superoxide dismutase in trophoblasts prior to 10 weeks [81,82]. This same effect, at a later gestational age, would have a contrasting effect to the larger embryo or fetus, providing biologic plausibility for the association with fetal loss at later gestations in the following studies. A large retrospective cohort study comparing 843 women with thrombophilia, of whom 571 had 1524 pregnancies, versus 541 control women, of whom 395 had 1019 pregnancies, noted a statistically significant association with stillbirth (OR 3.6, 95% CI 1.4–9.4) but not spontaneous abortion (OR 1.27, 95% CI 0.94–1.71) [29].

Rey *et al* found that FVL was significantly linked to both recurrent loss prior to 13 weeks (OR 2.01, 95% CI 1.13–3.58) and nonrecurrent FL (OR 1.73, 95% CI 1.18–2.54) [30]. One retrospective case–control study of over 2000 women with recurrent FL showed a striking association between FVL and stillbirth >22 weeks with an OR of 4.51 (95% CI 1.81–11.23) [83]. This finding was confirmed in a more contemporary prospective case–control trial of 5000 women in which stillbirth was defined as intrauterine demise of fetuses >500 g [84]. This study showed a significant association with FVL (OR 10.9, 95% CI 2.07–56.94). Rodger *et al* demonstrated a significant association between FVL and fetal loss (OR 1.52, 95% CI 1.06–2.19), but not between PGM and fetal loss (OR 1.13, 95% CI 0.64–2.01) [67]. Of note, the absolute risk of fetal loss in women with FVL was 4.2% as compared with 3.2% for FVL-negative women, representing a 52% higher risk of

fetal loss associated with FVL. Five of the seven prospective studies demonstrated no significant association [17,60,61,63,64] while two found a significant association [56,65]. Prior metaanalysis and systematic reviews evaluating the PGM have found a statistically significant link with ORs of 2.49 (95% CI 1.24–5) [85] and 2.3 (95% CI 1.1–4.8) [30]. However, the four prospective cohort studies [60,63,65,66] included in the latest metaanalysis demonstated no association between PGM and fetal loss [67].

Fewer data exist for the rarer inherited deficiencies of PS, PC, and AT. The metaanalysis by Rey *et al* reported an association between PS deficiency and recurrent late (>22 weeks or <25 weeks) FL (OR 14.7, 95% CI 1.0–218.0) as well as nonrecurrent FL at >22 weeks (OR 7.4, 95% CI 1.3–43) [30]. This relationship was strengthened by the metaanalysis of Alfirevic, which found that PS deficiency was associated with an increased risk of stillbirth (OR 16.2, 95% CI 5.0–52.3) [31]. Saade and McLintock reported an association between PS deficiency and late FL, with adjusted OR 41 (95% CI 4.8–359) [86]. In a systematic review, PS deficiency was associated with late FL, with OR 20.1 (95% CI 3.7–109) [85]. Regarding PC deficiency, Preston *et al* have reported that the risk of stillbirth is modestly increased (adjusted OR 2.3, 95% CI 0.6–8.3), but not miscarriage (OR 1.4, 95% CI 0.9–2.2) [29]. However, Alfirevic found no association between PC deficiency and stillbirth [31]. A relative paucity of data exists concerning obstetric complications and the rare condition of hereditary AT deficiency. In the largest retrospective cohort study, AT was associated with a significant increased risk of stillbirth at >28 weeks (OR 5.2, 95% CI 1.5–18.1) but a more modest association with FL <28 weeks (OR 1.7, 95% CI 1.0–2.8) [29].

For patients who have had a prior adverse pregnancy outcome and harbor an inherited thrombophilic condition such as FVL, PGM, or PS deficiency, the rate of recurrence is still being defined. According to the metaanalysis by Rey *et al* [30], the presence of PGM was associated with recurrent fetal loss before 25 weeks (n = 690 women; OR 2.56, 95% CI 1.04–6.29) and with nonrecurrent fetal loss after 20 weeks (five studies, n = 1299; OR 2.3, 95% CI 1.09–4.87). Rey *et al* also found that late fetal loss was associated with FVL mutation (n = 1888; OR 3.26, 95% CI 1.82–5.83), PGM (n = 1299; OR 2.30, 95% CI 1.09–4.87), PS deficiency (n = 878; OR 7.39, 95% CI 1.28–42.83) but not MTHFR, PC deficiency, or AT deficiency.

Recent larger prospective studies have suggested lower rates of recurrence. For example, women who suffered a first fetal loss and who were selected from two family cohorts of first-degree relatives of probands with FVL or PGM and a history of documented VTE or premature atherosclerosis were prospectively followed in a second pregnancy [87]. Their risk of loss of the subsequent pregnancy was higher than in women with a successful first pregnancy (25% versus 12%, RR 2.0, 95% CI 1.4–3.0]. The livebirth rate of the second pregnancy after an early first loss (<12 weeks of gestation) was 77% (95% CI 62–87) for carriers and 76% (95% CI 57–89) for noncarriers (RR 1.0, 95% CI 0.8–1.3). After a late first loss (>12 weeks), the livebirth rates were 68% (95% CI 46–85) and 80% (95% CI 49–94) for carriers and noncarriers, respectively (RR 0.9, 95% CI 0.5–1.3). In another prospective cohort study of 2480 patients with recurrent pregnancy loss, patients with FVL who had ≥ fetal loss had a favorable 98% livebirth rate in subsequent pregnancy [88].

Summary of inherited thrombophilias

While retrospective case–control and cohort studies suggest a link between inherited thrombophilias and placenta-mediated complications, large multicenter prospective studies have consistently failed to display such an association. Several factors affect studies concerning thrombophilia and PCMs, including the heterogeneity of the populations studied, small sample size, rarity of the endpoint evaluated, number of thrombophilias assayed for, detection methods employed, lack of consistent assessment of fetal thrombophilic status, as well as potential ascertainment biases [58,89]. These limitations have been confirmed in two independent studies on fetal genotype [90,91]. Other confounding factors are past pregnancy history and the severity of the pregnancy complication, which significantly affect the recurrence and occurrence of pregnancy complications in subsequent pregnancy, without considering thrombophilia [92].

The risk of composite pregnancy complications has also been assessed in prospective studies, and results have been mostly negative. One prospective cohort study of nulliparous women (n = 2034) demonstrated that the prothrombin gene mutation was associated with an increased risk of a composite of APO (OR 3.58, 95% CI 1.20–10.61) [65] but the majority of the remaining prospective cohort studies have not found such an association for FVL or PGM. The latest systematic review and metaanalysis comprising four prospective cohort studies demonstrated no significant association between FVL (OR 1.08, 95% CI 0.87–1.35) or PGM (OR 1.27, 95% CI 0.94–1.71) and a composite of PCMs [67].

Acquired thrombophilia

The well-characterized APAS has been defined by the combination of VTE, obstetric complications, and antiphospholipid antibodies (APA), commonly termed the Sapporo criteria for APAS [93]. Since 2005, revised criteria for the classification of APAS have been in place and are summarized in Box 15.1 [94]. Current accepted obstetric complications include at least one fetal death at

---

Box 15.1 Diagnosis of antiphospholipid antibody syndrome

Clinical criteria

Obstetric

History of three unexplained consecutive spontaneous abortions ≤10 weeks gestational age (GA), or History of one unexplained fetal death ≥10 weeks GA (morphologically and karyotypically normal), or History of preterm delivery <34 weeks GA, as a sequela of preeclampsia or uteroplacental insufficiency, including the following:
- Non-reassuring fetal testing indicative of fetal hypoxemia (e.g. abnormal Doppler flow)
- Oligohydramnios (Amniotic Fluid Index less than or equal to 5 cm)
- Intrauterine growth restriction less than the 10th percentile
- Placental abruption

Nonobstetric

Arterial thrombosis, including cerebrovascular accidents, transient ischemic attacks, myocardial infarction, amaurosis fugax Venous thromboembolism (VTE), including deep venous thrombosis (DVT), pulmonary emboli (PE), or small vessel thrombosis

Laboratory criteria

Should be present on two occasions, >12 weeks apart, and no more than 5 years prior to clinical manifestation.
- Anticardiolipin antibody
- IgG or IgM isotype, present in medium or high titers (i.e. 40 GPL or MPL, or >99th percentile), or anti-β2GPI antibody
- IgG or IgM isotype (>99th percentile), or lupus anticoagulant in plasma, utilizing one of the following tests:
  - Dilute Russell viper venom time (dRVVT)
  - Lupus anticoagulant

GPL, anticardiolipin antibody of IgG isotype; MPL. anticardiolipin antibody of IgM isotype.
Source: Miyakis *et al* [94].

---

or beyond the 10th week of gestation, or at least one premature birth before the 34th week as a sequela of preeclampsia or uteroplacental insufficiency, or at least three unexplained consecutive spontaneous abortions at or before the 10th week. The APA must be present on two occasions at least 12 weeks apart. The APA are immunoglobulins directed against proteins bound to negatively charged surfaces, usually anionic phospholipids [95]. The APA can be detected by screening for antibodies that:

• directly bind these protein epitopes (e.g. anti-β2-glycoprotein-1, prothrombin, annexin V, APC, protein S, protein Z, protein Z-related protease inhibitor (ZPI), high and low molecular weight kininogens, tPA, factors VII(a) and XII, the complement cascade constituents C4 and CH, and oxidized low-density lipoproteins antibodies

• are bound to proteins present in an anionic phospholipid matrix (e.g. anticardiolipin and phosphatidylserine antibodies

- exert downstream effects on prothrombin activation in a phospholipid milieu (i.e. lupus anticoagulants) [96]. Venous thrombotic events associated with APA include deep venous thrombosis (DVT) with or without acute pulmonary embolism (APE), while the most common arterial events include cerebral vascular accidents and transient ischemic attacks. At least half of patients with APA have systemic lupus erythematosus (SLE). The APA were associated with an OR of 2.17 (95% CI 1.51–3.11; 14 studies) for any thrombosis, OR 2.50 (95% CI 1.51–4.14) for DVT and APE, and OR 3.91 (95% CI 1.14–13.38) for recurrent VTE [97]. Patients with SLE and lupus anticoagulants (LAC) were at a sixfold greater risk for VTE compared with SLE patients without LAC, while SLE patients with APA had a twofold greater risk of VTE compared with SLE patients without these antibodies. The lifetime prevalence of arterial or venous thrombosis in affected patients with APA is approximately 30%, with an event rate of 1% per year [96]. These antibodies are present in up to 20% of individuals with VTE [98].

A review of 25 prospective, cohort, and case–control studies involving more than 7000 patients observed an OR range for arterial and venous thromboses in patients with LAC of 8.65–10.84 and 4.09–16.2, respectively, and 1–18 and 1–2.51 for APA [96]. Antiphosphatidylserine-dependent antiprothrombin IgG antibodies have been linked to second-trimester fetal loss [99]. However, data on clinical association of antiprothrombin antibodies, which include antibodies against prothrombin alone (aPT-A) and antibodies to the phosphatidylserine–prothrombin complex (aPS/PT), are not yet included in the classification criteria for APAS [94]. In a large, prospective cohort of 1155 women in whom a panel of APA was evaluated in the first trimester to determine their relationship to APO, the combinations of antiphosphatidylethanolamine IgG antibody plus ACA IgG (OR 17.5, 95% CI 4.7–66.7) or antiphosphatidylethanolamine IgG antibody plus LAC (OR 22.2, 95% CI 5.4–909) predicted severe preeclampsia with 30.8% sensitivity and 99.2% specificity [100].

There is a 5% risk of VTE during pregnancy and the puerperium among patients with APA despite treatment [101]. Recurrence risks of up to 30% have been reported in APA-positive patients with a prior VTE; thus, long-term prophylaxis is required in these patients. A severe form of APAS is termed catastrophic APS (CAPS), which is defined by potential life-threatening variant with multiple vessel thromboses leading to multiorgan failure [102]. In the Euro-Phospholipid Project Group (13 countries included), DVT, thrombocytopenia, stroke, pulmonary embolism, and transient ischemic attacks were found in 31.7%, 21.9%, 13.1%, 9.0%, and 7.0%, respectively.

The APA are associated with obstetric complications in approximately 15–20%, including fetal loss after 9 weeks' gestation, abruption, severe preeclampsia, and intrauterine growth restriction (IUGR). For LAC-associated fetal loss, reported OR range from 3.0 to 4.8 while ACA display a wider range of reported OR of 0.86–20.0 [95]. It is unclear whether APA are also associated with recurrent (three or more) early spontaneous abortions in the absence of stillbirth. Fifty percent or more of pregnancy losses in APA patients occur after the 10th week [103]. Patients with APA more often display initial fetal cardiac activity compared with patients with unexplained first-trimester spontaneous abortions without APA (86% versus 43%; P< 0.01) [104]. APA have been commonly found in the general obstetric population, with one survey demonstrating that 2.2% of such patients have either immunoglobulin M (IgM) or IgG ACA, with most such women having relatively uncomplicated pregnancies [105].

Other factors may have a role in the pathogenesis of APA. Potential mechanism(s) by which APA induce arterial and venous thrombosis as well as APO include APA-mediated impairment of endothelial thrombomodulin and APC-mediated anticoagulation; induction of endothelial tissue factor expression; impairment of fibrinolysis and AT activity; augmented platelet activation and/or adhesion; impairment of the anticoagulant effects of the anionic phospholipid binding proteins β2-glycoprotein-I and annexin V [106,107]. In the murine model, complement activation, namely C5 complement split product C5a, has been required for tissue factor expression of APA treated mice [108]. A specific anti-C5a monoclonal antibody was able to reverse the thrombogenicity of APA [109]. Heparin's inhibition of aberrant complement activation may explain its protective effects [110]. However, heparin does not completely prevent all APA-related obstetric complications, as has been demonstrated in clinical studies. One explanation may be that APA limit trophoblast migration by down-regulating interleukin-6 secretion and signal transducer and activator of transcription 3 (STAT 3), and heparin does not prevent these effects [111].

Prevention of adverse pregnancy outcomes in the setting of thrombophilia

Gris *et al* [45] compared administration of low-dose aspirin (LDA), 100 mg/day, with 40 mg/day enoxaparin from the 8th week of gestation in a cohort of patients with prior fetal loss after 10 weeks and the presence of heterozygous FVL, PGM, or PS deficiency. The authors found that 23/80 patients treated with LDA and 69/80 patients treated with enoxaparin had a successful pregnancy (OR 15.5, 95% CI 7–34; P <0.0001). Birthweights were higher and there were fewer SGA infants in the enoxaparin group. The study has been criticized for its randomization strategy [112].

A recent Cochrane review based upon an extensive literature search from 1966–2004 found only two trials involving either recurrent early pregnancy loss or fetal demise, and presence of inherited thrombophilia [113]. The other study besides the Gris trial was the trial reported by Tulppala *et al* [114] which involved 82 patients, and compared 50 mg LDA with placebo starting at the time of positive urine pregnancy test, in women with three or more unexplained consecutive losses. No differences were noted in the aspirin compared with the placebo group (RR 1.00 [0.78–1.29]).

Heparin and aspirin administration is the best strategy for the treatment of recurrent pregnancy loss associated with APAS, according to the Cochrane review of 2002 [115]. This approach has been associated with a 54% reduction in pregnancy loss and is better than aspirin alone. Steroid administration is associated with an excessive risk of prematurity, and therefore is not recommended as a first-line prevention strategy. However, the most recent evidence suggests that while unfractionated heparin and aspirin confers a significant benefit in livebirths in APAS, the efficacy of LMWH plus aspirin remains unproven, highlighting the urgent need for a large controlled trial [116].

Regarding prevention of recurrent fetal loss, two randomized, placebo-controlled trials have recently been completed. Kaandorp and colleagues conducted a randomized trial, in which these investigators enrolled 364 women between the ages of 18 and 42 years who had a history of unexplained recurrent miscarriage and were attempting to conceive or were less than 6 weeks pregnant [117]. Patients were randomly assigned to receive daily LDA 80 mg plus open-label subcutaneous nadroparin (at a dose of 2850 IU, starting as soon as a viable pregnancy was demonstrated), LDA 80 mg alone, or placebo. Livebirth rates did not differ significantly among the three study groups. The proportions of women who gave birth to a live infant were 54.5% in the group receiving LDA plus nadroparin (combination therapy group), 50.8% in the LDA-only group, and 57.0% in the placebo group (absolute difference in livebirth rate: combination therapy versus placebo, –2.6 percentage points; 95% CI –15.0 to 9.9; aspirin only versus placebo, –6.2 percentage points, 95% CI –18.8 to 6.4). Neither aspirin combined with nadroparin nor LDA alone improved the livebirth rate, as compared with placebo, among women with unexplained recurrent miscarriage, irrespective of thrombophilic status.

Clark and colleagues conducted a multicenter, randomized controlled trial in the United Kingdom and New Zealand to determine whether treatment with enoxaparin and LDA, along with intensive pregnancy surveillance, reduced rate of fetal loss compared with intensive pregnancy surveillance alone in women with history of two or more consecutive previous fetal losses [118]. Participants (n = 294) presenting for initial antenatal care at fewer than 7 weeks' gestation with history of two or more consecutive previous fetal losses at 24 or fewer weeks' gestation and no evidence of anatomic, endocrine, chromosomal, or immunologic abnormality were randomly assigned to receive either enoxaparin 40 mg subcutaneously and LDA 75 mg orally once daily along with intense pregnancy surveillance or intense pregnancy surveillance alone from random assignment until 36 weeks' gestation. All patients were advised to take folic acid 400 μg daily, beginning before conception and continuing until 10 weeks of gestation. Of the 147 participants receiving pharmacologic intervention, 32 (22%) fetal losses occurred, compared with 29 losses (20%) in the 147 subjects receiving intensive surveillance alone, giving an OR of 0.91 (95% CI 0.52–1.59) of having a successful pregnancy with pharmacologic intervention. These investigators observed no reduction in fetal loss rate with antithrombotic intervention in pregnant women with two or more consecutive previous fetal losses. Collectively, the results of these two studies confirm the need for well-conducted randomized trials in determining the optimal approach to the prevention of placenta-mediated complications.

In conclusion, these recent, well-conducted studies suggest that large-scale prospective association studies and clinical trials will provide the most robust evidence to guide practice patterns. Clinicians should await results of such studies before routinely obtaining inherited thrombophilic evaluations and placing patients on anticoagulation prophylaxis regimens solely to prevent placenta-mediated complications. The components of thrombophilia screening, when deemed indicated, are listed in Box 15.2.

Box 15.2 Screening for inherited and acquired thrombophilia

- Protein C (activity)
- Protein S (free antigen)
- Antithrombin (activity)
- Factor V Leiden (PCR)
- Prothrombin gene mutation 20210A (PCR)
- Homocysteine, fasting
- Platelet count
- Lupus anticoagulant
- Anticardiolipin antibody IgG, IgM, IgA
- β2-glycoprotein I IgG, IgM, IgA

PCR, polymerase chain reaction.

CASE PRESENTATION

The patient is a 30-year-old gravida 2, para 0010 who presented at 6 weeks with a viable singleton gestation. She experienced a PE and DVT on oral contraceptives 10 years ago. She was treated with therapeutic subcutaneous LMWH and then transitioned to oral warfarin therapy for 6 months. Two months following cessation of anticoagulation, a thrombophilia evaluation was performed and revealed the presence of heterozygous FVL. The remainder of the thrombophilia evaluation returned negative; namely, absence of PGM, fasting homocysteine 6.3 μmol/L, and no evidence of anticardiolipin IgG or IgM antibodies, a negative lupus anticoagulant screen, no β2-glycoprotein-I IgG or IgM antibodies, and normal free PS antigen and PS, PC and antithrombin activity.

At her first prenatal visit, baseline labs revealed prothrombin time (PT) of 10 sec, an APTT of 31 sec, and platelet count 209 × 1000/μL (normal). She was treated with prophylactic daily enoxaparin 40 mg subcutaneously until 35 weeks' gestation. One week after starting daily enoxaparin therapy, an anti-factor Xa level was obtained 4 h after her dose and returned 0.14 μ/mL, indicating a prophylactic level of anticoagulation. A repeat platelet count returned a platelet count of 199 × 1000/μL. At 35 weeks, she was switched to prophylactic unfractionated heparin 10,000 U subcutaneously every 12 h until she went into spontaneous labor at 39 5/7 weeks. First-trimester screening, anatomical survey, and fetal growth scans at 24 and 32 weeks were normal. Weekly nonstress testing and amniotic fluid volume assessments were instituted at 36 weeks. During labor, an epidural was placed for analgesia, 16 h after her last dose of unfractionated heparin. The patient delivered vaginally a healthy 3450 g male infant. The placenta delivered 15 min after delivery. The epidural catheter was removed after delivery of the placenta. Estimated blood loss was 450 mL. Twelve hours following delivery, prophylactic daily enoxaparin 40 mg subcutaneously was started and continued for 6 weeks postpartum. The patient was discharged on postpartum day 2. One week after reinstituting daily enoxaparin therapy, an anti-factor Xa level was obtained 4 h after her dose and returned 0.12 μ/mL and a repeat platelet count returned 175 × 1000/μL. The patient elected to breastfeed her infant. For contraception, a Mirena IUD was placed 2 months postpartum.

References

1. Bremme KA. Haemostatic changes in pregnancy. Best Pract Res Clin Haematol 2003;16:153–168.

2. Bremme K, Ostlund E, Almqvist I, Heinonen K, Blomback M. Enhanced thrombin generation and fibrinolytic activity in normal pregnancy and the puerperium. Obstet Gynecol 1992;80:132–137.

3. Paidas MJ, Ku DW, Lee MJ et al. Protein Z, protein S levels are lower in patients with thrombophilia and subsequent pregnancy complications. J Thromb Haemost 2005;3:497–501.

4. Schatz F, Lockwood CJ. Progestin regulation of plasminogen activator inhibitor type-1 in primary cultures of the endometrial stromal and decidual cells. J Clin Endocrinol Metab 1993;77:621–625.

5. Lockwood CJ, Krikun G, Schatz F. The decidua regulates hemostasis in the human endometrium. Semin Reprod Endocrinol 1999;17:45–51.

6. Erlich J, Parry GC, Fearns C et al. Tissue factor is required for uterine hemostasis and maintenance of the placental labyrinth during gestation. Proc Natl Acad Sci USA 1999;96: 8138–8143.

7. Egeberg O. Inherited antithrombin deficiency causing thrombophilia. Thromb Diath Haemorrh 1965;13:516–530.

8. Griffin JH, Evatt B, Zimmerman TS et al. Deficiency of protein C in congenital thrombotic disease. J Clin Invest 1981;68: 1370–1373.

9. Comp PC, Nixon RR, Cooper DW et al. Familial protein S deficiency is associated with recurrent thrombosis. J Clin Invest 1984;74:2082–2088.

10. American College of Obstetricians and Gynecologists. Clinical Updates in Women's Health: Thrombosis, Thrombophilia and Thromboembolism in Women. Washington, DC: American College of Obstetricians and Gynecologists, 2010.

11. Dahlback B. Inherited resistance to activated protein C, a major cause of venous thrombosis, is due to a mutation in the factor V gene. Haemostasis 1994;24:139–151.

12. Ridker PM, Miletich JP, Hennekens CH, Buring JE. Ethnic distribution of factor V Leiden in 4047 men and women. Implications for venous thromboembolism screening. JAMA 1997:277:1305–1307.

13. Lockwood CJ. Inherited thrombophilias in pregnant patients. Prenat Neonat Med 2001;6:3–14.

14. Voorberg J, Roeise J, Koopman R et al. Association of idiopathic venous thromboembolism with single point-mutation at Arg 506 of factor V. Lancet 1994;343:1535–1536.

15. Grandone E, Margaglione M, Colaizzo D et al. Genetic susceptibility to pregnancy related venous thromboembolism: roles of factor V Leiden, prothrombin G20210A, and methylenetetrahy-drofolate reductase mutations. Am J Obstet Gynecol 1998;179:1324–1328.

16. Zotz RB, Gerhardt A, Scharf RE. Inherited thrombophilia and gestational venous thromboembolism. Best Pract Res Clin Haematol 2003;16:243–259.

17. Dizon-Townson D, Miller C, Sibai B et al. The relationship of the factor V Leiden mutation and pregnancy outcomes for mother and fetus. Obstet Gynecol 2005;106:517–524.

18. Poort SR. A common genetic variation in the 3'-untranslated region of the prothrombin gene is associated with elevated plasma prothrombin levels and an increase in venous thrombosis. Blood 1996;88:3698–3703.

19. Franco R, Reitsma P. Genetic risk factors of venous thrombosis. Hum Genet 2001;109:369–384.

20. Gerhardt A, Eberhard Scharf R, Wilhelm Beckmann M et al. Prothrombin and factor V mutations in women with a history of thrombosis during pregnancy and the puerperium. N Engl J Med 2000;342:374–380.

21. Dahlback B. Protein S and C4b-binding protein: components involved in the regulation of the protein C anticoagulant pathway. Thromb Haemost 1991;66:49–61.

22. Mosnier LO, Meijers JCM, Bouma BN. The role of protein S in the activation of TAFI and regulation of fibrinolysis. Thromb Haemost 2001;86:1035–1039.

23. Dykes AC, Walker ID, McMahon AD et al. A study of protein S antigen levels in 3788 healthy volunteers: influence of age, sex and hormone use, and estimate for prevalence of deficiency state. Br J Haematol 2001;113:636.

24. Comp PC, Thurnau GR, Welsh J, Esmon CT. Functional and immunologic protein S levels are decreased during pregnancy. Blood 1986;68:881–885.

25. Cumming AM, Tait RC, Fildes S, Yoong A, Keeney S, Hay CRM. Development of resistance to activated protein C during pregnancy. Br J Haematol 1995;90:725–727.

26. Sugimura M, Kobayashi T, Kanayama N, Terao T. Detection of decreased response to activated protein C during pregnancy by an endogenous thrombin potential-based assay. Semin Thromb Hemost 1999;25:497–502.

27. Greenberg DL, Davie EW. Blood coagulation factors. In: Colman RW, Hirsh J, Marder VJ, Clowes AW, eds. Hemostasis and Thrombosis, Basic Principles and Clinical Practice, 4th edn. Philadelphia: Lippincott Williams and Wilkins, 2001.

28. Lockwood CJ. Inherited thrombophilias in pregnant patients: detection and treatment paradigm. Obstet Gynecol 2002;99: 333–341.

29. Preston FE, Rosendaal FR, Walker ID et al. Increased fetal loss in women with heritable thrombophilia. Lancet 1996;348: 913–916.

30. Rey E, Kahn SR, David M, Shrier I. Thrombophilic disorders and fetal loss: a meta-analysis. Lancet 2003;361:901–908.

31. Alfirevic Z. How strong is the association between maternal thrombophilia and adverse pregnancy outcome? A systematic review. Eur J Obstet Gynecol Reprod Biol 2002;101: 6–14.

32. Patnaik MM, Moll S. Inherited antithrombin deficiency: a review. Haemophilia 2008;14(6):1229–1239.

33. Weiler H, Isermann BH. Thrombomodulin. J Thromb Haemost 2003;1:1515–1524.

34. Paidas MJ, Ku DH, Lee MJ, Lockwood CJ, Arkel YS. Patients with thrombophilia and subsequent adverse pregnancy outcomes have a decreased first trimester response to thrombomodulin in an activated partial thromboplastin time (APTT) system. J Thromb Haemost 2004;2:840–841.

35. Han X, Fiehler R, Broze GJ Jr. Characterization of the protein Z-dependent protease inhibitor. Blood 2000;96:3049–3055.

36. Kemkes-Matthes B, Matthes KJ, Protein Z. Semin Thromb Hemost 2001;5:551–556.

37. Broze GJ Jr. Protein Z-dependent regulation of coagulation. Thromb Haemost 2001;86:8–13.

38. Broze GJ Jr. Protein-Z and thrombosis. Lancet 2001;357: 933–934.

39. Han X, Huang ZF, Fiehler R, Broze GJ Jr. The protein Z-dependent protease inhibitor is a serpin. Biochemistry 1999;38:11073–11078.

40. Yurdakok M, Gurakan B, Ozbag E, Vigit S, Dundar S, Kirazli S. Plasma protein Z levels in healthy newborn infants. Am J Hematol 1995;48:206–207.

41. Miletich JP, Broze GJ Jr. Human plasma protein Z antigen: range in normal subjects and effect of warfarin therapy. Blood 1987;69:1580–1586.

42. Kemkes-Matthes B, Nees M, Kuhnel G, Matzdorff A, Matthes KJ. Protein Z influences the prothrombotic phenotype in factor V Leiden patients. Thromb Res 2002;106:183–185.

43. McColl MD, Deans A, Maclean P, Tait RC, Greer IA, Walker ID. Plasma protein Z deficiency is common in women with antiphospholipid antibodies. Br J Haematol 2003;120: 913–914.

44. Gris JC, Quere I, Dechaud H et al. High frequency of protein Z deficiency in patients with unexplained early fetal loss. Blood 2002;99:2606–2608.

45. Gris JC, Mercier E, Quere I et al. Low-molecular-weight heparin versus low-dose aspirin in women with one fetal loss and a constitutional thrombophilic disorder. Blood 2004;103: 3695–3699.

46. Hunt LT, Dayhoff MO. A surprising new protein superfamily containing ovalbumin, antithrombin-III, and alpha-1 proteinase inhibitor. Biochem Biophys Res Commun 1980;95: 864–871.

47. Gettins P, Patston PA, Schapira M. Structure and mechanism of action of serpins. Hematol Oncol Clin North Am 1992;6: 1393–1408.

48. Andreasen PA, Georg B, Lund LR, Riccio A, Stacey SN. Plasminogen activator inhibitors: hormonally regulated serpins. Mol Cell Endocrinol 1990;68:1–19.

49. Kruithof EKO, Tran-Thang C, Gudinchet A et al. Fibrinolysis in pregnancy: a study of plasminogen activator inhibitors. Blood 1987;69:460–466.

50. Gilabert J, Estelles A, Aznar J et al. Contribution of platelets to increased plasminogen activator inhibitor type 1 in severe preeclampsia. Thromb Haemost 1990;63:361–366.

51. Astedt B, Lecander I, Ny T. The placental type plasminogen activator inhibitor, PAI-2. Fibrinolysis 1987;1:203–208.

52. Francis CW. Plasminogen activator inhibitor-1 levels and polymorphisms. Arch Pathol Lab Med 2002;126:1401–1404.

53. Rozen R. Genetic modulation of homocysteinemia. Semin Thromb Hemost 2000;26(3):255–261.

54. Foka ZJ, Lambropoulos AF, Saravelos H et al. Factor V leiden and prothrombin G20210A mutations, but not methylenetetrahydrofolate reductase C677T, are associated with recurrent miscarriages. Hum Reprod 2000;15:458–462.

55. Roque H, Paidas MJ, Funai EF, Kuczynski E, Lockwood CJ. Maternal thrombophilias are not associated with early pregnancy loss. Thromb Haemost 2004;91:290–295.

56. Murphy RP, Donoghue C, Nallen RJ et al. Prospective evaluation of the risk conferred by factor V Leiden and

thermolabile methylenetetrahydrofolate reductase polymorphisms in pregnancy. Arterioscler Thromb Vasc Biol 2000; 20:266–270.

57. Nelen WL, Blom HJ, Steegers EA et al. Hyperhomocysteinemia and recurrent early pregnancy loss: a meta-analysis. Fertil Steril 2000;74:1196.

58. Langhoff-Roos J, Paidas MJ, Ku DH, Arkel YS, Lockwood CJ. Inherited thrombophilias and early pregnancy loss. In: Mor G, ed. Immunology of Pregnancy. Georgetown, TX: Landes Bioscience, 2004.

59. Salomon O, Seligsohn U, Steinberg DM et al. The common prothrombotic factors in nulliparous women do not compromise blood flow in the feto-maternal circulation and are not associated with preeclampsia or intrauterine growth restriction. Am J Obstet Gynecol 2004;191(6):2002–2009.

60. Rodger M. Abstract: Factor V Leiden (FVL) and prothrombin gene variant (PGV) may be only weakly associated with placenta mediated pregnancy complications: a large prospective cohort study. J Thromb Haemost 2007;5:0S–054.

61. Clark P, Walker ID, Govan L, Wu O, Greer IA. The GOAL study: a prospective examination of the impact of factor V Leiden and ABO(H) blood groups on haemorrhagic and thrombotic pregnancy outcomes. Br J Haematol 2008;140(2): 236–240.

62. Dudding T, Heron J, Thakkinstian A et al. Factor V Leiden is associated with pre-eclampsia but not with fetal growth restriction: a genetic association study and meta-analysis. J Thromb Haemost 2008;6(11):1869–1875.

63. Karakantza M, Androutsopoulos G, Mougiou A, Sakellaropoulos G, Kourounis G, Decavalas G. Inheritance and perinatal consequences of inherited thrombophilia in Greece. Int J Gynaecol Obstet 2008;100(2):124–129.

64. Lindqvist PG, Svensson P, Dahlbäck B. Activated protein C resistance – in the absence of factor V Leiden – and pregnancy. J Thromb Haemost 2006;4(2):361–366.

65. Said JM, Higgins JR, Moses EK et al. Inherited thrombophilia polymorphisms and pregnancy outcomes in nulliparous women. Obstet Gynecol 2010;115(1):5–13.

66. Silver RM, Zhao Y, Spong CY et al. Prothrombin gene G20210A mutation and obstetric complications. Obstet Gynecol 2010;115(1):14–20.

67. Rodger MA, Betancourt MT, Clark P et al. The association of factor V Leiden and prothrombin gene mutation and placenta-mediated pregnancy complications: a systematic review and meta-analysis of prospective cohort studies. PLoS Med 2010;7(6):e1000292.

68. Infante-Rivard C, Rivard GE, Yotov WV et al. Absence of association of thrombophilia polymorphisms with intrauterine growth restriction. N Engl J Med 2002;347:19–25.

69. Howley HE, Walker M, Rodger MA. A systematic review of the association between factor V Leiden or prothrombin gene variant and intrauterine growth restriction. Am J Obstet Gynecol. 2005 Mar;192(3):694–708.

70. Grandone E, Margaglione M, Colaizzo D et al. Lower birth-weight in neonates of mothers carrying factor V G1691A and factor II A(20210) mutations. Haematologica 2002;87: 177–181.

71. Roque H, Paidas M, Rebarber A et al. Maternal thrombophilia is associated with second and third trimester fetal death [abstract]. Am J Obstet Gynecol 2001;184:S27.

72. Lindqvist PG, Svensson PJ, Marsaal K, Grennert L, Luterkort M, Dahlback B. Activated protein C resistance (FV:Q506) and pregnancy. Thromb Haemost 1999;81:532–537.

73. Kupferminc MJ, Many A, Bar-Am A, Lessing JB, Ascher-Landsberg J. Mid-trimester severe intrauterine growth restriction is associated with a high prevalence of thrombophilia. Br J Obstet Gynaecol 2002;109:1373–1376.

74. DeVries JI. Hyperhomocysteinaemia and protein S deficiency in complicated pregnancies. Br J Obstet Gynaecol 1997;104: 1248–1254.

75. Martinelli I. Familial thrombophilia and the occurrence of fetal growth restriction. Haematologica 2001;86:428–431.

76. Ananth CV, Smulian JC, Vintzileos AM. Incidence of placental abruption in relation to cigarette smoking and hypertensive disorders during pregnancy: a meta-analysis of observational studies. Obstet Gynecol 1999;93:622–628.

77. Addis A, Moretti ME, Ahmed Syed F, Einarson TR, Koren G. Fetal effects of cocaine: an updated meta-analysis. Reprod Toxicol 2001;15(4):341–369.

78. Kupferminc MJ, Eldor A, Steinman N et al. Increased frequency of genetic thrombophilia in women with complications of pregnancy. N Engl J Med 1999;340:9.

79. Ananth CV, Peltier MR, de Marco C et al. New Jersey-Placental Abruption Study Investigators. Associations between 2 polymorphisms in the methylenetetrahydrofolate reductase gene and placental abruption. Am J Obstet Gynecol 2007;197(4):385.

80. Rodesch F, Simon P, Donner C, Jauniaux E. Oxygen measurements in endometrial and trophoblastic tissues during early pregnancy. Obstet Gynecol 1992;80:283–285.

81. Jaffe R. Investigation of abnormal first-trimester gestations by color Doppler imaging. J Clin Ultrasound 1993;21: 521–526.

82. Watson AL, Skepper JN, Jauniaux E, Burton GJ. Susceptibility of human placental syncytiotrophoblastic mitochondria to oxygen-mediated damage in relation to gestational age. J Clin Endocrinol Metab 1998;83:1697–1705.

83. Gris J, Quéré I, Monpeyroux F et al. Case-control study of the frequency of thrombophilic disorders in couples with late foetal loss and no thrombotic antecedent – the Nîmes Obstetricians and Haematologists Study 5 (NOHA5). Thromb Haemost 1999;81:891–899.

84. Kocher O, Cirovic C, Malynn E et al. Obstetric complications in patients with hereditary thrombophilia identified using the LCx microparticle enzyme immunoassay: a controlled study of 5000 patients. Am J Clin Pathol 2007;127:68–75.

85. Robertson L, Wu O, Langhorne P et al, for the Thrombosis: Risk and Economic Assessment of Thrombophilia Screening (TREATS) study. Thrombophilia in pregnancy: a systematic review. Br J Haematol 2005;132(2):171–196.

86. Saade GR, McLintock C. Inherited thrombophilia and stillbirth. Semin Perinatol 2002;26(1):51–69.

87. Coppens M, Folkeringa N, Teune MJ et al. Outcome of the subsequent pregnancy after a first loss in women with the factor V Leiden or prothrombin 20210A mutations. J Thromb Haemost 2007;5(7):1444–1448.

88. Lindqvist PG, Merlo J. The natural course of women with recurrent fetal loss. J Thromb Haemost 2006;4(4):896–897.

89. Greer IA. Thrombophilia: implications for pregnancy outcome. Thromb Res 2003;109:73–81.

90. Stanley-Christian H, Ghidini A, Sacher R, Shemirani M. Fetal genotype for specific inherited thrombophilias is not associated with severe preeclampsia. J Soc Gynecol Invest 2005;12:198–201.

91. Vefring H, Lie RT, O'Degard R, Mansoor MA, Nilsen ST. Maternal and fetal variants of genetic thrombophilias and the risk of preeclampsia. Epidemiology 2004;15:317–322.

92. Lykke J, Paidas MJ, Langhoff-Roos J. Recurring complications in second pregnancy. Obstet Gynecol 2009;113(6):1217–1224.

93. Wilson WA, Gharavi AE, Koike T et al. International consensus statement on preliminary classification criteria for definite antiphospholipid syndrome. Arthritis Rheum 1999; 42:1309–1311.

94. Miyakis S, Lockshin MD, Atsumi T et al. International consensus statement on an update of the classification criteria for definite antiphospholipid syndrome (APS). J Thromb Haemost 2006;4:295–306.

95. Galli M, Barbui T. Antiphospholipid antibodies and thrombosis: strength of association. Hematol J 2003;4:180–186.

96. Galli M, Luciani D, Bertolini G, Barbui T. Anti-beta 2-glycoprotein I, antiprothrombin antibodies, and the risk of thrombosis in the antiphospholipid syndrome. Blood 2003;102:2717–2723.

97. Wahl DG, Guillemin F, de Maistre E, Perret C, Lecompte T, Thibaut G. Risk for venous thrombosis related to antiphospholipid antibodies in systemic lupus erythematosus: a meta-analysis. Lupus 1997;6:467–473.

98. Garcia-Fuster MJ, Fernandez C, Forner MJ, Vaya A. Risk factors and clinical characteristics of thromboembolic venous disease in young patients: a prospective study. Med Clin (Barc) 2004;123:217–219.

99. Yamada H, Atsumi T, Kato EH et al. Prevalence of diverse antiphospholipid antibodies in women with recurrent spontaneous abortion. Fertil Steril 2003;80:1276–1278.

100. Yamada H, Atsumi T, Kobashi G et al. Antiphospholipid antibodies increase the risk of pregnancy-induced hypertension and adverse pregnancy outcomes. J Reprod Immunol 2009;79(2):188–195.

101. Branch DW, Silver RM, Blackwell JL, Reading JC, Scott JR. Outcome of treated pregnancies in women with antiphospholipid syndrome: an update of the Utah experience. Obstet Gynecol 1992;80:614–620.

102. Cervera R, Piette JC, Font J et al. Euro-Phospholipid Project Group. Antiphospholipid syndrome: clinical and immunologic manifestations and patterns of disease expression in a cohort of 1,000 patients. Arthritis Rheum 2002;46:1019–1027.

103. Branch DW, Silver RM. Criteria for antiphospholipid syndrome: early pregnancy loss, fetal loss or recurrent pregnancy loss? Lupus 1996;5:409–413.

104. Rai RS, Clifford K, Cohen H, Regan L. High prospective fetal loss rate in untreated pregnancies of women with recurrent miscarriage and antiphospholipid antibodies. Hum Reprod 1995;10:3301–3304.

105. Lockwood C, Romero R, Feinberg R, Clyne L, Coster B, Hobbins J. The prevalence and biologic significance of lupus anticoagulant and anticardiolipin antibodies in a general obstetric population. Am J Obstet Gynecol 1989;161:369–373.

106. Rand JH, Wu XX, Andree HA et al. Pregnancy loss in the antiphospholipid-antibody syndrome: a possible thrombogenic mechanism. N Engl J Med 1997;337:154–160.

107. Field SL, Brighton TA, McNeil HP, Chesterman CN. Recent insights into antiphospholipid antibody-mediated thrombosis. Baillière's Best Pract Res Clin Haematol 1999;12: 407–422.

108. Redecha P, Tilley R, Tencati M et al. Tissue factor: a link between C5a and neutrophil activation in antiphospholipid antibody induced fetal injury. Blood 2007;110(7):2423–2431.

109. Pierangeli SS, Girardi G, Verga-Ostertag ME et al. Requirement of activation of complement C3 and C5 for antiphospholipid antibody-mediated thrombophilia. Arthritis Rheum 2005;52:2120–2124.

110. Girardi G, Redecha P, Salmon JE. Heparin prevents antiphospholipid antibody-induced fetal loss by inhibiting complement activation. Nat Med 2004;10:1222–1226.

111. Mulla MJ, Myrtolli K, Brosens JJ et al. Antiphospholipid antibodies limit trophoblast migration by reducing IL-6 production and STAT3 activity. Am J Reprod Immunol 2010;63(5):339–348. Erratum in: Am J Reprod Immunol 2011;65(1):88.

112. Rodger M. Important publication missing key information. Blood 2004;104(10):3413; author reply 3413–3414.

113. Nisio M, Peters LW, Middeldorp S. Anticoagulants for the treatment of recurrent pregnancy loss in women without antiphospholipid syndrome. Cochrane Database Syst Rev 2005;2:CD004734.

114. Tulppala M, Marttunen M, Soderstrom-Anttila V et al. Low-dose aspirin in prevention of miscarriage in women with unexplained or autoimmune related recurrent miscarriage: effect on prostacyclin and thromboxane A_2 production. Hum Reprod 1997;12:1567–1572.

115. Empson M, Lassere M, Craig JC, Scott JR. Recurrent pregnancy loss with antiphospholipid antibody: a systematic review of therapeutic trials. Obstet Gynecol 2002;99: 135–144.

116. Ziakas PD, Pavlou M, Voulgarelis M. Heparin treatment in antiphospholipid syndrome with recurrent pregnancy loss: a systematic review and meta-analysis.Obstet Gynecol 2010;115(6):1256–1262.

117. Kaandorp SP, Goddijn M, van der Post JA et al. Aspirin plus heparin or aspirin alone in women with recurrent miscarriage. N Engl J Med 2010;362(17):1586–1596.

118. Clark P, Walker ID, Langhorne P et al, for the Scottish Pregnancy Intervention Study (SPIN). A multicenter, randomized controlled trial of low-molecular-weight heparin and low-dose aspirin in women with recurrent miscarriage. Blood 2010;115(21):4162–4167.

Chapter 16
Thromboembolic Disorders

Christian M. Pettker and Charles J. Lockwood
Department of Obstetrics, Gynecology and Reproductive Sciences, Yale University School of Medicine, New Haven, CT, USA

Complicating 1 in 1000 to 1 in 2000 pregnancies, venous thromboembolism (VTE) is a leading cause of maternal morbidity and mortality [1–9]. Moreover, despite this seemingly low prevalence, pregnancy confers a nearly 6–10-fold increased risk of VTE in women of comparable child-bearing age. In one large retrospective cohort study, 94 of 127 (74.8%) pregnant women with documented deep venous thrombosis (DVT) developed their clot during the antepartum period, with half detected before 15 weeks and fewer than 30% diagnosed after 20 weeks [10]. In contrast, most cases of pulmonary embolism (PE) developed during the postpartum period (23 of 38; 60.5%) and PE was strongly associated with cesarean delivery. However, the *per diem* risk of VTE is approximately 3–8-fold higher in the puerperium than during an equivalent antepartum interval [9]. Pulmonary embolism is the leading cause of maternal mortality in the US, contributing to 19.6% of such deaths, and translating into 2.3 pregnancy-related deaths per 100,000 livebirths [11]. An untreated DVT presents a 25% risk of PE, with a mortality rate of approximately 15% if undetected and untreated [12]. On the other hand, if a DVT is promptly diagnosed and treated, the risk of PE is less than 5% and the risk of maternal mortality is less than 1% [13].

The increased risk of pregnancy-associated VTE reflects local and systemic mechanisms that mitigate the risk of hemorrhage during placentation and the third stage of labor. Appreciation of the thrombotic risk of pregnancy demands knowledge of the sophisticated systems of coagulation and fibrinolysis and their inhibitors.

Physiology of hemostasis

Platelet plug formation

Vasoconstriction and platelet aggregation are the initial constraints on hemorrhage following vascular disruption, particularly in arteries. Vasoconstriction limits total blood flow to promote platelet plug formation. It also limits the size of the plug required to obstruct blood flow through the vascular defect. Platelet adhesion is initially mediated through von Willebrand factor (vWF), which is synthesized by megakaryocytes and endothelial cells. It is constitutively secreted but the most active forms are stored in endothelial Weibel-Palade bodies or platelet α-granules where the molecule is released upon activation [14]. Upon vascular wall disruption and after binding to subendothelial collagen, vWF undergoes a conformational change. This change permits it to also bind to the platelet glycoprotein (GP) Ib/IX/V receptor to establish a hemostatic bridge between collagen in the damaged vessel wall and the platelet. The resultant GPIb/IX/V-vWF-collagen interaction facilitates platelet adhesion in the high-flow (shear stress) state induced by vasoconstriction. A second platelet–collagen interaction is mediated by the binding of collagen I and IV to the platelet GPIa/IIa (integrin α2β1) receptor in the low-flow settings created by the expanding platelet plug.

Following collagen-mediated attachment, a second platelet receptor, GPIIb/IIIa (integrin α-IIb/β-3), is now positioned to serve as an alternative extracellular matrix adhering site on platelet cell membranes, permitting attachment to subendothelial laminin, thrombospondin, fibronectin, vitronectin, and possibly also vWF. Moreover, GPIIb/IIIa-mediated platelet adhesion then triggers calcium-dependent protein kinase C (PKC) activation that induces thromboxane A_2 (TXA_2) synthesis and platelet granule release. Beside vWF, platelet α-granules also contain various other clotting factors while dense-granules contain adenosine diphosphate (ADP) and serotonin, which combine with TXA_2 to potentiate vasoconstriction and further promote platelet activation. Platelets can also be activated by thrombin, epinephrine, arachidonic acid, and platelet-activating factor. Platelet activation, in turn, releases more platelet surface GPIIb/IIIa receptors that promote aggregation by forming

Queenan's Management of High-Risk Pregnancy: An Evidence-Based Approach, Sixth Edition. Edited by John T. Queenan, Catherine Y. Spong, Charles J. Lockwood.

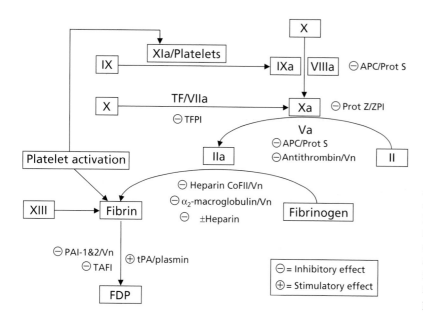

Figure 16.1 An outline of the mechanisms defining the careful balance of thrombosis and hemostasis versus anticoagulation and fibrinolysis. APC, activated protein C; FDP, fibrin degradation products; PAI-1, plasminogen activator inhibitor 1; TAFI, thrombin activatable fibrinolysis inhibitor; TF, tissue factor; TFPI, tissue factor pathway inhibitor; Vn, vitronectin; ZPI, protein Z-dependent protease inhibitor.

interplatelet fibrinogen, fibronectin, and vitronectin bridges [15]. Platelet aggregation in the setting of intact endothelium is prevented by active blood flow and prostacyclin, nitric oxide, and ADPase.

During the platelet activation process, anionic (negatively charged) phospholipids are exteriorized on the cell membrane, creating an ideal clotting surface (see below). Platelet and endothelial cell activation also induces release of P-selectins from platelet α-granules and endothelial Weibel-Palade bodies which embed in the cell walls to further promote platelet and enhance monocyte adherence. P-selectin binding also induces expression of the potent procoagulant, tissue factor (TF), on monocytes to further enhance clotting (see below). These steps underscore the critical role played by platelets, monocytes, and endothelial cells in promoting the classic coagulation cascade.

The coagulation cascade

Platelet plug aggregation in the absence of fibrin generation is inadequate to control the hemorrhage following significant vascular injury. Thus, adequate hemostasis also requires fibrin plug formation which follows exposure of circulating factor VII to perivascular TF (Fig. 16.1). The TF molecule is a cell membrane-bound glycoprotein, constitutively expressed by most nonendothelial extravascular cells and present in the blood in an encrypted (nonclotting) form [16]. This distribution reduces the likelihood of inappropriate activation of the clotting cascade in physiologic states, though obstetric sepsis can induce TF expression on monocytes and endothelial cells to generate thrombosis and disseminated intravascular coagulation (DIC) [16]. It is also highly induced by progesterone in perivascular decidualized endometrial stromal cells, first-trimester decidual cells, and term decidual

cells where it is positioned to promote perinatal hemostasis [17].

The high levels of TF in the decidua also account for the intense thrombin generation and DIC accompanying decidual hemorrhage (i.e. abruption) [18]. It is also present in high levels in the amniotic fluid, perhaps accounting for the coagulopathy observed in amniotic fluid embolism [19]. Following vascular injury, perivascular TF binds circulating factor VII which attaches to negatively charged phospholipids via divalent calcium ions. Factor VII is autoactivated after binding to TF and can be externally activated by thrombin, factors IXa, Xa, or XIIa [20]. (The activated form of clotting factors is denoted by the letter "a" after the Roman numeral.) The TF/VIIa complex can directly activate factor X (see Fig. 16.1) or indirectly activate Xa by activating factor IX (IXa) which then complexes with its co-factor, VIIIa, to activate factor X. In either case, factor Xa next complexes with its co-factor, Va, to convert prothrombin (factor II) to thrombin (factor IIa), which converts fibrinogen to fibrin, and actives platelets (see above). The co-factors V and VIII are activated by either thrombin or factor Xa. Thrombin, kallikrein-kininogen, and plasmin can each activate factor XII on the surface of platelets (see Fig. 16.1). Factor XIIa can activate factor XI, providing another route of factor IX activation. All of these reactions occur on negatively charged phospholipids and require ionized calcium. Ultimately, thrombin cleaves fibrinogen to fibrin monomers which self-polymerize and are cross-linked via thrombin-activated factor XIIIa.

Endogenous anticoagulants

There is evidence that the clotting system "idles" (i.e. is active at a low level) to optimize the immediate response to vascular injury [20]. This chronic basal level of thrombin activation underscores the critical role of the endogenous anticoagulant system in preventing thrombosis (see Fig. 16.1). The TF pathway inhibitor (TFPI) is the first agent in this system and acts on the factor Xa/TF/VIIa complex to inhibit TF-mediated clotting. The TFPI molecule is synthesized by endothelial cells and uses protein S as a co-factor (see below) [21]. Most TFPI (80%) is associated with the vessel wall, while the remainder circulates in plasma at a concentration of approximately 2.5 nM. However, factor XIa can bypass this TFPI-induced coagulation block and sustain clotting on the surface of activated platelets for some time. As a result, additional endogenous anticoagulant molecules are required to avoid thrombosis, including activated protein C, protein S, and protein Z.

Thrombin binds thrombomodulin on perturbed endothelial cell membranes, producing a conformational change that allows activation of protein C [22]. Activated protein C (APC) binds to anionic endothelial cell membrane phospholipids or to the endothelial cell protein C receptor (EPCR) to inactivate factors Va and VIIIa [23]. In addition to its potentiation role in the TFPI pathway, protein S also serves as a co-factor for both Va and VIIIa inactivation by APC. More than half of the total protein S exists in a high-affinity complex with C4b-binding protein, with the remainder circulating freely [24]. Protein Z-dependent protease inhibitor (ZPI) can also impede factor Xa activity. When bound to its co-factor, protein Z, the inhibitory activity of ZPI, is increased 1000-fold [25].

Serine protease inhibitors (SERPINs), which include heparin co-factor II, α2-macroglobulin and antithrombin, account for most of the thrombin inhibitory activity of plasma (see Fig. 16.1). Antithrombin alone accounts for 80% of plasma antithrombin activity and also inactivates factors IXa, Xa, and XIa [26]. Heparins and circulating vitronectin bind to SERPINs and together augment anticoagulant activity 1000-fold [27,28].

Fibrinolysis

Fibrinolysis is initiated by tissue-type plasminogen activator (tPA), embedded in fibrin, which cleaves plasminogen to generate plasmin. Plasmin, in turn, cleaves fibrin into fibrin degradation products (FDPs), which are often used clinically as indirect measures of fibrinolysis. These FDPs can also inhibit thrombin action, a salutary result when limited but when generated in excess can contribute to DIC. Inhibitors of fibrinolysis include α2-plasmin inhibitor and type 1 and 2 plasminogen activator inhibitors (PAI-1 and PAI-2) which inactivate tPA. The endothelium and uterine decidua are primary sources of PAI-1 while the placenta produces PAI-2 [29,30]. The thrombin-activatable fibrinolysis inhibitor (TAFI) modifies fibrin by cleaving carboxy-terminal lysine (Lys) residues from partially degraded fibrin. This in turn blocks tPA-mediated cleavage of plasminogen by preventing the formation of the tPA/plasminogen/fibrin complex. Thus, TAFI renders fibrin resistant to inactivation by plasmin [31]. Like activation of protein C, activation of TAFI by thrombin is greatly enhance by thrombin binding to thrombomodulin.

Pathophysiology of and risk factors for thrombosis in pregnancy

Risk factors for thrombosis not unique to pregnancy include age over 35 years, obesity, immobility, infection, smoking, nephrotic syndrome, hyperviscosity syndromes, malignancies, trauma, surgery, orthopedic procedures, and a prior history of VTE [32]. Pregnancy-specific risk factors include increased parity, endomyometritis, and cesarean and operative vaginal delivery.

All three components of Virchow's triad – vascular stasis, hypercoagulability, and vascular injury – are present in pregnancy. Stasis results from increases in deep vein capacitance secondary to increased circulating levels of estrogen and endothelial production of prostacyclin and nitric oxide, coupled with compression of the inferior vena cava and pelvic veins by the enlarging uterus [33–35]. Interestingly, over 85% of DVT cases in pregnancy are left-sided, likely due to compression of the left iliac vein by the right iliac artery and the gravid uterus [10,36].

Pregnancy-associated hypercoagulability results from changes in decidual and systemic hemostatic factors that likely meet the hemorrhagic challenges posed by vascular injury occurring in implantation, placentation, the third stage of labor and particularly cesarean delivery. Decidual TF and PAI-1 expression is increased in response to progesterone, and levels of placental PAI-2, which are negligible prior to pregnancy, increase until term [17,29,30]. By term, circulating levels of fibrinogen double and levels of factors VII, VIII, IX, X, XII, and vWF increase 20–1000% [37,38]. Additionally, levels of free protein S antigen and activity decrease by approximately 40% due to hormonal induction of C4b-binding protein, conferring overall resistance to APC [38]. Further reductions in free protein S concentrations are seen after cesarean delivery and in the context of infection, both of which augment C4b-binding protein levels, helping to explain the ninefold higher incidence of VTE after cesarean compared with vaginal delivery and why 80% of fatal PE episodes in pregnancy follow cesarean delivery [39,40]. In general, normalization of these coagulation parameters occurs by 6 weeks postpartum. While these mechanisms generally prevent puerperal hemorrhage, they predispose to thrombosis, a tendency aggravated by maternal thrombophilias.

Diagnosis of venous thromboembolism

Deep venous thrombosis

Clinical presentation

Chan and colleagues conducted a cross-sectional study over 7 years at five university-affiliated, tertiary care centers in Canada of 194 pregnant women with suspected DVT [41]. The prevalence of the disorder was 8.8% and the three most predictive clinical variables were left leg symptoms (adjusted odds ratio [adj OR] 44.3, 95% confidence interval [CI] 3.2–609.7), calf circumference difference of 2 cm or more (adj OR 26.9, 95% CI 6.1–118.5), and onset of presentation in the first trimester (adj OR 53.4, 95% CI 7.1–401). Among patients with a subsequently confirmed DVT, all had at least one variable, and 82.4% had two variables. Among patients without a confirmed DVT, half had no variables and only 5.7% had two or more variables. Conversely, none of the pregnant patients with suspected DVT who failed to manifest any of the three variables had subsequent documentation of a DVT, whereas when one or more variables were present, DVT was diagnosed in 16.4% and when two or three variables were present, DVT was diagnosed in 58.3% of cases (95% CI 35.8–75.5%).

D-dimer assays

D-dimer assays are useful, as in nonpregnant patients, as both screening tools and initial tests for DVT. The D-dimer is the product of degradation of fibrin by plasmin, and levels can be elevated in the setting of thrombosis. D-dimer testing employs monoclonal antibodies to D-dimer fragments with the most accurate and reliable tests being two rapid enzyme-linked immunosorbent assays (ELISAs) (Instant-IA D-dimer, Stago, Asniéres, France and VIDAS DD, bioMérieux, Marcy-l'Etoile, France) and a rapid whole-blood assay (SimpliRED D-dimer, Agen Biomedical, Brisbane, Australia).

Chan and associates evaluated the sensitivity and specificity of D-dimer measurements using the SimpliRED assay for diagnosing DVT in 149 at-risk pregnant women [42]. They tested whole blood for D-dimer elevations at initial presentation, and the results were correlated with compression venous ultrasonography (VUS). The prevalence of DVT was 8.7% and the sensitivity of the D-dimer assay was 100% (95% CI 77–100%) with a specificity of 60% (95% CI 52–68%), and a negative predictive value of 100% (95% CI 95–100%). Of note, pregnancy itself is associated with progressive elevations in D-dimer generation. Chan *et al* noted that the SimpliRED assay was "falsely" positive in 0% (95% CI 0–60%), 24% (95% CI 14–37%), and 51% (95% CI 40–61%) of women in the first, second, and third trimesters, respectively. Thus, D-dimer testing in pregnancy appears to have a higher negative predictive value than in the nonpregnant state, likely due

Table 16.1 Fetal radiation exposure of various ionizing modalities

Radiological modality	Fetal radiation exposure (rad)
Chest X-ray	0.01
Venography	
Limited, shielded	0.05
Full (unilateral), unshielded	0.31
Pulmonary angiography	
Brachial vein	0.05
Femoral vein	0.22–0.37
V/Q scan	
Ventilation scan	0.001–0.019
Perfusion scan	0.006–0.012
CTPA	0.013

CTPA, computed tomography pulmonary angiography; V/Q, ventilation/perfusion.
Source: Toglia and Weg [6].

to the higher rate of false-positive results. For this reason, we suggest that it may have a role in the initial triage of patients with suspected DVT for *ruling out* disease.

Venous imaging

Intravenous contrast venography is no longer used for the diagnosis of DVT in pregnancy since it has no greater diagnostic efficacy than VUS and is associated with appreciable radiation exposure (Table 16.1). Compression venous ultrasonography with or without color Doppler has emerged as the preferred initial imaging modality. It requires sonographic imaging of the common femoral vein at the inguinal ligament, and then assessment of the other major venous systems of the leg, including the greater saphenous, the superficial femoral, and the popliteal veins to the deep veins of the calf. Pressure is applied to the transducer to determine the compressibility of the vein lumen under duplex and color flow Doppler imaging [43]. The overall sensitivity and specificity of VUS approach 100% for proximal vein thromboses [44] with slightly less efficacy for detecting isolated calf vein DVT (sensitivity 92.5%, specificity 98.7%, and accuracy 97.2%) [45].

A metaanalysis of 14 studies comparing the efficacy of magnetic resonance (MR) venography with a reference standard in nonpregnant patients with suspected DVT showed a pooled sensitivity of 91.5% and a pooled specificity of 94.8%, with a higher sensitivity for proximal than distal DVT [46]. Thus, MR has equivalent sensitivity and specificity to VUS for the diagnosis of DVT. It may, however, be useful for detecting iliofemoral/pelvic vein thromboses which are poorly visualized by VUS and

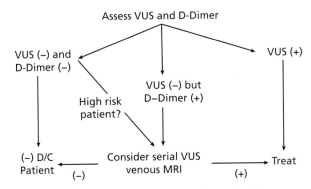

Patient with signs and symptoms of DVT

Figure 16.2 Diagnostic algorithm for the diagnosis of deep venous thrombosis in pregnant women. D/C, discharge; MRI, magnetic resonance imaging; VUS, venous ultrasonography.

account for 11% of DVT in pregnancy, compared with just 1% in the nonpregnant state [47].

Diagnostic algorithm for suspected deep venous thrombosis

Based on the available data, we propose the diagnostic algorithm in Figure 16.2 that allows the diagnosis of DVT with highest sensitivity and specificity. We suggest the initial use of a D-dimer assessment and VUS. If the patient has a negative D-dimer and VUS, the presence of a clinically significant DVT is remote and therapy is withheld. If such a patient is considered at very high risk because of a prior VTE, thrombophilia, the presence of all three characteristic clinical findings, or if the VUS is negative and the D-dimer is positive, consideration should be given to either repeating the evaluation in 3 and 7 days or carrying out MR interrogation of the leg and pelvic veins. If the VUS or MR is positive, initiate anticoagulation with low molecular weight heparin.

Pulmonary embolus

Clinical presentation

Gherman and colleagues analyzed the presenting signs and symptoms of pregnant women with confirmed PE and observed that 62% had shortness of breath, 55.3% had pleuritic chest pain, 23.7% cough, 18.4% diaphoresis, 7.9% hemoptysis, and 5.3% syncope [10]. In a retrospective cohort study of 304 pregnant and puerperal women consecutively evaluated for the clinical suspicion of PE, the most common signs and symptoms were dyspnea (60%), followed by tachycardia (54%) and desaturation to less than 95% (40%) [48]. However, none of these variables was significantly associated with subsequent documentation of a PE (i.e. all relative risks were nonsignificant). Factors significantly linked to a diagnosed PE included chest pain (relative risk [RR] 1.7, 95% CI 1.1–2.6) and a

PaO_2 less than 65 mmHg (RR 2.8, 95% CI 1.4–5.8), but neither was sufficiently predictive of PE to be useful clinically (positive likelihood ratios of <3). Presyncope and syncope are rare, although these symptoms may indicate a massive and potentially fatal PE [49].

Nonspecific studies

Nonspecific studies sometimes employed in the evaluation of patients with suspected PE include electrocardiogram (ECG), chest x-ray (CXR), and echocardiography. An abnormal ECG is present in 70–90% of nonpregnant patients with proven PE who do not have underlying cardiopulmonary disease, but these findings are generally nonspecific [50,51]. The classic ECG changes associated with PE are S1, Q3, and inverted T3, but other findings such as atrial fibrillation, nonspecific ST changes, right bundle branch block, or right axis deviation may also be present. These latter two findings are usually associated with cor pulmonale and right heart strain or overload, reflective of more serious cardiopulmonary compromise. The Urokinase Pulmonary Embolism Trial found that 26–32% of patients with a massive PE had the above ECG changes [50]. However, a lack of ECG changes should not reassure the physician when there is the clinical suspicion of PE.

Traditional CXR findings of pulmonary infarction, such as a wedge-shaped infiltrate ("Hampton hump") or decreased vascularity ("Westermark sign"), are rare [52]. The CXR may be valuable in ruling out other causes of hypoxemia, such as pulmonary edema or pneumonia. Thus, while a normal CXR in the setting of dyspnea, tachypnea, and hypoxemia in a patient without preexistent pulmonary or cardiovascular disease is suggestive of PE, a chest radiograph cannot confirm the diagnosis [52].

Large PE can create changes consistent with cor pulmonale and right heart strain, potentially identifiable on echocardiography. Abnormalities of right ventricular size or function on echocardiogram are seen in 30–80% of patients with PE although similar changes can be seen in exacerbations of chronic obstructive pulmonary disease [53–55]. Typical echocardiographic findings include a dilated and hypokinetic right ventricle or tricuspid regurgitation, in the absence of preexisting pulmonary arterial or left heart pathology. These findings indicate a large embolus and poor prognosis. Transesophageal echocardiography (TEE) improves the sensitivity of diagnosing main or right pulmonary artery emboli [56].

Pulmonary arteriography

Intravenous contrast pulmonary arteriography or angiography has been abandoned in the work-up of PE since it has a relative low sensitivity for smaller peripheral lesions [52,57,58], and is highly invasive, with a 0.5% mortality risk and a 3% complication rate, primarily as a result of the risks of contrast injection and catheter placement, including respiratory failure (0.4%), renal failure (0.3%), cardiac perforation (1%), and groin hematoma requiring transfusion (0.2%) [49,57,59,60].

D-dimer assays

Despite their utility in pregnant women as a "rule-out" test for DVT, there are reported false-negative D-dimer results in pregnant women with documented PE [61]. In a retrospective evaluation of 37 pregnant women with suspected PE undergoing both ventilation/perfusion (V/Q) scans and D-dimer testing, 13 women with low-probability V/Q scans were found to have D-dimer levels ranging from 0.25 to 2.2 mg/L, while 24 women with moderate-to-high probability V/Q results had D-dimer levels ranging from 0.31 to 1.74 mg/L [62]. The sensitivity and specificity of D-dimer as a test for suspected PE in pregnancy were 73% and 15%, respectively. Thus, D-dimer testing appears to be associated with an unacceptable false-negative rate in pregnancy and should not be used. The explanation for the paradoxical finding that D-dimer assays are less sensitive in pregnancy than in the nonpregnant state may be the combination of the small relative clot size compared with that found with lower-extremity DVT coupled with the 40% expansion in plasma volume found in pregnancy.

Ventilation/perfusion scanning versus spiral computed tomographic pulmonary angiography

Ventilation/perfusion scintigraphy (V/Q scan) involves comparative imaging of the pulmonary vascular bed and airspaces using intravenous and aerosolized radiolabeled markers [43]. The comparison of the resultant two images allows for differential diagnostic probabilities (high, intermediate, low, or normal). The Prospective Investigation of Pulmonary Embolism Diagnosis (PIOPED) study evaluated the accuracy of V/Q scanning in nearly 1000 nonpregnant adults with suspected PE [51]. Overall, high-probability V/Q scans correlated with PE in 87.2% of cases; however, only 41% of patients with PE had high-probability scans, yielding a sensitivity of 41% and a specificity of 97%. However, in young healthy pregnant women, without severe asthma or chronic lung disease, the diagnostic accuracy of V/Q scanning is expected to be optimal.

Computed tomographic pulmonary angiography (CTPA) scanning uses intravenous contrast injection to visualize the pulmonary vasculature during scanning with highly sensitive multidetector-row CT technology [52]. Sensitivity of this testing is high for large vessel emboli, but more limited for small subsegmental vessels or vessels oriented horizontally (e.g. in the right middle lobe). Given its broad diagnostic capabilities, CT can be helpful in detecting nonembolic etiologies for the patient's signs and symptoms, such as pneumonia or pulmonary edema.

Comparisons of spiral CT with V/Q scanning for patients with suspected PE indicate that when the CXR is normal, V/Q scanning is more accurate. In a retrospective cohort study, Cahill and associates evaluated 304 consecutive women who were either pregnant or within 6 weeks postpartum, with a clinical suspicion of PE [48]. Of these, 108 (35.1%) underwent initial CTPA and 196 (64.9%) initial V/Q/ scanning. In the subgroup of women with a normal CXR, CTPA was significantly more likely to produce a nondiagnostic result than V/Q scanning, even after adjusting for relevant confounding effects (30.0% compared with 5.6%; adj OR 5.4, 95% CI 1.4–20.1). In a smaller study, Ridge and associates compared the diagnostic accuracy of CTPA and V/Q scans in 28 and 25 pregnant patients with suspected PE, respectively [63]. They also found CTPA less reliable than V/Q scanning (inadequate diagnosis rate of 35.7% for CTPA versus 4% for V/Q scans, P <0.001). The authors also compared the relative efficiency of CTPA in pregnant versus nonpregnant women and noted that CTPA had a higher diagnostic inadequacy rate among pregnant compared with nonpregnant women (35.7% versus 2.1%) (P < 0.001). This was ascribed to more frequent interruption of contrast material by unopacified blood from the inferior vena cava in pregnancy, likely due to increased plasma volume.

Several other studies have also demonstrated that the quality of CTPA is lower in pregnancy. Andreou and colleagues compared contrast enhancement in 16 pregnant and 16 nonpregnant women and found significantly less pulmonary artery enhancement in the pregnancy group [64]. Similarly, U-King-Im and associates compared CTPA studies between 40 pregnant and 40 nonpregnant women and observed that pregnant women had more than triple the proportion of suboptimal studies (27.5% versus 7.5%, P = 0.015) [65]. Similar findings were noted by Litmanovich and colleagues [66]. Taken together, these studies strongly indicate that VQ is the preferred test in pregnant women with suspected PE when the CXR is normal and that CTPA should be reserved for at-risk pregnant women with abnormal CXRs.

In addition to its higher diagnostic accuracy, V/Q scanning also results in substantially lower breast and lung irradiation. It has been estimated that CTPA exposes the mother's breasts to about 150 times more radiation than V/Q scans [40]. This is particularly concerning given the increased glandularity and proliferative state of the gravid breast. Among women, the typical CT coronary angiogram delivers 50–80 mSV to the breast and 48–91 mSV to the lung, resulting in an increased lifetime attributable risk of all cancers in a 20-year-old woman of 1/114 and a lifetime attributable risk of breast cancer of 0.7% [67]. Breast shields and weight-based dose adjustment regimens may significantly lower this dose and should be considered when CTPA is chosen as the diagnostic modality.

By contrast, CTPA generates only slightly less fetal irradiation than V/Q scanning (see Table 16.1). Winer-Muram and associates calculated that the maximal fetal irradiation attributable to CTPA compared with V/Q scans was 131 μGy versus 370 μGy [68]. To put this dose in perspective, *in utero* radiation exposures of up to 50,000 μGy result in negligible increased childhood cancer risk, and fetal doses resulting from both CTPA and V/Q scanning are substantially less than the fetus receives from background radiation (1150–2550 μGy) [69]. Furthermore, lower dose perfusion scans without concomitant ventilation scans appear to have comparable diagnostic efficacy and can further lower reduce fetal radiation exposure.

Lower extremity venous ultrasonography evaluation

Reports in nonpregnant patients indicate that the prevalence of DVT among those with a documented PE ranges from 58% to 82% [70–72]. Metaanalysis suggests that in nonpregnant adults, the prevalence of DVT in those with suspected PE is 18% [73]. Le Gal and associates observed that VUS had a sensitivity of 39% and a specificity of 99% in nonpregnant patients with confirmed PE [74]. While it is uncertain whether comparable rates and diagnostic accuracy exist for pregnant women with co-existing DVT and PE, it seems reasonable to use this test first in stable patients with symptoms of both DVT and PE, as a positive VUS result would mandate the same treatment as a documented PE and would avoid breast and/or fetal irradiation.

Work-up of patients with suspected pulmonary embolism

Evaluation of patients with suspected PE should begin with assessment of their cardio-respiratory status. For stable patients with oxygen saturation levels above 80% and no hemodynamic instability, the assessment outlined in Figure 16.3 begins with an assessment of possible signs and symptoms of lower extremity thrombosis. The presence of left leg symptoms, calf circumference difference of 2 cm or more, and/or onset of presentation in the first trimester should prompt VUS, and if positive, anticoagulation should commence. If the VUS is negative or the patient has no suggestive leg symptoms, proceed to a CXR. If this is positive, CTPA should be the definitive test. If the CTPA is positive for PE, treatment is begun. If the CTPA is negative for PE, assess the patient for other pathologies that could be generating the signs and symptoms. These are often also discernible by chest CT.

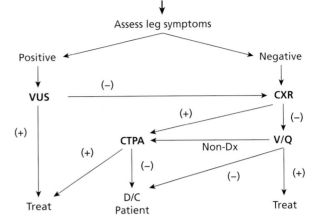

Figure 16.3 Diagnostic algorithm for the diagnosis of pulmonary embolism in hemodynamically stable pregnant women. CTPA, computed tomographic pulmonary angiography; CXR, chest x-ray; D/C, discharge; Dx, diagnostic; V/Q, ventilation/perfusion; VUS, venous ultrasonography.

If the CXR is negative, proceed to V/Q scan. If positive (high or moderate probability), treat the patient with anticoagulation. If negative or low probability in a low-risk patient (i.e. no prior VTE, no thrombophilia, no affected first-degree relative and no major clinical risk factors), anticoagulation can be withheld. If a low-probability V/Q result occurs in a high-risk patient, consider serial VUS or MR angiography with contrast. Though gadolinium crosses the placenta and enters the amniotic fluid after intravenous administration, the majority of animal studies suggest no carcinogenic, teratogenic or mutagenic effects and it is considered category C by the FDA.

In patients who are hypoxemic or displaying hemodynamic instability with signs and symptoms of PE, the protocol outlined in Figure 16.4 should be followed. Thus, anticoagulation is promptly initiated and a CXR obtained. The remainder of the work-up parallels that described above, except if no PE is documented by V/Q scan, consideration should be given to CTPA for further confirmation and to exclude other pulmonary, cardiac, and chest wall pathologies. Alternative causes of the hypoxia and/or hemodynamic instability must be excluded (e.g. sepsis with adult respiratory distress syndrome, pneumothorax, cardiomyopathy with pulmonary edema). Consideration should be given to performing a bedside echocardiogram (transthoracic or transesophageal, as appropriate) in very unstable patients as this is more likely to be diagnostic in this setting and avoids transporting a critically ill patient.

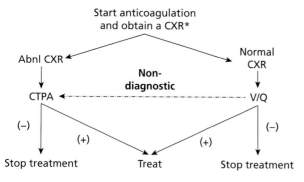

Patient with signs and symptoms of acute PE

Start anticoagulation
and obtain a CXR*

Abnl CXR   Normal CXR

Non-diagnostic

CTPA ◂┈┈┈┈┈┈┈┈┈┈┈┈ V/Q

(−)   (+)   (+)   (−)

Stop treatment   Treat   Stop treatment

*If hemodynamically unstable consider echocardiogram at bedside

Figure 16.4 Diagnostic algorithm for the diagnosis of pulmonary embolism in unstable pregnant women. CTPA, computed tomographic pulmonary angiography; CXR, chest x-ray; V/Q, ventilation/perfusion.

Conclusion

Avoidance of hemorrhage and thrombosis presents paradoxical challenges to the pregnant patient. Processes promoting hemostasis and endogenous anticoagulation are held in delicate equipoise, and the adaptations to and conditions of pregnancy predispose the gravid woman to increased risk of thromboembolic disease. Careful evaluation of risk of thromboembolic disease and elicitation of signs and symptoms are critical to making the diagnosis. The combination of VUS and D-dimer testing is a simple and effective strategy for ruling out DVT. Lower extremity VUS and/or the combination of CXR with either V/Q scan or CTPA are the mainstays of diagnosing PE in pregnancy and the puerperium.

CASE PRESENTATION 1

A 42-year-old gravida 1, para 0 infertility patient is status postovulation induction, *in vitro* fertilization, and transfer of three embryos resulting in a triplet gestation. Following several admissions for recurrent severe nausea and vomiting with weight loss, she has been resting at home for the past 4 days heavily sedated by her antiemetic regimen. She awakens late at night with left calf and thigh pain.

She is seen in her physician's office the following morning. She denies dyspnea but notes mild calf and posterior thigh tenderness to palpation, and has no other signs or symptoms of DVT. A VUS is ordered and she is found to have thrombosis involving the proximal thigh and calf veins. She is begun on therapeutic doses of low molecular weight heparin.

CASE PRESENTATION 2

A 27-year-old gravida 2, para 1 at 27 weeks' gestation complains of left calf pain which she believes began following the development of a painful muscle cramp which awoke her the night before. She is seen in her physician's office and has an unremarkable exam except for bilateral trace lower extremity edema. She is quite healthy, exer-

cises regularly, and has no personal or family history of thrombosis. A D-dimer and VUS are ordered which return negative. She is given instructions to call if the pain worsens or she develops unilateral lower extremity swelling, or dyspnea.

References

1. Ginsberg J, Brill-Edwards P, Burrows R et al. Venous thrombosis during pregnancy: leg and trimester of presentation. Thromb Haemost 1992;67:519–520.
2. Kierkegaard A. Incidence and diagnosis of deep vein thrombosis associated with pregnancy. Acta Obstet Gynecol Scand 1983;62:239–243.
3. Rutherford S, Montoro M, McGehee W, Strong T. Thromboembolic disease associated with pregnancy: an 11-year review (SPO Abstract). Obstet Gynecol 1991;164:286.
4. Simpson E, Lawrenson R, Nightingale A, Farmer R. Venous thromboembolism in pregnancy and the puerperium: incidence and additional risk factors from a London perinatal database. Br J Obstet Gynaecol 2001;108:56–60.
5. Stein P, Hull R, Jayali F et al. Venous thromboembolism in pregnancy: 21-year trends. Am J Med 2004;117:121–125.
6. Toglia M, Weg J. Venous thromboembolism during pregnancy. N Engl J Med 1996;335:108–114.
7. Treffers P, Huidekoper B, Weenink G, Kloosterman G. Epidemiological observations of thrombo-embolic disease during pregnancy and the puerperium, in 56,022 women. Intl J Gynaecol Obstet 1983;21:327–331.
8. James K, Lohr J, Deshmukh R, Cranley J. Venous thrombotic complications of pregnancy. Cardiovasc Surg 1996;4:777–782.

9. McColl M, Ramsay J, Tait R et al. Risk factors for pregnancy associated venous thromboembolism. Thromb Haemost 1997;78:1183–1188.

10. Gherman RB, Goodwin TM, Leung B, Byrne JD, Hethumumi R, Montoro M. Incidence, clinical characteristics, and timing of objectively diagnosed venous thromboembolism during pregnancy. Obstet Gynecol 1999; 94:730–734.

11. Chang J, Elam-Evans L, Berg C et al. Pregnancy-related mortality surveillance, United States, 1991–1999. MMWR Surveill Summ 2003;52:1–8.

12. Wessler S. Medical management of venous thrombosis. Annu Rev Med 1979;27:313–319.

13. Vallasanta U. Thromboembolic disease in pregnancy. Am J Obstet Gynecol 1965;93:142–160.

14. Löwenberg EC, Meijers JC, Levi M. Platelet-vessel wall interaction in health and disease. Neth J Med 2010; 68:242–251.

15. Pytela R, Pierschbacher M, Ginsberg M, Plow E, Ruoslahti E. Platelet membrane glycoprotein IIb/IIIa: member of a family of Arg-Gly-Asp-specific adhesion receptors. Science 1986;231: 1559–1562.

16. Mackman N.Role of tissue factor in hemostasis and thrombosis. Blood Cells Mol Dis 2006;36:104–107.

17. Lockwood CJ, Murk W, Kayisli UA et al. Progestin and thrombin regulate tissue factor expression in human term decidual cells. J Clin Endocrinol Metab 2009;94:2164–2170.

18. Lockwood CJ, Paidas M, Murk WK et al. Involvement of human decidual cell-expressed tissue factor in uterine hemostasis and abruption. Thromb Res 2009;124:516–520.

19. Lockwood C, Bach R, Guha A, Zhou X, Miller W, Nemerson Y. Amniotic fluid contains tissue factor, a potent initiator of coagulation. Am J Obstet Gynecol 1991;165:1335–1341.

20. Mackman N. The role of tissue factor and factor VIIa in hemostasis. Anesth Analg 2009;108:1447–1452.

21. Hackeng TM, Maurissen LF, Castoldi E, Rosing J. Regulation of TFPI function by protein S. J Thromb Haemost. 2009; 7(Suppl 1):165–168.

22. Esmon C. The protein C pathway. Chest 2003;124(3 Suppl): 26S–32S.

23. Dahlback B. Progress in the understanding of the protein C anticoagulant pathway. Int J Hematol 2004;79:109–116.

24. Dahlback B. The tale of protein S and C4b-binding protein, a story of affection. Thromb Haemost 2007;98:90–96.

25. Broze G. Protein Z-dependent regulation of coagulation. Thromb Haemost 2001;86:8–13.

26. Perry D. Antithrombin and its inherited deficiencies. Blood Rev 1994;8:37–55.

27. Preissner K, Zwicker L, Muller-Berghaus G. Formation, characterization and detection of a ternary complex between protein S, thrombin and antithrombin III in serum. Biochem J 1987;243:105–111.

28. Bouma B, Meijers J. New insights into factors affecting clot stability: a role for thrombin activatable fibrinolysis inhibitor. Semin Hematol 2004;41:13–19.

29. Schatz F, Lockwood C. Progestin regulation of plasminogen activator inhibitor type-1 in primary cultures of endometrial stromal and decidual cells. J Clin Endocrin Metab 1993;77: 621–625.

30. Lockwood C, Krikun G, Schatz F. The decidua regulates hemostasis in the human endometrium. Semin Reprod Endocrinol 1999;17:45–51.

31. Bouma BN, Mosnier LO. Thrombin activatable fibrinolysis inhibitor (TAFI) – how does thrombin regulate fibrinolysis? Ann Med 2006;38(6):378–388.

32. Girling J, de Swiet M. Inherited thrombophilia and pregnancy. Curr Opin Obstet Gynecol 1998;10:135–144.

33. Wright H, Osborn S, Edmunds D. Changes in the rate of flow of venous blood in the leg during pregnancy, measured with radioactive sodium. Surg Gynecol Obstet 1950;90:481.

34. Goodrich S, Wood J. Peripheral venous distensibility and velocity of venous blood flow during pregnancy or during oral contraceptive therapy. Am J Obstet Gynecol 1964;90:740.

35. Macklon N, Greer I, Bowman A. An ultrasound study of gestational and postural changes in the deep venous system of the leg in pregnancy. Br J Obstet Gynaecol 1997;104:191–197.

36. Ray JG, Chan WS. Deep vein thrombosis during pregnancy and the puerperium: a meta analysis of the period of risk and the leg of presentation, Obstet Gynecol Surv 1999;54: 265–271.

37. Hellgren M, Blomback M. Studies on blood coagulation and fibrinolysis in pregnancy, during delivery and in the puerperium. Gynecol Obstet Invest 1981;12:141–154.

38. Bremme K. Haemostatic changes in pregnancy. Baillière's Best Pract Res Clin Haematol 2003;16:153–168.

39. Macklon N, Greer I. Venous thromboembolic disease in obstetrics and gynecology: the Scottish experience. Scott Med J 1996;41:83–86.

40. Bourjeily G, Paidas M, Khalil H, Rosene-Montella K, Rodger M. Pulmonary embolism in pregnancy. Lancet 2010;375(9713):500–512.

41. Chan WS, Lee A, Spencer FA et al. Predicting deep venous thrombosis in pregnancy: out in "LEFt" field? Ann Intern Med 2009;151:85–92.

42. Chan WS, Chunilal S, Lee A, Crowther M, Rodger M, Ginsberg JS. A red blood cell agglutination D-dimer test to exclude deep venous thrombosis in pregnancy. Ann Intern Med 2007;147:165–170.

43. Hirsh J, Hoak J. Management of deep vein thrombosis and pulmonary embolism: a statement for healthcare professionals from the Council on Thrombosis (in Consultation with the Council on Cardiovascular Radiology), American Heart Association. Circulation 1996;93:2212–2245.

44. Kassai B, Boissel J, Cucherat M, Sonie S, Shah N, Leizorovicz A. A systematic review of the accuracy of ultrasound in the diagnosis of deep venous thrombosis in asymptomatic patients. Thromb Haemost 2004;91:655–666.

45. Gottlieb R, Widjaja J, Tian L, Rubens D, Voci S. Calf sonography for detecting deep venous thrombosis in symptomatic patients: experience and review of the literature. J Clin Ultrasound 1999;27:415–420.

46. Sampson FC, Goodacre SW, Thomas SM et al. The accuracy of MRI in diagnosis of suspected deep vein thrombosis: systematic review and meta-analysis. Eur Radiol 2007;17(1): 175–181.

47. James AH, Tapson VF, Goldhaber SZ. Thrombosis during pregnancy and the postpartum period, Am J Obstet Gynecol 2005;193:216–219.

48. Cahill AG, Stout MJ, Macones GA, Bhalla S. Diagnosing pulmonary embolism in pregnancy using computed-tomographic angiography or ventilation-perfusion. Obstet Gynecol 2009; 114:124–129.

49. Fedullo P, Tapson V. The evaluation of suspected pulmonary embolism. N Engl J Med 2003;349:1247–1256.

50. Urokinase Pulmonary Embolism Trial: a national cooperative study. Circulation 1973;47(Suppl II):1–108.

51. PIOPED Investigators. Value of the ventilation/perfusion scan in acute pulmonary embolism. Results of the prospective investigation of pulmonary embolism diagnosis (PIOPED). JAMA 1990;263:2653–2659.

52. Tapson V, Carroll B, Davidson B et al. The diagnostic approach to acute venous thromboembolism. Clinical practice guideline. American Thoracic Society. Am J Respir Clin Care Med 1999;160:1043–1066.

53. Come P. Echocardiographic evaluation of pulmonary embolism and its response to therapeutic interventions. Chest 1992;101:151S–62S.

54. Kasper W, Meinertz T, Kersting F, Lollgen H, Limbourg P, Just H. Echocardiography in assessing acute pulmonary hypertension due to pulmonary embolism. Am J Cardiol 1980;45:567–572.

55. Gibson N, Sohne M, Buller H. Prognostic value of echocardiography and spiral computed tomography in patients with pulmonary embolism. Curr Opin Pulm Med 2005;11:380–384.

56. Pruszczyk P, Torbicki A, Pacho R et al. Noninvasive diagnosis of suspected severe pulmonary embolism: transesophageal echocardiography vs spiral CT. Chest 1997;112:722–728.

57. Stein P, Athanasoulis C, Alavi A et al. Complications and validity of pulmonary angiography in acute pulmonary embolism. Circulation 1992;85:462–468.

58. Henry JW, Relyea B, Stein PD. Continuing risk of thromboemboli among patients with normal pulmonary angiograms. Chest 1995;107(5):1375–1378.

59. Mills S, Jackson D, Older R, Heaston D, Moore A. The incidence, etiologies, and avoidance of complications of pulmonary angiography in a large series. Radiology 1980;136:295–299.

60. Dalen J, Brooks H, Johnson L, Meister S, Szucs MJ, Dexter L. Pulmonary angiography in acute pulmonary embolism: indications, techniques, and results in 367 patients. Am Heart J 1971;81:175–185.

61. To MS, Hunt BJ, Nelson-Piercy C. A negative D-dimer does not exclude venous thromboembolism (VTE) in pregnancy. J Obstet Gynaecol 2008;28:222–223.

62. Damodaram M, Kaladindi M, Luckit J, Yoong W. D-dimers as a screening test for venous thromboembolism in pregnancy: is it of any use? J Obstet Gynaecol 2009;29:101–103.

63. Ridge CA, McDermott S, Freyne BJ, Brennan DJ, Collins CD, Skehan SJ. Pulmonary embolism in pregnancy: comparison of pulmonary CT angiography and lung scintigraphy. Am J Roentgenol 2009;193(5):1223–1227.

64. Andreou AK, Curtin JJ, Wilde S, Clark A. Does pregnancy affect vascular enhancement in patients undergoing CT pulmonary angiography? Eur Radiol 2008;18(12):2716–2722.

65. U-King-Im JM, Freeman SJ, Boylan T, Cheow HK. Quality of CT pulmonary angiography for suspected pulmonary embolus in pregnancy. Eur Radiol 2008;18(12):2709–2715.

66. Litmanovich D, Boiselle PM, Bankier AA, Kataoka ML, Pianykh O, Raptopoulos V. Dose reduction in computed tomographic angiography of pregnant patients with suspected acute pulmonary embolism. J Comput Assist Tomogr 2009;33:961–966.

67. Einstein AJ, Henzlova MJ, Rajagopalan S. Estimating risk of cancer associated with radiation exposure from 64-slice computed tomography coronary angiography. JAMA 2007;298(3):317–323.

68. Winer-Muram HT, Boone JM, Brown HL, Jennings SG, Mabie WC, Lombardo GT. Pulmonary embolism in pregnant patients: fetal radiation dose with helical CT. Radiology 2002;224(2):487–492.

69. Winer-Muram HT, Boone JM, and National Council on Radiation Protection. Exposure of the population in the United States and Canada to natural background radiation. Report No. 94. Bethesda, MD: National Council on Radiation Protection, 1987.

70. Yamaki T, Nozaki M, Sakurai H, Takeuchi M, Soejima K, Kono T. Presence of lower limb deep vein thrombosis and prognosis in patients with symptomatic pulmonary embolism: preliminary report. Eur J Vasc Endovasc Surg 2009;37:225–231.

71. Girard P, Musset D, Parent F, Maitre S, Phlippoteau C, Simonneau G. High prevalence of detectable deep venous thrombosis in patients with acute pulmonary embolism. Chest 1999;116:903–908.

72. Girard P, Sanchez O, Leroyer C et al. Deep venous thrombosis in patients with acute pulmonary embolism: prevalence, risk factors, and clinical significance. Chest 2005;128:1593–1600.

73. Van Rossum AB, van Houwelingen HC, Kieft G J, Pattynama PM. Prevalence of deep vein thrombosis in suspected and proven pulmonary embolism: a meta-analysis. Br J Radiol 1998;71:1260–1265.

74. Le Gal G, Righini M, Sanchez O et al. A positive compression ultrasonography of the lower limb veins is highly predictive of pulmonary embolism on computed tomography in suspected patients. Thromb Haemost 2006;95:963–966.

Chapter 17
Cardiac Disease

Stephanie R. Martin[1], Alexandria J. Hill[2], and Michael R. Foley[2]

[1]Department of Obstetrics and Gynecology, Baylor College of Medicine, Houston, TX, USA
[2]Department of Obstetrics and Gynecology, University of Arizona, Tucson, AZ, USA

Advances in diagnosis and treatment of congenital cardiac lesions have led to dramatically improved survival rates. Consequently, the predominant form of cardiac disease encountered during pregnancy has shifted from rheumatic to congenital heart disease [1,2]. During the mid-1950s, rheumatic heart disease during pregnancy was 16 times more common than congenital disease. By 1967, this ratio had reversed to 3:1 (congenital versus acquired) [1,2]. According to the National Center for Health Statistics, in 2004, the number of women postponing child bearing beyond age 40 had grown, thereby increasing the likelihood of other co-morbid conditions, including cardiac disease.

Despite complicating only 4% of all pregnancies in the United States, a disproportionate number of maternal deaths (34%) can be attributed to cardiac disease [3]. Approximately 15% of maternal intensive care unit (ICU) admissions are attributable to cardiac disease, but it accounts for up to 50% of all maternal deaths in the ICU [4]. Assessment of the pregnant patient with cardiac disease can be challenging, as many common complaints of normal pregnancy, such as dyspnea, fatigue, palpitations, orthopnea, and pedal edema, mimic symptoms of worsening cardiac disease. Obstetric patients with cardiac disease are susceptible to a number of potential complications resulting from significant physiologic changes associated with pregnancy and delivery. This chapter outlines the expected hemodynamic and physiologic changes occurring in pregnancy and reviews prognosis and management recommendations for obstetric patients with congenital and acquired cardiac lesions.

Physiologic changes

The adaptations that occur during pregnancy place substantial demands on maternal cardiac function. Table 17.1 [5,6] summarizes hemodynamic changes in pregnancy. The greatest impact on a compromised cardiovascular system results from four fundamental alterations: increased intravascular volume, increased cardiac output, decreased systemic vascular resistance, and hypercoagulability.

During pregnancy total blood and plasma volume increases by approximately 50%. However, red cell mass increases by only 33%, ultimately resulting in a decreased hemoglobin and hematocrit, as demonstrated in Figures 17.1 and 17.2. The heart is able to accommodate this increase in volume primarily because of decreased systemic vascular resistance. Consequently, systolic and diastolic blood pressures drop during pregnancy, reaching a nadir between 24 and 32 weeks' gestation. Cardiac output increases by 30–50% above prepregnant levels by the end of the third trimester and may increase by an additional 50% in the second stage of labor [5]. Strikingly, half of the increase in cardiac output occurs by 8 weeks' gestation [7]. Profound alterations in the coagulation cascade also occur, including increases in fibrinogen and factor VIII levels, resulting in a thrombophilic state that predisposes patients to the development of thromboembolic complications (Box 17.1). These changes will also affect the findings on various cardiovascular tests as outlined in Table 17.2 [8].

Counseling the patient

Functional status for patients with cardiac disease is commonly classified according to the New York Heart Association (NYHA) classification system as outlined in Box 17.2. The utility of this classification system during pregnancy is limited because it does not address specific lesions. However, as expected, patients with NYHA class I or II have less risk of complications compared with those in class III or IV. In the 1987 edition of *Critical Care Obstetrics*, a guideline was introduced that classified various cardiac abnormalities according to maternal death risk estimates (Box 17.3) [9]. Disorders associated

Queenan's Management of High-Risk Pregnancy: An Evidence-Based Approach, Sixth Edition. Edited by John T. Queenan, Catherine Y. Spong, Charles J. Lockwood.

Table 17.1 Expected cardiovascular changes in pregnancy

Measurement	Normal value	% Change in pregnancy
Heart rate (beats/min)	71 ± 10	10–20%
Stroke volume (mL)	73.3 ± 9	30%
Cardiac output (L/min)	4.3 ± 0.9	30–50%
Blood volume (L)	5	20–50%
Systemic vascular resistance (dyne/cm/s)	1530 ± 520	−20%
Mean arterial pressure (mmHg)	86.4 ± 7.5	Not significant
Oxygen consumption (mL/min)	250	20–30%

Source: Clark *et al* [5] and Elkayam and Gleicher [6].

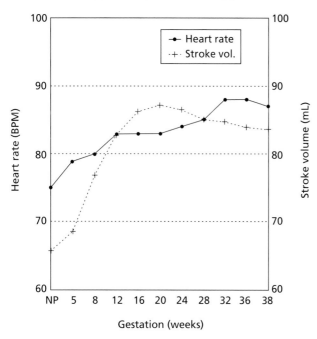

Figure 17.1 Alterations in stroke volume and heart rate during pregnancy. BPM, beats per minute.

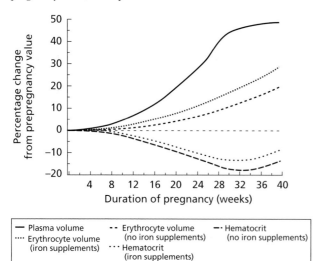

Figure 17.2 Changes in plasma volume, red cell volume, and hematocrit during pregnancy.

Table 17.2   Changes in cardiovascular tests during pregnancy

Cardiovascular exam	Findings in pregnancy
Chest x-ray	Cardiomegaly
	Enlarged left atrium
	Increased lung markings
	Small pleural effusions early postpartum
Electrocardiography	Left axis deviation by 15°
	Right bundle branch block
	Q waves in lead III and aVF
	T wave inversion in leads III, V2, and V3
	Shortening of PR and QT intervals
Echocardiography	Mild tricuspid regurgitation
	Pulmonary regurgitation
	Increased left atrial size by up to 14%
	Increased left ventricular end-diastolic dimensions by 6–10%
	Mitral regurgitation
	Pericardial effusion

Box 17.1 Clotting factor changes in pregnancy

Factor II (prothrombin)	Unchanged
Factors VII–X, XII	Increased
Fibrinogen	Increased
Platelets	Unchanged

Box 17.2 New York Heart Association (NYHA) functional classification

Class I: no limitations of physical activity. Ordinary physical activity does not precipitate cardiovascular symptoms such as dyspnea, angina, fatigue, or palpitations

Class II: slight limitation of physical activity. Ordinary physical activity does precipitate cardiovascular symptoms. Patients are comfortable at rest

Class III: less than ordinary physical activity precipitates cardiovascular symptoms. Patients are comfortable at rest

Class IV: unable to carry out physical activity without discomfort. Symptoms of cardiac insufficiency or angina are present at rest

with less than a 1% risk of death were considered minimal risk, moderate risk disorders carried a 5–15% risk of mortality, and major risk disorders were considered to have a mortality risk in excess of 25%. This classification system certainly provided more information with which to counsel patients; however, the patient's particular history is not taken into consideration.

In 1997, Siu *et al* [10] identified several independent risk factors for cardiac complications such as congestive heart failure, stroke, or arrhythmia, based on a series of 252 pregnant patients with a variety of cardiac diseases. The

Group 1: mortality < 1%

- Atrial septal defect
- Ventricular septal defect
- Patent ductus arteriosus
- Mitral stenosis: NYHA class I and II
- Pulmonic/tricuspid valve disease
- Corrected tetralogy of Fallot
- Bioprosthetic valve

Group 2: mortality 5–15%

Group 2A

- Mitral stenosis: NYHA class III and IV
- Aortic stenosis
- Coarctation of aorta without valvular involvement
- Uncorrected tetralogy of Fallot
- Previous myocardial infarction
- Marfan syndrome with normal aorta

Group 2B

- Mitral stenosis with atrial fibrillation
- Artificial valve

Group 3: mortality 25–50%

- Pulmonary hypertension
  - Primary
  - Eisenmenger
- Coarctation of aorta with valvular involvement
- Marfan syndrome with aortic involvement
- Peripartum cardiomyopathy with persistent left ventricular dysfunction

NYHA, New York Heart Association.
Source: Clark [9].

Table 17.3 Predicting adverse cardiac events during pregnancy

Number of risk factors	Risk of adverse event (%)
0	5
1	27
2 or more	75

Risk factors:
History of heart failure, transient ischemic attack, stroke or arrhythmia
Prepregnancy NYHA class II–IV or cyanosis
Left heart obstruction (mitral or aortic valve stenosis)
Ejection fraction <40%
Most common adverse events: pulmonary edema, arrhythmias.
NYHA, New York Heart Association.
Source: Siu *et al* [11].

most significant risk factors for complications include NYHA class III or IV, cyanosis, history of an arrhythmia, pulmonary vascular disease, ejection fraction of less than 40%, or significant mitral or aortic valve obstruction.

More recently, in the CARPREG study, Siu *et al* [11] prospectively evaluated 617 pregnancies complicated by maternal cardiac disease and identified four predictors of maternal complications.

- History of heart failure, transient ischemic attack, stroke, or arrhythmia.
- Prepregnancy NYHA class II–IV or cyanosis.
- Left heart obstruction (mitral valve area $< 2 \text{cm}^2$, aortic valve area $< 1.5 \text{cm}^2$, peak left outflow gradient $> 30 \text{mmHg}$).
- Ejection fraction less than 40%.

The risk of maternal complications was directly proportional to the number of risk factors identified. Five percent of patients with none of the four predictors developed a complication, whereas the addition of only one risk factor increased the adverse event rate to 27%. The incidence of complications increased to 75% in patients with more than one predictor (Table 17.3) [11]. Pulmonary edema and arrhythmias were the most commonly encountered complications. Route of delivery did not affect the complication rate. Six patients (1%) died secondary to stroke or cardiac decompensation. In that same study, the strongest predictors for neonatal complications were NYHA class II or above, heparin or warfarin (Coumadin) use during pregnancy, smoking, multiple gestation, and left heart obstruction. Twenty percent of the women in this study delivered small for gestational age (SGA) infants or delivered prematurely.

In a subsequent study, the same authors prospectively compared 300 pregnant women with cardiac disease against controls, primarily to evaluate neonatal and cardiac outcomes [12]. In this group of patients, 64% had congenital lesions, 28% had acquired lesions, and the remaining 8% had dysrhythmias. Forty-one percent of the gravidas had undergone previous surgical interventions. As expected, miscarriage and neonatal complications such as intraventricular hemorrhage, delivery before 34 weeks' gestation, and neonatal death occurred more commonly in gravidas with cardiac disease compared with controls. However, the addition of risk factors such as smoking, anticoagulant use, and multiple gestations in a patient with cardiac disease escalated the risk of neonatal complications to twice that of the control group. In this study, 17% of patients with cardiac disease had a cardiac complication, 94% of which were caused by cardiac failure or dysrhythmias. Moreover, delivery by cesarean section occurred more commonly in patients with cardiac disease (29% versus 23%), but preeclampsia and hemorrhage developed with equal frequency in study and control patients.

Significant congenital cardiac disease poses particular maternal and fetal risks. In a study of pregnant women with substantial congenital cardiac disease (repaired and unrepaired), 20% of patients experienced serious adverse cardiac events including death, congestive heart failure, myocardial infarction, stroke, urgent cardiac intervention, or arrhythmia. The majority of cardiac events (76%) occurred in the 6 weeks postpartum. In fact, in this group of patients, antepartum admission for a maternal cardiac indication was less common than admission for an obstetric reason such as preterm labor. Patients with intracardiac shunt physiology or conotruncal defects were at greatest risk. Obstetric complications developed in 45% of pregnancies and included preterm birth, fetal demise, growth restriction, and neonatal intensive care unit (NICU) admission [13].

Considering the patient's prior history of cardiac events and evaluation of functional status is important for accurate counseling regarding maternal and fetal risks. However, coronary artery disease, pulmonary hypertension, endocarditis, cardiomyopathy, and arrhythmias hold the greatest risk for maternal mortality [14].

Risk of fetal cardiac abnormalities

Patients with congenital cardiac abnormalities should also be counseled regarding the increased risk of fetal structural cardiac anomalies, which is estimated to be between 8.8% and 14.2%, versus the general population's risk of 0.08% of live births [15]. Paternal cardiac abnormalities also increase the risk of congenital cardiac disease; however, maternal disease poses the greatest risk by a factor of 3.5. Patients with aortic stenosis and ventricular septal defect appear to be at greatest risk for transmission; however, the lesion which develops may differ from that of the parent [16,17]. Therefore, fetal echocardiography is recommended for all patients with a congenital cardiac abnormality. Table 17.4 [18] outlines the risks of congenital cardiac disease by maternal disorder.

Valvular heart disease

Acquired valvular lesions are typically sequelae of rheumatic fever, yet valvular endocarditis secondary to

intravenous drug use is not uncommon. During pregnancy, most morbidity and mortality from these lesions is associated with dysrhythmias and congestive failure. The degree of risk for these complications depends on the specific lesion, number of valves involved, and the degree of valvular obstruction, particularly of the mitral and aortic valves. However, pregnancy does not appear to adversely affect long-term sequelae for women with rheumatic heart disease who survive the pregnancy. The American Heart Association 2007 recommendations do not recommend systemic bacterial endocarditis (SBE) prevention for vaginal delivery nor cesarean delivery unless infection is present, in which case the underlying infection should be treated [19]. If the cardiac condition is deemed severe enough, as listed in Box 17.4, then SBE therapy should be initiated. Box 17.5 [19] outlines the current antibiotic regimens for prevention of SBE in pregnant patients. Each valvular lesion will be addressed in the sections that follow. Table 17.5 [20] presents a summary of relative maternal and fetal risks in patients with valvular abnormalities.

Box 17.4 Cardiac lesions requiring SBE prophylaxis when delivery is associated with infection, based on the American Heart Association (AHA) and American College of Cardiology (ACC) Task Force recommendations

- Prosthetic cardiac valve or prosthetic material used for valve repair
- History of infective endocarditis
- Congenital heart diseases (CHD) listed below:
  - Unrepaired cyanotic CHD (includes palliative shunts, conduits)
  - Completely repaired CHD with prosthetic materials if repair <6 months old
  - Repaired CHD with residual defects

SBE, systemic bacterial endocarditis.
Source: American College of Obstetricians and Gynecologists [19].

Box 17.5 American College of Obstetricians and Gynecologists recommendations for antibiotic regimens for bacterial endocarditis

Regimen (administered 30–60 min prior to procedure)

- Ampicillin 2 g IV
- Cefazolin 1 g IV*
- Ceftriazone 1 g IV*
- Clindamycin 600 mg IV*
- Amoxicillin 2 g PO

*Does not cover enterococcus; for coverage vancomycin should be used.
IV, intravenous; PO, per os.
Source: American College of Obstetricians and Gynecologists [19].

Table 17.4 Risk of fetal congenital cardiac defects (%)

Cardiac lesion	Prior affected sibling	Father affected	Mother affected
Tetralogy of Fallot	2.5	1.5	2.6
Aortic coarctation			14.1
Atrial septal defect	2.5	1.5	4.6–11
Ventricular septal defect	3	2	90.5–15.6
Pulmonary stenosis	2	2	6.5
Aortic stenosis	2	3	15–17.9

Source: Lupton *et al* [18].

Table 17.5 Classification of valvular heart lesions according to maternal and fetal risks

Low maternal and/or fetal risks	High maternal and/or fetal risks
Asymptomatic AS with a low mean outflow gradient and normal LV systolic function (EF >50%)	Severe AS with or without symptoms NYHA III-IV and AR
NYHA I or II AR and normal LV systolic function	NYHA II-IV and MS
NYHA I or II MR and normal LV systolic function	NYHA III-IV and MR
MVP with no MR (if mild to moderate MR normal LV systolic function)	Marfan syndrome with or without AR
Mild MS without pulmonary hypertension	Aortic and/or mitral disease with pulmonary hypertension or LV systolic dysfunction (EF <40%)
Mild to moderate pulmonary stenosis	Mechanical prosthetic valve requiring anticoagulation

AR, aortic regurgitation; AS, aortic stenosis; EF, ejection fraction; LV, left ventricle; MR, mitral regurgitation; MS, mitral stenosis; MVP, mitral valve prolapse; NYHA, New York Heart Association. Adapted from ACC/AHA 2006 valvular guidelines [20].

Mitral stenosis

As mentioned above, rheumatic heart disease accounts for the majority of mitral valve disease. In fact, mitral stenosis is the most common rheumatic valvular lesion encountered in pregnancy [21]. The normal mitral valve area is 4–5 cm². As the mitral valve orifice narrows, filling of the left ventricle during diastole becomes progressively limited and cardiac output becomes fixed. The nonpregnant patient remains asymptomatic until the valve area falls below 2 cm². Moderate mitral stenosis is defined as a valve area measuring between 1 and 1.5 cm²; less than 1 cm² valve area defines severe mitral stenosis [22]. Patients with moderate-to-severe limitations of the valve area may not tolerate the normal pregnancy increases in cardiac output, blood volume, and heart rate, and they should ideally have the valve repaired prior to pregnancy. Patients who remain symptomatic despite conservative management may be candidates for surgical intervention during pregnancy. Case reports of over 100 women suggest that percutaneous balloon mitral valvuloplasty is a safe and effective procedure during pregnancy [23–25]. Mitral stenosis may be undiagnosed prior to pregnancy, becoming apparent only when challenged by normal physiologic changes of pregnancy. These patients may present with atrial fibrillation and/or pulmonary edema.

In a series of 80 pregnancies complicated by mitral stenosis, 38% of patients with moderate mitral stenosis

(valve area less than 1.5 cm²) and 67% of patients with severe mitral stenosis (valve area less than 1 cm²) experienced a cardiac event. Even patients with mild stenosis experienced complications in 11% of cases. The most common maternal complications were pulmonary edema and arrhythmias, primarily atrial fibrillation and supraventricular tachycardia. A history of prior cardiac events and moderate or severe stenosis were the strongest independent predictors of maternal complications. Sixty percent of patients experienced an initial episode of pulmonary edema during the antepartum period (mean gestational age of 30 weeks), and the most common neonatal complication was prematurity [26].

Management of patients with mitral stenosis should focus on prevention of tachycardia and maintenance of left ventricular filling (preload). As the heart rate increases, less time is allowed for the left atrium to adequately empty and fill the left ventricle during diastole. As a result, the left atrium may become overdistended, resulting in dysrhythmias (primarily atrial fibrillation, which increases the risk of thromboembolic complications), pulmonary edema, or both. Tachycardia is likely to develop as a result of pain, exertion, or anxiety or after administration of β-agonists such as terbutaline. Cardiac output can fall dramatically and lead to hypotension and/or sudden onset of pulmonary edema. Tachycardia can be avoided by aggressive pain management and avoidance of exertion during labor. Some patients may require therapy with β-blockers to maintain a heart rate below 90–100 beats/min. During labor, short-acting intravenous β-blockers, such as esmolol, are recommended in place of longer acting oral agents.

The second major consideration for patients with mitral valve stenosis is maintaining left ventricular filling (adequate preload). Overcoming the obstruction to left ventricular filling depends on high fluid volumes to maintain forward flow. Therefore, diuretics should be used cautiously to avoid inadvertent decreases in left ventricular filling and therefore decreases in cardiac output. Unlike in aortic stenosis, the utility of pulmonary artery catheterization to monitor left ventricular preload is limited, as pulmonary capillary wedge pressure may reflect a false increase in mean wedge pressure in the setting of mitral stenosis. Epidural anesthetic use is appropriate during labor to minimize tachycardia caused by pain or anxiety and therefore control fluctuations in cardiac output. Care should be taken to avoid sudden decreases in preload caused by abrupt sympathetic blockade from local anesthetics. Often intrathecal opioids are used, or an epidural will contain higher doses of opioids and lower concentrations of local anesthetics.

Medical management of the pregnant patient with mitral stenosis involves avoiding tachycardia with activity restriction or β-blockers, appropriate treatment of dysrhythmias if present, and careful diuretic use. The section on arrhythmias below addresses anticoagulation issues in patients with atrial fibrillation.

Pulmonic and tricuspid lesions

Pulmonary valve stenosis is a congenital lesion which, along with tricuspid valvular lesions, is more commonly caused by valvular endocarditis from intravenous drug use than by rheumatic heart disease in the adult population. The physiologic changes of pregnancy are tolerated well by patients with pulmonic or tricuspid valvular abnormalities. Patients with severe pulmonic obstruction (transvalvular pressure peak gradient exceeding 60 mmHg) are at highest risk for complications such as right heart failure. If symptomatic, pregnant women may be candidates for percutaneous valvuloplasty. Overall, most series indicate that maternal and fetal risks are minimal [27].

Mitral and aortic regurgitation

Mitral regurgitation is most commonly seen secondary to mitral valve prolapse in pregnant women [22] whereas aortic regurgitation is usually rheumatic in origin. The increased heart rate and decreased systemic vascular resistance that occur normally in pregnancy favor forward flow of blood; therefore both lesions are tolerated quite well in pregnancy. Patients with long-standing mitral or aortic insufficiency may have left ventricular dysfunction resulting from chronic ventricular dilation and thus are at increased risk for complications [28]. The decreased systemic vascular resistance that occurs following epidural placement is generally not problematic, but epidural placement should be undertaken with caution as one death has been reported [29]. Chronic mitral regurgitation may also lead to significant left atrial enlargement, which increases the risk for the development of atrial fibrillation. If this occurs, antiarrhythmic therapy is indicated and anticoagulation should be considered.

Mitral valve prolapse

Mitral valve prolapse is present in up to 3% of the general population but may be present in up to 17% of young women, making it one of the most common cardiac issues during pregnancy [30]. Because most women are asymptomatic, the diagnosis is generally made incidentally. The increased blood volume and decreased systemic vascular resistance of pregnancy improve the mitral valve function, so patients can be expected to tolerate pregnancy well. Occasionally palpitations will prompt therapy, usually with β-blockers. The incidence of antepartum and postpartum complications is no different from the general population, so no special precautions need to be taken during pregnancy or labor and delivery. Antibiotic prophylaxis for systemic bacterial endocarditis is not recommended for mitral valve prolapse [19].

Aortic stenosis

Aortic stenosis (AS) can develop as a consequence of rheumatic fever, in which case it usually involves other valvular abnormalities. However, congenital aortic stenosis is not uncommon, and when identified in younger patients, it is usually associated with a bicuspid aortic valve [22]. The hypervolemia and increased cardiac output of pregnancy are well tolerated by patients with mild disease (valve area > 1.5 cm^2, peak pressure gradient < 50 mmHg). However, as the orifice becomes progressively more stenotic, flow across the valve becomes progressively limited and the velocity of flow increases. This resistance serves as an impediment to increasing cardiac output but is not considered hemodynamically significant until the valve opening is decreased to one-quarter the normal diameter of 3–4 cm^2. These patients may be unable to maintain coronary or cerebral perfusion and can develop angina, myocardial infarction, syncope, or sudden death. A recent literature review of pregnant women greater than 20 weeks' gestation with congenital AS, repaired or unrepaired, reported the following maternal complications: arrhythmias, heart failure, and cardiovascular events such as myocardial infarction, stroke, and mortality from cardiovascular disease [31]. Patients with valve areas of less than 1 cm^2, mean gradients exceeding 40 mmHg, or ejection fractions below 40% have severe disease and should be evaluated for surgical correction, preferably prior to conception [22].

Complications arise in pregnant patients with AS primarily as a result of the inability to maintain cardiac output. The typical 40–50% increase in cardiac output is unlikely to result in pulmonary edema unless mitral valve disease co-exists. Labor and delivery or pregnancy termination is a particularly risky time. Pulmonary edema can result from the inability to increase cardiac output in response to increasing physical demands of delivery or termination. For this reason, judicious use of intravenous fluids is recommended. Any factor leading to diminished venous return (preload) will cause an increase in the valvular gradient, difficulty overcoming the obstruction, and ultimately diminished cardiac output. Diminished venous return may result from many common obstetric anesthetic complications including hypotension from blood loss or intravascular volume depletion, ganglionic blockade from regional anesthesia, or supine vena caval occlusion by the pregnant uterus. Exertion may place additional demands on cardiac output and may lead to coronary artery ischemia or inadequate cerebral perfusion which will manifest as angina, myocardial infarction, syncope, or sudden death. Limitation of physical activity is recommended for patients with severe disease. Because hypovolemia and decreased venous return present much higher risks for life-threatening complications to the patient than pulmonary edema, pulmonary artery catheterization may be indicated in patients with significant

AS to estimate intravascular volume accurately, and to maintain pulmonary artery wedge pressures mildly elevated in the range of 15–17 mmHg.

The risk of death in pregnant patients with AS has been reported to be as high as 17%. Fortunately, more recent data indicate that patients with AS, but without coronary artery disease, who receive adequate care have a minimal risk of dying [27]. In a series of 49 pregnancies complicated by congenital AS, cardiac complications occurred in 6% with severe disease, including one patient who required percutaneous valvuloplasty at 12 weeks' gestation. Prematurity and birth of SGA babies complicated 10% of pregnancies. Fifty percent of patients with severe AS required cardiac surgery in the first 4 years after delivery; however, it remains unclear whether the pregnancy intensified the need for surgical intervention [32]. In a series of 1000 pregnant women with cardiac disease, by contrast, 65% of those with moderate or severe AS experienced cardiac complications, including one maternal death [33]. In pregnant women with AS, severe AS (as defined above), with or without symptoms, and an ejection fraction less than 40% are the two greatest risk factors for maternal and/or fetal risk [22].

Mechanical heart valves

All patients with mechanical heart valves require life-long anticoagulation to decrease the risk of thromboembolic complications. In the nonpregnant population, warfarin is the recommended agent, with the therapeutic goal being to maintain an international normalized ratio (INR) between 2.0 and 3.5, depending on the type and location of the valve. Patients with biologic valves do not require anticoagulation beyond the initial 3 months post replacement unless they also have additional risk factors for thromboembolic disease, such as atrial fibrillation [22].

Recommendations for anticoagulation in pregnant women with mechanical heart valves are among the most controversial and challenging problems in obstetrics. The overall risk of maternal death reported in a 2000 meta-analysis of mothers treated with oral, subcutaneous, or a combination of the two anticoagulation therapies throughout pregnancy was 2.9% [34]. The three currently available medications are warfarin, unfractionated heparin (UFH), and low molecular weight heparin (LMWH). Warfarin crosses the placenta and can result in fetal malformations, including an embryopathy consisting of nasal/limb hypoplasia and epiphyseal stippling. The risk of anomalies appears to be greatest when exposure occurs between 6 and 12 weeks' gestation. Intracranial hemorrhage is also a concern if warfarin is taken during the second and third trimesters and is postulated to be the cause of rare central nervous abnormalities [35]. Spontaneous abortion rates and pregnancy loss rates are more common if warfarin is taken during the pregnancy and are highest (21% and 30%, respectively) if warfarin is taken in the first trimester and continued throughout gestation [34].

While warfarin is not effective at preventing all thromboembolic complications in pregnant patients with mechanical heart valves, studies with older generation heart valves have shown a lower risk of thromboembolic events when warfarin is used compared to addition of UFH use in the first trimester (3.9% versus 9.2%). Adjusted-dose UFH without warfarin use is associated with an even greater risk of maternal adverse outcomes: 25% risk of thromboembolic events and 6.7% risk of death [34]. Even when high-dose UFH is used in the first trimester, thromboembolic events remained higher in the UFH group (5% compared to 0.3%) [35].

Low molecular weight heparin is a third alternative for anticoagulation which, like UFH, does not cross the placenta. Advantages of using LMWH include potentially lower risk for osteoporosis, decreased risk of heparin-induced thrombocytopenia, and longer half-life [36]. In 2002 the manufacturer of one LMWH, Lovenox (enoxaparin sodium), issued a warning statement against the use of Lovenox for thromboprophylaxis in pregnant patients with prosthetic valves [37]. This statement was issued after two maternal and fetal deaths occurred in patients receiving Lovenox, 80 mg, twice daily as part of a clinical research trial. According to a recent review article, anti-Xa levels were monitored but not used to adjust dosage; the authors suggest that insufficient Lovenox dosing may have contributed to thromboses [38].

The ability to judge the effectiveness of UFH and LMWH at preventing thromboembolic phenomena is complicated by altered pharmacodynamics of these medications in the pregnant patient as a result of increased volume of distribution and alterations in the coagulation cascade [39]. These data suggest that monitoring of anticoagulant effect of UFH and LMWH should be accomplished with peak and/or trough anti-Xa measurements instead of utilizing the activated partial thromboplastin time (for UFH) or weight-based regimens (for LMWH).

In 2008, a focused update of the American College of Cardiology/American Heart Association Task Force on Practice Guidelines through the Committee on Management of Patients with Valvular Heart Disease addressed recommendations for the management of anticoagulation in pregnant patients with mechanical heart valves, as summarized in Box 17.6 [22]. It is imperative that patients with mechanical heart valves are restarted on their anticoagulation therapy approximately 4–6 h after delivery. If urgent cesarean delivery is necessary in a patient on anticoagulation, one must compare the risk of hemorrhage to that of thromboembolism. In doing so, it is important to know if the patient is therapeutically anticoagulated and decide if reversal of anticoagulation

Box 17.6 American Heart Association (AHA) and American College of Cardiology (ACC) recommendations for the management of anticoagulation in pregnant women with mechanical valve prostheses

First trimester

- Dose-adjusted LMWH or UFH

12–36 weeks

- Warfarin (goal INR 2.5–3.5)
- Continuous IV UFH
- Dose-adjusted SQ UFH (goal of APTT at least twice control)
- Dose-adjusted SQ LMWH (twice daily to keep anti-Xa between 0.7 and 1.2 U/mL 4 h after administration)

At 36 weeks

- If on warfarin, change to dose-adjusted LMWH or UFH

Prior to delivery

- If on LMWH and planning IOL, change to IV UFH at least 36 h prior to IOL
- UFH should be stopped 4–6 h prior to delivery

Postpartum

- UFH and LMWH can be restarted 4–6 h after delivery
- Warfarin can be restarted the same day

APTT, activated partial thromboplastin time; INR, international normalized ratio; IOL, induction of labor; IV, intravenous; LMWH, low molecular weight heparin; SQ, subcutaneous; UFH, unfractionated heparin.
Adpated from Bonow *et al* [22].

Box 17.7 Management of anticoagulated patients in need of urgent delivery

General recommendations

- Full reversal of anticoagulation is not necessary for either vaginal or cesarean delivery
- Partial reversal may be indicated (target INR of approximately 2.0) if the patient is supratherapeutic
- Full reversal is warranted in patients with life-threatening maternal hemorrhage

If patient on UFH or LMWH

- If time allows, discontinue therapy and delay delivery 4–6 h without protamine
- Vaginal delivery is preferred unless there are obstetric indications for cesarean delivery
- Consider protamine for emergency delivery (will only partially reverse the anticoagulant effects of LMWH)

If patient on warfarin with an elevated INR (therapeutic/ supratherapeutic) at the time of an urgent delivery

- Prefer cesarean delivery to reduce risks of fetal trauma/hemorrhage as fetus is also therapeutically anticoagulated
- If time allows, delay and/or administer small doses of vitamin K with goal INR of 2.0
- Administer FFP prior to emergency cesarean delivery to reach a target INR of 2.0
- If anticoagulation fully reversed at time of delivery, newborn may receive FFP and vitamin K

FFP, fresh frozen plasma; INR, international normalized ratio; LMWH, low molecular weight heparin; UFH, unfractionated heparin.
Adapted from Butchart *et al* [40].

is necessary [40]. Box 17.7 reviews management of anti-coagulated patients requiring urgent delivery.

Heparin resistance, defined as the need for greater than 35,000 units of heparin in a 24 h time period to reach a therapeutic partial thromboplastin time (PTT) value, is attributable to pregnancy-induced changes in the coagulation cascade, specifically elevation of factor VIII [39]. Therefore, anti-Xa is often used in pregnancy to monitor anticoagulation status because it is less affected by physiologic alterations of maternal clotting factors in gestation. The appropriate interval for checking anti-Xa levels is not known, but a review of expert opinion [38] recommended weekly anti-Xa levels during the first month of therapy to maintain anti-Xa between 0.5 and 1.0 units/mL. This range is generally accepted when LMWH is being used, with an anti-Xa range for the use of heparin being between 0.3 and 0.7 units/mL [41]. Of relevance to dosing, UFH made in the United States after 2009 is 10% less potent than before, given new reference standards [42]. Ultimately, the decision regarding an anticoagulation

regimen should be made after detailed discussion with the patient regarding the risks and benefits of each regimen to both the patient and the fetus.

Careful consideration of the timing of neuraxial needle placement for anesthesia purposes is important in the anticoagulated pregnant patient. With regard to the heparinized patient, it is recommended to stop UFH 4 h prior to insertion/removal of a neuraxial needle. Once the needle has been placed or removed, wait at least 1 h prior to the next dose of UFH. Patients on LMWH should receive their last dose 12 h prior to needle insertion if they are prophylactically dosed versus 24 h if they are therapeutically dosed. With either form of LMWH dosing, once neuraxial needle placement or removal has been performed, one should wait a minimum of 4 h before resuming the LMWH [43]. When using LMWH for postoperative thromboprophylaxis, it is recommended to wait at least 24 h postoperatively to administer the first dose if the patient will be dosed twice a day versus 6–8 h postoperatively if she will be dosed once a day. It is recommended that any indwelling catheter be removed in these patients prior to starting LMWH. However, if the catheter is maintained, the first dose of LMWH should be delayed until 2h after catheter removal. Although the anti-Xa level can be used to monitor anticoagulation status, it does not predict the risk of bleeding for patients receiving neuraxial needle placement [44].

Congenital cardiac abnormalities

Aortic coarctation

Aortic coarctation is a narrowing of the caliber of the aorta, usually distal to the left subclavian artery, which occurs in 6–8% of patients with congenital heart disease [45]. The presence of a significant blood pressure gradient between the upper and lower extremities (>20 mmHg) usually prompts evaluation for repair, which is accomplished surgically or with balloon angioplasty. Long-term survival following repair of aortic coarctation is quite good; however, the risks of recoarctation, aortic aneurysm, dissection, and rupture persist. Occasionally, patients will remain undiagnosed into adulthood (native coarctation).

While early reports of pregnancy in women with coarctation indicated mortality rates of 9.5%, more recent data suggest that pregnancy in women with a corrected or native coarctation is likely to be more successful [46]. Associated cardiac defects commonly co-exist with coarctation and may include bicuspid aortic valve, congenital aortic valvular stenosis, septal defects, and patent ductus arteriosus [47]. Intracranial aneurysms also occur with greater frequency in patients with aortic coarctation, compared with the general population (10% versus 2%). Preeclampsia is reported to complicate 2–22% of pregnancies in patients with coarctation [47,48].

In a large series studying pregnancy following coarctation repair, 98 pregnancies in 54 women ended in live birth without significant maternal complications. The cesarean delivery rate was 6%, with only one cesarean performed for a perceived maternal cardiovascular risk. Data on arm–leg blood pressure gradients or echocardiographic measurements were not available. Interestingly, the median gestational age at delivery was 40 weeks [47]. In a series of 118 pregnancies in women with repaired and native coarctation, one maternal death (patient with Turner syndrome who conceived twins through *in vitro* fertilization) resulting from aortic dissection was reported [49]. During pregnancy this patient had no evidence of hypertension, but expired suddenly at 36 weeks' gestation from an acute aortic dissection at a site apart from the previous repair. The remaining patients tolerated pregnancy well with good neonatal outcomes. Patients with significant coarctation were more likely to be hypertensive during pregnancy compared to those without

significant coarctation (58% versus 11%). The presence of hypertension in this group strongly suggested the presence of a significant coarctation. Delivery was accomplished by cesarean section in 36% of patients, primarily for perceived maternal cardiovascular risk. No difference was seen in maternal and neonatal outcomes between patients with repaired versus native coarctation in this cohort.

Concerns about the risk of aortic or intracranial aneurysm rupture and aortic dissection have prompted some physicians to recommend elective cesarean delivery. Coarctation of the aorta is associated with inherent abnormalities of the aorta which predispose patients to rupture, dilation, and dissection [50]. Other risk factors for rupture or dissection include Turner syndrome, bicuspid aortic valve, and aortic dilation [51]. Most patients will be able to have a successful vaginal delivery with careful management of pain using epidural anesthesia, control of blood pressure fluctuations, maintenance of adequate cardiac preload, and minimization of Valsalva efforts at delivery.

Ventricular septal defect

Although isolated ventricular septal defects (VSDs) account for approximately 15–20% of congenital cardiac abnormalities, most will close spontaneously in the first 2 years of life, making it an uncommonly encountered lesion in the pregnant patient [52]. Moderate to large-sized defects that remain patent or persist to adulthood may result in secondary pulmonary hypertension or congestive heart failure. Although blood flow across the shunt is usually left to right, reversal may occur and result in Eisenmenger syndrome, which is addressed in a later section. Isolated VSDs and corrected VSDs do not appear to increase the risk of adverse outcomes during pregnancy. However, echocardiography should be considered in a patient with a history of a VSD, repaired or unrepaired, to exclude underlying pulmonary hypertension which would substantially increase the risk of life-threatening complications [53].

Atrial septal defect

Atrial septal defects (ASDs) do not appear to pose substantial risk to the pregnant patient and are usually well tolerated [54]. Even if the defect is not repaired, complications such as arrhythmias and pulmonary hypertension generally do not occur during the child-bearing years [55]. Paradoxical embolism, presenting as a stroke, has been described during pregnancy and is possible in any patient with an intracardiac shunt [56].

Patent ductus arteriosus

Patent ductus arteriosus (PDA) is a commonly encountered lesion in neonates, particularly preterm neonates. PDA is generally repaired in childhood and is, therefore, very unusual during pregnancy. Pregnancy outcome following repair does not appear to be negatively affected [57]. However, patients with large unrepaired PDAs may develop secondary pulmonary hypertension, not unlike Eisenmenger syndrome.

Eisenmenger syndrome

Unrepaired congenital intracardiac shunts such as a VSD, ASD, or PDA lead to chronic overperfusion of the pulmonary vasculature. Over time, pulmonary hypertension results and may become significant enough to reverse the direction of flow across the shunt. This reversal of shunt flow to a right-to-left direction defines Eisenmenger syndrome. Correction of the septal defect or patent ductus before the development of pulmonary hypertension prevents the syndrome. Once the syndrome is established, the only surgical option is a heart-lung transplantation. Thirty-two percent of heart-lung transplants are performed for pulmonary hypertension secondary to congenital cardiac defects, making it the leading indication for this type of surgery [58].

Death is usually due to worsening hypoxia as a result of physiologic changes induced by pregnancy. For example, increased blood volume and lower right ventricular filling pressures that result from decreased systemic vascular resistance place increased demands on the right ventricle and may precipitate right heart failure if there is inability to overcome the elevated pulmonary pressures. Also, decreased systemic vascular resistance in pregnancy lowers the peripheral resistance relative to the pulmonary resistance, increasing the likelihood of shunt reversal and worsening hypoxia and cyanosis. Hypoxia, in turn, leads to pulmonary vasoconstriction and further increases in pulmonary artery pressures. The thrombophilic state induced by pregnancy also predisposes patients to thromboembolic phenomena, another common cause of death in Eisenmenger syndrome.

Although Eisenmenger syndrome may be a common cause of pulmonary hypertension in young women, it remains a rare complication of pregnancy. Therefore, data regarding outcomes, optimal route of delivery, and anesthetic risks are limited. The maternal mortality rate in Eisenmenger syndrome is estimated at 30–50%. In the most recent review, of 73 patients with pulmonary arterial hypertension from 1997 to 2007, overall mortality was 25% [59], a decrease from 38% mortality in a systematic review of similar patients from 1978 to 1996 [60]. Furthermore, a decrease in mortality for women with congenital heart disease associated pulmonary arterial hypertension was noted (36% versus 28%). Of the 18 patients who died, 83% died in the postpartum period, with the majority of deaths being within the first 6 days postpartum. Patients diagnosed or admitted to the hospital at later gestational ages were at much greater risk of death. Other factors historically associated with increased mortality include operative delivery and severe pulmonary hypertension. In both large series, the route of delivery did not appear to affect mortality rates.

Because of high maternal mortality rates, patients with Eisenmenger syndrome should be counseled to avoid pregnancy, and if pregnant, to consider termination. In ongoing pregnancies, therapies should be directed at minimizing cardiac demands, maximizing oxygenation, and avoiding excessive declines in systemic vascular resistance. Patients should be hospitalized at the end of the second trimester, prophylactically anticoagulated, and given supplemental oxygen. More recently, studies have utilized selective pulmonary artery vasodilators such as inhaled nitric oxide and IV epoprostenol (prostacyclin) during pregnancy with favorable results. Regional anesthetics must be used cautiously to avoid decreases in systemic vascular resistance and ventricular filling that may precipitate reversal of shunt flow and cyanosis. However, studies suggest that the cautious use of slow-onset epidural anesthetics may be associated with lower mortality rates than general anesthesia for cesarean section delivery [59].

In a recent retrospective review, nine patients with pulmonary hypertension all received epidural or combined spinal and epidural for anesthesia without complication [61]. This method of anesthesia was chosen given the adverse effects of intubation on positive pressure ventilation as well as pulmonary artery pressure. Avoidance of hypotensive events at any time during gestation, particularly during labor and delivery, is extremely important.

Accurate assessment of pulmonary artery pressure may be a challenge in many patients. Echocardiographic assessment of pulmonary artery pressures has been shown to be less accurate in the pregnant patient and pulmonary artery catheters have been associated with higher complication rates in the setting of Eisenmenger syndrome [62].

Ebstein anomaly

Ebstein anomaly is a congenital cardiac defect characterized by an apical displacement of the septal leaflet of the tricuspid valve. Tricuspid regurgitation is always present, leading to right atrial dilation. Right outflow tract obstruction can occur secondary to a fixed anterior leaflet of the tricuspid valve. ASD or patent foramen ovale co-exists in 50% of cases. Twenty-five percent will have an accessory conduction pathway such as Wolff–Parkinson–White syndrome [63]. Because it accounts for only 1% of all congenital cardiac disease, Ebstein anomaly is uncommonly encountered during pregnancy. Pregnancy appears to be well tolerated in patients with this lesion. In a series of 44 patients with 111 pregnancies, the live birth rate was 76% with no maternal complications reported [64]. In the neonates, prematurity (21%) and congenital cardiac abnormalities (6%) were noted.

Transposition of the great vessels

Complete transposition of the great vessels (TOGV) is uncommon in pregnant women. If it is uncorrected at birth, mortality rates approach 90% in the first year of life. Long-term survival rates are also diminished, with a reported 70–80% survival at 20–30 years post repair [65]. The most common corrective procedure for complete TOGV performed on patients of child-bearing age is the atrial switch (Mustard) procedure, in which blood is surgically redirected through the atria [63]. Right ventricular dysfunction and dysrhythmias such as atrial flutter are commonly encountered in patients who survive into adulthood. The most significant issue reported in a recent series of 28 pregnancies in 16 women with a prior Mustard operation was irreversible right ventricular dysfunction despite the fact that pregnancy itself was tolerated well [66] .

Tetralogy of Fallot

Tetralogy of Fallot refers to the cyanotic complex of VSD, over-riding aorta, right ventricular hypertrophy, and pulmonary stenosis. Most patients with tetralogy of Fallot undergo surgical correction in infancy and can expect excellent long-term survival rates [67]. Twenty years after surgical correction, approximately 10–15% will develop significant complications, including pulmonary insufficiency, which lead to right-sided heart failure and arrhythmias [68].

Most series report no adverse maternal events in pregnancy following surgical correction; however, in a recent literature review of 222 pregnant patients with tetralogy of Fallot, arrhythmia and heart failure were seen in 6.4% and 2.4% of patients, respectively [31]. Those patients with severe pulmonary regurgitation appear to be at greatest risk for these complications.

Marfan syndrome

Marfan syndrome is an inherited connective tissue disorder of autosomal dominant transmission which leads to defective fibrillin, an important component of all connective tissues. Therefore, patients have a 50% chance of passing the disorder to their children. The defective fibrillin results in cardiovascular, ocular, and musculoskeletal abnormalities, with 80% of patients having adverse cardiac effects [69]. Classic Marfan syndrome is estimated to occur in 4–6 per 100,000 people. Patients with Marfan syndrome have a shortened life expectancy (mean of 32 years if untreated), and more than 90% succumb to cardiac complications such as aortic dissection or rupture [70]. The weakened aortic media allows for progressive aortic dilation, which predisposes the individual to aortic rupture. The hemodynamic changes of pregnancy place additional stress on the dilated, weakened aorta, thereby increasing the risk of rupture.

Four population-based studies have been published which include a total of 107 women followed through 274 pregnancies [71–74]. The overall live birth rate was 80%, with 3.3% of patients experiencing an aortic dissection. One percent of patients died as a result of dissection. The degree of aortic dilation appears to correlate directly with risk for aortic dissection and rupture. Patients with an aortic root diameter more than 4.5 cm appear to be at greatest risk for aortic dissection and rupture. However, the exact threshold at which pregnancy termination should be advised is unclear. European and recently updated American College of Cardiology/American Heart Association guidelines recommend discouraging pregnancy if the aortic root is ≥4.0 cm whereas the Canadian guidelines recommend ≥4.5 cm as the threshold [22]. Elective valve replacement should be considered for patients with an aortic root diameter ≥4.7 cm, and updated 2010 guidelines state that prophylactic replacement is warranted if the patient is considering pregnancy [75].

It is important to assess the aortic root diameter preconception, if possible, to provide the patient with information regarding pregnancy risks. Echocardiography should be performed monthly or bimonthly to assess for worsening aortic dilation [75]. β-Blockers have been shown to improve long-term outcomes and should be continued throughout gestation [76]. Vaginal delivery is acceptable in patients with an aortic root < 4.0 cm and no signs of heart failure if pain is adequately managed with epidural anesthesia and Valsalva maneuvers are avoided. Cesarean delivery has been recommended in patients with severe aortic regurgitation, aortic distension, or an aortic root ≥ 4.0 cm [75].

Peripartum cardiomyopathy

Peripartum cardiomyopathy (PPCM) is defined as the development of heart failure in the last month of pregnancy or within 5 months of delivery, in the absence of an identifiable cause or preexisting heart disease. Additional criteria for diagnosing PPCM include evidence of left ventricular systolic dysfunction, as demonstrated by classic echocardiographic criteria: ejection fraction less than 45%, shortening fraction less than 30%, and left ventricular end-diastolic dimension more than 2.7 cm/m^2 body surface area [77]. Box 17.8 summarizes these diagnostic criteria.

The exact incidence of PPCM remains unknown; fortunately, it is relatively rare, occurring in only 1 in 5000 births [77]. Mortality rates have been reported to be as high as 56%; however, more recent studies suggest that mortality rates may be closer to 9% [78,79]. Despite this, PPCM accounts for 8% of all maternal deaths and is one of the few causes of maternal mortality that is rising [78]. Forty-eight percent of patients who succumb to PPCM will die in the first 6 weeks postpartum. Fifty percent of PPCM deaths occur in the ensuing year.

Classic risk factors for PPCM include multiparity, advanced maternal age, multifetal gestation (fourfold increased risk), preeclampsia, hypertension, and African descent (sixfold increased risk) [80]. The etiology of peripartum cardiomyopathy has not been determined, but the most current evidence suggests viral myocarditis. One study reported endomyocardial biopsies consistent with myocarditis in 76% of patients [81]. Evidence of autoantibodies against cardiac tissue proteins in patients with PPCM also supports a role for an autoimmune phenomenon.

Once PPCM is diagnosed, management is focused on reducing cardiac preload with diuretics (furosemide), reducing cardiac afterload with vasodilators (hydralazine, nitroglycerin, nitroprusside), and improving cardiac contractility with inotropic agents (dobutamine, digoxin). Diuresis should be undertaken cautiously in patients who are still pregnant at the time of diagnosis. Overaggressive fluid loss may result in decreased uterine perfusion and fetal compromise. Afterload reduction decreases the pressure against which the heart pumps and improves cardiac output. Stimulating cardiac output with inotropic agents is often necessary and will also improve uterine perfusion. Dobutamine, a selective β1-agonist and inotropic vasodilator, offers the advantage of selectively decreasing systemic vascular resistance but is primarily used as short-term therapy. Digoxin is useful for prolonged inotropic support but may require significantly higher doses and more frequent dosing intervals in pregnant patients. Dysrhythmias such as atrial fibrillation may occur as cardiac chamber distension worsens. Angiotensin-converting enzyme (ACE) inhibitors and angiotensin

receptor blockers (ARBs) are a standard part of heart failure management in nonpregnant patients but should be avoided in pregnant women. β-Blockers reduce myocardial oxygen requirements and may also be used if cardiac output does not improve satisfactorily with preload and afterload reduction.

Anticoagulation with UFH or LMWH should be considered to prevent thromboembolic events, especially in patients with dysrhythmias or markedly depressed ejection fractions. Warfarin may be used in postpartum patients and is compatible with breastfeeding. The risk of thrombus formation increases as the severity of ventricular dilation increases. Figure 17.3 outlines the approach to the patient with PPCM.

For pregnant patients diagnosed with PPCM, delivery poses particular concerns. In general, there is no evidence to suggest that cesarean delivery is beneficial, and it should be reserved for the usual obstetric indications. With careful monitoring, regional anesthesia is acceptable in patients with PPCM and is important for controlling pain, minimizing maternal effort, and reducing cardiac workload. An assisted second stage should be considered if contractions are insufficient to deliver the fetus without maternal pushing efforts. In the immediate postpartum period, decompensation may occur as third-space fluid reenters the intravascular space.

The prognosis for patients with PPCM is poor if left ventricular function does not normalize within 6 months of delivery. In this group, mortality rates approach 85% by 5 years [82]. Death usually results from dysrhythmias, thromboembolic phenomena, or progressive heart failure. Recent studies suggest that recovery of left ventricular function can be expected in 41–54% of patients [79]. However, predicting which patients are most likely to experience recovery has been challenging. Normalization of left ventricular function is significantly more likely in patients with an initial ejection fraction greater than 30% [79]. Other markers of ventricular size and function at initial diagnosis may also identify those less likely to recover.

Recurrent PPCM has been well described, even in patients whose left ventricular function has apparently returned to normal. This may be due to deficient contractile reserve, which may be demonstrated in response to a dobutamine challenge [83]. One author reported no adverse events in four pregnancies in patients with a history of PPCM [84]. In contrast, Elkayam *et al* [85] detailed outcomes in 35 ongoing pregnancies in women with a history of PPCM. Even in patients with apparently normal cardiac function at the onset as measured by an ejection fraction more than 50%, cardiac symptoms occurred in 6%, and 17% exhibited deteriorating cardiac function during gestation. Deterioration persisted after delivery in 9%, but no deaths occurred. Those with evidence of compromised left ventricular performance

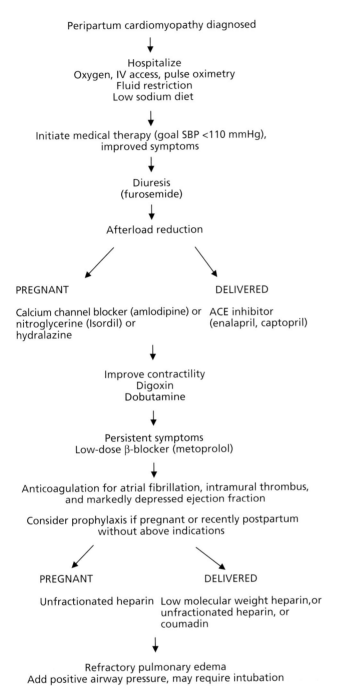

Peripartum cardiomyopathy diagnosed

↓

Hospitalize
Oxygen, IV access, pulse oximetry
Fluid restriction
Low sodium diet

↓

Initiate medical therapy (goal SBP <110 mmHg),
improved symptoms

↓

Diuresis
(furosemide)

↓

Afterload reduction

PREGNANT   DELIVERED

Calcium channel blocker (amlodipine) or   ACE inhibitor
nitroglycerine (Isordil) or   (enalapril, captopril)
hydralazine

↓

Improve contractility
Digoxin
Dobutamine

↓

Persistent symptoms
Low-dose β-blocker (metoprolol)

↓

Anticoagulation for atrial fibrillation, intramural thrombus,
and markedly depressed ejection fraction

Consider prophylaxis if pregnant or recently postpartum
without above indications

PREGNANT   DELIVERED

Unfractionated heparin   Low molecular weight heparin, or
                          unfractionated heparin, or
                          coumadin

↓

Refractory pulmonary edema
Add positive airway pressure, may require intubation

Figure 17.3 Management of peripartum cardiomyopathy. SBP, systolic blood pressure.

(ejection fraction less than 50%) suffered significant complications during gestation, with cardiac symptoms developing in 50%, deterioration of cardiac function in 33%, persistent decompensation in 42%, and death in 25% of women in this group. Habli *et al* identified 70 patients with documented PPCM and classified them into groups based on ejection fraction >25% (60%) or ≤25% (40%) [86]. Over half (57%) of the patients with an ejection fraction ≤25% had end-stage cardiac disease requiring

transplantation compared to no patients with an ejection fraction >25%. Other authors have reported similar findings in smaller series. Therefore, women with a history of PPCM and evidence of incomplete left ventricular recovery should be counseled to avoid pregnancy.

Acute myocardial infarction

Acute myocardial infarction (AMI) occurring during pregnancy and the puerperium is rare, affecting approximately 1 in 35,000 gravidas [87]. The incidence can be expected to increase as more women postpone childbearing into the fourth and fifth decades of life, when risk factors for coronary artery disease are more prevalent. In fact, a population-based study of AMI in pregnancies from 1991 to 2000 demonstrated an increasing incidence across the decade [87]. In this study of 151 patients, the mortality rate of AMI during pregnancy was 7.3%, significantly lower than reported in previous studies [88]. The three strongest predictors of AMI in this study were chronic hypertension, advancing maternal age, and diabetes. Sixty-six percent of the AMIs occurred in women older than 30 years. Only 21% of AMIs were diagnosed intrapartum; the remainder were evenly divided between the antepartum and postpartum periods, but no deaths occurred postpartum. Patients diagnosed with AMI intrapartum had the highest mortality rate and were more likely to have severe preeclampsia and eclampsia. Myocardial infarction occurring before or after labor was more likely to be related to diabetes, coronary artery disease, and lipid disorders [87].

A 2008 review summarized outcomes of 103 pregnant patients diagnosed with AMI [88]. The majority of myocardial infarctions occurred in women older than 30 years (72%), and location was most frequently found in the anterior wall (78%). In this review, the maternal death rate was 11% (twice as high if AMI was diagnosed in the peripartum period), and overall fetal mortality rate was 9%. Atherosclerotic disease was identified in 40% of patients, coronary thrombus in 8%, and apparently normal coronary arteries in 13%.

The acute treatment of AMI in pregnancy should adhere to the same management principles as for the nonpregnant patient: supplemental oxygen, aspirin (325 mg), narcotic analgesia, nitroglycerin, heparin, and β-blockers. The use of fibrinolytic agents during pregnancy (almost exclusively for the treatment of pulmonary emboli) is limited but has been associated with an increased rate of maternal hemorrhage, premature delivery, and fetal loss [88]. However, fibrinolytics such as streptokinase and reteplase are considered standard first-line therapy in nonpregnant patients to reduce mortality following AMI and should be considered based on maternal condition.

Given that only 10 of the 103 pregnancies reviewed in the aforementioned 2008 study delivered via cesarean section [88], vaginal delivery can safely be performed in these patients by minimizing myocardial demands, controlling heart rate, maintaining adequate blood pressure, and monitoring intravascular volume changes. Vaginal deliveries require aggressive pain management, supplemental oxygen, and minimization of maternal pushing efforts. The increased myocardial demand in labor may lead to cardiac decompensation in patients with a recent infarction. Some evidence exists suggesting that mortality is increased with cesarean delivery; however, the optimal route for delivery is controversial and should be individualized. Oxytocin, ergonovine, and prostaglandins have potential to cause coronary vasospasm and should be used with caution. Information regarding risks in subsequent pregnancies is very limited.

Arrhythmias

Interpretation of an electrocardiogram (ECG) in pregnant patients must take into account the common gestational changes, including increased heart rate, shortened PR and QT intervals, left axis deviation, and nonspecific ST changes. Asymptomatic arrhythmias occur with surprising frequency in laboring patients [89]. However, hemodynamically significant abnormalities and preexisting arrhythmias are less common. A history of supraventricular tachycardia (SVT) increases the risk of SVT during pregnancy [90]. The presence of atrial fibrillation or flutter should prompt evaluation for structural cardiac disease, hyperthyroidism, or electrolyte disturbances, as these arrhythmias are rare during pregnancy in the absence of one of these findings. Bradyarrhythmias are far less common in pregnancy than tachyarrhythmias and are generally well tolerated. Pacemakers may be placed safely during gestation, if necessary [90].

Pharmacologic management of arrhythmias in pregnancy is tailored to the specific diagnosis and is usually not altered by pregnancy. Many of these medications can also be used to treat fetal arrhythmias and pose minimal fetal risk in therapeutic doses. Table 17.6 [91] outlines many commonly used cardiac medications and their effect on pregnancy. Commonly used medications such as adenosine, β-blockers, digoxin, diltiazem, lidocaine, procainamide, and quinidine may be used safely in pregnancy but may require dosage adjustments to reach therapeutic levels as a result of increased maternal plasma volume, decreased protein binding, and increased renal excretion. Amiodarone has been associated with neonatal complications such as bradycardia as well as neurologic and thyroid abnormalities and should not be used during pregnancy. Patients with ventricular or supraventricular tachyarrhythmias resulting in hemodynamic instability that do not respond to medical management may safely undergo electrical cardioversion [92].

Ideally, patients with preexisting arrhythmias should be evaluated before conception to determine whether therapies such as radiofrequency ablation, pacemaker placement, or an implantable cardioverter-defibrillator (ICD) are appropriate, and to review the risks of fetal exposure to cardiac medications during pregnancy. Patients with ICDs appear to tolerate pregnancy well [93]. Anticoagulation should be considered for patients with chronic atrial fibrillation, particularly in the setting of rheumatic heart disease; this is reviewed elsewhere in the chapter.

Pregnancy after cardiac transplantation

The most common causes for cardiac transplantation in young women include cardiomyopathy, transposition of the great vessels, viral myocarditis, idiopathic dilated cardiomyopathy, and postpartum cardiomyopathy. Although cardiac transplantation is becoming more common (see Chapter 19), data on pregnancy after transplantation remain limited. Potential concerns regarding subsequent pregnancy consist of the ability of the denervated heart to respond adequately to the cardiovascular demands of pregnancy, the effect of pregnancy on rejection and mortality rates, and the potential complications for the neonate, particularly as a result of the immunosuppressive medications that are necessary to prevent rejection. Reports suggest that the transplanted heart retains its ability to adjust to hemodynamic changes before and during pregnancy, with the understanding that the denervated heart will at times maintain a fixed heart rate (sinus tachycardia is not uncommon given lack of parasympathetic innervation) and not respond adequately to indirect vasopressors like ephedrine [94,95].

In 2003, the National Transplantation Pregnancy Registry (NTPR) reported results on 20 pregnancies in 13 heart transplant recipients who underwent transplant before age 21. No deaths occurred during pregnancy, but rejection episodes developed in 57% of recipients during gestation. Most episodes were mild and graft outcome was considered "adequate." No graft losses occurred in the 2 years postpartum, but three patients died within 5.5 years of delivery. Forty-five percent experienced hypertension, and 11% met criteria for diagnosis of preeclampsia. No neonatal deaths were described, but prematurity was common (46%) [96]. This report is consistent with other case series published on the topic [94,97]. The most commonly encountered complications included hypertension, preeclampsia, preterm birth, and mild rejection episodes.

Table 17.6 Cardiovascular drugs commonly used in the obstetric intensive care setting and their effects on uterine blood flow and the fetus

Drug (safety category in pregnancy)	Dose	Uterine blood flow (UBF)	Fetal effects
Inotropic agents			
Digoxin (C)	Loading dose 0.5 mg IV over 5 min, then 0.25 mg IV q6 h × 2 Maintenance 0.125–0.375 mg IV/PO qday	No change	Placental transfer Higher maternal maintenance dose required for fetal effect Not teratogenic
Dopamine (C)	Initiate with 5 μg/kg/min and titrate by 5–10 μg/kg/min to max 50 μg/kg/min	Directly ↓ UBF May ↑UBF with improved maternal hemodynamics	No known adverse fetal effects
Dobutamine (B)	Initiate with 1.0 μg/kg/min and titrate up to 20 μg/kg/min	Same as dopamine	No known adverse fetal effects
Epinephrine (C)	Endotracheal, 0.5–1.0 mg q5 min; IV 0.5 mg bolus and follow with 2–10 μg/kg/min infusion	Same as dopamine	Not teratogenic
Vasodilators			
Nitroprusside (C)	Initiate with 0.3 μg/kg/min and titrate to 10 μg/kg/min	UBF unless significant ↓ in maternal BP	No known adverse fetal effects Potential for fetal cyanide toxicity Avoid prolonged use
Hydralazine (C)	5–10 mg IV q15–30 min Total dose 30 mg	Same as nitroprusside	Not teratogenic
Nitroglycerin (B)	0.4–0.8 mg sublingual 1–2 inches of dermal paste, IV infusion 10 μg/min, titrate up by 10–20 μg/min prn	Same as nitroprusside	Not teratogenic
β-Blockers			
Propranolol (C)	1 mg IV q2 min as needed	↓ UBF by ↑ uterine tone And/or ↓ maternal BP	Not teratogenic Readily crosses placenta Fetal bradycardia, IUGR (D) if used in 2nd/3rd trimester
Labetolol (C)	10–20 mg IV followed by 20–80 mg IV q10 min to total dose of 150 mg	Same as propranolol	Same as propranolol
Atenolol (D)	5 mg IV over 5 min, repeat in 5 min to a total dose of 15 mg	Same as propranolol	Same as propranolol
Metoprolol (C)	5 mg IV over 5 min; repeat in 10 min	Same as propranolol	Same as propranolol
Esmolol (C)	500 μg/kg IV over 1 min with infusion rate of 50–200 μg/kg/min	Same as propranolol	No known adverse fetal effects Rapid metabolism (half-life 11 min) also occurs in the fetus
Calcium channel blockers			
Verapamil (C)	2.5–5 mg IV bolus over 2 min, repeat in 5 min, then q 30 min prn to a max of 20 mg	Mild ↓ UBF	Not teratogenic
Nifedipine (C)	10 mg PO, repeat q6 h	Same as verapamil	Not teratogenic
Diltiazem (C)	20 mg IV bolus over 2 min, repeat in 15 min	Same as verapamil	Not teratogenic
Vasoconstrictors			
Ephedrine sulfate (C)	10–25 mg slow IV bolus, repeat q15 min prn ×3	No effect	Not teratogenic. 70% of maternal blood level in the fetus
Metaraminol (C)	Initiate with 0.1 mg/min and titrate to 2 mg/min	Mild ↓ UBF	No data available
Antiarrhythmic agents			
Lidocaine (B)	1 mg/kg bolus; repeat ½ bolus at 10 min as needed ×4; infusion at 1–4 mg/min; total dose 3 mg/kg	No effect	Not teratogenic Rapidly crosses placenta
Procainamide (C)	100 mg over 30 min, then 2–6 mg/min infusion Total dose 17 mg/kg	No effect	
Quinidine (C)	15 mg/kg over 60 min, then 0.02 mg/kg/min infusion	No effect	

(Continued)

Table 17.6 (*Continued*)

Drug (safety category in pregnancy)	Dose	Uterine blood flow (UBF)	Fetal effects
Bretylium (C)	5 mg/kg IV bolus, then 1–2 mg/min infusion	↓ UBF	Unknown
Phenytoin (D)	300 mg IV, then 100 mg every 5 min to a total of 1000 mg	No effect	Teratogenic "Fetal hydantoin syndrome"
Amiodarone (D)	5 mg/kg IV over 3 min, then 10 mg/kg/day	No effect	Teratogenic Transient bradycardia Prolonged QT
AV node blocking agents			
Adenosine	6 mg IV bolus over 1–3 sec, followed by 20 mL saline bolus; may repeat at 12 mg in 1–2 min × 2	↑ or ↓ UBF	No known adverse fetal effects
Verapamil	As stated above		
β-Blockers	As stated above		
Digoxin	As stated above		

AV, atrioventricular; BP, blood pressure; IUGR, intrauterine growth restriction; IV, intravenous; PO, per os; prn, pro re nata; q, every.
Reproduced from Hameed and Foley [91] with permission from McGraw-Hill.

Some of the commonly used immunosuppressive medications include corticosteroids, azathioprine (Imuran), cyclosporine A (Sandimmune), tacrolimus or FK506 (Prograf), and mycophenolate mofetil (CellCept). Although relatively few pregnancies in cardiac transplantation recipients have been reported, abundant data exist on the use of these medications to prevent graft rejection in pregnant renal transplant recipients. In general, patients can be reassured that the neonatal risks posed by these medications are minimal. Azathioprine has been associated with neonatal immunosuppression when used at high doses. Current protocols utilize relatively lower doses of this drug, and adverse neonatal events have not been reported. A recent clinical report identified seven documented cases of congenital anomalies (including cleft lip/palate, microtia, micrognathia) in mothers taking mycophenolate mofetil, and this drug has recently been classified as category D [98]. Given the high doses of immunosuppressive therapy and risk of rejection in the first year after transplant, pregnancy is discouraged within the first post-transplant year [99].

CASE PRESENTATION

A 20-year-old gravida 1, para 0 at 37 weeks' gestation, as determined by first-trimester ultrasound, presented to the obstetric triage unit with shortness of breath and irregular uterine contractions. She had been followed during the pregnancy for a repaired coarctation of her aorta and a bicuspid aortic valve. During initial assessment, her vital signs were blood pressure 131/76 mmHg, pulse 78 beats/min, oxygen saturation 99% on room air, respiratory rate 16/min, and temperature 98.7°F. Cardiopulmonary examination demonstrated no evidence of maternal cardiac decompensation. Her cervix was found to be 3 cm dilated, 80% effaced, with the fetus in vertex presentation at 0 station. The fetal heart rate pattern was a reassuring category I tracing.

The patient was admitted to the hospital for further evaluation. Review of her medical records revealed that her most recent echocardiogram showed mild aortic stenosis (as defined above), with an ejection fraction (EF) of 65%. An echocardiogram repeated in the hospital showed an EF of 66%, aortic diameter of 3.3 cm^2, and a peak gradient pressure of 11 mmHg. Subsequently, the patient experienced spontaneous rupture of membranes; oxytocin was initiated for labor augmentation. She received an epidural for pain control which was dosed slowly to prevent hypotension. Later that day, she developed chorioamnionitis. Intravenous ampicillin and gentamicin were started.

Upon achievement of complete dilation, and 3+ fetal station, an assisted second stage was attempted with forceps. When this failed, the patient underwent cesarean delivery of a viable 3200 g male with Apgars of 7 and 9 at 1 and 5 min, respectively. Clindamycin was added to the above antibiotic regimen for anaerobic coverage; antibiotics were discontinued postoperatively, after the woman remained afebrile for 24 h. Postpartum, her shortness of breath resolved and she was discharged home on postoperative day 4, with outpatient follow-up with her cardiologist and obstetrician.

Clinical points

A follow-up echocardiogram was performed because of new onset of symptoms. The patient's vital signs, physical examination, and fetal heart tracing were suggestive of sufficient maternal cardiac function, as confirmed by echocardiography.

A routine, though slowly dosed, epidural was appropriate, given mild aortic stenosis.

No antibiotic endocarditis prophylaxis was needed; antibiotics were administered to treat chorioamnionitis.

The second stage of labor was assisted to minimize maternal Valsalva efforts, which might have caused undue stress on the patient's coarctation repair.

References

1. Ullery JC. The management of pregnancy complicated by heart disease. Am J Obstet Gynecol 1954;67:834–866.

2. Szekely P, Turner R, Snaith L. Pregnancy and the changing pattern of rheumatic heart disease. Br Heart J 1973;35:1293–1303.

3. Chang C, Elam-Evans LD, Berg CJ et al. Pregnancy-related mortality surveillance, United States, 1991–1999. MMWR CDC Surveill Summ 2003;52:1–8.

4. Loverro G, Pansini V, Greco P, Vimercati A, Parisi AM, Selvaggi L. Indications and outcome for intensive care unit admission during puerperium. Arch Gynecol Obstet 2001;265:195–198.

5. Clark SL, Cotton DB, Lee W et al. Central hemodynamic assessment of normal term pregnancy. Am J Obstet Gynecol 1989;161:1439–1442.

6. Elkayam U, Gleicher N. Hemodynamics and cardiac function during normal pregnancy and the puerperium. In: Elkayam U, Gleicher N, eds. Cardiac Problems in Pregnancy, 3rd ed. New York: Wiley-Liss, 1998, pp.3–19.

7. Capeless EL, Clapp JF. Cardiovascular changes in early phase of pregnancy. Am J Obstet Gynecol 1989;161:1449–1453.

8. Gei AF, Hankins GD. Cardiac disease and pregnancy. Obstet Gynecol Clin North Am 2001;28:465–512.

9. Clark SL. Structural cardiac disease in pregnancy. In: Clark SL, Cotton DB, Phelan JP, eds. Critical Care Obstetrics. Oradell, NJ: Medical Economics Books, 1987, p.92.

10. Siu SC, Sermer M, Harrison DA et al. Risk and predictors for pregnancy-related complications in women with heart disease. Circulation 1997;96:2789–2794.

11. Siu SC, Sermer M, Colman JM et al. Prospective multicenter study of pregnancy outcomes in women with heart disease. Circulation 2001;104:515–521.

12. Siu SC, Colman JM, Sorensen S et al. Adverse neonatal and cardiac outcomes are more common in pregnant women with cardiac disease. Circulation 2002;105:2179–2184.

13. Ford AA, Wylie BJ, Waksmonski CA, Simpson LL. Maternal congenital cardiac disease: outcomes of pregnancy in a single tertiary care center. Obstet Gynecol 2008;112:828–833.

14. Dye TD, Gordon H, Held B, Tolliver NJ, Holmes AP. Retrospective maternal mortality case ascertainment in West Virginia, 1985 to 1989. Am J Obstet Gynecol 1992;167:72–76.

15. Montana E, Khoury MJ, Cragan JD, Sharma S, Dhar P, Fyfe D. Trends and outcomes after prenatal diagnosis of congenital cardiac malformations by fetal echocardiography in a well defined birth population, Atlanta, Georgia, 1990–1994. J Am Coll Cardiol 1996;28:1805–1809.

16. Driscoll DJ, Michels VV, Gersony WM et al. Occurrence risk for congenital heart defects in relatives of patients with aortic stenosis, pulmonary stenosis, or ventricular septal defect. Circulation 1993;87(Suppl):I114–120.

17. Teerlink JR, Foster E. Valvular heart disease in pregnancy: a contemporary perspective. Cardiol Clin 1998;16:573–598, x.

18. Lupton M, Oteng-Ntim E, Ayida G, Steer PJ. Cardiac disease in pregnancy. Curr Opin Obstet Gynecol 2002;14:137–143.

19. American College of Obstetricians and Gynecologists. Antibiotic Prophylaxis for Infective Endocarditis. ACOG Committee Opinion No. 421. Obstet Gynecol 2008;112:1193–1194.

20. Bonow RO, Carabello BA, Kanu C et al. ACC/AHA 2006 guidelines for the management of patients with valvular heart disease: a report of the American College of Cardiology/American Heart Association Task Force on Practice Guidelines (Writing Committee to Revise the 1998 Guidelines for the Management of Patients With Valvular Heart Disease): developed in collaboration with the Society of Cardiovascular Anesthesiologists: endorsed by the Society for Cardiovascular Angiography and Interventions and the Society of Thoracic Surgeons. Circulation 2006;114(5):e84–231.

21. Clark SL, Phelan JP, Greenspoon J, Aldahl D, Horenstein J. Labor and delivery in the presence of mitral stenosis: central hemodynamic observations. Am J Obstet Gynecol 1985;152:984–988.

22. Bonow RO, Carabello BA, Chatterjee K et al. Focused update incorporated into the ACC/AHA 2006 guidelines for the management of patients with valvular heart disease: a report of the American College of Cardiology/American Heart Association Task Force on Practice Guidelines (Writing Committee to Revise the 1998 Guidelines for the Management of Patients With Valvular Heart Disease): endorsed by the Society of Cardiovascular Anesthesiologists, Society for Cardiovascular Angiography and Interventions, and Society of Thoracic Surgeons. Circulation 2008;118:e523.

23. Iung B, Cormier B, Elias J et al. Usefulness of percutaneous balloon commissurotomy for mitral stenosis during pregnancy. Am J Cardiol 1994;73:398–400.

24. Kalra GS, Arora R, Khan JA, Nigam M, Khalillulah M. Percutaneous mitral commissurotomy for severe mitral stenosis during pregnancy. Catheter Cardiovasc Diagn 1994;33:28–30.

25. Sivadasanpillai H, Srinivasan A, Sivasubramoniam S et al. Long-term outcome of patients undergoing balloon mitral valvotomy in pregnancy. Am J Cardiol 2005;95:1504–1506.

26. Silversides CK, Colman JM, Sermer M, Siu SC. Cardiac risk in pregnant women with rheumatic mitral stenosis. Am J Cardiol 2003;91:1382–1385.

27. Hameed A, Karaalp IS, Tummala PP et al. The effect of valvular heart disease on maternal and fetal outcome of pregnancy. J Am Coll Cardiol 2001;37:893–899.

28. Sheikh F, Rangwala S, DeSimone C, Smith HS, O'Leary AM. Management of the parturient with severe aortic incompetence. J Cardiothorac Vasc Anesth 1995;9:575–577.

29. Alderson JD. Cardiovascular collapse following epidural anaesthesia for Caesarean section in a patient with aortic incompetence. Anaesthesia 1987;42:643–645.

30. Savage DD, Devereux RB, Garrison RJ et al. Mitral valve prolapse in the general population. 2. Clinical features: the Framingham Study. Am Heart J 1983;106:577–581.

31. Drenthen W, Pieper PG, Roos-Hesselink JW et al. Outcome of pregnancy in women with congenital heart disease: a literature review. J Am Coll Cardiol 2007;49(24):2303–2311.

32. Silversides CK, Colman JM, Sermer M, Farine D, Siu SC. Early and intermediate-term outcomes of pregnancy with congenital aortic stenosis. Am J Cardiol 2003;91:1386–1389.

33. Avila WS, Rossi EG, Ramires JA et al. Pregnancy in patients with heart disease: experience with 1000 cases. Clin Cardiol 2003;26:135–142.

34. Chan WS, Anand S, Ginsberg JS. Anticoagulation of pregnant women with mechanical heart valves: a systematic review of the literature. Arch Intern Med 2000;160:191–196.

35. Meschengieser SS, Fondevila CG, Santarelli MT, Lazzari MA. Anticoagulation in pregnant women with mechanical heart valve prostheses. Heart 1999;82(1):23–26.

36. Weitz JI. Low-molecular-weight heparins. N Engl J Med 1997;337:688–698.

37. Aventis Pharmaceuticals Inc. Lovenox injection, package insert. Bridgewater, NJ, 2002.

38. Seshadri N, Goldhaber SZ, Elkayam U et al. The clinical challenge of bridging anticoagulation with low-molecular-weight heparin in patients with mechanical prosthetic heart valves: an evidence-based comparative review focusing on anticoagulation options in pregnant and nonpregnant patients. Am Heart J 2005;150:27–34.

39. Raschke RA, Guidry JR, Foley MR. Apparent heparin resistance from elevated factor VIII during pregnancy. Obstet Gynecol 2000;96:804–806.

40. Butchart EG, Gohlke-Barwolf C, Antunes MJ et al. Recommendations for the management of patients after heart valve surgery. Eur Heart J 2005;26(22):2463–2471.

41. Hirsh J, Bauer KA, Donati MB et al. Parenteral anticoagulants: American College of Chest Physicians Evidence-Based Clinical Practice Guidelines (8th Edition). Chest 2008;133(6 Suppl):141S.

42. FDA Public Health Alert. Heparin: change in reference standard. www.fda.gov/Safety/MedWatch/SafetyInformation/SafetyAlertsforHumanMedicalProducts/ucm184687.htm.

43. Green L, Machin SJ. Managing anticoagulated patients during neuraxial anaesthesia. Br J Haematol 2010;149:195.

44. Horlocker TT, Wedel DJ, Rowlingson JC et al. Regional anesthesia in the patient receiving antithrombotic or thrombolytic therapy: American Society of Regional Anesthesia and Pain Medicine Evidence-Based Guidelines (Third Edition). Reg Anesth Pain Med 2010;35–64.

45. Hoffman JI, Kaplan S. The incidence of congenital heart disease. J Am Coll Cardiol 2002;39:1890–1900.

46. Deal K, Wooley CF. Coarctation of the aorta and pregnancy. Ann Intern Med 1973;78:706–710.

47. Vriend JW, Drenthen W, Pieper PG et al. Outcome of pregnancy in patients after repair of aortic coarctation. Eur Heart J 2005;26:2173–2178.

48. Saidi AS, Bezold LI, Altman CA, Ayres NA, Bricker JT. Outcome of pregnancy following intervention for coarctation of the aorta. Am J Cardiol 1998;82:786–788.

49. Beauchesne LM, Connolly HM, Ammash NM, Warnes CA. Coarctation of the aorta: outcome of pregnancy. J Am Coll Cardiol 2001;38:1728–1733.

50. Niwa K, Perloff JK, Bhuta SM et al. Structural abnormalities of great arterial walls in congenital heart disease: light and electron microscopic analyses. Circulation 2001;103:393–400.

51. Bonderman D, Gharehbaghi-Schnell E, Wollenek G, Maurer G, Baumgartner H, Lang IM. Mechanisms underlying aortic dilatation in congenital aortic valve malformation. Circulation 1999;99:2138–2143.

52. Myung K, Park MD, eds. Pediatric Cardiology for Practitioners, 4th edn. St Louis: Mosby, 2002.

53. Jackson GM, Dildy GA, Varner MW, Clark SL. Severe pulmonary hypertension in pregnancy following successful repair of ventricular septal defect in childhood. Obstet Gynecol 1993;82(Suppl):680–682.

54. Neilson G, Galea EG, Blunt A. Congenital heart disease and pregnancy. Med J Aust 1970;1:1086–1088.

55. Perloff JK. Congenital heart disease and pregnancy. Clin Cardiol 1994;17:579–587.

56. Kozelj M, Novak-Antolic Z, Grad A, Peternel P. Patent foramen ovale as a potential cause of paradoxical embolism in the postpartum period. Eur J Obstet Gynecol Reprod Biol 1999;84:55–57.

57. Actis Dato GM, Cavaglia M, Aidala E et al. Patent ductus arteriosus: follow-up of 677 operated cases 40 years later. Minerva Cardioangiol 1999;47:245–254.

58. Trulock EP, Edwards LB, Taylor DO et al. The Registry of the International Society for Heart and Lung Transplantation: twentieth official adult lung and heart-lung transplant report, 2003. J Heart Lung Transplant 2003;22:625–635.

59. Bedard E, Dimopoulos K, Gatzoulis MA. Has there been any progress made on pregnancy outcomes among women with pulmonary arterial hypertension? Eur Heart J 2009;30(3):256–265.

60. Weiss BM, Zemp L, Seifert B, Hess OM. Outcome of pulmonary vascular disease in pregnancy: a systematic overview from 1978 through 1996. J Am Coll Cardiol 1998;31:1650–1657.

61. Kiely DG, Condliffe R, Webster V et al. Improved survival in pregnancy and pulmonary hypertension using a multiprofessional approach. Br J Obstet Gynaecol 2010;117:565–574.

62. Penning S, Robinson KD, Major CA, Garite TJ. A comparison of echocardiography and pulmonary artery catheterization for evaluation of pulmonary artery pressures in pregnant patients with suspected pulmonary hypertension. Am J Obstet Gynecol 2001;184:1568–1570.

63. Webb GD, Smallhorn JF, Therrien J, Redington AN. Congenital heart disease. In: Zipes DP, Libby P, Bonow RO, Braunwald E, eds. Braunwald's Heart Disease: A Textbook of Cardiovascular Medicine, 7th edn. Philadelphia: Saunders, 2005.

64. Donnelly JE, Brown JM, Radford DJ. Pregnancy outcome and Ebstein's anomaly. Br Heart J 1991;66:368–371.

65. Wilson NJ, Clarkson PM, Barratt-Boyes BG et al. Long-term outcome after the Mustard repair for simple transposition of the great arteries: 28-year follow-up. J Am Coll Cardiol 1998;32:758–765.

66. Guedes A, Mercier LA, Leduc L, Berube L, Marcotte F, Dore A. Impact of pregnancy on the systemic right ventricle after a Mustard operation for transposition of the great arteries. J Am Coll Cardiol 2004;44:433–437.

67. Murphy JG, Gersh BJ, Mair DD et al. Long-term outcome in patients undergoing surgical repair of tetralogy of Fallot. N Engl J Med 1993;329:593–599.

68. Therrien J, Marx GR, Gatzoulis MA. Late problems in tetralogy of Fallot: recognition, management, and prevention. Cardiol Clin 2002;20:395–404.

69. Child AH. Marfan syndrome: current medical and genetic knowledge: how to treat and when. J Card Surg 1997; 12(Suppl):131–135.

70. Lalchandani S, Wingfield M. Pregnancy in women with Marfan's syndrome. Eur J Obstet Gynecol Reprod Biol 2003;110:125–130.

71. Lipscomb KJ, Smith JC, Clarke B, Donnai P, Harris R. Outcome of pregnancy in women with Marfan's syndrome. Br J Obstet Gynaecol 1997;104:201–206.

72. Meijboom LJ, Vos FE, Timmermans J, Boers GH, Zwinderman AH, Mulder BJ. Pregnancy and aortic root growth in the Marfan syndrome: a prospective study. Eur Heart J 2005; 26:914–920.

73. Pyeritz RE, McKusick VA. The Marfan syndrome: diagnosis and management. N Engl J Med 1979;300:772–777.

74. Rossiter JP, Repke JT, Morales AJ, Murphy EA, Pyeritz RE. A prospective longitudinal evaluation of pregnancy in the Marfan syndrome. Am J Obstet Gynecol 1995;173:1599–1606.

75. Hiratzka LF, Bakris GL, Beckman JA et al. ACCF/AHA/AATS/ACR/ASA/SCA/SCAI/SIR/STS/SVM Guidelines for the Diagnosis and Management of Patients With Thoracic Aortic Disease: A Report of the American College of Cardiology Foundation/American Heart Association Task Force on Practice Guidelines, American Association for Thoracic Surgery, American College of Radiology, American Stroke Association, Society of Cardiovascular Anesthesiologists, Society for Cardiovascular Angiography and Interventions, Society of Interventional Radiology, Society of Thoracic Surgeons, and Society for Vascular Medicine. Circulation 2010;121:e266.

76. Shores J, Berger KR, Murphy EA, Pyeritz RE. Progression of aortic dilatation and the benefit of long-term beta-adrenergic blockade in Marfan's syndrome. N Engl J Med 1994;330:1335–1341.

77. Pearson GD, Veille JC, Rahimtoola S et al. Peripartum cardiomyopathy: National Heart, Lung, and Blood Institute and Office of Rare Diseases (National Institutes of Health) workshop recommendations and review. JAMA 2000;283:1183–1188.

78. Tidswell M. Peripartum cardiomyopathy. Crit Care Clin 2004;20:777–788, xi.

79. Elkayam U, Akhter MW, Singh H et al. Pregnancy-associated cardiomyopathy: clinical characteristics and a comparison between early and late presentation. Circulation 2005;111:2050–2055.

80. Whitehead SJ, Berg CJ, Chang J. Pregnancy-related mortality due to cardiomyopathy: United States, 1991–1997. Obstet Gynecol 2003;102:1326–1331.

81. Midei MG, DeMent SH, Feldman AM, Hutchins GM, Baughman KL. Peripartum myocarditis and cardiomyopathy. Circulation 1990;81:922–928.

82. Sutton MS, Cole P, Plappert M, Saltzman D, Goldhaber S. Effects of subsequent pregnancy on left ventricular function in peripartum cardiomyopathy. Am Heart J 1991;121:1776–1778.

83. Lampert MB, Weinert L, Hibbard J, Korcarz C, Lindheimer M, Lang RM. Contractile reserve in patients with peripartum cardiomyopathy and recovered left ventricular function. Am J Obstet Gynecol 1997;176:189–195.

84. Sutton MS, Cole P, Plappert M, Saltzman D, Goldhaber S. Effects of subsequent pregnancy on left ventricular function in peripartum cardiomyopathy. Am Heart J 1991;121:1776–1778.

85. Elkayam U, Tummala PP, Rao K et al. Maternal and fetal outcomes of subsequent pregnancies in women with peripartum cardiomyopathy. N Engl J Med 2001;344:1567–1571.

86. Habli M, O'Brien T, Nowack E et al. Peripartum cardiomyopathy: prognostic factors for long-term maternal outcome. Am J Obstet Gynecol 2008;199:415.

87. Ladner HE, Danielsen B, Gilbert WM. Acute myocardial infarction in pregnancy and the puerperium: a population-based study. Obstet Gynecol 2005;105:480–484.

88. Roth A, Elkayam U. Acute myocardial infarction associated with pregnancy. J Am Coll Cardiol 2008;52(3):171–180.

89. Upshaw CB Jr. A study of maternal electrocardiograms recorded during labor and delivery. Am J Obstet Gynecol 1970;107:17–27.

90. Gowda RM, Khan IA, Mehta NJ, Vasavada BC, Sacchi TJ. Cardiac arrhythmias in pregnancy: clinical and therapeutic considerations. Int J Cardiol 2003;88:129–133.

91. Hameed AB, Foley MR. Cardiac disease in pregnancy. In: Foley MR, Strong TH Jr, Garite TJ, eds. Obstetric Intensive Care Manual, 2nd edn. New York: McGraw-Hill, 2004, pp.96–112.

92. Schroeder JS, Harrison DC. Repeated cardioversion during pregnancy. Treatment of refractory paroxysmal atrial tachycardia during 3 successive pregnancies. Am J Cardiol 1971;27:445–446.

93. Natale A, Davidson T, Geiger MJ, Newby K. Implantable cardioverter-defibrillators and pregnancy: a safe combination? Circulation 1997;96:2808–2812.

94. Scott JR, Wagoner LE, Olsen SL, Taylor DO, Renlund DG. Pregnancy in heart transplant recipients: management and outcome. Obstet Gynecol 1993;82:324–327.

95. Kim KM, Sukhani R, Slogoff S, Tomich PG. Central hemodynamic changes associated with pregnancy in a long-term cardiac transplant recipient. Am J Obstet Gynecol 1996;174:1651–1653.

96. Armenti VT, Radomski JS, Moritz MJ, Gaughan WJ, McGrory CH, Coscia LA. Report from the National Transplantation Pregnancy Registry (NTPR): outcomes of pregnancy after transplantation. Clin Transpl 2003;131–141.

97. Branch KR, Wagoner LE, McGrory CH et al. Risks of subsequent pregnancies on mother and newborn in female heart transplant recipients. J Heart Lung Transplant 1998;17: 698–702.

98. Perez-Aytes A, Ledo A, Boso V et al. In utero exposure to mycophenolate mofetil: a characteristic phenotype? Am J Med Genet Part A 2008;146A:1–7.

99. McKay DB, Josephson MA, Armenti VT et al. Reproduction and transplantation: report on the AST Consensus Conference on Reproductive Issues and Transplantation. Am J Transplant 2005;5(7):1592–1599.

Chapter 18
Renal Disease

David C. Jones

Department of Obstetrics, Gynecology and Reproductive Sciences, University of Vermont College of Medicine, Burlington, VT, USA

The presence of maternal renal disease during pregnancy carries risks for both the fetus and the mother. However, over the past 30 years, an improved understanding of the nature of those risks and how they can be best mitigated has led to a change in attitude. This change was summed up in the editorial comment "Children of women with renal disease used to be born dangerously or not at all – not at all if their doctors had their way" [1]. This has been replaced by the recognition that through careful management, the majority of affected women with all but the most severe renal disease have a high likelihood of a successful pregnancy.

Physiological changes in renal function during pregnancy

Renal function, water metabolism, and sodium homeostasis are among the systems undergoing physiologic changes during pregnancy, and it is important to understand these normal changes in order to identify pathologic changes. The volume expansion of pregnancy is characterized by an increase in extracellular fluid and peripheral vasodilation that begins in the first trimester and continues until delivery. Of the 6–8 L of body water accumulated during pregnancy, the majority is held in the extracellular compartment with about 1200 mL accounted for in the plasma volume and the rest distributed to the interstitial space. Plasma osmolality drops as the osmostat is reset from 280 mOsm/kg H_2O to about 270 mOsm/kg H_2O [2]. Although serum sodium levels subsequently drop by 3–4 mEq, there is actually an overall gain in total body sodium. Increases in serum progesterone and prostaglandins, and increases in the filtered load of sodium favor sodium excretion, while increased levels of aldosterone, deoxycorticosterone, and estrogen favor sodium reabsorption. While both sodium excretion and reabsorption are increased compared to the nonpregnant state, the net effect is an increase in body sodium during pregnancy of approximately 950 mg [3].

Vasopressin production is increased during pregnancy, but serum vasopressin levels remain unchanged due to a fourfold increase in metabolic clearance secondary to the placental production of vasopressinase, which rapidly degrades circulating vasopressin [4]. There is no change in the ability to concentrate urine or excrete water during pregnancy. However, in rare instances, diabetes insipidus develops near term due to failure to fully compensate for vasopressin degradation or excess vasopressinase production. The copious production of very dilute urine leads to hypernatremia, which can cause cerebral injury in the fetus or mother. While this condition occurs close to term when vasopressinase levels are at their peak, the etiology can be determined based on response to therapy. In the case of an inadequate central nervous system production of vasopressin, treatment with vasopressin corrects the insufficiency, leading to concentration of the urine and control of the loss of free water. In this case, pregnancy has unmasked a central defect, and recurrence in future pregnancies is likely. On the other hand, vasopressin replacement will not treat diabetes insipidus caused by excessive placental vasopressinase. In this case, therapy must consist of deamino arginine vasopressin (dDAVP), a vasopressin analog that is not cleaved by vasopressinase. Treatment with dDAVP will result in a rapid correction of urine concentration. Because this is the result of high vasopressinase production by that particular placenta, the condition is transient and unlikely to recur in future pregnancies.

Other changes are also noted in renal tubular function with regard to other electrolytes and nonelectrolyte solutes during pregnancy. These alterations result in an increase in the fractional excretion of glucose, amino acids, and small peptides [5]. It is not rare to see glycosuria in the face of normal serum glucose levels during pregnancy. Consequently, glycosuria is not a reliable

Queenan's Management of High-Risk Pregnancy: An Evidence-Based Approach, Sixth Edition. Edited by John T. Queenan, Catherine Y. Spong, Charles J. Lockwood.
© 2012 John Wiley & Sons, Ltd. Published 2012 by John Wiley & Sons, Ltd.

indicator of diabetes, and formal glucose tolerance testing or serum glucose levels are required to make the diagnosis. Protein excretion is also increased and can be double nongravid levels. Indeed, the mean 24-h urinary protein in pregnancy is 117 mg, and the upper 95% confidence limit is 259 mg, approaching the level of 300 mg/24 h that defines proteinuria [6]. While these findings suggest that there is a generalized reduction in the reabsorption of nonelectrolyte solutes during pregnancy, as was noted for sodium, there is a net retention of 350 mEq of potassium due to increased proximal tubular reabsorption [7].

Increases in both the renal plasma flow (RPF) and glomerular filtration rate (GFR) occur during pregnancy, with the RPF peaking in the second trimester at about 60–80% above baseline prepregnancy levels and then falling back to about 50–60% above baseline in the third trimester [1,8]. The GFR increases by about 30% during the first trimester and then to about 50% above baseline in the second trimester, a change that is sustained throughout the remainder of the pregnancy. Subsequently there is a reliable fall in the serum creatinine from an average of 0.67 ± 0.2 mg/dL in the nonpregnant state to about 0.5 ± 0.1 mg/dL during pregnancy. This dramatic fall is reliable to the point that a level above 0.8 mg/dL raises the possibility of mild renal insufficiency [9].

Recognizing physiologic changes promotes an understanding of the different cut-offs used during pregnancy when monitoring renal function for evidence of renal disease and insufficiency. Additionally, it has been long recognized that pooling of fluid in the lower extremities leads to a drop in urinary filtration [8]. Consequently, during the later stages of pregnancy, if an accurate measurement of the GFR is desired, the gravida should be well hydrated and lying on her left side during the measurement period, and it has been suggested that the measurements should be performed over two consecutive 1-h periods to reduce the influence of sequestered fluid in the lower extremities.

Anatomic changes in the urinary tract during pregnancy

The kidney increases in size during pregnancy by about 1–1.5 cm in length and about 30% in volume [10,11]. The urinary collecting system also dilates, with the right side more affected than the left [12,13]. The enlarging, dextrorotated uterus, the enlarged right ovarian vein plexuses and, to a lesser extent, hormonal influences, primarily from progesterone, play a role in creating the physiologic hydronephrosis and ureteric dilation of pregnancy. These anatomic changes must be borne in mind when interpreting imaging studies of the kidney in pregnant patients. Additionally, there is an increased incidence of

pyelonephritis complicating asymptomatic bacteriuria, with more infections noted on the right side, which, as noted, is usually more dilated than the left side.

Renal disease in pregnancy

Renal disease can be broadly characterized into primary and secondary, based on whether the disorder is inherent to the kidney or caused by some other systemic disease. This is true whether the patient is pregnant or not; however, pregnancy adds a number of secondary causes of renal disease. When assessing a pregnant patient with apparent renal disease, the most important questions to start with relate to whether there was evidence of renal disease prior to the pregnancy and, if not, what was the gestational age of the pregnancy when the first signs of renal disease were noted? While it is possible that renal disease unrelated to pregnancy could coincidentally arise during the pregnancy, the later in the pregnancy it is seen, the more likely it is to be a pregnancy-related renal condition. Conversely, when renal disease is diagnosed before 20 weeks' gestation, it is very rarely related to a pregnancy-associated condition such as preeclampsia.

The main markers for renal disease during pregnancy are the same markers identified outside of pregnancy: proteinuria and renal insufficiency as manifest by an elevated serum creatinine. Unfortunately, in many cases, neither prepregnancy nor early pregnancy measurements of serum creatinine and proteinuria are available, since these are not checked routinely in early pregnancy or preconception.

Proteinuria
Proteinuria is defined as urinary protein excretion greater than 300 mg/24 h. Proteinuria is usually indicative of renal disease and can be characterized based on the site of the injury – glomerular or tubulointerstitial. While this distinction is not always critical to management of the disease, it can be. When the excretion is >2.0 g/24 h, the injury is usually glomerular. As the amount of proteinuria increases, so do symptoms. Although excretion <3.0 g/24 h is usually asymptomatic, above that level, there may be edema formation due to the retention of sodium and water. Nephrotic syndrome is defined as proteinuria >3.0 g/24 h with a serum albumin level <3.0 g/dL. Edema can only develop in the presence of hypoalbuminemia, and when this is present, edema will form when the sodium intake exceeds the maximum capacity for sodium excretion. Edema formation with nephrotic syndrome can be profound, affecting not only the legs but also the arms and vulva. Edema in the carpal tunnel can cause carpal tunnel syndrome. Vulvar edema can make the patient extremely uncomfortable and may increase the likelihood of vaginal lacerations at the time of delivery.

While some women may enter into a pregnancy with nephrotic syndrome range proteinuria secondary to known renal disease, it may also be caused by intrinsic renal disease that is unmasked by the pregnancy, the most common being minimal change disease (MCD), also referred to as nil disease or lipoid nephrosis. In this condition, proteinuria is generally detected on routine urine dipstick analysis, leading to further investigation. Proteinuria may also result from renal disease that is secondary to a chronic systemic disease such as diabetes, and it may also be related to pregnancy complications. The most common cause for the new onset of proteinuria in pregnancy is preeclampsia, a condition defined by new-onset hypertension (blood pressure >140/90 on two occasions at least 6h apart) and a 24-h urine protein collection >300 mg. Proteinuria >5000 mg/24 h is one of the findings that would classify the disease as severe preeclampsia.

In women with known renal disease or those with systemic disease that has the potential to cause renal disease (e.g. diabetes, poorly controlled chronic hypertension), it is of value to obtain a 24-h urine collection early in the pregnancy as a baseline. While baseline proteinuria can worsen simply due to the pregnancy itself, such baseline measurements are useful for comparison to collections later in the pregnancy when the clinician may need to attempt to distinguish an exacerbation of underlying renal disease from preeclampsia. While this may be difficult and perhaps impossible in some cases, the presumed diagnosis affects clinical management. In pregnancies affected by renal disease without renal failure that are otherwise uncomplicated, the goal is to carry the pregnancy to term. In nonsevere (mild) preeclampsia, the goal is generally to carry to 37 weeks' gestation. In severe preeclampsia, the pregnancy is rarely carried beyond 34 weeks' gestation.

After nephrotic syndrome has been diagnosed, management is focused on limiting edema formation. Dietary sodium restriction is the primary means available, and intake should be limited to 1.5 g sodium daily. Bedrest in the lateral recumbent position is helpful in promoting an increase in sodium excretion. While clinicians tend to emphasize the left lateral recumbent position, which is the best side for enhancing return of blood to the heart from the lower part of the body, the right recumbent position also promotes blood returned compared to the supine position and may offer women a different position should lying on the left side become uncomfortable. In general, diuretics are best avoided during pregnancy due to the potential to reduce intravascular volume, decreasing uterine blood flow and subsequently decreasing perfusion of the placental bed. However, in cases of severe edema causing excessive discomfort or severe carpal tunnel syndrome, low doses of loop diuretics or hydrochlorthiazide may be used every other day, to reduce edema while minimizing the risk of excessive reduction of plasma volume. Note that the reduced circulating plasma volume that characterizes preeclampsia generally precludes using diuretics in the setting of edema secondary to proteinuria in severe preeclampsia. It should also be noted that in patients with preexisting renal disease, the degree of proteinuria does not appear to be predictive of outcome [14].

Renal insufficiency

Renal insufficiency is diagnosed based on the serum creatinine. As noted previously, levels that may be consistent with normal function outside pregnancy suggest renal disease when measured during pregnancy [9]. The severity of renal insufficiency during pregnancy is classified based on the creatinine at initial presentation or a serum creatinine within 6 months of conception if the patient presents for care late in her pregnancy. Mild insufficiency is defined as serum creatinine >0.8 to ≤1.4 mg/dL, moderate as >1.4 to ≤2.5 mg/dL, and severe as >2.5 mg/dL.

Mild renal insufficiency

It has been recognized for over 20 years that women with mild renal insufficiency can be expected to have relatively uncomplicated pregnancies. In the first large series examining pregnancy complicated by mild renal insufficiency, it was shown that new-onset hypertension or exacerbation of hypertension was seen in about 25% but returned to prepregnancy levels after delivery. Severe or significantly increased proteinuria was seen in 47% of the women, with 68% of them being in the nephrotic range. In 63% of the women with prepregnancy urinary protein measurements, the proteinuria occurred for the first time in pregnancy. Decreases in renal function were seen in 16% but were small and generally reversible [15]. Several other authors documented similar findings [16–18]. Indeed, there is no evidence that pregnancy alters the long-term natural course of renal disease in these cases. Infant survivals have been quite high, about 90% or higher, and are expected to be even better today given that most of these reports were from the 1980s. However, studies of women with moderate and severe disease have not been quite as favorable.

Moderate and severe renal insufficiency

Early reports of pregnancies in women with moderate and severe renal disease suggested that pregnancy accelerated progression of the natural history of the renal disease in about 50% of cases [19,20]. However, with improvements in management of hypertension, recent reports have been more encouraging. Two small series suggested that about one-third of women with moderate renal insufficiency would experience a permanent deterioration in their renal function that was higher than the rate of deterioration they had prior to their pregnancy [21,22]. The decline in renal function was further

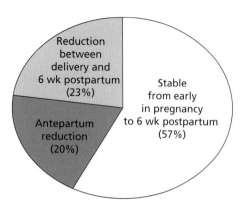

Glomerular filtration rate during pregnancy

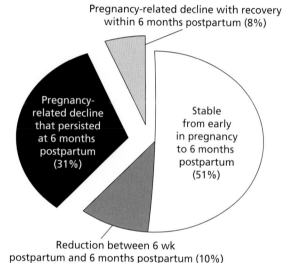

Glomerular filtration rate 6 months postpartum

Figure 18.1 Changes in the glomerular filtration rate in women with primary renal disease before pregnancy and after delivery. Reproduced from Jones and Hayslett [23] with permission from Massachusetts Medical Society.

characterized in a series of 82 pregnancies complicated by moderate and severe renal insufficiency, as shown in Figure 18.1 [23]. Over half (57%) of the pregnancies had stable renal function during the pregnancy, with 20% showing a reduction during the pregnancy itself and the remaining 23% showing a reduction in function during the postpartum interval. The majority of women with stable renal function through the 6-week postpartum visit remained stable at 6 months postpartum (84%) (Fig. 18.2). The majority of women with a pregnancy-related decline in renal function (i.e. a decline during the pregnancy or within 6 weeks after delivery) had a persistent loss at 6 months postpartum, with only 21% of those women recovering their renal function to prepregnancy levels.

Among pregnant women with moderate and severe renal insufficiency, <10% of the pregnancies showed a decline to end-stage disease within 12 months of delivery (see Fig. 18.2) [23]. Significantly, the risk appeared to be low for women with baseline creatinine <2.0 mg/dL, with only 2% of these women showing an accelerated decline in renal function. The risk of a rapid decline to end-stage disease was significantly higher for women with baseline creatinine levels between 2.0 and 2.5 mg/dL, with 33% showing an accelerated decline related to pregnancy. Among women with only moderate renal insufficiency, the most common maternal complications were worsening hypertension (24%), worsening proteinuria (29%), preterm delivery (55%) and intrauterine growth restriction (IUGR) (31%). In this setting, preeclampsia is difficult to diagnose, and no data on the frequency of that diagnosis were reported. In the subset of women with severe disease (creatinine >2.5 mg/dL), 33% had an accelerated decline in renal function and obstetric complications were more frequent. Hypertension was noted to worsen in 62%, preterm delivery occurred in 73%, and IUGR affected 57%.

In the entire cohort with moderate and severe renal disease, infant outcomes were relatively good owing to advances in neonatal medicine. Despite the preterm birth rate of 59% and IUGR noted in 37%, perinatal mortality (neonatal deaths plus stillbirths) was only 7%. Another report that included 11 women with severe renal insufficiency found a higher rate of preterm birth (86%) and lower rate of IUGR (43%) [24]. A comparison of outcomes for pregnancies complicated by moderate and severe renal disease is shown in Table 18.1.

In summary, while neonatal outcomes are generally good for women with moderate and severe renal insufficiency, these pregnancies carry significant risks of obstetric and maternal complications, including a risk of accelerated loss of renal function, particularly for women with baseline creatinine levels >2.0 mg/dL.

Chronic hypertension with renal insufficiency

Chronic hypertension frequently complicates renal insufficiency. As has been noted above, exacerbations of chronic hypertension are common during pregnancy. The report of the National High Blood Pressure Education Working Group on High Blood Pressure in Pregnancy, published in 2000, noted that "hypertensive disorders during pregnancy are the second leading cause, after embolism, of maternal mortality in the United States" and goes on to state that these disorders "contribute significantly to stillbirths and neonatal morbidity and mortality" [25]. While the treatment of stage 1–2 hypertension (140–160 mmHg systolic or 90–109 mmHg diastolic, respectively) has not been shown to have a dramatic impact on the frequency of superimposed preeclampsia, preterm delivery, abruption or perinatal death compared to untreated groups, there is evidence that treatment prevents the exacerbation of chronic hypertension to severe hypertension. The authors suggest that as blood pressures drop in the first half of

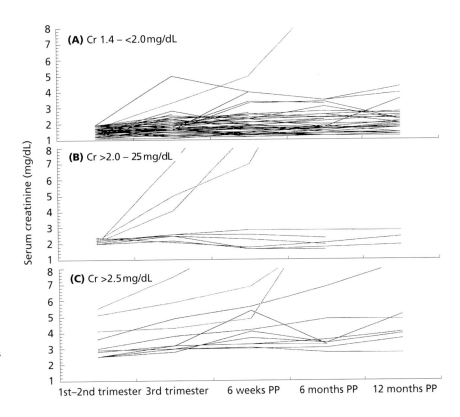

Figure 18.2 Serum creatinine concentrations in women with primary renal disease during and after pregnancy, according to the concentration measured early in gestation. Reproduced from Jones and Hayslett [23] with permission from Massachusetts Medical Society. PP, postpartum.

Table 18.1 Comparison of outcomes in pregnancies complicated by moderate and severe renal disease

Author	Antepartum renal decline (%)	Perinatal mortality (%)	Worsening hypertension (%)	Worsening proteinuria (%)	Preeclampsia (%)	Preterm delivery (%)	SGA/IUGR (%)
Hou[21]*		16	56			61	37
Cunningham[24]†	19	15			58	30	35
Jones[23]†	21	7	24	29		55	31
Cunningham[24]‡	10	0			64	86	43
Jones[23]‡	17	0	38	15		73	57

*Study reporting on moderate renal insufficiency.
†Subset from study, women presenting with serum creatinine level <2.5 mg/dL.
‡Subset from study, women presenting with serum creatinine level ≥2.5 mg/dL.
IUGR, intrauterine growth restriction; SGA, small for gestational age.
Modified from Jones DC. Pregnancy complicated by chronic renal disease. Clin Perinatol 1997;24:483–496, with permission from Elsevier.

pregnancy, medications may be tapered or discontinued on the basis of blood pressures; however, blood pressures must be adequately controlled in women with renal insufficiency.

Although obstetricians have traditionally preferred to use α-methyldopa as their antihypertensive of choice due to its long track record of safety for the fetus, other medications have been gaining in popularity, particularly labetolol and, to a lesser extent, calcium channel blockers. Diltiazem has been proposed as an appropriate antihypertensive medication to use in pregnant women with renal disease, as it decreases proteinuria and preserves renal structure and function [26]. A small series suggested trends towards improved pregnancy outcomes in women

treated with diltiazem compared to no therapy, but there were no statistically significant findings. Consequently, it is usually most appropriate to leave a pregnant woman on the medication that was controlling her blood pressure, with the exception of angiotensin-converting enzyme (ACE) inhibitors and angiotensin receptor blockers (ARB) since they are fetotoxic. Poorly controlled blood pressure has been shown to be a major factor implicated in the progressive decline in renal function in women with chronic renal disease [27]. Given the increased vulnerability of the kidney during pregnancy due to renal vascular dilation, it is critical to maintain blood pressure control during pregnancy in the normal to slightly high normal range.

Special cases

The guidelines for managing renal disease in pregnancy are mostly independent of the etiology of the renal disease, with the exception of renal disease secondary to diabetes and lupus. In the case of diabetes, control of maternal blood sugar levels is critical for both pregnancy outcome and long-term renal function. While "good control" once meant serum glucose levels adequate to keep the patient out of the emergency room, control that merely avoids hypoglycemic coma and diabetic ketoacidosis has now been recognized as inadequate. This is particularly true in pregnancy, and maternal-fetal medicine specialists were among the first to recognize this and for years found themselves explaining to patients why they wanted significantly better control during pregnancy than a patient's regular physician accepted outside pregnancy. The situation has improved greatly, and the value of tight control in and out of pregnancy is now well accepted.

The other form of renal disease deserving special mention is lupus nephritis. Pregnancy outcomes are clearly better when women delay pregnancy until after an interval of disease quiescence. A recent report of women with lupus compared three groups: lupus without renal involvement, lupus with renal involvement but at least 6 months' quiescence, and lupus with active renal involvement at first pregnancy visit [28]. The authors found a higher fetal loss rate and a higher preterm birth rate in the active nephritis group (35%, $P = 0.031$ and 52%, $P = 0.007$ respectively) but not the quiescent lupus group (25%, $P = 0.28$ and 30%, $P = 0.39$) compared to the group of women without lupus nephritis (9% and 19%). One recent review stated that women with lupus nephritis should be in remission for at least 12–18 months prior to trying to conceive, which is considerably longer than the 6 months suggested by many other authors [29].

Renal dialysis

When renal disease has progressed to the point that dialysis is required, pregnancies are far less common, but they can occur and be managed with both peritoneal dialysis and hemodialysis. In the largest series of pregnancies from a single center, 52 pregnancies were followed with hemodialysis [30]. Forty-seven of 54 fetuses survived (two sets of twins) with four stillbirths and three neonatal deaths for a perinatal mortality of 13%. The preterm delivery rate was 85% with a mean gestational age at delivery of 32.7 weeks. The authors found that preeclampsia was diagnosed in 19% of pregnancies, but these pregnancies accounted for a disproportionate share of the other obstetric complications, including 70% of the fetuses born prior to 30 weeks and 57% of the perinatal losses. Another small series reporting on women undergoing nocturnal hemodialysis suggested that dramatically increasing time on dialysis improves pregnancy outcomes [31]. The authors followed seven pregnancies in five women who were treated with an average dialysis time of 36h/wk prior to conception and 48h/wk during pregnancy. One pregnancy was terminated due to suspicion of a molar pregnancy; however, all six of the others survived with a mean gestational age at delivery of 36 weeks. Peritoneal dialysis has also been described during pregnancy.

A recent review suggested that the overall survival from published reports is over 75%, and the authors proposed that patients on dialysis, rather than being strictly counseled to avoid pregnancy, should be counseled on the "success rate, risks to the mother, demands on the daily life of the pregnant patient, and long-term results" so that they can make an informed choice about whether to pursue pregnancy [32]. These women often have anemia, and erythropoietin is often required. Also, since dialysis removes water-soluble vitamins, pregnant women require extra supplementation. In particular, folic acid intake should be increased about fourfold.

While the overall experience with pregnant women maintained on renal dialysis is very limited, it is clear that the numbers will be increasing in the future.

Renal transplantation

Successful pregnancy after renal transplantation was first reported in 1958 and since that time, over 10,000 pregnancies have been reported among women with renal transplants. Those that survive the first trimester are successful over 90% of the time. The common obstetric complications seen in women with renal disease are again increased in women with transplants. Hypertension is seen in about 70% and preeclampsia in 30% [33]. Over 50% of these pregnancies are delivered preterm with a mean gestational age of about 36 weeks. While about half of these infants weigh <2500g, it is not clear from the reports whether this represents normally grown preterm infants or growth-restricted infants. Urinary tract infections are seen in 40%.

Graft rejection is a problem that is unique to this population, and it affects 2–4% of pregnancies in women with renal transplants [34]. It does not appear that pregnancy decreases long-term graft survival. As might be expected, pregnancy outcomes are better (96% fetal survival) for transplant recipients with creatinine levels ≤1.4mg/dL, but fetal survival is about 75%, even with moderate renal insufficiency. A number of immunosuppressants are used, but discussion of their use is beyond the scope of this chapter. It is considered appropriate to avoid pregnancy until at least 2 years have passed since a transplant, and the best candidates are normotensive women who are otherwise in good health with no or minimal proteinuria and stable renal function without evidence of graft rejection on maintenance immunosuppression.

Management of pregnancies complicated by renal disease

These pregnancies are followed more closely than those of healthy women and are ideally managed at a tertiary care hospital with a level III neonatal intensive care unit by a maternal-fetal medicine specialist and a nephrologist. Surveillance is increased starting at the first visit with the addition of baseline labs including a 24-h urine protein collection, serum creatinine, blood urea nitrogen (BUN), albumin, cholesterol, and creatinine clearance. The patient is generally seen biweekly until 32 weeks when weekly visits begin. The blood pressure should be checked at each visit, and in women with hypertension should be checked regularly at home. The goal is to maintain the blood pressure between 120/70 mmHg and 140/90 mmHg. Lower blood pressures are associated with an increased risk of IUGR while higher pressures may lead to renovascular damage and abruption. Ongoing assessment of the renal disease includes serum creatinine and 24-h urine protein measurements every 4–6 weeks. Nephrotic syndrome is a risk factor for thromboembolism due to loss of antithrombin, and at least one author has recommended routine thromboprophylaxis when proteinuria exceeds 1g/24h [35]. Urine culture to assess for possible urinary tract infection should be performed monthly. Monthly urinalysis is also performed, and if hematuria is identified, a microscopic urinalysis should be performed, as red cell casts could indicate active renal parenchymal disease. Anemia is common in women with renal disease, and the hemoglobin should be monitored to keep it above 10g/dL. If it falls below this level, iron supplementation should be initiated, and treatment with erythropoietin may be necessary if the level cannot be brought up.

Fetal surveillance consists of ultrasounds to assess fetal growth starting at 28–32 weeks and then every 4 weeks as well as weekly biophysical profiles, or weekly or semiweekly nonstress tests, starting at 32–34 weeks.

Finally, two routine practices in pregnancies must be handled with caution. First, maternal serum aneuploidy screening has been shown to be less accurate in women with an elevated serum creatinine, producing an increased screen positive rate [36,37]. In these and other studies, a direct correlation was noted between the multiples of the mean of the serum human chorionic gonadotropin (hCG) and the maternal serum creatinine. One recent study suggested that total hCG was less affected than free β-hCG [38]. These reports suggest that it is probably better to rely on first-trimester nuchal translucency screening alone than combined first-trimester screening with serum and nuchal translucency. The other routine practice that must be modified is the use of magnesium sulfate for seizure prophylaxis in preeclamptic patients. Since magnesium is excreted by the kidney, dosing must be modified downward or else toxicity may quickly ensue. However, the loading dose of magnesium sulfate is minimally affected, and a 4g loading dose is reasonable. Patients may be managed on maintenance doses of 1g/h or less, and dosing based on the creatinine and followed with serum magnesium levels is crucial.

Conclusion

In summary, although women with renal disease have a considerable chance of having a successful pregnancy, significant risks remain for both fetus and mother, especially when maternal serum creatinine levels are >2.0 mg/dL. Women with severe renal insufficiency must be counseled and consider such issues as whether carrying a pregnancy to term is worth the risk of an accelerated decline to end-stage renal disease or whether it might make sense, in some cases, to wait until after a renal transplant has been carried out and her condition stabilized to conceive. The best time to consider these questions is prior to conception, but frequently the pregnancy predates these considerations. Integrated care by a team of specialists can maximize the chance of a healthy infant at the smallest risk to the mother.

Acknowledgment
The author thanks Dana Damron MD for sharing two of the case reports provided in this chapter.

CASE PRESENTATION 1

A 28-year-old woman with Sjögren syndrome was referred for care during her first pregnancy. She had renal tubular acidosis with a baseline serum creatinine that ran from 1.5 to 1.7 mg/dL. During pregnancy, her creatinine fell to 1.0 mg/dL. She was maintained on azathioprine and prednisone, which was continued during the pregnancy. Her fetus developed IUGR and she was followed with weekly biophysical profiles and umbilical artery Doppler studies as well as ultrasound for growth every 3 weeks. She was ultimately induced at 39 weeks. She had a normal vaginal delivery with a good outcome and an infant weighing 2722g.

This case illustrates a good outcome despite a fetal complication that is typical of the patient with moderate renal insufficiency. It also shows how the serum creatinine drops during pregnancy to a level that would be seen as high-normal in the nonpregnant setting, so when seeing a pregnant patient with a "high-normal" creatinine, you must consider the possibility that she has an underlying renal disease.

CASE PRESENTATION 2

A 21-year-old gravida 1 presented at 11 weeks' gestation with a history of chronic renal disease secondary to diffuse proliferative lupus nephritis. Five years before presentation, she developed a facial rash and arthralgias, and the diagnosis of lupus was made after laboratory testing. About 1 year prior to presentation, she became quite ill and was hospitalized and required ICU care. She developed acute renal failure, but recovered after treatment with plasmapheresis. At presentation, she was being treated with labetolol 100 mg bid, prednisone 10 mg daily, and azathioprine 50 mg bid. She was begun on aspirin 81 mg daily. At 17 weeks' gestation, she was noted to have hypertension: 148/98 and 162/97. Upon evaluation, the patient admitted she had discontinued the labetalol and azathioprine. Labs revealed creatinine 4.3 mg/dL, potassium 4.8 mg/dL, urine 4+ protein, and a urinary protein:creatinine ratio of 5.2. An obstetric ultrasound was performed, which identified a fetal demise. She was admitted to the hospital for induction of labor with misoprostol. Her lupus nephritis flare was treated with high-dose steroids and IV cyclophosphamide. Her serum creatinine peaked at 5.6 mg/dL, after which hemodialysis was started. She was later discharged from the hospital and required maintenance with home continuous ambulatory peritoneal dialysis.

This case illustrates the danger and unpredictability of a lupus flare as well as some of the risks inherent in pursuing pregnancy in the face of lupus nephritis.

CASE PRESENTATION 3

A 28-year-old gravida 1 with type I diabetes since age 5 and diabetic nephropathy presented for care in the first trimester. She was managed with an insulin pump and in the first trimester had a serum creatinine 1.3 mg/dL, 24-h urinary protein excretion of 630 mg, and HbA$_{1c}$ 8.6%. Her pregnancy proceeded with improved control and without complications until she developed preeclampsia at 36 weeks. She was diagnosed with severe preeclampsia based on systolic blood pressures ≥160. Her 24° was 3.7 g and her serum creatinine was 1.4 mg/dL. She was induced but developed an arrest of dilation and was delivered by cesarean section. Her infant girl weighed 2726 g and did well. At the time of discharge, the patient's creatinine was 1.3 mg/dL. She presented to the office about 1 year later for a preconception visit. Her HbA$_{1c}$ was 7.8% and her creatinine was 1.6 mg/dL. She had developed hypertension, which was being treated with a β-blocker. She was counseled to try to improve her glycemic control prior to her next pregnancy.

This case illustrates the generally good outcomes that can be expected with mild renal insufficiency, even in the face of diabetes. It shows the importance of sound diabetic control and the mild drop in creatinine that can be seen between pregnancies, reflecting the natural history of the underlying disease.

References

1. Pregnancy and renal disease. Lancet 1975;2:801–802.
2. Davison JM, Shiells EA, Philips PR, Lindheimer MD. Serial evaluation of vasopressin release and thirst in human pregnancy. Role of human chorionic gonadotrophin in the osmoregulatory changes of gestation. J Clin Invest 1988;81:798–806.
3. Lindheimer MD, Barron WM, Durr J, Davison JM. Water homeostasis and vasopressin release during rodent and human gestation. Am J Kidney Dis 1987;9:270–275.
4. Davison JM, Sheills EA, Barron WM, Robinson AG, Lindheimer MD. Changes in the metabolic clearance of vasopressin and in plasma vasopressinase throughout human pregnancy. J Clin Invest 1989;83:1313–1318.
5. Davison JM, Hytten FE. The effect of pregnancy on the renal handling of glucose. Br J Obstet Gynaecol 1975;82:374–381.
6. Higby K, Suiter CR, Phelps JY, Siler-Khodr T, Langer O. Normal values of urinary albumin and total protein excretion during pregnancy. Am J Obstet Gynecol 1994;171:984–989.
7. Lindheimer MD, Richardson DA, Ehrlich EN, Katz AI. Potassium homeostasis in pregnancy. J Reprod Med 1987;32:517–522.
8. Davison JM, Hytten FE. Glomerular filtration during and after pregnancy. J Obstet Gynaecol Br Commonw 1974;81:588–595.
9. Lindheimer MD, Katz AI. Current concepts. The kidney in pregnancy. N Engl J Med 1970;283:1095–1097.
10. Bailey RR, Rolleston GL. Kidney length and ureteric dilatation in the puerperium. J Obstet Gynaecol Br Commonw 1971;78:55–61.
11. Christensen T, Klebe JG, Bertelsen V, Hansen HE. Changes in renal volume during normal pregnancy. Acta Obstet Gynecol Scand 1989;68:541–543.
12. Fried AM, Woodring JH, Thompson DJ. Hydronephrosis of pregnancy: a prospective sequential study of the course of dilatation. J Ultrasound Med 1983;2:255–259.
13. Schulman A, Herlinger H. Urinary tract dilatation in pregnancy. Br J Radiol 1975;48:638–645.

14. Bar J, Ben-Rafael Z, Padoa A, Orvieto R, Boner G, Hod M. Prediction of pregnancy outcome in subgroups of women with renal disease. Clin Nephrol 2000;53:437–444.

15. Katz AI, Davison JM, Hayslett JP, Singson E, Lindheimer MD. Pregnancy in women with kidney disease. Kidney Int 1980;18:192–206.

16. Jungers P, Forget D, Henry-Amar M et al. Chronic kidney disease and pregnancy. Adv Nephrol Necker Hosp 1986;15: 103–141.

17. Abe S, Amagasaki Y, Konishi K, Kato E, Sakaguchi H, Iyori S. The influence of antecedent renal disease on pregnancy. Am J Obstet Gynecol 1985;153:508–514.

18. Barceló P, López-Lillo J, Cabero L, del Río G. Successful pregnancy in primary glomerular disease. Kidney Int 1986;30: 914–919.

19. Bear RA. Pregnancy in patients with renal disease. A study of 44 cases. Obstet Gynecol 1976;48:13–18.

20. Kincaid-Smith P, Fairley KF, Bullen M. Kidney disease and pregnancy. Med J Aust 1967;2:1155–1159.

21. Hou SH, Grossman SD, Madias NE. Pregnancy in women with renal disease and moderate renal insufficiency. Am J Med 1985;78:185–194.

22. Imbasciati E, Pardi G, Capetta P et al. Pregnancy in women with chronic renal failure. Am J Nephrol 1986;6:193–198.

23. Jones DC, Hayslett JP. Outcome of pregnancy in women with moderate or severe renal insufficiency. N Engl J Med 1996;335:226–232.

24. Cunningham FG, Cox SM, Harstad TW, Mason RA, Pritchard JA. Chronic renal disease and pregnancy outcome. Am J Obstet Gynecol 1990;163:453–459.

25. Report of the National High Blood Pressure Education Program Working Group on High Blood Pressure in Pregnancy. Am J Obstet Gynecol 2000;183:S1–S22.

26. Khandelwal M, Kumanova M, Gaughan JP, Reece EA. Role of diltiazem in pregnant women with chronic renal disease. J Matern Fetal Neonat Med 2002;12:408–412.

27. Zucchelli P, Zuccala A, Borghi M et al. Long-term comparison between captopril and nifedipine in the progression of renal insufficiency. Kidney Int 1992;42:452–458.

28. Wagner SJ, Craici I, Reed D et al. Maternal and foetal outcomes in pregnant patients with active lupus nephritis. Lupus 2009;18:342–347.

29. Kong NC. Pregnancy of a lupus patient – a challenge to the nephrologist. Nephrol Dial Transplant 2006;21:268–272.

30. Luders C, Castro MC, Titan SM et al. Obstetric outcome in pregnant women on long-term dialysis: a case series. Am J Kidney Dis 2010;56:77–85.

31. Barua M, Hladunewich M, Keunen J et al. Successful pregnancies on nocturnal home hemodialysis. Clin J Am Soc Nephrol 2008;3:392–396.

32. Piccoli GB, Conijn A, Consiglio V et al. Pregnancy in dialysis patients: is the evidence strong enough to lead us to change our counseling policy? Clin J Am Soc Nephrol 2010;5:62–71.

33. Fuchs KM, Wu D, Ebcioglu Z. Pregnancy in renal transplant recipients. Semin Perinatol 2007;31:339–347.

34. Mastrobattista JM, Gomez-Lobo V. Pregnancy after solid organ transplantation. Obstet Gynecol 2008;112:919–932.

35. Williams D, Davison J. Chronic kidney disease in pregnancy. BMJ 2008;336:211–215.

36. Cararach V, Casals E, Martinez S et al. Abnormal renal function as a cause of false-positive biochemical screening for Down's syndrome. Lancet 1997;350:1295.

37. Karidas CN, Michailidis GD, Spencer K, Economides DL. Biochemical screening for Down syndrome in pregnancies following renal transplantation. Prenat Diagn 2002;22: 226–230.

38. Benachi A, Dreux S, Kaddioui-Maalej S et al. Down syndrome maternal serum screening in patients with renal disease. Am J Obstet Gynecol 2010;203:60.

Chapter 19
Pregnancy in Transplant Patients

James R. Scott

Department of Obstetrics and Gynecology, University of Utah, Salt Lake City, UT, USA

Chronic renal failure or end-stage renal disease affects over 20 million people in the USA alone. These patients have only two treatment options for survival: dialysis or a kidney transplant. Kidney transplantation leads to a longer life than dialysis, restores many patients to near normal lifestyles, and is cost-effective for the health-care system. The donor kidney is surgically placed extraperitoneally in the recipient's iliac fossa. The procedure is accomplished by anastomosing the donor renal artery to the proximal end of the divided hypogastric artery and the donor renal vein to the external iliac vein, as illustrated in Figure 19.1A, or anastomosing the donor renal artery directly to the external iliac artery, as shown in Figure 19.1B. The donor ureter is then attached to the recipient's bladder by ureteroneocystostomy. Transplantation has also evolved as the treatment of choice or only option for many women of reproductive age with end-stage liver, heart, and lung disease.

It has been over 50 years since the first child was born to a renal allograft recipient, and women with virtually all types of organ transplants have now had successful pregnancies. Nevertheless, it is clear that these are high-risk pregnancies that require expert obstetric care [1]. All transplant patients have underlying medical disorders that can adversely affect pregnancy outcome. Problems can occur unpredictably, and each organ has its own specific issues. This combination of factors presents a unique management challenge to the obstetrician. There are no randomized trials that have investigated pregnancy management options for transplant patients, but a great deal has been learned through experience.

Prepregnancy assessment and counseling

Preconception counseling is indicated for all female transplant recipients at the pretransplant evaluation and before a pregnancy is attempted [1,2]. Any woman contemplating pregnancy should be in good health with no evidence of graft rejection (Box 19.1). Serious medical problems such as diabetes mellitus, cardiovascular or pulmonary disease, recurrent infections, and major side-effects from immunosuppressive drugs may make pregnancy inadvisable. The ideal time for pregnancy is between 2 and 5 years after transplantation when allograft function has stabilized and immunosuppressive medication has been reduced to moderate doses. An assessment of the patient's family and spouse support as well as a tactful but honest discussion of her life expectancy and potential pregnancy problems are important. The medical literature and media tend to be overly optimistic about pregnancy outcomes and long-term prognosis, which can give patients unrealistic expectations. Long-term organ allograft survival rates are not 100%, and the transplant recipient may not live to raise her child to adulthood.

Antepartum care

Kidney transplantation is the prototype, but prenatal care is similar with essentially all other organ allografts. Early diagnosis of pregnancy is important, and a first-trimester ultrasound examination is essential to establish an accurate date of delivery. Antenatal management should be meticulous with frequent prenatal visits and serial assessment of maternal allograft function and prompt diagnosis and treatment of infections, anemia, hypertension, and preeclampsia. Nausea and vomiting or hyperemesis gravidarum can lead to decreased absorption and inadequate immunosuppression. Close fetal surveillance for preterm labor is necessary, and the known risk for fetal growth restriction is monitored by serial ultrasound examinations.

The incidence of intraepithelial and invasive cancer of the genital tract in patients taking immunosuppressive

Queenan's Management of High-Risk Pregnancy: An Evidence-Based Approach, Sixth Edition. Edited by John T. Queenan, Catherine Y. Spong, Charles J. Lockwood.

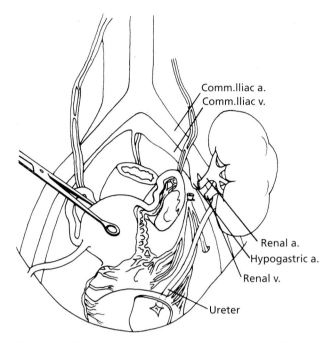

Figure 19.1 The usual technique of renal transplantation. The renal artery is anastomosed to the hypogastric artery, and all branches of the iliac vein are ligated and tied. The periurethral tissue is left intact and the ureter is placed into the bladder through a tunnel. Reproduced from Norton and Scott [44] with permission from Elsevier.

Box 19.1 Factors associated with optimum pregnancy outcome in transplant patients. Pregnancies outside these guidelines need to be evaluated on a case-by-case basis

- Good general health and prognosis
- No evidence of rejection in the past year
- Serum creatinine < 1.5 mg/dL
- Stable immunosuppressive regimen
- No or minimal hypertension and proteinuria
- Spouse and family support
- Established medical compliance

drugs is increased, and regular cervical cytology and screening for malignancies are vital components of clinical care [3]. Condyloma and human papillomavirus (HPV) are common in transplant patients, but if the patient is negative for HPV, she should receive the HPV vaccine. Skin cancer is the most common malignancy and affects the majority of patients eventually, with 30–70% of patients developing squamous cell carcinoma, melanoma, and basal cell carcinoma within 20 years [4].

Urinary tract infections are particularly common in kidney transplant patients, with up to a twofold increase in the incidence of pyelonephritis. Asymptomatic bacteriuria should be treated for 2 weeks with follow-up urine cultures, and suppressive doses of antibiotics may be needed for the rest of the pregnancy. Other bacterial and fungal infections associated with immunosuppression include endometritis, wound infections, skin abscesses, and pneumonia, often with unusual organisms.

Some patients have become Rh sensitized from the allograft, and commonly acquired viral infections such as cytomegalovirus (CMV), herpes genitalis (HSV), HPV, human immunodeficiency virus (HIV), and hepatitis B (HBV) and C (HCV) pose a risk for both the mother and her fetus. The transplanted graft is a source of CMV, and patients typically receive prophylaxis against CMV for 1–3 months postoperatively when the risk of infection is highest. The greatest risk of congenital infection in the fetus is with primary CMV infection during pregnancy, but recurrent CMV infection in immunosuppressed women has also caused congenital CMV in the infant [5]. HBV and HCV are usually acquired through dialysis and blood transfusions prior to transplantation. Hepatitis B immunoglobulin (HBIG) and HBV vaccine should be given to the newborn and are 90% effective in preventing chronic hepatitis. Acyclovir as prophylaxis or treatment of HSV can be used safely during pregnancy.

Immunosuppressive agents

Obstetricians are not usually familiar with this class of drugs, but it is important that they understand their impact on pregnancy and the potential side-effects. Most maintenance antirejection regimens in transplant patients include combinations of daily corticosteroids, azathioprine, cyclosporine, and, more recently, tacrolimus. However, new agents continually become available, and multiple drug regimens are common.

Lack of information about the teratogenic effects of some of these drugs is a serious practical problem for the obstetrician. New antimetabolites raise substantial theoretical concern because rapidly dividing cells in the embryo may be susceptible to damage by these inhibitors of DNA and RNA synthesis. The potential fetal risks for each drug as presently categorized by the US Food and Drug Administration are shown in Table 19.1.

Prednisone is the usual maintenance corticosteroid used in transplant patients, and intravenous glucocorticoids are used to treat acute rejection reactions. Because prednisone is largely metabolized by placental 11-hydroxygenase to the relatively inactive 11-keto form, the fetus is exposed to only 10% of the maternal dose of the active drug. Most patients are maintained on moderate doses of prednisone (10–30 mg/day) which are relatively safe with few fetal effects.

Azathioprine, and its more toxic metabolite 6-mercaptopurine, is a purine analog whose principal action is to decrease delayed hypersensitivity and cellular cytotoxicity. The primary maternal hazards of

Table 19.1 Classification of fetal risk for immunosuppressive drugs used in transplantation

	Pregnancy category
Corticosteroids (prednisone)	B
Azathioprine (Imuran)	D
Cyclosporine (Sandimmune, Neoral, Gengraf)	C
Tacrolimus (Prograf)	C
Sirolimus (Rapamune)	C
Mycophenolate mofetil (CellCept, Myfortic)	D
Antithymocyte globulin (ATGAM, ATG, thymoglobulin)	C
Muromonab-CD3 (Orthoclone OKT3)	C
Basilizimab (Simulect)	B
Daclizumab (Zenapax)	C
Leflunomide (Avara)	X

Category A, controlled studies, no risk; Category B, no evidence of risk in humans; Category C, risk cannot be ruled out; Category D, positive evidence of risk; Category X, contraindicated in pregnancy.

azathioprine administration are an increased risk of infection and neoplasia. Maternal liver toxicity and bone marrow supression have occurred but usually resolve with a decrease in dosage. Between 64% and 90% of azathioprine crosses the placenta in human pregnancies, but the majority is the inactive form thiouric acid. Classification of azathioprine as Category D is based largely on two early series which reported an incidence of congenital anomalies of 9% and 6.4% [6]. No specific pattern has emerged, and experience has shown that azathioprine is not associated with more congenital malformations than seen in the normal population [7–12].

Cyclosporine, a fungal metabolite whose major inhibitory effect is on T-cell-mediated responses by preventing formation of interleukin (IL)-2, is a calcineurin inhibitor. It became a standard component of many immunosuppressant regimens. The drug has a propensity for nephrotoxicity and hypertension. Other side-effects include hirsutism, tremor, gingival hyperplasia, hyperuricemia, viral infections, hepatotoxicity, and an increased risk for neoplasia such as lymphomas. Cyclosporine readily crosses the placenta, but there is no evidence of teratogenicity in humans [7–12].

Tacrolimus is a macrolide that is now widely used in solid organ transplantation, replacing some of the older immunosuppressant agents. There are currently over 90,000 transplant recipients being treated with tacrolimus in the USA, and it is prescribed to the majority of new kidney and liver transplant recipients worldwide [7–12]. There is an increase in glucose intolerance and new-onset diabetes mellitus among recipients treated with tacrolimus, but control of blood glucose levels can usually be achieved by decreasing the dosage. Nephrotoxicity and hyperkalemia develop in many patients, and

neurotoxicities such as headache, tremor, changes in motor function, mental status, or sensory function have also been described. Cord blood concentrations are approximately 50% of maternal levels. Neonatal complications reported include hyperkalemia and cardiomyopathy, but there has been no proven association with congenital malformations [13–16].

Mycophenolic acid is a reversible inhibitor of isonine monophosphate dehydrogenase which blocks *de novo* purine synthesis that has become widespread in transplantation. Maternal complications have included bone marrow suppression leading to leukopenia, anemia from pure red cell aplasia, gastrointestinal bleeding, and progressive multifocal leukoencephalopathy. A distinctive mycophenolate mofetil embryopathy is now recognized [17,18]. The specific structural anomalies in these newborns are microtia, auditory canal atresia, cleft lip and palate, micrognathia, hypertelorism, ocular coloboma, short fingers and hypoplastic nails (Plate 19.1). The FDA has notified physicians of an increased risk of miscarriage and congenital malformations with mycophenolate mofetil exposure *in utero*, and the pregnancy category has been changed from C to D. Patients taking this agent should use two effective methods of contraception beginning 4 weeks before starting treatment and continue use for 6 weeks after the last dose. These women should also be switched to a less teratogenic agent preconceptionally.

New classes of immunosuppressant agents are becoming available, but less is known about their teratogenic potential or safety during pregnancy [15]. Sirolimus is an orally administered macrolide that inhibits cytokine-stimulated T-lymphocyte activation and proliferation. The major adverse effects have been hypercholesterolemia, hypertriglyceridemia, thrombocytopenia, and leukopenia. It has been linked with small for gestational age (SGA) infants and delayed skeletal ossification but has not been associated with specific fetal malformations. Basilizimab and dacliximab are genetically engineered "humanized" mouse IgG1 antibodies that block the IL-2 receptor. Lefluomide is a pyrimidine synthesis inhibitor of dihydroorotate dehydrogenase which is required for the biosynthesis of pyrimidines, and therefore of DNA and RNA. It has teratogenic and fetotoxic effects in animal studies, and 7/90 babies from full-term pregnancies have been born with congenital malformations [8,19–21].

Kidney transplant patients

Approximately 1 in 20 women of child-bearing age with a functioning renal allograft becomes pregnant [22–24], and it is estimated that more than 15,000 pregnancies have now occurred (Fig. 19.2). Many women have now had more than one pregnancy, and some have

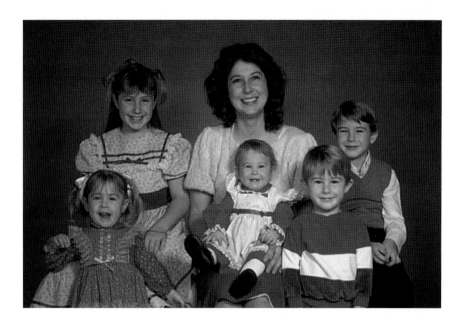

Figure 19.2 Renal transplant recipient with her five children all born after her transplant. These pregnancies were all managed at the University of Utah Medical Center.

successfully delivered twins and triplets. One of our patients has had five livebirths with no deleterious effect on the kidney [25].

If preconception graft function is adequate, as evidenced by a plasma creatinine of less than 1.5 mg/dL, the pregnancy can be expected to progress normally until near term. The transplanted kidney usually functions satisfactorily during gestation, but most patients do not have the increased glomerular filtration rate (GFR) seen in normal pregnant women. GFR instead typically decreases during the third trimester. Proteinuria also occurs in 40% of renal transplant patients in the third trimester, but this characteristically resolves postpartum. If there are no signs of preeclampsia, this proteinuria requires no specific treatment.

In contrast, pregnancy is almost always more complicated in patients with elevated creatinine levels or chronic rejection episodes [23]. Deterioration of renal function, rejection, and even maternal death have occurred. Rejection is characterized by fever, oliguria, deteriorating renal function, enlargement of the kidney, and tenderness to palpation. This diagnosis can be difficult because the findings overlap with other disorders such as pyelonephritis, preeclampsia, and nephrotoxicity from immunosuppressant drugs. Nevertheless, it is crucial to establish the diagnosis of rejection before initiating additional antirejection therapy. Imaging studies such as ultrasound are useful to detect changes in the kidney indicative of rejection. If the diagnosis is still unclear, renal biopsy is sometimes necessary.

Chronic hypertension and preeclampsia are the most common complications in these patients and contribute to the increase in preterm births, fetal growth restriction, and perinatal death [22–26]. Hypertension is present in at least half of these pregnancies, and almost one-third develop preeclampsia. In a transplant patient with a blood pressure greater than 140/90 mmHg, antihypertensive medications should be continued during pregnancy. However, angiotensin-converting enzyme (ACE) inhibitors should not be used because of adverse effects on the fetus, including oligohydramnios, pulmonary hypoplasia, and long-lasting neonatal anuria. Calcium channel blockers are the preferred agents, and an additional beneficial effect appears to be in countering the vasoconstrictive effect of cyclosporine. Preeclampsia should be anticipated, and the management is the same as with nontransplant patients.

Other organ transplant patients

Pancreas

Whole or segmental cadaveric pancreas transplantation, usually combined with kidney transplantation, is now a treatment option for patients with juvenile-onset insulin-dependent (type 1) diabetes mellitus. One-year graft survival rate is approximately 80%, with a 5-year graft survival rate of 60%. The 10-year probability of insulin independence is approximately 90% if the patient has a functioning graft at 5 years [27]. Most cases of pancreas transplantation are performed in patients who already have or will receive a kidney allograft at the same time they receive the pancreas (Fig. 19.3).

Although renal transplantation allows women with diabetes to become pregnant, immunosuppression adds to the complexity of management [27,28,43]. Because many issues are the same, antepartum and intrapartum management is similar to that for kidney transplant

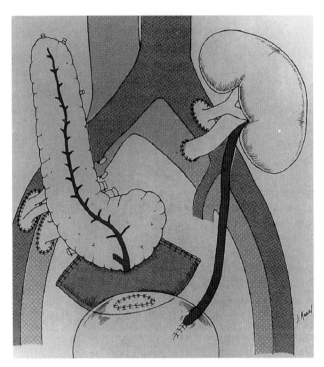

Figure 19.3 Combined pancreas–kidney transplantation with duodenal segment technique. Reproduced from Sollinger HW, Stegall, MD. Pancreas transplantation. In: Sabiston DC, ed. Textbook of Surgery, 14th edn. Philadelphia: WB Saunders, 1991, with permission from Elsevier.

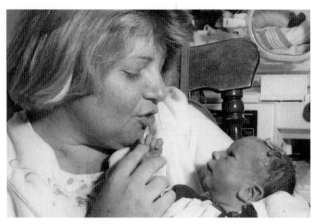

Figure 19.4 Heart transplant recipient holding her newborn, delivered at the University of Utah Medical Center 6 years after transplant. Reproduced from *American Journal of Transplantation* with permission from Wiley-Blackwell.

patients. However, the diabetogenic effects of pregnancy, corticosteroids, cyclosporine, and other immunosuppressive drugs can all lead to or aggravate hyperglycemia, macrosomia, and other sequelae in pancreas transplant patients. Euglycemia should be achieved preconception, and glucose tolerance testing (GTT) is warranted prior to 20 weeks. If hypoglycemia is present, diet and insulin therapy should be instituted at that time. If the GTT screen is normal, it should be repeated at 24–28 weeks as with any pregnant patient. Most pancreas transplant patients have maintained euglycemia throughout pregnancy and labor, but complications have included osteoporosis, fractures, diabetic neuropathy, chronic vascular insufficiency, maternal death, stillbirth, neonatal hypocalcemia, and hypoglycemia.

Liver

Improvements in immunosuppressant drug therapy and surgical techniques have resulted in longer life expectancy and many pregnancies have been reported in women with liver allografts [29,30]. Currently, 11% of all patients receiving liver transplants are women of reproductive age, and an additional 15% are younger patients who will survive beyond the child-bearing age. Of particular concern is HCV, because it is the most common indication for liver transplantation, and the rate of maternal-to-fetal

transmission is unknown. Clinical signs suggestive of liver rejection are fever, right upper quadrant pain, leukocytosis, and elevated serum bilirubin and aminotransferase levels. Because these tests are nonspecific, suspected graft rejection needs biopsy confirmation. Most rejection episodes can be managed by adjusting the drug regimen. Maternal complications have included elevated liver function tests, rejection, recurrent hepatitis, decreased renal function, urinary tract infection, adrenal insufficiency, and endometritis [29,30]. There is also an increased rate of fetal growth restriction, preeclampsia, hemolysis, elevated liver enzymes, and low platelet count (HELLP) syndrome, premature rupture of membranes, preterm birth, and neonatal infections. These complications are in part dependent on maternal health before pregnancy, and management is similar to that in renal transplant patients.

Heart

More than 5000 women in North America have undergone heart transplants at a current rate of more than 500 per year (Fig. 19.4). The transplanted heart must adapt to the physiologic changes of pregnancy. Arrhythmias may be present, and the denervated heart may not respond to some vasopressors in a predictable way. Only direct-acting vasoactive drugs have an effect, and the transplanted heart may be more sensitive to β-adrenergic agonists because of an increase in β-receptors [31].

One-third of patients have tricuspid regurgitation 1 year post transplant, and it may worsen with the increased blood volume associated with pregnancy. Almost one-third of cardiac transplant patients have atherosclerotic coronary vessel stenosis by 3 years after the transplant and up to 50% have atherosclerosis at 5 years [32]. Because myocardial ischemia does not cause chest pain as there is no afferent innervation, paroxysmal dyspnea may be the only presenting symptom. Maternal graft rejection episodes occur in 20–30% of pregnancies, but most are not clinically evident and are diagnosed by routine surveillance biopsies. These biopsies are obtained from the right ventricle guided by either fluoroscopy or echocardiography. Rejection episodes are usually successfully managed by increasing the immunosuppression regimen. The increased incidence rates of hypertension, preeclampsia, prematurity, and low birthweight are similar to those of other transplant patients [33,34]. It is good to involve an anesthesiologist to formulate a well-organized plan for labor and delivery because these patients have an increased sensitivity to hypovolemia and catecholamines.

Lung

The most frequent indications for heart-lung or lung transplants are congenital heart disease with Eisenmenger syndrome, primary pulmonary hypertension, and, less commonly, cystic fibrosis and emphysema [35–37]. One-year survival rate for heart-lung recipients is 63%, and this decreases to approximately 40% at 5 years. In addition to the management issues related to heart transplant patients, there are specific issues to be considered in the pregnant lung transplant recipient. Diagnosing chronic rejection of the lung allograft may be challenging, but one of the first symptoms is often a mild cough with subsequent deterioration in pulmonary function. During the transplant, there is a loss of pulmonary innervation, bronchial arterial supply, and pulmonary lymphatics. This denervation leads to compromise of the cough reflex and difficulty protecting the airway. Decreased lung compliance may result in a persistent alveolar–arterial oxygen gradient. Pulmonary edema is a definite possibility in these patients, and excess intravenous hydration should be avoided. Two patients have died postpartum from complications of obliterative bronchiolitis.

Intrapartum management

The timing of delivery is often dependent on events such as premature labor, premature ruptured membranes, or severe preeclampsia. The extraperitoneal location of the transplanted kidney in the iliac fossa usually does not interfere with vaginal delivery (Fig. 19.5). There are no particular contraindications to induction, labor, or vaginal delivery in organ graft recipients. Because of an increased susceptibility to infection, vaginal examinations should be kept to a minimum and artificial rupture of membranes and internal monitoring performed only when specifically indicated.

Cesarean delivery should be based on accepted obstetric indications. Operative deliveries in these patients are managed with prophylactic antibiotics and additional

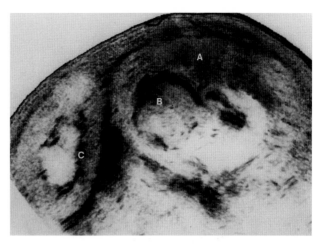

Figure 19.5 Transverse sonogram at 22 weeks' gestation below the level of the iliac crest showing anterior placenta (A), fetal trunk (B), and mild hydronephrosis of the transplanted kidney (C). Reproduced from Norton PA, Scott JR. Gynecologic and obstetric problems in renal allograft recipients. In: Buchsbaum H, Schmidt J, eds. Gynecologic and Obstetric Urology, 3rd edn. Philadelphia: WB Saunders, 1993, with permission from Elsevier.

glucocorticoids, and require strict asepsis and careful attention to hemostasis. A lower midline vertical incision provides the greatest exposure and avoids the region of the transplanted kidney. A low transverse uterine incision is almost always possible, but the obstetrician should be aware of the anatomic alterations associated with the transplanted kidney in order to avoid inadvertent damage to the blood supply, urinary drainage, or bladder damage.

Obstetric emergencies

Acute emergencies may arise in pregnant transplant patients with severe consequences that require aggressive management and intensive care. These are best managed in a tertiary setting where the transplant surgeon, obstetrician, nephrologist, and other subspecialists and intensivists can work together. Most difficult is severe and chronic rejection or allograft vasculopathy with loss of graft function which threatens the life of the mother and fetus. Renal allograft patients with deteriorating function may have to be placed back on dialysis therapy for the remainder of the pregnancy, and other organ recipients need a variety of supportive measures or retransplantation. Sepsis and overwhelming infections are also a constant threat in these women, and patients have died of meningitis, pneumonia, gastroenteritis, HCV and HBV, and AIDS [1,2,23,24]. With the high incidence of hypertension and preeclampsia, it is not surprising that HELLP syndrome, stroke, and eclampsia have occurred [1,2,23,24]. Other causes of morbidity that have required emergency surgery include rupture of renal vessel anastomosis,

CASE PRESENTATION

A 26-year-old primigravida underwent heart transplantation for idiopathic dilated cardiomyopathy and intractable congestive heart failure. When she conceived 4 years after the transplant, she was receiving conventional doses of cyclosporine, azathioprine, and prednisone.

The patient was followed from 7 weeks' gestation with frequent antepartum visits and serial sonograms for fetal growth. Right heart catheterizations and cardiac biopsies showed stable cardiac function throughout pregnancy. The pregnancy progressed normally until 33 weeks. At that time, she developed pruritus, slight icterus, and a blood pressure of 130/90 mmHg. Admission laboratory tests were normal except for a hematocrit of 28.5%, platelet count 99,000/μL, alkaline phosphatase 12 mg/dL, lactic dehydrogenase 345 mg/dL, and total bilirubin 2.8 mg/dL. Despite bedrest, her blood pressure gradually rose to 150/100 mmHg, and she developed proteinuria. A diagnosis of preeclampsia was made, and labor was induced at 34 weeks' gestation. The patient delivered a healthy 2500 g female infant.

Over the first 4 postpartum days, the mother had three intermittent episodes of sudden vaginal bleeding, which were treated with uterine massage, intravenous oxytocin, intramuscular prostaglandin $F_{2\alpha}$, uterine curettage, and blood transfusions. Persistent uterine bleeding on the fifth postpartum day prompted an abdominal hysterectomy. The uterus contained an unusual arteriovenous malformation which was most likely unrelated to her heart transplant. She had an uneventful postoperative course and her infant did well.

The patient developed coronary artery arteriosclerosis and gradual compromise of cardiac function over the next decade. She was otherwise in relatively good health except for chronic vulvar condylomata unresponsive to multiple therapeutic regimens. At age 35, 14 years after her transplant and 9 years after her delivery, a vulvar biopsy revealed invasive vulvar carcinoma which was treated with a radical vulvectomy and bilateral inguinal lymphadenectomy. One year later, her allograft vasculopathy was progressing and she was hospitalized and treated for an acute myocardial infarction and a pulmonary embolism. She was again admitted to the intensive care unit 3 weeks later with herpes encephalitis, where she developed acute tachycardia, severe hypoxia despite intubation, rapidly deteriorated, and died. She is survived by her husband and her daughter, who is now 14 years old.

This case illustrates short- and long-term problems that commonly occur in transplant patients of reproductive age.

mechanical obstruction of the ureter, antepartum bleeding, uterine rupture, small bowel injury at cesarean delivery, severe postpartum hemorrhage, abdominal wound dehiscence, and pelvic abscess .

The baby

All immunosuppressive drugs cross the placental barrier and diffuse into the fetal circulation. Because there is no convincing evidence that prednisone, azathioprine, cyclosporine, or tacrolimus produces congenital abnormalities in the human fetus, they are the drugs of choice during pregnancy. Other than fetal growth restriction and preterm birth, most offspring born to these mothers have had relatively uncomplicated neonatal courses. Mothers are usually empirically advised against breastfeeding, but the dosage of immunosuppressive drugs detected in breastmilk and delivered to the infant is small. Breastfeeding in these patients should no longer be viewed as absolutely contraindicated [1].

Most neonates have progressed normally through childhood [38,39]. Concerns have recently been raised about the possibility of delayed adverse effects in adulthood such as later development of fertility problems, autoimmune disorders, and neoplasia [40–42,44]. Thus, it is important that all offspring exposed to these agents have long-term follow-up.

References

1. McKay DB, Josephson MA. Reproduction and transplantation: report on the consensus conference on reproductive issues and transplantation. Am J Transplant 2005;5:1592–1599.
2. Mastrobattista JM, Gomez-Lobo V. Pregnancy after solid organ transplantation. Obstet Gynecol 2008;112(4):919–932.
3. Dantal J, Soulillou J-P. Immunosuppressive drugs and the risk of cancer after organ transplantation. N Engl J Med 2005; 352:1271–1273.
4. Hampton T. Skin cancer's ranks rise. Immunosuppression to blame. JAMA 2005;294:1476–1480.
5. American College of Obstetricians and Gynecologists. Perinatal viral and parasitic infections. ACOG Pract Bulletin No. 20, September 2000. Int J Gynaecol Obstet 2002;76(1):95–107.
6. Registration Committee of the European Dialysis and Transplant Association. Successful pregnancies in women treated by dialysis and kidney transplantation. Br J Obstet Gynaecol 1980;87:839–845.

7. Rizzoni G, Ehrich JHH, Broyer M. Successful pregnancies in women on renal replacement therapy: report from the EDTA Registry. Nephrol Dial Transplant 1992;7:279–287.

8. Lau RJ, Scott JR. Pregnancy following renal transplantation. Clin Obstet Gynecol 1985;23:339–350.

9. Bumgardner GL, Matas AJ. Transplantation and pregnancy. Transplant Rev 1992;6:139–162.

10. Armenti VT, Moritz MJ, Radomski JS et al. Pregnancy and transplantation. Graft 2000;3:59–63.

11. Kallen B, Westgren M, Aberg A, Olaussen PO. Pregnancy outcome after maternal organ transplantation in Sweden. Br J Obstet Gynaecol 2005;112:904–909.

12. Sims CJ. Organ transplantation and immunosuppressive drugs. Clin Obstet Gynecol 1991;34:100–111.

13. Pirsch JD, Miller J, Deierhoi MH, Vincenti D, Filo RS. A comparison of tacrolimus (FK506) and cyclosporine for immunosuppression after cadaveric renal transplantation. FK506 kidney transplant study group. Transplantation 1997;63:977–983.

14. Kainz A, Harabacz I, Cowlrick IS, Gadgil D, Hagiwara D. Review of the course and outcome of 100 pregnancies in 84 women treated with tacrolimus. Transplantation 2000;70:1718–1721.

15. Vincenti F. A decade of progress in kidney transplantation. Transplantation 2004;77:S52–61.

16. Miller J, Mendez R, Pirsch JD, Jensik SC. Safety and efficacy of tacrolius in combination with mycophenolate mofetil (MMF) in cadaveric renal transplant recipients. FK506/MMF dose ranging kidney transplant study group. Transplantation 2000;69:875–880.

17. Merlo B, Stahl B, Klinger G. Tetrada of the possible mycophenolate mofetil embryopathy: a review. Reprod Toxicol 2009;28(1):105–108.

18. Perez-Aytes A, Ledo A, Boso V et al. In utero exposure to mycophenolate mofetil: a characteristic phenotype? Am J Med Genet 2008;146A:1–7.

19. DeSantis M, Straface G, Cavaliere A, Carducci B, Caruso A. Paternal and maternal exposure to leflunomide: pregnancy and neonatal outcome. Ann Rheum Dis 2005;64:1096–1097.

20. Ostensen M. Disease specific problems related to drug therapy in pregnancy. Lupus 2004;13:746–750.

21. Winkler ME, Niessart S, Ringe B, Pichlmayr R. Successful pregnancy in a patient after liver transplantation maintained on FK 506. Transplantation 1993;56:751.

22. Alston PK, Kuller JA, McMahon MJ. Pregnancy in transplant recipients. Obstet Gynecol Surv 2001;56:289–295.

23. Norton PA, Scott JR. Gynecologic and obstetric problems in renal allograft recipients. In: Buchsbaum H, Schmidt J, eds. Gynecologic and Obstetric Urology, 3rd edn. Philadelphia: WB Saunders, 1993, pp.657–674.

24. Scott JR. Pregnancy in transplant recipients. In: Coulam CB, Faulk WP, McIntyre JA, eds. Immunology and Obstetrics. New York: WW Norton, 1992, pp.640–644.

25. Scott JR, Branch DW, Kochenour NK, Larkin RM. The effect of repeated pregnancies on renal allograft function. Transplantation 1986;42:694–695.

26. Davidson JM. Towards long-graft survival in renal transplantation in pregnancy. Nephrol Dial Transplant 1995;10:85–89.

27. Sutherland DER, Gruessner A. Long-term function (>5 years) of pancreas grafts from the International Pancreas Transplant Registry database. Transplant Proc 1995;27:2977.

28. Barrou BM, Gruessner AC, Sutherland DER, Gruessner RWG. Pregnancy after pancreas transplantation in the cyclosporine era: report from the International Pancreas Transplant Registry. Transplantation 1998;65:524–527.

29. Casele HL, Laifer SA. Pregnancy after liver transplantation. Semin Perinatol 1998;22:149–155.

30. Armenti VT, Wilson GA, Radomski JS, Moritz MJ, McGrory CH, Coscia LA. Report from the National Transplantation Pregnancy Registry (NTPR). Outcomes of pregnancy after transplantation. In: Cecka JM, Terasaki PI, eds. Clinical Transplants. Los Angeles: UCLA Immunogenetics Center, 1999, pp.111–119.

31. Camann WR, Goldman GA, Johnson MD, Moore J, Greene M. Cesarean delivery in a patient with a transplanted heart. Anesthesiology 1989;71:618–620.

32. Uretsky BF, Murali S, Reddy PS et al. Development of coronary disease in cardiac transplant patients receiving immunosuppressive therapy with cyclosporine and prednisone. Circulation 1987;76:827–834.

33. Scott JR, Wagoner LE, Olsen SL, Taylor DO, Renlund DG. Pregnancy in heart transplant recipients. Management and outcome. Obstet Gynecol 1993;82:324–327.

34. Branch KR, Wagoner LE, McGrory CH et al. Risks of subsequent pregnancies on mother and newborn in female heart transplant recipients. J Heart Lung Transplant 1998;17:698–702.

35. Parry D, Hextall A, Banner N, Robinson V, Yacoub M. Pregnancy following lung transplantation. Transplant Proc 1997;29:629.

36. Trouche V, Ville Y, Fernandez H. Pregnancy after heart or heart-lung transplantation: a series of 10 pregnancies. Br J Obstet Gynaecol 1998;105:454–458.

37. Rigg CD, Bythell VE, Bryson MR, Halshaw J, Davidson JM. Caesarean section in patients with heart-lung transplants: a report of three cases and review. Int J Obstet Anesth 2000;9:125–132.

38. Willis FR, Findlay CA, Gorrie MJ, Watson MA, Wilkinson AG, Beattie TJ. Children of renal transplant recipient mothers. J Pediatr Child Health 2000;36:230–235.

39. Scott JR. Development of children born to mothers with connective tissue diseases. Lupus 2002;11:655–660.

40. Classen BJ, Shevach EM. Evidence that cyclosporine treatment during pregnancy predisposes offspring to develop autoantibodies. Transplantation 1991;51:1052–1057.

41. Scott, JR, Branch DW, Holman J. Autoimmune and pregnancy complications in the daughter of a kidney transplant patient. Transplantation 2002;73:815–816.

42. Garovoy MR, Vincenti F, Amend WJC et al. Renal Transplantation, the Modern Era. New York: Gower Medical, 1987.

43. Sollinger HW, Knechtle SJ. The current status of combined kidney-pancreas transplantation. In: Sabiston DC, ed. Textbook of Surgery, Update 6. Philadelphia: WB Saunders, 1990.

44. Norton PA, Scott JR. Gynecologic and obstetric problems in renal allograft recipients. In: Buchsbaum H, Schmidt J, eds. Gynecologic and Obstetric Urology, 3rd edn. Philadelphia: WB Saunders, 1993.

Chapter 20
Gestational Diabetes Mellitus

Deborah L. Conway

Department of Obstetrics and Gynecology, University of Texas School of Medicine, San Antonio, TX, USA

Normal pregnancy is a state of insulin resistance. To spare glucose for the developing fetus, the placenta produces several hormones that antagonize maternal insulin, shifting the principal energy source from glucose to ketones and free fatty acids. Most pregnant women maintain normal blood glucose levels despite the increased insulin resistance through enhanced insulin production and release by the pancreas, both in the basal state, and in response to meals.

Gestational diabetes mellitus (GDM) is a state of carbohydrate intolerance that develops or is first recognized during pregnancy. In some women, β-cell production of insulin cannot keep pace with the resistance to insulin produced by the diabetogenic hormones from the placenta. The prevalence of GDM in the USA is 2–5%, and is proportional to the prevalence of type 2 diabetes in the population under examination, because they share a similar pathophysiology [1]. The prevalence of GDM, along with the prevalence of type 2 diabetes, appears to be increasing [2]. It is the most common medical complication of pregnancy and is clearly linked to several maternal and fetal complications including fetal macrosomia with operative delivery and birth trauma, preeclampsia and hypertensive disorders, metabolic complications in the neonate including hypoglycemia, hypocalcemia, and hyperbilirubinemia, prematurity, and perinatal mortality.

Screening for diabetes in pregnancy

Rigorous identification followed by effective treatment of women with diabetes minimizes the occurrence of pregnancy complications that can result from maternal hyperglycemia [3,4]. Selecting the threshold glucose values that warrant treatment poses a problem, as it appears that the frequency of complications associated with GDM increases with rising levels of glycemia, with no clear cut point [5].

With guidelines for diagnostic algorithms for GDM currently under review and revision, most experts agree that all pregnant women should undergo screening for GDM. However, "screening" does not necessarily involve universal laboratory testing for hyperglycemia. In risk factor-based screening, women who meet all the criteria listed in Box 20.1 are deemed "low risk" for GDM, and may forego laboratory glucose testing. In a retrospective comparison, over 18,000 women were screened for GDM with the 1-h 50 g glucose challenge test (GCT) [7]. If only those with risk factors had undergone laboratory testing, just 3% of women with GDM would have been undetected. However, in this population, only 10% of women were "low risk" by all criteria, and thus able to forego the 1-h GCT. Therefore, in clinical settings with a high burden of GDM and type 2 diabetes, a risk factor-based screening algorithm is unlikely to be either cost or time efficient.

The most commonly employed cut-off value for the GCT is 140 mg/dL, which results in an approximately 15% test positive rate. By reducing the cut-off to 130 mg/dL, the sensitivity of the test (i.e. the proportion of women with GDM who have a "positive" screen) improves to nearly 100%, at the expense of specificity [8]. In a low-risk population (i.e. one with a low burden of type 2 diabetes), the actual number of extra cases identified with this increase in sensitivity is greatly outweighed by the number of false-positive screens between 130 and 140 mg/dL. Conversely, in a high-risk population in which type 2 diabetes is common, the number missed by using the higher cut-off may be unacceptable. Therefore, the population characteristics should be taken into consideration when selecting the appropriate cut-off for gestational diabetes screening.

Queenan's Management of High-Risk Pregnancy: An Evidence-Based Approach, Sixth Edition. Edited by John T. Queenan, Catherine Y. Spong, Charles J. Lockwood.

Box 20.1 Criteria for avoiding laboratory screening for gestational diabetes*

- Age less than 25 years
- Not a member of an ethnic group with an increased prevalence of type 2 DM
- BMI of ≤ 25
- No prior history of glucose intolerance (GDM, DM, IGT, or IFG)
- No prior history of obstetric outcomes associated with GDM (macrosomia, stillbirth, malformations)
- No known diabetes in a first-degree relative

*All criteria must be met for a patient to be considered "low risk" and glucose testing avoided.
DM, diabetes mellitus; GDM, gestational diabetes mellitus; IFG, impaired fasting glucose; IGT, impaired glucose tolerance.
Source: American Diabetes Association [6].

Table 20.1 Diagnostic thresholds for gestational diabetes using the 3-h 100 g glucose tolerance test

Time	ADA/Carpenter & Coustan thresholds* [10] (mg/dL)	NDDG thresholds* [11] (mg/dL)
Fasting	95	105
1-h	180	190
2-h	155	165
3-h	140	145

ADA, American Diabetes Association; NDDG, National Diabetes Data Group.
*If two or more values *meet or exceed* these thresholds, the diagnosis of gestational diabetes is made.

For women at low risk for GDM, screening should occur between 24 and 28 weeks, because insulin resistance during pregnancy increases as a function of increasing gestational age until approximately 32 weeks' gestation. Women who are at high risk should be tested upon entry to prenatal care. Women at high risk for GDM include those with GDM, macrosomia, stillbirth, or congenital anomaly in a prior pregnancy, those with a first-degree relative with type 2 diabetes, as well as women with polycystic ovarian syndrome or a history of glucose intolerance or "prediabetes" prior to the current pregnancy.

After a positive screening test result is obtained, a diagnostic 3-h oral glucose tolerance test (OGTT) should be performed. This test involves a 100 g oral glucose load after a fasting plasma glucose level is drawn. Plasma glucose levels are then obtained at 1, 2, and 3 h post glucose load. There is no difference in OGTT results with or without carbohydrate "loading" in the days prior to the test [9]. There are two different sets of values commonly used that define a positive result. According to the

recommendations by the American Diabetes Association's Fourth International Workshop Conference on Gestational Diabetes, the Carpenter and Coustan modification of O'Sullivan and Mahan's original values should be used [10]. These values are more stringent than the values cited by the National Diabetes Data Group (NDDG) (Table 20.1) [11].

The testing algorithm for GDM is expected to change over the next few years. These changes will be based on the evidence from the Hyperglycemia and Adverse Pregnancy Outcome Study [5] in combination with the results of two randomized clinical trials showing maternal and fetal benefits from treating mild GDM [3,4]. It is likely that the screening GCT will be eliminated in favor of one-step screening and diagnosis with a 2-h, 75 g OGTT, with diagnostic thresholds selected to identify pregnancies at increased risk for excessive fetal size and adiposity, and fetal hyperinsulinemia [12].

Therapeutic modalities in gestational diabetes

Medical management of GDM aims to optimize glycemic control to prevent or minimize the complications associated with the disease, while avoiding ketosis and poor nutrition. A multidisciplinary approach (involving, for example, obstetricians, perinatologists, dietitians, diabetes educators, internists, and endocrinologists) is very valuable. Diet, exercise, patient education, and, if need be, medical therapies should be utilized.

The cornerstone of care of a pregnancy complicated by diabetes is diet. Medical nutrition therapy for GDM is aimed at optimizing metabolic outcomes and improving health by encouraging healthy food choices, while addressing personal and cultural preferences and providing adequate energy and nutrients for optimal pregnancy outcomes [13]. Elements of dietary therapy include total calorie allocation, calorie distribution, and nutritional component management. Total daily calorie intake is based on ideal bodyweight, with overweight and obese women allocated fewer kilocalories per kilogram of pre-pregnancy bodyweight than normal and underweight women. For example, overweight and obese women can be given approximately 25 kcal/kg, up to a total of 2800–3000 kcal/day. Women with normal prepregnancy Body Mass Index (BMI) receive approximately 30 kcal/kg, with a minimum intake of 1800 kcal/day. These calories are typically distributed between three meals and 2–4 snacks during the day. Smaller, more frequent meals lead to better satiety, improved compliance with the diet, and reduced magnitude of postprandial peak glucose levels.

Postprandial glucose measurements are directly influenced by the amount of carbohydrate in the consumed food. A traditional diet for diabetics typically contains 55–60% carbohydrate. Major *et al* [14] described their success with a diet containing 40–42% carbohydrate. Mild carbohydrate restriction resulted in improved glycemic control, less need for insulin, and fewer large-for-gestational-age (LGA) infants.

Exercise is another key component in diabetes care. Cardiovascular exercise reduces insulin resistance [15]. Fasting and postprandial glucose levels are lower in women with GDM who exercise, possibly avoiding the need for insulin treatment in some women [16]. The physiologic and anatomic constraints of pregnancy should be taken into consideration when counseling pregnant women about exercise.

There is no established standard as to how frequently glucose levels should be checked in patients with GDM. The goal of monitoring is to identify whether or not glycemic targets are being met. Commonly used targets include fasting values below 95 mg/dL and 2-h postprandial values below 120 mg/dL Alternatively, 1-h postprandial values may be used, with a target below 130–140 mg/dL. Many experts recommend daily monitoring with a meter that has built-in memory, so that results can be verified, analyzed, and reviewed with the patient during clinic visits. The benefits of an "intensified" approach to care of diabetes during pregnancy have been reported [17]. One essential component of this regimen is frequent daily readings (seven times per day) that provide information on the effectiveness of the current treatment regimen. Using this intensified approach, rates of macrosomia, shoulder dystocia, cesarean delivery, and neonatal hypoglycemia were reduced compared with those women monitored less frequently with weekly fasting and 2-h postprandial readings. One randomized trial suggested that monitoring postprandial glucose determinations was more effective than preprandial values in managing women with GDM on insulin [18]. The women randomized to postprandial readings had significantly less fetal overgrowth, fewer cesarean deliveries for cephalopelvic disproportion, and less neonatal hypoglycemia, compared with women who checked their glucose levels before meals.

Ultimately, some women with GDM will not be able to meet glycemic targets with diet therapy alone and will require medical intervention with insulin or an oral antidiabetic medication. This can usually be determined once dietary therapy has been in place for 2 weeks [19]. Insulin dosage is calculated according to bodyweight, starting in the range of 0.7–1.0 units/kg of current bodyweight, usually given in the form of short- and intermediate-acting human insulin, in split doses. Two-thirds of the total calculated dose is given with breakfast and one-third in the evening.

The pregnant woman with diabetes demonstrates both insulin resistance and relative insulin deficiency; thus, it is typical to require large doses of insulin to achieve adequate glycemic control [20]. It is important to remember that with advancing gestational age, the patient will become more insulin resistant and therefore insulin requirements will increase. The insulin dose can be adjusted as frequently as every 3–4 days and can be increased 10–20% depending on the corresponding values obtained from patient monitoring.

Another treatment option for women who are not adequately controlled on diet alone is the sulfonylurea drug glyburide. In the past, there was concern over transplacental passage of sulfonylurea drugs leading to fetal and neonatal hypoglycemia. Studies using human placental models demonstrated that the transplacental passage of glyburide is negligible [21]. In a randomized trial comparing insulin with glyburide in women with GDM, no differences were found between groups in terms of mean maternal blood glucose, LGA infants, macrosomia (greater than 4000 g), lung complications, hypoglycemia, or cord blood insulin levels. In addition, no glyburide could be detected in the cord blood of infants born to women treated with that agent [22]. The initial dose of glyburide is usually 2.5 mg, given in the morning if daytime control is required or at bedtime if fasting hyperglycemia is present. The dosage can be adjusted upward by 2.5–5 mg on a weekly basis, to a maximum of 20 mg/day (10 mg twice daily). Although maternal hypoglycemia is a potential complication of glyburide therapy, it occurs less often than in insulin-treated women [22].

Metformin has also been shown in a randomized trial to be a relatively effective alternative to insulin in the treatment of GDM [23]. Approximately half the women randomized to metformin treatment required addition of insulin to achieve glycemic targets. In addition, it is likely that metformin readily crosses the placenta, and the long-term effects of this exposure for the infant are as yet unknown [24].

Antenatal testing

Documenting fetal well-being during the antepartum period is important for any woman whose pregnancy is complicated by pregestational diabetes (White class B or higher). However, there is no unified opinion regarding the need for antepartum fetal assessment in women with well-controlled, uncomplicated preexisting and gestational diabetes [25]. The American College of Obstetricians and Gynecologists (ACOG) recommends that antenatal testing be performed on all women with pregestational diabetes, GDM with poor glycemic control, or GDM with another pregnancy complication such as hypertension or abnormal fetal growth [26]. The method of testing (e.g. nonstress testing, biophysical profile) is left to the discretion of the provider, guided by local practice. In addition, all women with GDM should be instructed to perform fetal kick counts daily, beginning in the third trimester, and to notify their care provider promptly if fetal movements are diminished.

Delivery: when and how to deliver

Timing of delivery is a delicate balance in a pregnancy complicated by diabetes. Once term has been reached, ongoing pregnancy exposes the fetus to the risk of stillbirth and continued *in utero* growth that may make delivery more risky. On the other hand, needless intervention places women at risk for the complications associated with long labors and operative deliveries. Very few prospective trials have been undertaken with regard to optimizing delivery outcomes in diabetics. What has been consistently shown is that the cesarean delivery rate is higher in women with diabetes than in women without diabetes [27], even when careful antenatal care has achieved near normal rates of fetal overgrowth [28].

An additional consideration in the optimal timing of delivery is that infants of mothers with diabetes may have delayed pulmonary maturity and are at increased risk of respiratory distress syndrome (RDS). Poorly controlled diabetes is associated with fetal pulmonary immaturity, but the risk in well-controlled pregnancies parallels that of a nondiabetic population [29]. Other investigators have found that the risk of RDS becomes equal to that of pregnancies without diabetes at 38.5 weeks' gestation [30]. In one study [29], no cases of RDS occurred after 37 weeks' gestation, despite "immature" results on the amniotic fluid tests for fetal lung maturity. Lung maturity testing in the setting of diabetes might only be necessary if preterm delivery is considered, if glucose control has been very poor, or if gestational age is uncertain. Furthermore, tests for lung maturity should only be obtained in cases where delay in delivery is prudent even if the test suggests an immature surfactant profile.

Indications for delivery at any time after approximately 38 weeks' gestation include inability to achieve adequate glucose control, poor compliance with visits or prescribed treatment, prior stillbirth, and presence of chronic hypertension. Women with well-controlled GDM, good compliance with care, and an appropriately grown fetus are allowed to enter spontaneous labor, until 40–41 weeks' gestation is reached. Comparison of this approach to planned labor induction at 38 weeks' gestation in a randomized trial women with class A2 and B diabetes showed that expectant management prolonged gestation by 1 week, and resulted in a doubling in the rate of macrosomic

infants [31]. The women managed expectantly had a similar cesarean delivery rate to those induced at 38 weeks, although half of the expectant management group underwent labor induction. The most frequent indication for induction was abnormal antepartum testing.

Macrosomia and shoulder dystocia occur more frequently in pregnancies complicated by diabetes than in the general obstetric population. Based on the observation that most cases of shoulder dystocia in diabetic women occur when birthweight is above 4000 g [32], we recommend cesarean delivery without a trial of labor to women with an estimated fetal weight above 4250 g who have diabetes. By implementing this practice, our shoulder dystocia rate in women with diabetes has been reduced by 80%, and shoulder dystocia rates among macrosomic infants (birthweight over 4000 g) fell from 19% to 7% after implementing this practice. There was a small but significant increase in the cesarean delivery rate [33]. We use a threshold of 4250 g to account for ultrasound error in order to minimize unnecessary operative delivery. Shoulder dystocia remains most often an unpredictable and unpreventable obstetric emergency. The ACOG recommends that planned cesarean delivery to prevent shoulder dystocia may be considered for suspected fetal macrosomia with estimated fetal weight exceeding 4500 g in women with diabetes [34].

Postpartum considerations

Gestational diabetes may be the first signal of inherent insulin resistance. Women with GDM need to have glucose tolerance reassessed in the postpartum period. Use of the 2-h OGTT permits identification of both impaired glucose tolerance and overt diabetes. Twenty to thirty percent of women with GDM will have abnormal values when tested early in the postpartum period [35,36]. The factors that increase the risk of abnormal OGTT postpartum included diagnosis of GDM at an earlier gestational age, higher glucose values on GTT during pregnancy, increased age, increased parity, increased BMI, and increased birthweight [36]. All these risk factors suggest a higher degree of insulin resistance.

The importance of postpartum testing cannot be overstated. Within 5–6 years after a pregnancy complicated with GDM, up to 50% of women will have type 2 diabetes [37]. Early identification of impaired glucose tolerance affords the opportunity to institute therapeutic measures such as exercise, diet, and weight control, perhaps preventing progression to diabetes. Identification and treatment of overt diabetes early in the course of the disease offer the best opportunity to delay or avoid the micro- and macrovascular complications associated with the disease.

CASE PRESENTATION

A 27-year-old woman, gravida 2, para 1001, at 12 weeks' gestation presents for initial prenatal care. She denies a history of GDM. Her first child, born by uncomplicated spontaneous vaginal delivery, weighed 4100 g at 38 weeks' gestation. Her records indicate that the 3-h GTT performed at 25 weeks in her first pregnancy had the following values: fasting 96 mg/dL, 1-h 191 mg/dL, 2-h 152 mg/dL, 3-h 122 mg/dL. Her mother and her older sister have type 2 diabetes mellitus.

A 50 g GCT is performed with her initial prenatal laboratory tests, and it is abnormal. A 3-h GTT performed at 13 weeks' gestation is normal (96/177/148/125). However, repeat testing at 25 weeks reveals she has GDM (99/202/168/141). In initiating treatment, she is prescribed medical nutrition therapy which provides 40–45% carbohydrates, 30–35% protein, and 25% fat. Total energy supplied is calculated to be 2500 kcal/day, based on her prepregnancy weight of 100 kg (BMI 35 obese, 25 kcal/kg). She is instructed to perform self-monitored blood glucose readings. After 1 week of therapy, her fasting glucose levels are consistently above 95 mg/dL, and more than 50% of her postprandial glucose values are also above target range. Insulin is initiated, but despite increasing doses over the subsequent weeks, she remains poorly controlled as term approaches. Her fundal height at 38 weeks measures 41 cm, and an ultrasound reveals a fetal weight estimate of 4600 g, with a head circumference:abdominal circumference ratio of 0.85. Given these findings, in the setting of poorly controlled GDM, the patient is counseled about and accepts a cesarean delivery. The infant's birthweight is 4450 g, and the neonatal course is complicated by hypoglycemia that requires intravenous glucose infusion.

At the time of the postpartum visit, a 2-h GTT is obtained and indicates impaired glucose tolerance (fasting 97 mg/dL, 2-h 178 mg/dL). Lifestyle modifications are recommended to prevent progression to type 2 diabetes mellitus, and annual screening for diabetes is suggested.

References

1. Engelgau MM, Herman WH, Smith PJ, German RR, Aubert RE. The epidemiology of diabetes and pregnancy in the US, 1988. Diabetes Care 1995;18:1029–1033.

2. Hunt KJ, Schuller KL. The increasing prevalence of diabetes in pregnancy. Obstet Gynecol Clin North Am 2007;34(2): 173–199.

3. Crowther CA, Hiller JE, Moss JR et al, for the ACHOIS Trial Group. Effect of treatment of gestational diabetes mellitus on pregnancy outcomes. N Engl J Med 2005;352(24):2477–2486.

4. Landon MB, Spong CY, Thom E et al, for the Eunice Kennedy Shriver NICHD Maternal-Fetal Medicine Units Network. A multicenter, randomized trial of treatment for mild gestational diabetes. N Engl J Med 2009;361:1339–1348.

5. HAPO Study Cooperative Research Group. Hyperglycemia and adverse pregnancy outcomes. N Engl J Med 2008; 358(19):1991–2002.

6. American Diabetes Association. Diagnosis and classification of diabetes mellitus. Diabetes Care 2010;33(Suppl 1):S62–69.

7. Danilenko-Dixon DR, van Winter JT, Nelson RL, Ogburn PL Jr. Universal versus selective gestational diabetes screening: application of 1997 American Diabetes Association recommendations. Am J Obstet Gynecol 1999;181:798–802.

8. Coustan DR, Widness JA, Carpenter MW, Rotondo L, Pratt DC, Oh W. Should the fifty-gram one-hour glucose screening test for gestational diabetes be administered in the fasting or fed state? Am J Obstet Gynecol 1986;154:1031–1035.

9. Crowe SM, Mastrobattista JM, Monga M. Oral glucose tolerance test and the preparatory diet. Am J Obstet Gynecol 2000;182:1052–1054.

10. Carpenter MW, Coustan DR. Criteria for screening tests for gestational diabetes. Am J Obstet Gynecol 1982;144:768–773.

11. National Diabetes Data Group. Classification and diagnosis of diabetes mellitus and other categories of glucose intolerance. Diabetes 1979;28:1039–1057.

12. IADPSG Consensus Panel. International Association of Diabetes and Pregnancy Study Group recommendations on the diagnosis and classification of hyperglycemia in pregnancy. Diabetes Care 2010;33(3):676–682.

13. American Diabetes Association. Nutrition principles and recommendations in diabetes. Diabetes Care 2004;27(Suppl 1):S36–S46.

14. Major CA, Henry MJ, de Veciana M, Morgan MA. The effects of carbohydrate restriction in patients with diet-controlled gestational diabetes. Obstet Gynecol 1998;91:600–604.

15. Horton ES. Exercise in the treatment of NIDDM. Applications for GDM? Diabetes 1991;40(Suppl 2):175–178.

16. Jovanovic-Peterson L, Durak EP, Peterson CM. Randomized trial of diet versus diet plus cardiovascular conditioning on glucose levels in gestational diabetes. Am J Obstet Gynecol 1989;161:415–419.

17. Langer O, Rodriquez DA, Xenakis EM, McFarland MB, Berkus MD, Arrendondo F. Intensified versus conventional management of gestational diabetes. Am J Obstet Gynecol 1994; 170:1036–1047.

18. De Veciana M, Major CA, Morgan MA et al. Postprandial versus preprandial glucose monitoring in women with gestational diabetes mellitus requiring insulin therapy. N Engl J Med 1995;333:235–246.

19. McFarland MB, Langer O, Conway DL, Berkus MD. Dietary therapy for gestational diabetes: how long is long enough? Am J Obstet Gynecol 1999;93:978–982.

20. Langer O, Anyaegbunam A, Brustman L, Guidetti D, Mazze R. Gestational diabetes: insulin requirements in pregnancy. Am J Obstet Gynecol 1987;157:669–675.

21. Elliot BD, Langer O, Schenker S, Johnson RF. Insignificant transfer of glyburide occurs across the human placenta. Am J Obstet Gynecol 1991;165:807–812.

22. Langer O, Conway DL, Berkus MD, Xenakis EM, Gonzales O. A comparison of glyburide and insulin in women with gestational diabetes mellitus. N Engl J Med 2000;343:1134–1138.

23. Rowan JA, Hague WM, Gao W, Battin MR, Moore MP, MiG Trial Investigators. Metformin versus insulin for the treatment of gestational diabetes. N Engl J Med 2008;358(19):2003–2015.

24. Elliott BD, Langer O, Schuessling F. Human placental glucose uptake and transport are not altered by the oral antihyperglycemic agent metformin. Am J Obstet Gynecol 1997;176:527–530.

25. Landon MB, Vickers S. Fetal surveillance in pregnancy complicated by diabetes mellitus: is it necessary? J Matern Fetal Neonat Med 2002;12:413–416.

26. American College of Obstetricians and Gynecologists. Gestational diabetes. ACOG Practice Bulletin No. 30. Obstet Gynecol 2001;98(3):525–538.

27. Jacobson JD, Cousins L. A population-based study of maternal and perinatal outcome in patients with gestational diabetes. Am J Obstet Gynecol 1989;161:981–986.

28. Naylor CD, Sermer M, Chen E, Sykora K. Cesarean delivery in relation to birth weight and gestational glucose tolerance: pathophysiology or practice style? JAMA 1996;275:1165–1170.

29. Piper JM, Xenakis EM, Langer O. Delayed appearance of pulmonary maturation markers is associated with poor glucose control in diabetic pregnancies. J Matern Fetal Med 1998;7:148–153.

30. Kjos SL, Walther FJ, Montoro M, Paul RH, Diaz F, Stabler M. Prevalence and etiology of respiratory distress in infants of diabetic mothers: predictive value of fetal lung maturation tests. Am J Obstet Gynecol 1990;163:898–903.

31. Kjos SL, Henry OA, Montoro M, Buchanan TA, Mestman JH. Insulin-requiring diabetes in pregnancy: a randomized trial of active induction of labor and expectant management. Am J Obstet Gynecol 1993;169:611–615.

32. Langer O, Berkus MD, Huff RW, Samueloff A. Shoulder dystocia: should the fetus weighing greater than or equal to 4000 grams be delivered by cesarean section? Am J Obstet Gynecol 1991;165:831–837.

33. Conway DL, Langer O. Elective delivery of infants with macrosomia in diabetic women: reduced shoulder dystocia versus increased cesarean deliveries. Am J Obstet Gynecol 1998;178:922–925.

34. American College of Obstetricans and Gynecologists. Shoulder dystocia. ACOG Practice Bulletin No. 40. Int J Gynaecol Obstet 2003;80(1):87–92.

35. Kjos SL, Buchanan TA, Greenspoon JS, Montoro M, Bernstein GS, Mestman JH. Gestational diabetes mellitus: the prevalence of glucose intolerance and diabetes mellitus in the first two months postpartum. Am J Obstet Gynecol 1990;163:93–98.

36. Conway DL, Langer O. Effects of new criteria for type 2 diabetes on the rate of postpartum glucose intolerance in women with gestational diabetes. Am J Obstet Gynecol 1999;181:610–614.

37. Kjos SL, Peters RK, Xiang A, Henry OA, Montoro M, Buchanan TA. Predicting future diabetes in Latino women with gestational diabetes: utility of early postpartum glucose tolerance testing. Diabetes 1995;44:586–591.

Chapter 21
Diabetes Mellitus

George Saade

Department of Obstetrics and Gynecology, University of Texas Medical Branch, Galveston, TX, USA

As more women with diabetes are contemplating pregnancy and more women are delaying pregnancy, healthcare providers should expect to see more pregnant women with pregestational as well as gestational diabetes. Management of these women should follow accepted guidelines in order to decrease maternal and perinatal morbidity and mortality. To that end, the central goal is to decrease the risk for congenital anomalies secondary to preconception hyperglycemia, as well as to guide the pregnant woman through pregnancy in order to reach term without maternal complications such as preeclampsia or fetal complications such as uteroplacental insufficiency, fetal death, macrosomia, birth injury, and postnatal hypoglycemia. This can be achieved by a combination of frequent glucose monitoring, dietary and pharmacologic interventions, diligent fetal surveillance, appropriate timing of delivery, and judicious choice of delivery route. In most cases, patients with diabetes can be brought to term, and perinatal mortality from stillbirth, prematurity, and birth injury can be markedly reduced. It is important that the obstetrician who occasionally manages patients with diabetes is familiar with the uses and limitations of established treatments. This chapter concentrates on the pregestational patient with diabetes. For discussion of gestational diabetes, see Chapter 20.

At present, the leading cause of perinatal mortality in pregnancies complicated by insulin-dependent diabetes mellitus is congenital malformation. The risk of major malformations in such pregnancies is increased 3–4-fold over the 2–3% incidence noted in the general population. There is good evidence that these anomalies are a result of marked alterations in maternal glycemic control during the critical period of fetal embryogenesis, at 5–8 weeks' gestation. Patients whose diabetes is poorly regulated are also at greater risk for a spontaneous abortion.

There is a direct correlation between maternal glycosylated hemoglobin (hemoglobin [Hb] A_{1c}) levels and the risk for spontaneous abortion and fetal anomalies [1] (Table 21.1). In one study, the risks of spontaneous abortion and major malformations were 12.4% and 3.0%, respectively, with first-trimester HbA_{1c} ≤9.3%, versus risks of 37.5% and 40%, respectively, with HbA_{1c} >14.4% [2]. Preconception care in diabetic women is associated with fewer maternal hospitalizations, less use of neonatal intensive care, and a reduction in major congenital anomalies and perinatal deaths [3]. The aim should be to maintain HbA_{1c} less than 7%. For this reason, treatment of the woman with insulin-dependent diabetes who is considering a pregnancy should be initiated before conception [4]. In addition, the preconception patient should be placed on 4mg/day folic acid supplementation in order to reduce the risk for neural tube defect. Thorough evaluation should be undertaken to detect evidence of maternal retinopathy, nephropathy, or coronary artery disease. For the most recent classification and diagnostic criteria for pregestational diabetes, refer to the report of the Expert Committee of the American Diabetes Association [5] and the American College of Obstetricians and Gynecologists (ACOG) technical bulletin addressing pregestational diabetes [6].

Initial evaluation

For women with previously diagnosed diabetes, it is important to take a careful history and perform a physical examination as soon as pregnancy is diagnosed, paying special attention to the following.
- Careful dating of the pregnancy by history, ultrasound and physical signs.
- Evaluation for presence of other co-morbid conditions.
- Progress and outcome of any previous pregnancies.
- Careful fundoscopic examination for the presence of retinopathy.

Queenan's Management of High-Risk Pregnancy: An Evidence-Based Approach, Sixth Edition. Edited by John T. Queenan, Catherine Y. Spong, Charles J. Lockwood.

Table 21.1 Risk of major malformation in fetuses of women with insulin-dependent diabetes according to HbA$_{1c}$ levels based on a compilation of seven studies of 1405 women

	Moderate HbA$_{1c}$	High HbA$_{1c}$	Highest HbA$_{1c}$
Major malformations	2.2%	8.6%	26.6%

The studies included used various methods to measure HbA$_{1c}$, resulting in different cut-offs. In general, comparing to current standards, moderate levels would correspond to less than 7, high would correspond to 7–10, and highest would correspond to more than 10.
Source: Kitzmiller *et al* [1].

• Findings of urinalysis and culture, as well as 24-h urine collection for creatinine clearance and protein.
• Baseline blood pressure measurement, electrocardiogram (ECG), and thyroid function tests.
• Baseline glycosylated hemoglobin measurement.
• Review of insulin dosage, nutrition, physical activity, and logs of home glucose monitoring.

Regulating maternal glycemia

Careful control of maternal glucose levels significantly improves perinatal outcome. Except during brief periods after meals, glucose should normally remain below 100 mg/dL. Maternal hyperglycemia and rapid fluctuations in blood glucose produce similar changes in the fetal compartment. Fetal hyperglycemia leads to β-cell hyperplasia and hyperinsulinemia. Also, there is a significant correlation between maternal glucose levels and subsequent adiposity in the infant. Ketoacidosis at any time during pregnancy may lead to death *in utero*. Management of diabetic ketoacidosis includes aggressive fluid and electrolyte replacement, in addition to insulin administration.

Maintenance of euglycemia depends not only on diligent regulation of diet and insulin, but also on strict attention to physical activity and stress. Patients should eat three meals and three snacks each day, adding up to 30–35 cal/kg of ideal bodyweight.

The most successful regimen of insulin administration usually includes two injections daily of both NPH and regular insulin. The amount of NPH insulin given in the morning generally exceeds that of regular insulin by a 2:1 ratio. In the evening, equal amounts of NPH and regular insulin are given. If several fasting or postprandial glucose levels are not acceptable (usually more than one-third of values), insulin doses are increased by 20%. Several days are then allowed to pass before further changes are made. The use of other insulin types or administration routes (e.g. short- or long-acting, insulin pump), as well as oral hypoglycemic agents, should be individualized and reserved for special circumstances [7]. Limited evidence suggests that pregestational women with diabetes who continue oral hypoglycemics when they become pregnant are at higher risk for complications [8]. Generally pregestational women with diabetes are best switched to and managed with insulin during pregnancy [9]. During labor, a continuous insulin infusion is best to stabilize maternal glucose levels and reduce neonatal hypoglycemia. The goal is to maintain hourly glucose levels at less than 110 mg/dL.

Glycemic control cannot be accurately assessed by random blood glucose determinations or by testing urine specimens for glucose. The patient should be taught to assess her capillary glucose levels by using reagent strips and a blood glucose reflectance meter. Determinations should be made in the fasting state and 2 h after meals. The goal of therapy is to maintain capillary whole-blood glucose levels as close to normal as possible, including a fasting glucose level of 95 mg/dL or less, and 2-h postprandial values of 120 mg/dL or less. When using a meter, it is imperative to determine whether it tests whole blood, serum or plasma, as results may vary (plasma levels approximately 10 mg/dL higher than whole blood). A blood glucose sample drawn 80 min after breakfast correlates well with the mean amplitude of glycemic excursions throughout the day. Measurements made before lunch, dinner, and bedtime may also be helpful; these premeal values should be 100 mg/dL or less. Some prefer to monitor 1-h postpartum glucose levels which should be at 140 mg/dL or less.

A useful parameter for assessing control over a prolonged period (4–8 weeks) is HbA$_{1c}$, a minor variant of HbA, produced by the addition of a single glucose moiety to the terminal valine of the β-chain. This glycosylated hemoglobin is synthesized throughout the red blood cell's life cycle in amounts that reflect the degree of chronic hyperglycemia present. Levels correlate significantly with mean fasting glucose, mean daily glucose, and highest daily glucose values. In normal pregnancy, glycosylated hemoglobin declines during the first and second trimesters, returning to baseline levels at term. To convert the HbA$_{1c}$ level to the mean glucose level, one can use the "rule of 8s." An HbA$_{1c}$ level of 8% reflects a mean glucose level of 180 mg/dL in most laboratories. Each change of 1% in the HbA$_{1c}$ value indicates a change of 30 mg/dL in mean glucose. There is a direct correlation between maternal third-trimester HbA$_{1c}$ levels and increased birthweight [10]. HbA$_{1c}$ should be checked every trimester.

The insulin requirement postpartum decreases dramatically (usually by 50%) and thus must be carefully monitored. Patients with type 1 diabetes are at increased risk for postpartum thyroiditis, so a high index of suspicion should be maintained.

Management during pregnancy

Major fetal malformations occur in around 5% of women with type 1 diabetes. Diabetes is not associated with an increase in the risk of fetal chromosomal abnormalities. During the second trimester, a careful evaluation for fetal malformations includes obtaining a maternal serum α-fetoprotein level at 16 weeks (helpful in detecting neural tube defects), a targeted ultrasound at 18–20 weeks, and fetal echocardiography at 20 weeks [11]. In addition, the rate of fetal growth, development of early signs of preeclampsia, and incidence of infection of the urinary tract or other sites are closely monitored. By accurately assessing fetal health and maturity, clinicians can prevent intrauterine deaths while safely prolonging pregnancy to avoid the hazards of iatrogenic prematurity.

At 28 weeks, daily maternal assessment of fetal activity is started. Twice-weekly nonstress tests (NSTs) are ordered at 32 weeks, or earlier if there are other maternal or fetal complications (e.g. hypertension, growth restriction) [12]. A nonreactive NST must be followed by a biophysical profile or contraction stress test. Antepartum heart rate testing using the twice-weekly NSTs has proved to be a reliable index of fetal well-being in a metabolically stable patient [13]. Timing of delivery should be individualized and depends on glycemic control, presence of associated maternal complications, and fetal status [14]. Ideally, the pregnant patients with diabetes should not go beyond 40 weeks' gestation. In general, presence of co-morbidity (hypertension), complications of diabetes (vasculopathy, nephropathy), poor glycemic control, or fetal growth abnormalities would favor earlier delivery, while absence of any of these factors would favor expectant management until the expected date of delivery. Presence of more than one of these factors would tip the balance further toward earlier delivery.

Unless indicated for obstetric (preeclampsia, abruptio) or fetal (nonreassuring surveillance) reasons, delivery of the patient with diabetes prior to 39 weeks requires confirmation of fetal lung maturity by amniocentesis. Traditionally, presence of phosphatidylglycerol was required to confirm fetal lung maturity in women with diabetes. However, fetal lung maturity levels >70 mg/g are now accepted as evidence of fetal lung maturity [15,16].

Finally, in order to avoid birth injury from fetal macrosomia, a liberal attitude toward cesarean delivery (CD) should be employed in such cases. Sonographic assessment of estimated fetal weight and growth of the abdominal circumference is of value in detecting fetal macrosomia. If the estimated fetal weight exceeds 4500 g, delivery by elective CD should be considered. A macrosomic fetus, particularly in the presence of polyhydramnios, is usually an indication of poor glycemic control. These patients may be delivered at 38 weeks after documentation of fetal lung maturity [17].

Management of insulin during labor

When delivery is scheduled, the usual dose of insulin should be given at bedtime and the morning dose should be withheld [6]. The patient should be admitted early in the morning and a saline infusion started. Glucose levels should be checked hourly, and the infusion changed to 5% dextrose if the glucose level drops below 70 mg/dl. The rate of glucose infusion should be adjusted to keep the glucose level at about 100 mg/dl. If the glucose level is above 100 mg/dl on saline infusion, then infusion of regular insulin is needed. Regular short-acting insulin can be started at 1 U/h and titrated to keep the glucose level below 100 mg/dL. When the delivery is unscheduled, then the patient's usual intermittent insulin doses should be withheld and she should be managed similar to the scheduled patient. If the patient is on subcutaneous insulin pump, she may continue her basal rate.

Insulin requirements decrease rapidly after delivery. The patient can be restarted on half of her predelivery insulin dose as soon as she is eating regular food. For postoperative patients, sliding scale insulin regimen may be instituted until the patient is tolerating regular food.

CASE PRESENTATION

A 30-year-old gravida 4, para 3 was first seen at 18 weeks' gestation. Her past obstetric history included the vaginal delivery of a 4100 g baby boy, who suffered a fractured humerus during delivery. The patient's mother had diabetes mellitus. Plasma glucose was obtained 1 h after a 50 g oral glucose load and was found to be 175 mg/dL. A 3-h OGTT was then ordered. The results were as follows: fasting, 110 mg/dL; 1 h, 243 mg/dL; 2 h, 176 mg/dL; and 3 h, 154 mg/dL. Pregestational diabetes was suspected.

The patient was started on a 2200-calorie diet with strict avoidance of concentrated sweets. Fasting and postprandial capillary glucose determinations were obtained daily. The fasting values ranged from 100 to 110 mg/dL, so she was started on split-dose insulin. Fetal growth was normal, and the patient remained normotensive. Antepartum fetal evaluation was initiated with twice-weekly nonstress testing initiated at 32 weeks. Her glucose levels remained within the acceptable range. At 40 weeks, the estimated fetal weight was 4600 g. A cesarean delivery was performed. A 2-h OGTT performed at 6 weeks postpartum confirmed type 2 diabetes.

References

1. Kitzmiller JL, Buchanan TA, Kjos S et al. Preconception care of diabetes, congenital malformations, and spontaneous abortions. Diabetes Care 1996;19:514–541.
2. Greene MF, Hare JW, Cloherty JP, Benacerraf BR, Soeldner JS. First-trimester hemoglobin A1 and risk for major malformation and spontaneous abortion in diabetic pregnancy. Teratology 2002;65:97–101.
3. Korenbrot CC, Steinberg A, Bender C, Newberry S. Preconception care: a systematic review. Matern Child Health J 2002;6:75–88.
4. American Diabetes Association. Preconception care of women with diabetes. Diabetes Care 2004;27(Suppl 1):S76–78.
5. Expert Committee on the Diagnosis and Classification of Diabetes Mellitus, American Diabetes Association. Report of the Expert Committee on the Diagnosis and Classification of Diabetes Mellitus. Diabetes Care 2003;26(Suppl 1):S5–20.
6. American College of Obstetricians and Gynecologists. Pregestational diabetes mellitus. ACOG Practice Bulletin No. 60. Obstet Gynecol 2005;105:675–685.
7. Siebenhofer A, Plank J, Berghold A et al. Short acting insulin analogues versus regular human insulin in patients with diabetes mellitus. Cochrane Metabolic and Endocrine Disorders Group. Cochrane Database Syst Rev 2006;2:CD003287.
8. Hughes RC, Rowen JA. Pregnancy in women with type 2 diabetes: who takes metformin and what is the outcome? Diabet Med 2006;23:318–322.
9. Ekpebegh CO, Coetzee EJ, van der Merwe L, Levitt NS. A 10-year retrospective analysis of pregnancy outcome in pregestational type 2 diabetes: comparison of insulin and oral glucose-lowering agents. Diabet Med 2007;24(3):253–258.
10. Widness JA, Schwartz HC, Thompson D et al. Glycohemoglobin (HbA$_{1c}$): a predictor of birth weight in infants of diabetic mothers. J Pediatr 1978;92:8.
11. Albert TJ, Landon MB, Wheller JJ et al. Prenatal detection of fetal anomalies in pregnancies complicated by insulin-dependent diabetes mellitus. Am J Obstet Gynecol 1996;174:1424–1428.
12. Landon MB, Langer O, Gabbe SG et al. Fetal surveillance in pregnancies complicated by insulin-dependent diabetes mellitus. Am J Obstet Gynecol 1992;167:617–621.
13. Gabbe SG, Graves CR. Management of diabetes mellitus complicating pregnancy. Obstet Gynecol 2003;102:857–868.
14. Boulvain M, Stan C, Irion O. Elective delivery in diabetic pregnant women. Cochrane Pregnancy and Childbirth Group. Cochrane Database Syst Rev 2006;2:CD000451.
15. Del Valle GO, Adair CD, Ramos EE, Gaudier FL, Sanchez-Ramos L, Morales R. Interpretation of the TDx-FLM fluorescence polarization assay in pregnancies complicated by diabetes mellitus. Am J Perinatol 1997;14(5):241–244.
16. Livingston EG, Herbert WN, Hage ML, Chapman JF, Stubbs TM. Use of the TDx-FLM assay in evaluating fetal lung maturity in an insulin-dependent diabetic population. The Diabetes and Fetal Maturity Study Group. Obstet Gynecol 1995;86(5):826–829.
17. American College of Obstetricians and Gynecologists. Macrosomia. ACOG Practice Bulletin No. 22. Washington, DC: ACOG; 2000.

Chapter 22
Hypothyroidism and Hyperthyroidism

Brian Casey

Department of Obstetrics and Gynecology, University of Texas Southwestern Medical Center, Dallas, TX, USA

Hypothyroidism

Overview

Hypothyroidism complicates 1–3 in 1000 pregnancies. Women with overt hypothyroidism are at increased risk for complications such as early pregnancy failure, preeclampsia, placental abruption, low birthweight, and stillbirth [1,2]. Treatment of women with hypothyroidism has been associated with improved pregnancy outcomes. Subclinical hypothyroidism affects 2–3% of pregnant women [3,4] and has recently been implicated in impaired neurologic development in offspring [5], as well as an increase in pregnancy complications such as preterm birth, placental abruption, and fetal death [4,6]. These findings have prompted calls for routine thyroid screening during pregnancy for subclinical hypothyroidism. One study has even suggested that such screening would be cost-effective under a wide range of circumstances [7]. However, there have been no randomized clinical trials confirming the efficacy of early pregnancy treatment and/or screening for subclinical hypothyroidism and this topic remains an area of controversy.

The most common cause of primary hypothyroidism in pregnancy is chronic autoimmune thyroiditis (Hashimoto thyroiditis). This is a painless inflammation with progressive enlargement of the thyroid gland which is characterized by diffuse lymphocytic infiltration, fibrosis, parenchymal atrophy, and eosinophilic change. Other important causes of primary hypothyroidism include endemic iodine deficiency and a history of either ablative radio-iodine therapy or thyroidectomy. Secondary hypothyroidism is pituitary in origin. For example, Sheehan syndrome resulting from prior obstetric hemorrhage is characterized by pituitary ischemia and necrosis, with subsequent deficiencies in some or all pituitary responsive hormones. Other etiologies of secondary hypothyroidism include lymphocytic hypophysitis and a history of a hypophysectomy. Tertiary or hypothalamic hypothyroidism is very rare.

Presentation

Clinical hypothyroidism is often characterized by vague, nonspecific signs or symptoms which are insidious in onset. Initial symptoms include fatigue, constipation, cold intolerance, and muscle cramps. These may progress to insomnia, weight gain, carpal tunnel syndrome, hair loss, voice changes, and intellectual slowness. The presence of an enlarged thyroid gland is dependent upon the etiology of hypothyroidism. Specifically, women in areas of endemic iodine deficiency and those with Hashimoto thyroiditis are much more likely to have a goiter. Other signs of hypothyroidism include periorbital edema, dry skin, and prolonged relaxation phase of deep tendon reflexes.

The diagnosis of clinical hypothyroidism during pregnancy is especially difficult because many of the signs or symptoms listed above may be attributed to the pregnancy itself. For example, pregnancy is accompanied by moderate enlargement of the thyroid gland from hyperplasia of glandular tissue and increased vascularity. By definition, subclinical hypothyroidism occurs in asymptomatic women whose thyroid-stimulating hormone (TSH) concentration is above the statistically defined upper limit of normal while their serum free thyroxine (fT_4) concentration is within its reference range [3].

Diagnosis

The diagnosis of hypothyroidism is generally established by an elevated serum TSH and a low serum fT_4. If the free thyroxine concentration is low in the presence of a normal or depressed TSH, then pituitary (central) hypothyroidism should be suspected. The nonpregnancy reference ranges for serum TSH and fT_4 concentration are

Queenan's Management of High-Risk Pregnancy: An Evidence-Based Approach, Sixth Edition. Edited by John T. Queenan, Catherine Y. Spong, Charles J. Lockwood.

0.4–4.5 mIU/L and 0.7–1.8 ng/dL, respectively. During pregnancy, maternal serum chorionic gonadotropin (hCG) peaks at approximately 10 weeks' gestation and has some thyroid stimulating activity as a result of its structural homology with TSH. This results in a decrease in the maternal serum TSH and a modest increase in fT_4 during the first trimester [8].

These physiologic changes confound the laboratory diagnosis of hypothyroidism during pregnancy and underscore the need for gestational age-specific TSH and possibly fT_4 thresholds. Such TSH thresholds have been established from a large population-based screening study of pregnant women in Dallas [9]. From these data, the upper limit of the statistically defined normal range for TSH (97.5th percentile) in the first half of pregnancy was 3.0 mU/L. A more recent study of 4000 Italian women has demonstrated that those with a first-trimester TSH between 2.5 and 5.0 mIU/L were at increased risk for pregnancy loss [10]. This led the authors to conclude that the upper limit of normal in the first trimester should be redefined as 2.5 mIU/L. Similar gestational age-specific fT_4 thresholds have been derived for the cohort from Dallas [11]. Even though pregnancy is associated with significant shifts in free thyroxine, overall, fT_4 levels remain within the nonpregnancy reference range [8].

Finally, it may be helpful to confirm the presence of either antimicrosomal or antithyroglobulin antibodies in cases where autoimmune thyroiditis is suspected. Specifically, the presence of antithyroid antibodies may identify a population of women at particular risk for pregnancy complications or progression to symptomatic disease. For example, in one recent study, more than 47% of women who tested positive for thyroid peroxidase antibodies early in pregnancy developed postpartum thyroid dysfunction [12].

Management and treatment

The goal of treatment for pregnant women with overt hypothyroidism is clinical and biochemical euthyroidism. Levothyroxine sodium is the treatment of choice for routine management of hypothyroidism. Starting doses usually range from 1.6 to 1.8 μg/kg/day. Serum TSH is then measured at 4–6-week intervals and thyroxine is adjusted by 25–50 μg increments. Women who have hypothyroidism at the time of conception should have a serum TSH evaluated at their first prenatal visit. An increased requirement for thyroid replacement in hypothyroid women during pregnancy has been demonstrated [13]. Because of the risks for early pregnancy failure and the potential for neurodevelopmental impairment in offspring, some have recommended that hypothyroid women increase levothyroxine dose by 30% when pregnancy is confirmed [13]. However, the etiology of hypothyroidism is very important in determining the timing and magnitude of these adjustments [14].

Moreover, this practice has not been shown to be beneficial and thyroid treatment is probably best guided through evaluation of thyroid function studies. Therefore, it is recommended that serum TSH be measured at least each trimester during pregnancy. Notably, several drugs may interfere with levothyroxine absorption (e.g. cholestyramine, ferrous sulfate, aluminum hydroxide in antacids) or its metabolism (e.g. phenytoin, carbamazepine, and rifampin).

Treatment of women with subclinical hypothyroidism is controversial. A report has linked subclinical hypothyroidism during pregnancy with subsequent neurodevelopmental complications in offspring [5]. These findings have led to recommendations for treatment of subclinical hypothyroidism to restore the TSH to the reference range [15]. Importantly, however, there are no published intervention trials assessing the safety or efficacy of screening and treatment to improve neuropsychologic performance in such offspring. Currently, routine screening and treatment of subclinical hypothyroidism during pregnancy are not recommended by the American College of Obstetricians and Gynecologists [16].

Follow-up

After completion of pregnancy, the levothyroxine dose should be restored to the prepregnancy value and a TSH should be checked 6–8 weeks postpartum. Breastfeeding is not contraindicated in women treated for hypothyroidism. Levothyroxine is excreted into breastmilk but levels are too low to alter thyroid function in the infant or to interfere with neonatal thyroid screening programs [17]. Periodic monitoring of hypothyroidism with an annual serum TSH concentration is advised because of the impact of changing weight and age on thyroid function. Women with subclinical hypothyroidism, particularly those with thyroid autoantibodies, are at an increased risk for developing clinical disease within 5 years. While treatment of these women is not recommended, yearly evaluation for the development of clinically apparent disease is recommended.

Hyperthyroidism

Overview

Hyperthyroidism complicates approximately 1–2 in 1000 pregnancies. The overwhelming cause of hyperthyroidism during pregnancy is Graves disease or autoimmune thyrotoxicosis. Pregnant women with hyperthyroidism are at increased risk for congestive heart failure, thyroid storm, preterm labor, preeclampsia, fetal growth restriction, and perinatal mortality. Treatment of hyperthyroid women to achieve adequate metabolic control will result in improved pregnancy outcomes. However, overtreatment may result in maternal or fetal hypothyroidism. Gestational transient thyrotoxicosis (GTT) is 10 times more prevalent than Graves disease and may be caused by the elevated hCG values typically observed with hyperemesis gravidarum. Subclinical hyperthyroidism affects 1.7% of pregnant women and has only recently been introduced into clinical practice because of the development of extremely sensitive serum TSH assays. Subclinical hyperthyroidism is not associated with any adverse maternal pregnancy outcomes [18]. Treatment of the latter two clinical entities has not been shown to be beneficial.

Graves disease is an organ-specific autoimmune process in which thyroid-stimulating autoantibodies attach to and activate TSH receptors. Other less common causes include toxic multinodular goiter, subacute thyroiditis, adenoma, or iodine-induced thyrotoxicosis. Thyrotropin receptor activation by hCG, which has some cross-reactivity with TSH, explains the biochemical and occasional clinical findings of thyrotoxicosis in women with hyperemesis gravidarum and gestational trophoblastic decrease.

Presentation

As with hypothyroidism, clinical features of hyperthyroidism can be easily confused with physiologic symptoms of pregnancy. Suggestive complaints or findings include nervousness, heat intolerance, palpitations, goiter, failure to gain weight or weight loss, and exophthalmos. GTT usually occurs in women with hyperemesis gravidarum. Subclinical hyperthyroidism, defined as a serum TSH concentration below the statistically defined lower limit of normal with a serum concentration of fT_4 within the reference range, is typically identified in asymptomatic women.

Diagnosis

In women with a depressed serum TSH level (<0.4 mIU/L), clinical hyperthyroidism is confirmed by an elevation in fT_4 (>1.8 ng/dL) concentration. As is true for the diagnosis of hypothyroidism, one must consider the impact of pregnancy on TSH and possibly fT_4. Rarely, hyperthyroidism is caused by abnormally high serum triiodothyronine values (T_3 thyrotoxicosis). In women with depressed TSH yet normal fT_4, evaluation of fT_3 or free T_3 index may explain a patient's hypermetabolic symptoms. Also, evaluation of TSH receptor antibodies may be helpful in evaluation of women with Graves disease to identify those at risk for delivery of an infant with fetal or neonatal hyperthyroidism.

Management and treatment

Thyrotoxicosis during pregnancy can nearly always be controlled by thioamide drugs and treatment has been associated with improved pregnancy outcomes [19,20]. Some clinicians prefer propylthiouracil because it inhibits peripheral conversion of T_4 to T_3 and it crosses the placenta less readily than methimazole. Methimazole used in early pregnancy has also been associated with esophageal and choanal atresia as well as aplasia cutis [21–24]. Transient leukopenia occurs in approximately 10% of women treated with thioamides, but this does not require cessation of therapy. In approximately 0.2%, agranulocytosis develops suddenly, is not dose related, and, because of its acute onset, serial leukocyte counts during therapy are not helpful. Rather, if fever or sore throat develops, patients should be instructed to discontinue medication immediately and report for a complete blood count.

The dose of propylthiouracil is empirical, and the American Thyroid Association recommends an initial daily dose of 100–600 mg for propylthiouracil or 10–40 mg for methimazole [25]. Women with overt hyperthyroidism diagnosed during pregnancy may require a higher initial dose between 300 and 450 mg/day. The starting daily dose of methimazole is 20–40 mg. The goal of therapy is clinical euthyroidism with free thyroxine in the upper range of normal [26]. The median time to normalization of thyroid function tests is 6–8 weeks, but TSH levels may remain suppressed beyond normalization of fT_4. Once euthyroidism is achieved, serial measurement of TSH and fT_4 during each trimester is recommended.

There is currently no convincing evidence that subclinical hyperthyroidism should be treated in nonpregnant individuals [18]. In fact, it should be considered contraindicated during pregnancy because maternal antithyroid drugs cross the placenta and may cause fetal thyroid suppression. There are other alternatives for treatment of overt hyperthyroidism which are rarely undertaken during pregnancy. For example, although thyroidectomy is typically reserved for treatment outside pregnancy, pregnant women who cannot adhere to medical therapy or in whom therapy is toxic may benefit from surgical management [27]. Ablative radio-active iodine is contraindicated in pregnancy as it can cause fetal thyroid destruction.

Thyroid storm

Thyroid storm and heart failure are rare and acute life-threatening exacerbations of thyrotoxicosis. Women with thyroid storm classically present with fever, tachycardia, nausea, diarrhea, dehydration, and delirium or coma. Treatment of thyrotoxic storm or heart failure is similar and should be carried out in an intensive care setting. Specific treatment consists of 1 g propylthiouracil (PTU) given orally or crushed and placed through a nasogastric tube. PTU is continued in 200 mg doses every 6 h. An hour after initial PTU dosing, iodide is given to inhibit thyroid release of T_3 and T_4. It is given every 8 h intravenously as 500–1000 mg sodium iodide or it can be given orally as five drops of supersaturated solution of potassium iodide

(SSKI) or as 10 drops of Lugol solution every 8 h. With a history of iodine-induced anaphylaxis, lithium carbonate, 300 mg every 6 h, is given instead. Dexamethasone can be used to further block peripheral conversion of T_4 to T_3 and may be given intravenously as 2 mg every 6 h for a total of four doses. β-Blocker therapy such as propranolol, labetalol, and esmolol to control tachycardia have all been used successfully intrapartum.

Follow-up

Women with Graves disease should be followed closely after delivery because recurrence or aggravation of symptoms is not uncommon in the first few months postpartum. Asymptomatic women should have a TSH and fT_4 performed approximately 6 weeks postpartum. Both PTU and methimazole are excreted in breastmilk, PTU less so than methimazole. PTU is largely protein bound and does not seem to pose a significant risk to the breastfed infant. Methimazole has been found in breastfed infants of treated women in amounts sufficient to cause thyroid dysfunction; however, at low doses (10–20 mg/day) methimazole does not appear to pose a major risk to the nursing infant [28]. The American Academy of Pediatrics considers both compatible with breast-feeding [29].

Postpartum thyroiditis

Transient autoimmune thyroiditis has been identified in up to 10% of women during the first year after childbirth [30,31]. The likelihood of developing postpartum thyroiditis antedates pregnancy and is related to increasing serum levels of thyroid autoantibodies. Women with high antibody titers in early pregnancy are most commonly affected [32]. In clinical practice, postpartum thyroiditis is infrequently diagnosed because it typically develops months after delivery and has vague and nonspecific symptoms. These include depression, carelessness, and memory impairment [33]. Risk factors other than antithyroid antibodies include previous thyroid dysfunction or a family history of thyroid or other autoimmune disease. For example, 25% of women with type 1 diabetes develop postpartum thyroid dysfunction [34].

There are two recognized clinical phases of postpartum thyroiditis. Between 1 and 4 months after delivery, approximately 4% of all women develop transient thyrotoxicosis from excessive release of hormone caused by glandular disruption [35]. The onset is abrupt, and a small, painless goiter is commonly found. Fatigue and palpitations are the most common complaints in women with early postpartum thyroiditis. Antithyroid medications such as thioamides are typically ineffective and approximately two-thirds of these women spontaneously return to a euthyroid state. Between 4 and 8 months postpartum, 2–5% of women develop hypothyroidism [30,35]. However, hypothyroidism can even develop within 1 month of the onset of thyroiditis. Thyromegaly and other symptoms are common and more prominent than during the thyrotoxic phase. Thyroxine replacement is recommended for at least 6–12 months. Importantly, women who experience either type of postpartum thyroiditis have an approximately 30% risk of developing permanent hypothyroidism [36].

CASE PRESENTATION

A 32-year-old woman who was previously diagnosed with hypothyroidism and currently taking 100 µg levothyroxine presented for prenatal care at 12 weeks' gestation. At that time her TSH was 7.8 mU/L and her fT_4 was 0.54 ng/dL. Her levothyroxine dose was increased to 125 µg and thyroid function testing was planned for 4 weeks hence. Repeat thyroid studies were TSH 2.3 mU/L and fT_4 1.0 ng/dL. Normal ranges for TSH and fT_4 were 0.4–4.5 mU/L and 0.7–1.8 ng/dL, respectively. Further thyroid function testing was performed at 24 weeks' gestation (TSH 1.8 mU/L and fT_4 1.1 ng/dL) and 32 weeks' gestation (TSH 2.2 mU/L and fT_4 0.9 ng/dL). No further change in therapy was prescribed.

During a routine prenatal care visit at 37 weeks' gestation, she was found to have a blood pressure of 144/98 mmHg. Laboratory evaluation revealed an aspartate aminotransferase (AST) of 92 U/L, a platelet count of $236 × 10^3$/L and 3 proteinuria. A labor induction for severe preeclampsia with magnesium sulfate seizure prophylaxis was initiated. Hydralazine was given during the intrapartum period for severe hypertension. A cesarean delivery for fetal distress was performed. The infant weighed 3205 g and Apgar scores were 7 and 9 at 1 and 5 min. There was no evidence of placental abruption. The postpartum course was further complicated by a postpartum hemorrhage with a total estimated blood loss of 2000 mL, for which the patient received a blood transfusion. Upon discharge, she was instructed regarding the safety of breastfeeding while taking levothyroxine and to resume taking 100 µg levothyroxine each day. Repeat thyroid function testing was scheduled for 6 weeks postpartum.

References

1. Davis LE, Leveno KJ, Cunningham FG. Hypothyroidism complicating pregnancy. Obstet Gynecol 1988;72:108.

2. Leung AS, Millar LK, Koonings PP, Montoro M, Mestman JH. Perinatal outcome in hypothyroid pregnancies. Obstet Gynecol 1993;81:349–353.

3. Surks MI, Ortiz E, Daniels GH et al. Subclinical thyroid disease, scientific review and guidelines for diagnosis and management. JAMA 2004;291:228–238.

4. Casey BM, Dashe JS, Wells CE et al. Pregnancy outcomes in women with subclinical thyroid insufficiency. Obstet Gynecol 2005;105:239–245.

5. Haddow JE, Palomaki GE, Allan WC et al. Maternal thyroid deficiency during pregnancy and subsequent neuropsychological development of the child. N Engl J Med 1999;341:1549–1555.

6. Allan WC, Haddow JE, Palomaki GE et al. Maternal thyroid deficiency and pregnancy complications: implications for population screening. J Med Screen 2000;7:127–130.

7. Thung SF, Funai EF, Grobman WA. The cost-effectiveness of universal screening in pregnancy for subclinical hypothyroidism. Am J Obstet Gynecol 2009;200:267.

8. Glinoer D, de Nayer P, Bourdoux P et al. Regulation of maternal thyroid during pregnancy. J Clin Endocrinol Metab 1990;71:276–287.

9. Dashe JS, Casey BM, Wells CE et al. Thyroid-stimulating hormone in singleton and twin pregnancy: importance of gestational age-specific reference ranges. Obstet Gynecol 2005;106:753–757.

10. Negro R, Schwartz A, Gismondi R, Tinelli A, Mangieri T, Stagnaro-Green A. Increased pregnancy loss rate in thyroid antibody negative women with TSH levels between 2.5 and 5.0 in the first trimester of pregnancy. J Clin Endocrinol Metab 2010;95:E44–E48.

11. Casey BM, Dashe JS, Spong CY, McIntire DD, Leveno KL, Cunningham GF. Perinatal significance of isolated maternal hypothyroxinemia identified in the first half of pregnancy. Obstet Gynecol 2007;109:1129–1135.

12. Premawardhana LD, Parkes AB, John R, Harris B, Lazarus JH. Thyroid peroxidase antibodies in early pregnancy: utility for prediction of postpartum thyroid dysfunction and implications for screening. Thyroid 2004;14:610–615.

13. Alexander EK, Marqusee E, Lawrence J, Jarolim P, Fischer GA, Larsen PR. Timing and magnitude of increases in levothyroxine requirements during pregnancy in women with hypothyroidism. N Engl J Med 2004;351:241–249.

14. Loh JA, Wartofsky L, Jonklaas J, Burman KD. The magnitude of increased levothyroxine requirements in hypothyroid pregnant women depends upon the etiology of the hypothyroidism. Thyroid 2009;19:269–275.

15. Gharib H, Tuttle RM, Baskin HJ, Fish LH, Singer PA, McDermott MT. Consensus Statement No 1. Subclinical Thyroid Dysfunction: a joint statement on management from the American Association of Clinical Endocrinologists, the American Thyroid Association, and the Endocrine Society. Thyroid 2005;15:24–28.

16. American College of Obstetricians and Gynecologists. Thyroid disease in pregnancy. ACOG Practice Bulletin No. 37. Obstet Gynecol 2002;100:387–396.

17. Franklin R, O'Grady C, Carpenter L. Neonatal thyroid function: comparison between breast-fed and bottle-fed infants. J Pediatr 1985;106:124–126.

18. Casey BM, Dashe JS, Wells CE, McIntire DD, Leveno KJ, Cunningham FG. Subclinical hyperthyroidism and pregnancy outcomes. Obstet Gynecol 2006;107:337–341.

19. Davis LE, Lucas MJ, Hankins GD, Roark ML, Cunningham FG. Thyrotoxicosis complicating pregnancy. Am J Obstet Gynecol 1989;160:63–70.

20. Millar KJ, Wing DA, Leung AS, Koonings PP, Montoro MN, Mestman JH. Low birth weight and preeclampsia in pregnancies complicated by hyperthyroidism. Obstet Gynecol 1994;84:946–949.

21. Milham S Jr, Elledge W. Maternal methimazole and congenital defects in children. Teratology 1972;5:125.

22. Clementi M, di Gianantonio E, Pelo E, Manni I, Basile RT, Tenconi R. Methimazole embryopathy: delineation of the phenotype. Am J Med Genet 1999;83:43–46.

23. Di Gianantino E, Schaefer C, Mastroiacovo P et al. Adverse effects of prenatal methimazole exposure. Teratology 2001;64:262–266.

24. Mandel S, Cooper D. The use of antithyroid drugs in pregnancy and lactation. J Clin Endocrinol Metab 2001;86:2354–2359.

25. Singer PA, Cooper DS, Levy EG et al. Treatment guidelines for patients with hyperthyroidism and hypothyroidism. JAMA 1995;273:808–812.

26. Brent GA. Graves' disease. N Engl J Med 2008;358:2594–2595.

27. Davison S, Lennard TWJ, Davison H et al. Management of a pregnant patient with Graves' disease complicated by thionamide-induced neutropenia in the first trimester. Clin Endocrinol 2001;54:559.

28. Cooper DS. Antithyroid drugs: to breast-feed or not to breast-feed. Am J Obstet Gynecol 1987;157:234–235.

29. American Academy of Pediatrics Committee on Drugs. The transfer of drugs and other chemicals into human milk. Pediatrics 2001;108:776–789.

30. Jansson R, Dahlberg PA, Karlsson FA. Postpartum thyroiditis. Baillière's Clin Endocrinol Metab 1988;2:619–635.

31. Muller AF, Drexhage HA, Berghout A. Postpartum thyroiditis and autoimmune thyroiditis in women of childbearing age: recent insights and consequences for antenatal and postnatal care. Endo Rev 2001;22:605–630.

32. Premawardhana LD, Parkes AB, Ammari F et al. Postpartum thyroiditis and long-term thyroid status: prognostic influence of thyroid peroxidase antibodies and ultrasound echogenicity. J Clin Endocrinol Metab 2000;85:71–75.

33. Amino N, Tada H, Hidaka Y, Izumi Y. Postpartum autoimmune thyroid syndrome. Endocr J 2000;47:645–655.

34. Alvarez-Marfany M, Roman SH, Drexler AJ, Robertson C, Stagnaro-Green A. Long-term prospective study of postpartum thyroid dysfunction in women with insulin dependent diabetes mellitus. J Clin Endocrinol Metab 1994;79:10–16.

35. Pearce EN, Farwell AP, Braverman LE. Thyroiditis. N Engl J Med 2003;348:2646–2655.

36. Dayan CM, Daniels GH. Chronic autoimmune thyroiditis. N Engl J Med 1996;335:99–107.

Chapter 23
Asthma

Michael Schatz
Department of Allergy, Kaiser Permanente Medical Center, San Diego, CA, USA

Recent data suggest that asthma affects 4–8% of pregnant women [1], making it probably the most common, potentially serious medical problem to complicate pregnancy. Moreover, the prevalence of asthma during pregnancy appears to be increasing [1,2]. Although data have been conflicting, the largest recent studies [3–6] have suggested that maternal asthma increases the risk of perinatal mortality, preeclampsia, preterm birth, and low-birthweight infants. More severe asthma is associated with increased risks [3,5], while better controlled asthma is associated with decreased risks [7–11]. The course of asthma may also change during pregnancy; some women improve while others worsen [12]. This chapter reviews the definition and diagnosis of asthma and the interrelationships between asthma and pregnancy as a prelude to discussing the management of asthma in pregnant women.

Definition of asthma

Asthma is an inflammatory disease of the airways that is associated with reversible airway obstruction and airway hyperreactivity to a variety of stimuli. Although the cause of asthma is unknown, a number of clinical triggering factors exist, including viral infections, allergens, exercise, sinusitis, reflux, weather changes, and stress.

Airway obstruction in asthma can be produced by varying degrees of mucosal edema, bronchoconstriction, mucus plugging, and airway remodeling. In acute asthma, these changes can lead to ventilation/perfusion imbalance and hypoxia. Although early acute asthma is typically associated with hyperventilation and hypocapnea, progressive acute asthma can cause respiratory failure with associated carbon dioxide retention and acidosis.

Effect of pregnancy on the course of asthma

Clinical observations

A metaanalysis of 14 studies evaluating the effect of pregnancy on the course of asthma, which included 1658 patients, came to the conclusion that asthma severity improves in one-third of women, worsens in one-third, and remains unchanged in one-third [12]. However, a more recent and critical review of the literature found only three studies of 54 women that were prospective, enrolled women before the third trimester, and assessed their patients with objective measures of asthma severity or validated severity scales [13]. In a recent large prospective study of 1739 pregnant asthmatic women, severity classification (based on symptoms, pulmonary function, and medication use) worsened in 30% and improved in 23% of patients during pregnancy [14]. Asthma appears to be more likely to be more severe or to worsen during pregnancy in women who have more severe asthma before becoming pregnant [12,15].

The course of asthma may vary by stage of pregnancy. The first trimester is generally well tolerated in asthmatics, with infrequent acute episodes [16–18]. Increased symptoms and more frequent exacerbations have been reported to occur between weeks 17 and 36 of gestation [16–18]. In contrast, asthmatic women in general tend to experience fewer symptoms and less frequent asthma exacerbations during weeks 37–40 of pregnancy than during any earlier 4-week gestational period [17,18]. These studies suggest that the first trimester and the last month of pregnancy are relatively free of asthma exacerbations and that the second and earlier third trimester have more potential for increased asthma symptoms.

The variable effect of pregnancy on the course of asthma appears to be more than just random fluctuation in the

Queenan's Management of High-Risk Pregnancy: An Evidence-Based Approach, Sixth Edition. Edited by John T. Queenan, Catherine Y. Spong, Charles J. Lockwood.

natural history of the disease, because pregnancy-associated changes usually revert toward the prepregnancy state by 3 months postpartum [17]. It is also of interest that the course of asthma is often consistent in an individual woman during successive pregnancies [17,19].

Mechanisms

The mechanisms responsible for the altered clinical course of asthma during pregnancy are unknown and represent a fertile area for additional research. There are multiple biochemical and physiologic changes during pregnancy that could potentially ameliorate or exacerbate gestational asthma [20]. However, it is not clear which, if any, of these factors are actually important in determining the course of asthma during pregnancy.

There are additional factors that may contribute to the clinical course of asthma during pregnancy. Pregnancy may be a source of stress for many women, and this stress can aggravate asthma. Adherence to therapy can change during pregnancy with a corresponding change in asthma control. Most commonly observed is decreased adherence as a result of a mother's concerns about the safety of medications for the fetus.

Physician reluctance to treat may also affect the severity of asthma during pregnancy. A surveillance study identified 51 pregnant women and 500 nonpregnant women presenting to the emergency department with acute asthma [21]. Although asthma severity appeared to be similar in the two groups based on peak flow rates, pregnant women were significantly less likely to be treated with systemic steroids in the emergency department (44% versus 66%) and significantly less likely to be discharged on oral steroids (38% versus 64%). Presumably related to this undertreatment, pregnant women were three times more likely than nonpregnant women to report an ongoing exacerbation 2 weeks later (P = 0.02).

Infections during pregnancy can certainly affect the course of gestational asthma. Some degree of decrease in cell-mediated immunity may make the pregnant patient more susceptible to viral infections, and upper respiratory tract infections have been reported to be the most common precipitants of asthma exacerbations during pregnancy [19,22]. Sinusitis, a known asthma trigger, has been shown to be six times more common in pregnant compared with nonpregnant women [23]. In addition, pneumonia has been reported to be greater than five times more common in asthmatic than nonasthmatic women during pregnancy [24].

Finally, changes in specific immunoglobulin E (IgE) or environmental exposure may influence the gestational asthma course. Most pregnant asthmatic patients are atopic. A positive correlation between levels of specific IgE against cockroach antigen and gestational asthma severity has been described in pregnant inner-city women [25].

Effect of asthma on pregnancy

Clinical observations

Controlled studies that have evaluated outcomes of pregnancy in asthmatic compared with nonasthmatic women were reviewed in detail [26], with only a few important relevant articles published since [6,27–30]. The largest single comprehensive study [4] described the outcomes of pregnancy in 36,985 women identified as having asthma in either the Swedish Medical Birth Registry and/or the Swedish Hospital Discharge Registry. These outcomes were compared with the total of 1.32 million births that occurred in the Swedish population during the years of the study (1984–95). Significantly increased rates of preeclampsia (odds ratio [OR] 1.15), perinatal mortality (OR 1.21), preterm births (OR 1.15), and low-birthweight infants (OR 1.21), but not congenital malformations (OR 1.05), were found in the pregnancies of asthmatic versus control women. The risks appeared to be greater in patients with more severe asthma, which was confirmed in a more recent Swedish Birth Registry report [29].

In contrast to older studies and retrospective studies, more recent prospective cohort studies [27,31–33] have not generally reported increased risks of perinatal complications in the pregnancies of women with asthma, suggesting either a previous ascertainment bias or that prospective asthma management may reduce perinatal risks. Two recent case–control studies have reported marginal increased risks of congenital malformations in infants of mothers with versus without asthma (OR 1.2, 95% confidence interval [CI] 1.0–1.3 [34]; OR 1.1, 95% CI 1.0–1.2 [35]) and a recent large cohort study reported a marginal increased risk in infants of mothers with asthma (defined as those receiving asthma medications) compared to infants of mothers without asthma [36]. In addition to fetal morbidity and mortality, severe asthma during pregnancy may be a cause of maternal mortality [37].

Mechanisms

Definition of the mechanism(s) of maternal asthma's adverse effect on pregnancy outcomes reported in some studies should allow institution of optimal intervention strategy. Mechanisms postulated to explain these increased perinatal risks have included:
• hypoxia and other physiologic consequences of poorly controlled asthma
• medications used to treat asthma
• demographic or pathogenic factors *associated with* asthma but not actually caused by the disease or its treatment.

The latter would imply that asthma and adverse perinatal outcomes may share the same underlying pathogenetic mechanism (such as a predisposition to inflammation) or demographic associations (such as smoking), but that inadequately controlled asthma or asthma treatment is not causally related to the adverse perinatal outcome [25].

Data supporting specific mechanisms for the most common specific adverse outcomes have been reviewed [21,25]. The published data do not fully define the mechanism(s) of maternal asthma's potential adverse effects on pregnancy and the infant reported in some studies. Available information, however, suggests that inadequate asthma control, as defined by symptoms [38–40], pulmonary function [10,11], or acute exacerbations [8,9,28,40], may be the most remedial factor and supports the important generalization that adequate asthma control during pregnancy is important in improving maternal-fetal outcome. Oral corticosteroids have also been associated with increased risks of preeclampsia [41,42] and prematurity [7,38,43] in pregnant asthmatic women. However, whether this represents a drug effect, an effect of inadequately controlled asthma, or a marker for common pathogenesis factors associated with more severe asthma is not clear from the data.

Maternal use of bronchodilators has been associated with an increased risk of infant cardiac defects [35,44] and gastroschisis [45]. However, since women experiencing asthma exacerbations during the first trimester of pregnancy have been reported to have an increased risk of congenital malformations in their infants compared to infants of asthmatic women not experiencing exacerbations [46], the reported relationships between congenital malformations and bronchodilators may be confounded by severe asthma episodes.

Diagnosis of asthma during pregnancy

Many patients with asthma during pregnancy will already have a physician diagnosis of asthma. A new diagnosis of asthma is usually suspected on the basis of typical symptoms — wheezing, chest tightness, cough, and associated shortness of breath — which tend to be episodic or at least fluctuating in intensity and are typically worse at night. Identification of the characteristic triggers described above further supports the diagnosis. Wheezing may be present on auscultation of the lungs, but the absence of wheezing on auscultation does not exclude the diagnosis. The diagnosis is ideally confirmed by spirometry which shows a reduced forced expiratory volume in 1 sec (FEV$_1$; <80% predicted) with an increase in FEV$_1$ of 12% or more after an inhaled short-acting bronchodilator.

It is sometimes difficult to demonstrate reversible airway obstruction in patients with mild or intermittent asthma. Although methacholine challenge testing may be considered in nonpregnant patients with normal pulmonary function to confirm asthma, such testing is not recommended during pregnancy. Exhaled nitric oxide (eNO) is elevated in nonpregnant patients with asthma and has also been shown to be elevated in pregnant patients with asthma [47]. If available, an elevated eNO (>25 ppb) would support a diagnosis of asthma during pregnancy. If eNO is not available for women with suspected but unconfirmed asthma during pregnancy, therapeutic trials of asthma therapy should generally be used. Improvement with asthma therapy supports the diagnosis, which can then be confirmed postpartum with additional testing if necessary.

The most common differential diagnosis is dyspnea of pregnancy, which may occur in early pregnancy in approximately 70% of women. This dyspnea is differentiated from asthma by its lack of association with cough, wheezing, or airway obstruction.

Management

The National Asthma Education and Prevention Program (NAEPP) first published guidelines on the management of asthma during pregnancy in 1993 [48], and an update on pharmacologic treatment was published in 2005 [49]. An updated set of NAEPP guidelines for all patients with asthma, the Expert Panel Report 3, was published in 2007 [59]. The guidelines describe the management of asthma in four categories.
- Assessment and monitoring
- Control of factors contributing to severity
- Patient education
- Pharmacologic therapy

Assessment and monitoring

Once the diagnosis of asthma is considered confirmed, the next step is assessment of severity (in patients not already on controller medications) or assessment of control (in patients already on controller medications). Severity is assessed in untreated patients based on the frequency of daytime and nighttime symptoms and pulmonary function (ideally spirometry, minimally peak flow rate) (Table 23.1). Based on this severity assessment, controller therapy is initiated (if indicated).

In treated patients (either initially or with follow-up), it is important to determine whether their asthma is controlled [51] (Table 23.2). Like severity, assessment of control depends on frequency of symptoms, nighttime awakening, inteference with normal activity, exacerbations and pulmonary function [50,51]. Therapy is adjusted based on this assessment of control (see below). Patients with persistent asthma should be monitored monthly for asthma control. This is in part because, as described above, the course of asthma changes in approximately two-thirds of women during pregnancy. Home peak flow monitoring should be considered for

Table 23.1 Stepwise approach for managing asthma during pregnancy in patients not on controllers

Clinical features before treatment	Symptoms/day ——————— Symptoms/night	PEFR or FEV$_1$	Medications required to maintain long-term control Daily medications
Severe persistent	Continual Frequent	≤60%	• Preferred treatment: – High-dose inhaled corticosteroid *and* – Long-acting inhaled β2-agonist *and*, if needed, – Corticosteroid tablets or syrup long term (starting at 1 mg/kg/day, reducing systemic corticosteroid to lowest effective dose) • Alternative treatment: – High-dose inhaled corticosteroid *and* – Sustained release theophylline to serum concentration of 5–12 µg/mL
Moderate persistent	Daily >1 night/week	>60–<80%	• Preferred treatment: *either* – Low-dose inhaled corticosteroid and long-acting β2-agonist *or* – Medium-dose inhaled corticosteroid If needed (particularly in patients with recurring severe exacerbations): – Medium-dose inhaled corticosteroid and long-acting inhaled β2-agonist • Alternative treatment: – Low-dose inhaled corticosteroid and either theophylline or leukotriene receptor antagonist. If needed: – Medium-dose inhaled corticosteroid and either theophylline or leukotriene receptor antagonist
Mild persistent	>2 days/week but <daily >2 nights/month	>80%	• Preferred treatment: – Low-dose inhaled corticosteroid • Alternative treatment: leukotriene receptor antagonist *or* sustained-release theophylline to serum concentration of 5–12 µg/mL
Mild intermittent	≤2 days/week ≤2 nights/month	≥80%	• No daily medication needed • Severe exacerbations may occur, separated by long periods of normal lung function and no symptoms

FEV$_1$, forced expiratory volume in 1 sec; PEFR, peak expiratory flow rate.

Table 23.2 Assessment of asthma control in pregnant women

Components of control	Classification of control[a]		
	Well controlled	Not well controlled	Very poorly controlled
Symptoms	≤2 days/week	>2 days/week	Throughout the day
Nighttime awakening	≤2 times/month	1–3 times/week	≥4 times/week
Interference with normal activity	None	Some limitation	Extremely limited
Short-acting β2-agonist use for symptom control	≤2 days/week	>2 days/week	Several times per day
FEV$_1$ or peak flow	>80%[b]	60–80%[b]	<60%[b]
Exacerbations requiring systemic corticosteroids	0–1 in past 12 months	≥2 in past 12 months	

[a]The level of control is based on the most severe category. Assess symptom frequency and impact by patient's recall of previous 2–4 weeks.
[b]Predicted or personal best.
Reproduced from Schatz and Dombrowsk [51] with permission from Massachusetts Medical Society.

patients with moderate-to-severe asthma, especially for those who have difficulty perceiving signs of worsening asthma.

Because asthma has been associated with intrauterine growth restriction and preterm birth in some studies, pregnancy dating should be established accurately by first-trimester ultrasound where possible [49]. All patients should be instructed to be attentive to fetal activity. The intensity of antenatal testing of fetal well-being should be considered on the basis of the severity and control of the asthma as well as other high-risk features of the pregnancy that may be present [49]. Evaluation of fetal activity and growth by serial ultrasounds should be considered for women:

- who have suboptimally controlled asthma
- with moderate-to-severe asthma (starting at 32 weeks)
- who are recovering from a severe asthma exacerbation [49].

Control of factors contributing to asthma severity

Identifying and avoiding asthma triggers can lead to improved maternal well-being with less need for medications. In previously untested patients, *in vitro* tests (radioallergosorbent test [RAST], enzyme-linked immunosorbent assay [ELISA]) should be performed to identify relevant allergens, such as mite, animal dander, mold, and cockroach, for which specific environmental control instructions can be given. Smokers must be encouraged to discontinue smoking, and all patients should try to avoid exposure to environmental tobacco smoke and other potential irritants as much as possible. Effective allergen immunotherapy can be continued during pregnancy, but risk/benefit considerations do not generally favor beginning immunotherapy during pregnancy [48].

Sinusitis and reflux are relatively common co-morbidities during pregnancy that may exacerbate asthma. A high index of suspicion should be maintained for sinusitis, for which symptoms and signs during pregnancy may be subtle [23]. Although reflux is common during pregnancy and may not require pharmacologic treatment, reflux treatment should be considered in symptomatic patients with difficult-to-control asthma during pregnancy or those with very troublesome reflux symptoms.

Patient education

Pregnant women should have access to information about asthma in general as well as regarding the interrelationships between asthma and pregnancy. Controlling asthma during pregnancy is important for the well-being of the fetus as well as for the mother's well-being, and the pregnant woman must understand that it is safer to be treated with asthma medications than it is to have uncontrolled symptoms, reduced pulmonary function, or exacerbations. She should also understand how she can reduce her exposure to or otherwise control the asthma triggers that contribute to her asthma severity.

The pregnant woman should be instructed regarding optimal inhaler technique, and she should be asked to demonstrate this technique to assure its correctness. She must be able to recognize symptoms of worsening asthma and know what to do about them. She should be given an individualized action plan that defines:

- maintenance medication
- symptoms (and possibly peak flow levels) that indicate exacerbations
- rescue therapy and increases in maintenance medications in response to her level of exacerbation
- how and when to contact her asthma clinician for uncontrolled symptoms.

Pharmacologic therapy

Asthma medicines are classified into two types: relievers and long-term controllers. Relievers provide quick relief of bronchospasm and include short-acting β-agonists (albuterol is preferred during pregnancy, 2–4 puffs every 3–4 h when required) and the anticholinergic bronchodilator ipratropium (generally used as second-line therapy for acute asthma — see below). Long-term control medications are described in Table 23.3. Inhaled corticosteroids (Table 23.4) are the most effective controller asthma medications.

Chronic asthma

Patients with intermittent asthma do not need controller therapy. In patients with persistent asthma not already on controller therapy, it should be initiated as shown in Table 23.1. Controller therapy should be progressed in steps (Table 23.5) until adequate control is achieved, as defined above. Therapy should be increased one step for patients whose asthma is not well controlled despite attention to the nonpharmacologic strategies described above. A two-step increase, a course of oral corticosteroids, or both should be recommended for women whose asthma is very poorly controlled.

Once control is achieved and sustained for several months, a stepdown to less intensive therapy is encouraged for nonpregnant patients to identify the minimum therapy necessary to maintain control. Although a similar stepdown approach can be considered for pregnant patients, it should be undertaken cautiously and gradually to avoid compromising the patient's asthma control [48]. For some patients it may be prudent to postpone attempts to reduce therapy that is effectively controlling the woman's asthma until after the infant's birth [48].

Inhaled corticosteroids are the mainstay of controller therapy during pregnancy. Because it has the most published reassuring human gestational safety data, budesonide is considered the preferred inhaled corticosteroid for asthma during pregnancy. It is important to note that no data indicate that the other inhaled corticosteroid preparations are unsafe. Therefore, inhaled corticosteroids other than budesonide may be continued in patients who were well controlled by these agents prior to pregnancy, especially if it is thought that changing formulations may jeopardize asthma control. Based on longer duration of availability in the USA, salmeterol is considered the

Table 23.3 Long-term control medications for asthma during pregnancy

Medication	Dosage form	Adult dose	Use during pregnancy
Inhaled corticosteroids		See Table 23.4	First-line controller therapy
Systemic corticosteroids		Short course "burst" to achieve	Burst therapy for severe acute
Methylprednisolone	2,4,8,16,32 mg tablets	control: 40–60 mg/day as single	symptoms
Prednisolone	5 mg tablets, 5 mg/mL, 15 mg/mL	or divided doses for 3–10 days	
Prednisone	1, 2.5, 5, 10, 20, 50 mg tablet		Maintenance therapy for severe
	5 mg/mL, 5 mg/5 mL	7.5–60 mg/day in a single dose in	asthma uncontrolled by other
		AM or qod., taper to lowest	means
		effective dose	
Long-acting β-agonists			Add-on therapy in patients not
Salmeterol	DPI 50 μg/blister	1 blister q12h	controlled by low–medium-dose
Formoterol	DPI 12 μg/single-use capsule	1 capsule q12h	inhaled corticosteroids
Leukotriene receptor anagonists			Alternative therapy for persistent
Montelukast	10 mg tablets	10 mg q HS	asthma in patients who have
Zafirlukast	10 or 20 mg tablets	20 mg bid	shown good response prior to
			pregnancy
Theophylline	Liquids, sustained-release tablets,	400–800 mg/day to achieve serum	Alternative therapy for persistent
	and capsules	concentration of 5–12 μg/mL	asthma during pregnancy

HS, bedtime; q, every.
Source: National Asthma Education and Prevention Program Working Group [49].

Table 23.4 Clinically comparable doses of inhaled corticosteroids

Drug	Low daily dose (μg)	Medium daily dose (μg)	High daily dose (μg)
[tb]Beclomethasone HFA MDI	80–240	>240–480	>480
Budesonide DPI	200–600	>600–1200	>1200
Ciclesonide HFA MDI	160–320	>320–640	>640
Flunisolide			
CFC MDI	500–1000	>1000–2000	>2000
HFA MDI	320	>320–640	>640
Fluticasone			
HFA MDI	88–264	>264–440	>440
DPI	100–300	>300–500	>500
Momethasone DPI	220	440	>440
Triamcinolone acetonide CFC MDI	300–750	>750–1500	>1500

CFC MDI, chlorofluorocarbon-propelled metered dose inhaler; DPI, dry powder inhaler; HFA MDI, hydrofluoroalkaline-propelled metered dose inhaler.
Source: Kelly [52].

long-acting β-agonist of choice during pregnancy. As described in Table 23.3, theophylline (primarily because of increased side-effects compared with alternatives) and leukotriene receptor antagonists (because of the limited published human gestational data for these drugs) are considered by the NAEPP to be alternative, but not preferred, treatments for persistent asthma during pregnancy. Although oral corticosteroids have been associated with possible increased risks during pregnancy, such as oral clefts [53], preeclampsia, and prematurity as described above, if needed during pregnancy, they should be used because these risks are less than the potential risks of severe uncontrolled asthma, which include maternal mortality, fetal mortality, or both.

Table 23.5 Steps of asthma therapy during pregnancy

Step	Preferred controller medication	Alternative controller medication
1	None	–
2	Low-dose ICS	LTRA, theophylline
3	Medium-dose ICS	Low-dose ICS + either LABA, LTRA or theophylline
4	Medium-dose ICS + LABA	Medium-dose ICS + LTRA or theophylline
5	High-dose ICS + LABA	–
6	High-dose ICS + LABA + oral prednisone	–

ICS, inhaled corticosteroids; LABA, long-acting β-agonists; LTRA, leukotriene receptor antagonists.
Source: Schatz and Dombrowski [51].

Acute asthma

A major goal of chronic asthma management is the prevention of acute asthmatic episodes. When increased asthma does not respond to home therapy, expeditious acute management is necessary for the health of both the mother and fetus.

As a result of progesterone-induced hyperventilation, normal blood gases during pregnancy reveal a higher PO_2 (100–106 mmHg) and a lower PCO_2 (28–30 mmHg) than in the nonpregnant state. The changes in blood gases that occur secondary to acute asthma during pregnancy will be superimposed on the "normal" hyperventilation of pregnancy. Thus, a $PCO_2 > 35$ or a $PO_2 < 70$ associated with acute asthma will represent more severe compromise during pregnancy than will similar blood gases in the nongravid state.

The recommended pharmacologic therapy of acute asthma during pregnancy is summarized in Box 23.1 [48]. Intensive fetal monitoring as well as maternal monitoring is essential. In addition to pharmacologic therapy, supplemental oxygen (initially 3–4 L/min by nasal cannula) should be administered, adjusting fraction of inspired oxygen (FiO_2) to maintain at $PO_2 \geq 70$ and/or O_2 saturation by pulse oximetry >95%. Intravenous fluids (containing glucose if the patient is not hyperglycemic) should also be administered, initially at a rate of at least 100 mL/h.

Systemic corticosteroids (approximately 1 mg/kg) are recommended for patients who do not respond well (FEV_1 or peak expiratory flow rate [PEFR] $\geq 70\%$ predicted) to the first β-agonist treatment as well as for patients who have recently taken systemic steroids and for those who present with severe exacerbations (FEV_1 or PEFR $\leq 50\%$ predicted). Patients with good responses to emergency therapy (FEV_1 or PEFR $\geq 70\%$ predicted) can be discharged home, generally on a course of oral corticosteroids. Inhaled corticosteroids should also be continued or initiated upon discharge until review at medical

Box 23.1 National Asthma Education and Prevention Program (NAEPP) recommendations for the pharmacologic management of acute asthma during pregnancy

1 Initial therapy

A FEV_1 or PEFR $\geq 50\%$ predicted or personal best
  1 Short-acting inhaled β2-agonist by metered dose inhaler or nebulizer, up to three doses in first hour
  2 Oral systemic corticosteroid if not immediate response or if patient recently took oral systemic corticosteroid

B FEV_1 or PEFR $< 50\%$ predicted or personal best (severe exacerbation)
  1 High-dose short-acting inhaled β2-agonist by nebulization every 20 min or continuously for 1 h plus inhaled ipratropium bromide
  2 Oral systemic corticosteroid

2 Repeat assessment

A Moderate exacerbation (FEV_1 or PEFR 50–80% predicted or personal best, moderate symptoms)
  1 Short-acting inhaled β2-agonist every 60 min
  2 Oral systemic corticosteroid (if not already given)
  3 Continue treatment 1–3 h, provided there is improvement

B Severe (FEV_1 or PEFR <50% predicted or personal best, severe symptoms at rest)
  1 Short-acting inhaled β2-agonist hourly or continuously plus inhaled ipratropium bromide
  2 Systemic corticosteroid (if not already given)

3 Response and disposition

A Good (FEV_1 or PEFR $\geq 70\%$ predicted or personal best, no distress, response sustained 60 min after last treatment). Discharge home

B Incomplete (FEV_1 or PEFR $\geq 50\%$ predicted or personal best but <70%, mild or moderate symptoms). Individualize decision regarding discharge home versus admit to hospital ward

C Poor (FEV_1 or PEFR <50% predicted or personal best, $PCO_2 > 42$ mmHg, severe symptoms, drowsiness, confusion). Admit to hospital intensive care

FEV_1, forced expiratory volume in 1 sec; PEFR, peak expiratory flow rate.
Source: National Asthma Education and Prevention Program [49].

follow-up. Hospitalization should be considered for patients with an incomplete response (FEV_1 or PEFR $\geq 50\%$ but <70% predicted). Admission to an intensive care unit should be considered for patients with persistent FEV_1 or PEFR <50% predicted, $PCO_2 > 42$, or sensorium changes.

Management during labor and delivery

Asthma medications should be continued during labor and delivery. If systemic corticosteroids have been used in the previous 4 weeks, then stress-dose steroids (e.g. 100 mg hydrocortisone every 8 h IV) should be administered during labor and for the 24-h period after delivery to prevent maternal adrenal crisis [48].

Prostaglandin (PG) E_2 or E_1 can be used for cervical ripening, the management of spontaneous or induced abortions, or postpartum hemorrhage [49]. However, 15-methyl-PGF$_2$-α and methylergonovine can cause bronchospasm [48]. There is no contraindication to the use of oxytocin for postpartum hemorrhage [48]. Magnesium sulfate and β-adrenergic agents, which are bronchodilators, can be used to treat preterm labor [49]. Indomethacin can induce bronchospasm in the aspirin-sensitive patient and thus must be avoided in such patients [49].

Epidural anesthesia has the additional benefit of reducing oxygen consumption and minute ventilation during labor [49]. If a general anesthetic is necessary, preanesthetic use of atropine and glycopyrrolate may provide bronchodilation [48]. Ketamine is the agent of choice for induction of anesthesia because it decreases airway resistance and can prevent bronchospasm [48]. Low concentrations of halogenated anesthetics are recommended as inhalation anesthetic agents in pregnant asthmatic patients because they also cause bronchodilation [48].

Conclusion

Asthma is a common medical problem during pregnancy. Optimal diagnosis and management of asthma during pregnancy should maximize maternal and fetal health.

CASE PRESENTATION

The patient is a 23-year-old gravida 2, para 1 woman who is seen during her first trimester for asthma. Her asthma was first diagnosed at age 15. She has not been hospitalized for asthma, but did require an emergency department visit for asthma 6 months previously. She was worse during her prior pregnancy 2 years ago. She is currently having daily asthma symptoms, nocturnal symptoms twice a week, and using her albuterol inhaler 3–4 times per day. She was given a steroid inhaler, but was afraid to use it while she was pregnant. She has noticed that cleaning the house triggers her asthma. She has had a cat at home for 1 year, has been worse over this time period, but does not think the cat affects her asthma. She has had some daily sneezing and nasal congestion since childhood, which she considers mild. She does not smoke cigarettes, has not been previously evaluated for allergies, and denies any other significant medical history.

Auscultation of the lungs was normal, and examination of the nose revealed mild mucosal edema. Spirometry showed an FEV$_1$ of 70% predicted. The diagnostic impression was moderate persistent asthma with a probable mite and dander allergy component and mild allergic rhinitis. The initial plan included education regarding asthma and pregnancy, an allergy evaluation (*in vitro* tests), environmental control instructions based on the testing, initiation of medium-dose inhaled budesonide with instructions on inhaler technique, provision of a symptom-based home action plan, and scheduled follow-up in 1 month.

References

1. Kwon HL, Belanger K, Bracken MB. Asthma prevalence among pregnant and childbearing-aged women in the United States: estimates from national health surveys. Ann Epidemiol 2003;13:317–324.
2. Berg CJ, MacKay AP, Qin C, Callaghan WM. Overview of maternal morbidity during hospitalization for labor and delivery in the United States. Obstet Gynecol 2009;113:1075–1081.
3. Demissie K, Breckenridge MB, Rhoads GG. Infant and maternal outcomes in the pregnancies of asthmatic women. Am J Respir Crit Care Med 1998;158:1091–1095.
4. Kallen B, Rydhstroem H, Aberg A. Asthma during pregnancy: a population based study. Eur J Epidemiol 2000;16:167–171.
5. Wen SW, Demissie K, Liu S. Adverse outcomes in pregnancies of asthmatic women: results from a Canadian population. Ann Epidemiol 2001;11:7–12.
6. Sheiner E, Mazor M, Levy A et al. Pregnancy outcome of asthmatic patients: a population-based study. J Mat-Fet Neonat Med 2005;18:237–240.
7. Perlow JH, Montgomery D, Morgan MA, Towers CV, Porto M. Severity of asthma and perinatal outcome. Am J Obstet Gynecol 1992;167:963–967.
8. Greenberger, Patterson R. The outcome of pregnancy complicated by severe asthma. Allergy Proc 1988;9:539–543.
9. Jana N, Vasishta K, Saha SC, Khunnu B. Effect of bronchial asthma on the course of pregnancy, labour and perinatal outcome. J Obstet Gynaecol 1995;21:227–223.
10. Schatz, M, Zeiger RS, Hoffman CP et al. Intrauterine growth is related to gestational pulmonary function in pregnant asthmatic women. Chest 1990;98:389–392.
11. Schatz M, Dombrowski MP, Wise R et al. Spirometry is related to perinatal outcomes in pregnant asthmatic women. Am J Obstet Gynecol 2006;194:120–126.
12. Juniper EF, Newhouse MT. Effect of pregnancy on asthma: a systematic review and meta-analysis. In: Schatz M, Zeiger RS,

Claman HN, eds. Asthma and Immunological Diseases in Pregnancy and Early Infancy. New York: Marcel Dekker, 1998, pp.401–427.

13. Kwon HL, Belanger K, Bracken MB. Effect of pregnancy and stage of pregnancy on asthma severity: a systematic review. Am J Obstet Gynecol 2004;190:1201–1210.

14. Schatz M, Dombrowski MP, Wise R et al. Asthma morbidity during pregnancy can be predicted by severity classification. J Allergy Clin Immunol 2003;112:283–288.

15. Belanger K, Hellenbrand ME, Holford TR, Bracken M. Effect of pregnancy on maternal asthma symptoms and medication use. Obstet Gynecol 2010;115:559–567.

16. Gluck JC, Gluck PA. The effects of pregnancy on asthma: a prospective study. Ann Allergy 1976;37:164–168.

17. Schatz M, Harden K, Forsythe A et al. The course of asthma during pregnancy, post-partum, and with successive pregnancies: a prospective analysis. J Allergy Clin Immunol 1988;81:509–517.

18. Stenius-Aarniala BSM, Hedman J, Teramo KA. Acute asthma during pregnancy. Thorax 1996;51:411–414.

19. Williams DA. Asthma and pregnancy. Acta Allergol 1967;22:311–323.

20. Gluck JC, Gluck PA. The effect of pregnancy on the course of asthma. Immunol Allergy Clin North Am 2000;20:729–743.

21. Cydulka RK, Emerman CL, Schreiber D, Molander KH, Woodruff PG, Camargo C. Acute asthma among pregnant women presenting to the emergency department. Am J Respir Crit Care Med 1999;160:887–892.

22. Murphy VE, Gibson P, Talbot P, Clifton VL. Severe asthma exacerbations during pregnancy. Obstet Gynecol 2005;106:1046–1054.

23. Sorri M, Hartikanen-Sorri A-L, Karja J. Rhinitis during pregnancy. Rhinology 1980;18:83–86.

24. Munn MB, Groome LJ, Atterbury JL et al. Pneumonia as a complication of pregnancy. J Matern Fetal Med 1999;8:151–154.

25. Henderson CE, Ownby DR, Trumble A, DerSimonian R, Kellner LH. Predicting asthma severity from allergic sensitivity to cockroaches in pregnant inner city women. J Reprod Med 2000;45:341–344.

26. Murphy VE, Gibson PG, Smith R, Clifton VL. Asthma during pregnancy: mechanisms and treatment implications. Eur Respir J 2005;25:731–750.

27. Tata LJ, Lewis SA, McKeever TM et al. A comprehensive analysis of adverse obstetric and pediatric complications in women with asthma. Am J Respir Crit Care Med 2007;175:991–997.

28. Enriquez R, Griffin MR, Carroll KN et al. Effect of maternal asthma and asthma control on pregnancy and perinatal outcomes. J Allergy Clin Immunol 2007;120:625–630.

29. Kallen B, Olausson PO. Use of anti-asthma drugs during pregnancy. 2. Infant characteristics excluding congenital malformations. Eur J Clin Pharmacol 2007;63:375–881.

30. Breton M-C, Beauchesne M-F, Lemiere C et al. Risk of perinatal mortality associated with asthma during pregnancy. Thorax 2009;64:101–106.

31. Schatz M, Zeiger RS, Hoffman CP et al. Perinatal outcomes in the pregnancies of asthmatic women: a prospective controlled analysis. Am J Respir Crit Care Med 1995;151:1170–1174.

32. Stenius-Aarniala BSM, Hedman J, Teramo KA. Acute asthma during pregnancy. Thorax 1996;51:411–414.

33. Dombrowski MP, Schatz M, Wise R et al. Asthma during pregnancy. Obstet Gynecol 2004;103:5–12.

34. Tamasi L, Somoskovi A, Muller V et al. A population-based case-control study on the effect of bronchial asthma during pregnancy for congenital abnormalities of the offspring. J Asthma 2006;43:81–86.

35. Tata LJ, Lewis SA, McKeever TM et al. Effect of maternal asthma, exacerbations and asthma medication on congenital malformations in offspring: a UK population-based study. Thorax 2008;63:981–987.

36. Kallen B, Olausson PO. Use of anti-asthmatic drugs during pregnancy. 3. Congenital malformations. Eur J Clin Pharmacol 2007;63:383–388.

37. Schatz M, Dombrowski M. Outcomes of pregnancy in asthmatic women. Immunol Allergy Clin North Am 2000;20:715–727.

38. Bracken MB, Triche EW, Belanger K et al. Asthma symptoms, severity, and drug therapy: a prospective study of effects on 2205 pregnancies. Obstet Gynecol 2003;102:739–752.

39. Triche EW, Saftlas AF, Belanger K et al. Association of asthma diagnosis, severity, symptoms, and treatment with risk of preeclampsia. Obstet Gynecol 2004;104:585–593.

40. Bakhireva LN, Schatz M, Jones KL et al. Asthma control during pregnancy and the risk of preterm delivery or impaired fetal growth. Ann Allergy Asthma Immunol 2008;101:137–143.

41. Schatz M, Zeiger RS, Harden K et al. The safety of asthma and allergy medications during pregnancy. J Allergy Clin Immunol 1997;100:301.

42. Martel M-J, Rey E, Beauchesne M-F et al. Use of inhaled corticosteroids during pregnancy and risk of pregnancy-induced hypertension: nested case–control study. BMJ 2005;330:230–235.

43. Schatz M, Dombrowski MP, Wise R. The relationship of asthma medication use to perinatal outcomes. J Allergy Clin Immunol 2004;113:1040–1045.

44. Lin S, Herdt-Losavio M, Gensburg L et al Maternal asthma, asthma medication use, and the risk of congenital heart defects. Birth Defects Research (Part A) 2009;85:161–168.

45. Lin S, Munsie JPW, Herdt-Losavio M et al. Maternal asthma medication use and the risk of gastroschisis. Am J Epidemiol 2008;168:73–79.

46. Blais L, Forget A. Asthma exacerbations during the first trimester of pregnancy and the risk of congential malformations among asthmatic women. J Allergy Clin Immunol 2008;121:1379–1384

47. Tamasi L, Bohacs A, Bikov A et al. Exhaled nitric oxide in pregnant healthy and asthmatic women. J Asthma 2009;46:786–791.

48. National Asthma Education Program Report of the Working Group on Asthma and Pregnancy. Management of asthma during pregnancy. NIH Publication 93-3279A. Bethesda, MD: National Institutes of Health, 1993.

49. National Asthma Education and Prevention Program Working Group Report on Managing Asthma During Pregnancy. Recommendations for pharmacologic treatment. Update 2004. NIH Publication 05-5236. Bethesda, MD: National Institutes of Health, 2005.

50. National Asthma Education and Prevention Program Expert Panel Report 3. Guidelines for the diagnosis and management of asthma. Summary Report 2007. J Allergy Clin Immunol 2007;120:S93–S138.

51. Schatz M, Dombrowski MP. Asthma in pregnancy. N Engl J Med 2009;360:1862–1869.

52. Kelly HW. Comparison of inhaled corticosteroids: an update. Ann Pharmacother 2009;43(3):519–527.

53. Park-Wyllie L, Mazzotta P, Pastuszak A et al. Birth defects after maternal exposure to corticosteroids: prospective cohort study and meta-analysis of epidemiological studies. Teratology 2000;62:385–392.

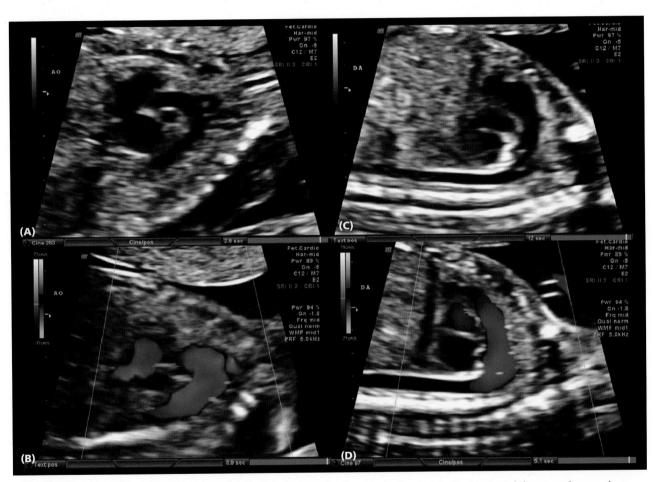

Plate 6.1 (A) Two-dimensional image of the aortic arch demonstrating head and neck vessels. The aortic arch has a candy cane shape. (B) Same image with color Doppler demonstrating forward flow through the aortic arch (*blue*). (C) Two-dimensional image of the ductal arch which has the shape of a hockey stick. (D) Color flow mapping of the ductal arch showing normal antegrade flow (*blue*).

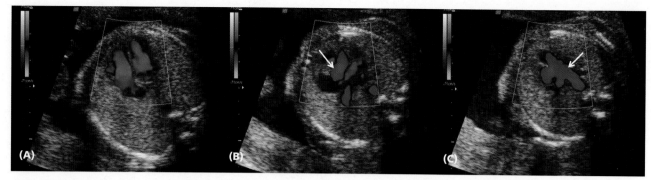

Plate 6.2 (A) Color Doppler demonstrating forward flow from the atria to the ventricles across the atrioventricular valves (*red*). The atrioventricular valves are open and the interventricular septum appears to be intact. (B) Long-axis view of the left ventricular outflow tract demonstrating normal antegrade flow across the aortic valve (*blue*). (C) Color flow mapping showing forward flow in the right ventricular outflow tract (*blue*). Note that the main pulmonary artery crosses over the ascending aorta as it exits the right ventricle.

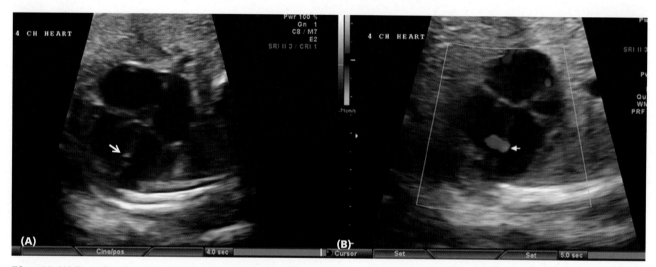

Plate 6.3 (A) Four-chamber view suspicious for an apical muscular ventricular septal defect (VSD) based on an echogenic spot on the interventricular septum (*arrow*). (B) Muscular VSD confirmed on color Doppler which demonstrated right-to-left flow during systole (*blue; arrow*).

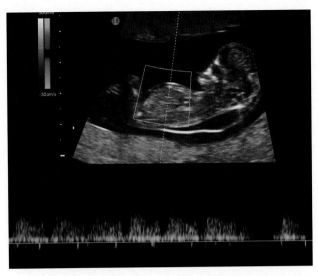

Plate 7.1 Septated cystic hygroma at 11 weeks' gestation: midsagittal view demonstrating increased NT space extending along the entire length of the fetus. The ductus venosus shows positive a-wave. Chorionic villus sampling revealed normal male karyotype. The pregnancy proceeded to full term with the delivery of a healthy infant.

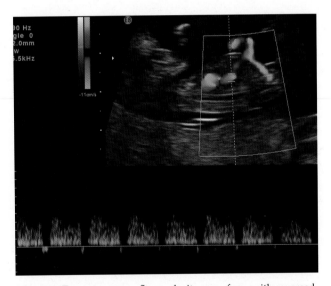

Plate 7.2 Ductus venosus flow velocity waveform with reversed a-wave. The Doppler gate is placed in the ductus venosus between the umbilical venous sinus and the inferior vena cava. Subsequent CVS confirmed a fetus affected by trisomy 21.

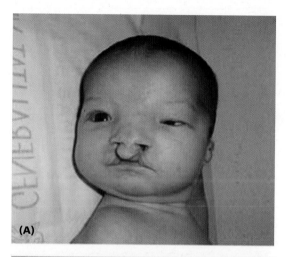

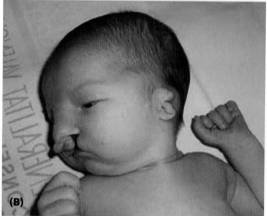

Plate 19.1 (A) Frontal view of the newborn presenting ptosis of the left eyelid, upper cleft lip, hypertelorism, and micrognathia. (B) Lateral view of the newborn with microtia with the absence of the external auditory duct. Reproduced from Perez-Aytes *et al* [18] with permission from Wiley-Blackwell.

Chapter 24
Epilepsy

Autumn M. Klein and Page B. Pennell
Department of Neurology, Brigham and Women's Hospital and Harvard Medical School, Boston, MA, USA

Epilepsy is a chronic brain disorder of various etiologies characterized by recurrent, unprovoked seizures. A seizure is caused by paroxysmal abnormal cerebral neuronal discharges. Clinical manifestations are stereotyped, episodic alterations in behavior or perception. Epilepsy can begin at any age of life, and two-thirds of cases are idiopathic. The prevalence is approximately 0.64% in the United States [1]. Epilepsy is the most common neurologic disorder that requires continuous treatment during pregnancy, and antiepileptic drugs (AEDs) are one of the most frequent chronic teratogen exposures [2,3]. Over one million women with epilepsy in the United States are in their active reproductive years and give birth to over 24,000 infants each year. However, it is estimated that the total number of children in the United States exposed *in utero* to AEDs is nearly twice that amount with the emergence of AED use for other illnesses including headache, chronic pain, and mood disorders [4]. Many of the principles outlined below about AED use during pregnancy can be extrapolated to women with any disorder treated with these agents. Although some of the other disorders may allow for discontinuation of the AED during pregnancy unlike most epilepsy cases, pregnancies are often not identified until after organogenesis occurs.

The vast majority of women with epilepsy will have a normal pregnancy with a favorable outcome, but there are increased maternal and fetal risks compared to the general population. Careful management of any pregnancy in a woman with epilepsy is essential to minimize these risks, ideally beginning with preconceptional planning. The initial visit between the physician and a woman with epilepsy of child-bearing age should include a discussion about family planning. Topics should include effective birth control, the importance of planned pregnancies with AED optimization and folate supplementation prior to conception, obstetric complications, and teratogenicity of AEDs versus the risks of seizures during pregnancy. The goal is effective control of maternal seizures with the least risk to the fetus. In 2009, the American Academy of Neurology (AAN) and the American Epilepsy Society (AES) published Practice Parameter updates on the pregnant woman with epilepsy [5–7]. These guidelines reviewed medications, teratogenicity, obstetric outcomes, vitamins, breastfeeding, and other management issues in the pregnant woman with epilepsy. These guidelines will be reviewed in this chapter.

Birth control for women on antiepileptic drugs

Many of the AEDs induce the hepatic cytochrome P450 system, the primary metabolic pathway of the sex steroid hormones. This leads to rapid clearance of steroid hormones and may allow ovulation in women taking oral contraceptives or other hormonal forms of birth control [8,9]. The 1998 guidelines by the American Academy of Neurology recommend use of an estradiol dose of 50 μg or its equivalent for 21 days of each cycle when using oral contraceptive agents with the enzyme-inducing AEDs [10]. While no studies have looked at contraceptive efficacy, this is still not entirely adequate protection against pregnancy, and a back-up barrier method is recommended. Table 24.1 lists effects of the individual AEDs on hormonal contraceptive agents [9,11,12]. Lamotrigine (LTG) is a commonly used AED, and estrogens can lower its serum level. Therefore, when taking estrogens with LTG, serum levels should be checked. The newer transdermal patch and vaginal ring formulations also have higher failure rates with these AEDs.

Fetal anticonvulsant syndrome

Offspring of women with epilepsy on AEDs are at increased risk for intrauterine growth retardation, minor

Queenan's Management of High-Risk Pregnancy: An Evidence-Based Approach, Sixth Edition. Edited by John T. Queenan, Catherine Y. Spong, Charles J. Lockwood.
© 2012 John Wiley & Sons, Ltd. Published 2012 by John Wiley & Sons, Ltd.

Table 24.1 AED effects on hormonal contraceptive agents

Lowers hormone levels	No significant effects
Phenobarbital	Ethosuximide
Phenytoin	Valproate
Carbamazepine	Gabapentin
Primidone	Lamotrigine
Topiramate	Tiagabine
Oxcarbazepine	Levetiracetam
Rufinamide	Zonisamide
	Lacosamide
	Pregabalin

Table 24.2 Major malformations in infants of women with epilepsy

	General population	Infants of women with epilepsy
Congenital heart	0.5%	1.52%
Cleft lip/palate	0.15%	1.4%
Neural tube defect	0.06%	1–3.8% (VPA)
		0.5–1% (CBZ)
Urogenital defects	0.7%	1.7%

CBZ, carbamazepine; VPA, valproic acid.

Table 24.3 Relative timing and developmental pathology of certain malformations

Tissues	Malformations	Postconceptional age
Central nervous system	Neural tube defect	28 days
Heart	Ventricular septal defect	42 days
Face	Cleft lip	36 days
	Cleft maxillary palate	47–70 days

Adapted from Yerby [71] and Moore [82].

anomalies, major congenital malformations, cognitive dysfunction, microcephaly, and infant mortality [13,14]. The term "fetal anticonvulsant syndrome" includes various combinations of these findings and has been described with virtually all of the AEDs [15,16].

Minor anomalies

Minor anomalies are defined as structural deviations from the norm that do not constitute a threat to health. Minor anomalies affect 6–20% of infants born to women with epilepsy, an approximately 2.5-fold increase compared to the general population [14]. Minor anomalies seen in infants of mothers on AEDs include distal digital and nail hypoplasia and midline craniofacial anomalies, including broad nasal bridge, ocular hypertelorism, epicanthal folds, short upturned nose, altered lips, and low hairline [17,18].

Major congenital malformations

The reported major congenital malformation (MCM) rates in the general population vary between 1.6% and 3.2% [19] and women with a history of epilepsy but on no AEDs show similar MCM rates. The average MCM rates among all AED exposures vary between 3.1% and 9%, or approximately 2–3-fold higher than the general population. Reported MCM rates in monotherapy exposures are 2.3–7.8%, while AED polytherapy exposures carry an average MM rate of 6.5–18.8% [16]. Monotherapy use of AEDs is preferred to polytherapy during pregnancy and should be achieved during the preconception planning phase [17]. The 2009 AAN/AES Practice Parameter updates found that there was probably an increased risk of MCMs with AED exposure in the first trimester, but it could not be determined if the risk was from one AED or several [6]. They determined that AED polytherapy probably contributes to an increased rate of MCMs as compared to monotherapy. Information on malformations and AEDs comes from drug company and physician and/or patient registries based in North America, Europe, the United Kingdom, Australia, and India.

Major congenital malformations most commonly associated with AED exposure include congenital heart disease, cleft lip/palate, urogenital defects, and neural tube defects (Table 24.2) [16,17]. The congenital heart defects can involve almost any structural abnormality, and the urogenital defects commonly involve glandular hypospadias. The neural tube defects (NTD) are usually lower defects, but tend to be severe open defects frequently complicated by hydrocephaly and other midline defects [20]. Some studies have identified spina bifida aperta (an open defect with failure of the neural tube to close over the spinal cord) as the NTD most commonly associated with valproic acid (VPA) or carbamazepine (CBZ) exposure. The abnormal neural tube closure usually occurs between the third and fourth weeks of gestation. By the time most women realize they are pregnant, it is too late to make medication adjustments to avoid malformations (Table 24.3).

Antiepileptic drug monotherapies during pregnancy

Although features of the fetal anticonvulsant syndrome have been described in association with virtually all of the AEDs, there are some notable differences in the likelihood of specific malformations with the different AEDs [16,21].

A comparison between two cohorts highlighted differences in fetal MCM with changes in prescribing practices over time [20]. The older cohort (1972–9) had more women taking phenobarbital (PB), primidone, and phenytoin

(PHT); the newer cohort (1981–5) represented more monotherapy with VPA or CBZ. The features of the older cohort were congenital heart defects, facial clefts, and minor anomalies. The MCM identified most frequently with the newer cohort were neural tube defects and glandular hypospadias. The relative risk for neural tube defects with valproate is at least 20 times that of the general population [22]. One analysis pooling data from five prospective studies suggested that the absolute risk with valproate monotherapy may be as high as 3.8% for neural tube defects, and that offspring of women receiving >1000 mg/day of valproate were especially at increased risk [23].

Recent prospective data from the North American AED Pregnancy Registry are available for PB, VPA, and LTG. Of 77 women receiving PB monotherapy, five of the infants had confirmed major malformations (6.5%; 95% confidence interval [CI] 2.1–14.5%). Major malformations in exposed infants included one cleft lip and palate and four heart defects [24]. In first-trimester VPA monotherapy exposures (n = 149), major birth defects occurred in 10.7% of infants, as compared with 1.6% in external control infants (relative risk [RR] to controls 7.3, 95% CI 4.4–12.2). Birth defects included cardiac anomalies, neural tube defects, hypospadias, polydactyly, bilateral inguinal hernia, dysplastic kidney, and equinovarus club foot [25]. Perhaps more relevant to the prescribing physician is the relative risk compared to the internal comparison group. The internal comparison group was the major congenital malformation rate (2.9%) of three other AED monotherapy regimens; the relative risk of VPA for malformations compared to this group was 4.0 (95% CI 2.1–7.4).

The UK Epilepsy and Pregnancy Register has collected prospective, full outcome data on 3607 cases [26]. Comparisons between monotherapy regimens did reveal a statistically significant increased MCM rate for pregnancies exposed to VPA (6.2%, 95% CI 4.6–8.2%) compared to those exposed to CBZ (2.2%, 95% CI 1.4–3.4%, adjusted OR 2.97, P < 0.001). Although a lower MCM rate was identified for pregnancies exposed to LTG (3.2%, 95% CI 2.1–4.9), the adjusted OR 0.59 compared to the VPA group was not statistically significant (P = 0.064) [26]. The Australian Pregnancy Registry has enrolled over 800 women [27,28]. Significantly greater risk for MCM on VPA monotherapy was demonstrated (17.1%) compared to other AED monotherapy exposures (2.4%) and no AED exposures (2.5%). The MCM rate increased with increasing VPA dosage (P < 0.05) with a MCM rate of >30% for doses >1100 mg/day. Other MCM rates reported were PHT 4.7%, CBZ 4.5%, and LTG 5.6% for monotherapy exposures. The findings of these large prospective pregnancy registries scattered across different regions of the world reveal a consistent pattern of amplified risk for the development of MCM in pregnancies exposed to VPA.

The newer generation of AEDs consists of a large number of structurally diverse compounds, most of which have demonstrated teratogenic effects in preclinical animal experiments and MCM in offspring of women on these AEDs. With the possible exception of LTG, none have sufficient human pregnancy experience to assess their safety or teratogenicity. The reported rates for MCM with LTG use during the first trimester are consistently moderately low across several studies, varying between 2.0% and 3.2% [26,29,30]. The reported MCM rate for LTG use from the North American AED Pregnancy Registry was 2.7% (95% CI 1.5–4.3%), but a significantly increased risk for nonsyndromic cleft lip/cleft palate was noted [29].

The 2009 AAN/AES Practice Parameter update drew several conclusions [6]. Compared to CBZ, it is highly probable that first-trimester exposure to VPA has higher risk of MCMs, and compared to PHT or LTG, it is possible that VPA has higher risk of MCMs. Compared to untreated women with epilepsy (WWE), it is probable that polytherapy that includes VPA and possible that monotherapy with VPA contributes to the development of MCMs. The authors also reported that AED polytherapy compared to monotherapy regimens probably contributes to the development of MCMs. There is insufficient evidence to know if LTG or other AEDs increase the risk. Recommendations were to avoid VPA in monotherapy or in polytherapy in the first trimester if possible in order to decrease the risk of MCMs. Since the Pratice Parameters were published, subsequent studies have suggested that limiting the doses of VPA and LTG during the first trimester should be considered to decrease the risk of MCMs [31].

Prenatal screening

While there were no recommendations from the 2009 AAN Practice Parameter updates, women on AEDs during pregnancy should undergo adequate prenatal screening to detect any fetal major congenital malformations. In addition to routine screening measures, ultrasonographic measurements of nuchal lucency in combination with levels of placenta-associated pregnancy protein A, α-fetoprotein, human chorionic gonadotropin, and estriol can be performed to determine risk of congenital malformations. If not routinely done, a detailed anatomic ultrasound at 16–18 weeks can be performed to further evaluate for any malformations, and if there are any cardiac concerns, fetal echocardiography should also be done. Amniocentesis (with measurements of amniotic fluid α-fetoprotein and acetylcholinesterase) is not performed routinely but should be offered if any screening tests are equivocal, increasing the sensitivity for detection of neural tube defects to greater than 99%. If the patient's weight gain and fundal growth do not appear appropriate, serial sonography should be performed to assess fetal size and amniotic fluid [32].

Neurodevelopmental outcome

Studies investigating cognitive outcome in children of women with epilepsy report an increased risk of mental deficiency, affecting 1.4–6% of children of women with epilepsy, compared to 1% of controls [13,33,34]. Verbal scores on neuropsychometric measures may be selectively more involved [4]. A variety of factors contribute to the cognitive problems of children of mothers with epilepsy, but AEDs appear to play a role [4].

Studies of particular AEDs have reported that the child's level of IQ is negatively correlated with *in utero* exposure to VPA [35,36], PRM [37], PB [38], PHT [36,39], CBZ [36,40,41], polytherapy [35–37,42], and seizures [43]. Exposure during the last trimester may actually be the most detrimental [38].

Several studies have suggested a notably higher risk of VPA for the neurodevelopment of children exposed *in utero*, often with lower verbal IQ scores [35,42,44,45]. Additionally, greater than five convulsive seizures during pregnancy had a negative effect on verbal IQ [45]. The AAN Practice Parameter updates recommend that avoiding VPA, PHT, and PB in pregnancy should be considered due to the risk of poor cognitive outcomes [6] and similar to prior recommendations, monotherapy should be considered to reduce the risk of adverse cognitive outcomes.

Since publication of the AAN/AES Practice Parameter updates, results from the Neurodevelopmental Effects of Antiepileptic Drugs (NEAD) Study Group have further confirmed these findings [46]. This study looked at cognitive outcomes of offspring born to WWE taking monotherapy of one of four AEDs – CBZ, LTG, VPA, and PHT. When corrected for maternal IQ, maternal age, AED dose, gestational age at birth and preconception folate, on average, verbal IQ at 3 years of age was significantly lower in the VPA group compared to each of the other three AEDs studied and this effect was dose related. The suggestion of the authors was to consider avoiding VPA in women of reproductive age, especially when there are now proven safer AED options. These findings should be considered in light of the concern that third-trimester exposure may have the greatest impact on cognitive development, and therefore VPA, PHT, or PB should not be added to the patient's regimen during the second or third trimester without consideration of the effect on fetal brain development.

Microcephaly has been associated with *in utero* AED exposure [13,14] and most often with polytherapy, PB, and primidone [47]. The risk of epilepsy in children of WWE is higher (RR 3.2) compared to controls [48]. Interestingly, this same increased risk has not been demonstrated for children of fathers with epilepsy.

Mortality

Fetal death (fetal loss at greater than 20 weeks' gestational age) may be another increased risk for women with epilepsy. Previous reports showed that stillbirth rates vary between 1.3% and 14.0% compared to rates of 1.2–7.8% for women without epilepsy [13], and perinatal death rates were also up to twofold higher for women with epilepsy (1.3–7.8%) compared to controls (1.0–3.9%) [13]. Based on a few studies, the AAN Practice Parameter update stated that WWE have no substantially increased risk of perinatal death [6]. One study published since the guidelines showed that there is an increase in perinatal death from 0.3% in controls to 2.2% in WWE [49]. Figures for spontaneous abortions (<20 weeks' gestational age) vary considerably [10,50,51] and the AAN guidelines concluded that there was insufficient evidence to draw any conclusions [5].

Potential mechanisms

The causes of the "anticonvulsant embryopathy" are likely multifactorial. However, recent studies have supported the anticonvulsant drugs as the most significant offending factor, more so than actual traits carried by mothers with epilepsy, environmental factors, or possibly even seizures during pregnancy [52–54]. Teratogenicity by AEDs is likely mediated by several mechanisms, including antifolate effects and reactive intermediates of AEDs. Almost all AEDs are associated with folate deficiency or interference with folate metabolism [55–57]. Although the beneficial effects of folic acid supplementation are clear for lowering the risk of neural tube defects in women without epilepsy [58,59], it is not as clear in women with epilepsy on AEDs. Older AEDs such as CBZ, PHT, PB, and primidone lower serum folic acid levels, so folic acid supplementation in women taking AEDs is encouraged. The AAN Practice Parameter updates concluded that the risk of MCMs in offspring of WWE was possibly reduced by folic acid supplementation and they recommend consideration of folic acid supplementation in WWE [7]. The ideal amount of folic acid supplementation needed for women taking AEDs is unknown. The Canadian Obstetrics and Gynecologists organization recommends 5 mg per day in WWE [60] and a 5 mg folic acid tablet is formulated in Europe and has been in use for many years. In the United States, to approximate 5 mg, epileptologists suggest 4 mg in addition to a regular prenatal vitamin.

Seizures during pregnancy

The physiologic changes and psychosocial adjustments that accompany pregnancy can alter seizure frequency,

Table 24.4 Alterations of AED clearance and/or concentrations during pregnancy

AED	Reported increases in clearance	Reported decreases in total concentrations	Reported changes in free AED or metabolites
PHT	19–150%	60–70%	Free PHT clearance increased in TM3 by 25%; free PHT concentration decreased by 16–40% in TM3
CBZ	−11 to +27%	0–12%	No change
PB	60%	55%	Decrease in free PB concentration by 50%
PRM	Inconsistent	Inconsistent	Decrease in derived PB concentrations, with lower PB:PRM ratios
VPA	Increased by TM2 and TM3		No change in clearance of free VPA. Free fraction increased by TM2 and TM3
ESX	Inconsistent	Inconsistent	
LTG	65–230%, substantial interindividual variability		89% increase in clearance of free LTG
OXC		MHD & active moiety decreased by 36–61%	
LEV	243%	60% by TM3	

AED, antiepileptic drug; CBZ, carbamazepine; ESX, ethosuximide; LEV, levetiracetam; LTG, lamotrigine; MHD, monohydroxy derivative of oxcarbazepine; OXC, oxcarbazepine; PB, phenobarbital; PHT, phenytoin; PRM, primidone; TM, trimester; VPA, valproic acid.
Source: Pennell and Hovinga [68].

including changes in sex hormone concentrations, changes in AED metabolism, sleep deprivation, and new stresses. Noncompliance with medications is common during pregnancy and is in large part due to the strong message that any drugs taken during pregnancy are harmful to the fetus. Teratogenic effects of AEDs are well described, but risks to the fetus are often exaggerated or misrepresented. Proper education about the risks of AEDs versus the risks of seizures can be very helpful in assuring compliance during pregnancy. The AAN Practice Parameter updates concluded that there was insufficient evidence to state whether or not there was a change in seizure frequency in pregnant WWE [5]. Two studies have shown that if WWE are well controlled for the 9 months prior to conception, they have a 84–92% chance of remaining seizure free during pregnancy [61,62].

Generalized tonic-clonic seizures (GTCS) can cause maternal and fetal hypoxia and acidosis [13,63]. After a single GTCS, fetal intracranial hemorrhages [64], miscarriages, and stillbirths have been reported [55]. A single brief tonic-clonic seizure has been shown to cause depression of fetal heart rate for more than 20 min [65], and longer or repetitive tonic-clonic seizures are incrementally more hazardous to the fetus as well as the mother.

Status epilepticus is an uncommon complication of pregnancy, and older studies showed that it carried a high maternal and fetal mortality rate [66] but this is no longer the case with improved medical care. In the EURAP study, 36 of 1956 pregnancies had status, with only 12 convulsive. Of these, only one had stillbirth [67]. No studies, however, compare the risk of status epilepticus in the pregnant WWE versus the nonpregnant WWE.

It is not as clear what the effects of nonconvulsive seizures are on the developing fetus. Many types of seizures can cause trauma, which can result in ruptured fetal membranes with an increased risk of infection, premature labor, and even fetal death [18]. If the woman is still having seizures, restrictions on driving and climbing heights should be reinforced with her, with special emphasis on the risk to the fetus.

Antiepileptic drug management

Management of AEDs during pregnancy can be complex. Clearance of virtually all of the AEDs increases during pregnancy, resulting in a decrease in serum concentrations (Table 24.4) [68]. Clearance of most of the AEDs normalizes gradually over the first 2–3 postpartum months. Lamotrigine metabolism, however, undergoes an exaggerated increase throughout pregnancy, and quickly converts back to baseline clearance within the first few weeks postpartum [31,69,70].

Several physiologic factors contribute to the decline in AED levels during pregnancy (Table 24.5). The greater extent of increased LTG clearance during pregnancy probably reflects its distinctive metabolic pathway of glucuronidation. The changes in AED levels during pregnancy can vary widely and are not predictable for an individual. The ratio of free to bound drug may increase during pregnancy for many of the older AEDs, but the amount of free AED still usually declines [68]. The optimal approach to monitoring AED levels during pregnancy is one that measures free levels of any AED that is highly or moderately protein bound [10]. Total levels are sufficient for AEDs that are minimally protein bound. The ideal

Table 24.5 Physiologic changes during pregnancy: effects on drug disposition

Parameter	Consequences
↑ Total body water, extracellular fluid	Altered drug distribution
↑ Fat stores	↓ Elimination of lipid-soluble drugs
↑ Cardiac output	↑ Hepatic blood flow leading to ↑ elimination
↑ Renal blood flow and glomerular flow rate	↑ Renal clearance of unchanged drug
Altered cytochrome P450 activity	Altered systemic absorption and hepatic elimination
↓ Maternal albumin	Altered free fraction; increased availability of drug for hepatic extraction

Source: Pennell [83].

AED (free) level(s) need to be established for each individual patient prior to conception, and should be the level at which seizure control is the best possible for that patient without debilitating side-effects. Levels should be obtained at least at baseline prior to conception and repeated at the beginning of each trimester and again in the last 4 weeks of pregnancy [10,32]. Some authors recommend monthly monitoring given the possibility of rapid and unpredictable decreases in AED levels in an individual patient [68]. The 2009 AAN Practice Parameter update concluded that pregnancy probably reduces the levels of LTG, CBZ, and PHT and so recommends that monitoring levels of these AEDs during pregnancy should be considered [7].

Obstetric complications

Women with epilepsy may have an increased risk of certain obstetric complications such as peripartum hemorrhage, preterm delivery, hypertensive disorders of pregnancy, and cesarean delivery. The AAN Practice Parameter updates determined that there is probably no substantially increased risk (greater than two times) of cesarean delivery or late pregnancy bleeding and that for WWE who smoke as compared to those who do not, there is a substantially increased risk of premature contractions and preterm labor [5]. They did not find sufficient evidence to comment on whether or not there was an increased risk of preeclampsia, pregnancy-induced hypertension, or spontaneous abortion in WWE.

There have since been several other studies evaluating obstetric outcomes. Using the Medical Birth Registry of Norway, only one-third of WWE were taking AEDs, and they had an increased risk of mild preeclampsia, gestational hypertension, vaginal bleeding, and delivery before

34 weeks, whereas the WWE not taking AEDs had no increased risk of these adverse outcomes [72]. In a study using a national database, WWE were found to have increased rates of hospitalization during pregnancy, intra-uterine growth restriction, and cesarean delivery but not increased rates of hypertension in pregnancy or premature rupture of membranes [73]. While these studies are useful in guiding obstetric care, more detailed prospective studies will be needed to differentiate the extent of these outcomes.

Neonatal vitamin K deficiency

Many of the AEDs can inhibit vitamin K transport across the placenta [13,74–76]. Infant mortality from this hemorrhagic disorder is very high at greater than 30% and is usually due to bleeding in the abdominal and pleural cavities leading to shock. Older AAN 1998 guidelines recommend prophylactic treatment with vitamin K administered orally as 10 mg to the mother during the last month of pregnancy and 1 mg administered intramuscularly or intravenously to the newborn at birth [10]. The 2009 AAN Practice Parameter updates compared studies looking at newborns of WWE on AEDs to newborns of women without epilepsy where all newborns got intramuscular vitamin K and the WWE did not have prentatal vitamin K supplementation. Their conclusion was that there was not enough evidence to determine if there was an increased risk of hemorrhagic disease of the newborn in WWE taking AEDs [7]. Since all newborns are now given intramuscular vitamin K at birth and fewer WWE are on older enzyme-inducing medications, administration of vitamin K during pregnancy is no longer widely practiced.

Labor and delivery

The majority of WWE will not experience seizures during labor and delivery. Reports of women with seizures during labor and the first 24 h postpartum are 2%, and may be as high as 12.5% of women with primary generalized epilepsy syndromes [77,78]. A more recent large study showed that 3.5% of women had seizures during delivery, with most of these occurring in women who had active epilepsy [67]. Sleep deprivation may provoke seizures and obstetric anesthesia may be used to allow for some rest prior to delivery if sleep deprivation has been prolonged. The specific analgesic meperidine should be avoided because of its potential to lower seizure threshold.

During a prolonged labor, oral absorption of AEDs may be erratic and any emesis will confound the problem. Phenobarbital, (fos)phenytoin, and VPA can be given intravenously at the same maintenance dosage. Convulsive seizures and repeated seizures during labor should be treated promptly with parenteral lorazepam (1–4 mg) or valium (5–10 mg) [77]. Benzodiazepines can cause neonatal respiratory depression, decreased heart rate, and maternal apnea if given in large doses, and these potential side-effects need to be monitored closely. Administration of another, longer-acting AED is controversial due to the inhibitory effects on myometrial contractions [77]. If convulsive seizures occur, oxygen should be administered to the patient and she should be placed on her left side to increase uterine blood flow and decrease the risk of maternal aspiration [32]. Prompt cesarean delivery should be performed when repeated GTCS cannot be controlled during labor or when the mother is unable to cooperate during labor because of impaired awareness during repetitive absence or complex partial seizures [77].

Postpartum care

Most of the AED levels gradually increase after delivery and plateau by 10 weeks postpartum. AED levels may need to be followed closely during this postpartum period [10]. Lamotrigine levels, however, increase immediately and plateau within 2–3 weeks postpartum. In order to avoid toxicity, adjustments in LTG doses need to be made on an anticipatory basis beginning within the first few days after delivery [79]. One prospective study demonstrated a significantly reduced risk for postpartum toxicity if an empiric LTG taper over the first 10–14 days postpartum was followed, with return to preconception dose or slightly above preconception dose (to provide extra protection from seizures during sleep deprivation) [31].

Perinatal lethargy, irritability, and feeding diffculties have been attributed to intrauterine exposure to benzodiazepines and barbiturates, and breastfeeding on these medications may prolong sedation and feeding problems. The 2009 AAN Practice Parameter update found no articles addressing symptomatic effects of AEDs on the newborn and acknowledged that this may lead to anxiety for the mother on an AED considering breastfeeding [7]. Despite this, most infants of WWE can successfully breastfeed without complications. The concentrations of the different AEDs in breastmilk are considerably less than those in maternal serum (Table 24.6). The infant's serum concentration is determined by this factor as well as the AED elimination half-life in neonates, which is usually more prolonged than that in adults [68]. The benefits of breastfeeding are believed to outweigh the small risk of adverse effects of AEDs [10,80] and parents should be advised to watch for signs of increased lethargy to a degree that interferes with normal growth and development.

Table 24.6 Antiepileptic drug exposure through breastmilk

AED	Breast milk/maternal concentration	Adult half-life	Neonate half-life
CBZ	0.36–0.41	8–25	8–36
PHT	0.06–0.19	12–15	15–105
PB	0.36–0.46	75–125	100–500
ESX	0.86–1.36	32–60	32–38
PRM	0.72	4–12	7–60
VPA	0.01–0.1	6–20	30–60
LTG	0.5–0.77	30	–
ZNS	0.41–0.93	63	61–109
TPM	0.86	21	24
GBP	0.7–1.3	7–9	14
OXC	0.5–0.65	19.3	17–22
LEV	0.8–1.3	6–8	16–18

AED, antiepileptic drug; CBZ, carbamazepine; ESX, ethosuximide; LEV, levetiracetam; LTG, lamotrigine; OXC, oxcarbazepine; PB, phenobarbital; PHT, phenytoin; PRM, primidone; TPM, topiramate; VPA, valproic acid; ZNS, zonisamide.
Source: Hovinga and Pennell [84].

The Neurodevelopmental Effects of Antiepileptic Drugs study examined potential effects of breastfeeding on cognitive development when the mother was on an AED [81]. The mothers were on one of four AEDs in monotherapy (VPA, PHT, LTG, CBZ). When comparing breast-fed children to children who did not breastfeed, the IQs for breast-fed children did not differ from nonbreast-fed children, for all AEDs combined and for each AED monotherapy group. These findings provide reassurance that women taking AEDs are not further harming their children's development by exposing them to AEDs via breastmilk.

Summary of management of epilepsy and pregnancy

Improving maternal and fetal outcomes for women with epilepsy involves effective preconceptional counseling and preparation. The importance of planned pregnancies with effective birth control should be emphasized, with consideration of the effects of the enzyme-inducing AEDs on lowering efficacy of hormonal contraceptive medications.

Before pregnancy occurs, the patient's diagnosis and treatment regimen should be reassessed. Once the diagnosis of epilepsy is confirmed, it is important to verify whether that individual patient continues to need medications and whether she is on the most appropriate AED to balance control of her seizures against teratogenic risks. For most women with epilepsy, withdrawal of all AEDs prior to pregnancy is not a realistic option. In the vast majority of cases requiring continued

AED therapy, monotherapy at the lowest effective dose should be employed. If large daily doses are needed, then frequent smaller doses or extended-release formulations may be helpful to avoid high peak levels. Some of the newest information about differential risks between AEDs should also be considered. The woman's AED regimen should be optimized and folate supplementation should begin prior to pregnancy. Given that 50% of pregnancies in the United States are unplanned, folate supplementation should be encouraged in all women of child-bearing age on any AED and for any indication. Dosing recommendations vary between 0.4 mg and 5 mg daily.

If a woman with epilepsy presents after conception on a single AED that is effective, her medication should usually not be changed. Exposing the fetus to a second agent during a cross-over period of AEDs only increases the teratogenic risk, and seizures are more likely to occur with any abrupt medication changes. If a woman is on polytherapy, it may be possible to safely switch to monotherapy. Maintaining seizure control during pregnancy is important, and monitoring of serum AED levels can help achieve that goal. Seizure control prior to pregnancy predicts good seizure control during pregnancy.

Prenatal screening can detect major malformations in the first and second trimesters. Postpartum care should focus on safety and medication monitoring and adjustment.

Although women on AEDs for epilepsy, or for other indications, do have increased risks for maternal and fetal complications, these risks can be considerably reduced with effective preconceptional planning and careful multidisciplinary management during pregnancy and the postpartum period.

CASE PRESENTATION

A 32 year-old, gravida 1, para 0 right-handed Caucasian female suffered a closed head injury with loss of consciousness in 1988 during a motor vehicle accident. Five years later, she developed her first seizure, which presented as an aura followed by a generalized tonic-clonic (grand mal) seizure. Her second seizure occurred in 1994, with similar semiology. She was diagnosed with epilepsy and started on phenytoin. Two years later, because of interference with birth control pills, her phenytoin was switched to valproic acid, 500 mg PO bid of the extended-release formulation. She had no further grand mal seizures but still had occasional auras with dizziness and wave-like vision, once per year. The patient stopped her birth control in 2005 with eager anticipation of pregnancy. She was not counseled about specific risks of her medication and was not on any vitamin supplementation.

She presented to our clinic at 17 weeks' gestational age for a second opinion regarding her epilepsy management in the setting of recent ultrasound diagnosis of multiple fetal congenital malformations, including meningomyelocele, severe hydrocephalus, and heart calcifications. Folic acid at 4 mg daily and a prenatal vitamin were pre-scribed. She was referred to a maternal-fetal medicine specialist and chose to undergo therapeutic dilation and evacuation. She returned to the neurology clinic 6 weeks later with her husband and they were given information on specific reported risks of MCM for lamotrigine monotherapy compared to valproate monotherapy. A gradual cross-over of her medication from valproic acid to lamotrigine was prescribed. A baseline, trough lamotrigine serum concentration measurement 1 month after the transition to lamotrigine monotherapy was ordered. She was counseled to wait until 6 months after the cross-over was complete before trying to conceive again, to assure medication tolerability and efficacy.

Following conception, monthly serum lamotrigine levels were obtained for therapeutic drug monitoring to maintain her individualized target concentration through dosage adjustments. She remained seizure free, and delivered a healthy 7 lb 13 oz baby boy. She breastfed her son until he was 1 year old. She returned to clinic the next year, planning for another pregnancy, and she delivered a full-term healthy 7 lb 10 oz baby girl following another uneventful seizure-free pregnancy with therapeutic drug monitoring of lamotrigine.

References

1. Hauser WA, Hersdorffer DC. Epilepsy: Frequency, Causes, and Consequences. New York: Demos, 1990.
2. Holmes LB. The teratogenecity of anticonvulsant drugs: a progress report. J Med Genet 2002;39(4):245–247.
3. Fairgrieve SD, Jackson M, Jonas P et al. Population based, prospective study of the care of women with epilepsy in pregnancy. BMJ 2000;321(7262):674–675.
4. Meador KJ, Zupanc ML. Neurodevelopmental outcomes of children born to mothers with epilepsy. Cleveland Clin J Med 2004;71(Suppl 2):S38–S40.
5. Harden CL, Hopp J, Ting TY et al. Practice Parameter update: management issues for women with epilepsy – focus on pregnancy (an evidence-based review): obstetrical complications and change in seizure frequency: Report of the Quality Standards Subcommittee and Therapeutics and Technology Subcommittee of the American Academy of Neurology and American Epilepsy Society. Neurology 2009;73(2):126–132.

6. Harden CL, Meador KJ, Pennell PB et al. Practice Parameter update: management issues for women with epilepsy – focus on pregnancy (an evidence-based review): teratogenesis and perinatal outcomes. Report of the Quality Standards Subcommittee and Therapeutics and Technology Subcommittee of the American Academy of Neurology and American Epilepsy Society. Neurology 2009;73(2):133–141.

7. Harden CL, Meador KJ, Pennell PB et al. Practice Parameter update: management issues for women with epilepsy – focus on pregnancy (an evidence-based reiview): vitamin K, folic acid, blood levels, and breastfeeding. Report of the Quality Standards Subcommittee and Therapeutics and Technology Subcommittee of the American Academy of Neurology and American epilepsy Society. Neurology 2009;73(2):142–149.

8. Janz D, Schmidt D. Anti-epileptic drugs and failure of oral contraceptives. Lancet 1974;1:113.

9. Guberman A. Hormonal contraception and epilepsy. Neurology 1999;53(Suppl 1):S38–S40.

10. Report of the Quality Standards Subcommittee of the American Academy of Neurology. Practice parameter: management issues for women with epilepsy (summary statement). Neurology 1998;51:944–948.

11. Krauss G, Brandt J, Campbell M, Plate C, Summerfield M. Antiepileptic medication and oral contraceptive interactions: a national survey of neurologists and obstetricians. Neurology 1996;46:1534–1539.

12. Rosenfeld W, Doose D, Walker S, Nayak R. Effect of topiramate on the pharmacokinetics of an oral contraceptive containing norethindrone and ethinyl estradiol in patients with epilepsy. Epilepsia 1997;38:317–323.

13. Yerby MS. Quality of life, epilepsy advances, and the evolving role of anticonvulsants in women with epilepsy. Neurology 2000;55(5):21–31.

14. Hvas C, Henriksen T, Ostergaard J, Dam M. Epilepsy and pregnancy: effect of antiepileptic drugs and lifestyle on birthweight. Br J Obstet Gynaecol 2000;107:896–902.

15. Arpino C, Brescianini S, Robert E et al. Teratogenic effects of antiepileptic drugs: use of an international database on malformations and drug exposure (MADRE). Epilepsia 2000;41:1436–1443.

16. Pennell PB. Pregnancy in women who have epilepsy. Neurol Clin 2004;22(4):799–820.

17. Morrell M. Guidelines for the care of women with epilepsy. Neurology 1998;51(Suppl 5):S21–S27.

18. Yerby M, Devinsky O. Epilepsy and pregnancy. In: Devinsky O, Feldmann E, Hainline B, eds. Advances in Neurology: Neurological Complications of Pregnancy. New York: Raven Press, 1994, pp.45–63.

19. Honein MA, Paulozzi LJ, Cragan JD, Correa A. Evaluation of selected characteristics of pregnancy drug registries. Teratology 1999;60:356–364.

20. Lindhout D, Meinardi H, Meijer J, Nau H. Antiepileptic drugs and teratogenesis in two consecutive cohorts: changes in prescription policy paralleled by changes in pattern of malformations. Neurology 1992;42(Suppl 5):94–110.

21. Barrett C, Richens A. Epilepsy and pregnancy: report of an Epilepsy Research Foundation Workshop. Epilepsy Res 2003;52(3):147–187.

22. Lindhout D, Schmidt D. In-utero exposure to valproate and neural tube defects. Lancet 1986;2:1392–1393.

23. Samren E, van Duijn C, Koch S et al. Maternal use of antiepileptic drugs and the risk of major congenital malformations: a joint European prospective study of human teratogenesis asssociated with maternal epilepsy. Epilepsia 1997;38:981–990.

24. Holmes LB, Wyszynski DF, Lieberman E. The AED (antiepileptic drug) pregnancy registry: a 6-year experience. Arch Neurol 2004;61(5):673–678.

25. Wyszynski DF, Nambisan M, Surve T, Alsdorf RM, Smith CR, Holmes LB. Increased rate of major malformations in offspring exposed to valproate during pregnancy. Neurology 2005;64(6):961–965.

26. Morrow J, Russell A, Guthrie E et al. Malformation risks of antiepileptic drugs in pregnancy: a prospective study from the UK Epilepsy and Pregnancy Register. J Neurol Neurosurg Psychiatry 2006;77(2):193–198.

27. Vajda FJ, O'Brien TJ, Hitchcock A, Graham J, Lander C, Eadie MJ. The Australian registry of anti-epileptic drugs in pregnancy: experience after 30 months. J Clin Neurosci 2003;10(5):543–549.

28. Vajda F, O'Brien T, Hitchcock A, Graham J, Lander C, Eadie MJ. Critical relationship between sodium valproate dose and human teratogenicity: results of the Australian register of anti-epileptic drugs in pregnancy. J Clin Neurosci 2004;1(8):854–858.

29. Holmes LB, Wyszynski DF, Baldwin EJ et al. Increased frequency of isolated cleft palate in infants exposed to lamotrigine during pregnancy. Neurology 2008;70(22 Pt 2):2152–2158.

30. Sabers A, Dam M, Rogvi-Hansen B et al. Epilepsy and pregnancy: lamotrigine as main drug used. Acta Neurol Scand 2004;109(1):9–13.

31. Pennell PB, Peng L, Newport DJ et al. Lamotrigine in pregnancy: clearance, therapeutic drug monitoring, and seizure frequency. Neurology 2008;70:2130–2136.

32. Committee on Educational Bulletins of the American College of Obstetricians and Gynecologists. Seizure disorders in pregnancy. Int J Gynecol Obstet 1997;56:279–286.

33. Leavitt A, Yerby M, Robinson N, Sells C, Erickson D. Epilepsy in pregnancy: developmental outcome of offspring at 12 months. Neurology 1992;42(4 Suppl 5):141–143.

34. Ganstrom M, Gaily E. Psychomotor development in children of mothers with epilepsy. Neurology 1992;42(Suppl 5):144–148.

35. Adab N, Jacoby A, Smith D, Chadwick D. Additional educational needs in children born to mothers with epilepsy. J Neurol Neurosurg Psychiatry 2001;70:15–21.

36. Dean J, Hailey H, Moore S, Lloyd D, Turnpenny P, Little J. Long term health and neurodevelopment in children exposed to antiepileptic drugs before birth. J Med Genet 2002;39(4):251–259.

37. Koch S, Titze K, Zimmerman R, Schroder M, Lehmkuhl U, Rauh H. Long-term neuropsychological consequences of maternal epilepsy and anticonvulsant treatment during pregnancy for school-age children and adolescents. Epilepsia 1999;40:1237–1243.

38. Reinisch J, Sanders S, Mortensen E, Rubin D. In utero exposure to phenobarbital and intelligence deficits in adult men. JAMA 1995;724:1518–1525.

39. Vanoverloop D, Schnell R, Harvey E, Holmes L. The effects of prenatal exposure to phenytoin and other anticonvulsants on

intellectual function at 4 to 8 years of age. Neurotoxicol Teratol 1992;14(5):329–335.

40. Ornoy A, Cohen E. Outcome of children born to epileptic mothers treated with carbamazepine during pregnancy. Arch Dis Child 1996;75(6):517–520.

41. Matalon S, Schechtman S, Goldzweig G, Ornoy A. The teratogenic effect of carbamazepine: a meta-analysis of 1255 exposures. Reprod Toxicol 2002;16(1):9–17.

42. Adab N, Tudor-Smith C, Vinten J, Winterbottom J. A systematic review of long term developmental outcomes in children exposed to antiepileptic drugs in utero. Epilepsia 2002;43(Suppl 7):230–231.

43. Leonard G, Andermann E, Ptito A. Cognitive effects of antiepileptic drug therapy during pregnancy on school-age offspring [abstract]. Epilepsia 1997;38(Suppl 3):170.

44. Gaily E, Kantola-Sorsa E, Hiilesmaa V et al. Normal intelligence in children with prenatal exposure to carbamazepine. Neurology 2004;62(1):28–32.

45. Vinten J, Adab N, Kini U, Gorry J, Gregg J, Baker GA. Neuropsychological effects of exposure to anticonvulsant medication in utero. Neurology 2005;64(6):949–954.

46. Meador KJ, Baker GA, Browning N et al. Cognitive function at 3 years of age after fetal exposure to antiepileptic drugs. N Engl J Med 2009;360(16):1597–1605.

47. Battino D, Kaneko S, Andermann E et al. Intrauterine growth in the offspring of epileptic women: a prospective multicenter study. Epilepsy Res 1999;36:53–60.

48. Annegers J, Hauser W, Elveback L, Anderson V, Kurland L. Congenital malformations and seizure disorders in the offspring of parents with epilepsy. Int J Epidemiol 1978;7:241–247.

49. Mawer G, Briggs M, Baker GA et al. Pregnancy with epilepsy: obstetric and neonatal outcome of a controlled study. Seizure 2010;19(2):112–119.

50. Yerby M, Cawthon M. Fetal death, malformations and infant mortality in infants of mothers with epilepsy. Epilepsia 1996;37(Suppl 5):98.

51. Yerby M, Collins S. Teratogenecity of antiepileptic drugs. In: Engel J, Pedley T, eds. Epilepsy, A Comprehensive Textbook. Philadelphia: Lippincott-Raven, 1997, pp.1195–1203.

52. Canger R, Battino D, Canerini M et al. Malformations in offspring of women with epilepsy: a prospective study. Epilepsia 1999;40:1231–1236.

53. Holmes LB, Harvey EA, Coull BA et al. The teratogenicity of anticonvulsant drugs. N Engl J Med 2001;344(15):1132–1138.

54. Holmes LB, Rosenberger PB, Harvey EA, Khoshbin S, Ryan L. Intelligence and physical features of children of women with epilepsy. Teratology 2000;61(3):196–202.

55. Zahn CA, Morrell MJ, Collins SD, Labiner DM, Yerby MS. Management issues for women with epilepsy: a review of the literature. Neurology 1998;51(4):949–956.

56. Dansky L, Rosenblatt D, Andermann E. Mechanisms of teratogenesis: folic acid and antiepileptic therapy. Neurology 1992;42:32–42.

57. Wegner C, Nau H. Alteration of embryonic folate metabolism by valproic acid during organogenesis: implications for mechanisms of teratogenesis. Neurology 1992;42(Suppl 5):17–24.

58. Botto L, Moore C, Khoury M, Erickson J. Medical progress: neural-tube defects. N Engl J Med 1999;341:1509–1519.

59. MRC Vitamin Study Research Group. Prevention of neural-tube defects: results of the Medical Research Council Vitamin Study. Lancet 1991;338:131–137.

60. De Wals P, Tairou F, van Allen MI et al. Reduction in neural-tube defects after folic acid fortification in Canada. N Engl J Med 2007;357(2):135–142.

61. Gjerde IO, Strandjord RE, Ulstein M. The course of epilepsy during pregnancy: a study of 78 cases. Acta Neurol Scand 1988;78(3):198–205.

62. Tomson T, Lindbom U, Ekqvist B, Sundqvist A. Epilepsy, and pregnancy: a prospective study of seizure control in relation to free and total plasma concentrations of carbamazepine and phenytoin. Epilepsia 1994;35(1):122–130.

63. Stumpf D, Frost M. Seizures, anticonvulsants, and pregnancy. Am J Dis Child 1978;132:746–748.

64. Minkoff H, Schaffer R, Delke I, Grunevaum A. Diagnosis of intracranial hemorrhage in utero after a maternal seizure. Obstet Gynecol 1985;65(Suppl):22S–24S.

65. Teramo K, Hiilesmaa V, Bardy A et al. Fetal heart rate during a maternal grand mal epileptic seizure. J Perinat Med 1979;7:3–5.

66. Teramo K, Hiilesmaa V. Pregnancy and fetal complications in epileptic pregnancies: review of the literature. In: Janz D, Bossi L, Dam M et al, eds. Epilepsy, Pregnancy and the Child. New York: Raven Press, 1982, pp.53–59.

67. EURAP Study Group. Seizure control and treatment in pregnancy: observations from the EURAP Epilepsy Pregnancy Registry. Neurology 2006;66(3):354–360.

68. Pennell PB, Hovinga CA. Antiepileptic drug therapy in pregnancy I: gestation-induced effects on AED pharmacokinetics. Int Rev Neurobiol 2008;83:227–240.

69. Pennell P, Montgomery J, Clements S, Newport D. Lamotrigine clearance markedly increases during pregnancy. Epilepsia 2002;43(Suppl 7):234.

70. Tran TA, Leppik IE, Blesi K, Sathanandan ST, Remmel R. Lamotrigine clearance during pregnancy. Neurology 2002;59(2):251–255.

71. Yerby MS. Clinical care of pregnant women with epilepsy: neural tube defects and folic acid supplementation. Epilepsia 2003;44:33–40.

72. Borthen I, Eide MG, Veiby G, et al. Complications during pregnancy in women with epilepsy: population-based cohort study. Br J Obstet Gynaecol 2009;116(13):1736–1742.

73. Kelly VM, Nelson LM, Chakravarty EF. Obstetric outcomes in women with multiple sclerosis and epilepsy. Neurology 2009;73(2):1831–1836.

74. Howe A, Oakes D, Woodman P, Webster W. Prothrombin and PIVKA-II levels in cord blood from newborn exposed to anticonvulsants during pregnancy. Epilepsia 1999;40:980–984.

75. Srinivasan G, Seeler RA, Tiruvury A et al. Maternal anticonvulsant therapy and hemorrhagic disease of the newborn. Obstet Gynecol 1982;59:250–252.

76. Nelson KB, Ellenber JH. Maternal seizure disorder, outcomes of pregnancy, and neurologic abnormalities in the children. Neurology 1982;32:1247–1254.

77. Delgado-Escueta A, Janz D. Consensus guidelines: preconception counseling, management, and care of the pregnant woman with epilepsy. Neurology 1992;42:149–160.

78. Katz JM, Devinsky O. Primary generalized epilepsy: a risk factor for seizures in labor and delivery? Seizure 2003;12(4): 217–219.

79. Pennell PB, Newport DJ, Stowe ZN, Helmers SL, Montgomery JQ, Henry TR. The impact of pregnancy and childbirth on the metabolism of lamotrigine. Neurology 2004;62(2):292–295.

80. Pschirrer E, Monga M. Seizure disorders in pregnancy. Obstet Gynecol Clin 2001;28(3):601–611.

81. Meador KJ, Baker GA, Browning N et al, for the NEAD Study Group. Effects of breastfeeding in children of women taking antiepileptic drugs. Neurology 2010;75(22):1954–1960.

82. Moore K. The Developing Human: Clinically Oriented Embryology, 4th edn. Philadelphia: WB Saunders, 1988.

83. Pennell PB. Antiepileptic drug pharmacokinetics during pregnancy and lactation. Neurology 2003;61(6 Suppl 2): S35–S42.

84. Hovinga CA, Pennell PB. Antiepileptic drug therapy in pregnancy II: fetal and neonatal exposure. Int Rev Neurobiol 2008;83:241–258.

Chapter 25
Chronic Hypertension

Heather A. Bankowski and Dinesh M. Shah
Department of Obstetrics and Gynecology, University of Wisconsin Medical School, Madison, WI, USA

Hypertensive disorders are one of the most serious complications in pregnancy because of the potential to cause serious maternal and perinatal morbidity and mortality. Although a substantial number of hypertensive patients have relatively good outcomes, difficulty in differentiating between various hypertensive conditions, inability to predict which patients are at highest risk, and variability in the progression of preeclampsia make these disorders one of the greatest medical challenges in obstetrics.

Diagnosis

Chronic hypertension in pregnancy is diagnosed if there is a sustained elevation of arterial blood pressure of 140/90 mmHg or greater prior to the 20th week of gestation, or if hypertension existed prior to pregnancy [1]. The diagnosis of chronic hypertension in pregnancy may be missed because of the physiologic decline in blood pressure as a result of the vascular relaxation of pregnancy. As a result, chronic hypertension may be diagnosed as gestational hypertension in the third trimester. Chronic hypertension should be suspected if first-trimester diastolic pressures of 80 mmHg or higher are present, especially in a multiparous patient, or in a patient with a family history of chronic hypertension [2]. Patients who develop hypertension in more than one pregnancy most likely have chronic hypertension [3,4]. The rates of adverse perinatal and maternal outcomes increase when preeclampsia develops in a patient with underlying hypertension [5]. Patients with preeclampsia, in general, have a greater risk of cardiovascular mortality later in life [6]. Associated conditions involving the kidneys, such as systemic lupus erythematosus and diabetes mellitus, help make the diagnosis of secondary hypertension.

Classification

Although during pregnancy hypertension is commonly classified as mild (≥140/90 mmHg) or severe (≥160/105–110 mmHg), chronic hypertension outside pregnancy can be categorized as prehypertension, stage I and II hypertension, depending on the absolute level of blood pressure with or without evidence of end-organ damage [7]. The National High Blood Pressure Working Group has recommended that blood pressure be taken in the sitting position after 10 min of rest. Diastolic measurement is the pressure at Korotkoff phase V, when the sound disappears [1]. If automated blood pressure monitors are used, the diastolic pressure will be between the fourth and fifth Korotkoff sounds. To reduce inaccurate readings, an appropriate size cuff should be used (length 1.5 times upper arm circumference or a cuff with a bladder that encircles 80% or more of the arm). The patient should not use tobacco or caffeine for 30 min preceding the measurement [8]. Uterine size and compression of the inferior vena cava and aorta are factors (especially in the supine position) that alter blood pressure readings as the uterus enlarges.

Preconceptional therapy guidelines

Preconceptional counseling is important for the woman who has chronic hypertension. It is important to establish baseline data on this patient, and to teach her self-blood pressure monitoring prior to conception. Medication should be changed to one that would be acceptable during pregnancy. If she is taking a diuretic, the dosage should be diminished gradually and preferably eliminated prior to conception. Angiotensin-converting enzyme (ACE) inhibitors and angiotensin receptor blockers (ARB) are both associated with fetal hypocalvaria, lung hypoplasia

Queenan's Management of High-Risk Pregnancy: An Evidence-Based Approach, Sixth Edition. Edited by John T. Queenan, Catherine Y. Spong, Charles J. Lockwood.
© 2012 John Wiley & Sons, Ltd. Published 2012 by John Wiley & Sons, Ltd.

renal anomalies, and renal failure which may not be reversible, which is why these medications are contraindicated after the first trimester [9,10]. They are also contraindicated in the periconceptual period and the first trimester, as they have been associated with cardiac and central nervous system (CNS) anomalies with an overall risk ratio of 2.7 (95% confidence interval [CI] 1.7–4.3; actual anomaly rate 7.1% versus 2.6%) [11].

Evaluation

When hypertension is present or suspected, additional testing should be carried out based on clinical considerations. If a practitioner has not had extensive experience with hypertension during pregnancy, consultative advice should be sought from a subspecialist (i.e. maternal-fetal medicine).

Reasonable assessment for all patients may include urinalysis for protein and microscopic examination for sediment, especially if significant proteinuria is detected by the dipstick method. Baseline assessments of complete blood count with platelet count, serum creatinine, liver function testing (aspartate aminotransferase [AST], alanine aminotransferase [ALT]), uric acid, lactate dehydrogenase (LDH) should also be performed. A 24-h collection for total protein and creatinine clearance should be performed early in the pregnancy for patients with overt or suspected chronic hypertension. We suggest repeating this testing around 26–28 weeks' gestation to define a new baseline, because of the pregnancy-associated increase in renal blood flow that may physiologically increase proteinuria. Such an increase, if proportionate to increased glomerular filtration rate, should be interpreted as a physiologic change. This assists the practitioner's management if superimposed preeclampsia develops later in gestation.

Other tests to consider are based on clinical presentation. Consideration should be given to the possibility of systemic lupus erythematosus in patients with proteinuria disproportionate to the degree of hypertension, and one should check antinuclear antibodies (ANA) and anti-double-stranded DNA. Generally, the presence of diabetes mellitus is known, but in patients with proteinuria this should remain a consideration. If the hypertension is severe and gestation is less than 20 weeks, one should check serum electrolytes to evaluate for hyperaldosteronism or consider evaluation for a molar pregnancy. Cushing syndrome is rare and difficult to evaluate during pregnancy. If the patient has paroxysmal hypertension, frequent "hypertensive crises," seizures, and/or anxiety attacks, a 24-h collection of urine for vanillylmandelic acid, metanephrines, or unconjugated catecholamines should be performed to evaluate for pheochromocytoma [12]. A toxicology screen should be obtained in all patients with severe and/or accelerated hypertension to examine for illicit substance abuse, such as cocaine or methamphetamine.

If the hypertension has been present for several years, additional consideration should be given to ordering an electrocardiogram, echocardiogram, or ophthalmologic examination. Furthermore, the sleep apnea syndrome should be suspected and appropriate referral for evaluation should be undertaken in obese women with hypertension who snore loudly while asleep, awake with headache, and fall asleep inappropriately during the day. For patients with an elevated creatinine, a renal ultrasound may occasionally be useful. A young woman with severe hypertension (especially with no family history) may also require Doppler flow studies or magnetic resonance angiography to evaluate for renal artery stenosis, but this is generally detected before the patient has seen the obstetrician. Furthermore, negative results from renal ultrasonography do not rule out renal artery stenosis.

Differential diagnosis

Preexisting hypertension should be suspected in the absence of proteinuria and other corroborative laboratory findings of preeclampsia, family history of hypertension, obesity, multiparity, or other diseases known to affect the kidney. One should review medical records from prior healthcare visits to ascertain prepregnancy blood pressure measurements.

Preexisting hypertension, secondary to renal disease, should be suspected when proteinuria is disproportionate to the degree of hypertension, especially when the patient is multiparous or presents with hypertension prior to 34 weeks [13].

Forty-three percent of multiparous women presenting with preeclampsia had renal biopsies showing evidence of preexisting renal parenchymal or vascular disease [14]. Of women with preeclampsia diagnosed prior to 34 weeks, 70% had laboratory or renal biopsy evidence of preexisting renal disease [15].

Therapy during pregnancy

Home blood pressure monitoring permits the patient to be her own advocate and further reinforces the control of her environmental situation. Home blood pressure data are preferable, and correct calibration should be confirmed. Self-monitoring can reduce the use of antihypertensive medication and the need for hospitalization [16,17].

Bedrest has been suggested as therapy for women who have chronic hypertensive diseases of pregnancy. Uterine

Table 25.1 Antihypertensive medications for chronic hypertension

Medication	Dose	Important side-effects	Comment
Methyldopa	250 mg bid to 500 mg qid	Lethargy, fever, hepatitis, hemolytic anemia, positive Coombs test	Centrally acting α-agonist
Labetalol	100 mg bid to 800 mg tid; maximum dose 2400 mg/day	Tremulousness, flushing, headache; agents may lead to decreased placental perfusion	β-Blocker with α-blocking activity
Nifedipine	30 mg XL qd to 90 mg XL bid; 190 mg/day. We recommend bid dosing	Headache, tachycardia, orthostatic hypotension; avoid use in the setting of coronary artery disease	Calcium channel blocker
Thiazide diuretics	12.5–25 mg/day	May be harmful in volume-contracted states such as preeclampsia; initial effect is to decrease plasma volume	Limit use to fluid overload only
Hydralazine	5–10 mg IV	May cause fetal distress; flushing, headache, tachycardia, lupus syndrome	Vasodilator used in hypertensive emergencies

bid, twice a day; IV, intravenous; qd, every day; tid, three times a day; XL extended release.

blood flow is increased when the woman is in the left lateral recumbent position.

Antihypertensive therapy should be considered when the blood pressure exceeds 140/90 mmHg in the office or 135/85 mmHg on home monitoring [18]. The National High Blood Pressure Education Program Working Group on High Blood Pressure in Pregnancy recommends that antihypertensive therapy should be initiated or increased if the systolic blood pressure exceeds 150–160 mmHg or the diastolic pressure exceeds 100–110 mmHg. A table of commonly used antihypertensive medications is included for reference (Table 25.1).

Antihypertensive therapy has not been shown to improve fetal condition or to prevent preeclampsia [19]. However, such therapy controls acceleration of blood pressure, reduces antepartum hospitalizations due to severe hypertension, and should help prevent maternal stroke from uncontrolled hypertension. While the most extensively studied antihypertensive agent is methyldopa, it is currently rarely used in pregnant women. Labetalol and long-acting nifedipine, though introduced as second-line agents, are commonly used as first-line agents for control of hypertension in pregnancy [20]. Nifedepine is an ideal first-line antihypertensive agent in pregnancy due to its low maternal side-effect profile and steady blood pressure control with twice-daily extended-release dosing. The effect of calcium channel blockade is vasodilation and it may have a salutary effect on the uterine blood flow similar to its effect on renal blood flow.

Labetalol is an alternative medication that has α-adrenergic and central β-blocking effects. Other β-blocking medications do not have this dual effect, which may explain why these other β-blockers are associated with intrauterine growth restriction [21].

Oral hydralazine is a mild vasodilator and may be associated with a lupus-like reaction. Diuretics should be considered only as adjuvant therapy and preferably infrequently used. These medications should be reserved for patients with excessive fluid retention and for fluid overload. We would not recommend diuretic use for extremity edema of pregnancy.

Furthermore, various antihypertensive medications have been used to treat severe hypertension in pregnancy. Magee *et al*, in a metaanalysis, found that hydralazine was associated with a trend towards less persistent severe hypertension than labetalol, but more severe hypertension than nifedipine or isradipine [22]. Though there was significant heterogeneity in outcomes and in methodological qualities, they found that hydralazine was associated with more maternal hypotension, more maternal oliguria, and more frequent adverse effects on the fetus. They concluded that the results of these studies do not support the use of hydralazine as the first-line agent for treatment of severe hypertension in pregnancy. Magee *et al* performed another metaanalysis of randomized control trials that showed that nifedipine appears to be a reasonable agent for treatment of acute severe hypertension in pregnancy [23].

All of the aforementioned drugs probably cross the placenta and enter the fetal circulation, but have not been known to cause birth defects. As mentioned above, antihypertensive medications that work through the renin–angiotensin system (ARB and ACE inhibitors) are associated with various congenital anomalies and subsequent renal defects, oligohydramnios, and skeletal deformities and are contraindicated immediately before and during pregnancy.

One should avoid using two antihypertensive medications of the same class whenever a patient needs more than one agent to control the hypertension. This is most likely to occur for agents acting on the adrenergic system (e.g. avoid combining methyldopa with labetalol).

Antepartum fetal evaluation

Antepartum fetal evaluation should include sonography for the establishment of gestational age. Careful dating of gestation is important in the hypertensive pregnancy so that fetal growth may be assessed accurately and appropriate timing of delivery planning may be undertaken. Serial sonograms should be performed at 4-week intervals. If interval growth is not appropriate or estimated fetal weight is below the 10th percentile, umbilical artery Doppler velocimetry should be assessed. Intrauterine growth restriction is usually not seen until after 30–32 weeks' gestation in the majority of patients with mild hypertension not requiring pharmacotherapy.

Even uncomplicated patients with chronic hypertension or gestational hypertension carry an increased risk of perinatal mortality. Therefore, we recommend twice-weekly antepartum fetal testing beginning at 32 weeks' gestational age for all patients who carry a diagnosis of hypertension in pregnancy. Twice-weekly antenatal testing should consist of modified biophysical profile with either a full biophysical profile (BPP) or a contraction stress test [24]. Patients should be instructed on performing fetal movement assessment at home. It is generally recommended that patients assess fetal movement by counting the number of perceived movements that occur in 1h, or the length of time required for 10 movements [25]. Patients with hypertension complicated by fetal growth restriction, diabetes mellitus, preexisting renal disease, or preeclampsia comprise a higher risk patient population and may benefit from antepartum testing as early as 24–26 weeks or when fetal intervention is deemed to be appropriate.

Indications for delivery

Most pregnant patients with mild chronic hypertension remain stable. Delivery should be considered whenever any of the following exist.

• Superimposed preeclampsia at term.
• Severe preeclampsia or eclampsia at any gestational age [26].
• Evidence of fetal compromise in the context of gestational age and administration of betamethasone for fetal lung maturation if indicated: low biophysical profile, persistently nonreactive nonstress testing (NST), repetitive late decelerations at any gestational age, absent or reversed end-diastolic flow on fetal umbilical artery velocimetry.
• Documentation of fetal lung maturity.
• Severe hypertension (diastolic blood pressures persistently equal to or greater than 100mmHg) at or beyond 37 weeks' gestation.

Expert opinion suggests that pregnancy in patients with chronic hypertension should not be allowed to advance beyond 40 weeks. Delivery should be undertaken upon completion of the 38th week and no later than 39 weeks' gestation. Chronic hypertension is associated with a doubling in the rate of abruptio placentae. The risk for abruption is 0.7–1.4% among those with mild chronic hypertension, but increases to 5–10% for women with severe hypertension [19].

If the patient develops preeclampsia, hospitalization and early delivery may be indicated. Expectant management in selected cases of severe preeclampsia prior to 34 weeks' gestation may be considered to maximize perinatal outcome, within the bounds of maternal safety in consultation with a maternal-fetal medicine specialist. Stable patients may be delivered before 37 weeks after documentation of fetal lung maturity.

Postpartum follow-up

Women who have chronic hypertension usually do well during pregnancy, although 5–10% with severe hypertension have major catastrophic events [19]. Many of these women have completed their child bearing and can be offered a permanent form of contraception. Oral contraceptives are not contraindicated and can be prescribed postpartum. Other temporary contraceptive options that may be considered include intrauterine device (levonorgestrel or copper), contraceptive vaginal ring, etonogestrel contraceptive implant, or a barrier method. Long-term follow-up includes referral to an appropriate primary care physician who can facilitate routine monitoring of blood pressure, appropriate laboratory studies and lifestyle interventions to maximize cardiovascular health and decrease hypertension-related morbidity and mortality.

CASE PRESENTATION

A physician must be diligent when evaluating hypertension during pregnancy. The initial steps in diagnostic evaluation require careful consideration of the clinical history of the patient.

A 40-year-old gravida 3, para 2 presented to her physician in the second trimester with systolic blood pressures 130–140 mmHg and diastolic measurements of 90–100 mmHg. A 24-h urine collection revealed 351 mg/24 h of protein and creatinine clearance of 162 mL/min. The remaining laboratory findings were in the accepted normal range of reference for the laboratory. Because she had evidence of end-organ damage, antihypertensive medications were started.

The patient had persistent hypertension and proteinuria that would suggest preeclampsia. However, she also had hypertension in a prior pregnancy. This should raise suspicion that her hypertension is related to essential hypertension. She subsequently presented at 37 weeks with an increase in her blood pressure despite antihypertensive medication and 930 mg protein in 24 h. Labor was induced. She stopped her medication during the postpartum period and 12 weeks after delivery still had blood pressures greater than 140/90 mmHg. She should be followed by a primary care physician for long-term management of hypertension and to address her cardiovascular health and lifestyle modifications.

References

1. Report of the National High Blood Pressure Education Program Working Group on High Blood Pressure in Pregnancy. Am J Obstet Gynecol 2000;183(1):S1–S22.
2. MacGillivray I. Pre-Eclampsia: The Hypertensive Disease of Pregnancy. Baltimore, MD: WB Saunders, 1983, p.214.
3. Chesley LC. Remote prognosis after eclampsia. Perspect Nephrol Hypertens 1976;5:31–40.
4. Chesley LC, Annitto JE, Cosgrove RA. The remote prognosis of eclamptic women. Sixth periodic report. Am J Obstet Gynecol 1976;124(5):446–459.
5. Sibai BM, Lindheimer M, Hauth J et al. Risk factors for preeclampsia, abruptio placentae, and adverse neonatal outcomes among women with chronic hypertension. National Institute of Child Health and Human Development Network of Maternal-Fetal Medicine Units. N Engl J Med 1998;339(10): 667–671.
6. Funai EF, Friedlander Y, Paltiel O et al. Long-term mortality after preeclampsia. Epidemiology 2005;16(2):206–215.
7. Chobanian AV, Bakris G, Black H et al. The Seventh Report of the Joint National Committee on Prevention, Detection, Evaluation, and Treatment of High Blood Pressure: the JNC 7 report. JAMA 2003;289(19):2560–2572.
8. Sixth Report of the Joint National Committee on Prevention, Detection, Evaluation, and Treatment of High Blood Pressure. Arch Intern Med 1997;157:2413–2446.
9. Martinovic J, Benachi A, Laurent D et al. Fetal toxic effects and angiotensin-II-receptor antagonists. Lancet 2001;358(9277): 241–242.
10. Piper JM, Ray WA, Rosa FW. Pregnancy outcome following exposure to angiotensin-converting enzyme inhibitors. Obstet Gynecol 1992;80(3 Pt 1):429–432.
11. Cooper WO, Hernandez-Diaz S, Arbogast PG et al. Major congenital malformations after first-trimester exposure to ACE inhibitors. N Engl J Med 2006;354(23): 2443–2451.
12. Botchan A, Hauser R, Kupfermine M et al. Pheochromocytoma in pregnancy: case report and review of the literature. Obstet Gynecol Surv 1995;50(4):321–327.
13. Browne JC, Veall N. The maternal placental blood flow in normotensive and hypertensive women. J Obstet Gynaecol Br Emp 1953;60(2):141–147.
14. Fisher KA, Luger A, Spargo B, Lindheimer M. Hypertension in pregnancy: clinical-pathological correlations and remote prognosis. Medicine (Baltimore) 1981;60(4):267–276.
15. Ihle BU, Long P, Oats J. Early onset pre-eclampsia: recognition of underlying renal disease. BMJ(Clin Res Ed) 1987;294(6564): 79–81.
16. Rayburn WF, Zuspan FP, Piehl EJ. Self-monitoring of blood pressure during pregnancy. Am J Obstet Gynecol 1984;148(2): 159–162.
17. Symonds EM. Bed rest in pregnancy. Br J Obstet Gynaecol 1982;89(8):593–595.
18. O'Brien E, Asmar R, Beilin L et al. European Society of Hypertension recommendations for conventional, ambulatory and home blood pressure measurement. J Hypertens 2003; 21(5):821–848.
19. Sibai BM. Chronic hypertension in pregnancy. Obstet Gynecol 2002;100(2):369–377.
20. Creasy RK, Resnik R, Iams JD, Lockwood CJ. Creasy and Resnik's Maternal-Fetal Medicine: Principles and Practice, 6th edn. Philadelphia: Saunders Elsevier, 2009.
21. Bayliss H, Churchill D, Beevers M, Beevers D. Anti-hypertensive drugs in pregnancy and fetal growth: evidence for "pharmacological programming" in the first trimester? Hypertens Pregnancy 2002;21(2):161–174.
22. Magee LA, Cham C, Waterman E et al. Hydralazine for treatment of severe hypertension in pregnancy: meta-analysis. BMJ 2003;327(7421):955–960.
23. Magee LA, Cote AM, von Dadelszen P. Nifedipine for severe hypertension in pregnancy: emotion or evidence? J Obstet Gynaecol Can 2005:27(3):260–262.
24. Freeman RK. Antepartum testing in patients with hypertensive disorders in pregnancy. Semin Perinatol 2008;32(4): 271–273.
25. Chesley LC. Hypertensive Disorders in Pregnancy. Norwalk, CT: Appleton-Century-Crofts, 1978, pp.482–483.
26. Sibai BM. Management of pre-eclampsia remote from term. Eur J Obstet Gynecol Reprod Biol 1991;42(Suppl):S96–101.

Chapter 26
Systemic Lupus Erythematosus

Christina S. Han and Edmund F. Funai
Department of Obstetrics and Gynecology, The Ohio State University College of Medicine, Columbus, OH, USA

Systemic lupus erythematosus (SLE) is a chronic autoimmune disorder characterized by periods of disease flares and remissions. It is a heterogeneous disorder with a variety of clinical and laboratory manifestations. Affected patients can have a relatively benign course, affecting only the skin and musculoskeletal system, or be affected by aggressive, life-threatening visceral involvement.

Systemic manifestations include arthralgias, rashes, renal abnormalities, neurologic complications, thromboemboli, myocarditis, and serositis [1]. Box 26.1 outlines the revised diagnostic criteria put forth by the American College of Rheumatology [2,3]. Patients must fulfil at least four of the 11 criteria at some point in the course of their disease, although not necessarily concurrently. These criteria have been found to be 96% sensitive and 96% specific for the diagnosis of SLE [2].

Epidemiology

The prevalence of SLE varies with the population studied but is generally 5–125 per 100,000 and affects approximately 1% of pregnancies [4]. The lifetime risk of a woman developing SLE is 1 in 700, with a peak incidence at age 30 [5]. The prevalence of SLE is affected by sex, race, and geography. Lupus affects women 3–10 times as often as men, and disproportionately affects African-Americans, Afro-Caribbeans, Asians, and Hispanics [1,5]. In addition, the disease appears to be more prevalent in urban populations compared to rural populations [6].

Etiology

The etiology of SLE is multifactorial and many studies have suggested a combination of genetic, epigenetic, and environmental factors. Major advances in human genome-wide linkage analyses have identified several independently replicated SLE linkage regions, which may contribute to specific clinical or immunologic features of SLE. Key candidate genes with strong evidence for a role in pathogenesis of SLE include MHC, ITGAM, IRF5, BLK, STAT4, PTPN22, and FCGR2A [7]. Specific genes on different chromosomes are associated with clinical subsets of SLE, such as nephritis (2q34), hemolytic anemia (11q14), or development of specific autoantibodies, such as anti-double-stranded DNA (19p13.2). Although these genetic factors influence risk of SLE, additional factors are necessary to trigger onset of the disease [8].

Hormonal and environmental factors have been shown to contribute to the disease process. Early menarche, estrogen-containing contraceptive use, and hormone replacement therapy are associated with increased risk of SLE [9]. Viral infections, ultraviolet light, and medications have also all been implicated in the disease process [10,11].

Pathogenesis

Pathogenesis of SLE begins with recognition of autoantigens and activation of the innate immune system. Dysregulated response to initial cytokine signals from both the innate and adaptive immune systems results in an overactive, proinflammatory response to the autoantigens [7].

Autoantibodies in SLE include antinuclear antibodies (ANA), anti-double-stranded DNA (anti-dsDNA), anti-Smith (anti-Sm), anti-ribonucleoprotein (anti-RNP), anti-Ro/SSA, and anti-La/SSB antibodies. These autoantibodies carry diagnostic and prognostic implications, and contribute to the wide spectrum of clinical manifestations. ANA is the most common antibody for screening for autoimmune syndromes. However, 10% of asymptomatic pregnant women without autoimmune disease have ANA antibodies compared to 2% of nonpregnant controls

Queenan's Management of High-Risk Pregnancy: An Evidence-Based Approach, Sixth Edition. Edited by John T. Queenan, Catherine Y. Spong, Charles J. Lockwood.
© 2012 John Wiley & Sons, Ltd. Published 2012 by John Wiley & Sons, Ltd.

Box 26.1 Criteria for diagnosis of SLE

1 Malar rash

Fixed erythema, flat or raised, over the malar eminences, tending to spare the nasolabial folds

2 Discoid rash

Erythematous raised patches with adherent keratotic scaling and follicular plugging; atrophic scarring may occur in older lesions

3 Photosensitivity

Skin rash as a result of unusual reaction to sunlight, by patient history or physician observation

4 Oral ulcers

Oral or nasopharyngeal ulceration, usually painless, observed by a physician

5 Arthritis

Nonerosive arthritis involving two or more peripheral joints, characterized by tenderness, swelling, or effusion

6 Serositis

(a) Pleuritis: convincing history of pleuritic pain or rub heard by a physician or evidence of pleural effusion

or

(b) Pericarditis: documented by ECG or rub or evidence of pericardial effusion

7 Renal disorder

Persistent proteinuria greater than 0.5 g/day or greater than 3+ proteinuria if quantitation is not performed

or

Cellular casts: may be red cell, hemoglobin, granular, tubular, or mixed

8 Neurologic disorder

Seizures, in the absence of offending drugs or known metabolic derangements (e.g. uremia, ketoacidosis, or electrolyte imbalance)

or

Psychosis, in the absence of offending drugs or known metabolic derangements (e.g. uremia, ketoacidosis, or electrolyte imbalance)

9 Hematologic disorder

Hemolytic anemia, with reticulocytosis

or

Leukopenia: less than 4000/mm^3 on 2 or more occasions

or

Lymphopenia: less than 1500/mm^3 on 2 or more occasions

or

Thrombocytopenia: less than 100,000/mm^3 in the absence of offending drugs

10 Immunologic disorder

Anti-ds DNA antibody

or

Anti-Sm antibody

or

Positive findings of antiphospholipid antibodies based on:

(i) Abnormal serum level of IgG or IgM anticardiolipin antibodies

or

(ii) Positive test result for lupus anticoagulant

or

(iii) False-positive serologic test for syphilis known to be positive for at least 6 months and confirmed by *Treponema pallidum* immobilization or fluorescent treponemal antibody absorption test

11 Antinuclear antibody

An abnormal titer of antinuclear antibody by immunofluorescence or an equivalent assay at any point in time and in the absence of drugs known to be associated with "drug-induced lupus" syndrome

A person is classified as having SLE if any 4 of the 11 criteria are present (serially or simultaneously) during any interval of the evaluation.

Adapted from Tan *et al* [2] and Hochberg [55].

[12]. Because of the high prevalence in the general population, ANA is used mainly as a screening test for lupus.

Anti-dsDNA and anti-Sm are highly specific for lupus. Anti-dsDNA has been correlated with disease activity, particularly lupus nephritis. Renal damage is secondary to immune complex deposition, complement activation, and inflammation and subsequent fibrosis [1].

Anti-RNP can be found in SLE, mixed connective tissue disease, and scleroderma, and is associated with myositis, Raynaud phenomenon, and less severe lupus. Anti-Ro/SSA and anti-La/SSB are more often associated with Sjögren syndrome, but are also found in 20–40% of women with SLE. Anti-Ro/SSA and anti-La/SSB are of particular significance in pregnancy due to the association with neonatal lupus syndrome [13,14]. Lastly, antiribosomal P protein is associated with lupus cerebritis and neuropsychiatric manifestations [15].

Lupus flares are difficult to characterize, as they represent worsening of a heterogeneous disease process. A variety of scoring systems has been developed to measure SLE disease status and to aid the diagnosis of a flare. In one retrospective study, flares occurred in 68% of SLE pregnancies, the majority of which were mild to moderate [16]. Symptoms of flares include fatigue, fever, arthralgias, myalgias, weight loss, rash, renal deterioration, serositis, lymphadenopathy, and central nervous system symptoms. The titer of autoantibodies to Sm, RNP, Ro/SSA, or La/SSB may or may not fluctuate in parallel with disease flares. However, rising titers of anti-dsDNA (particularly in the setting of falling complement levels) may suggest an impending flare of disease and thus should trigger closer surveillance of the patient [17].

Patients with SLE may also form antibodies to cell membrane phospholipids. Approximately 30% of women with SLE have antiphospholipid antibodies (APA), which increase the risk for thrombosis and adverse pregnancy outcomes [18]. Antiphospholipid antibody syndrome (APS) will be discussed separately below.

Placentas from women with SLE demonstrate characteristic changes: reduction in size, placental infarctions, intraplacental hemorrhage, deposition of immunoglobulin and complement, and thickening of the trophoblast basement membrane [19,20]. These changes appear to be responsible for many of the effects of SLE on pregnancy outlined below (e.g. increased rates of preeclampsia, intrauterine growth restriction [IUGR], preterm delivery).

Differential diagnosis

The main differential diagnosis for SLE is between other rheumatologic and connective tissue disorders. Many of these autoimmune diseases share common diagnostic criteria and it may take time for the varied manifestations of these diseases to appear for ultimate diagnosis. Additionally, because of the varied nature of the criteria for diagnosis, patients presenting with several of the criteria could have other local or systemic disorders.

Differentiation of SLE from normal pregnancy symptoms can be challenging, given the frequency of vague musculoskeletal complaints or symptoms of fatigue in both processes. In addition, differentiation of SLE flare from preeclampsia can be even more challenging. The difficult diagnosis results from a high rate of chronic hypertension and disproportionately high rate of preeclampsia in SLE pregnancies. In one population, chronic hypertension was reported in 28% of SLE patients, with preeclampsia developing in 23% of nonhypertensive pregnancies and in 32% of the hypertensive pregnancies, although this was not found to be statistically significant [21].

Lupus flares often feature inflammatory arthritis, significant leukopenia or thrombocytopenia, inflammatory rashes, pleuritis, and fevers. Many of the manifestations of SLE flare can be similar to preeclampsia (hypertension, proteinuria, activation of the coagulation cascade) although the treatment for each is very different. The treatment for severe preeclampsia often involves delivery, while lupus flares can be treated conservatively while continuing a pregnancy. A rising anti-dsDNA titer, active urinary sediment, and low complement levels (C3, C4, and CH50) suggest a lupus flare [17,22,23]. In general, complement levels rise in pregnancy and are unaffected by uncomplicated preeclampsia.

Conversely, rising uric acid levels or a greater coagulopathy suggest severe preeclampsia and HELLP (hemolysis, elevated liver enzymes, and low platelet count) syndrome. As the pregnancy approaches term, efforts at discriminating between the two are not likely to be worthwhile: delivery will cure preeclampsia and if the symptoms do not improve, treatment of lupus flare can be initiated.

Table 26.1 Systemic lupus erythematosus and pregnancy

Effect of SLE on pregnancy	Effect of pregnancy on SLE
Increased stillbirth rate (25 times baseline)	Worsening of renal status if nephropathy present
	Increased flare rates (higher if active at start of pregnancy)
Increased preeclampsia rate (20–30%)	
Increased growth restriction rate (12–32%)	
Increased preterm delivery rate (50–60%)	
Increased PPROM rate	
Neonatal lupus (1–2% if anti-SSA/SSB present)	

PPROM, preterm premature rupture of membranes.

Morbidity

General morbidity and mortality

Because of the effect of SLE on multiple organ systems, patients with this disease have significantly increased morbidity and mortality. Women with SLE are more prone to cardiovascular disease, thromboembolic phenomena, infection, and renal disease [4]. With better understanding of the disease process and potential complications, survival rates have improved with 5-, 10-, 15-, and 20-year survival rates of 93%, 85%, 79%, and 68%, respectively [24]. Risk factors for mortality include renal damage, thrombocytopenia, lung involvement, high disease activity at diagnosis, and age ≥50 at diagnosis [24]. A summary of the effects of SLE on pregnancy and pregnancy on SLE can be found in Table 26.1.

Effects of pregnancy on systemic lupus erythematosus

The effect of pregnancy on SLE is widely debated in the literature. A shift in cytokines from a type 1 helper T response (Th1) to a type 2 helper T response (Th2) pattern is seen in pregnancy, with predominance of the antiinflammatory and pro-B-cell cytokines interleukin (IL)-4 and IL-10 [5]. Because the autoimmunity in SLE is largely humorally mediated, one might expect that this cytokine shift may worsen the disease process or increase the rate of lupus flares in pregnancy [5].

The reported incidence of lupus flares in pregnancy, however, ranges from 13% to 74% [25–28]. The discrepancies in reported rates can be attributed to variations in criteria for diagnosing lupus flares and the inherent heterogeneity of patients [5].

Ruiz-Irastorza *et al* [29] found that flare rates were higher in pregnancy than nonpregnant controls. When the pregnant women were followed for the year postpartum, it was found that they flared more frequently during pregnancy compared to the year following their deliveries. However, the flares during pregnancy were no more severe than those experienced by the nonpregnant controls or postpartum. Other authors have found equivalent rates of flares in pregnancy compared with nonpregnant controls [30,31].

It is generally believed that the risk for flare in pregnancy is increased if women are not in remission prior to becoming pregnant [5,30]. Approximately 35% of flares occur in the second trimester with another 35% occurring postpartum [26,29]. The majority of flares are minor and do not require immunosuppressive therapy; however, serious manifestations can occur.

Lupus nephropathy is the end-result of autoimmune-mediated inflammation and renal damage. Pregnancy causes a worsening in renal function in approximately 20% of women with nephropathy but is reversible 95% of the time [24]. The risk of renal deterioration is directly correlated with prepregnancy renal status.

The impact of pregnancy on postpartum damage accrual in SLE was reported in 2006 by Andrade *et al* [32]. The Systemic Lupus International Collaborating Clinics Damage Index (SDI) score was strongly associated with longer pregnancy duration (P = 0.006), disease activity (P = 0.001), damage prior to pregnancy (P <0.001), and total disease duration (P = 0.039) by multivariable analyses [32].

Effects of systemic lupus erythematosus on pregnancy

Systemic lupus erythematosus in pregnancy can affect both the mother and offspring. Maternal and obstetric sequelae include hypertension, preeclampsia, worsening renal disease, and thrombosis. Fetal effects include stillbirth, IUGR, abnormal fetal testing, neonatal lupus erythematosus (NLE), and preterm birth (both iatrogenic and spontaneous).

Adverse pregnancy outcomes are seen more frequently in women with SLE than in controls or in women who later develop SLE [33]. Preeclampsia occurs in 20–30% of women with SLE, with higher rates seen in women with underlying hypertension, renal disease, or APS [20,34,35]. IUGR has been reported in 12–32% of lupus pregnancies, which was higher than control populations [27,35,36]. Preterm birth is increased in SLE pregnancies, with rates as high as 50–60% resulting from preeclampsia, IUGR, abnormal fetal testing, and preterm premature rupture of membranes (PPROM) [27,36,37]. Rupture of membranes in women with SLE is more common in preterm and term pregnancies when compared with controls and appears to be unrelated to disease status, treatment, or serology [37]. Factors that were associated with premature delivery included prednisone use at conception (relative risk [RR] 1.8), the use of antihypertensive medications (RR 1.8), and a severe flare during pregnancy (RR 2.0) [16].

Pregnancy outcome and risk of stillbirth are related to the baseline disease status prior to pregnancy and do not appear to be affected by the presence or absence of flares in pregnancy [38]. Fewer pregnancies among women with high-activity lupus ended with livebirths compared to those with low-activity lupus (77% versus 88%, P = 0.063) [39]. Stillbirth rates in women with SLE have been found to be 150 per 1000 births, 25 times the national average [35]. Much of the effect of SLE on fetal loss rates has been attributed to concomitant APS [38,40]. If initial diagnosis of SLE is made during pregnancy, complication rates and fetal loss rates are further increased.

Risk factors for pregnancy loss that can be identified in the first trimester include secondary APS (adjusted odds ratio [OR] 3.4, 95% confidence interval [CI] 1.1–10.5), thrombocytopenia (adjusted OR 4.4, 95% CI 1.4–13.4), and hypertension (adjusted OR 3.0, 95% CI 1.1–8.5) [41]. In women with active renal disease, stillbirth rates are as high as 30%, and for women with more advanced renal disease, fetal loss rates approach 60%. Active renal disease also prognosticates risks of hypertensive disorders of pregnancy, IUGR, and premature birth. However, women with stable lupus nephritis, plasma creatinine values less than 1.5 mg/dL, proteinuria less than 2 g/24 h, and no hypertension have lower risks of adverse pregnancy outcome [34].

Neonatal lupus erythematosus (NLE) occurs in 1–2% of women with anti-Ro/SSA or anti-La/SSB antibodies regardless of whether they also have SLE [14]. The pathophysiology is thought to be transplacental passage of autoantibodies that target the developing fetus with resulting inflammation. The syndrome is most commonly characterized by fetal and neonatal congenital heart block (CHB), dermatologic findings, and occasionally thrombocytopenia, anemia, and hepatitis [14].

Approximately 50% of women whose fetuses or infants have CHB are asymptomatic, but more than 85% are anti-Ro/SSA or anti-La/SSB positive [14,42]. Approximately half of these women will eventually develop symptoms of a rheumatic disease, most commonly Sjögren syndrome. These women should be reassured that they do not have SLE in the absence of other clinical features, and have less than 50% likelihood of developing SLE in the future.

While other manifestations are transient humorally mediated effects with resolution in the first few months of life, CHB is a permanent condition. The anti-Ro/SSA and anti-La/SSB maternal antibodies cross the placenta and can damage the fetal atrioventricular conducting system, which results in varying degrees of heart block and, less often, fetal myocarditis. Fetal CHB is most commonly diagnosed between 18 and 24 weeks' gestation [43]. These autoantibodies may act via apoptosis [44] or by direct interference with cardiac conduction through calcium channels [45].

The risk of CHB in women with anti-Ro/SSA antibodies and no prior affected infants is 1–2% [13,14] but increases to 19% with a prior affected child [42]. Although third-degree or "complete" CHB is permanent, there are some observational data that first- or second-degree disease can be reversed with antenatal fluorinated steroid therapy, and that progression to more severe forms of heart block may be prevented [46]. Additionally, steroid therapy has shown some reversal of hydropic features in fetuses with CHB and evidence of cardiac failure [46]. At present, there is no evidence supporting the routine use of prophylactic steroid therapy in women with anti-Ro/SSA or anti-La/SSB antibodies to prevent the onset of CHB [44].

Management during pregnancy

Management of SLE during pregnancy begins with preconceptional counseling and a multidisciplinary approach. Prior to conception, maternal disease status should be assessed and risks of pregnancy discussed. Evaluation for any preexisting renal disease is performed with a 24-h urine collection and serum creatinine to measure proteinuria and creatinine clearance. Remission for 6 months prior to pregnancy reduces adverse outcomes.

Early pregnancy assessment should include assessment of maternal disease status including 24-h urine collection, plasma creatinine, complete blood count, anti-Ro/SSA antibody, anti-La/SSB antibody, anti-dsDNA antibody, C3, and C4 levels. Baseline presence of lupus anticoagulant (LAC), anticardiolipin antibody (ACA), and anti-β_2-glycoprotein-I (anti-β_2GPI) antibody should also be evaluated.

In addition, routine obstetric management plays an integral role. Early ultrasound and establishment of reliable dating are particularly important given the risks of premature delivery. In patients with severe disease which may be affected by a pregnancy, early genetic risk assessment may expedite the diagnosis of nonviable genetic abnormalities, for which a patient may revise her desires on continuation of a pregnancy.

Repeat anti-dsDNA, 24-h urine collection, plasma creatinine, C3, and C4 levels to monitor disease status may be considered each trimester. LAC, ACA, and anti-β_2GPI antibody can also be repeated in the second trimester to screen for development of APS.

Medication regimens should be adjusted by rheumatologists prior to conception in order to achieve optimal disease status with minimal teratogenicity. Medication classes used in the management of lupus include nonsteroidal antiinflammatory drugs (pregnancy class B), antimalarials (pregnancy class C), glucocorticoids (pregnancy class C), and immunosuppressive agents (pregnancy categories D and X). If APS is also present, anticoagulation can reduce the associated complications [4].

Prepregnancy drug regimens, if safe in pregnancy, should be continued in pregnancy to maintain remission. Nonsteroidal antiinflammatory agents are contraindicated after 28 weeks' gestation because of the risk of closure of the fetal ductus arteriosus. Hydroxychloroquine, an antimalarial medication used to treat SLE, is often maintained during pregnancy. Glucocorticoids are also safe in pregnancy, although stress-dose steroids should be given at delivery for patients requiring chronic use. Azathioprine (pregnancy class D) is an immunosuppressive agent that is metabolized to 6-mercaptopurine and is a cytotoxic purine analog. Most investigators have found azathioprine to be acceptable in pregnancy although there is a risk of growth restriction and fetal immunosuppression. Other cytotoxic agents such as cyclophosphamide (pregnancy class D) and methotrexate (pregnancy class X) are contraindicated in pregnancy and are to be avoided. Amenorrhea and infertility may be present in patients with exposure to prior immunosuppressive therapy or chronic steroid administration. A summary of medications used in the management of SLE is given in Table 26.2.

Fetal growth assessment as a measure of fetal well-being is performed at 4-week intervals in the third trimester, with more frequent assessment if IUGR is suspected. Doppler evaluation is reserved for assessment of fetal well-being if estimated fetal weight is less than the 10th percentile. Weekly nonstress testing with assessment of amniotic fluid can begin at 30–32 weeks. Additional surveillance with mechanical P-R intervals should be initiated at regular intervals if maternal anti-Ro/SSA or anti-La/SSB is present.

Making the diagnosis of lupus flare in pregnancy requires excluding the other diagnoses as outlined above. Flares can be managed conservatively with adjustment of medication regimen as outlined above or addition of analgesics such as acetaminophen. Glucocorticoid therapy can be initiated for more severe flares [20]. The exact treatment of the flare will vary with the nature and severity of the flare, and should be undertaken with the assistance of the rheumatology and/or nephrology services.

When women are followed in an intensive multidisciplinary clinic with pregnancies initiated during disease quiescence and treatment of underlying disease, fetal outcomes appear to be improved. Diagnosis and treatment of APS further decrease fetal loss rates.

Antiphospholipid antibodies

Antiphospholipid antibodies can be present alone or in conjunction with APS. APS has specific diagnostic criteria, which was revised by an international consensus

Table 26.2 Systemic lupus erythematosus therapeutic agents

Drug	Safety in pregnancy	Comments
Hydroxychloroquine	Generally considered safe Pregnancy class C	Antimalarial. Reduces disease flares
NSAIDs	Pregnancy class B	Association with oligohydramnios and ductus arteriosus closure. Avoid after 28 weeks
Glucocorticoids	Safe Pregnancy class C	Association with growth restriction at high dose, need stress-dose steroids at delivery or for medical illnesses if chronic use through pregnancy. Increased risk of PPROM and preterm delivery
Azathioprine	Pregnancy class D	Risk of fetal growth restriction and immunosuppression. Use as second-line agent
Cyclophosphamide	Unsafe Pregnancy class D	Alkylating agent. Skeletal and palate defects, also defects in eyes and limbs
Methotrexate	Unsafe Pregnancy class X	Folic acid antagonist. Abortifacient and teratogen

NSAIDs, nonsteroidal anti-inflammatory drugs; PPROM, preterm premature rupture of membranes.

conference in 2006 [47]. The clinical and laboratory criteria are listed in Box 26.2.

Clinical complications of APS include thrombosis, adverse pregnancy outcome (including IUGR and third-trimester fetal death), and recurrent pregnancy loss [47]. Prospective studies of women with APS without treatment have shown fetal loss rates as high as 50–90% [48]. APA and LAC are found in 1–5% of asymptomatic pregnant women but are higher in SLE patients (12–30% and 15–34%, respectively) [18].

The laboratory component for diagnosis of APS tests for ACA, LAC, and anti-β_2GPI antibody. ACA and LAC bind to β_2GPI, other phospholipid-associated proteins, or the phospholipids themselves. β_2GPI and annexin V are associated with phospholipids in the cell membrane and inhibit platelet and clotting cascade activation. Both molecules are found endogenously in high concentrations on the endothelium and syncytiotrophoblast and are thought to provide a protective layer. ACA, LAC, and anti-β_2GPI antibodies disrupt this protective layer, activating the clotting cascade and allowing complement-mediated injury to the placental vasculature to occur [49].

LAC is detected by the prolongation of various clotting assays with failure to normalize with the addition of control plasma (to exclude factor deficiencies). One common test is the dilute Russell viper venom test (dRVVT), and is reported as present or absent. ACA are detected by direct β_2GPI-dependent immunoassays and are reported by antibody class and low or high titer. Medium or high titers of IgG or IgM (i.e. >40 GPL or MPL, respectively, or >99th percentile) are clinically relevant [50]. Although LAC and ACA are frequently concordant and sometimes share epitope specificity, they are distinct entities. The presence of LAC is more specific for APS than ACA. Anti-β_2GPI antibodies are considered positive if they are >99th percentile.

Box 26.2 Criteria for the classification of antiphospholipid antibody syndrome. Presence of at least one clinical criterion and one laboratory criterion necessary for the diagnosis of APAS

Clinical criteria

1 Nonobstetric morbidity: thrombosis in any tissue, diagnosed via objective validated criteria, such as diagnostic imaging or histopathologic diagnosis.
   (a) Arterial thrombosis, including: cerebrovascular accidents, transient ischemic attacks, myocardial infarction, amaurosis fugax
   (b) Venous thromboembolism, including: deep venous thrombosis, pulmonary emboli, or small vessel thrombosis
2 Obstetric morbidity
   (a) Unexplained IUFD at ≥10 weeks in a morphologically and karyotypically normal fetus
   (b) Three or more unexplained spontaneous abortions at ≤10 weeks
   (c) History of preterm delivery < 34 weeks, as a sequela of preeclampsia or uteroplacental insufficiency, including the following:
       (i) Nonreassuring fetal testing indicative of fetal hypoxemia (e.g. abnormal Doppler flow velocimetry waveform)
       (ii) Oligohydramnios
       (iii) IUGR <10th percentile
       (iv) Placental abruption

Laboratory criteria

Positive testing for APA is required on two occasions, at least 12 weeks apart, and no more than 5 years prior to clinical manifestations.
1 Anticardiolipin antibody (ACA): IgG or IgM isotype, present in moderate or high titers (i.e. >40 GPL or MPL, or >99th percentile)
2 Anti-β_2-glycoprotein-I (anti-β_2GPI): IgG or IgM isotype (>99th percentile)
3 Presence of lupus anticoagulant (LAC)

APA, antiphospholipid antibody; GPL, IgG phospholipid units; Ig, immunoglobulin; IUFD, intrauterine fetal death; MPL, IgM phospholipid units.
Source: Miyakis *et al* [47].

Treatment goals for APS include improvement of fetal outcomes and reduction in risk for maternal thrombosis. Current accepted therapies include heparin anticoagulation and low-dose aspirin (LDA). Heparin has been shown to prevent both thromboembolic events and pregnancy loss. Either unfractionated heparin (UFH, pregnancy class C) and low molecular weight heparin (LMWH, pregnancy class B) can be used. Multiple mechanisms of action for heparin in treatment of APS have been proposed. UFH potentiates the effects of antithrombin, increases levels of factor Xa inhibitor, and inhibits platelet aggregation. Heparins may also render APA inactive via binding [51]. LMWH *in vitro* has been shown to counteract APA-induced trophoblast inflammation. However, in the absence of APA, LMWH *in vitro* induces potentially detrimental pro-inflammatory and anti-angiogenic profile in the trophoblast. Therefore, anticoagulation should only be used when truly indicated [52].

A meta-analysis showed that the livebirth rate was improved by 54% with heparin and aspirin therapy [53]. One cautionary note is that despite anticoagulation, 20–30% of women with APS have fetal losses, which may be explained by the *in vitro* effects of the medications on trophoblast function [52]. Intravenous immunoglobulin (IVIG) has been shown to be effective, although the cost and side-effects currently limit it to women with severe APS or those who have been refractory to heparin therapy.

Aspirin therapy can be initiated at the first positive pregnancy test and heparin therapy can be initiated at 5–7 weeks' gestation. As there is no maternal blood flow through the placenta prior to 5–7 weeks, heparin is not necessary before this point and may exacerbate implantation bleeding. Heparin therapy can either be therapeutic (i.e. 1 mg/kg enoxaparin every 12 h with maintenance of anti-Xa levels between 0.5 and 1.0) or prophylactic (i.e. 40 mg/day enoxaparin). It is not our practice to follow anti-Xa levels in those women receiving prophylactic heparin treatment. Although heparin-induced thrombocytopenia is a rare occurrence with LMWH, a platelet count should be obtained within 2 weeks of initiation of therapy. Because of the 1–2% risk of osteoporosis and fracture with UFH anticoagulation in pregnancy [54], we recommend daily calcium, vitamin D supplementation, and daily weight-bearing exercise as tolerated. Data suggest that LMWH anticoagulation during pregnancy does not significantly affect bone mineral density [55]. At 36 weeks, aspirin can be discontinued and LMWH switched to UFH to facilitate anticoagulation management at delivery. Postpartum anticoagulation (if indicated) can be with either warfarin or LMWH.

Treatment of APS during pregnancy with active fetal surveillance has shown improved outcomes. Nonetheless, antepartum complications remain common with elevated rates of preeclampsia, growth restriction, and premature birth [5].

CASE PRESENTATION

The patient is a 32-year-old gravida 5, para 1 at 7 weeks' gestation with a history of a term vaginal delivery 7 years ago of an infant with second-degree heart block. She had three subsequent miscarriages at approximately 10 weeks' gestation. An evaluation revealed the presence of anti-Ro/SSA antibodies, positive ANA, positive dRVVT, as well as high-titer ACA IgG. She also complains of periodic arthralgias and has had persistent proteinuria. What is her diagnosis and what therapy recommendations and prognosis can be given for her current pregnancy?

The patient can be diagnosed with APS because of her high-titer ACA and recurrent first-trimester miscarriages.

Additionally, she meets the criteria for SLE (ANA, ACA, arthralgias, renal disease). She has a 19% chance of another child with CHB and a substantial risk of miscarriage given her prior losses. Additionally, she has increased risk for preeclampsia, IUGR, PPROM, and preterm delivery. She can be offered aspirin and heparin therapy for her APS and close fetal surveillance to monitor for the development of heart block or IUGR. Therapy for SLE should be reviewed and optimized for her pregnancy. Her baseline renal status should be assessed and a baseline cardiac evaluation including electrocardiography would not be unreasonable.

References

1. Mills JA. Systemic lupus erythematosus. N Engl J Med 1994;330:1871–1879.
2. Tan EM, Cohen AS, Fries JF et al. The 1982 revised criteria for the classification of systemic lupus erythematosus. Arthritis Rheum 1982;25:1271–1277.
3. Hochberg MC. Updating the American College of Rheumatology revised criteria for the classification of systemic lupus erythematosus. Arthritis Rheum 1997;40:1725.
4. Ruiz-Irastorza G, Khamashta MA, Castellino G, Hughes GR. Systemic lupus erythematosus. Lancet 2001;357:1027–1032.
5. Buyon JP. The effects of pregnancy on autoimmune diseases. J Leukoc Biol 1998;63:281–287.
6. Chakravarty EF, Bush TM, Manzi S et al. Prevalence of adult systemic lupus erythematosus in California and Pennsylvania in 2000: estimates obtained using hospitalization data. Arthritis Rheum 2007; 56:2092.
7. Rhodes B, Vyse TJ. The genetics of SLE: an update in the light of genome-wide association studies. Rheumatology 2008;47(11):1603–1611.

8. Sestak AL, Nath SK, Sawalha AH, Harley JB. Current status of lupus genetics. Arthritis Res Ther 2007;9(3):210.

9. Costenbader KH, Feskanich D, Stampfer MJ, Karlson EW. Reproductive and menopausal factors and risk of systemic lupus erythematosus in women. Arthritis Rheum 2007;56(4): 1251–1262.

10. Cooper GS, Dooley MA, Treadwell EL et al. Risk factors for the development of systemic lupus erythematosus: allergies, infections, and family history. J Clin Epidemiol 2002; 55(10):982–9

11. Lehmann P, Holzle E, Kind P et al. Experimental reproduction of skin lesions in lupus erythematosus by UVA and UVB radiation. J Am Acad Dermatol 1990;22(2 Pt 1):181–187.

12. Farnam J, Lavastida MT, Grant JA, Reddi RC, Daniels JC. Antinuclear antibodies in the serum of normal pregnant women: a prospective study. J Allergy Clin Immunol 1984;73: 596–599.

13. Gladman G, Silverman ED, Yuk L et al. Fetal echocardiographic screening of pregnancies of mothers with anti-Ro and/or anti-La antibodies. Am J Perinatol 2002;19:73–80.

14. Lee LA. Neonatal lupus erythematosus. J Invest Dermatol 1993;100:9S–13S.

15. Schneebaum AB, Singleton JD, West SG et al. Association of psychiatric manifestations with antibodies to ribosomal P proteins in systemic lupus erythematosus. Am J Med 1991;90(1):54–62.

16. Chakravarty EF, Colon I, Langen ES et al. Factors that predict prematurity and preeclampsia in pregnancies that are complicated by systemic lupus erythematosus. Am J Obstet Gynecol 2005;192(6):1897–1904.

17. Repke JT. Hypertensive disorders of pregnancy: differentiating preeclampsia from active systemic lupus erythematosus. J Reprod Med 1998;43:350–354.

18. Levine JS, Branch DW, Rauch J. The antiphospholipid syndrome. N Engl J Med 2002;346:752–763.

19. Hanly JG, Gladman DD, Rose TH, Laskin CA, Urowitz MB. Lupus pregnancy: a prospective study of placental changes. Arthritis Rheum 1988;31:358–366.

20. Lockshin MD, Sammaritano LR. Lupus pregnancy. Autoimmunity 2003;36:33–40.

21. Egerman RS, Ramsey RD, Kao LW et al. Hypertensive disease in pregnancies complicated by systemic lupus erythematosus. Am J Obstet Gynecol 2005;193:1676.

22. Buyon JP, Tamerius J, Ordorica S, Young B, Abramson SB. Activation of the alternative complement pathway accompanies disease flares in systemic lupus erythematosus during pregnancy. Arthritis Rheum 1992;35:55–61.

23. Abramson SB, Buyon JP. Activation of the complement pathway: comparison of normal pregnancy, preeclampsia, and systemic lupus erythematosus during pregnancy. Am J Reprod Immunol 1992;28:183–187.

24. Abu-Shakra M, Urowitz MB, Gladman DD, Gough J. Mortality studies in systemic lupus erythematosus. Results from a single center. II. Predictor variables for mortality. J Rheumatol 1995;22:1265–1270.

25. Lockshin MD. Pregnancy does not cause systemic lupus erythematosus to worsen. Arthritis Rheum 1989;32:665–670.

26. Carmona F, Font J, Cervera R, Munoz F, Cararach V, Balasch J. Obstetrical outcome of pregnancy in patients with systemic lupus erythematosus: a study of 60 cases. Eur J Obstet Gynecol Reprod Biol 1999;83:137–142.

27. Mintz G, Niz J, Gutierrez G, Garcia-Alonso A, Karchmer S. Prospective study of pregnancy in systemic lupus erythematosus: results of a multidisciplinary approach. J Rheumatol 1986;13:732–739.

28. Nossent HC, Swaak TJ. Systemic lupus erythematosus. VI. Analysis of the interrelationship with pregnancy. J Rheumatol 1990;17:771–776.

29. Ruiz-Irastorza G, Lima F, Alves J et al. Increased rate of lupus flare during pregnancy and the puerperium: a prospective study of 78 pregnancies. Br J Rheumatol 1996;35:133–138.

30. Urowitz MB, Gladman DD, Farewell VT, Stewart J, McDonald J. Lupus and pregnancy studies. Arthritis Rheum 1993;36: 1392–1397.

31. Lockshin MD, Reinitz E, Druzin ML, Murrman M, Estes D. Lupus pregnancy: case–control prospective study demonstrating absence of lupus exacerbation during or after pregnancy. Am J Med 1984;77:893–898.

32. Andrade RM, McGwin G Jr, Alarcon GS et al. Predictors of post-partum damage accrual in systemic lupus erythematosus: data from LUMINA, a multiethnic US cohort (XXXVIII). Rheumatology (Oxford) 2006;45:1380.

33. Kiss E, Bhattoa HP, Bettembuk P, Balogh A, Szegedi G. Pregnancy in women with systemic lupus erythematosus. Eur J Obstet Gynecol Reprod Biol 2002;101:129–134.

34. Hayslett JP, Lynn RI. Effect of pregnancy in patients with lupus nephropathy. Kidney Int 1980;18:207–220.

35. Simpson LL. Maternal medical disease: risk of antepartum fetal death. Semin Perinatol 2002;26:42–50.

36. Lima F, Buchanan NM, Khamashta MA, Kerslake S, Hughes GR. Obstetric outcome in systemic lupus erythematosus. Semin Arthritis Rheum 1995;25:184–192.

37. Johnson MJ, Petri M, Witter FR, Repke JT. Evaluation of preterm delivery in a systemic lupus erythematosus pregnancy clinic. Obstet Gynecol 1995;86:396–399.

38. Faussett MB, Branch DW. Autoimmunity and pregnancy loss. Semin Reprod Med 2000;18:379–392.

39. Clowse ME, Magder LS, Witter F, Petri M. The impact of increased lupus activity on obstetric outcomes. Arthritis Rheum 2005;52:514.

40. Ginsberg JS, Brill-Edwards P, Johnston M et al. Relationship of antiphospholipid antibodies to pregnancy loss in patients with systemic lupus erythematosus: a cross-sectional study. Blood 1992;80:975–980.

41. Clowse ME, Magder LS, Witter F, Petri M. Early risk factors for pregnancy loss in lupus. Obstet Gynecol 2006;107:293.

42. Buyon JP, Rupel A, Clancy RM. Neonatal lupus syndromes. Lupus 2004;13:705–712.

43. Buyon JP, Waltuck J, Kleinman C, Copel J. In utero identification and therapy of congenital heart block. Lupus 1995;4: 116–121.

44. Buyon JP, Clancy RM. Maternal autoantibodies and congenital heart block: mediators, markers, and therapeutic approach. Semin Arthritis Rheum 2003;33:140–154.

45. Boutjdir M. Molecular and ionic basis of congenital complete heart block. Trends Cardiovasc Med 2000;10:114–122.

46. Saleeb S, Copel J, Friedman D, Buyon JP. Comparison of treatment with fluorinated glucocorticoids to the natural history of autoantibody-associated congenital heart block: retrospective review of the research registry for neonatal lupus. Arthritis Rheum 1999;42:2335–2345.

47. Miyakis S, Lockshin MD, Atsumi T et al. International consensus statement on an update of the classification criteria for definite antiphospholipid syndrome (APS). J Thromb Haemost 2006;4:295–306.

48. Warren JB, Silver RM. Autoimmune disease in pregnancy: systemic lupus erythematosus and antiphospholipid syndrome. Obstet Gynecol Clin North Am 2004;31:345–372, vi–vii.

49. Salmon JE, Girardi G, Holers VM. Activation of complement mediates antiphospholipid antibody-induced pregnancy loss. Lupus 2003;12:535–538.

50. Silver RM, Porter TF, van Leeuween I, Jeng G, Scott JR, Branch DW. Anticardiolipin antibodies: clinical consequences of "low titers". Obstet Gynecol 1996;87:494–500.

51. Franklin RD, Kutteh WH. Effects of unfractionated and low molecular weight heparin on antiphospholipid antibody binding in vitro. Obstet Gynecol 2003;101(3):455–462.

52. Han CS, Mulla MJ, Brosens JJ et al. Aspirin and heparin effect on basal and antiphospholipid antibody modulation of trophoblast function. Obstet Gynecol 2011; in press.

53. Empson M, Lassere M, Craig JC, Scott JR. Recurrent pregnancy loss with antiphospholipid antibody: a systematic review of therapeutic trials. Obstet Gynecol 2002;99:135–144.

54. Dahlman TC. Osteoporotic fractures and the recurrence of thromboembolism during pregnancy and the puerperium in 184 women undergoing thromboprophylaxis with heparin. Am J Obstet Gynecol 1993;168:1265–1270.

55. Pettila V, Leinonen P, Markkola A, Hiilesmaa V, Kaaja R. Postpartum bone mineral density in women treated for thromboprophylaxis with unfractionated heparin or LMW heparin. Thromb Haemost 2002;87:182–186.

56. Hochberg MC. Updating the American College of Rheumatology revised criteria for the classification of systemic lupus erythematosus (letter). Arthritis Rheum 1997;40(9):1725.

Chapter 27
Perinatal Infections

Jeanne S. Sheffield
Department of Obstetrics and Gynecology, University of Texas Southwestern Medical Center, Dallas, TX, USA

Perinatal infections continue to plague pregnancies both in the United States and worldwide. Most perinatal infections are asymptomatic in the mother but may have devastating consequences to the fetus. In the last decade, many advances in maternal and fetal diagnosis as well as treatment have occurred and will be addressed.

Parvovirus B$_{19}$

Parvovirus B$_{19}$, a single-stranded DNA virus, is the only parvovirus causing human disease (erythema infectiosum or fifth disease). It is an endemic viral infection predominantly seen in preschool and school-age children; by adulthood only 40% of women tested are susceptible. The annual seroconversion rate is 1–2%. Though often asymptomatic in the mother, parvovirus B$_{19}$ replicates in rapidly proliferating cells such as euthyroid progenitor cells, leading to severe anemia in the fetus, young child and adults with erythrocyte membrane abnormalities or chronic hemolytic anemias.

Transmission
Transmission of parvovirus B$_{19}$ occurs predominantly through respiratory droplets via person-to-person contact. The virus can also be transmitted parenterally through blood or blood product transfusion, or vertically from mother to fetus. Vertical transmission to the fetus occurs in an estimated one-third of pregnancies when the mother is infected [1,2].

Parvovirus B$_{19}$ infections occur sporadically or in outbreaks in school systems during late winter and early spring. The incubation period is between 4 and 14 days (as high as 20 days in rare instances) and the secondary attack rate among susceptible household contacts approaches 50%. Patients with erythema infectiosum (EI) are infectious before the onset of the rash and remain contagious for only 1–2 days after the rash develops. In contrast, women with transient aplastic crisis are infectious prior to the onset of clinical symptoms through the subsequent week. There is no reactivation phase for parvovirus.

Clinical manifestations
There are a number of clinical manifestations of parvovirus B$_{19}$ infection, depending on age and co-morbid conditions. Asymptomatic infection occurs in 20–30% of adult cases. Erythema infectiosum or fifth disease, characterized by mild systemic "flu-like" symptoms, fever and headache, may occur in the initial phase of symptomatic infection. In children, facial erythema or a "slapped cheek" rash then develops followed by a lacy reticular rash on the trunk and extremities. Adults often do not develop the facial rash but develop a rash on the trunk and extremities and frequently acute symmetric polyarthralgias and arthritis that may persist for several weeks. Myocarditis is rarely seen.

Chronic euthyroid hypoplasia and transient aplastic crisis may occur in women with immunodeficiency or chronic hemolytic anemias. Occasionally this is accompanied by thrombocytopenia and neutropenia.

Fetal infection has been associated with abortion, fetal death, and nonimmune hydrops [2–6]. Fetal loss rates as high as 15% have been reported though the actual risk is debated. Infection <20 weeks' gestation is associated with an overall increased risk of death as compared to late second- and third-trimester infection [7]. Parvovirus is the most common infectious etiology of nonimmune hydrops. Fetal hydrops develops in only 1.1% of infected women overall and frequently resolves within 4–6 weeks without intervention [7,8]. Intrauterine transfusion for the severely anemic fetus may improve survival (see below).

Diagnosis
A pregnant woman suspected of having parvovirus B$_{19}$ because of symptoms or, more commonly, secondary to

---

Queenan's Management of High-Risk Pregnancy: An Evidence-Based Approach, Sixth Edition. Edited by John T. Queenan, Catherine Y. Spong, Charles J. Lockwood.
© 2012 John Wiley & Sons, Ltd. Published 2012 by John Wiley & Sons, Ltd.

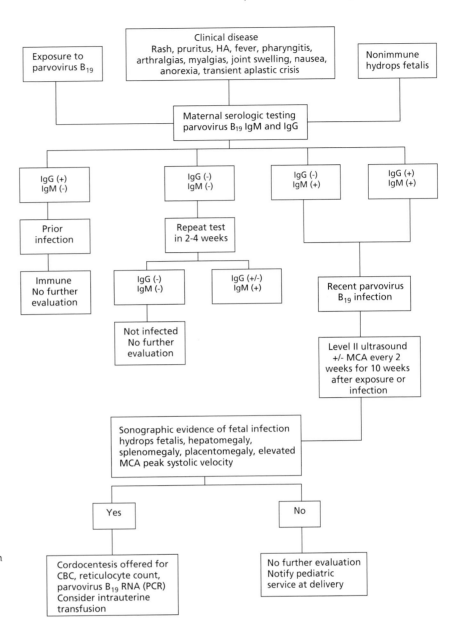

Figure 27.1 Algorithm for evaluation and management of parvovirus B₁₉ infection in pregnancy. CBC, complete blood count; HA, headache; MCA, middle cerebral artery Doppler measurements; PCR, polymerase chain reaction.

exposure to an infected child should have serologic testing performed. A serologic assay for the presence of immunoglobulin (Ig)G and IgM parvovirus-specific antibodies by enzyme-linked immunosorbent assay (ELISA) or radio-immunoassay will determine past and recent infection. IgM develops within days of infection and persists for 2–3 months (up to 6 months in rare cases) [9,10]. IgG develops several days later. The absence of IgM and IgG indicates no prior infection and a susceptible individual. Early infection, prior to antibody formation, may also result in this combination and serology should be repeated 1–2 weeks later. IgG alone indicates prior infection and immunity. IgM alone indicates very recent infection, and IgM and IgG both present indicates recent infection 1 week to 6 months previously (Fig. 27.1).

Fetal parvovirus infection should be considered if nonimmune hydrops is detected on sonography. DNA amplification techniques for parvovirus B₁₉ using amniotic fluid or fetal blood samples are now the diagnostic test of choice, as they are more sensitive and specific than fetal serology. Fetal (and maternal) viral loads do not, however, predict fetal morbidity and mortality. Fetal IgM is not recommended for diagnosis; the fetus <22 weeks is relatively immunocompetent and may not form a detectable IgM response.

Management of parvovirus B₁₉ in pregnancy

Figure 27.1 details the evaluation and management of human parvovirus B₁₉ infection in pregnancy. The vast majority of fetal parvovirus-associated hydrops occurs in the first 10 weeks after infection; serial sonography should be performed every 2 weeks in women with evidence of recent infection. Middle cerebral artery (MCA) Doppler evaluation may also be used to predict fetal anemia [11,12]. If evidence of fetal infection is noted, a cordocentesis is offered to assess the degree of anemia and confirm infection via DNA or RNA amplification techniques.

At the time of cordocentesis and depending on gestational age, an intrauterine transfusion may be performed. If a transfusion is performed and the fetus survives, 94% will recover within 6–12 weeks. The overall mortality rate is <10% [8,13,14]. Most fetuses require only one transfusion as fetal hematopoiesis resumes as the parvovirus infection resolves. Long-term neurodevelopmental outcomes of children following intrauterine transfusion for parvovirus infection have been reported. No significant delay was noted on standard neurodevelopmental testing, despite severe fetal anemia and intrauterine transfusion [15]. However, a recent review of 25 intrauterine transfusions for fetal parvovirus infection noted abnormal long-term neurodevelopment in 32% of survivors, attributed to the infection itself [16].

Rubella

Rubella, or German measles, though usually causing a minor maternal illness, is one of the most teratogenic infections known. Fortunately, since the introduction of the rubella vaccine, the incidence of rubella and congenital rubella syndrome has decreased substantially. The number of reported cases in the United States has declined more than 99% over the last three decades, though globally it remains a major issue. Less than 200 cases per year are now seen in the United States.

Pathogenesis and transmission
Rubella is an RNA togavirus with no extra-human reservoir. Following exposure to the virus via nasopharyngeal secretions, almost 80% of susceptible individuals become infected. Replication occurs in the nasopharynx and regional lymph nodes, with viremia developing 5–7 days after exposure. It is this viremia that results in placental and fetal infection. Adults are infectious during the viremia through 5–7 days of the rash. Subclinical rubella reinfection has been reported during outbreaks, though resultant fetal infection is rare. The peak incidence is in late winter and spring.

Clinical manifestations
After an incubation period of 12–23 days, a prodrome of low-grade fever and malaise, headache, arthralgias, arthritis, pharyngitis, and conjunctivitis may develop. A maculopapular rash beginning on the face and spreading to the trunk and extremities occurs in 50–80% of infected women. Posterior cervical, postauricular, and occipital lymphadenopathy is common. Rarely, thrombocytopenia purpura, neuritis, and encephalitis complicate maternal infection. Up to a third of women are asymptomatic.

Congenital rubella syndrome is a devastating consequence of maternal infection. The risk of fetal infection varies depending on when in gestation maternal infection occurs. Eighty-five to 90% of pregnant women with rubella in the first trimester have a fetus with congenital infection. As gestation extends beyond 20 weeks, the risk of congenital infection drops markedly. Congenital rubella syndrome may result in abortion and fetal death along with severe infant morbidity. The most common defects are sensorineural deafness, cataracts, heart defects, microcephaly, developmental delay, and mental retardation, though all organs may be affected. Congenitally infected infants shed virus from the throat for 6–12 months following birth and are infectious to susceptible contacts [16].

As many as a third of neonates asymptomatic at birth will develop late sequelae from fetal infection. Type 1 diabetes, thyroid disease, ocular damage, and progressive panencephalitis all may present during the second decade of life [17].

Diagnosis
Though rubella can be isolated from the nasopharynx, urine, and cerebrospinal fluid, the diagnosis of maternal rubella infection usually relies on serologic analysis. Detection of rubella-specific IgM indicates recent infection, though reexposure to rubella may induce an amnestic response resulting in reappearance of low-titer IgM. Following a primary rubella infection, IgM can be detected within 5–7 days and may persist up to 2 months. Specific IgG develops by 2 weeks and persists for life; reexposure may increase IgG titers transiently. Rubella IgG avidity assays are now available and may be useful in determining the acuity of the infection [18].

As up to 10% of US adults are seronegative and susceptible to infection, rubella immune status should be assessed at initiation of prenatal care. Susceptible women should be counseled regarding prevention strategies and be vaccinated postpartum.

Women with confirmed maternal rubella in the first 20 weeks of pregnancy should be assessed for fetal infection. Sonography is not a sensitive or specific diagnostic modality. However, cerebral ventriculomegaly, intracranial calcifications, meconium peritonitis, cardiac malformations, hepatosplenomegaly, microcephaly, fetal growth restriction, and microphthalmia have all been found in fetuses subsequently diagnosed with congenital rubella. Diagnosis of fetal rubella using DNA amplification techniques has been reported in a few small series but false-positive and false-negative tests have been noted [19].

Management and prevention

There is no treatment for rubella; supportive care should be offered. Droplet precautions are recommended for 7 days after the onset of the rash. Passive immunization using immunoglobulin is not recommended. Primary prevention of rubella relies on comprehensive vaccination programs. The (measles, mumps, rubella) MMR vaccine should be offered to susceptible women of child-bearing age. Pregnancy should be avoided for 4 weeks after vaccination as the vaccine is a live-attenuated virus with a theoretical malformation risk of 0.5–1.7%. However, if inadvertent vaccination of a pregnant woman does occur, pregnancy termination is no longer recommended as the observed risk to the fetus is minimal. After vaccination, at least 95% of women will seroconvert, developing long-term immunity [20]. Women delivering and who are rubella nonimmune should be offered MMR vaccine prior to discharge. Breastfeeding is safe in those women vaccinated postpartum.

Syphilis

Despite the description of syphilitic infection for more than 500 years and the availability of adequate therapy for more than 60 years, syphilis in the adult and neonate remains a nemesis for public health providers. In the United States in 2006 alone, there were 3.3 per 100,000 new cases of syphilis reported, an increase of 13.8% from 2005. Although pregnancy itself does not alter the clinical course of syphilis, it is important to diagnose syphilis in pregnancy to ensure prevention of congenital infection and adequate treatment.

Pathogenesis and transmission

Treponema pallidum, the causative agent of syphilis, is acquired in women primarily by intimate contact with an infected partner. Minute abrasions in the vaginal mucosa provide a portal of entry for the spirochete. The cervical changes associated with pregnancy, including eversion, hyperemia, and friability, increase the risk of spirochete entry. Local replication then occurs and lymphatic dissemination leads to the systemic findings of secondary syphilis. The incubation period averages 3 weeks (3–90 days), depending on inoculum load and host factors [21]. The early stages of syphilis, namely primary, secondary, and early latent, are associated with the highest spirochete loads and transmission rates of 30–50% [22,23]. Transmission rates in late-stage disease are much lower.

Fetal acquisition of syphilitic infection may occur by several means. Transplacental passage is the most common. *T. pallidum* has been isolated in the placenta, umbilical cord, and amniotic fluid [24–28]. Transmission may also occur across the membranes or by direct contact with the lesions at delivery. The risk of fetal infection increases as pregnancy advances but infection may occur at any gestational age.

Risk factors associated with maternal syphilis include young age, black and Hispanic ethnicity, single, low socio-economic status, less education, inadequate prenatal care and screening, prostitution, and substance abuse [29–32].

Clinical manifestations

Pregnancy has little effect on the clinical course of syphilis. Syphilis, however, has a major impact on pregnancy. Preterm delivery, stillbirth, spontaneous abortion, neonatal demise, and congenital infection are all increased. The fetal risk is directly related to the stage of disease and level of maternal spirochetemia. Maternal syphilis infection is staged according to disease duration and clinical features. Primary syphilis is the initial stage – the chancre is the characteristic lesion. The chancre is usually painless with a smooth base and a red, raised firm border. The painless nature of the chancre and its location may explain why women often are not diagnosed until later stages. If untreated, it will resolve in 3–8 weeks and the woman will progress to the secondary stage.

Secondary syphilis is the time of systemic dissemination that involves many major organ systems. Ninety percent of women with secondary syphilis have dermatologic manifestations. A diffuse macular rash will develop on the trunk and proximal extremities. Plantar and palmar maculopapular target-like lesions commonly are seen. Patchy alopecia may result when hair follicles are involved. Mucosal lesions called mucous patches will develop in 35% of women. These manifest as silver-gray painless superficial erosions of the genital, anal, or oral mucosa. They are highly infectious, with very high spirochete loads.

Genital tract involvement will occur in 20% of women at this stage. Condyloma lata (white-gray raised plaques) develop along with generalized lymphadenopathy. Constitutional symptoms are also common in secondary syphilis (70%), with low-grade fever, malaise, anorexia, headache, arthralgias, and myalgias most common. Finally, 40% of women will have cerebrospinal fluid abnormalities, though only 1–2% will develop aseptic meningitis.

Again, if untreated, the lesions will resolve and the woman will enter the latent stages of syphilis. Early latent syphilis is latent syphilis of less than 12 months' duration. During this stage 20–25% of women will relapse. Late latent syphilis is diagnosed after being asymptomatic for greater than 12 months. The woman is still infectious during latent stages, though the risk decreases with time. Eventually, 20–30% of untreated women will progress to tertiary syphilis. Tertiary syphilis, involving the integument, cardiovascular, and neurologic systems, is rarely seen in reproductive-age women.

Table 27.1 Oral desensitization protocol for penicillin-allergic patients

Dose*	Phenoxymethyl penicillin (units/mL)†	Dose (units)	Cumulative dose (units)
1	1000	100	100
2	1000	200	300
3	1000	400	700
4	1000	800	1500
5	1000	1600	3100
6	1000	3200	6300
7	1000	6400	12,700
8	10,000	12,000	24,700
9	10,000	24,000	48,700
10	10,000	48,000	96,700
11	80,000	80,000	176,000
12	80,000	160,000	336,700
13	80,000	320,000	636,700
14	80,000	640,000	1,296,700

Observe for 30 min prior to parenteral benzathine penicillin G.
*15-min intervals.
†250 mg/5 mL equals 80,000 units/mL.
Reproduced from Wendel *et al* [34] with permission from Lippincott Williams and Wilkins.

Congenital syphilis is rare before 18 weeks' gestation. Common findings of congenital syphilis in the nursery include hepatosplenomegaly, rash, reticuloendothelial abnormalities, osteochondritis, periostitis, rhinitis, and central nervous system (CNS) involvement. Late congenital syphilis, presenting after 2 years of life and often in early adolescence, includes Hutchinson teeth, interstitial keratitis, and eighth nerve deafness (Hutchinson triad) as well as mental retardation, seizures, saddle nose deformity, frontal bossing, saber shins, and cranial nerve palsies. Congenital syphilis is one of the sexually transmitted diseases infecting a neonate that can be prevented or treated *in utero*.

Diagnosis

Diagnosis of maternal syphilis is commonly performed using a nontreponemal serologic screening test with a treponemal serologic test used for confirmation. Pregnant women should be screened at the initial visit, at 28–32 weeks and again at delivery. The screening tests used are the rapid plasma reagin (RPR) or the Venereal Disease Research Laboratory (VDRL) test. They can be quantitated and usually become negative with adequate therapy, allowing them to be used for follow-up. However, the false-positive rate is approximately 1%, so a positive test must be confirmed using a treponemal test. The treponemal tests used are the fluorescent treponemal antibody absorption (FTA-Abs) test, the microhemagglutination assay for antibodies to *T. pallidum* (MHA-TP), and the

T. pallidum passive particle agglutination (TP-PA) test. Rapid "point of care" tests are currently in development [33].

The diagnosis of congenital syphilis prenatally is difficult. Sonographic findings may include hydrops fetalis, hepatomegaly, placental thickening and hydramnios, but often the infected fetus will have a normal sonogram. Polymerase chain reaction (PCR) can be performed using infected amniotic fluid. Serologic testing of cord blood at delivery is difficult to interpret. Treponemal tests reflect maternal infection. The nontreponemal tests need cord blood titers to be at least fourfold higher than maternal titers. A nonreactive RPR or VDRL does not exclude infection.

Management

Penicillin remains the drug of choice for the treatment of syphilis in pregnancy. The 2006 CDC guidelines recommend 2.4 million units IM of benzathine penicillin G for primary, secondary, and early latent syphilis (some experts recommend repeating this dose 1 week later). Late latent syphilis or syphilis of unknown duration is treated with benzathine penicillin G 2.4 million units IM weekly for three doses. No other antimicrobial agent is recommended in pregnancy. If a woman reports a penicillin allergy, a skin test for major or minor determinant antigens of penicillin should be performed if possible. If reactive, penicillin desensitization should be performed orally (Table 27.1) or intravenously [34]. Up to 50% of women treated for early-stage syphilis will have a systemic reaction called the Jarisch–Herxheimer reaction. Though transient with only mild constitutional symptoms, preterm labor and fetal distress may complicate treatment. Treatment after 20 weeks' gestation should be preceded by an ultrasound to assess possible fetal infection. If abnormal, antepartum fetal heart rate monitoring should accompany treatment. In fetuses at or near term, delivery with treatment of the mother and infant postpartum may be warranted.

Careful follow-up after treatment should be performed to determine treatment failure (rare) or reinfection. Nontreponemal tests should be performed every month during pregnancy because the consequence of a treatment failure or reinfection in these high-risk women is a congenitally infected infant.

Toxoplasmosis

Toxoplasma gondii, a ubiquitous protozoon transmitted in infected cat feces, undercooked raw meat, and transplacentally, causes an estimated 400–4000 cases of congenital toxoplasmosis in the United States every year [35]. Acute infections, in often times asymptomatic pregnant women, can cause severe illness in the fetus or neonate (mental retardation, epilepsy, and blindness). Approximately 15–30% of women in the US are immune and the incidence of new infection ranges from 0.5 to 8.1 per 1000 in susceptible pregnancies [35,36].

Pathogenesis and transmission

Toxoplasma gondii exists in three forms or stages: (1) the tachyzoite, which is the acute phase in which the organism invades and replicates; (2) the bradyzoite, in the latent phase when tissue cysts are formed; and (3) the oocyst sporozoite, which may survive in the environment for months. The cat is the definitive host and thus the main reservoir of infection. Infected cats excrete several million oocytes a day which then sporulate and become infectious. Ingestion of these sporulated oocytes is the predominant mode of transmission in humans. They may be ingested in raw or undercooked infected meat or in uncooked foods in contact with infected meat or soil, or inadvertently ingested from cat litter.

Transplacental passage of toxoplasmosis occurs when a woman becomes infected during a pregnancy. The risk of developing congenital toxoplasmosis increases as the gestation advances. The incidence of transmission is 10–25% if infection occurs in the first trimester and highest (60%) in the third trimester. Conversely, however, disease severity is worse if infection occurs during the first trimester. Infection prior to pregnancy confers immunity with little risk of vertical transmission.

Clinical manifestations

Maternal toxoplasmosis is often asymptomatic. If symptoms do occur, fatigue, fever, malaise, and lymphadenopathy (particularly posterior cervical) are usually reported. Photophobia, maculopapular rash, and headache are less common. Most women recover within a few weeks without therapy or sequelae. Women who are immunocompromised, however, may have more severe disease, complicated by encephalitis, pneumonitis and chorioamnionitis. *T. gondii* infection is one of the AIDS-defining criteria.

Congenital toxoplasmosis has been associated with spontaneous abortion, stillbirth, and intrauterine growth restriction. Though many infected fetuses are born with no evidence of toxoplasmosis, the majority (up to 80%) develop learning and visual disturbances later in life [37,38]. Chorioretinitis is the most common clinical finding among infected newborns. Hydrocephaly, intracerebral calcifications, cataracts, microphthalmia, glaucoma, hepatosplenomegaly, anemia and petechiae, jaundice, and seizures may also manifest in the nursery or over time.

Diagnosis

The parasite is rarely detected in body fluids or tissue; diagnosis is based on serologic evaluation or DNA amplification. A combination of serologic tests is now used to determine recent and past infection. Toxoplasma IgG develops within 1–2 weeks after acquisition, peaks at 1–2 months, and usually persists for life. Avidity testing may help discriminate between recent and past infection. IgM antibodies appear by 10 days after infection and usually become negative within a few months. However, occasionally IgM may be detected in chronic infection and persist for years. The IgM tests available have low specificity and should not be used alone to diagnose acute toxoplasmosis. IgA and IgE antibodies are also used to help diagnose acute infection. IgA persist longer than IgE antibodies. Because of the difficulty in running and interpreting serologic data, the Toxoplasma Serology Laboratory in Palo Alto, California, can be consulted. They use a Toxoplasma Serologic Profile (TSP) and provide the clinician with a detailed interpretation of results [39].

Prenatal diagnosis of toxoplasmosis can now be performed using a number of techniques. DNA amplification by PCR of toxoplasmosis from amniotic fluid or blood is becoming a standard modality with improved sensitivity over standard isolation techniques [40]. Sonographic evidence of hydrocephaly and intracranial calcifications, placental thickening, liver calcifications, hyperechoic bowel, ascites, and growth restriction have all been reported prenatally. Toxoplasma-specific IgM and IgA may be found in amniotic fluid or cordocentesis samples but their absence does not indicate lack of infection. When neonatal serology is performed, IgA and IgM may confirm a diagnosis of congenital infection; however, about 20% of infected neonates will have nondetectable IgM at birth. The placenta should be evaluated in suspected cases as almost half will have evidence of *T. gondii* cysts.

Management and prevention

Currently toxoplasma screening is not recommended in the US pregnant population (excepting immunocompromised women). Prevalence rates in the US are low, and equivocal or false-positive tests high in this setting. Areas where toxoplasmosis is more common, e.g., France and Austria, have screening programs in place and have reported a decline in congenital disease.

Treatment of toxoplasmosis in infected pregnant women is variable, depending on maternal immune status, gestational age, and presence of fetal infection. Spiramycin can be obtained from the Food and Drug Administration (FDA) to treat laboratory-confirmed acute maternal infection. If fetal infection is documented, a combination of pyrimethamine, folinic acid and a sulfonamide (usually sulfadiazine) is recommended. The effectiveness of prenatal treatment remains controversial.

Prevention of toxoplasmosis in pregnant women is paramount. Women should be counseled to avoid close contact with cat feces (avoid changing cat litter or wear gloves), cook meat to safe temperatures, wash fruits and vegetables thoroughly prior to eating, wear gloves when gardening, and wash hands after contact with soil and raw meats.

Herpes simplex infection

Genital herpes has become the most prevalent sexually transmitted disease with over 1.6 million new herpes simplex virus (HSV) infections per year in the United States alone. It is estimated that over 50 million adolescents and adults are currently affected. Though the majority of women are unaware of their status, 24.2% of women overall in the US are seropositive for HSV-2, with higher rates reported in high-risk populations [41–43]. As most cases of HSV are transmitted by persons unaware of their infection or who are asymptomatic, containing this worsening public health problem has become a major concern.

Pathogenesis and transmission

There are two serotypes of this DNA virus: HSV-1 and HSV-2. There is a large amount of DNA sequence concordance between the two viruses and prior infection with one type attenuates a new infection with the other type. Transmission occurs secondary to intimate contact with an infected partner or vertically to a fetus/neonate. The incubation period averages 3–6 days.

Following a mucocutaneous infection, the virus travels retrograde along sensory nerves and remains latent in cranial nerves or dorsal spinal ganglia. The frequency of mucocutaneous recurrences is variable. HSV-1, originally localized to orolabial areas, now causes 5–30% of initial genital herpes. This is probably due to an increase in orogenital sexual practices. HSV-2 occurs almost entirely in the genital region. The majority (>90%) of recurrent genital herpes is secondary to HSV-2. Recurrences are most frequent in the first years after infection but may continue for many years.

Neonatal infection may occur transplacentally or via ascending infection at any time during pregnancy, but over 85% of neonatal herpes results by direct contact with the birth canal [44]. It occurs in 1 in 3200 to 1 in 30,000 livebirths [45,46]. Risk factors for neonatal HSV include the presence of HSV in the genital tract (often asymptomatic shedding), the type of HSV (HSV-1 > HSV-2, though usually skin/eye/mouth disease, not CNS infection), invasive obstetric procedures, and stage of maternal infection. Women acquiring HSV late in the third trimester have the highest likelihood of transmission to the neonate. This is due to high viral loads and the neonate having no protective antibodies acquired transplacentally.

Clinical manifestations

There are four classifications of clinical HSV. A *first episode primary infection* occurs when HSV-1 or HSV-2 is isolated from a genital lesion in the absence of any HSV antibodies in serum. Many women with new infections are asymptomatic. However, this group is the one with the highest likelihood of having clinical symptoms. Focal painful vesicles may be present or the lesions may appear as painful abraded areas. Inguinal lymphadenopathy, fever, malaise, dysuria, and vulvar pruritus are all more common in this group, though only noted in approximately one-third of newly acquired infections. Hepatitis, encephalitis, meningitis or pneumonia are uncommon. Viral shedding and symptomatology usually last 1–4 weeks.

First episode nonprimary infection is diagnosed when HSV-2 is isolated from the genital tract in the presence of preexisting HSV-1 serum antibodies. These infections have a shorter clinical course with less severe symptoms and fewer lesions. Transmission risk to a partner or fetus/neonate is much lower in this group. *Recurrent infection* or *reactivation* occurs when HSV-1 or HSV-2 is isolated from the genital tract in the presence of same serotype antibodies. Reactivation disease has a much shorter course with few lesions and rare systemic symptoms. During pregnancy, 5–10% of women with a history of HSV will have a symptomatic recurrence. The risk of transmission is very low. Finally, *asymptomatic viral shedding* is the presence of HSV on the surface of the skin and mucosa in the absence of signs and symptoms. Most women will shed virus asymptomatically throughout life and the majority of HSV transmission occurs during a period of asymptomatic viral shedding (up to 70%).

Neonatal HSV is acquired predominantly intrapartum when the fetus comes into contact with virus shed from the cervix or lower genital tract [47]. Infants born to mothers with a first episode of genital HSV near delivery have the highest risk of acquiring HSV. Neonatal infection may manifest as localized infection of the skin, eyes, and mucous membranes. Localized CNS encephalitis may also occur. Finally disseminated disease with involvement of multiple organs, predominantly liver and lungs, may occur and has the highest reported mortality rate [48].

Diagnosis

History and clinical examination are useful in the diagnosis of HSV but as genital HSV often has a nonclassic presentation or is asymptomatic, laboratory testing should be performed. Viral culture is best when performed early in an outbreak. The lesion should be unroofed and the fluid cultured. The sensitivity drops markedly as the vesicular lesions ulcerate and then crust over. PCR is more sensitive but not yet approved by the FDA.

Type-specific serology (distinguishing HSV-1 from HSV2) is now available and proves useful for screening and determining classification of disease for counseling purposes. The best tests available are based on antibodies formed to type-specific G-glycoproteins. Sensitivity approaches 80–90% and specificity >96% [33,49,50]. If new infection is suspected and antibody testing is negative, repeat the serologic tests in 4–6 weeks.

Management and prevention

Women with symptomatic first episode HSV infection during pregnancy can be treated with systemic acyclovir, valacyclovir or famcyclovir for 7 days. Treatment will attenuate symptoms but not eradicate the latent virus. Severe recurrent disease may also benefit from antiviral therapy, but mild recurrent disease will not. These antiviral medications are pregnancy Category B.

Acyclovir or valacyclovir therapy in the latter part of pregnancy (36 weeks' gestation until delivery) has been shown to decrease HSV outbreaks at term, decreasing the need for cesarean delivery. They have also been shown to decrease asymptomatic HSV shedding at delivery. The American College of Obstetricians and Gynecologists (ACOG) states that prophylactic antiviral therapy should be considered, especially in the setting of a first episode of HSV during the current pregnancy.

Upon presentation for delivery, a woman with a known history of HSV should be questioned regarding prodromal symptoms (vulvar itching, burning) and recent HSV lesions. A careful examination of the vulva, vagina, and cervix should be performed for herpetic lesions. Suspicious lesions should be cultured. Women with any evidence of prodromal or active HSV should be offered a cesarean delivery. Of note, 10–15% of infants with HSV are born to women undergoing a cesarean delivery – counseling should reflect a decreased risk of HSV transmission with a cesarean delivery but not a negative risk. A nongenital lesion should be covered and vaginal delivery allowed. If a woman presents at term with an HSV lesion and ruptured membranes, regardless of rupture duration, a cesarean delivery should be effected. If the infant is preterm, expectant management should be offered as the risk of prematurity outweighs the unknown benefit of delivery. If, at the time of labor, the lesion has resolved, vaginal delivery is allowed.

Women with active HSV may breastfeed as long as there is no HSV lesion on the breast. Strict handwashing should be performed before contact with the neonate. Acyclovir may be used in the postpartum period as excretion into breastmilk is low.

Though screening for HSV is not recommended at this time, a woman known to be HSV seropositive at her first prenatal visit should be counseled regarding safe sexual practices [51]. Avoid intercourse with a partner known to have or suspected of having HSV, particularly in the third trimester. Condom use is effective in preventing most, but not all, HSV transmission.

Cytomegalovirus

Cytomegalovirus (CMV) remains the most common cause of perinatal infection in the United States, infecting 0.5–2% of all neonates [52,53]. Fifty-five percent of reproductive-age women in high socio-economic classes are seropositive, compared to 85% of women in the lower socio-economic classes. The risk of seroconversion for a susceptible pregnant woman is 1–4% during the pregnancy – those women acquiring primary CMV during pregnancy are at highest risk to transmit to the neonate.

Pathogenesis and transmission

Cytomegalovirus is a ubiquitous DNA herpesvirus. As with other herpesviruses, it has a latent phase with periodic reactivation despite antibody formation. Transmission occurs with contact from infected nasopharyngeal secretions, urine, saliva, semen or cervical secretions (sexual contact), blood, or tissue.

Though neonates may acquire infection secondary to passage through the maternal genital tract or from breastfeeding, the majority are infected transplacentally via hematogenous dissemination. Congenital CMV may occur after either primary or nonprimary maternal infection. In a series of elegant reports of CMV in pregnancy, Stagno and colleagues defined outcomes of CMV infection depending on the type of maternal infection [52–55]. These findings are summarized in Figure 27.2.

Women with primary CMV infections during pregnancy will transmit the virus to the fetus 40% of the time. In contrast, of women with recurrent infection, only 0.15–1% will transmit the virus to the fetus. The risk of clinically apparent disease or sequelae in the neonate is higher in those infants infected during a primary maternal infection. As with many other congenital infections, perinatal transmission is more likely in the third trimester, but outcomes are more severe the earlier in gestation transmission occurs. Recent evidence has shown that reinfection with a different strain of CMV can also lead to intrauterine transmission [56,57].

Clinical manifestations

The majority of adults infected with CMV are asymptomatic. Fifteen percent of infected pregnant women with primary CMV will develop a mononucleosis-like illness with malaise, headache, fever, lymphadenopathy, pharyngitis, and arthritis. Immunocompromised women may develop more severe complications such as interstitial pneumonitis, myocarditis, hepatitis, retinitis, gastrointestinal disease, and meningoencephalitis, though these are

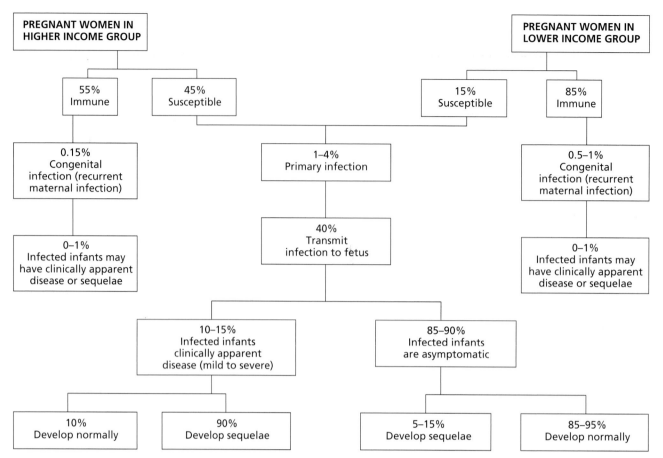

Figure 27.2 Characteristics of CMV infection in pregnancy. Reproduced from Stagno and Whitley [54] with permission from the Massachusetts Medical Society.

uncommon. Reactivation episodes with CMV are usually asymptomatic, though viral shedding is common.

Congenital CMV infection may present with hepatosplenomegaly, thrombocytopenia, jaundice, and petechiae ("blueberry muffin"). Low birthweight, microcephaly, intracranial calcifications, chorioretinitis, hearing deficits, pneumonitis, microphthalmia, and seizures are also not uncommon. Though the majority of infected infants are asymptomatic at birth, some will develop late-onset sequelae. These commonly include psychomotor retardation, hearing loss, neurologic deficits, chorioretinitis, and learning disabilities.

Diagnosis

Primary maternal CMV infection, if symptomatic, often presents similarly to Epstein–Barr virus. However, heterophile antibody testing will be negative. CMV IgM is detected within a few days of infection but is only found in 75–90% of women with acute infection [55]. CMV IgM may remain positive for 4–8 months and reemerge with recurrent infection, making it problematic for diagnosis of acute disease. CMV IgG testing is more reliable – a fourfold rise in paired acute and convalescent sera

indicates acute infection. CMV viral culture remains the gold standard for diagnosis though a minimum of 21 days is required for a culture to be reported as negative. Avidity testing is now available to determine disease acuity [33].

Perinatal infection may be suspected when certain findings on ultrasound are noted. Though nonspecific, fetal hydrops, intrauterine growth restriction, microcephaly, ventriculomegaly, hepatomegaly, cerebral calcifications, hyperechoic bowel, and amniotic fluid abnormalities have all been described. If suspected, amniotic fluid for DNA amplification testing has become the gold standard, though a negative result does not exclude fetal infection [58,59]. Finally, amniotic fluid for CMV culture may be useful but requires a long incubation period.

Management and prevention

The management of an immunocompetent pregnant woman with primary or recurrent CMV is limited. There are no current treatment regimens available for these women beyond symptomatic treatment. If recent primary infection is diagnosed, invasive testing can be offered to identify infected fetuses. Counseling then is performed regarding the stage of infection and gestational age, understanding that the majority of fetuses develop normally. Pregnancy termination may be an option in rare cases.

Routine serologic screening for CMV is not recommended. Preventive measures including handwashing and minimizing exposure to CMV from high-risk areas such as day-care centers and nurseries are the mainstays of preventing primary CMV infection. A CMV vaccine is not available currently for use in pregnancy.

Varicella zoster virus

Varicella zoster virus (VZV) is the most contagious viral infection complicating pregnancy. Fortunately, more than 95% of adults have serologic evidence of immunity with only 0.1–0.4 cases per 1000 pregnant women occurring each year in the United States. Though it is uncommon in the pregnant population, if infected, the morbidity for an adult is much greater than that for an infected child.

Pathogenesis and transmission

Varicella zoster virus is a double-stranded DNA herpesvirus that causes clinical infection only in humans. The primary infection, varicella or chicken pox, presents predominantly as a rash with systemic symptoms (see Clinical manifestations, below). The virus then becomes latent, with occasional reactivation (herpes zoster or shingles) occurring in certain individuals. Both primary and reactivation diseases are infectious, though viral shedding is less with reactivation. In temperate climates, varicella occurs predominantly in late winter and early spring.

Transmission of VZV occurs primarily by direct contact with an infected individual, though transmission also may occur by inhalation of virus from respiratory droplets or airborne virus particles from skin lesions (predominantly with zoster). The virus usually enters the mucosa of the upper respiratory tract or the conjunctiva. Transplacental passage of the virus may occur, causing congenital varicella in up to 2% of maternal varicella infections prior to 20 weeks' gestation (highest risk 13–20 weeks). Neonatal infection occurs secondary to exposure of the fetus or newborn 5 days prior to delivery to 2 days postpartum before protective maternal antibodies develop.

A susceptible individual has a 60–95% risk of becoming infected after exposure. The incubation period is 10–21 days with a mean of 15 days. An infected person is then contagious from one day before the onset of the rash until lesions are crusted over. Once infected, lifelong immunity to reinfection develops in the immunocompetent individual, though subclinical reinfections have been reported. Reactivation disease (shingles) occurs sporadically with an often unknown inciting event.

Clinical manifestations

Varicella or chicken pox often presents in an adult with a 1–2-day prodrome of fever, malaise, headache, and myalgias. Lesions then appear initially as papules, rapidly progressing to superficial clear vesicles surrounded by a halo of erythema. The head and trunk are affected first, spreading then sporadically to the lower abdomen and extremities. The vesicles are intensely pruritic and appear in crops over 3–7 days. The lesions begin to crust during the outbreak. A typical varicella outbreak has at any one time all stages of lesions. Once all the lesions have crusted, the patient is no longer considered infectious.

The risk of varicella pneumonia is increased in adults and may be increased again by pregnancy. In a reported series of varicella in pregnancy [60], 5.2% of women with varicella were diagnosed as having pneumonia. Risk factors for developing pneumonia included current smoking and >100 skin lesions. The mortality, reportedly as high as 40% in early series, has now decreased to <2% with aggressive antiviral use and intensive care facilities. Pneumonia usually develops 2–4 days after the onset of rash, and may present with minimal symptoms (often only a mild cough). A chest x-ray should be performed on all pregnant women presenting with varicella.

Congenital varicella, usually following maternal infection between 12–20 weeks, often presents with limb abnormalities such as cutaneous scarring, limb hypoplasia, and muscle atrophy. Microphthalmia, chorioretinitis, microcephaly, seizures, cortical atrophy, and mental retardation may also occur. Neonatal varicella, occurring secondary to exposure near or around delivery, carries a 25–50% attack rate and mortality rate near 25%. Clinical manifestations include pneumonia, disseminated mucocutaneous lesions, and visceral infection.

Herpes zoster infection, or shingles, occurs upon reactivation of the VZV virus in 1–3 sensory nerve dermatomes. Pain along the infected dermatome heralds the appearance of papules and then vesicles. These vesicles may coalesce, rupture, and then crust over. Systemic symptoms are uncommon.

Diagnosis

The diagnosis of varicella is usually made clinically. The characteristic rash in susceptible individuals allows for accurate diagnosis in the majority of cases. If the diagnosis is not readily apparent, VZV can be isolated by scraping the base of the vesicles during the acute phase of the infection. Tzanck smear, tissue culture, and direct fluorescent antibody testing (DFA) are all available to test the vesicle specimen. DNA amplification techniques of body fluid or tissue are very sensitive and are rapidly becoming the gold standard. Seroconversion can be documented by antibody assay using acute and convalescent sera. VZV IgM develops rapidly and will remain positive for 4–5 weeks and may be useful in the acute setting.

Fetal varicella can be diagnosed using DNA amplification techniques on amniotic fluid specimens, though it often does not correlate with clinical disease [61].

Management and prevention

The pregnant woman with primary VZV infection should be isolated from other pregnant women and evaluated for evidence of pneumonia. Chest x-ray is useful. Hospitalization and antiviral therapy are reserved for those women complicated by pneumonia or those with systemic symptoms severe enough to require intravenous fluids and symptomatic relief. If antiviral therapy is required, acyclovir is the drug of choice. Acyclovir ($500\,mg/m^2$ or $10–15\,mg/kg$ every 8 h) should be started as soon as possible. No fetal side-effects have been reported from acyclovir use in pregnancy. Antiviral use to prevent or treat congenital infection has not been studied.

Prevention is the mainstay of population-based VZV management. The infected individual should be isolated from other susceptible individuals. An exposed pregnant woman should be evaluated as to past disease – if no history of varicella infection, an IgG titer can be rapidly performed. At least 70% of individuals without reported history of VZV actually have VZV IgG. An exposed pregnant woman who is deemed susceptible may be given passive immunity using varicella zoster immune globulin (VariZIG). This is a human globulin fraction produced in Canada and available under an expanded access protocol. Contact information is at www.cdc.gov [62]. VariZIG should be given within 96 h of exposure to maximize the effect. As VariZIG is limited in quantity and is expensive, IgG testing is essential to limit the number of women requiring its administration.

The varicella vaccine currently available is a live-attenuated vaccine (Varivax). It is not recommended in pregnancy and pregnancy should be avoided within 1 month of administration. To date, there have been no adverse outcomes in women inadvertently receiving the vaccine immediately before or during pregnancy.

CASE PRESENTATION

The patient is a 30-year-old accountant who presents to your office in January at 26 weeks' gestation. She states that her 6-year-old son was sent home from school that day with a fever and a facial rash with a "slapped cheek" appearance. The pediatrician correctly diagnoses her son with parvovirus B_{19} and is concerned for her fetus. She has never had parvovirus B_{19}, which you confirm with IgG serologic testing.

As she is susceptible, you counsel her on the clinical manifestations in adults including fever, headache, truncal rash, and polyarthralgias. The incubation period is 4–14 days so you repeat the IgM and IgG testing in 3 weeks. Although she is asymptomatic, her parvovirus B_{19} IgM is now positive. A level II ultrasound with MCA Doppler is performed with no evidence of hydrops fetalis or other signs of fetal infection. She undergoes sonographic evaluation every 1–2 weeks for 10–12 weeks after exposure, and the fetus develops hepatosplenomegaly, ascites, and an elevated MCA peak systolic velocity consistent with fetal anemia.

She undergoes cordocentesis which reveals a fetal hemoglobin of 6.2 g/dL. Parvovirus B_{19} RNA testing is positive. An intrauterine transfusion is performed at the time of the cordocentesis without complication. Weekly follow-up sonographic evaluation notes a slow resolution of the fetal ascites with normalization of the MCA Doppler findings. No further transfusions are required and she delivers a healthy male infant at term.

References

1. Public Health Laboratory Service Working Party on Fifth Disease. Prospective study of human parvovirus (B19) infection in pregnancy. BMJ 1990;300:1166–1170.
2. De Jong EP, de Haan TR, Kroes AC et al. Parvovirus B19 infection in pregnancy. J Clin Virol 2006;36:1.
3. Harger JH, Adler SP, Koch WC et al. Prospective evaluation of 618 pregnant women exposed to parvovirus B19: risks and symptoms. Obstet Gynecol 1998;91:413–420.
4. Rodis JF, Quinn DL, Garry GW et al. Management and outcomes of pregnancies complicated by human B19 parvovirus infection: a prospective study. Am J Obstet Gynecol 1990;163:1168–1171.
5. Brown T, Anand A, Ritchie LD. Intrauterine parvovirus infection associated with hydrops fetalis. Lancet 1984;2:1033–1034.
6. Goldenberg RL, Thompson C. The infectious origins of stillbirth. Am J Obstet Gynecol 2003;189:861.
7. Crane J. Parvovirus B19 infection in pregnancy. J Obstet Gynaecol Can 2002;24:727.
8. Enders M, Weidner A, Zoellner I et al. Fetal morbidity and mortality after acute human parvovirus B19 infection in pregnancy: prospective evaluation of 1018 cases. Prenat Diagn 2004;24:513–518.
9. Enders M, Schalasta G, Baisch C et al. Human parvovirus B19 infection during pregnancy – value of modern molecular and serological diagnosis. J Clin Virol 2006;35:400.

10. Butchko AR, Jordan JA. Comparison of three commercially available serologic assays used to detect human parvovirus B19-specific immunoglobulin M (IgM) and IgG antibodies in sera of pregnant women. J Clin Microbiol 2004;42:3191.

11. Delle Chiaie L, Buck G, Grab D et al. Prediction of fetal anemia with doppler measurement of the middle cerebral artery peak systolic velocity in pregnancies complicated by maternal blood group alloimmunization or parvovirus B_{19} infection. Ultrasound Obstet Gynecol 2001;18:232–236.

12. Cosmi E, Mari G, delle Chiaie L et al. Noninvasive diagnosis by doppler ultrasonography of fetal anemia resulting from parvovirus infection. Am J Obstet Gynecol 2002;187: 1290–1293.

13. Schild RL, Bald R, Plath H et al. Intrauterine management of fetal parvovirus B19 infection. Ultrasound Obstet Gynecol 1999;13:161–166.

14. Von Kaisenberg CS, Jonat W. Fetal parvovirus B19 infection. Ultrasound Obstet Gynecol 2001;18:280–288.

15. Dembinski J, Haverkamp F, Hansmann M et al. Neurodevelopmental outcome after intrauterine red cell transfusion for parvovirus B_{19}-induced fetal hydrops. Br J Obstet Gynaecol 2002;109:1232–1234.

16. Nagel HT, de Haan TR, Vandenbussche FP et al. Long-term outcome after fetal transfusion for hydrops associated with parvovirus B19 infection. Obstet Gynecol 2007;109(1):42.

17. Webster WS. Teratogen update: congenital rubella. Teratology 1998;58:13–23.

18. Mubareka S, Richards H, Gray M et al. Evaluation of commercial rubella immunoglobulin G avidity assays. J Clin Microbiol 2007;45:231.

19. Tang JW, Aarons E, Hesketh LM et al. Prenatal diagnosis of congenital rubella infection in the second trimester of pregnancy. Prenat Diagn 2003;6:509–512.

20. Haas DM, Flowers CA, Congdon CL. Rubella, rubeola, and mumps in pregnant women. Obstet Gynecol 2005;106:295.

21. Larsen SA, Hunter EF, McGrew BE. Syphilis. In: Wentworth BB, Judson FN, eds. Laboratory Methods for the Diagnosis of Sexually Transmitted Diseases. Washington, DC: American Public Health Association, 1984, pp.1–42.

22. Sanchez PJ, Wendel GD. Syphilis in pregnancy. Clin Perinatol 1997;24:71–90.

23. Maruti S, Hwany LY, Ross M et al. The epidemiology of early syphilis in Houston, TX, 1994–1995. Sex Transm Dis 1997;24: 475–480.

24. Wendel GE, Sanchez PJ, Peters MT et al. Identification of *Treponema pallidum* in amniotic fluid and fetal blood from pregnancies complicated by congenital syphilis. Obstet Gynecol 1991;78:890–895.

25. Qureshi F, Jacques SM, Reyes MP. Placental histopathology in syphilis. Human Pathol 1993;24:779–784.

26. Genest DR, Choi-Hong SR, Tate JE et al. Diagnosis of congenital syphilis from placental examination. Human Pathol 1996;27:366–372.

27. Grimprel E, Sanchez PJ, Wendel GD et al. Use of polymerase chain reaction and rabbit infectivity testing to detect *Treponema pallidum* in amniotic fluids, fetal and neonatal sera, and cerebrospinal fluid. J Clin Microbiol 1991;29:1711–1718.

28. Wendel GD, Maberry MC, Christmas JT et al. Examination of amniotic fluid in diagnosing congenital syphilis with fetal death. Obstet Gynecol 1989;74:967–970.

29. Johnson HL, Erbelding EJ, Zenilman JM et al. Sexually transmitted diseases and risk behaviors among pregnant women attending inner city public sexually transmitted diseases clinics in Baltimore, MD, 1996–2002. Sex Transm Dis 2007; 34:991.

30. Trepka MJ, Bloom SA, Zhang G et al. Inadequate syphilis screening among women with prenatal care in a community with a high syphilis incidence. Sex Transm Dis 2006;33:670.

31. Taylor MM, Mickey T, Browne K et al. Opportunities for the prevention of congenital syphilis in Maricopa County, Arizona. Sex Transm Dis 2008;35:341.

32. Wilson EK, Gavin NI, Adams EK et al. Patterns in prenatal syphilis screening among Florida Medicaid enrollees. Sex Transm Dis 2007;34:378.

33. Greer L, Wendel GD. Rapid diagnostic methods in sexually transmitted infections. Infect Dis Clin North Am 2008;22:601.

34. Wendel GD, Stark BJ, Jamison RB et al. Penicillin allergy and desensitization in serious infections during pregnancy. N Engl J Med 1985;312:1229–1232.

35. Centers for Disease Control and Prevention. CDC recommendations regarding selected conditions affecting women's health. MMWR 2000;49(RR-2):59–75.

36. Jones JL, Kruszon-Moran D, Wilson M. Toxoplasma gondii infection in the United States, 1999–2000. Emerg Infect Dis (serial online) 2003. www.cdc.gov/ncidod/EID/vol9no11/03-0098.htm.

37. Carter AO, Frank JW. Congenital toxoplasmosis: epidemiologic features and control. Can Med Assoc J 1986;135: 618–623.

38. Wilson CB, Remington JS, Stagno S et al. Development of adverse sequelae in children born with subclinical congenital *toxoplasma* infection. Pediatrics 1980;66:767–774.

39. Montoya JG. Laboratory diagnosis of *Toxoplasma gondii* infection and toxoplasmosis. J Infect Dis 2002;185(Suppl 1): 573–582.

40. Thalib L, Gras L, Roman S et al. Prediction of congenital toxoplasmosis by polymerase chain reaction analysis of amniotic fluid. Br J Obstet Gynaecol 2005;11:567.

41. Fleming D, McQuillan G, Johnson R et al. Herpes simplex virus type 2 in the United States, 1976 to 1994. N Engl J Med 1997;337:1105–1011.

42. Xu F, Markowitz LE, Gottlieb SL et al. Seroprevalence of herpes simplex virus types 1 and 2 in pregnant women in the United States. Am J Obstet Gynecol 2007;196:43.

43. Xu F, Sternberg MR, Kottiri BJ et al. Trends in herpes simplex virus type 1 and type 2 seroprevalence in the United States. JAMA 2006;30:964.

44. Brown ZA, Wald A, Morrow RA et al. Effect of serologic status and cesarean delivery on transmission rates of herpes simplex virus from mother to infant. JAMA 2003;289:203–209.

45. Mahnert N, Roberts SW, Laibl VR et al. The incidence of neonatal herpes infection. Am J Obstet Gynecol 2007;196: e55.

46. Whitley R, Davis EA, Suppapanya N. Incidence of neonatal herpes simplex virus infections in a managed-care population. Sex Transm Dis 2007;34:704.

47. Kimberlin DW, Rouse DJ. Genital herpes. N Engl J Med 2004;350:1970–1977.

48. Kimberlin DW. Neonatal herpes simplex infection. Clin Microbiol Rev 2004;17:1–13.

49. Anzivino E, Fioriti D, Mischitelli M et al. Herpes simplex virus infection in pregnancy and in neonate: status of art of epidemiology, diagnosis, therapy and prevention. Virol J 2009;6:40.

50. Laderman EI, Whitworth E, Dumaual E et al. Rapid, sensitive, and specific lateral-flow immunochromatographic point-of-care device for detection of herpes simplex virus type 2-specific immunoglobulin G antibodies in serum and whole blood. Clin Vaccine Immunol 2008;15:159.

51. American College of Obstetricians and Gynecologists. Management of herpes in pregnancy. Practice Bulletin No. 82. Obstet Gynecol 2007;109:1489–1498.

52. Stagno S, Pass RF, Dworsky ME et al. Congenital cytomegalovirus infection. The relative importance of primary and recurrent maternal infection. N Engl J Med 1982;306:945–949.

53. Stagno S, Cloud G, Pass RF et al. Primary cytomegalovirus infections in pregnancy: incidence, transmission to the fetus and clinical outcome. JAMA 1986;256:1904–1908.

54. Stagno S, Whitley RJ. Herpesvirus infections of pregnancy. Part I: Cytomegalovirus and Epstein–Barr virus infections. N Engl J Med 1985;313:1270–1274.

55. Stagno S, Tinker MK, Irod C et al. Immunoglobulin M antibodies detected by enzyme-linked immunosorbent assay and radioimmunoassay in the diagnosis of cytomegalovirus infections in pregnant women and newborn infants. J Clin Microbiol 1985;21:930–935.

56. Yamamoto AY, Mussi-Pinhata MM, Boppana SB et al. Human cytomegalovirus reinfection is associated with intrauterine transmission in a highly CMV immune maternal population. Am J Obstet Gynecol 2010;202(3):297.

57. Ross SA, Arora N, Novak Z, Fowler KB, Britt WJ, Boppana SB. Cytomegalovirus reinfections in healthy seroimmune women. JID 2010;201:386–389.

58. Revello MG, Genna G. Pathogenesis and prenatal diagnosis of human cytomegalovirus infection. J Clin Virol 2004;29: 71–83.

59. Liesnard C, Donner C, Brancart F et al. Prenatal diagnosis of congenital CMV infection: prospective study of 237 pregnancies at risk. Obstet Gynecol 2000;95:881–888.

60. Harger JH, Ernest JM, Thurnau GR et al. Risk factors and outcome of varicella-zoster virus pneumonia in pregnancy women. J Infect Dis 2002;185:422–427.

61. Mendelson E, Aboundy Y, Smetana Z et al. Laboratory assessment and diagnosis of congenital viral infections: rubella, cytomegalovirus (CMV), varicella-zoster virus (VZV), herpes simplex virus (HSV), parvovirus B19 and human immunodeficiency virus (HIV). Reprod Toxicol 2006;21:350.

62. Centers for Disease Control aand Prevention. A new product (VariZIG) for postexposure prophylaxis of varicella available under an investigational new drug application expanded access protocol. MMWR 2006;55:209.

Chapter 28
Malaria

Richard M.K. Adanu
Department of Obstetrics and Gynaecology, University of Ghana Medical School, Accra, Ghana

Malaria is a disease caused by the protozoon *Plasmodium* which is transmitted through the bite of the female *Anopheles* mosquito. The four species of *Plasmodium* responsible for malaria are *P. falciparum*, *P. vivax*, *P. ovale*, and *P. malariae*. *Plasmodium falciparum* is responsible for most of the cases of malaria worldwide. It has been reported that, worldwide, there are about 400 million cases of malaria annually with 1–3 million deaths [1,2]. Malaria in pregnancy is responsible for 75,000–200,000 infant deaths per year [1]. Over 90% of malaria cases occur in sub-Saharan Africa [2].

Clinical features

Malaria usually begins with a nonspecific flu-like reaction. The patient usually complains of fever, headaches, and general malaise. Others might complain of abdominal pains and vomiting. This stage of the disease is usually missed in holoendemic areas where residents have developed some level of immunity to the disease. Visitors to such areas, however, display a more severe version of this stage of the disease. Immunocompromised patients might even develop mild jaundice and hepatosplenomegaly.

Malaria is characterized by febrile paroxysms which last for 6–10 h and are characterized by three stages. The patient first experiences a cold stage in which there is intense shivering. The next stage is the occurrence of a high-grade fever which later breaks and brings on the sweating stage of the febrile paroxysm. After the resolution of these stages, symptoms subside for a time and then the cycle is repeated within 36–48 h.

Clinical examination of a pregnant woman with malaria during a febrile paroxysm usually reveals a woman who is febrile with a temperature of 38°C or higher. Depending on whether the disease has been going on for some time and on the hemoglobin level of the woman before the start of the disease, pallor of the mucous membranes may be present. The degree of pallor is worst in women who suffer from hemoglobinopathies such as sickle cell disease. Other signs that could be present in malaria are jaundice and splenomegaly. Jaundice and splenomegaly are usually found in people who live outside holoendemic areas and thus who have no immunity to malaria, and also in patients with preexisting hemoglobinopathies. Women living in holoendemic areas usually only have fever as the sign that is noted on clinical examination.

Diagnosis

To successfully diagnose malaria in pregnancy outside holoendemic areas, the clinician needs to have a high index of suspicion. A history of travel to a malaria-endemic area should lead to malaria being considered when a fever occurs. In holoendemic areas, however, there is a risk of clinicians overdiagnosing malaria from clinical signs and symptoms. Because malaria is a common condition in such places, a thorough work-up on the cause of a fever is often overlooked.

To diagnose malaria correctly, there is the need to confirm the clinical diagnosis with laboratory investigations. The microbiological test for malaria is a thick or thin peripheral blood film for microscopic examination. The thick blood film is used for low parasitemias and the thin blood film for high parasitemias [2,3]. The level of parasitemia as well as the species of *Plasmodium* responsible for the condition is revealed by microscopic examination. Microscopy is the gold standard for routine laboratory diagnosis of malaria and is a very reliable way of diagnosing the condition [3].

In areas where malaria cases are not commonly seen, leading to reduced skill in microscopy for malaria, polymerase chain reaction (PCR) procedures are more accurate for making the diagnosis even though this method is more expensive and takes longer to arrive at a

Queenan's Management of High-Risk Pregnancy: An Evidence-Based Approach, Sixth Edition. Edited by John T. Queenan, Catherine Y. Spong, Charles J. Lockwood.
© 2012 John Wiley & Sons, Ltd. Published 2012 by John Wiley & Sons, Ltd.

diagnosis. In areas where there is no laboratory support for the clinician, rapid diagnostic tests which are designed to determine the presence of plasmodial antigens can be used [4].

Treatment

The medications that can be used in the treatment of malaria in pregnancy depend on the stage of pregnancy at which the disease is diagnosed and the general condition of the patient.

A combination of quinine and clindamycin is recommended when malaria is diagnosed in the first trimester. Quinine can be used alone if clindamycin in unavailable or unaffordable [5]. In the second and third trimesters, artemisinin-based combination therapy (ACT) is used for treatment. The recommended forms of ACT are artemether-lumefantrine, artesunate plus amodiaquine, artesunate plus mefloquine, and artesunate plus sulfadoxine-pyrimethamine [5].

There are limited data on the safety of ACT in the first trimester even though it is recommended that ACT be used in the first trimester if it is the only available treatment [5].

Antiemetics and analgesics are used to manage severe vomiting, headaches, and myalgia associated with malaria in pregnancy. In severe cases of vomiting, patients are unable to take oral medication and are also unable to eat. These patients are managed with fluid and electrolyte replacement therapy, parenteral quinine and parenteral antiemetic agents. Oral medication is commenced once the vomiting stops.

Complications

Malaria affects both the mother and the fetus. Malaria has been reported to cause severe anemia leading to cardiac failure. It can lead to acute renal failure as a result of infected red blood cells causing endothelial damage and resultant reduced blood flow to the kidneys. It also causes hypoglycemia leading to central nervous complications of cerebral malaria characterized by seizures and loss of consciousness. Malaria causes maternal mortality through these complications.

Malaria causes miscarriages when it occurs in the first trimester. Intrauterine growth restriction and intrauterine fetal death from malaria are caused by the reduction in oxygen and nutrient delivery due to placental malaria. Malaria causes low birthweight because of the associated maternal anemia and the intrauterine growth restriction. Intrauterine infection of the fetus with malaria – congenital malaria – results from placental malaria. The febrile paroxysms due to malaria could precipitate preterm labor and prematurity.

Prevention

In holoendemic areas, malaria in pregnancy is prevented by the following measures.
- Intermittent preventive treatment [6]
- Use of insecticide-treated nets [7]
- Effective case management of malaria and anemia

Intermittent preventive treatment is the use of antimalarial medications at specific intervals during the pregnancy in the absence of clinical malaria. The World Health Organization recommends that all pregnant women in holoendemic areas should receive three doses of sulfadoxine-pyrimethamine at monthly intervals after quickening. The first dose should not be administered earlier than 16 weeks' gestation and the last dose should not be after 36 weeks' gestation [5].

Pregnant women in holoendemic areas are advised to sleep under insecticide-treated bed-nets in order to reduce the frequency of mosquito bites.

Effective diagnosis and treatment of malaria will prevent the occurrence of maternal and fetal complications.

CASE PRESENTATION

A 26-year-old primigravida at 33 weeks' gestation presented to the clinic with complaints of recurrent lower abdominal pain radiating to her back and thighs. She also complained of a mild fever and chills but no dysuria.

On examination, the patient appeared to be in moderate pain but did not appear acutely ill. She was warm to touch with a temperature of 38°C. She was neither pale nor jaundiced. Examination of her abdomen showed a uterus that was appropriate for dates. She had a singleton pregnancy in cephalic presentation with a normal fetal heart rate. She was having two contractions in 10 min with each contraction lasting about 20 sec. Speculum examination showed that her cervix was about 3 cm long and not dilated.

Laboratory tests ordered were urine microscopy, biochemistry and culture, complete blood count, blood film for malaria parasites, and an ultrasound scan.

The urine tests were normal; hemoglobin level was 9.5 g/dL; thick film smear for malaria parasites showed 2+ parasitemia. The ultrasound examination did not show any abnormalities.

A diagnosis of malaria complicated by preterm contractions was made. She was put on a course of artemether-lumefantrine and the dosage of her regular hematinic was doubled. She was admitted for observation because of the preterm contractions.

By the second day of admission, she was feeling better and the contractions had stopped. She was discharged home to complete the antimalarial treatment. On her return visit a week later, she was in a very good state of health with no complaints.

References

1. Lagerberg RE. Malaria in pregnancy: a literature review. J Midwifery Womens Health 2008;53(3):209–215.
2. World Health Organization. World Malaria Report 2008. Geneva: World Health Organization, 2008.
3. World Health Organization. Role of Laboratory Diagnosis to Support Malaria Disease Management. Report of a WHO Consultation. Geneva: World Health Organization, 2006.
4. World Health Organization. The Use of Malaria Rapid Diagnostic Tests, 2nd edn. Geneva: World Health Organization, 2006.
5. World Health Organization. Guidelines for the Treatment of Malaria. Geneva: World Health Organization, 2006.
6. Kayentao K, Kodio M, Newman RD et al. Comparison of intermittent preventive treatment with chemoprophylaxis for the prevention of malaria during pregnancy in Mali. J Infect Dis 2005;191(1):109–116.
7. Kabanywanyi AM, Macarthur JR, Stolk WA et al. Malaria in pregnant women in an area with sustained high coverage of insecticide-treated bed nets. Malar J 2008;7:133.

Chapter 29
Group B Streptococcal Infection

Ronald S. Gibbs

Department of Obstetrics and Gynecology, University of Colorado School of Medicine, Denver, CO, USA

In the 1970s, group B streptococci (GBS) dramatically became the leading cause of neonatal infection and an important cause of maternal genital tract infection and septicemia [1–4]. After the implementation of nationally used prevention guidelines first instituted in 1996, there was a decrease in neonatal deaths of over 70%. New guidelines released in 2002 recommended the single strategy of universal culture-based screening at 35–37 weeks' gestation, and extensively changed antibiotic recommendations. The most recent set of guidelines was released in late 2010 [5].

Epidemiology of group B streptococci perinatal infection

Twenty to 30% of all pregnant women are colonized rectogenitally with GBS. Prenatal screening at 35–37 weeks' gestation is currently recommended in the USA. Early-onset neonatal disease occurs within the first week of life; late-onset disease occurs after the first week. Because of the dramatic decrease in early-onset disease, the incidence of early- and late-onset neonatal disease is now equivalent (at approximately 0.4 cases/1000 births). Meningitis is much more common in late-onset disease. For term infants with GBS sepsis, survival is approximately 98%, but for preterm infants the survival is 90% for cases at 34–36 weeks and 70% for cases at ≤33 weeks. These suboptimal outcomes led to effective prevention strategies. Risk factors for early-onset disease include maternal GBS colonization, prolonged rupture of membranes, preterm delivery, GBS bacteriuria during pregnancy, birth of a previous infant with invasive GBS disease, and maternal fever in labor.

In pregnant women, GBS can cause urinary tract infection, chorioamnionitis, endometritis, bacteremia, puerperal wound infection, and stillbirth.

Isolation of group B streptococci

To optimize detection of GBS in rectogenital tract specimens, selective media that suppress the growth of competing bacteria should be used. Commercially available selective media include Todd–Hewitt broth (a nutritive broth for gram-positive organisms) supplemented with gentamicin plus nalidixic acid or colistin plus nalidixic acid. Nucleic acid amplification tests such as polymerase chain reaction (PCR) can also be used after enrichment by incubation of the specimen for 18–24 h [5].

Recommended antibiotics for prophylaxis

Resistance to penicillin or ampicillin has not been detected in GBS. Because of its universal activity against GBS and narrow spectrum of activity, penicillin remains the antibiotic of choice for GBS prophylaxis, with ampicillin remaining an alternative [5].

Resistance to clindamycin and erythromycin has increased among GBS isolates in the last 15 years. The prevalence of resistance in the USA and Canada was in the range 25–32% for erythromycin and 13–20% for clindamycin in studies published in the last 5 years [5]. Resistance to cefoxitin has also been reported [5]. It has been recognized that GBS isolates which show susceptibility to clindamycin but resistance to erythromycin by traditional *in vitro* testing may demonstrate inducible resistance to clindamycin. Use of the D-zone test can detect inducible resistance [5].

Rising resistance to clindamycin and erythromycin is a key element in recommendations for GBS chemoprophylaxis in penicillin-allergic women (Fig. 29.1). The 2002 guidelines recommended clindamycin or erythromycin only if a patient's GBS isolate has been shown to

---

Queenan's Management of High-Risk Pregnancy: An Evidence-Based Approach, Sixth Edition. Edited by John T. Queenan, Catherine Y. Spong, Charles J. Lockwood.

have *in vitro* susceptibility to both. Vancomycin is recommended for women at high risk of penicillin allergy colonized by clindamycin-resistant or erythromycin-resistant isolates. Vancomycin is recommended even if an isolate shows *in vitro* resistance to either clindamycin or erythromycin because of possible inducible resistance.

Prevention of perinatal group B streptococci infection

Use of intrapartum antibiotics is the only effective intervention available against perinatal GBS disease.

For indications for prophylaxis under the 2010 Centers for Disease Control (CDC) GBS guidelines, see Figure 29.1. In addition, women who have had a previous infant with invasive GBS disease or who have GBS bacteriuria during pregnancy should receive intrapartum

prophylaxis. Women with unknown culture status at the time of labor should receive intrapartum antibiotic prophylaxis if they present with the risk factors outlined in Figure 29.1. Figure 29.1 also outlines some common circumstances in which intrapartum prophylaxis is not indicated. Women undergoing a planned cesarean delivery in the absence of labor or membrane rupture do not require GBS prophylaxis.

Recommended antibiotics for intrapartum prophylaxis are shown in Figure 29.1.

Preterm premature rupture of the membranes

Preterm premature rupture of the membranes (PPROM) places the fetus or newborn at special risk for GBS sepsis. The 2010 guidelines provide separate algorithms for

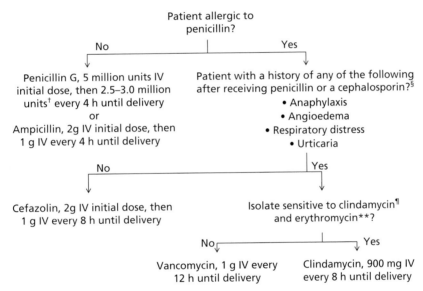

Figure 29.1 Recommended regimens for intrapartum antibiotic prophylaxis for prevention of early-onset group B streptococcal (GBS) disease [5].

*Broader spectrum agents, including an agent active against GBS, might be necessary for treatment of chorioamnionitis.

†Doses ranging from 2.5 to 3.0 million units are acceptable for the doses administered every 4 hours following the initial dose. The choice of dose within that range should be guided by which formulations of penicillin G are readily available to reduce the need for pharmacies to specially prepare doses.

§Penicillin-allergic patients with a history of anaphylaxis, angioedema, respiratory distress, or urticaria following administration of penicillin or a cephalosporin are considered to be at high risk for anaphylaxis and should not receive penicillin, ampicillin, or cefazolin for GBS intrapartum prophylaxis. For penicillin-allergic patients who do not have a history of those reactions, cefazolin is the preferred agent because pharmacologic data suggest it achieves effective intraamniotic concentrations. Vancomycin and clindamycin should be reserved for penicillin-allergic women at high risk for anaphylaxis.

¶If laboratory facilities are adequate, clindamycin and erythromycin susceptibility testing should be performed on prenatal GBS isolates from penicillin-allergic women at high risk for anaphylaxis. If no susceptibility testing is performed, or the results are not available at the time of labor, vancomycin is the preferred agent for GBS intrapartum prophylaxis for penicillin-allergic women at high risk for anaphylaxis.

**Resistance to erythromycin is often but not always associated with clindamycin resistance. If an isolate is resistant to erythromycin, it may have inducible resistance to clindamycin, even if it appears susceptible to clindamycin. If a GBS isolate is susceptible to clindamycin, resistant to erythromycin, and D-zone testing for inducible resistance has been performed and is negative (no inducible resistance), then clindamycin can be used for GBS intrapartum prophylaxis instead of vancomycin.

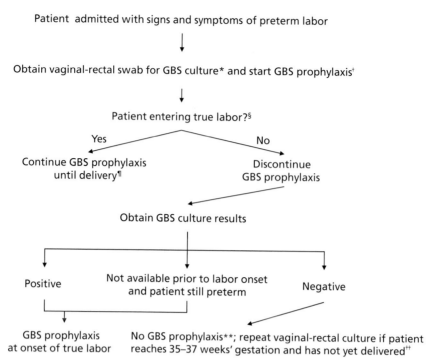

Figure 29.2 Algorithm for group B streptococcus (GBS) intrapartum prophylaxis for women with preterm labor (PTL) [5].
*If patient has undergone vaginal-rectal GBS culture within the preceding 5 weeks, the results of that culture should guide management. GBS-colonized women should receive intrapartum antibiotic prophylaxis. No antibiotics are indicated for GBS prophylaxis if a vaginal-rectal screen within 5 weeks was negative.
†See Figure 29.1 for recommended antibiotic regimens.
§Patient should be regularly assessed for progression to true labor; if the patient is considered not to be in true labor, discontinue GBS prophylaxis.
¶If GBS culture results become available prior to delivery and are negative, then discontinue GBS prophylaxis. **Unless subsequent GBS culture prior to delivery is positive.
††A negative GBS screen is considered valid for 5 weeks. If a patient with a history of PTL is readmitted with signs and symptoms of PTL and had a negative GBS screen >5 weeks before, she should be rescreened and managed according to this algorithm at that time.

preterm labor and preterm premature rupture of membranes (Figs 29.2, 29.3).

Bacteriuria

The 2010 GBS guidelines recommend that all women with GBS bacteriuria, defined as GBS isolated from the urine at $\geq 10^4$ colonies/mL, should receive intrapartum prophylaxis. These women do not require late antenatal screening. Symptomatic or asymptomatic GBS urinary tract infections should be treated according to usual standards.

CASE PRESENTATION

A 20-year-old primigravida reports a "penicillin allergy" at her first prenatal visit. Details confirm that she had an immediate hypersensitivity reaction including urticaria, hives, and wheezing.

What testing should be performed on the GBS isolate? Because the patient should be given neither penicillin nor a cephalosporin, this isolate must be tested for susceptibility to both clindamycin and erythromycin. In addition, if the isolate is resistant to erythromycin but susceptible to clindamycin, by traditional *in vitro* testing, the isolate

should be tested for inducible clindamycin resistance by the D-zone test.

What antibiotics should be used for intrapartum prophylaxis? If the isolate is sensitive to both clindamycin and erythromycin, and if there is no inducible clindamycin resistance, clindamycin should be used for prophylaxis. Erythromycin is no longer recommended. However, if the isolate is resistant to either (or both) clindamycin or erythromycin, then vancomycin must be used.

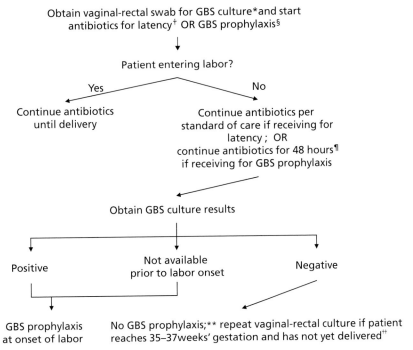

Figure 29.3 Algorithm for group B streptococcus (GBS) intrapartum prophylaxis for women with preterm premature rupture of membranes (PPROM) [5].

*If patient has undergone vaginal-rectal GBS culture within the preceding 5 weeks, the results of that culture should guide management. GBS-colonized women should receive intrapartum antibiotic prophylaxis. No antibiotics are indicated for GBS prophylaxis if a vaginal-rectal screen within 5 weeks was negative.

†Antibiotics given for latency in the setting of pPROM that include ampicillin 2 g IV × 1, followed by 1 g IV q6h for at least 48 h are adequate for GBS prophylaxis. If other regimens are used, GBS prophylaxis should be initiated in addition.

§See Figure 29.1 for recommended antibiotic regimens.

¶GBS prophylaxis should be discontinued at 48 h for women with PPROM who are not in labor. If results from a GBS screen performed on admission become available during the 48-h period and are negative, GBS prophylaxis should be discontinued at that time.

**Unless subsequent GBS culture prior to delivery is positive.

††A negative GBS screen is considered valid for 5 weeks. If a patient with PPROM is entering labor and had a negative GBS screen >5 weeks before, she should be rescreened and managed according to this algorithm at that time.

References

1. Gibbs RS, Schrag S, Schuchat A. High risk pregnancy series: an expert's view. Perinatal infections due to group B streptococci. Obstet Gynecol 2004;104:1062–1076.
2. Sweet RL, Gibbs RS. Group B streptococci. In: Sweet RL, Gibbs RS, eds. Infectious Diseases of the Female Genital Tract, 4th edn. Philadelphia: Lippincott Williams and Wilkins, 2002, pp.31–46.
3. Centers for Disease Control and Prevention. Prevention of perinatal group B streptococcal disease. Revised guidelines from CDC. MMWR 2002;51(RR-11):1–22.
4. Centers for Disease Control and Prevention. Prevention of perinatal group B streptococcal disease: a public health perspective. MMWR 1996;45(RR-7):1–24.
5. Centers for Disease Control and Prevention. Prevention of perinatal group B streptococcal disease: revised guidelines from CDC. MMWR 2010;59(RR-10):1–36.

Chapter 30
Hepatitis

Patrick Duff

Department of Obstetrics and Gynecology, University of Florida College of Medicine, Gainesville, FL, USA

The purpose of this chapter is to review six different types of viral hepatitis: A, B, C, D, E, and G; describe the diagnostic tests for each of these infections; and define the perinatal complications associated with the various forms of viral hepatitis (Table 30.1). I have grouped the infections in terms of their epidemiology rather than simply listing them alphabetically.

Hepatitis A

Hepatitis A is the second most common form of viral hepatitis in the United States. The infection is caused by an RNA virus that is transmitted by fecal–oral contact. The incubation period ranges from 15 to 50 days. Infections in children are usually asymptomatic; infections in adults are usually symptomatic. The disease is most prevalent in areas of poor sanitation and crowded living [1]. The typical clinical manifestations of hepatitis A include low-grade fever, malaise, anorexia, right upper quadrant pain and tenderness, jaundice, and acholic stools. The diagnosis is most easily confirmed by detection of IgM antibody specific for the hepatitis A virus.

Hepatitis A does not cause a chronic carrier state. Perinatal transmission virtually never occurs, and, therefore, the infection does not pose a major risk to either the mother or baby unless the mother develops fulminant hepatitis and liver failure, which is extremely rare [1].

Hepatitis A can be prevented by administration of an inactivated vaccine. Two monovalent formulations of the vaccine are available: Vaqta® and Havrix® [2]. Both vaccines require an initial intramuscular injection, followed by a second dose 6–12 months later. The vaccine should be offered to the following individuals.
- International travelers
- Children in endemic areas
- Intravenous drug users

- Individuals who have occupational exposure, e.g. workers in a primate laboratory
- Residents and staff of chronic care institutions
- Individuals with liver disease
- Homosexual men
- Individuals with clotting factor disorders

The vaccine can also be given in a bivalent form in combination with hepatitis B vaccine.

Standard immunoglobulin provides reasonably effective passive immunization for hepatitis A if it is given within 2 weeks of exposure. The standard intramuscular dose of immunoglobulin is 0.02 mg/kg. Interestingly, however, Victor *et al* [3] recently demonstrated that the hepatitis A vaccine also provided effective postexposure prophylaxis. In fact, it offered several advantages over immunoglobulin.
- It was readily available and comparable in cost to immunoglobulin.
- It provided both short-term and long-term protection against hepatitis A.
- It was less painful to administer.
- It did not interfere with other vaccination schedules.

Accordingly, in my opinion, hepatitis A vaccine should now be the agent of choice for both pre- and postexposure prophylaxis.

Hepatitis E

Hepatitis E is caused by an RNA virus. The epidemiology of hepatitis E is quite similar to that of hepatitis A. The incubation period averages 45 days. The disease is quite rare in the US but is endemic in developing countries of the world. In these countries, maternal infection with hepatitis E often has an alarmingly high mortality, in the range of 10–20%. This high mortality is probably less the result of the virulence of the microorganism and more

Queenan's Management of High-Risk Pregnancy: An Evidence-Based Approach, Sixth Edition. Edited by John T. Queenan, Catherine Y. Spong, Charles J. Lockwood.
© 2012 John Wiley & Sons, Ltd. Published 2012 by John Wiley & Sons, Ltd.

Table 30.1 Viral hepatitis in pregnancy: summary of key facts

Infection	Mechanism of transmission	Best diagnostic test	Carrier state	Perinatal transmission	Vaccine	Remarks
A	Fecal–oral	Antibody detection	No	No	Yes	Pre- or postexposure prophylaxis – either standard immunoglobulin or hepatitis A vaccine
E	Fecal–oral	Antibody detection	No	Rare	No	High maternal mortality in developing countries. No immunoprophylaxis is available
B	Parenteral/sexual contact	Antigen detection	Yes	Yes	Yes	Postexposure prophylaxis – hepatitis B immunoglobulin (HBIG) and booster dose of hepatitis B vaccine
D	Parenteral/sexual contact	Antibody detection	Yes	Yes	Prevented by hepatitis B vaccine	Virus cannot replicate in absence of hepatitis B infection
C	Parenteral/sexual contact	Antibody detection	Yes	Yes	No	No immunoprophylaxis is available. High risk of co-infection with hepatitis B and HIV
G	Parenteral/sexual contact	Antibody detection	Yes	Yes	No	Infection has no clinical significance

related to poor nutrition, poor general health, and lack of access to modern medical care [1].

The clinical presentation of acute hepatitis E is similar to that of hepatitis A. The diagnosis can be established by using electron microscopy to identify viral particles in the stool of infected patients. The most useful diagnostic test, however, is serology.

Hepatitis E does not cause a chronic carrier state. Perinatal transmission can occur but is extremely rare [4].

Hepatitis B

Hepatitis B is caused by a DNA virus that is transmitted parenterally and via sexual contact. The infection also can be transmitted perinatally from an infected mother to her infant.

Acute hepatitis B occurs in approximately 1–2 per 1000 pregnancies in the United States. The chronic carrier state is more frequent, occurring in 6–10 per 1000 pregnancies. The infection is particularly likely to occur in association with hepatitis C and HIV infection [5]. Worldwide, over 400 million individuals are chronically infected with hepatitis B virus. In the US, approximately 1.25 million individuals are chronically infected. Hepatitis B infection accounts for 4000–5500 deaths annually in the US and 1 million deaths worldwide from cirrhosis, liver failure, and hepatocellular carcinoma [6].

Approximately 90% of patients who acquire hepatitis B mount an effective immunologic response to the virus and completely clear their infection. Less than 1% of infected patients develop fulminant hepatitis and die. Approximately 10% of patients develop a chronic carrier state. As noted, some individuals with chronic hepatitis B infection ultimately develop severe chronic liver disease

such as chronic active hepatitis, chronic persistent hepatitis, cirrhosis, or hepatocellular carcinoma [1].

The diagnosis of hepatitis B is best confirmed by serologic tests. Patients with acute hepatitis B are positive for the hepatitis B surface antigen and positive for IgM antibody to the core antigen. Patients with chronic hepatitis B are positive for the surface antigen and positive for IgG antibody to the core antigen. Infected patients may or may not be positive for the hepatitis B*e* antigen. When this latter antigen is present, it denotes active viral replication and a high level of infectivity [7].

In the absence of intervention, approximately 20% of mothers who are seropositive for the hepatitis B surface antigen alone will transmit infection to their neonates. Approximately 90% of mothers who are positive for both the surface antigen and the *e* antigen will transmit infection. Fortunately, we now have excellent immunoprophylaxis for prevention of perinatal transmission of hepatitis B infection, and, therefore, all pregnant women should be routinely screened for hepatitis B during pregnancy. Infants delivered to seropositive mothers should receive hepatitis B immunoglobulin within 12 h of birth. Prior to their discharge from the hospital, these infants also should begin the three-dose hepatitis B vaccination series. Infants delivered to seronegative women require only the hepatitis B vaccine [1,7,8].

Of special note, immunoprophylaxis is approximately 90% effective in preventing perinatal transmission of hepatitis B infection to the infants of asymptomatic hepatitis B carriers who are positive for either the hepatitis B surface antigen or the surface antigen and *e* antigen. The most common cause for failure of immunoprophylaxis is transplacental infection during pregnancy. Intrauterine infection is most likely to occur in women who have higher viral loads, defined as greater than 10^3 copies/mL.

Recently, two additional interventions have been proven effective in reducing the risk of intrauterine infection in such patients. One strategy is to administer hepatitis B immunoglobulin, 200 international units intramuscularly monthly, from 28 weeks' gestation to delivery. A second strategy is to administer lamivudine, 100 mg orally each day, from 28 weeks' gestation until 1 month after delivery. The latter strategy is probably preferable because, in combination with conventional immunoprophylaxis, it further reduces the risk of mother-to-infant transmission after birth. In this limited dose, lamivudine appears to be very safe for mother and infant [9].

The hepatitis B vaccine should also be offered to all women of reproductive age who are not already infected. This is an inactivated vaccine that is prepared by recombinant technology from yeast cells. The vaccine is safe for administration during pregnancy and in lactating women [5,7,8].

Hepatitis D (delta virus infection)

Hepatitis D is an RNA virus which depends upon co-infection with hepatitis B for replication. Therefore, the epidemiology of hepatitis D is essentially identical to that of hepatitis B. Patients with hepatitis D may have two types of infection. Some may have acute hepatitis D and hepatitis B (co-infection). These individuals typically clear their infection and have a good long-term prognosis. Others may have chronic hepatitis D infection superimposed upon chronic hepatitis B infection (superinfection). These women are particularly likely to develop chronic liver disease [1].

The diagnosis of hepatitis D can be established by identifying the delta antigen in liver tissue or serum. However, the most useful diagnostic tests are detection of IgM and/or IgG antibody in serum.

As noted, hepatitis D can cause a chronic carrier state in conjunction with hepatitis B infection. Perinatal transmission of hepatitis D occurs, but it is uncommon. Moreover, the immunoprophylaxis outlined above for hepatitis B is highly effective in preventing transmission of hepatitis D [1].

Hepatitis C

Hepatitis C is caused by an RNA virus. The virus may be transmitted parenterally, via sexual contact, and perinatally. In many patient populations, hepatitis C is actually as common, if not more common, than hepatitis B. Approximately 2.7 million people (1–2% of the population) in the US have hepatitis C. About 33,000 new cases occur annually, and almost 10,000 individuals die of the disease each year. The disease occurs in about 1% of pregnant patients. The prevalence is significantly higher in women who are co-infected with hepatitis B or HIV or who are intravenous drug users. In the latter group, the prevalence approaches 70–95%. Chronic hepatitis C infection is now the most common reason for liver transplantation in the US [1,10–12].

The disease is usually asymptomatic. The diagnosis is best confirmed by serologic testing. The initial screening test should be an enzyme immunoassay (EIA). The confirmatory test is a recombinant immunoblot assay (RIBA). Seroconversion may not occur for up to 16 weeks following infection [1].

In patients who have a low serum concentration of hepatitis C RNA and who do not have co-existing HIV infection, the risk of perinatal transmission of hepatitis C is less than 5%. If the patient's serum concentration of hepatitis C RNA is high and/or she has HIV infection, the perinatal transmission rate may approach 25% [13,14].

Unfortunately, there is no vaccine or hyperimmune globulin for hepatitis C. Moreover, although there are new drugs that are reasonably effective in treating hepatitis C [15], they have not been shown to affect the rate of perinatal transmission. Some small nonrandomized, uncontrolled cohort studies (level II evidence) [16,17] support elective cesarean delivery prior to the onset of labor and rupture of membranes in women who have detectable hepatitis C virus RNA or who are co-infected with HIV. Other studies do not show an advantage for elective cesarean delivery [18]. No study has demonstrated that breastfeeding is harmful in infected women.

Hepatitis G

Hepatitis G is caused by an RNA virus which is related to the hepatitis C virus. Hepatitis G is more prevalent but less virulent than hepatitis C. Many patients who have hepatitis G are co-infected with hepatitis A, B, C, and HIV. Interestingly, co-infection with hepatitis G does not adversely affect the prognosis of these other infections [19–22].

Most patients with hepatitis G are asymptomatic. The diagnosis is best established by detection of virus by polymerase chain reaction and by detection of antibody by enzyme-linked immunosorbent assay (ELISA).

Hepatitis G may cause a chronic carrier state, and perinatal transmission has been documented. However, the clinical effect of infection in the mother and baby appears to be minimal. Accordingly, patients should not routinely be screened for this infection. There is no antiviral agent, vaccine, or hyperimmune globulin for hepatitis G, and no special treatment is indicated even if infection is confirmed.

CASE PRESENTATION

A 32-year-old woman, gravida 3, para 1102, at 18 weeks' gestation is found to be seropositive for hepatitis B surface antigen. Additional testing shows that she also is positive for hepatitis C and D and seronegative for HIV infection. There is no evidence of gonorrhea, chlamydia, or syphilis.

1. What additional testing is indicated in this patient? *Answer*: Patients who are co-infected with hepatitis B, C, and D are particularly likely to develop chronic liver disease such as chronic active hepatitis, chronic persistent hepatitis, and cirrhosis. In some individuals, the liver disease may progress to hepatocellular carcinoma and/or frank hepatic failure. Therefore, this patient should have a battery of liver function tests and a coagulation profile. She should have a determination of hepatitis B viral load. If the viral load is >1000 copies/mL, she should be offered treatment with oral lamivudine from 28 weeks' gestation through the first month after delivery. In addition, near term she should have a test to determine the serum concentration of hepatitis C virus RNA. In selected instances, patients with high hepatitis C viral loads may be candidates for a scheduled cesarean delivery before the onset of labor.

2. What interventions are appropriate for her sexual partner? *Answer*: The patient's sexual partner should be tested for hepatitis B, C, and D. If he is seronegative for hepatitis B, he should receive an injection of hepatitis B immunoglobulin and begin the hepatitis B vaccine series. This immunoprophylaxis will also protect against hepatitis D infection.

3. What type of immunoprophylaxis is indicated for this patient's neonate? *Answer*: Unfortunately, there is no immunoprophylaxis for hepatitis C. However, effective immunoprophylaxis against hepatitis B and D is available. The infant should receive hepatitis B immunoglobulin within 12 h of birth. Prior to discharge from hospital, the infant should receive the first dose of hepatitis B vaccine. A second and third dose should be administered at 1 month of age and 6 months of age.

4. Is it safe for the baby to breastfeed? *Answer*: Yes. The immunoprophylaxis described above is very effective in preventing transmission of hepatitis B and D. Fortunately, even in the absence of immunoprophylaxis, breastfeeding does not appear to increase the risk of hepatitis C in the neonate.

References

1. Duff P. Hepatitis in pregnancy. Semin Perinatol 1998;22: 277–283.
2. Duff B, Duff P. Hepatitis A vaccine: ready for prime time. Obstet Gynecol 1998;91:468–471.
3. Victor JC, Monto AS, Surdina TY et al. Hepatitis A vaccine versus immune globulin for postexposure propylaxis. N Engl J Med 2007;357:1685–1694.
4. Khuroo MS, Kamili S, Jameel S. Vertical transmission of hepatitis E virus. Lancet 1995;345:1025–1026.
5. Koziel MJ, Peters MG. Viral hepatitis in HIV infection. N Engl J Med 2007;356:1445–1454.
6. Dienstag JL. Hepatitis B virus infection. N Engl J Med 2008;359:1486–1500.
7. Hepatitis B virus: a comprehensive strategy for eliminating transmission in the United States through universal childhood vaccination. MMWR 1991;40:1–25.
8. Poland GA, Jacobson RM. Prevention of hepatitis B with the hepatitis B vaccine. N Engl J Med 2004;351: 2832–2838.
9. Shi Z, Yang Y, Ma L et al. Lamivudine in late pregnancy to interrupt in utero transmission of hepatitis B virus. A systematic review and meta-analysis. Obstet Gynecol 2010;116: 147–159.
10. Leikin EL, Reirus JF, Schnell E et al. Epidemiologic predictors of hepatitis C virus infection in pregnant women. Obstet Gynecol 1994;84:529–534.
11. Bohman VR, Stettler W, Little BB et al. Seroprevalence and risk factors for hepatitis C virus antibody in pregnant women. Obstet Gynecol 1992;80:609–613.
12. Berkley EMF, Lesliek KK, Arora S, Qualls C, Dunkelberg JC. Chronic hepatitis C in pregnancy. Obstet Gynecol 2008;112: 304–310.
13. Ohto H, Terazawa S, Sasaki N et al. Transmission of hepatitis C virus from mothers to infants. N Engl J Med 1994;330: 744–750.
14. Steininger C, Kundi M, Jatzko G et al. Increased risk of mother-to-infant transmission of hepatitis C virus by intrapartum infantile exposure to blood. J Infect Dis 2003;187: 345–351.
15. Hoofnagle JH. A step forward in therapy for hepatitis C. N Engl J Med 2009;360:1899–1901.
16. Gibb DM, Goodall RL, Dunn DT et al. Mother-to-child transmission of hepatitis C virus: evidence for preventable peripartum transmission. Lancet 2000;356:904–907.
17. Zanetti AR, Paccagnini S, Principi N et al. Mother-to-infant transmission of hepatitis C virus. Lancet 1995;345: 289–291.
18. European Paediatric Hepatitis C Virus Network. A significant sex – but not elective cesarean section – effect on

mother-to-child transmission of hepatitis C virus infection. J Infect Dis 2005;192:1872–1879.

19. Jarvis LM, Davidson F, Hanley JP et al. Infection with hepatitis G virus among recipients of plasma products. Lancet 1996;348:1352–1355.

20. Kew MC, Kassionides C. HGV: hepatitis G virus or harmless G virus. Lancet 1996;348(Suppl):10.

21. Alter MJ, Gallagher M, Morris TT et al. Acute non-A-E hepatitis in the United States and the role of hepatitis G infection. N Engl J Med 1997;336:741–746.

22. Miyakawa Y, Mayuma M. Hepatitis G virus – a true hepatitis virus or an accidental tourist? N Engl J Med 1997;336:795–796.

Chapter 31
HIV Infection

Howard L. Minkoff
Department of Obstetrics and Gynecology, Maimonides Medical Center, New York, NY, USA

The HIV epidemic is now 30 years old, with well-defined epidemiology and pathophysiology, and with many effective therapeutic regimens available for use. However, the epidemic is far from contained. In many parts of the world, most notably sub-Saharan Africa where about 90% of the world's 500,000 infected infants are born annually, the disease continues to exact a frightening toll. There are cities in the US (e.g. Washington, DC) where the prevalence rivals that seen in several endemic countries. An increasing number of infected individuals are women, the overwhelming majority of whom are of reproductive age. Thus, obstetricians worldwide continue to play a pivotal role. While the care of HIV-infected women is more successful than ever and the rates of mother-to-child transmission of HIV are lower than ever (at least in communities with access to therapy), management is also more complex than ever. This chapter is designed to provide guidance to the obstetrician who must identify and treat infected women, and act to reduce rates of HIV transmission and drug toxicity while optimizing pregnant women's health.

Identifying infected patients

Approximately 25% of HIV-infected persons in the United States are unaware of their status [1]. Despite remarkable improvements in the potency and tolerability of antiretroviral regimens, women can only avail themselves of their benefits after their serostatus is known. Because of the remarkable improvement in outcomes associated with antiretroviral therapy, and the reduction in stigma associated with the diagnosis, obstetric and public health organizations have become strong advocates of prenatal HIV screening. Previously protocols for screening reflected the social and medical environment that was extant at the time that tests first became available and informed written consents preceded by detailed

counseling were required. Those protocols resulted in low testing rates, in part because the process itself contained a stigma, and because some providers only screened women they perceived to be at risk. Finally in 1998, the Institute of Medicine proposed, and the American College of Obstetricians and Gynecologists (ACOG) subsequently endorsed, a process referred to as "opt-out," a process AOCG now believes should be widely employed [2].

In the "opt-out" process, HIV testing is "routinized." Women are told that testing is part of the standard battery of prenatal tests for all pregnant women and that the test will be performed unless the woman objects. Hence, the "opt-out" policy is also referred to as "informed right of refusal." When "opt-out" is utilized, women are no longer required to sign an informed consent in order to find out their serostatus, but they retain the right to refuse the test if they so desire. This approach, in the settings in which it has been adopted, has resulted in improved testing rates. A table detailing the status of the laws in various states can be found at www.nccc.ucsf.edu/consultation_library/state_hiv_testing_laws/.

The actual laboratory procedure for standard (as distinct from "rapid") testing may involve the detection of antigen from the virus itself, antibodies to portions of the virus, viral nucleic acid or, less commonly, culture of the virus. The most widely used method (enzyme-linked immunosorbent assay [ELISA] confirmed by Western blot) involves the detection of antibodies to virus in the patient's sera. If a woman has a positive ELISA but a negative Western blot, she is considered to have a negative test.

In the US, a disproportionate share of infection among pregnant women has always occurred among those with late or no prenatal care [3] and many nonpregnant women have emergency rooms as their only contact with the healthcare system. Therefore there is a need to rapidly identify women who are infected and who initially present for care in labor or in an emergency setting.

Queenan's Management of High-Risk Pregnancy: An Evidence-Based Approach, Sixth Edition. Edited by John T. Queenan, Catherine Y. Spong, Charles J. Lockwood.
© 2012 John Wiley & Sons, Ltd. Published 2012 by John Wiley & Sons, Ltd.

Several rapid HIV tests have been approved by the FDA including:
• OraQuick (and its newer version OraQuick Advance) Rapid HIV-1/2 Antibody Test (OraSure Technologies, Inc., Bethlehem, PA)
• Reveal™ (and its newer version Reveal™ G2) Rapid HIV-1 Antibody Test (MedMira, Halifax, Nova Scotia)
• Uni-Gold Recombigen HIV Test (Trinity BioTech, Bray, Ireland)
• Multispot HIV-1/HIV-2 Rapid Test (Bio-Rad Laboratories, Redmond, WA)[4].
Rapid HIV testing has been compared with the standard enzyme immunoassay (EIA), which is still utilized extensively by blood transfusion services which perform most of the HIV tests worldwide (although always backed up by a Western blot assay), and they have been found to be comparable, with specificities over 99.5%. A reactive result from any of the four rapid HIV tests is interpreted as a "preliminary positive" and requires confirmation by a more specific assay, typically a Western blot (WB) or immunofluorescent assay (IFA).

Posttest counseling of seropositive women

Once an individual's serostatus is determined, there is an acute need to provide appropriate posttest counseling. This counseling must address psychosocial as well as medical aspects of the diagnosis. From a patient education standpoint, it is important to draw a clear distinction between HIV infection and AIDS. The patient should be instructed in ways to avoid transmitting the virus to others: safe sex practices, no sharing of razors, and the like. Treatment with antiretrovirals should also be considered a prevention strategy. The natural history of HIV disease and long-term follow-up plans should also be incorporated into the counseling. At the current time, advances in the treatment of HIV warrant an air of optimism in these initial conversations, an optimism that may be necessary to dispel the many myths that are still associated with the diagnosis of HIV. Perinatal counseling focuses on the potential consequences of pregnancy on HIV disease and the impact of HIV disease status on pregnancy outcome, particularly current estimates of HIV transmission rates. There are no convincing data that demonstrate that pregnancy has an untoward effect on HIV disease [5]. However, pregnancy may have indirect effects: if obstetricians are reluctant to utilize the latest pharmacologic interventions then the woman's disease course may indeed be compromised [6]. However, this does not usually happen any longer in the US.

Perhaps the most important component of counseling relates to the success that obstetricians have had in preventing mother-to-child transmission of HIV with the use of appropriate antiretroviral therapies and cesarean delivery as indicated (see below). Women should be informed of these therapies, as well as risks that may be associated with their use and should be assured that they will have access to these if they so desire.

Although a focus of attention during pregnancy will be on the prevention of mother-to-child transmission of HIV, care begins with a focus on the health of the mother. A baseline CD4 count and viral load provide a reliable picture of the patient's status, the likelihood of progression to clinical illness, and the need for instituting antiviral therapy. Baseline liver and renal function tests should be obtained. If the mother needs medication for her own well-being then therapy should be instituted, although modifications of standard regimens may sometimes be necessary. It is also important to screen for infections that may be prevalent in these women, and whose course might be modified by HIV infection (e.g. hepatitis B and C, and syphilis). Appropriate management of co-infections can be achieved by co-management with an infectious disease specialist.

Resistance testing in infected pregnant women should be performed for the same indications as for nonpregnant persons:
• those with acute infection
• those who have virologic failure with persistently detectable HIV-1 RNA levels while receiving antenatal therapy, or suboptimal viral suppression after initiation of antiretroviral therapy
• those with a high likelihood of having resistant virus based on community prevalence of resistant virus, known drug resistance in the woman's sex partner, or other source of infection
• those who are about to start therapy.
In essence, any pregnant woman with detectable virus should have resistance testing at her first visit.
Below we discuss, in sequence, care of the mother for her own well-being, and the steps needed to minimize the rates of mother-to-child transmission of HIV.

Care of seropositive women in general

Obtaining a CD4 count and a viral load provides the clinician with a useful snapshot of the patient's status and medication needs when she is first encountered. The threshold for treatment continues to evolve with a clear trend toward earlier and earlier starting points (i.e. at higher CD4 counts) [7,8]. Some organizations now recommend treatment even if the CD4 count is under $500\,mm/mL^3$, with some suggestion that there is an advantage for treating when the CD4 count is even higher (e.g. all women at diagnosis) [9]. If a nonpregnant woman were not considered a candidate for therapy even with the new, more liberalized criteria, she would still be a candidate when pregnant. In that circumstance, the treatment would be for the prevention of mother-to-child transmission. The therapy should be a highly active antiretroviral therapy (HAART) regimen. HAART regimens are medication combinations that are capable of providing sustained reductions in the viral load. It is anticipated that the viral load will decrease by more than 1 log/month, and reach an undetectable level within 6 months. If not, further studies and/or changing regimens are appropriate.

There are several possible regimens that can be used. Currently there are seven major classes of antiretroviral drugs: nucleoside analog reverse transcriptase inhibitor (NRTI), nonnucleoside reverse transcriptase inhibitor (NNRTI), protease inhibitor (PI), fusion inhibitor, chemokine co-receptor antagonist (consisting of two subclasses: CCR5 antagonist and CXCR4 antagonist), integrase inhibitors and maturation inhibitors. Most HAART regimens are composed of agents from two different classes of antiretroviral therapy; the most commonly used classes in pregnancy are NRTIs, NNRTIs, and PIs). Most regimens are composed of two NRTIs and either an NNRTI or a PI (sometimes two PIs are used with one acting as a "booster" of the second). If the chosen regimen fails, the possibility of poor adherence, viral resistance, or both, must be considered. Resistance testing should be performed before the failing regimen is discontinued lest wild-strain viruses overgrow resistant strains and mask the identity of the mutated strain. In the latter circumstance, the utility of the resistance test for assisting in the selection of the optimal salvage regimen would be compromised.

Finally, women whose CD4 counts drop below $200 \, mm/mL^3$ are at risk of developing opportunistic infection. Therefore, PCP prophylaxis (e.g. Bactrim-DS daily) should be given if the CD4 count drops below $200 \, mm/mL^3$, and *Mycobacterium avium* complex prophylaxis (azithromycin, 1200 mg/week) should be initiated when the CD4 count equals $50 \, mm/mL^3$. Therapy can be discontinued when CD4 rises above $200 \, mm/mL^3$ for 3 months.

Care of seropositive women in pregnancy

The basic tenets of care are not substantively altered by pregnancy. The goal remains optimizing the health of the mother. However, during pregnancy an additional goal is to minimize the rate of mother-to-child transmission of HIV. Table 31.1 provides a list of antiretroviral drugs and recommendations for use in pregnant HIV-infected women. In pregnancy the virologic and immunologic triggers for therapy, the timing of initiation, and the choice of components of antiviral therapy may need to be adjusted [7]. For example, as noted above, even if a woman does not meet the criteria for treatment when nonpregnant, because of her pregnancy, HAART would be recommended in order to minimize the risk of transmission. In fact, many providers would start HAART in any pregnant woman regardless of viral load or CD4 count in order to reduce transmission to the child and to decrease the rate at which resistance develops in the mother.

Usually, when HAART is used it is started as soon as criteria for therapy are met. However, if it is being given for the purpose of preventing mother-to-child transmission, therapy may be delayed until the start of the second trimester because there is no immediate threat to the mother's health from delay in initiation, and caution would dictate that fetal exposure to these agents be delayed until beyond embryogenesis. The three-part zidovudine (ZDV) chemoprophylaxis regimen, initiated after the first trimester, would be recommended, as it is for all pregnant women with HIV-1 infection, regardless of antenatal HIV-1 RNA copy number. The regimen consists of oral administration of 300 mg ZDV bid, initiated at 14–34 weeks' gestation and continued throughout the pregnancy. During labor, intravenous administration of ZDV is a 1-h initial dose of 2 mg/kg bodyweight, followed by a continuous infusion of 1 mg/kg bodyweight/h until delivery. Finally, oral administration of ZDV is given to the newborn (ZDV syrup at 2 mg/kg bodyweight/ dose every 6 h) for the first 6 weeks of life, beginning at 8–12 h after birth. The ZDV regimen would be but one component of a therapeutic "cocktail."

There are additional pregnancy-specific considerations related to the other agents that might be added to the ZDV. For example, there are several antiretroviral medications that should be avoided in pregnancy. These include efavirenz (Sustiva), which is a class D drug that has been associated with neural tube defects and which should not be used in the first trimester and should only be used thereafter if other alternatives are not available. Another potentially dangerous medication is nevirapine (Viramune), which should be avoided as a component of HAART in pregnant women with CD4 counts $>250 \, mm^3$ because of the high risk of rapidly progressive and potentially nonreversible liver toxicity (this has not been reported in conjunction with its use in single-dose peripartum regimens) [10]. Additionally, because pregnancy itself can mimic some of the early symptoms of the lactic acidosis or hepatic steatosis syndrome or be associated with other disorders of liver metabolism, physicians caring for HIV-1-infected pregnant women receiving nucleoside analog drugs should be alert for early signs of this syndrome. Pregnant women receiving nucleoside analog drugs should have hepatic enzymes and electrolytes assessed more frequently during the last trimester of pregnancy, and any new symptoms should be evaluated thoroughly. Additionally, because of potential mitochondrial toxicity and reports of several cases

Table 31.1 Antiretroviral drug use in pregnant HIV-infected women: pharmacokinetic and toxicity data in human pregnancy and recommendations for use in pregnancy

Antiretroviral drug	Pharmacokinetics in pregnancy	Concerns in pregnancy	Recommendations for use in pregnancy
NRTIs/NtRTIs			NRTIs are recommended for use as part of combination regimens, usually including two NRTIs with either an NNRTI or one or more PIs. Use of single or dual NRTIs alone is not recommended for treatment of HIV infection
Recommended agents			
Lamivudine*	Pharmacokinetics not significantly altered in pregnancy; no change in dose indicated	No evidence of human teratogenicity. Well-tolerated, short-term safety demonstrated for mother and infant. If hepatitis B co-infected, possible hepatitis B flare if drug stopped postpartum	Because of extensive experience with lamivudine in pregnancy in combination with zidovudine, lamivudine plus zidovudine is the recommended dual NRTI backbone for pregnant women
Zidovudine*	Pharmacokinetics not significantly altered in pregnancy; no change in dose indicated	No evidence of human teratogenicity Well-tolerated, short-term safety demonstrated for mother and infant	Preferred NRTI for use in combination antiretroviral regimens in pregnancy based on efficacy studies and extensive experience. Zidovudine should be included in the antenatal antiretroviral regimen unless there is severe toxicity, stavudine use, documented resistance, or the woman is already on a fully suppressive regimen
Alternative agents			
Abacavir*	Pharmacokinetics not significantly altered in pregnancy; no change in dose indicated	No evidence of human teratogenicity. Hypersensitivity reactions occur in ~5–8% of nonpregnant persons; fatal reactions occur in a much smaller percentage of persons and are usually associated with rechallenge. Rate of hypersensitivity reactions in pregnancy is unknown. Testing for HLA-B*5701 identifies patients at risk of reactions and should be done and documented as negative before starting abacavir. Patient should be educated regarding symptoms of reactions	Alternative NRTI for dual nucleoside backbone of combination regimens#
Didanosine	Pharmacokinetics not significantly altered in pregnancy; no change in dose indicated	Cases of lactic acidosis, some fatal, have been reported in pregnant women receiving didanosine and stavudine together	Alternative NRTI for dual nucleoside backbone of combination regimens. Didanosine should not be used with stavudine
Emtricitabine†	Pharmacokinetic study shows slightly lower levels in third trimester compared to postpartum. No clear need to increase dose	No evidence of human teratogenicity	Alternative NRTI for dual nucleoside backbone of combination regimens
Stavudine	Pharmacokinetics not significantly altered in pregnancy; no change in dose indicated	No evidence of human teratogenicity. Cases of lactic acidosis, some fatal, have been reported in pregnant women receiving didanosine and stavudine together	Alternative NRTI for dual nucleoside backbone of combination regimens. Stavudine should be not used with didanosine

Table 31.1 *(Continued)*

Antiretroviral drug	Pharmacokinetics in pregnancy	Concerns in pregnancy	Recommendations for use in pregnancy
Use in special circumstances			
Tenofovir†	Limited studies in human pregnancy; data indicate AUC lower in third trimester than postpartum but trough levels similar	No evidence of human teratogenicity. Studies in monkeys at doses approximately 2-fold higher than dosage for human therapeutic use show decreased fetal growth and reduction in fetal bone porosity. Clinical studies in humans (particularly children) show bone demineralization with chronic use; clinical significance unknown. Significant placental passage in humans. If hepatitis B co-infected, possible hepatitis B flare if drug stopped postpartum	Alternate NRTI for dual NRTI backbone of combination regimens. Would be a preferred NRTI in combination wit 3TC or FTC in women with chronic HBV. Monitor renal function
NNRTIs		Hypersensitivity reactions, including hepatic toxicity, and rash more common in women; unclear if increased in pregnancy	NNRTIs are recommended for use in combination regimens with 2 NRTI drugs
Recommended agents			
Nevirapine	Pharmacokinetics not significantly altered in pregnancy; no change in dose indicated	No evidence of human teratogenicity. Increased risk of symptomatic, often rash-associated, and potentially fatal liver toxicity among women with CD4 counts >250/mm³ when first initiating therapy; unclear if pregnancy increases risk	Nevirapine should be initiated in pregnant women with CD4 counts >250 cells/mm³ only if benefit clearly outweighs risk, due to the increased risk of potentially life-threatening hepatotoxicity in women with high CD4 counts. Women who enter pregnancy on nevirapine regimens and are tolerating them well may continue therapy, regardless of CD4 count
Use in special circumstances			
Efavirenz†	Small study of 600 mg once daily; postpartum peak levels during lactation were 61% higher than previously reported in HIV-infected nonpregnant individuals at that dose. AUC decreased in third trimester but no change in dosage necessary	FDA pregnancy class D; significant malformations (anencephaly, anophthalmia, cleft palate) were observed in 3 (15%) of 20 infants born to cynomolgus monkeys receiving efavirenz during the first trimester at a dose giving plasma levels comparable to systemic human therapeutic exposure. There are 6 retrospective case reports and 1 prospective case report of neural tube defects in humans with first-trimester exposure; relative risk unclear	Use of efavirenz should be avoided in the first trimester. Use after the first trimester can be considered if, after consideration of other alternatives, this is the best choice for a specific woman. If efavirenz is to be continued postpartum, adequate contraception must be assured. Women of child-bearing potential must be counseled regarding the teratogenic potential of efavirenz and avoidance of pregnancy while on the drug
Insufficient data to recommend use			
Etravirine	No pharmacokinetic studies in human pregnancy	No experience in human pregnancy	Safety and pharmacokinetics in pregnancy data are insufficient to recommend use during pregnancy
Protease inhibitors (PIs)		Hyperglycemia, new onset or exacerbation of diabetes mellitus, and diabetic ketoacidosis reported with PI use; unclear if pregnancy increases risk. Conflicting data regarding preterm delivery in women receiving PIs	PIs are recommended for use in combination regimens with 2 NRTI drugs

(Continued)

Table 31.1 (*Continued*)

Antiretroviral drug	Pharmacokinetics in pregnancy	Concerns in pregnancy	Recommendations for use in pregnancy
Recommended agents			
Lopinavir/ritonavir	AUC decreased in second and third trimester with standard dosing	No evidence of human teratogenicity (can rule out 2-fold increase in overall birth defects). Well-tolerated, short-term safety demonstrated in Phase I/II studies	Some experts would administer standard dosing (2 tablets twice daily) throughout pregnancy and monitor virologic response and lopinavir drug levels, if available. Recent data suggest increasing the dose of the tablet formulation during the second and third trimester (from 2 to 3 tablets twice daily), returning to standard dosing postpartum
Alternative agents			
Atazanavir (recommended to be combined with low-dose ritonavir boosting)	Two of three intensive pharmacokinetic studies of atazanavir with ritonavir boosting during pregnancy suggest that standard dosing results in decreased plasma concentrations compared to nonpregnant adults. However, for most pregnant women (not on interacting concomitant medications) no dose adjustment was needed	No evidence of human teratogenicity. Transplacental passage is low. Theoretical concern re increased indirect bilirubin levels exacerbating physiologic hyperbilirubinemia in the neonate not observed in clinical trials to date	Alternative PI for use in combination regimens in pregnancy. Should give as low-dose ritonavir-boosted regimen, may use once-daily dosing. In treatment-naïve patients unable to tolerate ritonavir, 400 mg once-daily dosing without ritonavir boosting may be considered, although there are no data describing atazanavir concentrations or efficacy under these circumstances. If co-administered with tenofovir, atazanavir must be given with low-dose ritonavir boosting
Indinavir (combined with low-dose ritonavir boosting)	Two small studies of women receiving indinavir 800 mg three times daily showed markedly lower levels during pregnancy compared to postpartum, although suppression of HIV RNA was seen. In a study of ritonavir-boosted indinavir (400 mg indinavir/100 mg ritonavir twice daily), 82% of women met the target trough level	No evidence of human teratogenicity. Theoretical concern re increased indirect bilirubin levels, which may exacerbate physiologic hyperbilirubinemia in the neonate, but minimal placental passage. Use of unboosted indinavir during pregnancy is not recommended	Because of twice daily dosing, pill burden, and potential for renal stones, Indinavir should only be used when preferred and alternative agents cannot be used
Nelfinavir	Adequate drug levels are achieved in pregnant women with nelfinavir 1250 mg given twice daily. In one study women in the third trimester had lower concentration of nelfinavir than women in the second trimester. In a study of the new 625 mg tablet formulation dosed at 1250 mg twice daily, lower AUC and peak levels were observed during the third trimester of pregnancy than postpartum	No evidence of human teratogenicity. Well-tolerated, short-term safety demonstrated for mother and infant	Given pharmacokinetic data and extensive experience with use in pregnancy, nelfinavir is an alternative PI for combination regimens in pregnant women receiving combination antiretroviral drugs only for perinatal prophylaxis. In clinical trials of initial therapy in nonpregnant adults, nelfinavir-based regimens had a lower rate of viral response compared to lopinavir-ritonavir or efavirenz-based regimens but similar viral response to atazanavir- or nevirapine-based regimens
Ritonavir	Phase I/II study in pregnancy showed lower levels during pregnancy compared to postpartum	Limited experience at full dose in human pregnancy; has been used as low-dose ritonavir boosting with other PIs	Given low levels in pregnant women when used alone, recommended for use in combination with second PI as low-dose ritonavir "boost" to increase levels of second PI

Table 31.1 (*Continued*)

Antiretroviral drug	Pharmacokinetics in pregnancy	Concerns in pregnancy	Recommendations for use in pregnancy
Saquinavir HGC (combined with low-dose ritonavir boosting)	Limited pharmacokinetic data on saquinavir HGC and the new 500 mg tablet formulation suggest that 1000 mg saquinavir HGC/100 mg ritonavir given twice daily achieves adequate saquinavir drug levels in pregnant women	Well-tolerated, short-term safety demonstrated for mother and infant for saquinavir in combination with low-dose ritonavir	Only limited pharmacokinetic data on saquinavir HGC and the new tablet formulation in pregnancy. Ritonavir-boosted saquinavir HGC or saquinavir tablets are alternative PIs for combination regimens in pregnancy and are alternative initial antiretroviral recommendations for nonpregnant adults. Must give as low-dose ritonavir-boosted regimen

Insufficient data to recommend use

Antiretroviral drug	Pharmacokinetics in pregnancy	Concerns in pregnancy	Recommendations for use in pregnancy
Darunavir (combined with low-dose ritonavir boosting)	No pharmacokinetic studies in human pregnancy.	No experience in human pregnancy	Safety and pharmacokinetics in pregnancy data are insufficient to recommend use during pregnancy. Must give as low-dose ritonavir-boosted regimen
Fosamprenavir (recommended to be combined with low-dose ritonavir boosting)	No pharmacokinetic studies in human pregnancy.	Limited experience in human pregnancy	Safety and pharmacokinetics in pregnancy data are insufficient to recommend use during pregnancy. Recommended to be given as low-dose ritonavir-boosted regimen
Tipranavir (combined with low-dose ritonavir boosting)	No pharmacokinetic studies in human pregnancy.	No experience in human pregnancy	Safety and pharmacokinetics in pregnancy data are insufficient to recommend use during pregnancy. Must give as low-dose ritonavir-boosted regimen

Entry inhibitors
Insufficient data to recommend use

Antiretroviral drug	Pharmacokinetics in pregnancy	Concerns in pregnancy	Recommendations for use in pregnancy
Enfuvirtide	No pharmacokinetic studies in human pregnancy.	Minimal data in human pregnancy	Safety and pharmacokinetics in pregnancy data are insufficient to recommend use during pregnancy
Maraviroc	No pharmacokinetic studies in human pregnancy.	No experience in human pregnancy	Safety and pharmacokinetics in pregnancy data are insufficient to recommend use during pregnancy

Integrase inhibitors
Insufficient data to recommend use

Antiretroviral drug	Pharmacokinetics in pregnancy	Concerns in pregnancy	Recommendations for use in pregnancy
Raltegravir	Standard dose appears appropriate in pregnancy	No experience in human pregnancy	Safety and pharmacokinetics in pregnancy data are insufficient to recommend use during pregnancy

AUC, area under the curve; HGC, hard gel capsule; NNRTI, nonnucleoside reverse transcriptase inhibitor; NRTI, nucleoside reverse transcriptase inhibitor; NtRTI, nucleotide reverse transcriptase inhibitor; PI, protease inhibitor.

*Zidovudine and lamivudine are included as a fixed-dose combination in Combivir; zidovudine, lamivudine, and abacavir are included as a fixed-dose combination in Trizivir; lamivudine and abacavir are included as a fixed-dose combination in Epzicom.

†Emtricitabine and tenofovir are included as a fixed-dose combination in Truvada; emtricitabine, tenofovir, and efavirenz are included as a fixed-dose combination in Atripla.

#Triple NRTI regimens including abacavir have been less potent virologically compared to PI-based combination antiretroviral drug regimens. Triple NRTI regimens should be used only when an NNRTI- or PI-based combination regimen cannot be used (e.g. due to significant drug interactions).

Modified from AIDSinfo.nih.gov, a service of the US DHHS.

of maternal mortality secondary to lactic acidosis with prolonged use of the combination of d4T and ddI, clinicians should not prescribe this antiretroviral combination during pregnancy. HAART regimens in general may be associated with a slight increase in rates of preterm birth though the finding has not been uniformly reported across cohorts.[11]

In addition, the CDC recommends that infected women in the USA refrain from breastfeeding to avoid postnatal transmission of HIV-1 to their infants. In the developing world new strategies involving prolonged ART for mothers or infants have been shown to reduce transmission from breastfeeding [12]. Women who must temporarily discontinue therapy because of pregnancy-related hyperemesis should not resume therapy until sufficient time has elapsed to ensure that the drugs will be tolerated. To reduce the potential for emergence of resistance, if therapy requires temporary discontinuation for any reason during pregnancy, all drugs should be stopped and reintroduced simultaneously.

HIV-1-infected women who are receiving antiretroviral therapy and whose pregnancy is identified after the first trimester should continue therapy. ZDV should be a component of the antenatal antiretroviral treatment regimen whenever possible, although this may not always be feasible. Women receiving antiretroviral therapy whose pregnancy is recognized during the first trimester should be counseled regarding the benefits and potential risks of antiretroviral administration during this period, and continuation of therapy should be generally recommended. If therapy is discontinued during the first trimester, all drugs should be stopped and reintroduced simultaneously to avoid the development of drug resistance. Regardless of the antepartum antiretroviral regimen, ZDV administration is recommended during the intrapartum period and for the newborn.

All HIV-infected women who have labor or ruptured membranes and have not received antepartum antiretroviral therapy should have intravenous ZDV started immediately [7]. In general, ZDV and other NRTI drugs as well as NNRTI drugs cross the placenta well, PI drugs do not. Intravenous intrapartum ZDV followed by oral ZDV for 6 weeks for the infant significantly reduces transmission but new evidence suggests that in this circumstance ZDV alone is not adequate for the child. Intrapartum prophylaxis alone, without an infant postexposure prophylaxis component, is not effective. Several intrapartum/neonatal prophylaxis regimens have been found to be effective including oral ZDV/lamivudine during labor followed by 1 week of pediatric oral ZDV/lamivudine and single-dose intrapartum/newborn nevirapine. Some experts feel additional drugs may be warranted. One option is to add the single-dose intrapartum/newborn nevirapine regimen to the intravenous/6-week infant ZDV regimen. However, that may be associated

with the development of nevirapine-resistant virus. Nevirapine resistance can be substantially reduced by using a short postpartum course of antiretroviral agents from alternate classes (a "tail"). There is no current consensus about the exact duration or composition of the tail. In the United States the use of maternal postpartum ZDV/lamivudine for at least 7 days is suggested as a reasonable tail after intrapartum single-dose nevirapine use.

Studies have consistently shown that cesarean delivery performed before onset of labor and rupture of membranes is associated with a significant decrease in perinatal HIV-1 transmission compared with other types of delivery, with reductions ranging from 55% to 80%. The ACOG Committee on Obstetric Practice, after reviewing these data, issued a Committee Opinion concerning route of delivery, recommending consideration of scheduled cesarean delivery for HIV-1-infected pregnant women with HIV-1 RNA levels >1000 copies/mL near the time of delivery [13]. However, those studies were performed at a time when HAART was not in use. More recent observational data from PACTG 367 [14] and the European Collaborative Study [15], which considered HIV RNA levels and maternal antiretroviral therapy as well as mode of delivery, do not demonstrate an additive benefit from scheduled cesarean delivery if women are on HAART and have a low HIV RNA level. Data are not as clear in regard to woman on HAART but with higher HIV RNA levels. If cesarean delivery is chosen as the delivery option, the procedure should be scheduled at 38 weeks' gestation, based on the best available clinical information. Amniocentesis for fetal lung maturity should not be performed because, in animal models, contamination of amniotic fluid has been shown to be a vector for fetal infection.

For a scheduled cesarean delivery, intravenous ZDV should begin 3 h before surgery, using the standard dosage regimen. Other antiretroviral medications taken during pregnancy should not be interrupted near the time of delivery, regardless of route of delivery. Because maternal infectious morbidity is potentially increased, clinicians should consider perioperative antimicrobial prophylaxis.

In the immediate postpartum period, the woman should have appropriate assessments (e.g. CD4+ count and HIV-1 RNA copy number) to determine whether antiretroviral therapy is recommended for her own health.

Ethical and legal considerations

Obstetricians are acutely aware of the fact that in the course of their professional lifetimes, exigencies of law and ethical issues will often influence the practice of medicine, and there are many other highly controversial areas of law and ethics that attend the care of HIV-infected women. Among the areas that continue to defy consensus are confidentiality, including charting, the appropriateness of "routine" (right of refusal) prenatal HIV testing, and the duty to warn HIV-infected patients' sexual partners of the index patient's seropositive status.

Clinicians should be aware of the relevant statutes within their own jurisdiction. Regardless of statute, it is important that clinicians accept the primacy of their fiduciary responsibility to their patients. They should attempt to limit knowledge of a patient's serostatus to those with a medical need to know and advocate on their behalf in all circumstances; discrimination in housing and jobs has waned but has not disappeared.

The clinician also has an obligation to try to persuade the seropositive patient to notify her sex partner(s). The physician will often have the option of contacting exposed partners or utilizing the local health department. A consultation with local health authorities may provide useful information to the provider.

Conclusion

In the 21st century, in the developed world and many parts of the developing world, HIV has become a treatable infection whose transmission from mother to child can be rendered a rare occurrence. However, the remarkable progress in the care of the HIV-infected pregnant woman has been purchased at the price of increasing therapeutic complexity. Obstetricians must be prepared to offer their patients the best prognosis that modern medicine permits by determining women's serostatus as early in pregnancy as possible, assessing their infected patients' immunologic and virologic status, recommending the most efficacious and safest antiretroviral regimens, monitoring their response assiduously, and then choosing the optimum time and method of delivery. By taking those steps, and coordinating their patients' care with experts in the field of HIV, obstetricians can contribute to the diminishing number of HIV-infected children born in this country and to the improved prognosis of their mothers. For providers in regions with fewer resources, the words of Lynn Mofenson are most apt:

Debate about which intervention is optimal and most effective should not be used to justify inaction. Success will be tied less to what regimen is provided than to the integration of services for the identification, care, and treatment of women with HIV-1 infection and their infants. The implementation of these new options for the perinatal prevention of HIV-1 infection in resource-limited countries offers a unique opportunity to link prevention and treatment efforts . . . We now have the tools to make a considerable difference in controlling the pediatric HIV-1 epidemic. A generation of children awaits our actions [16].

CASE PRESENTATION

The patient is a 27-year-old para 0010 at 8 weeks' gestation who underwent routine HIV testing at her first prenatal visit. The ELISA test was repeatedly positive, as was the confirmatory Western blot. When the patient was informed of the results she was unable to recall any specific risk behavior, never having used intravenous drugs or having a sexual partner known to have HIV, and having had only three lifetime sexual partners. The initial evaluation included a CD4 count that was 380 mm^3 and a viral load of 8000 copies. She was informed that those results would now be seen as indications for the initiation of antiretroviral therapy. Additionally, because she was pregnant, therapy would also reduce the likelihood of transmission to her child. However, because her condition was good, the initiation of therapy could be deferred until she was beyond the first trimester. When she was 14 weeks pregnant she was started on a HAART regimen of twice-daily Combivir (ZDV + 3TC) and Kaletra (lopinavir + ritonovir). Baseline liver function tests, CBC, hepatitis serologies, viral resistance studies and routine prenatal blood studies were obtained and appropriate vaccinations (influenza, etc.) given. She was scheduled to return for repeat viral load testing in a month. Within 2 months her viral load was undetectable and her CD4 count had risen to 440/mm^3. At 36 weeks' gestation, when a decision was to be made about mode of delivery, her viral load was still undetectable and a decision was made to allow a trial of labor. When she arrived in labor an intravenous infusion of ZDV was begun and she continued her other medications orally. Immediately after delivery all medications were restarted. At follow-up, the patient remained well and was referred for ongoing care to a specialist in HIV infection. Her child was uninfected.

References

1. Centers for Disease Control and Prevention. Rapid HIV testing in outreach and other community settings – United States, 2004–2006. MMWR 2007;56:1233–1237.

2. American College of Obstetricians and Gynecologists. Routine human immunodeficiency virus screening. ACOG Committee Opinion No. 411. Obstet Gynecol 2008;112:401–403.

3. Birkhead GS, Pulver WP, Warren BL, Hackel S, Rodríguez D, Smith L. Acquiring human immunodeficiency virus during pregnancy and mother-to-child transmission in New York: 2002–2006. Obstet Gynecol 2010;115(6):1247–1255.

4. Greenwald JL, Burstein GR, Pincus J, Branson B. A rapid review of rapid HIV antibody tests. Curr Infect Dis Rep 2006;8:125–131.

5. Minkoff H, Hershow R, Watts H et al. The relationship of pregnancy to disease progression. Am J Obstet Gynecol 2003;189:552–559.

6. Minkoff H, Ahdieh L, Watts HD. The relationship of pregnancy to the use of highly active antiretroviral therapy. Am J Obstet Gynecol 2001;184:1221–1227.

7. Guidelines for Perinatal care of HI. AIDSinfo.nih.gov.

8. Thomson MA, Aberg JA, Cahn P et al. Antireroviral treatment of adult HIV-infection: 2010 recommendations of the International AIDS Society-USA panel. JAMA 2010;304: 321–333.

9. Kitahata MM, Gange SJ, Abraham AG et al, for the NA-ACCORD Investigators. Effect of early versus deferred antiretroviral therapy for HIV on survival. N Engl J Med 2009;360(18): 1815–1826.

10. Baylor MS, Johann-Liang R. Hepatotoxicity associated with nevirapine use. J Acquir Immune Defic Syndr 2004;35: 538–539.

11. Townsend C, Schulte J, Thorne C et al, for the Pediatric Spectrum of HIV Disease Consortium, the European Collaborative Study and the National Study of HIV in Pregnancy and Childhood. Antiretroviral therapy and preterm delivery – a pooled analysis of data from the United States and Europe. Br J Obstet Gynaecol 2010;117(11):1399–1410.

12. Chasela CS, Hudgens MG, Jamieson DJ et al, for the BAN Study Group. Maternal or infant antiretroviral drugs to reduce HIV-1 transmission. N Engl J Med 2010;362(24):2271–2281.

13. American College of Obstetricians and Gynecologists. Scheduled cesarean delivery and the prevention of vertical transmission of HIV infection. ACOG Committee Opinion No. 234. Obstet Gynecol 2000;95(5).

14. Shapiro D, Tuomala R, Pollack H et al. Mother-to-child HIV transmission risk according to antiretroviral therapy, mode of delivery, and viral load in 2895 US women (PACTG 367). Oral presentation at the 11th Conference on Retroviruses and Opportunistic Infections, San Francisco, CA, February, 2004 (Abstract 99).

15. European Collaborative Study. Mother-to-child transmission of HIV infection in the era of highly active antiretroviral therapy. Clin Infect Dis 2005;40:458–465.

16. Mofenson LM. Protecting the next generation – eliminating perinatal HIV-1 infection. N Engl J Med 2010;362:2316–2318.

Other recommended reading

Best BM, Stek AM, Mirochnick M et al, for the International Maternal Pediatric Adolescent AIDS Clinical Trials Group 1026s Study Team. Lopinavir tablet pharmacokinetics with an increased dose during pregnancy. J Acquir Immune Defic Syndr 2010;54(4):381–388.

Freeman AF, Holland SM. Antimicrobial prophylaxis for primary immunodeficiencies.

Curr Opin Allergy Clin Immunol 2009;9(6):525–530.

International Perinatal HIV Group. The mode of delivery and the risk of vertical transmission of human immunodeficiency virus type 1: a meta-analysis of 15 prospective cohort studies. N Engl J Med 1999;340:977–987.

Mofenson LM, Centers for Disease Control and Prevention. US Public Health Service Task Force recommendations for use of antiretroviral drugs in pregnant HIV-1-infected women for maternal health and interventions to reduce perinatal HIV-1 transmission in the United States. MMWR Recomm Rep 2002;51(RR-18):1–38.

Shapiro R, Hughes M, Ogwu A et al. Antiretroviral regimens in pregnancy and breast-feeding in Botswana. N Engl J Med 2010;362:2282–2294.

Sperling RS, Shapiro DE, Coombs RW et al. Maternal viral load, zidovudine treatment and the risk of transmission of human immunodeficiency virus type 1 from mother to infant. N Engl J Med 1996;335:1621–1629.

Sturt AS, Dokubo EK, Sint TT. Antiretroviral therapy (ART) for treating HIV infection in ART-eligible pregnant women. Cochrane Database Syst Rev 2010;3:CD008440.

Tuomala RE, Shapiro D, Mofenson LM et al. Antiretroviral therapy during pregnancy and the risk of an adverse outcome. N Engl J Med 2002;346:1863–1870.

Chapter 32
Pregnancy in Women with Physical Disabilities

Caroline C. Signore

Eunice Kennedy Shriver National Institute of Child Health and Human Development, National Institutes of Health, United States Department of Health and Human Services, Bethesda, MD, USA

According to United States census data, more than 11% of women of reproductive age report some type of disability, with mobility limitations most frequently cited [1]. Among women aged 18–44 years, 1.1 million use a cane, wheelchair or other mobility aid and 1.1 million have a disabling condition serious enough to cause difficulty with activities of daily living. The incidence of spinal cord injury (SCI) among women is increasing, and with today's improved management, growing numbers of women survive acute traumatic SCI each year [2]. Multiple sclerosis rates are also increasing, with peak incidence in women of child-bearing age [3]. Improved survival of very preterm infants and infants with congenital anomalies is translating into increasing numbers of women with cerebral palsy and spina bifida reaching their reproductive years. Most women with disabilities do not have impaired fertility, and many want to be mothers. Thus, practitioners should expect increasing numbers of women with disabilities presenting for pregnancy care. There is, however, an unfortunate paucity of data to inform counseling and guide management of pregnancy in women with physical disabilities. This chapter will summarize current evidence on pregnancy risks and outcomes among women with disabilities.

General considerations

Urinary tract infections

Bladder dysfunction and urinary tract infections (UTIs) are common among women with physical disabilities; these problems may be exacerbated by pregnancy. Spinal cord injury, multiple sclerosis, and spina bifida are frequently associated with neurogenic bladder. Most women with SCI, for example, rely on permanent indwelling catheters (40% urethral, 11% suprapubic) or intermittent catheterization (28%) for urinary management [4]. Women with SCI who had recurrent UTIs prior to pregnancy are more likely to have UTIs during pregnancy [5]. The American College of Obstetricians and Gynecologists (ACOG) recommends frequent monitoring for UTI in pregnant women with SCI, and suggests that chronic antibiotic suppression may be appropriate [6]. In one small study, a weekly oral cyclic antibiotic regimen significantly decreased the incidence of UTI in pregnancy as compared to prepregnancy incidence in women with SCI [7]. There is no consensus in the literature about the optimal management of bacteriuria or UTI in pregnant women with physical disabilities.

Venous thromboembolic disease

The prothrombotic combination of pregnancy and impaired mobility raises concern for heightened risk of venous thromboembolic disease, and limited data suggest this is the case. In a survey of 24 women with SCI who had completed 37 pregnancies, a thrombotic event occurred in three (8%) pregnancies [8]. The use of routine thromboprophylaxis during pregnancy in women with paralysis or other mobility disorders has not been tested in clinical trials and the risk:benefit ratio of anticoagulation is unclear. Nevertheless, this therapy is instituted with some regularity; in the study mentioned above, 19% of all women with SCI received thromboprophylaxis during pregnancy [8]. There are no data specifically examining the risks and benefits of postpartum thromboprophylaxis in women with physical disabilities.

Weight gain, mobility, and skin integrity

For women with impaired mobility, the weight gain and alterations in body mechanics associated with advancing pregnancy can pose special problems. Increased weight may make it difficult for women to propel a manual wheelchair, prevent them from accomplishing transfers (for example, from wheelchair to bed) independently, or

Queenan's Management of High-Risk Pregnancy: An Evidence-Based Approach, Sixth Edition. Edited by John T. Queenan, Catherine Y. Spong, Charles J. Lockwood.
© 2012 John Wiley & Sons, Ltd. Published 2012 by John Wiley & Sons, Ltd.

increase risk for falls. Additionally, extra weight increases the risk for decubitus ulcers and frequent skin inspection, weight-shifting maneuvers, and adjustments in wheelchair seating and cushioning may be needed to prevent this complication. Women who are ambulatory may experience increased fatigue carrying pregnancy weight, or may find that their altered center of gravity makes ambulation more difficult and increases risk for injury from falls. Obesity is common among women with physical disabilities [9] but there are no data on which to base recommendations for appropriate gestational weight gain in these women.

Psychosocial risk factors

All women are at risk for psychosocial concerns during pregnancy; however, a higher background prevalence of some psychosocial problems among women with disabilities suggests that careful screening is warranted.

Approximately two-thirds of women with physical disabilities have experienced some form of physical violence or abuse [10] though it is not known whether pregnancy affects the risk or form of abuse of women with disabilities. Beyond the threat of bodily harm (e.g. kicking, slapping), abuse may take the form of refusal to provide needed assistance, withholding of medication or adaptive equipment, or neglect. Frequently, abuse is perpetrated by personal attendants and healthcare providers [10]. Women with mobility impairments may find it difficult or impossible to extract themselves from abusive situations, and thus are at risk for prolonged exposure to abuse compared to able-bodied women [10]. A simple tool for screening for abuse among women with disabilities is available [11].

Compared to nondisabled women, women with disabilities report higher levels of perceived stress [12] and feelings of sadness, unhappiness, or depression [13]. Self-reported rates of depression among nonpregnant women with disabilities are as high as 75%, but little is known about rates of depression in pregnancy. Women with disabilities may be at increased risk for postpartum depression, which was reported by 35% of women in one study [8].

Illicit drug use is more common among women with disabilities than in the general population, with risk factors including chronic pain, use of prescription drugs, social adjustment difficulties, and being a victim of substance abuse-related violence [14]. Most reports indicate that women with disabilities consume alcohol at rates and amounts similar to those of women in general [15] but smoking is more common among people with disabilities than the general public. Beyond the well-known adverse pregnancy effects of smoking, for women with physical disabilities and mobility impairment, tobacco use increases the risk of decubitus ulcer formation and impairs wound healing.

Antepartum consultation

Depending upon the nature and severity of a woman's disability and condition, antepartum care could require coordination of care and consultation with a number of appropriate specialists. Obstetrician gynecologists in general practice may seek consultation with maternal-fetal medicine specialists to plan obstetric management and monitor maternal and fetal well-being. All maternity care providers should seek and maintain contact with women's primary care providers (physiatrists, neurologists, rheumatologists, etc.) to collaboratively monitor the status of the disabling condition, development or progression of secondary conditions, any medication use or changes, and to plan strategies for prevention and management of complications. Antepartum consultation with an obstetric anesthesiologist is recommended. For women who have had abdominal surgeries such as urinary diversion procedures or ventriculoperitoneal shunting, prenatal consultation with the urologist or neurosurgeon is advisable; if cesarean delivery is required, these colleagues could be invited to assist at the time of surgery.

Medication use

Many women with physical disabilities use medication regularly for treatment of the underlying disorder or prevention and management of secondary conditions. Ideally, medication use should be evaluated preconceptionally, and regimens modified or discontinued as appropriate. The effects of many drugs on fetal development may not be well understood. Women who must continue medications during pregnancy should be counseled about potential risks and fetal effects to the extent possible. Medications commonly used by women with disabilities are presented in Table 32.1. It is also important to consider how newly prescribed therapies may affect the health and quality of life of women with physical disabilities. Chronic constipation is a common problem, which may be exacerbated by iron supplementation, for example. Drugs with significant gastrointestinal side-effects, particularly those causing diarrhea, can be especially difficult to tolerate for women with mobility and bowel control limitations.

Barriers to care

The Americans with Disabilities Act of 1990 ushered in an era of improved access and participation in society for people with disabilities. Nevertheless, barriers remain, taking diverse forms, such as limitations in access to transportation, lack of health insurance or underinsurance, difficulty with physical access within healthcare facilities, and fragmented care delivered by multiple providers [16].

In the office, women with disabilities may have difficulty completing lengthy medical history forms, or

Table 32.1 Medications commonly used by women with physical disabilities

Medication	Indication/use	FDA pregnancy category
Anticholinergics (e.g. oxybutinin)	Bladder relaxation	B
Baclofen	Spasticity	C
Copolymer-1	Disease-modifying agent, MS	B
Dantrolene	Spasticity	C
Gabapentin	Neuropathic pain, spasticity	C
Glatiramer acetate	Disease-modifying agent, MS	B
Interferon β-1B	Disease-modifying agent, MS	C
Leflunomide	DMARD	X
Methenamine	UTI prevention	C
Methotrexate	DMARD	X
Plaquenil	DMARD	C
Prednisone	Antiinflammatory, immunosuppressant	C
Propantheline	Bladder relaxation	C
Sulfasalazine	DMARD	B

FDA, Food and Drug Administration; DMARD, disease-modifying antirheumatic drug; MS, multiple sclerosis; UTI, urinary tract infection.

require assistance to collect a urine specimen. Very few offices have a platform scale designed to weigh women seated in wheelchairs, thus making impossible one of the most fundamental assessments in prenatal care. Many women who use wheelchairs could transfer to an exam table independently but are prevented from doing so if the table will not lower to wheelchair height (17–20 inches). Joint contractures or neuromuscular spasticity may make achieving and maintaining position for a pelvic exam difficult or impossible without adaptations.

Women with disabilities report being troubled by perceived negative attitudes from healthcare providers. When presenting for prenatal care, some women feel that their practitioners do not consider them capable or qualified to parent and that they are thought to be irresponsible for becoming pregnant with a disability. Another attitudinal barrier may arise in discussions of prenatal screening and genetic counseling. Some women with disabilities may view these measures as devaluing and consider them an offensive attempt by society to eliminate people with bodily or mental differences.

Parenting may indeed pose extra challenges for women with physical disabilities, but with proper planning and adaptive aids, most women are fully capable of being loving and nurturing mothers. During pregnancy, a multidisciplinary team of medical providers, social workers, nurses, physical and occupational therapists, and lactation consultants should coordinate care and begin preparations for the transition to parenthood. A number of internet-based resources for parenting with disabilities are available [17,18].

Pregnancy outcomes

Most women with physical disabilities can expect largely uneventful pregnancies and normal birth outcomes. Nevertheless, current evidence suggests that risks for certain complications are higher among women with disabilities compared to their nondisabled counterparts. The reasons for these increased risks are not well understood, but may involve interactions between the pregnant state and the medical condition causing the physical disability. Existing data have important limitations, however, such as small sample sizes, retrospective study designs, and outcome ascertainment through self-report and administrative databases.

Spinal cord injury

Acute traumatic injury of the spinal cord occurs in approximately 2400 women per year in the United States [2]. The most common cause of injury is motor vehicle accident (42%), followed by falls (27%) and violence (15%). Approximately half of all injuries are to the cervical spinal cord, resulting in varying degrees of tetraplegia (weakness in all four limbs); the remainder are to the thoracic, lumbar, or sacral regions of the cord, resulting in paraplegia (weakness of the lower limbs).

Acute SCI during pregnancy should be managed in either a high-risk obstetrics or trauma unit by a team including obstetricians, trauma surgeons, anesthesiologists, and critical care nursing [19]. Acute SCI is associated with rapid loss of sympathetic tone and peripheral vasodilation, termed neurogenic or spinal shock, which lasts approximately 1–3 weeks [19,20]. Acute management consists of volume resuscitation and pressor support. For women at or beyond the second trimester, left lateral tilt positioning is recommended to avoid aortocaval compression by the gravid uterus [19]. Incident venous thromboembolic disease among nonpregnant patients with acute SCI occurs in 67–100%, with highest risk in the first 8–12 weeks after injury [21]. While neither the incidence of thromboembolism nor the optimal management of thrombotic risk in pregnancy and acute SCI has been investigated thoroughly, prophylactic anticoagulation for at least 8–12 weeks post injury has been recommended [19,21]. A recent metaanalysis of randomized trials in nonpregnant patients with acute SCI found low molecular weight heparin to be more effective than unfractionated heparin for the prevention of deep vein thrombosis [21]. Data on birth outcomes among women who sustain a SCI during pregnancy are limited to case reports.

For women who become pregnant after SCI, existing data, though limited, suggest that pregnancy outcomes are favorable. Jackson and Wadley surveyed 472 women with SCI, 246 of whom had had preinjury pregnancies and 66 of whom had had at least one pregnancy after injury [4]. Compared to preinjury pregnancies, there were no differences in the proportions of livebirths, miscarriages, or stillbirths in pregnancies after SCI.

Women with SCI are at increased risk for several potential antenatal complications. UTIs are common, with rates as high as 51% [8]. Baseline respiratory function may be compromised by posttraumatic kyphoscoliosis and weakened inspiratory musculature; the gravid uterus may exacerbate problems with respiratory reserve. Some experts recommend routine incentive spirometry or serial peak flow or vital capacity measurement [22]. Decubitus ulcers occur in 6–12% [4,5] and are a preventable condition that can cause substantial morbidity.

Autonomic dysreflexia (ADR) is one of the most feared complications of pregnancy and SCI. Characterized by acute onset of extreme hypertension, this syndrome is caused by unchecked sympathetic outflow in response to a stimulus below the level of the spinal cord lesion. ADR largely affects individuals with injuries at T6 and above, but occurs rarely with lower level lesions [23,24]. Common precipitants include dilation of a hollow viscus (e.g. bladder distension), skin injury, or other noxious stimuli. Labor is a potent inciting event. The literature is mixed on the incidence of ADR during pregnancy and delivery, with rates of 12–80% reported [4,25–27]. Signs and symptoms of ADR include marked hypertension, reflex bradycardia or other cardiac rhythm disturbances, severe headache, sweating, flushing, piloerection, and general apprehension. Left untreated, ADR can result in fetal distress, maternal intracranial hemorrhage, coma, seizures, and death. Care must be taken to distinguish ADR from preeclampsia. One key difference is that in ADR, blood pressure rises and falls with contractions, while in preeclampsia blood pressure is unrelated to contractions. The key to management of ADR is prevention. Women with SCI should have epidural anesthesia instituted early in labor to block labor pain. Vital signs must be monitored frequently throughout labor, with pharmacologic control of refractory hypertension with rapid-acting agents such as nitroglycerin, nitroprusside, or labetalol as indicated [28].

Preterm birth (<37 weeks) occurs in 18–27% [4,5,8] of women with SCI, and data from one study indicate that the majority (77%) are spontaneous preterm deliveries. Inability to perceive contractions among women with injuries at T10 or above may contribute to this risk. In one study, 80% of women who delivered preterm could not feel contractions. Women can be taught to palpate uterine

contractions and monitor for other unique symptoms of labor such as ADR, increased spasticity, or bladder spasms [4]. Some suggest routine cervical examination after 28 weeks [19] or serial ultrasonographic assessment of cervical length [8] but neither practice has been tested in women with SCI.

Women with SCI are capable of vaginal delivery, which is achieved by 33–78%, and in most cases is spontaneous [4,5,8]. Cesarean delivery rates as high as 67% have been reported [4,5,8] although it is not clear whether this reflects a true elevation in obstetrical indications for operative delivery.

Multiple sclerosis

This autoimmune demyelinating disorder most commonly affects women of child-bearing age, with features including muscular weakness and spasticity, disrupted coordination and balance, disturbances of sensation, visual changes, and bowel and bladder dysfunction. The pregnancy course of multiple sclerosis (MS) resembles that of other autoimmune diseases. A large European prospective cohort study showed that MS flare rates tend to decrease during pregnancy, but rise during the first 3 months postpartum, occurring in approximately 30% [29].

A number of studies have indicated increased risk of adverse pregnancy outcomes in women with MS. In a study of administrative data on more than 10,000 women with MS, Kelly and colleagues reported significantly higher rates of fetal growth restriction (odds ratio [OR] 1.7, 95% confidence interval [CI] 1.2–2.4), antenatal hospitalization (OR 1.3, 95% CI 1.2–1.5), and cesarean delivery (OR 1.3, 95% CI 1.1–1.4)), but not hypertensive disorders or premature rupture of membranes [30]. A smaller study (n = 174) from Taiwan confirmed an increased risk of impaired fetal growth and cesarean delivery, and also found a more than twofold increase in preterm birth (<37 weeks). It is not clear whether the excess cesarean and preterm deliveries were the result of obstetric or fetal indications.

Rheumatoid arthritis

As with other autoimmune conditions, rheumatoid arthritis (RA) disease activity has traditionally been thought to decrease substantially during pregnancy and then flare in the postpartum period. However, more recent data suggest that in the third trimester, fewer than 25% of women are in remission and 10–20% have high disease activity [31,32].

Analysis of administrative data on 1425 delivery hospitalizations in US women with RA demonstrated an increased risk of intrauterine growth restriction (OR 2.2, 95% CI 1.2–4.1) and cesarean delivery (OR 1.5, 95% CI 1.2–1.9) compared to controls [33]. Preterm birth rates of 6.4–26% have been reported, and are positively associated with disease activity and systemic steroid use [34–36]. Again, it is not clear whether excess preterm births are spontaneous or indicated.

Cerebral palsy

Women with cerebral palsy (CP) experience varying degrees of movement and posture disorders, spasticity, and joint contractures, with the lower extremities most often affected. Data on pregnancy outcomes for women with CP are inconclusive. In one small descriptive study, pregnancies among women with CP were complicated by preeclampsia (17.9%), cesarean delivery (33%, most often for cephalopelvic disproportion and abnormal fetal position), and preterm birth (7.8%) [37]. Another study found a similar rate of cesarean delivery, but preeclampsia occurred in only 5% [38]. Difficulties in labor and delivery due to spasticity or joint contractures did not occur, but a small proportion of women reported increased physical disability postpartum [37].

Spina bifida

Conditions associated with spina bifida (SB) include deformity of the spine or pelvis, spasticity, bowel and bladder dysfunction, ileal conduits and ventriculoperitoneal shunting for management of hydrocephalus. Allergy to latex is common, occurring in about 23% [39].

Offspring of mothers with SB have a 4–7% rate of neural tube defects [40]. Women with SB considering pregnancy should begin folic acid supplementation before conception. The precise dose needed to reduce fetal neural tube defect risk in mothers with SB is unknown, but 4 mg daily has been recommended for women at high risk [41].

There are scant data on the course and outcomes of pregnancy in women with SB. A survey of 17 women who had had 23 pregnancies revealed frequent antepartum admissions, recurrent UTIs, worsening pressure sores, and stomal problems [42]. Hypertensive disorders occurred in 26%, preterm birth in 35%, cesarean delivery in 50%, and small for gestational age infants in 47% of pregnancies. Regional anesthesia was rare, and 92% of cesareans were performed under general anesthesia.

Conclusion

Most women with physical disabilities can expect an uneventful pregnancy and delivery of a healthy baby. Maternal care providers should be aware of problems that may arise more frequently in women with mobility impairments as compared to their able-bodied peers. These include urinary tract infections, venous thromboembolic disease, respiratory compromise, decline in mobility, substance misuse, stress and depression, and limitations in access to care. Pregnancy course and outcomes depend on the nature and severity of the disabling condition. Though the mechanisms are unclear, limited data suggest that women with a range of physical disabilities are at increased risk of low-birthweight infants and cesarean delivery. Management of these pregnancies should be undertaken by a multidisciplinary team, with vigilance for common complications and marshaling of necessary supports for the transition to motherhood.

CASE PRESENTATION

The patient was a 29-year-old primigravida who sustained a complete thoracic (T4) SCI at age 19 and presented for antenatal care at 10 weeks' gestation. She was using a manual wheelchair for mobility, and aside from occasional episodes of autonomic dysreflexia related to bladder distension and frequent UTIs (3–5 per year), she had no health complaints or complications from her injury. Bladder management was by clean intermittent catheterization, which she was able to perform independently. Her last known weight, 3 years ago, was 131 lb, corresponding to a BMI of 23.3 kg/m². She was married, worked part time at a nonprofit organization, and did not smoke or use drugs or alcohol. Current medications were oxybutinin for bladder relaxation and oral baclofen for management of mild spasticity. Examination was unremarkable with the exception of bilateral 2+ pitting edema

in the lower extremities. Compression stockings were recommended.

Routine prenatal labs were normal except for mild anemia (Hct 36.3); the patient refused oral iron supplementation for fear of constipation. Her pregnancy progressed uneventfully through the second trimester with the exception of a UTI treated with a 10-day course of nitrofurantoin. At 28 weeks, the patient was seen by an obstetric anesthesiologist to develop a plan for early induction of epidural anesthesia upon presentation for labor. Additionally, referrals to physical and occupational therapy were made to assist with current mobility and begin planning for adaptations for baby care after delivery. She was instructed on abdominal/uterine palpation to detect contractions. At 30 weeks' gestation, she experienced an episode of ADR because she found she

Continued

was unable to self-cath; the ADR resolved when the bladder spontaneously emptied. After discussion, a Foley catheter was inserted, to remain until after delivery. Antibiotic suppression was started. By 32 weeks, she required assistance with transfers and propelling her wheelchair.

One evening at 35 weeks, she noted a substantial increase in spasticity, headache, skin tingling, and profuse sweating above the level of her injury. Upon presentation at labor and delivery, her blood pressure was 230/120, with heart rate of 55 bpm. Urine dipstick for protein was negative. She was placed in a seated upright position with a wedge under her right hip and examined for the source of the presumed ADR. Her catheter was draining normally, there was no evidence of skin injury, and tocodynamometer revealed contractions occurring every 4 min. Fetal heart rate tracing (FHT) was 120–130 bpm, with decreased variability and occasional late decelerations. Cervical exam was 3/70/-3 and she was admitted for labor and urgent epidural placement. Under epidural anesthesia to the T10 level, her blood pressure, heart rate, and FHT normalized and remained stable throughout labor. She was delivered via spontaneous vaginal delivery of a 2515 g infant with Apgars of 7 and 9. A second-degree laceration was repaired. The infant was monitored for 2 days in the NICU. The patient's postpartum course was unremarkable, and she was discharged on postpartum day 2 with instructions to continue Foley catheterization, avoid ice or heat to the perineum, and continue working with her lactation consultant.

References

1. Centers for Disease Control and Prevention. Prevalence and most common causes of disability among adults – United States, 2005. MMWR 2009;58(16):421–426.

2. National Spinal Cord Injury Statistical Center. Spinal Cord Injury Facts and Figures at a Glance. Birmigham, AL: University of Alabama, 2009.

3. Koch-Henriksen N, Sorensen PS. The changing demographic pattern of multiple sclerosis epidemiology. Lancet Neurol 2010;9(5):520–532.

4. Jackson AB, Wadley V. A multicenter study of women's self-reported reproductive health after spinal cord injury. Arch Phys Med Rehabil 1999;80(11):1420–1428.

5. Westgren N, Hultling C, Levi R, Westgren M. Pregnancy and delivery in women with a traumatic spinal cord injury in Sweden, 1980–1991. Obstet Gynecol 1993;81(6): 926–930.

6. American College of Obstetricians and Gynecologists, Committee on Obstetric Practice. Obstetric management of patients with spinal cord injuries. ACOG Committee Opinion No. 275. Int J Gynaecol Obstet 2002;79(2):189–191.

7. Salomon J, Schnitzler A, Ville Y et al. Prevention of urinary tract infection in six spinal cord-injured pregnant women who gave birth to seven children under a weekly oral cyclic antibiotic program. Int J Infect Dis 2009;13(3):399–402.

8. Ghidini A, Healey A, Andreani M, Simonson MR. Pregnancy and women with spinal cord injuries. Acta Obstet Gynecol Scand 2008;87(10):1006–1010.

9. Nosek MA, Hughes RB, Petersen NJ et al. Secondary conditions in a community-based sample of women with physical disabilities over a 1-year period. Arch Phys Med Rehabil 2006;87(3):320–327.

10. Young ME, Nosek MA, Howland C, Chanpong G, Rintala DH. Prevalence of abuse of women with physical disabilities. Arch Phys Med Rehabil 1997;78(12 Suppl 5):S34–S38.

11. McFarlane J, Hughes RB, Nosek MA, Groff JY, Swedlend N, Dolan MP. Abuse assessment screen-disability (AAS-D): measuring frequency, type, and perpetrator of abuse toward women with physical disabilities. J Womens Health Gend Based Med 2001;10(9):861–866.

12. Hughes RB, Taylor HB, Robinson-Whelen S, Nosek MA. Stress and women with physical disabilities: identifying correlates. Womens Health Issues 2005;15(1):14–20.

13. Hughes RB, Robinson-Whelen S, Taylor HB, Petersen NJ, Nosek MA. Characteristics of depressed and nondepressed women with physical disabilities. Arch Phys Med Rehabil 2005;86(3):473–479.

14. Li L, Ford JA. Illicit drug use by women with disabilities. Am J Drug Alcohol Abuse 1998;24(3):405–418.

15. Ford JA, Glenn MK, Li L, Moore DC. Substance abuse and women with disabilities. In: Welner SL, Haseltine F, eds. Welner's Guide to the Care of Women with Disabilities. Philadelphia: Lippincott Williams and Wilkins, 2004.

16. Coughlin TA, Long SK, Kendall S. Health care access, use, and satisfaction among disabled Medicaid beneficiaries. Health Care Financ Rev 2002;24(2):115–136.

17. Through the Looking Glass. www.lookingglass.org/.

18. Parents with Disabilities Online. www.disabledparents.net/.

19. Pereira L. Obstetric management of the patient with spinal cord injury. Obstet Gynecol Surv 2003;58(10):678–87.

20. Gilson GJ, Miller AC, Clevenger FW, Curet LB. Acute spinal cord injury and neurogenic shock in pregnancy. Obstet Gynecol Surv 1995;50(7):556–560.

21. Ploumis A, Ponnappan RK, Maltenfort MG et al. Thromboprophylaxis in patients with acute spinal injuries: an evidence-based analysis. J Bone Joint Surg Am 2009;91(11): 2568–2576.

22. Rouse D. Pregnancy and women with spinal cord injuries. Obstet Gynecol Surv 2009;64:141–142.

23. Gimovsky ML, Ojeda A, Ozaki R, Zerne S. Management of autonomic hyperreflexia associated with a low thoracic spinal cord lesion. Am J Obstet Gynecol 1985;153(2):223–224.

24. Yaginuma Y, Kawamura M, Ishikawa M. Pregnancy, labor and delivery in a woman with a damaged spinal cord. J Obstet Gynaecol 1995;21(3):277–279.

25. Cross LL, Meythaler JM, Tuel SM, Cross AL. Pregnancy, labor and delivery post spinal cord injury. Paraplegia 1992;30(12): 890–902.

26. McGregor JA, Meeuwsen J. Autonomic hyperreflexia: a mortal danger for spinal cord-damaged women in labor. Am J Obstet Gynecol 1985;151(3):330–333.

27. Wanner MB, Rageth CJ, Zach GA. Pregnancy and autonomic hyperreflexia in patients with spinal cord lesions. Paraplegia 1987;25(6):482–490.

28. Baschat AA, Weiner CP. Chronic neurologic diseases and disabling conditions in pregnancy. In: Welner SL, Haseltine F, eds. Welner's Guide to the Care of Women with Disabilities. Philadelphia: Lippincott Williams and Wilkins, 2004, pp.145–158.

29. Vukusic S, Hutchinson M, Hours M et al. Pregnancy and multiple sclerosis (the PRIMS study): clinical predictors of postpartum relapse. Brain 2004;127(Pt 6):1353–1360.

30. Kelly VM, Nelson LM, Chakravarty EF. Obstetric outcomes in women with multiple sclerosis and epilepsy. Neurology 2009;73(22):1831–1836.

31. De Man YA, Hazes JM, van de Geijn FE, Krommenhoek C, Dolhain RJ. Measuring disease activity and functionality during pregnancy in patients with rheumatoid arthritis. Arthritis Rheum 2007;57(5):716–722.

32. De Man YA, Dolhain RJ, van de Geijn FE, Willemsen SP, Hazes JM. Disease activity of rheumatoid arthritis during pregnancy: results from a nationwide prospective study. Arthritis Rheum 2008;59(9):1241–1248.

33. Chakravarty EF, Nelson L, Krishnan E. Obstetric hospitalizations in the United States for women with systemic lupus erythematosus and rheumatoid arthritis. Arthritis Rheum 2006;54(3):899–907.

34. Chambers CD, Johnson DL, Jones KL. Pregnancy outcome in women exposed to anti-TNF-alpha medications: the OTIS Rheumatoid Arthritis in Pregnancy Study [abstract]. Arthritis Rheum 2004;50:S479–S480.

35. De Man YA, Hazes JM, van der Heide H et al. Association of higher rheumatoid arthritis disease activity during pregnancy with lower birth weight: results of a national prospective study. Arthritis Rheum 2009;60(11):3196–3206.

36. Skomsvoll JF, Ostensen M, Irgens LM, Baste V. Obstetrical and neonatal outcome in pregnant patients with rheumatic disease. Scand J Rheumatol 1998;107(Suppl):109–112.

37. Winch R, Bengtson L, McLaughlin J, Fitzsimmons J, Budden S. Women with cerebral palsy: obstetric experience and neonatal outcome. Dev Med Child Neurol 1993;35(11):974–982.

38. Foley J. The offspring of people with cerebral palsy. Dev Med Child Neurol 1992;34(11):972–978.

39. Jackson AB, Mott PK. Reproductive health care for women with spina bifida. Sci World J 2007;7:1875–1883.

40. Jackson AB, Sipski ML. Reproductive issues for women with spina bifida. J Spinal Cord Med 2005;28(2):81–91.

41. Cheschier N. Neural tube defects. ACOG Practice Bulletin No. 44. (Replaces Committee Opinion No. 252, March 2001). Int J Gynaecol Obstet 2003;83(1):123–133.

42. Arata M, Grover S, Dunne K, Bryan D. Pregnancy outcome and complications in women with spina bifida. J Reprod Med 2000;45(9):743–748.

Chapter 33
Recurrent Spontaneous Abortion

Charles J. Lockwood

Department of Obstetrics, Gynecology and Reproductive Sciences, Yale University School of Medicine, New Haven, CT, USA

Patients with recurrent spontaneous abortion (SAB) are among the most challenging to manage. The history of care for these patients has been strewn with nonevidence-based, anecdotal, and occasionally dangerous management approaches. The nomenclature of recurrent SAB is confusing, with myriad different definitions extant. Prevalence estimates are compromised by the high background rate of pregnancy wastage in the general population which exceeds 50% when losses from conception through discernible embryonic development are included [1]. A generally accepted number is that 1% of couples suffer two or more consecutive pregnancy losses prior to the third trimester [2].

Sporadic miscarriage and maternal age

Approximately 50–60% of sporadic miscarriages are associated with aneuploidy [1]. The most frequent causes are trisomy (most commonly trisomy 16 or 22), followed by polyploidy and monosomy X [1]. Maternal age is strongly associated with the risk of both SAB and aneuploidy. A prospective cohort study, derived from the FASTER trial, assessed SAB rates in over 36,000 women stratified into three age groups: less than 35 years, 35–39 years, and 40 years or older [3]. Multivariable logistic regression analysis adjusting for race, parity, Body Mass Index, education, marital status, smoking, medical history, use of assisted reproductive technologies, and study site noted that compared to women less than 35 years, those aged 35–39 were at increased risk for SAB with an adjusted odds ratio (adjOR) of 2.0 (95% confidence interval [CI] 1.5–2.6) while those 40 years or older had an adjOR for SAB of 2.4 (95% CI 1.6–3.6). The association of conceptus chromosomal abnormalities with these two age groups produced adjORs of 4.0 (95% CI 2.5–6.3) and 9.9 (95% CI 5.8–17.0), respectively. Moreover, a large prospective Danish cohort tracking 634,272 women through 1,221,546 pregnancies

found rates of SAB of less than 12% for women 20–29 years, 15% for those 30–34 years, 24.6% for those 35–39 years, 51% for ages 40–44, and 93.4% for women over 44 years [4]. Thus, maternal age is the single strongest epidemiologic predictor of SAB, the majority of which are linked to aneuploidy.

While there is no accepted explanation for the increased rate of aneuploidy associated with advanced maternal age, chronic oxidative stress and progressive shortening of oocyte telomere length are among the possible causes [5]. Shortened telomeres lead to abnormal chiasma formation and nondisjunction [6]. Unfortunately, most current "treatments" for recurrent early SAB do not take into account the substantially older age among affected patients and the worsening of subsequent livebirth rates with aging [7]. Proposed treatments must also be judged against the high spontaneous remission rate in such patients, as the probability of a livebirth after four successive SABs is about 40% [8].

Etiologies of recurrent spontaneous abortion

Genetic abnormalities

Aneuploidy
While it is difficult to assess the precise rate of aneuploidy in recurrent abortus specimens, as initial losses are usually not karyotyped, estimates range from 25% to 57% [9,10]. Data gleaned from preimplantation genetic diagnosis employed at the time of *in vitro* fertilization (IVF) suggest that patients with recurrent SAB have far higher rates of abnormal embryos compared with controls (70.7% versus 45.1%; P < 0.0001) [11]. Unfortunately, the etiology of recurrent miscarriage resulting from repetitive chromosomal abnormalities is not adequately understood. Abnormalities that arise during the oocyte's first meiotic

Queenan's Management of High-Risk Pregnancy: An Evidence-Based Approach, Sixth Edition. Edited by John T. Queenan, Catherine Y. Spong, Charles J. Lockwood.

division account for the majority of cases. The association of recurrent SAB with increasing maternal age suggests that, as in maternal age-associated sporadic miscarriage, oxidative stress and reduced oocyte telomere length may be factors [5]. Alternatively, it has been proposed that because aging is associated with an ever-shrinking oocyte pool, there is a progressive depletion of the number of oocytes available at the requisite stage of maturation for completion of normal meiosis [12]. Supporting this thesis is the observation that women who have lost at least one trisomic fetus have diminished ovarian reserve and enter the menopause at an earlier age than those with no such history [13,14].

An argument has been put forward that patients with recurrent miscarriage resulting from advanced maternal age-related aneuploidy should be managed through IVF with preimplantation genetic screening (PGS) for chromosomal abnormalities commonly found in abortus specimens. The argument suggests that since such losses are stochastic, recruitment of large numbers of embryos with subsequent selection and transfer of those deemed putatively euploid following PGS will increase the likelihood of a livebirth.

A number of randomized controlled trials have examined the outcome of IVF with PGS for common aneuploidies in women of advanced reproductive age. Hardarson *et al* compared 56 and 53 patients over 37 years of age randomized to PGS versus control and observed a decreased clinical pregnancy rate in the PGS group (8.9%, 95% CI 2.9–19.6%, versus 24.5%, 95% CI 13.8–38.3%) [15]. Similarly, Mastenbroek and colleagues conducted a randomized, double-blind, controlled trial comparing three cycles of IVF with and without PGS in 408 women aged 35–41 years [16]. The primary outcome measure was ongoing pregnancy at 12 weeks of gestation. They noted a lower ongoing pregnancy rate in the PGS versus control group (25% [52/206] versus 37% [74/ 202]; rate ratio 0.69, 95% CI 0.51–0.93). Similarly the PGS group had a lower livebirth rate (24% [49/206] versus 35% [71/202]; rate ratio 0.68, 95% CI 0.50–0.92).

While PGS methodological arguments have challenged the validity of these findings, there is no consensus that IVF with PGS improves livebirth rates or reduces SAB rates in women of advanced reproductive age or those with recurrent miscarriage. In the latter case, if affected patients are fertile, it is quite possible that "natural" selection of optimal oocytes during the ovulation process is a far more efficient and far less expensive option than IVF with or without PGS. Moreover, by the time recurrent aborters become infertile, they likely have few remaining viable oocytes, and donor egg IVF, rather than IVF with their own oocyte with or without PGS, is likely a far more cost-effective option.

Low folate levels have been linked to aneuploidy-induced SAB (OR 1.95, 95% CI 1.09–3.48) but not when the fetal karyotype is normal (OR 1.11, 95% CI 0.55–2.24) [17]. Folate deficiency may also have a role in meiotic nondisjunction. In addition, metaanalysis suggests that fasting hyperhomocysteinemia is modestly associated with recurrent pregnancy loss (<16 weeks) [18]. Thus, given its low cost and toxicity, it would seem prudent to treat patients experiencing recurrent miscarriage with periconceptional folate supplementation (1–4 mg/day).

Fragile sites on chromosomes have been linked to an increased risk of malignancy and various developmental disorders but may also be associated with recurrent SAB [19]. Chromosomal mosaicisms and deletions [20], as well as both large pericentric and paracentric chromosomal inversions [21,22], have also been associated with recurrent miscarriages. However, there are limited data in the literature to establish the strength of these, likely rare, causes of recurrent SAB. Skewed inactivation of the X chromosome was thought to be linked to recurrent SAB due to either trisomies or unmasking of an X-linked dominant or germline developmentally lethal mutation on the X chromosome but recent studies have refuted such an association [23,24].

There is a 30-fold increase in the occurrence of balanced translocations among couples with recurrent SAB with a prevalence of 3.6% [25]. Up to a 29% rate of miscarriage has been observed among clinically recognized pregnancies in couples bearing a balanced translocation, with 36% of the abortuses found to have an unbalanced translocation [26]. Thus, high-resolution parental karyotyping should be performed in couples with unexplained recurrent SAB. There is controversy as to whether IVF with PGS reduces loss rates in affected couples [27,28].

Single gene defects

Single gene defects may also promote recurrent miscarriage. These may be X-linked, autosomal recessive or germline mutations involving loss of heterozygosity for developmentally lethal genes. With advances in genomic technology, it may be feasible in the future to inexpensively sequence the genome of miscarriage samples to discover these putative single gene causes which will likely involve developmentally relevant genes such as those in the Tbx, HOX, SOX, and FOX gene families. Most examples of known single gene causes of recurrent loss are associated with second-trimester miscarriages. For example, lethal multiple pterygium syndromes are a collection of autosomal recessive and X-linked recessive disorders that are associated with fetal death at 14–20 weeks with variable features including arthrogryposis, hydrocephalus, hydrops, and cystic hygromas [29]. Incontinentia pigmenti is an X-linked disorder usually lethal in males [30]. Affected males may also develop hydrops and/or cystic hygromas while affected females have dental anomalies and cutaneous manifestations [30].

Unfortunately, until the advent of inexpensive and rapid whole-genome screening, there is no simple way to identify such mutations. However, aberrant regulation of trophoblast growth resulting from developmental abnormalities often results in the formation of trophoblast inclusions – abnormal invaginations of the villous surface which on section appear as inverted islands of trophoblast [31]. Thus, careful examination of the placenta may provide valuable clues as to a developmental etiology of recurrent intermittent losses.

Infectious diseases

Acute severe bacterial, parasitic, and viral infections can cause isolated SABs. However, there are no unequivocal data establishing an association between chronic genital tract carriage of bacteria and recurrent SAB. Moreover, there is no evidence that the presence of *Chlamydia trachomatis*, *Ureaplasma urealyticum*, *Mycoplasma hominis*, human cytomegalovirus (HCMV), adeno-associated virus (AAV), and human papilloma viruses (HPV) are associated with even isolated first-trimester SAB [32]. *Ureaplasma urealyticum* (serotype 4) is more commonly isolated from women with recurrent miscarriage than controls [33]. Moreover, nonrandomized trials suggest that treatment of genital tract mycoplasma with doxycycline may reduce early loss rates [34]. However, there is no evidence from appropriately conducted randomized clinical trials that eradication of mycoplasma species reduces miscarriage rates. There is also no convincing link between either recovery of genital tract *Chlamydia trachomatis* or the presence of antichlamydial antibodies and recurrent miscarriage [35–37]. The presence of bacterial vaginosis (BV) has been linked to early isolated SAB (adjOR 2.67, 95% CI 1.26–5.63) [38]. However, the link between BV and recurrent miscarriage and the benefits of treatment has yet to be firmly established. Moreover, it is second-, not first-trimester pregnancy loss that appears to be more strongly associated with BV [39].

Celiac disease

Bustos *et al* compared the prevalence of various autoantibodies in 118 otherwise healthy women with three or more SABs with the prevalence in 125 fertile, multiparous control women who were without SABs [40]. The authors observed an increased prevalence of celiac disease-related antibodies for antigliadin type IgA as well as IgG and IgA antitransglutaminase antibodies among cases versus controls (P < 0.04). In contrast, Greco and associates observed antihuman IgA class anti-tissue transglutaminase (TGASE) antibodies as well as endomysial antibodies (EMA) in 51 of 5055 pregnant women but found no higher rate of SAB among affected women [41]. Kotze compared 76 adult celiac patients to 84 adult controls with irritable bowel syndrome and observed a higher prevalence of SABs among the former (24.4% versus

11.6%) (P = 0.003) [42]. Moreover, when pregnancy outcomes in 12 adult celiac patients were compared before the diagnosis of celiac disease and after treatment, the number of SABs decreased (38.9% versus 5.6%) (P = 0.045). Similar findings have been noted by other investigators [43,44]. Thus, symptomatic celiac disease has been linked to recurrent miscarriage and treatment appears to improve livebirth rates. In contrast, it is unclear whether related autoantibodies and occult disease are associated with recurrent SAB. Thus, screening for occult celiac disease is not currently recommended in the work-up of recurrent SAB.

Endocrinopathies

While poorly controlled diabetes and thyroid disease are linked to recurrent miscarriage, there is no evidence of such a link with either subclinical diabetes or thyroid disease [45,46]. However, antithyroid peroxidase and antithyroglobulin antibodies are more commonly found in recurrent aborters [47]. Moreover, nonrandomized studies have suggested that levothyroxine therapy may decrease SAB rates in euthyroid, thyroid antibody-positive women. There were initial reports that polycystic ovarian syndrome (PCOS) was associated with recurrent miscarriage. However, recent studies have found no such link [48,49]. Moreover, treatment with metformin does not appear to reduce SAB rates. Legro and colleagues randomized 626 infertile women with PCOS to receive clomiphene citrate plus placebo, extended-release metformin plus placebo, or a combination of metformin and clomiphene for up to 6 months and observed livebirth rates of 22.5%, 7.2% and 26.8%, respectively [50]. In addition, the rate of first-trimester SAB did not differ significantly among the groups. Thus, screening for PCOS appears to have little value in the work-up of fertile recurrent SAB patients.

Progesterone plays a crucial role in the maintenance of endometrial hemostasis and architectural integrity [51]. Conversely, the antiprogestin RU 486 can induce menstruation and early abortion by inhibiting these salutary effects of progesterone [52,53]. These observations provide biological plausibility to the theory that luteal-phase defects could promote early pregnancy loss. Indeed, the prevalence of luteal-phase defects among recurrent miscarriage patients is reported to be 10–30% [54,55]. However, among recurrent aborters, those with documented luteal-phase defects actually had lower SAB rates in a subsequent pregnancy than those without such a defect [56]. Moreover, there are no definitive diagnostic criteria because the condition is intermittent [57]. Moreover, metaanalysis of trials of progesterone therapy for recurrent SAB have not demonstrated a benefit [58].

Among recurrent aborters with hyperprolactinemia, treatment with bromocryptine appears to improve livebirth rates [59]. Thus, although data are limited. it may be

Table 33.1 Müllerian duct anomalies and their association with miscarriage

Müllerian Anomaly	Proportion of all müllerian anomalies (%)	Risk of SAB (<20 weeks) (%)
Septum	55	65
Unicornuate uterus	20	51
Uterus didelphys	5–7	43
Bicornuate uterus	10	32

useful to obtain prolactin levels in such patients and a trial of therapy in hyperprolactinemic women with recurrent SAB may improve livebirth rates.

Uterine abnormalities

The traditional association between müllerian tract anomalies and recurrent SAB is based on older descriptive, small observational studies replete with potential ascertainment and selection biases. Salim and colleagues [60] compared women with and without a history of three or more consecutive unexplained pregnancy losses before 14 weeks using three-dimensional (3-D) ultrasound, and found major uterine congenital anomalies in 23.8% of women with losses compared with 5.3% in controls. However, in both groups the most common anomalies were minor, arcuate and subseptate uteri, which accounted for more than 90% of cases. In other studies, the former uterine anomaly does not appear to be associated with a higher rate of recurrent abortion, and may represent a normal variant [61]. The prevalence of major uterine anomalies has been reported to be 6.9% in women with recurrent SAB compared with 1.7% in controls [61]. Table 33.1 lists the relative distribution of the major anomalies and their associated miscarriage rates (see reference [62] for details).

Various theories have been promulgated to account for the association of uterine anomalies with recurrent SAB, including decreased vascularity in the septum, increased inflammation, and a reduction in sensitivity to steroid hormones [62]. However, there is no substantive evidence to support any of these putative etiologies. There are also no controlled randomized clinical trials of pregnancy outcome following resection of uterine septae, although reductions in recurrent loss have been reported in several large series [63,64]. Open metroplasty is rarely recommended for bicornuate or didelphys uteri because of the attendant risks of infertility and uterine rupture during pregnancy as well as their generally more favorable associated pregnancy outcomes.

While pregnancy outcomes are generally believed to be relatively unaffected by the presence of myomas [65], submucous myomas that distort the uterine cavity have been posited as causes of recurrent miscarriage and reduced IVF success rates [66]. Hysteroscopic resection may improve fertility, livebirth rates, and bleeding patterns [67]. Other uterine defects such as Asherman syndrome and polyps have been proposed as causes of recurrent SAB, and descriptive series suggest improvements in pregnancy outcomes following hysteroscopic resection [68]. Thus, based on expert opinion, it would seem reasonable to offer patients with recurrent miscarriage screening for uterine defects by sonohysterography. Subsequent magnetic resonance imaging (MRI) or concomitant use of 3-D ultrasound allows differentiation of bicornuate from septate uteri. Operative hysteroscopy can then be employed for the treatment of submucous fibroids, polyps, septae, and synechiae. However, these recommendations are not based upon randomized clinical trials.

Thrombophilias

Inherited thrombophilias

The possible link between inherited thrombophilias and recurrent SAB has become a highly contentious issue. Such an association was initially suggested by retrospective, generally small, case–control studies. The most robust data were available for the factor V Leiden (FVL) mutation as it represents the most common major inheritable thrombophilia. It is present in about 5% of European-derived populations and 3% of African-Americans but is virtually absent in nonwhite Africans and Asians [69]. It arises from a point mutation in the factor V gene causing the substitution of a glutamine for an arginine at position 506, the site of cleavage by activated protein C. It accounts for the vast majority of cases of activated protein C resistance. A metaanalysis of 31 studies reported a modest link between FVL and first-trimester SAB with OR 2.01 (95% CI 1.13–3.58) but a stronger association with late (>19 weeks) nonrecurrent fetal loss (OR 3.26, 95% CI 1.82–5.83) [70]. A large case–control study of patients with recurrent stillbirths beyond 22 weeks showed an even stronger association with FVL (OR 7.83, 95% CI 2.83–21.67) [71]. Moreover, Dudding and Attia [72] conducted a metaanalysis of the link between FVL and adverse pregnancy events and noted no association with first-trimester SAB but a strong association with two or more second- or third-trimester fetal losses (OR 10.7, 95% CI 4.0–28.5).

A similar pattern holds for inherited thrombophilias in general. The European Prospective Cohort on Thrombophilia (EPCOT) retrospectively compared pregnancy outcomes among 571 women with thrombophilias having 1524 pregnancies with 395 controls having 1019 pregnancies and reported an association between inherited thrombophilias and stillbirth (OR 3.6, 95% CI 1.4–9.4) but not with SAB (OR 1.27, 95% CI 0.94–1.71) [73]. Roque and colleagues assessed a cohort of 491 patients with a history of various adverse pregnancy outcomes and noted that maternal thrombophilia was protective against recurrent SAB at less than 10 weeks (OR 0.55, 95% CI 0.33–0.92) [74]. In contrast, these authors observed a modest association between maternal thrombophilias and losses at 10 weeks or more (OR 1.76, 95% CI 1.05–2.94) and a stronger association with fetal loss after 14 weeks (OR 3.41, 95% CI 1.90–6.10). Consistent with this protective effect of FVL on early pregnancy are the reports that IVF livebirth and/or implantation rates were higher among FVL carriers than among noncarriers [75,76]. Indeed, extravillous endovascular trophoblast occlude spiral arteries to minimize uteroplacental blood flow before 10 weeks' gestation, accounting for the low intervillous oxygen partial pressures prior to 10 weeks compared with after 12 weeks (17 ± 6.9 versus 60.7 ± 8.5 mmHg) [77,78]. Thus, there is no *a priori* reason why thrombophilias would promote early pregnancy loss.

Recent prospective studies have now cast doubt on the association between FVL and the other common inherited thrombophilias and later SABs, stillbirth, and other adverse pregnancy outcomes. Dizon-Townson and associates assessed the prevalence and clinical significance of FVL among pregnant women with singleton gestations and no history of thromboembolism who were less than 14 weeks of gestation [79]. They noted that the mutation was present in 2.7% of the 4885 women tested and a nested case–control analysis found no differences in pregnancy loss, preeclampsia, placental abruption, or small for gestational age births between FVL carriers and noncarriers. Similarly, Silver and colleagues tested the same cohort for the prothrombin G20210A mutation (PGM) and found that the 3.8% of women who were heterozygous for PGM had similar rates of pregnancy loss and other adverse pregnancy outcomes compared with noncarriers [80]. Lindqvist *et al* tested 2480 women for activated protein C resistance/FVL in early pregnancy and also observed no association between this condition and fetal loss, preeclampsia or fetal growth restriction [81]. Similarly, Clark *et al* found no association between FVL and fetal loss or other adverse pregnancy outcomes among 4250 pregnant women screened between 7 and 16 weeks' gestation [82].

In contrast, the prospective study by Murphy and associates observed a modestly higher number of pregnancy losses among FVL carriers (3 of 27; 11.1%) compared with noncarriers (24 of 572; 4.2%) controls [83]. However, the very low rate of losses amongst controls and overall small sample size of FVL carriers reduce the interpretative strength of this association. Said and associates screened 2034 healthy nulliparous women for various thrombophilias before 22 weeks [84]. They found a modest association between PGM and a primary composite outcome of severe preeclampsia, fetal growth restriction, placental abruption, stillbirth, or neonatal death (adjOR 3.58, 95%

CI 1.20–10.61). However, this association was almost entirely accounted for by a higher rate of placental abruption among PGM carriers in a small (n = 9) number of patients. Univariate analysis detected an association between FVL and an increased risk of stillbirth (OR 8.85, 95% CI 1.60–48.92) but again the total number of affected patients was very small (n = 6).

Thus, retrospective studies do not demonstrate an association between inherited thrombophilias and early (<10 week) pregnancy loss and prospective studies in low-risk populations do not suggest an association between inherited thrombophilias and later losses or other adverse pregnancy events.

It is also unclear whether anticoagulation therapy prevents recurrent fetal loss among such patients. Gris and colleagues conducted a clinical trial of the low molecular weight heparin (LMWH) enoxaparin versus low-dose aspirin in 160 women with one unexplained fetal loss at more than 10 weeks who were heterozygous for FVL or PGM or had protein S deficiency [85]. They reported that enoxaparin therapy resulted in greater numbers of healthy livebirths (86.2%) than low-dose aspirin (28.8%; P < 0.0001) (OR 15.5, 95% CI 7–34). However, this study has been criticized both on methodological grounds and because of the far lower than expected livebirth rate in the aspirin-treated group. In contrast, Kaandorp and colleagues conducted a randomized clinical trial among 364 women with a history of unexplained recurrent SAB comparing the efficacy of 80 mg of aspirin plus LMWH (nadroparin at a dose of 2850 IU), 80 mg of aspirin alone, or placebo and observed no difference in livebirth rates among the three study groups (54.5%. 50.8%, and 57.0%, respectively) [86]. Moreover, they found no significant benefits among the 16% of women with an inherited thrombophilia.

Given these findings, there is no apparent value to establishing the diagnosis of inherited thrombophilia in patients with recurrent early pregnancy loss. There is also no consensus on the utility of such evaluations among patients with later pregnancy losses and other adverse pregnancy outcomes. Finally, there is no clear evidence that treatment with anticoagulation improves pregnancy outcomes among such patients.

Antiphospholipid antibody (APA) syndrome

The antiphospholipid antibody (APA) syndrome is defined by the combination of a prior deep venous or arterial thrombosis, characteristic obstetric complications, or thrombocytopenia associated with laboratory confirmation of APA [87]. Laboratory criteria include the presence of medium to high titer IgG/IgM anticardiolipin antibodies (ACA), IgG/IgM anti-β_2-glycoprotein-I antibodies at levels ≥99th percentile, or a lupus anticoagulant (LAC) on ≥2 occasions at least 12 weeks apart. Obstetric complications include at least one fetal death at 10 weeks' or more gestation, at least one premature birth before

35 weeks, or at least three consecutive SABs before 10 weeks. All other causes of pregnancy morbidity must be excluded.

The APAs are immunoglobulins directed against proteins bound to negatively charged (anionic) phospholipids [88]. They can be detected by screening for antibodies binding directly to protein epitopes (e.g. β_2-glycoprotein-1, prothrombin, annexin V) or by indirectly detecting antibodies reacting to proteins present in an anionic phospholipid matrix (e.g. cardiolipin and phosphatidylserine) or by evaluating the "downstream" coagulation effects of these antibodies on *in vitro* prothrombin activation (i.e. lupus anticoagulants) [89].

Persistently high levels of APAs are associated with obstetric complications in about 15–20% of affected patients, including fetal loss after 9 weeks' gestation, abruption, severe preeclampsia, and intrauterine growth restriction (IUGR). Between 5% and 15% of women with recurrent SAB have documented APA compared with 2–5% of the general obstetric population [90]. The most consistent association with fetal loss is seen with LAC which has reported ORs for pregnancy loss of 3.0–4.8 while ACAs display a wider range of reported ORs of 0.86–20.0 [88]. There is controversy over whether APA are also associated with recurrent (three or more) SABs at less than 10 weeks in the absence of associated stillbirth. Compared with patients having unexplained first-trimester losses without APA, those with antibodies more often have documented fetal cardiac activity prior to a loss (86% versus 43%; P < 0.01) [91]. In addition, a metaanalysis of seven studies reported no significant association between APA and either clinical pregnancy (OR 0.99, 95% CI 0.64–1.53) or livebirth rates (OR 1.07, 95% CI 0.66–1.75) in patients undergoing IVF [92].

Suggested pathogenic mechanism(s) by which APA induce fetal loss include impairment of the anticoagulant effects of placental anionic phospholipid binding proteins β_2-glycoprotein-I and annexin V [93,94], and APA induction of decidual and placental bed complement activation [95]. Treatment includes LMWH and low-dose aspirin. Mak and associates performed a metaanalysis of randomized clinical trials comparing the efficacy of heparin/LMWH plus aspirin to aspirin alone in patients with APA and recurrent pregnancy loss [96]. Data were available from five trials involving 334 patients. Livebirth rates were 74.3% and 55.8%, respectively. Moreover, the combination of heparin and aspirin modestly increased the likelihood of a livebirth compared with aspirin alone (relative risk [RR] 1.3, 95% CI 1.0–1.6, number needed to treat = 5.6 per livebirth). No significant differences were noted in the prevalence of preeclampsia, or preterm labor between the two groups. While there are reports that aspirin alone is equally efficacious [97,98], these studies may be affected by inclusion of patients with low APA levels, fewer thrombotic co-morbidities and small sample sizes.

Immunologic causes

Two principal theories have been espoused to account for possible maternal immunologically mediated recurrent SAB: absence of so-called "blocking" antibodies, and excessive decidual natural killer (NK) cell activity. The nature of the putative blocking antibodies was maternal antipaternal lymphocytoxic antibodies. The theory was that excessive human leukocyte antigen (HLA) sharing by prospective parents would lead to the absence of such antibodies. This, in turn, would expose placental antigens to a more cytotoxic maternal immune response. Proponents of this theory advocated treatment of recurrent SAB patients lacking such antibodies with infusions of their partner's or third party leukocytes or extracts of placental trophoblast to induce antibody production. However, metaanalyses of such approaches failed to support efficacy [99]. Ober *et al* conducted a double-blind, placebo-controlled, multicenter, randomized, clinical trial in which 91 recurrent miscarriage patients were assigned to immunization with paternal mononuclear cells, and 92 to sterile saline injections [100]. These investigators found higher numbers of viable pregnancies in the placebo compared with treatment groups (41/85 [48%] versus 31/86 [36%]; OR 0.60, 95% CI 0.33–1.12). Ultimately, the US Food and Drug Administration moved to constrain such treatment.

The link between elevated NK cell activity and recurrent SAB has been suggested by several small studies. The underlying theory is that excess decidual NK cell activity may damage the implanting blastocyst or derange early placentation to promote SAB. Yamada and colleagues reported that elevated peripheral blood preconception NK cell activity (>46%, RR 3.6, 95% CI 1.6–8.0) and percentages of circulating NK cells (>16.4%, RR 4.9, 95% CI 1.7–13.8) predicted subsequent biochemical pregnancy and SAB with normal karyotype in the next pregnancy among recurrent aborters [101]. These findings have been supported by other [102,103] but not all investigators [104].

It is now understood that measurement of circulating NK cell cytotoxic activity is unlikely to provide insights into the decidual NK cell phenotype since the mRNA repertoire of circulating NK cells is far different from that of decidual NK cells [105]. This calls into question the logic and biologic plausibility of measuring peripheral blood NK cell activity as a proxy for decidual and placental bed NK cell activity. In addition, there is evidence that decidual NK cells are actually crucial to normal endovascular trophoblast invasion despite the fact that these cells are replete with potentially cytotoxic factors which likely permit them to fight pathogens [106].

However, aberrant interactions between decidual NK cells and trophoblast antigens may active this cytotoxic capability to promote adverse pregnancy outcomes. For example, decidual NK cells at the site of placentation express killer cell immunoglobulin-like receptors (KIR) that can bind to HLA-C molecules on trophoblast cells. While this process normally appears to trigger elaboration of salutary growth and angiogenic factors by NK cells that promote trophoblast invasion, the presence of KIR AA haplotypes on decidual NK cells, particularly the activating KIR for HLA-C2 groups (KIR2DS1), coupled with HLA-C2 bearing trophoblast may modestly promote both preeclampsia and recurrent loss [107,108]. This is an active area of research but at this point there is absolutely no support for measuring NK cell activity in patients with recurrent abortion nor for treating those with putatively increased activity.

Evidence-based evaluation of couples experiencing recurrent spontaneous abortion

A number of social and anthropomorphic factors are modestly associated with the occurrence of isolated and recurrent miscarriage. These include cigarette smoking, heavy caffeine use, and obesity [109,110]. Thus, smoking cessation, reduction in caffeine use, exercise, and diet are all prudent interventions in affected patients.

The focus of the evaluation of a patient with recurrent first-trimester SABs should be on the identification of genetic factors. Thus, parental karyotypes, aggressive karyotyping of abortus specimens, and assessment of the placental pathology for trophoblast inclusions would appear reasonable diagnostic studies. The latter are particularly appropriate when no prior abortus' karyotypes were obtained and/or when there are intermittent euploid losses at around the same gestational ages. In the near future, genotyping abortus specimens will likely become an option and this process will undoubtedly identify both autosomal and X-linked recessive and germline loss of heterozygosity for developmentally lethal mutations. Treatment of patients with recurrent early losses should include nutritional supplementation with folate. However, the utility of IVF with preimplantational screening for common aneuploidies remains an unproven therapy in patients with recurrent aneuploid losses because of advanced maternal age or parental chromosomal abnormalities.

It is still a standard approach to search for uterine anatomic abnormalities, which should be conducted with sonohysterography and 3-D ultrasound. Remediable defects should be corrected prior to attempting a subsequent pregnancy. In addition, a work-up for APA should be performed. If the patient meets the criteria for APA syndrome, treat with LMWH and low-dose aspirin. Assessing prolactin levels and screening for antithyroid antibodies, and providing appropriate treatment with bromocriptine and levothyroxine, respectively, for those found affected may also be reasonable strategies but these approaches require further study.

Further complicating care, these patients have high rates of subsequent depression, and repetitive miscarriage may increase risks of posttraumatic stress disorders [111]. As a consequence, they are highly suggestible and more easily accepting of unorthodox treatments. Thus, couples experiencing recurrent miscarriage should be screened for depression and posttraumatic stress disorder, and appropriate psychological support provided. Finally, patients should be reassured of the high spontaneous remission rate.

CASE PRESENTATION 1

A 39-year-old gravida 5, para 0050 presents with five consecutive miscarriages in the past 2 years. She has unremarkable past medical, surgical, and gynecological histories, and a 15 pack-year smoking history. Her menses are regular although her cycle has lengthened in the past 18 months from 28 to 34 days. She also notes recent onset of occasional hot flushes and night sweats that disturb her sleep. All losses occurred at <9 weeks. Two consisted of chemical pregnancies. Three required curettage. The products of conception of her last loss were karyotyped and revealed trisomy 22.

1. What is the most likely etiology of these losses?
2. What additional diagnostic studies are indicated?
3. What treatment regimen would you recommend?

CASE PRESENTATION 2

A 28-year-old gravida 5, para 2032 presents with a history of two term births of healthy unaffected female infants following uncomplicated pregnancies. She also had three losses each at around 12 weeks' gestation in her initial, middle, and last pregnancies. She has no medical complications, does not smoke or abuse caffeine. Karyotype of her last loss revealed 46 XY. Parental karyotypes were normal. Placental pathology reports of her losses each revealed no evidence of ischemia, decidual vasculopathy, thrombosis, or inflammation but made mention of multiple trophoblast inclusions.

1. What is the most likely etiology of these losses?
2. Are there any diagnostic studies indicated?
3. How should she be counseled?

References

1. Rai R, Regan L. Recurrent miscarriage. Lancet 2006;368: 601–611.

2. Regan L. Recurrent miscarriage. BMJ 1991;302:543–544.

3. Cleary-Goldman J, Malone FD, Vidaver J et al, for the FASTER Consortium. Impact of maternal age on obstetric outcome. Obstet Gynecol 2005;105:983–990.

4. Nybo Andersen AM, Wohlfahrt J, Christens P, Olsen J, Melbye M. Maternal age and fetal loss: population based register linkage study. BMJ 2000;320:1708–1712.

5. Keefe DL, Marquard K, Liu L. The telomere theory of reproductive senescence in women. Curr Opin Obstet Gynecol 2006;18:280–285.

6. Liu L, Franco S, Spyropoulos B, Moens PB, Blasco MA, Keefe DL. Irregular telomeres impair meiotic synapsis and recombination in mice. Proc Natl Acad Sci USA 2004;101: 6496–6501.

7. Habayeb OM, Konje JC. The one-stop recurrent miscarriage clinic: an evaluation of its effectiveness and outcome. Hum Reprod 2004;19:2952–2958.

8. Stirrat GM. Recurrent miscarriage. Lancet 1990;336:673–675.

9. Nybo Andersen AM, Wohlfahrt J, Christens P, Olsen J, Melbye M. Maternal age and fetal loss: population based register linkage study. BMJ 2000;320:1708–1712.

10. Stern JJ, Dorfmann AD, Gutierrez-Najar AJ, Cerrillo M, Coulam CB. Frequency of abnormal karyotypes among abortuses from women with and without a history of recurrent spontaneous abortion. Fertil Steril 1996;65:250–253.

11. Rubio C, Simon C, Vidal F et al. Chromosomal abnormalities and embryo development in recurrent miscarriage couples. Hum Reprod 2003;18:182–188.

12. Warburton D. The effect of maternal age on the frequency of trisomy: change in meiosis or in utero selection? Prog Clin Biol Res 1989;311:165–181.

13. Freeman SB, Yang Q, Allran K, Taft LF, Sherman SL. Women with a reduced ovarian complement may have an increased risk for a child with Down syndrome. Am J Hum Genet 2000;66:1680–1683.

14. Kline J, Kinney A, Levin B, Warburton D. Trisomic pregnancy and earlier age at menopause. Am J Hum Genet 2000;67: 395–404.

15. Hardarson T, Hanson C, Lundin K et al. Preimplantation genetic screening in women of advanced maternal age caused a decrease in clinical pregnancy rate: a randomized controlled trial. Hum Reprod 2008;23:2806–2812.

16. Mastenbroek S, Twisk M, van Echten-Arends J et al. In vitro fertilization with preimplantation genetic screening. N Engl J Med 2007;357:9–17.

17. George L, Mills JL, Johansson AL et al. Plasma folate levels and risk of spontaneous abortion. JAMA 2002;288: 1867–1873.

18. Nelen WL, Blom HJ, Steegers EA, den Heijer M, Eskes TK. Hyperhomocysteinemia and recurrent early pregnancy loss: a meta-analysis. Fertil Steril 2000;74:1196–1199.

19. Toncheva D. Fragile sites and spontaneous abortions. Genet Couns 1991;2:205–210.

20. Sachs ES, Jahoda MG, van Hemel JO, Hoogeboom AJ, Sandkuyl LA. Chromosome studies of 500 couples with two or more abortions. Obstet Gynecol 1985;65:375–378.

21. Wolf GC, Mao J, Izquierdo L, Joffe G. Paternal pericentric inversion of chromosome 4 as a cause of recurrent pregnancy loss. J Med Genet 1994;31:153–155.

22. Turczynowicz S, Sharma P, Smith A, Davidson AA. Paracentric inversion of chromosome 14 plus rare 9p variant in a couple with habitual spontaneous abortion. Ann Genet 1992;35: 58–60.

23. Warburton D, Kline J, Kinney A, Yu CY, Levin B, Brown S. Skewed X chromosome inactivation and trisomic spontaneous abortion: no association. Am J Hum Genet 2009;85: 179–193.

24. Pasquier E, Bohec C, de Saint Martin L et al. Strong evidence that skewed X-chromosome inactivation is not associated with recurrent pregnancy loss: an incident paired case control study. Hum Reprod 2007;22:2829–2833.

25. Fryns JP, van Buggenhout G. Structural chromosome rearrangements in couples with recurrent fetal wastage. Eur J Obstet Gynecol Reprod Biol 1998;81:171–176.

26. Stephenson MD, Sierra S. Reproductive outcomes in recurrent pregnancy loss associated with a parental carrier of a structural chromosome rearrangement. Hum Reprod 2006;21: 1076–1082.

27. Sugiura-Ogasawara M, Suzumori K. Can preimplantation genetic diagnosis improve success rates in recurrent aborters with translocations? Hum Reprod 2005;20: 3267–3270.

28. Fischer J, Colls P, Escudero T, Munné S. Preimplantation genetic diagnosis (PGD) improves pregnancy outcome for translocation carriers with a history of recurrent losses. Fertil Steril 2010;94:283–289.

29. Lockwood C, Irons M, Troiani J, Kawada C, Chaudhury A, Cetrulo C. The prenatal sonographic diagnosis of lethal multiple pterygium syndrome: a heritable cause of recurrent abortion. Am J Obstet Gynecol 1988;159:474–476.

30. Odent S, Le Marec B, Smahi A et al. Spontaneous abortion of male fetuses with incontinentia pigmenti (apropos of a family). J Gynecol Obstet Biol Reprod (Paris) 1997;26: 633–636.

31. Kliman HJ, Segel L. The placenta may predict the baby. J Theor Biol 2003;225:143–145.

32. Matovina M, Husnjak K, Milutin N, Ciglar S, Grce M. Possible role of bacterial and viral infections in miscarriages. Fertil Steril 2004;81:662–669.

33. Naessens A, Foulon W, Breynaert J, Lauwers S. Serotypes of Ureaplasma urealyticum isolated from normal pregnant women and patients with pregnancy complications. J Clin Microbiol 1988;26:319–322.

34. Quinn PA, Shewchuk AB, Shuber J et al. Efficacy of antibiotic therapy in preventing spontaneous pregnancy loss among couples colonized with genital mycoplasmas. Am J Obstet Gynecol 1983;145:239–244.

35. Sozio J, Ness RB. Chlamydial lower genital tract infection and spontaneous abortion. Infect Dis Obstet Gynecol 1998;6: 8–12.

36. Paukku M, Tulppala M, Puolakkainen M, Anttila T, Paavonen J. Lack of association between serum antibodies to Chlamydia trachomatis and a history of recurrent pregnancy loss. Fertil Steril 1999;72:427–430.

37. Sugiura-Ogasawara M, Ozaki Y, Nakanishi T, Kumamoto Y, Suzumori K. Pregnancy outcome in recurrent aborters is not

influenced by Chlamydia IgA and/or G. Am J Reprod Immunol 2005;53:50–53.

38. Ralph SG, Rutherford AJ, Wilson JD. Influence of bacterial vaginosis on conception and miscarriage in the first trimester: cohort study. BMJ 1999;319:220–223.

39. Oakeshott P, Hay P, Hay S, Steinke F, Rink E, Kerry S. Association between bacterial vaginosis or chlamydial infection and miscarriage before 16 weeks' gestation: prospective community based cohort study. BMJ 2002;325:1334.

40. Bustos D, Moret A, Tambutti M et al. Autoantibodies in Argentine women with recurrent pregnancy loss. Am J Reprod Immunol 2006;55:201–207.

41. Greco L, Veneziano A, di Donato L et al. Undiagnosed celiac disease does not appear to be associated with unfavourable outcome of pregnancy. Gut 2004;53:149–151.

42. Kotze LM. Gynecologic and obstetric findings related to nutritional status and adherence to a gluten-free diet in Brazilian patients with celiac disease. J Clin Gastroenterol 2004;38:567–574.

43. Tata LJ, Card TR, Logan RF, Hubbard RB, Smith CJ, West J. Fertility and pregnancy-related events in women with celiac disease: a population-based cohort study. Gastroenterology 2005;128:849–855.

44. Ciacci C, Cirillo M, Auriemma G, di Dato G, Sabbatini F, Mazzacca G. Celiac disease and pregnancy outcome. Am J Gastroenterol 1996;91:718–722.

45. Mills JL, Simpson JL, Driscoll SG et al. Incidence of spontaneous abortion among normal women and insulin-dependent diabetic women whose pregnancies were identified within 21 days of conception. N Engl J Med 1988;319:1617–1623.

46. Rushworth FH, Backos M, Rai R, Chilcott IT, Baxter N, Regan L. Prospective pregnancy outcome in untreated recurrent miscarriers with thyroid autoantibodies. Hum Reprod 2000;15:1637–1639.

47. Stagnaro-Green A, Glinoer D. Thyroid autoimmunity and the risk of miscarriage. Best Pract Res Clin Endocrinol Metab 2004;18:167–181.

48. Rai R, Backos M, Rushworth F, Regan L. Polycystic ovaries and recurrent miscarriage: a reappraisal. Hum Reprod 2000;15:612–615.

49. Liddell HS, Sowden K, Farquhar CM. Recurrent miscarriage: screening for polycystic ovaries and subsequent pregnancy outcome. Aust N Z J Obstet Gynaecol 1997;37:402–406.

50. Legro RS, Barnhart HX, Schlaff WD et al, for the Cooperative Multicenter Reproductive Medicine Network. Clomiphene, metformin, or both for infertility in the polycystic ovary syndrome. N Engl J Med 2007;356:551–566.

51. Lockwood CJ, Krikun G, Rahman M, Caze R, Buchwalder L, Schatz F. The role of decidualization in regulating endometrial hemostasis during the menstrual cycle, gestation, and in pathological states. Semin Thromb Hemost 2007;33:111–117.

52. Lockwood CJ, Krikun G, Papp C, Aigner S, Nemerson Y, Schatz F. Biological mechanisms underlying RU 486 clinical effects: inhibition of endometrial stromal cell tissue factor content. J Clin Endocrinol Metab 1994;79:786–789.

53. Lockwood CJ, Krikun G, Hausknecht VA, Papp C, Schatz F. Matrix metalloproteinase and matrix metalloproteinase inhibitor expression in endometrial stromal cells during progestin-initiated decidualization and menstruation-related progestin withdrawal. Endocrinology 1998;139:4607–4613.

54. Lessey BA, Fritz MA. Defective luteal function. In: Fraser JS, Jansen RPS, Lobo RA, Whitehead MI, eds. Estrogens and Progestogens in Clinical Practice. Philadelphia: W.B. Saunders, 1998, pp.437–453.

55. Potdar N, Konje JC. The endocrinological basis of recurrent miscarriages. Curr Opin Obstet Gynecol 2005;17:424–428.

56. Ogasawara M, Kajiura S, Katano K, Aoyama T, Aoki K. Are serum progesterone levels predictive of recurrent miscarriage in future pregnancies? Fertil Steril 1997;68:806–809.

57. Dawood MY. Corpus luteal insufficiency. Curr Opin Obstet Gynecol 1994;6:121–127.

58. Oates-Whitehead RM, Haas DM, Carrier JAK. Progestogen for preventing miscarriage (Cochrane Review). In: The Cochrane Library, Issue 3, 2004. Oxford: Update Software.

59. Hirahara F, Andoh N, Sawai K, Hirabuki T, Uemura T, Minaguchi H. Hyperprolactinemic recurrent miscarriage and results of randomized bromocriptine treatment trials. Fertil Steril 1998;70:246–252.

60. Salim R, Regan L, Woelfer B, Backos M, Jurkovic D. A comparative study of the morphology of congenital uterine anomalies in women with and without a history of recurrent first trimester miscarriage. Hum Reprod 2003;18:162–166.

61. Raga F, Bauset C, Remohi J, Bonilla-Musoles F, Simon C, Pellicer A. Reproductive impact of congenital Mullerian anomalies. Hum Reprod 1997;12:2277–2281.

62. Devi Wold AS, Pham N, Arici A. Anatomic factors in recurrent pregnancy loss. Semin Reprod Med 2006;24:25–32.

63. Daly DC, Maier D, Soto-Albors C. Hysteroscopic metroplasty: six years' experience. Obstet Gynecol 1989;73:201–205.

64. De Cherney AH, Russell JB, Graebe RA, Polan ML. Resectoscopic management of mullerian fusion defect. Fertil Steril 1986;45:726–728.

65. Vergani P, Ghidini A, Strobelt N et al. Do uterine leiomyomas influence pregnancy outcome? Am J Perinatol 1994;11: 356–358.

66. Bajeckal N, Li TC. Fibroids, infertility and pregnancy wastage. Hum Reprod 2000;6:614–620.

67. Fernandez H, Sefrioui O, Virelizier C, Gervaise A, Gomel V, Frydman R. Hysteroscopic resection of submucosal myomas in patients with infertility. Hum Reprod 2001;6:1489–1492.

68. Sanders B. Uterine factors and infertility. J Reprod Med 2006;51:169–176.

69. Franco RF, Reitsma PH. Genetic risk factors of venous thrombosis. Hum Genet 2001;109:369–384.

70. Rey E, Kahn SR, David M, Shrier I. Thrombophilic disorders and fetal loss: a meta-analysis. Lancet 2003;361:901–908.

71. Gris JC, Quere I, Monpeyroux F et al. Case–control study of the frequency of thrombophilic disorders in couples with late foetal loss and no thrombotic antecedent: the Nimes Obstetricians and Haematologists Study5 (NOHA5). Thromb Haemost 1999;81:891–899.

72. Dudding TE, Attia J. The association between adverse pregnancy outcomes and maternal factor V Leiden genotype: a meta-analysis. Thromb Haemost 2004;91:700–711.

73. Preston FE, Rosendaal FR, Walker ID et al. Increased fetal loss in women with heritable thrombophilia. Lancet 1996;348: 913–916.

74. Roque H, Paidas MJ, Funai EF, Kuczynski E, Lockwood CJ. Maternal thrombophilias are not associated with early pregnancy loss. Thromb Haemost 2004;91:290–295.

75. Gopel W, Ludwig M, Junge AK, Kohlmann T, Diedrich K, Moller J. Selection pressure for the factor V Leiden mutation and embryo implantation. Lancet 2001;358:1238–1239.

76. Rudick B, Su HI, Sammel MD, Kovalevsky G, Shaunik A, Barnhart K. Is factor V Leiden mutation a cause of in vitro fertilization failure? Fertil Steril 2009;92:1256–1259.

77. Rodesch F, Simon P, Donner C, Jauniaux E. Oxygen measurements in endometrial and trophoblastic tissues during early pregnancy. Obstet Gynecol 1992;80:283–285.

78. Jaffe R. Investigation of abnormal first-trimester gestations by color Doppler imaging. J Clin Ultrasound 1993;21:521–526.

79. Dizon-Townson D, Miller C, Sibai B et al, for the National Institute of Child Health and Human Development Maternal-Fetal Medicine Units Network. The relationship of the factor V Leiden mutation and pregnancy outcomes for mother and fetus. Obstet Gynecol 2005;106:517–524.

80. Silver RM, Zhao Y, Spong CY et al, for the Eunice Kennedy Shriver National Institute of Child Health and Human Development Maternal-Fetal Medicine Units (NICHD MFMU) Network. Prothrombin gene G20210A mutation and obstetric complications. Obstet Gynecol 2010;115:14–20.

81. Lindqvist PG, Svensson PJ, Marsaál K, Grennert L, Luterkort M, Dahlbäck B. Activated protein C resistance (FV:Q506) and pregnancy. Thromb Haemost 1999;81:532–537.

82. Clark P, Walker ID, Govan L, Wu O, Greer IA. The GOAL study: a prospective examination of the impact of factor V Leiden and ABO(H) blood groups on haemorrhagic and thrombotic pregnancy outcomes. Br J Haematol 2008;140:236–240.

83. Murphy RP, Donoghue C, Nallen RJ et al. Prospective evaluation of the risk conferred by factor V Leiden and thermolabile methylenetetrahydrofolate reductase polymorphisms in pregnancy. Arterioscler Thromb Vasc Biol 2000;20:266–270.

84. Said JM, Higgins JR, Moses EK et al. Inherited thrombophilia polymorphisms and pregnancy outcomes in nulliparous women. Obstet Gynecol 2010;115:5–13.

85. Gris JC, Mercier E, Quere I et al. Low-molecular-weight heparin versus low-dose aspirin in women with one fetal loss and a constitutional thrombophilic disorder. Blood 2004;103:3695–3699.

86. Kaandorp SP, Goddijn M, van der Post JA et al. Aspirin plus heparin or aspirin alone in women with recurrent miscarriage. N Engl J Med 2010;362:1586–1596.

87. Miyakis S, Lockshin MD, Atsumi T et al. International consensus statement on an update of the classification criteria for definite antiphospholipid syndrome (APS). J Thromb Haemost 2006;4:295–306.

88. Galli M, Barbui T. Antiphospholipid antibodies and thrombosis: strength of association. Hematol J 2003;4:180–186.

89. Galli M, Luciani D, Bertolini G, Barbui T. Anti-beta 2-glycoprotein I, antiprothrombin antibodies, and the risk of thrombosis in the antiphospholipid syndrome. Blood 2003;102:2717–2723.

90. Branch DW, Gibson M, Silver RM. Clinical practice. Recurrent miscarriage. N Engl J Med 2010;363:1740–1747.

91. Rai RS, Clifford K, Cohen H, Regan L. High prospective fetal loss rate in untreated pregnancies of women with recurrent miscarriage and antiphospholipid antibodies. Hum Reprod 1995;10:3301–3304.

92. Hornstein M, Davis O, Massey J, Paulson R, Collins J. Antiphospholipid antibodies and in vitro fertilization success: a meta-analysis. Fertil Steril 2000;73:330–333.

93. Field SL, Brighton TA, McNeil HP, Chesterman CN. Recent insights into antiphospholipid antibody-mediated thrombosis. Baillière's Best Pract Res Clin Haematol 1999;12:407–422.

94. Rand JH, Wu XX, Andree HA et al. Pregnancy loss in the antiphospholipid-antibody syndrome: a possible thrombogenic mechanism. N Engl J Med 1997;337:154–160.

95. Girardi G, Redecha P, Salmon JE. Heparin prevents antiphospholipid antibody-induced fetal loss by inhibiting complement activation. Nat Med 2004;10:1222–1226.

96. Mak A, Cheung MW, Cheak AA, Ho RC. Combination of heparin and aspirin is superior to aspirin alone in enhancing live births in patients with recurrent pregnancy loss and positive anti-phospholipid antibodies: a meta-analysis of randomized controlled trials and meta-regression. Rheumatology (Oxford) 2010;49:281–288.

97. Laskin CA, Spitzer KA, Clark CA et al. Low molecular weight heparin and aspirin for recurrent pregnancy loss: results from the randomized, controlled HepASA Trial. J Rheumatol 2009;36:279–287.

98. Farquharson RG, Quenby S, Greaves M. Antiphospholipid syndrome in pregnancy: a randomized, controlled trial of treatment. Obstet Gynecol 2002;100:408–413.

99. Porter TF, LaCoursiere Y, Scott JR. Immunotherapy for recurrent miscarriage. Cochrane Database Syst Rev 2006;2:CD000112.

100. Ober C, Karrison T, Odem RR et al. Mononuclear-cell immunisation in prevention of recurrent miscarriages: a randomised trial. Lancet 1999;354:365–369.

101. Yamada H, Morikawa M, Kato EH, Shimada S, Kobashi G, Minakami H. Pre-conceptional natural killer cell activity and percentage as predictors of biochemical pregnancy and spontaneous abortion with normal chromosome karyotype. Am J Reprod Immunol 2003;50:351–354.

102. Aoki K, Kajiura S, Matsumoto Y et al. Preconceptional natural-killer-cell activity as a predictor of miscarriage. Lancet 1995;345:1340.

103. Shakhar K, Ben-Eliyahu S, Loewenthal R, Rosenne E, Carp H. Differences in number and activity of peripheral natural killer cells in primary versus secondary recurrent miscarriage. Fertil Steril 2003;80:368–375.

104. Shimada S, Iwabuchi K, Kato EH et al. No difference in natural-killer-T cell population, but Th2/Tc2 predominance in peripheral blood of recurrent aborters. Am J Reprod Immunol 2003;50:334–339.

105. Koopman LA, Kopcow HD, Rybalov B et al. Human decidual natural killer cells are a unique NK cell subset with immunomodulatory potential. J Exp Med 2003;198:1201–1212.

106. Kalkunte S, Chichester CO, Gotsch F, Sentman CL, Romero R, Sharma S. Evolution of non-cytotoxic uterine natural killer cells. Am J Reprod Immunol 2008;59:425–432.

107. Hiby SE, Walker JJ, O'shaughnessy KM et al. Combinations of maternal KIR and fetal HLA-C genes influence the risk of preeclampsia and reproductive success. J Exp Med 2004;200:957–965.

108. Hiby SE, Regan L, Lo W, Farrell L, Carrington M, Moffett A. Association of maternal killer-cell immunoglobulin-like

receptors and parental HLA-C genotypes with recurrent miscarriage. Hum Reprod 2008;23:972–976.

109. George L, Granath F, Johansson AL, Olander B, Cnattingius S. Risks of repeated miscarriage. Paediatr Perinat Epidemiol 2006;20:119–126.

110. Lashen H, Fear K, Sturdee DW. Obesity is associated with increased risk of first trimester and recurrent miscarriage: matched case–control study. Hum Reprod 2004;19: 1644–1646.

111. Neugebauer R, Kline J, Shrout P et al. Major depressive disorder in the 6 months after miscarriage. JAMA 1997;277: 383–388.

Further reading

American College of Obstetricians and Gynecologists. Inherited thrombophilias in pregnancy. ACOG Practice Bulletin No. 113. Obstet Gynecol 2010;116(1):212–222.

American College of Obstetricians and Gynecologists. Antiphospholipid syndrome. ACOG Practice Bulletin No. 118. Obstet Gynecol 2011;117(1):192–199.

1.

Branch DW, Gibson M, Silver RM. Clinical practice. Recurrent miscarriage. N Engl J Med 2010;363(18):1740–1747.

Oates-Whitehead RM, Haas DM, Carrier JA. Progestogen for preventing miscarriage. Cochrane Database Syst Rev 2003;4: CD003511.

Porter TF, LaCoursiere Y, Scott JR. Immunotherapy for recurrent miscarriage. Cochrane Database Syst Rev 2006;2:CD000112.

Chapter 34
Cervical Insufficiency

John Owen

Department of Obstetrics and Gynecology, University of Alabama at Birmingham, AL, USA

Although the term "cervical incompetence" was first used in *The Lancet* in 1865, the contemporary concept was not widely accepted until the middle of the 20th century, after Palmer and Lacomme [1] in 1948 and Lash and Lash [2] in 1950 independently described interval repair of anatomic cervical defects associated with recurrent spontaneous midtrimester birth. Soon thereafter, Shirodkar [3] in 1955, McDonald [4] in 1957, and later Benson and Durfee [5] in 1965 described the cerclage procedures utilized in contemporary obstetric practice. Nevertheless, the literature on cervical *insufficiency* (the preferred contemporary term) has largely been a chronicle of surgical methods to correct often posttraumatic anatomic disruption of the internal os, in women who had experienced recurrent painless dilation and midtrimester birth. Evidence-based guidelines for many aspects of the diagnosis and management are still lacking.

Syndrome of spontaneous preterm birth

Spontaneous preterm birth is a syndrome composed of several anatomic components [6]. These include the uterus and its contractile function (i.e. preterm labor), loss of chorio-amnion integrity (i.e. preterm rupture of membranes), and, finally, diminished cervical competence, either from an anatomic cervical defect or from early pathologic cervical ripening, a functional deficit. In any pregnancy, a single feature may appear to predominate, even though it is more likely that most cases of spontaneous preterm birth result from the interaction of multiple stimuli and functional pathways. Importantly, the manifestation and relative contributions of each of these components may vary, not only among different women but also in successive pregnancies of the same woman.

Biologic continuum of cervical competence

As early as 1962, Danforth and Buckingham [7] suggested that cervical competence was not an all-or-nothing phenomenon as traditionally taught. Rather, it comprised degrees of insufficiency, and combinations of factors could cause "cervical failure." In their proposed classification, one group of patients had ostensibly normal cervical tissue, whose integrity as a fibrous ring had been previously damaged as the result of antecedent obstetric trauma. This might even be concealed by a normal-appearing external os and ectocervix. The second group possessed an abnormally low collagen:muscle ratio that would compromise its mechanical function and lead to premature dilation. The third group comprised women who had no history of antecedent trauma and who also had normal collagen:muscle ratios, but whose obstetric histories mimicked those of groups 1 and 2, presumably from premature triggering of other factors (e.g. cervical ripening). These biochemical and ultrastructural findings support the variable, and often unpredictable, clinical course of women with a history of cervical insufficiency [8].

Although the traditional paradigm has depicted the cervix as either competent or insufficient, recent evidence, including clinical data [9–12] and interpretative reviews [13–15], suggests that, as with most other biologic processes, cervical competence is rarely an all-or-nothing phenomenon, and it functions along a continuum of reproductive performance. Although some women have tangible anatomic evidence of poor cervical integrity, most women with a clinical diagnosis of cervical insufficiency have ostensibly normal cervical anatomy. In a proposed model of cervical competence as a continuum, a poor obstetric history results from a process of premature cervical ripening, induced by infection, inflammation,

Queenan's Management of High-Risk Pregnancy: An Evidence-Based Approach, Sixth Edition. Edited by John T. Queenan, Catherine Y. Spong, Charles J. Lockwood.

and local or systemic hormonal effects, probably modulated by genetic predisposition.

Diagnosis of cervical insufficiency

The incidence of cervical insufficiency in the general obstetric population is reported to vary between approximately 1 in 100 and 1 in 2000 [16–18]. This wide disparity is likely because of differences among study populations, reporting bias, and the diagnostic criteria used to establish the diagnosis. Most of what is known about cervical insufficiency and its treatment indicates that it is a *clinical diagnosis*, characterized by recurrent painless dilation and spontaneous midtrimester birth, usually of a living fetus. Associated characteristics, such as antecedent fetal demise, painful uterine contractions, bleeding, overt infection (especially chorioamnionitis), or premature rupture of membranes, would shift the cause of spontaneous preterm birth away from cervical insufficiency and better support other components of the preterm birth syndrome.

Because cervical insufficiency is likely part of a broader syndrome, the clinical diagnosis is retrospective and suggested only after poor obstetric outcomes have occurred (or, occasionally, are in evolution). Because there are no proven objective criteria, other than a rare, gross cervical malformation, a careful history and review of the past obstetric records are crucial to making an accurate diagnosis. However, records may be incomplete or unavailable, and many women cannot provide an accurate history. Even with excellent records and history, clinicians might reasonably disagree on the clinical diagnosis in all but the most classic presentations. Confounding factors in the history, medical records, or current physical assessment might be utilized to either support or refute the diagnosis, based on their perceived importance. It is crucial to realize that the physician managing a patient who experiences a spontaneous midtrimester birth is in the best position to assess and document whether and which clinical criteria for cervical insufficiency were present. Women with cervical insufficiency often have some premonitory symptoms such as increased pelvic pressure, vaginal discharge, and urinary frequency. These symptoms, although neither specific nor uncommon in a normal pregnancy, should not be ignored, particularly in women with risk factors for spontaneous preterm birth.

Because of its unproven efficacy in randomized clinical trials, and the attendant surgical risks, the recommendation for *history-indicated* (a.k.a. prophylactic) cerclage should be limited to women with recurrent spontaneous preterm birth syndrome, after a careful history or physical examination suggests a dominant cervical component. Unless the physical examination confirms a significant

cervical anatomic defect, consistent with disruption of its circumferential integrity, the clinician should assess the history for other components of the preterm birth syndrome. Although some authorities consider cervical insufficiency to be a diagnosis of exclusion, it is plausible that premature silent cervical dilation might occur, consistent with functional insufficiency, which would predispose to early membrane rupture or ascending genital tract infection with intact membranes, either of which might cause overt labor and be utilized to refute the diagnosis. It is also plausible that intrauterine subclinical infection could contribute to local effects responsible for the pathologic dilation.

"Risk factors" for cervical insufficiency

While the historic concept of the diagnosis and treatment of cervical insufficiency often includes women with past cervical trauma from birth-associated lacerations, forced dilation, operative injury, or cervical amputation, the prevalence of these antecedent events appears to be decreasing in contemporary US practice. More common in contemporary practice are patients who have undergone prior treatment of cervical dysplasia using cold-knife cone, laser cone, or a loop electrosurgical excision procedure (LEEP). These cervical procedures are plausible risk factors for cervical insufficiency. Numerous studies have confirmed that most women with prior LEEP, laser ablation, or cone biopsy do not appear to have a clinically significant rate of second-trimester loss or even preterm birth [19–21]. However, women in whom a large cone specimen was removed or destroyed (including cervical amputations), or who have undergone multiple prior procedures do have an increased risk of spontaneous preterm birth [22,23]. Whether prophylactic cerclage is an effective strategy in these at-risk women remains speculative. The available clinical trial data [24] do not suggest a benefit from history-indicated cerclage in women with these risk factors, and so they may be followed clinically.

A similar controversy arises over the management of women with *in utero* diethylstilbestrol (DES) exposure. Because many women exposed to DES *in utero* were the products themselves of complicated gestations and were born to women with poor reproductive histories, it is plausible that at least a portion of the presumed DES effect may simply be of genetic origin [25]. Because the use of DES was effectively curtailed in the early 1970s, this congenital risk factor should comprise a steadily diminishing group of patients and will soon be of no clinical concern. Currently, no controlled data support the efficacy of history-indicated cerclage in these patients.

Management

Most of what is known about the management of the cervical insufficiency is based on case series that reported surgical correction of the presumed underlying mechanical defect in the cervical stroma. Branch [26] in 1986 and Cousins [27] in 1980 collectively tabulated over 25 case series of cerclage efficacy published between 1959 and 1981. Branch [26] estimated a precerclage perinatal survival range of 10–32% versus a range of 75–83% in the same cohorts of women managed with Shirodkar cerclage. Similarly, case series that utilized McDonald cerclage reported a cohort perinatal survival range of 7–50% before and 63–89% using cerclage. Cousins [27] estimated a "mean" survival before Shirodkar cerclage of 22% versus 82% post therapy, and 27% and 74%, respectively, for investigators who utilized the McDonald technique. In total, over 2000 patients have been reported in these historic cohort comparisons. However, interpretation of these series is problematic.

- Diagnostic criteria were not consistent or always reported.
- Definitions of treatment success were inconsistent (but generally recorded as perinatal survival, as opposed to a gestational age-based endpoint).
- Treatment approaches were not always detailed and might involve multiple combinations of surgery, medication, bedrest, and other uncontrolled therapies.
- Cases were not subcategorized according to etiology (i.e. anatomic defects versus a presumed functional cause) [27]. Nevertheless, based on compelling but potentially biased efficacy data, placement of a history-indicated cerclage in women with clinically defined cervical insufficiency has become standard practice.

Once a patient has been properly evaluated and deemed a suitable candidate for a history-indicated cerclage, a surgical method is chosen. In the presence of normal cervical anatomy and no prior failed cerclage procedures (or a prior successful McDonald cerclage), a McDonald procedure is the technique of choice, because it is technically easier to perform and appears to be similarly effective to the Shirodkar technique [28]. Shirodkar cerclage should be reserved for women with anatomic deformities such as an unrepaired cervical laceration or a hypoplastic cervix where a McDonald cerclage is felt to be technically inadvisable. For example, a Shirodkar cerclage should be considered whenever there is less than 1 cm of visible cervix below the vaginal fornix.

A patient with a prior failed McDonald cerclage occasionally presents for subsequent obstetric care or preconception counseling. If the prior pregnancy failure is believed to have been the result of cervical insufficiency (as opposed to other components of the spontaneous preterm birth syndrome), the patient might be considered a candidate for either a Shirodkar or cervicoisthmic procedure. Because few patients are appropriate candidates, and few physicians have surgical experience with the cervicoisthmic procedure, it would seem prudent to relegate the decision to place a cerclage via the abdominal approach, and the procedure itself, to a tertiary center.

The chief advantage to history-indicated cerclage is that it can be offered in the early second trimester, after most spontaneous abortions have occurred. It also permits a sonographic evaluation to rule out many fetal anomalies and the potential for first-trimester screening; prenatal diagnosis using chorionic villus sampling can be performed prior to surgery. Many clinicians recommend obtaining cervicovaginal cultures for common pathogens and treating positive cultures prior to placing a cerclage. Active cervicitis is considered a contraindication to cerclage placement, and should be successfully treated before surgery. Other contraindications to cerclage include ruptured membranes, certain (e.g. lethal) fetal anomalies, suspected or confirmed intrauterine infection, vaginal bleeding, and labor.

McDonald cerclage

To place a McDonald cerclage, the anesthetized patient is placed in the dorsal lithotomy position. At least one assistant is required to provide exposure using right angle or medium-sized Deaver retractors. After an antiseptic vaginal prep, the anterior ectocervix is grasped with a sponge forceps or similar nontraumatic instrument, which is used to provide countertraction. The urinary bladder is generally emptied prior to the procedure, although some recommend leaving some urine in the bladder to better define the position of the bladder as it reflects onto the cervix.

Most surgeons utilize a permanent synthetic material such as No 1 or 2 Prolene or Mersilene. Mersilene 5 mm tape has also been proposed, but is more difficult to pull through the stroma and requires more tissue traction and manipulation. For right-handed surgeons, the first tissue bite is taken at the 11–12:00 position on the cervix, exiting at around the 10:00 position. When placing the anterior stitch, the surgeon must avoid the bladder mucosa that can be identified by moving the cervix in and out, and noting where the vaginal mucosa folds in as it reflects off the ectocervix. As the descending branches of the uterine artery are found at 3:00 and 9:00, this area should also be avoided when placing the stitches high near the lateral fornices.

The last tissue bite should exit in close proximity to the original entry site. Another variation of the original procedure uses two sutures placed several millimeters apart [29]. This has the theoretic advantage of spreading the suture tension over a larger area and may help prevent the more cephalic stitch from becoming displaced. A second stitch should be considered if the first suture was not optimally placed at the bladder reflection anterior or as high as possible in the posterior vaginal fornix. It is necessary to record how many stitches were placed and where the knots were tied to facilitate their later removal.

After the cerclage stitch has been placed, it is important to take up any slack introduced with the multiple tissue bites, utilizing a "laundry bag" technique, whereby traction is applied to each side of the exiting suture while holding countertraction at the exit site with two fingers of the opposite hand. Once this is accomplished, the suture is tied down firmly but should not cause visible blanching of the surrounding tissue. In order to facilitate later identification and removal, a long tag should be left above the knot. After placement, a digital examination will confirm a closed endocervical canal that is not overly constricted. However, it should not admit a gloved finger.

Figure 34.1 shows a short cervix by ultrasound before cerclage placement, and Figure 34.2 shows the suture visible after ultrasound-indicated cerclage placement.

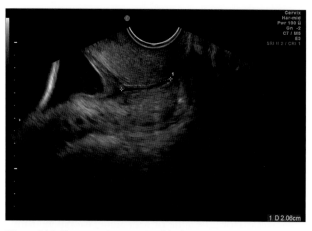

Figure 34.1 Short cervix, measured before cerclage (2.06 cm).

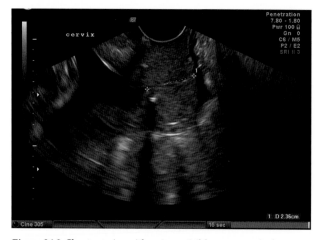

Figure 34.2 Short cervix, with suture visible, measured after ultrasound-indicated cerclage (2.36 cm).

Acute cervical insufficiency

On occasion, a woman will present with symptoms and physical findings that support an antepartum diagnosis of cervical insufficiency. This syndrome, however, comprises a wide spectrum of clinical expression. Women who present with acute cervical insufficiency, generally defined as: (1) midtrimester cervical dilation of at least 2 cm, (2) membranes prolapsing to or beyond the external os, and (3) no other predisposing cause (e.g. labor, infection, abruption), are often considered for *physical examination-indicated* (a.k.a. emergency) cerclage.

Aarts *et al* [30] reviewed eight case series published between 1980 and 1992 comprising 249 patients who received an emergency midtrimester cerclage and estimated a mean neonatal survival rate of 64% (range 22–100%). Smaller, uncontrolled reports of cerclage suggested no benefit [31] or some benefit [32]. Although these reports are not of sufficient scientific quality on which to base firm management recommendations, collectively they demonstrated several important concepts. The earlier the gestational age at presentation and the more advanced the cervical dilation, the greater the risk of poor neonatal outcome. The finding of membrane prolapse into the vagina is also a significant risk factor for poor outcome [33].

Althuisius and colleagues [34] reported the results of a randomized clinical trial of physical exam-indicated cerclage plus bedrest versus bedrest alone in 23 women (singletons and twins) who presented with nonlabor cervical dilation and prolapsing membranes prior to 27 weeks' gestation. They observed a longer mean interval from presentation to delivery (54 versus 20 days; P = 0.046) in the cerclage group. Neonatal survival was 9/16 with cerclage and 4/14 in the bedrest group. Although the survival differences were not statistically significant, there was significantly lower neonatal composite morbidity (including death) in the cerclage group (10/16 versus 14/14; P = 0.02).

Other reports show that women who present with acute cervical insufficiency have an appreciable (nominal 50%) incidence of bacterial colonization of their amniotic fluid, including other markers of subclinical chorioamnionitis [35–37] or proteomic markers of inflammation or bleeding [38]. Women with abnormal amniotic fluid markers have a much shorter presentation-to-delivery interval, regardless of whether they receive cerclage or are managed expectantly with bedrest. Of interest, a sonographic marker of intrauterine subclinical infection has been demonstrated [39].

Thus, the optimal management of women who present with acute cervical insufficiency remains indefinite. Although emergency cerclage may confer some benefit, patient selection remains largely empiric. While not standard care, the evaluation of amniotic fluid markers of infection and inflammation appears to have important prognostic value, although it is still unclear whether and to what extent the results should direct patient management.

Should cervical insufficiency become a sonographic diagnosis?

Numerous investigators have asserted that cervical insufficiency can be diagnosed by midtrimester sonographic evaluation of the cervix. Various sonographic findings, including shortened cervical length, funneling at the internal os, and dynamic response to provocative maneuvers (e.g. fundal pressure), have been utilized to select women for treatment, generally cerclage. In most of these earlier reports, the sonographic evaluations were not blinded, leading to uncontrolled interventions and difficulty determining their effectiveness. In many instances, the sonographic criteria for cervical insufficiency were only qualitatively described and thus were not reproducible.

Currently, five randomized trials of cerclage for sonographic indications have been published [40–44]. Althuisius *et al* [40] in The Netherlands enrolled patients whose history or symptoms suggested cervical insufficiency. Of the 19 assigned to cerclage, there was no preterm birth <34 weeks versus a 44% preterm birth rate in the no cerclage–home rest group (P = 0.002); none of the women who maintained a cervical length of at least 25 mm experienced a preterm birth. Rust *et al* [41] enrolled 138 women who had various risk factors for preterm birth (including 12% with multiple gestations) and randomly assigned them to receive McDonald cerclage or no cerclage after their cervical length shortened to <25 mm or they developed funneling >25%. Rates of preterm birth <34 weeks were 35% in the cerclage group versus 36% in the control group.

In a multinational trial comprising 12 hospitals in six countries, To *et al* [42] screened 47,123 unselected women at 22–24 weeks' gestation with vaginal ultrasound to identify 470 with a shortened cervical length of 15 mm or less. Of these 470, 253 participated in a randomized trial whose primary outcome was the intergroup rates of delivery prior to 33 weeks' gestation. Women assigned to the (Shirodkar) cerclage group (n = 127) had a similar rate of preterm birth to the control population (n = 126), 22% versus 26% (P = 0.44). Berghella *et al* [43] screened women with various risk factors for spontaneous preterm birth (prior preterm birth, curettage, cone biopsy, DES exposure) with vaginal scans every 2 weeks from 14 to 23 weeks' gestation and randomly assigned 61 with a cervical length <25 mm or funneling >25% to McDonald cerclage or to a no-cerclage control group. Preterm birth <35 weeks was observed in 45% of the cerclage group and 47% of the control group. More recently, a patient-level metaanalysis of these four randomized trials uncovered a relationship between pregnancy history and cerclage

efficacy [45]: intervention was only effective in singleton pregnancies (there was a statistically significant *harm* in multiples), and ultrasound-indicated cerclage was especially effective in women who had a prior preterm birth (adjusted odds ratio, 0.6).

The fifth randomized trial, performed by a consortium of 15 US centers, was recently published [44] and included only women who had at least one prior spontaneous preterm birth at 17–34 weeks' gestation, who were followed with serial vaginal scans beginning at 16 weeks. As long as the cervical length was at least 30 mm, scans were scheduled every 2 weeks, but increased to weekly if the measured length was 25–29 mm. Those who developed a shortened cervical length <25 mm between 16 and $22^{6/7}$ weeks were assigned to McDonald cerclage or no cerclage. These investigators observed a statistically significant decrease in previable births <24 weeks (6% versus 14%), perinatal mortality (9% versus 16%) and birth <37 weeks (45% versus 60%), but a nonsignificant decrease in the comparative rates of preterm birth <35 weeks (32% versus 42%), which was the trial's primary outcome. Cerclage benefit was closely linked to cervical status, and women with cervical length <15 mm accrued a much greater benefit than those women who were randomized with a cervical length of 15–24 mm, suggesting that shorter lengths are more likely associated with a primary cervical etiology and more amenable to mechanical support. The results of this trial confirmed the findings of the metaanalysis described above and established the utility of screening and ultrasound-indicated cerclage in selected women based on their *obstetric history*. Establishing the "optimal" cervical length for recommending cerclage in women with a prior spontaneous preterm birth and short cervix was not a primary goal of the trial, and will be the subject of future investigations.

Ultrasound-indicated versus history-indicated cerclage

Since a woman may present with a history consistent with the spontaneous preterm birth syndrome (and may have even undergone prior cerclage even though review of her prior pregnancy(ies) did not confirm a clinical diagnosis of insufficiency), investigators have questioned whether these patients fare better using vaginal ultrasound versus obstetric history as the chief indication for surgery. A systematic review by Blickman and colleagues [46] addressed this issue and included a thorough literature search and the selection of six relevant studies with various methodologies including cohort, case–control, and randomized designs. In none of these six reports was either strategy favored for preventing preterm birth at various gestational age cut-offs ranging from <24 to <37 weeks. In the ultrasound-indicated groups, cerclage was avoided in 40–68% of women who underwent ultrasound surveillance.

A more recent multicenter randomized trial [47] of women with at least one prior spontaneous birth <34 weeks demonstrated similar preterm birth outcomes <34 weeks in the history (15%) and ultrasound (15%) groups; however, in this trial fewer cerclage procedures were performed (19% versus 32%) in the history-indicated group. Women were randomly assigned to the history or ultrasound arm prior to clinician's assessment of the history and the diagnosis of insufficiency. While this trial confirmed the systematic review in that neither history nor ultrasound cerclage indication yields superior outcomes, the indications for cerclage in the history group were not thoroughly described (and reproducible), but rather left solely to clinician judgment.

In summary, when evaluating a patient with a history of spontaneous preterm birth in whom the indication for cerclage is questioned, ultrasound surveillance appears to decrease surgical interventions while yielding similar outcomes as history-indicated cerclage.

Postcerclage management

There are a number of empiric recommendations regarding physical activity after discharge. A limited interval (24–48 h) of mandatory bedrest is often advised in the immediate postoperative period. Pelvic rest and sexual abstinence for the remainder of gestation are widely prescribed. Because the use of bedrest in pregnancy as an effective therapy has been questioned [48], it seems reasonable to individualize this recommendation based on a patient's symptoms and physical findings. However, because women with cervical insufficiency and cerclage are still at increased risk for preterm birth, physically demanding occupations or prolonged standing should be curtailed.

In the absence of indications for earlier removal, the stitch should be removed around 37 weeks' gestation. Often performed in an outpatient setting, elective removal at term may be complicated by hemorrhage or difficulty locating the suture, which may have become embedded in the cervical stroma. Because it is generally buried under the bladder reflection, removal of a Shirodkar cerclage may be particularly troublesome. Difficult removal increases patient discomfort, and, at times, light conscious sedation may be required. Hemorrhage from the suture track may occur, but it can usually be controlled with direct pressure.

Because many women with clinically defined cervical insufficiency and cerclage remain at high risk for developing other components of the spontaneous preterm birth syndrome, indications for cerclage removal remote from term may develop. Patients with cerclage should be instructed on the symptoms of preterm labor and be able to present early for evaluation. Women with cerclage and preterm labor can be managed with tocolytic medications and should receive corticosteroids according to published guidelines. Nevertheless, if labor is progressive, the cerclage must be removed. This decision is made by the managing obstetrician based on serial examination of the cervix and lower uterine segment.

Preterm premature rupture of membranes (PPROM) complicates 25–30% of pregnancies managed with cerclage [18,37]. Uncontrolled retrospective series have demonstrated that, when the cerclage is removed on admission, perinatal outcomes are indistinguishable from similar cases of PPROM with no antecedent cerclage [49–51]. Other series have addressed the question of whether the cerclage should be left in place or removed immediately after spontaneous membrane rupture [52–54]. While these retrospective series cannot define optimal management, in the absence of clinical trial data confirming a benefit from leaving the cerclage in place after PPROM, the current weight of evidence suggests that the cerclage should be removed. Women with a periviable pregnancy might question whether cerclage removal is indicated, believing that it will maintain the pregnancy. In the absence of a well-controlled trial confirming harm from leaving the stitch *in situ*, individualization should be permitted.

Cerclage complications

The perceived simplicity and safety of transvaginal cerclage have made this treatment subject to empiric use, in spite of the risk of associated complications [55]. The most commonly reported complications associated with cerclage are membrane rupture and intrauterine infection. Bleeding may occur, but serious hemorrhage is generally limited to the cervicoisthmic procedure. Essentially all transvaginal cerclage procedures are performed under regional anesthesia, which has a low complication rate.

Harger [55] tabulated cerclage-associated complications reported in the past 40 years. Chorioamnionitis complicated 0.8–8% of elective (i.e. history-indicated) cerclage procedures and 9–37% of emergency procedures. Membrane rupture attributed to history-indicated cerclage was observed in 1–18% and was associated with up to 65% of emergency cases. Ultrasound-indicated cerclage has been associated with low rates of perioperative complications [44]. Whether cerclage alone can precipitate overt preterm labor seems doubtful. However, the foreign body might lower the threshold for uterine activity because of local inflammatory effects. Uterine activity often occurs in proximity to cerclage placement and women who have undergone cerclage are more likely to receive tocolytic agents during their gestation [24].

Adjunctive management strategies for cervical insufficiency

Alternative therapies for cervical insufficiency can be broadly classified as either providing mechanical support or administering pharmacologic measures to reduce inflammation and infection in order to maintain uterine quiescence. A review of older case series of cerclage indicated that progesterone (usually 17α-hydroxyprogesterone caproate) and, more recently, various tocolytic agents (usually indomethacin) and various prophylactic antibiotic regimens are widely prescribed adjuncts to cerclage. Whether these agents alone or in combination offer any therapeutic value is unknown, because none has been proved effective in controlled intervention trials. A recent retrospective analysis suggested that indomethacin was not effective in prolonging gestation when administered in the perioperative period as an adjunct to ultrasound-indicated cerclage [56]. Of the agents commonly prescribed in this clinical setting, progesterone appears to be the most promising [57–59]; however, it may not confer additional benefit to women undergoing ultrasound-indicated cerclage for short cervix [60].

Investigators in Europe and the USA have studied vaginal pessaries for the treatment of the incompetent cervix [61]. In 1961, Vitsky [62] proposed the mechanism whereby a lever pessary (Smith, Hodge, or Risser design) might be an effective treatment for the incompetent cervix. A vaginal pessary would displace the cervix posteriorly and shift the gravitational effects of the expanding uterine contents off the internal os and onto the anterior lower uterine segment. Interpretation of the clinical research in this area has been hampered by the frequent use of historic-control study designs, similar to those utilized in most series espousing the efficacy of cerclage. Likewise, the reported success rates of vaginal pessaries closely mirror those observed with cerclage and nominal success rates are in the 80–90% range [61]. Only one randomized trial has been located, and this was a German study published in 1986 by Forster *et al* [63]. In this trial, 250 women with cervical change suggesting insufficiency were randomized to cerclage or pessary (the type was not stated). The cerclage group and pessary group had term delivery rates of 69% and 62%, respectively. Another recent retrospective analysis of 36 women with midtrimester cervical shortening, managed either expectantly or with a Smith–Hodge pessary, showed a significant decrease in the incidence of preterm birth <35 weeks (0% versus 40%; P = 0.03) [64]. Although further comparative efficacy trials are needed, it would seem reasonable to recommend a trial of vaginal pessary in women with unclear histories or those who demonstrate progressive cervical change on serial midtrimester evaluations.

Conclusion

Contemporary lines of evidence indicate that cervical insufficiency is rarely a distinct and well-defined clinical entity, but only one component of a larger and more complex syndrome of spontaneous preterm birth. The original paradigm of obstetric and gynecologic trauma as a common antecedent of cervical insufficiency has been replaced by the recognition of *functional*, as opposed to *anatomic* deficits as the more prevalent etiology. Cervical *competence* functions along a continuum, influenced by both endogenous and exogenous factors that interact through various pathways with other recognized components of the preterm birth syndrome: uterine contractions and decidual activation/membrane rupture. Thus, the convenient term *cervical insufficiency* may actually represent an oversimplified, incomplete version of the broader pathophysiologic process.

CASE PRESENTATION

History

A 24-year-old para 0201 is seen for preconception counseling. Her obstetric history includes two prior spontaneous preterm births at 27 and 23 weeks' gestation. More careful questioning and review of records show that both deliveries were preceded by premature rupture of membranes. In her first pregnancy she was admitted at 26 weeks' gestation with PPROM and managed expectantly with prophylactic antibiotics, corticosteroids, and fetal surveillance. At 27 weeks she developed chorioamnionitis and underwent induction of labor. In her second pregnancy she experienced PPROM at 21 weeks and labor at 23 weeks. The liveborn infant succumbed to respiratory failure. Review of the placental pathology report showed chorioamnionitis, although she did not have puerperal fever.

Physical examination

Normal cervical anatomy with no palpable defect around the circumference. The cervical length to palpation is 1.5 cm. The external os appears parous but is firmly closed.

Assessment

Preterm birth syndrome (recurrent).

Plan

Discuss history-indicated cerclage versus serial cervical length assessment and ultrasound-indicated cerclage for cervical shortening. Adjunctive weekly progesterone (Delalutin) is also recommended beginning at 16 weeks.

Continued

Follow-up

In her next pregnancy, she develops cervical shortening (16 mm) at 21 weeks and undergoes McDonald cerclage. At 30 weeks she experiences PPROM; the cerclage is removed and the patient is managed expectantly in the hospital with antibiotics and corticosteroids. At 32 weeks she develops regular contractions, and the cervix is found to be 6 cm dilated. She undergoes a low transverse cesarean for breech presentation. The infant has a 3-week neonatal ICU course, but survives with no long-term sequelae.

References

1. Palmer R, Lacomme M. La béance de l'orifice interne, cause d'avortements à répétition? Une observation de déchrure cervico-isthmique répareeé chirurgicalement, avec gestation à terme consécutive. Gynecol Obstet 1948;47:905–906.

2. Lash AF, Lash SR. Habitual abortion: the incompetent internal os of the cervix. Am J Obstet Gynecol 1950;59:68–76.

3. Shirodkar VN. A new method of operative treatment for habitual abortions in the second trimester of pregnancy. Antiseptic 1955;52:299–300.

4. McDonald IA. Suture of the cervix for inevitable miscarriage. J Obstet Gynecol Br Empire 1957;64:346–353.

5. Benson RC, Durfee RB. Transabdominal cervico-uterine cerclage during pregnancy for the treatment of cervical incompetency. Obstet Gynecol 1965;25:145–155.

6. Romero R, Espinoza J, Kusanovic JP et al. The preterm parturition syndrome. Br J Obstet Gynaecol 2006;113(Suppl 3):17–42.

7. Danforth DN, Buckingham JC. Cervical incompetence: a re-evaluation. Postgrad Med 1962;32:345–351.

8. Dunn LJ, Dans P. Subsequent obstetrical performance of patients meeting the historical criteria for cervical incompetence. Bull Sloan Hosp Women 1962;7:43–45.

9. Iams JD, Johnson FF, Sonek J, Sachs L, Gebauer C, Samuels P. Cervical competence as a continuum: a study of ultrasonography cervical length and obstetric performance. Am J Obstet Gynecol 1995;172:1097–1106.

10. Iams JD, Goldenberg RL, Meis PJ et al. The length of the cervix and the risk of spontaneous premature delivery. N Engl J Med 1996;334:567–572.

11. Buckingham JC, Buethe RA, Danforth DN. Collagen–muscle ratio in clinically normal and clinically incompetent cervixes. Am J Obstet Gynecol 1965;91:232–237.

12. Ayers JWR, DeGrood RM, Compton AA, Barclay M, Ansbacher R. Sonographic evaluation of cervical length in pregnancy: diagnosis and management of preterm cervical effacement in patients at risk for premature delivery. Obstet Gynecol 1988;71:939–944.

13. Craigo SD. Cervical incompetence and preterm delivery [editorial]. N Engl J Med 1996;334:595–596.

14. Olah KS, Gee H. The prevention of preterm delivery: can we afford to continue to ignore the cervix? Br J Obstet Gynaecol 1992;99:278–280.

15. Romero R, Gomez R, Sepulveda W. The uterine cervix, ultrasound and prematurity [editor's comments]. Ultrasound Obstet Gynecol 1992;2:385–388.

16. Barter RH, Dusbabek JA, Riva HL, Parks J. Surgical closure of the incompetent cervix during pregnancy. Am J Obstet Gynecol 1958;75:511–524.

17. Jennings CL. Temporary submucosal cerclage for cervical incompetence: report of forty-eight cases. Am J Obstet Gynecol 1972;113:1097–1102.

18. Kuhn R, Pepperell R. Cervical ligation: a review of 242 pregnancies. Aust N Z J Obstet Gynaecol 1977;17:79–83.

19. Ferenczy A, Choukroun D, Falcone T, Franco E. The effect of cervical loop electrosurgical excision on subsequent pregnancy outcome: North American experience. Am J Obstet Gynecol 1995;172:1246–1250.

20. Althuisius SM, Shornagel GA, Dekker GA, van Geijn HP, Hummel P. Loop electrosurgical excision procedure of the cervix and time of delivery in subsequent pregnancy. Int J Gynecol Obstet 2001;72:31–34.

21. Weber T, Obel E. Pregnancy complications following conization of the uterine cervix. Acta Obstet Gynecol Scand 1979;58:259.

22. Raio L, Ghezzi F, di Naro E, Gomez R, Luscher K. Duration of pregnancy after carbon dioxide laser conization of the cervix: influence of cone height. Obstet Gynecol 1997;90:978–982.

23. Sadler L, Saftlas A, Wang W, Exeter M, Whittaker J, McCowan L. Treatment for cervical intraepithelial neoplasia and risk of preterm delivery. JAMA 2004;291:2100–2106.

24. Final report of the Medical Research Council/Royal College of Obstetrics and Gynaecology multicentre randomized trial of cervical cerclage. Br J Obstet Gynaecol 1993;100:516–523.

25. Mangan CE, Borow L, Burtnett-Rubin MM, Egan V, Giuntoi RL, Mijuta JJ. Pregnancy outcome in 98 women exposed to diethylstibestrol in utero, their mothers, and unexposed siblings. Obstet Gynecol 1982;59:315–319.

26. Branch DW. Operations for cervical incompetence. Clin Obstet Gynecol 1986;29:240–254.

27. Cousins JM. Cervical incompetence: 1980. A time for reappraisal. Clin Obstet Gynecol 1980;23:467–479.

28. Cardwell MS. Cervical cerclage: a ten-year review in a large hospital. South Med J 1988;81:15.

29. Hofmeister FJ, Schwartz WR, Vondrak BF, Martens W. Suture reinforcement of the incompetent cervix. Am J Obstet Gynecol 1968;101:58–65.

30. Aarts JM, Jozien T, Brons J, Bruinse HW. Emergency cerclage: a review. Obstet Gynecol Surv 1995;50:459–469.

31. Novy MJ, Gupta A, Wothe DD, Gupta S, Kennedy KA, Gravett MG. Cervical cerclage in the second trimester of pregnancy: a historical cohort study. Am J Obstet Gynecol 2002;186:594–596.

32. Olatunbosun OA, AL-Nuaim L, Turnell RW. Emergency cerclage compared with bed rest for advanced cervical dilatation in pregnancy. Int Surg 1995;80:170–174.

33. Kokia E, Dor J, Blankenstein J et al. A simple scoring system for treatment of cervical incompetence diagnosed during the second trimester. Gynecol Obstet Invest 1991;31: 12–16.

34. Althuisius SM, Dekker GA, Hummel P, van Geijn HP. Cervical incompetence prevention randomized cerclage trial: emergency cerclage with bed rest versus bed rest alone. Am J Obstet Gynecol 2003;189:907–910.

35. Romero R, Gonzalez R, Sepulveda W et al. Infection and labor. VIII. Microbial invasion of the amniotic cavity in patients with suspected cervical incompetence: prevalence and clinical significance. Am J Obstet Gynecol 1992;167:1086–1091.

36. Mays JK, Figuerioa R, Shah J, Khakoo H, Kaminsky S, Tejani N. Amniocentesis for selection before rescue cerclage. Obstet Gynecol 2000;95:652–655.

37. Treadwell MC, Bronsteen RA, Bottoms SF. Prognostic factors and complication rates for cervical cerclage: a review of 482 cases. Am J Obstet Gynecol 1991;165:555–558.

38. Weiner CP, Lee KY, Buhimschi CS, Christner R, Buhimschi IA. Proteomic biomarkers that predict the clinical success of rescue cerclage. Am J Obstet Gynecol 2005;192:710–718.

39. Romero R, Kusamovic JP, Espinoza J et al. What is amniotic fluid "sludge"? Ultrasound Obstet Gynecol 2007;30: 793–798.

40. Althuisius SM, Dekker GA, van Geijn HP, Bekedam DJ, Hummel P. Cervical Incompetence Prevention Randomized Cerclage Trial (CIPRACT): study design and preliminary results. Am J Obstet Gynecol 2000;183:823–829.

41. Rust OA, Atlas RO, Reed J, van Gaalen J, Balducci J. Revisiting the short cervix detected by transvaginal ultrasound in the second trimester: why cerclage may not help. Am J Obstet Gynecol 2001;185:1098–1105.

42. To MS, Alfirevic Z, Heath VCF et al, on behalf of the Fetal Medicine Foundation Second Trimester Screening Group. Cervical cerclage for prevention of preterm delivery in women with short cervix: randomised controlled trial. Lancet 2004;363:1849–1853.

43. Berghella V, Odibo AO, Tolosa JE. Cerclage for prevention of preterm birth in women with a short cervix found on transvaginal ultrasound: a randomized trial. Am J Obstet Gynecol 2004;191:1311–1317.

44. Owen J, Hankins G, Iams JD et al. Multicenter randomized trial of cerclage for preterm birth prevention in high-risk women with shortened midtrimester cervical length. Am J Obstet Gynecol 2009;201:375.

45. Berghella V, Odibo AO, To MS, Rust OA, Althuisius SM. Cerclage for short cervix on ultrasonography, meta-analysis of trials using individual patient-level data. Obstet Gynecol 2005;106(1):181–189.

46. Blickman MJC, Le T, Bruinese HW, Geert JM, van der Heijden MG. Ultrasound-predicted versus history-predicated cerclage in women at risk of cervical insufficiency: a systematic review. Obstet Gynecol Surv 2008;63:803–812.

47. Simcox R, Seed PT, Bennett P, Teoh TG, Poston L, Shennan AH. A randomized controlled trial of cervical scanning vs history to determine cerclage in women at high risk of preterm birth (CIRCLE trial). Am J Obstet Gynecol 2009; 200:623.

48. Goldenberg RL, Cliver SP, Bronstein J, Cutter GR, Andrews WA, Mennemeyer ST. Bed rest in pregnancy. Obstet Gynecol 1994;84:131–136.

49. Blickstein I, Katz Z, Lancet M, Molgilner BM. The outcome of pregnancies complicated by preterm rupture of the membranes with and without cerclage. Int J Obstet Gynecol 1989;28:237–242.

50. Yeast JD, Garite TR. The role of cervical cerclage in the management of preterm premature rupture of the membranes. Am J Obstet Gynecol 1988;158:106–110.

51. McElrath TF, Norwitz ER, Lieberman ES, Heffner LJ. Perinatal outcome after preterm premature rupture of membranes with in situ cervical cerclage. Am J Obstet Gynecol 2002;187: 1147–1152.

52. Ludmir J, Bader T, Chen L, Lindenbaum C, Wong G. Poor perinatal outcome associated with retained cerclage in patients with premature rupture of membranes. Obstet Gynecol 1994;84:823–826.

53. Jenkins TM, Berghella V, Shlossman PA et al. Timing of cerclage removal after preterm premature rupture of membranes: maternal and neonatal outcomes. Am J Obstet Gynecol 2000; 183:847–852.

54. McElrath TF, Norwitz ER, Lieberman ES, Heffner LJ. Management of cervical cerclage and preterm premature rupture of the membranes: should the stitch be removed? Am J Obstet Gynecol 2000;183:840–846.

55. Harger JH. Cerclage and cervical insufficiency: an evidenced-based analysis. Obstet Gynecol 2002;100:1313–1327.

56. Visintine J, Airoldi J, Berghella V. Indomethacin administration at the time of ultrasound-indicated cerclage: is there an association with a reduction in spontaneous preterm birth? Am J Obstet Gynecol 2008;198(6):643.

57. Sherman AI. Hormonal therapy for control of the incompetent os of pregnancy. Obstet Gynecol 1966;28:198–205.

58. Keirse MJNC. Progesterone administration in pregnancy may prevent preterm delivery. Br J Obstet Gynaecol 1990;97: 149–154.

59. Meis PJ for the NICHD MFMU Network. Prevention of recurrent preterm delivery by 17 alpha-hydroxyprogesterone caproate prevents recurrent preterm birth. N Engl J Med 2003;348:2379–2385.

60. Berghella V, Figueroa D, Szychowski JM et al, for the Vaginal Ultrasound Trial Consortium. 17-alpha-hydroxyprogesterone caproate for the prevention of preterm birth in women with prior preterm birth and a short cervical length. Am J Obstet Gynecol 2010;202(4):351.

61. Newcomer J. Pessaries for the treatment of incompetent cervix and premature delivery. Obstet Gynecol Surv 2000; 55:443–448.

62. Vitsky M. Simple treatment of the incompetent cervical os. Am J Obstet Gynecol 1961;81:1194–1197.

63. Forster F, Dunng R, Schwarzlus G. Therapy of cervix insufficiency: cerclage or support pessary? Zentralbl Gynaekol 1986;108:230–237.

64. Broth R, Pereira L, Slepian J, Berghella V. Role of pessary in management of patients with cervical shortening [Abstract 211]. Am J Obstet Gynecol 2002;187:S118.

Chapter 35
Gestational Hypertension, Preeclampsia, and Eclampsia

Labib M. Ghulmiyyah and Baha M. Sibai
Department of Obstetrics and Gynecology, University of Cincinnati College of Medicine, Cincinnati, OH, USA

Hypertension is the most common medical disorder arising during pregnancy [1]. Approximately 70% of women diagnosed with hypertension during pregnancy will have gestational hypertension/preeclampsia. The term "preeclampsia" is used to describe a wide spectrum of patients who may have only mild elevation in blood pressure (BP) or severe hypertension with end-organ dysfunction, including acute gestational hypertension, preeclampsia, eclampsia, and hemolysis, elevated liver enzymes, low platelet count (HELLP) syndrome.

Gestational hypertension

Gestational hypertension is defined as a systolic BP of at least 140 mmHg and/or a diastolic BP of at least 90 mmHg on at least two occasions at least 4–6 h apart after the 20th week of gestation in women known to be normotensive before pregnancy and before 20 weeks' gestation. The BP recordings used to establish the diagnosis should be obtained no more than 7 days apart [2]. Gestational hypertension is considered severe if there are sustained elevations in systolic BP to at least 160 mmHg and/or in diastolic BP to at least 110 mmHg for at least 6 h [1,3]. Some women with gestational hypertension will subsequently progress to preeclampsia. The rate of progression depends on gestational age at time of diagnosis; the rate reaches 50% when gestational hypertension develops before 30 weeks' gestation [4].

Preeclampsia

Preeclampsia is primarily defined as gestational hypertension plus proteinuria (greater than 300 mg/24-h period) [1]. If a 24-h urine collection is not available, then proteinuria is defined as a concentration of at least 30 mg/dL (at least +1 on dipstick) in at least two random urine samples collected at least 6 h apart. The urine measurements used to establish proteinuria should be taken no more than 7 days apart [2].

The concentration of urinary protein in random urine samples is highly variable. Recent studies have found that urinary dipstick determinations correlate poorly with the amount of proteinuria found in 24-h urine determinations in women with gestational hypertension [5]. Therefore, the definitive test to diagnose proteinuria is a quantitative protein excretion in a 24-h period. Severe proteinuria is defined as protein excretion of at least 5 g/24-h period, but in clinical practice this may be difficult to ascertain. Urine dipstick values should not be used to diagnose severe proteinuria [1,6]. In the absence of proteinuria, preeclampsia should be considered when gestational hypertension is associated with persistent cerebral symptoms, epigastric or right upper quadrant pain with nausea or vomiting, thrombocytopenia or abnormal liver enzymes. These women are considered to have atypical preeclampsia [7].

Preeclampsia is considered severe if there is severe gestational hypertension in association with abnormal proteinuria or if there is hypertension in association with severe proteinuria (at least 5 g/24-h period). In addition, preeclampsia is considered severe in the presence of multiorgan involvement such as pulmonary edema, seizures, oliguria (i.e. urine output less than 500 mL/24-h period), thrombocytopenia (platelet count less than 100,000/mm^3), abnormal liver enzymes in association with persistent epigastric or right upper quadrant pain, or persistent severe central nervous system symptoms (altered mental status, headaches, blurred vision, or blindness) [1].

Queenan's Management of High-Risk Pregnancy: An Evidence-Based Approach, Sixth Edition. Edited by John T. Queenan, Catherine Y. Spong, Charles J. Lockwood.
© 2012 John Wiley & Sons, Ltd. Published 2012 by John Wiley & Sons, Ltd.

Perinatal outcomes

Gestational hypertension

In general, the majority of cases of mild gestational hypertension develop at or beyond 37 weeks' gestation, and thus pregnancy outcome is similar to that seen in women with normotensive pregnancies. On the other hand, maternal and perinatal morbidities are substantially increased in women with severe gestational hypertension. Indeed, these women have higher morbidities than women with mild preeclampsia. The rates of abruptio placentae, preterm delivery (at less than 37 and 35 weeks), and small for gestational age (SGA) infants in women with severe gestational hypertension are similar to those seen in women with severe preeclampsia. Therefore, these women should be managed as if they had severe preeclampsia [1,8].

Preeclampsia

The perinatal death rate and rates of preterm delivery, SGA infants, and abruptio placenta in women with mild preeclampsia are similar to those of normotensive pregnancies. The rate of eclampsia is less than 1%, but the rate of cesarean delivery is increased to 40–50% because of increased rates of induction of labor. In contrast, perinatal mortality and morbidities as well as the rates of abruptio placentae are substantially increased in women with severe preeclampsia. The rate of neonatal complications is markedly increased in those who develop severe preeclampsia in the second trimester (80–90%), whereas it is minimal in those with severe preeclampsia beyond 35 weeks' gestation (10–20%).

Severe preeclampsia is also associated with increased risk of maternal mortality (0.2%) and increased rates of maternal morbidities (5%) such as convulsions, pulmonary edema, acute renal or liver failure, liver hemorrhage, disseminated intravascular coagulopathy, and stroke. These complications are usually seen in women who develop preeclampsia before 32 weeks' gestation and in those with preexisting medical conditions [1,9].

Etiology and pathophysiology

The etiology of preeclampsia remains an obstetric enigma. Some of the suggested causes include inadequate endovascular remodeling of uterine spiral arteries, immunologic intolerance between fetoplacental and maternal tissues, maladaptation to cardiovascular changes, excess inflammatory changes of pregnancy, abnormal angiogenesis, and genetic abnormalities [8]. Some reported pathophysiologic abnormalities of preeclampsia include placental ischemia, generalized vasospasm, abnormal hemostasis with activation of the coagulation system, vascular endothelial dysfunction, abnormal nitric oxide

and lipid metabolism, leukocyte activation, and changes in various cytokines and growth factors. There is substantial evidence suggesting that the pathophysiologic abnormalities of preeclampsia are caused by abnormal angiogenesis, particularly an imbalance in the soluble fms-like tyrosine kinase-1 (sFlt-1):placental growth factor (PLGF) ratio [10]. In addition, serum levels of endoglin are also elevated before and after the onset of preeclampsia. Moreover, some authors have reported that soluble endoglin contributes to the pathogenesis of preeclampsia by amplifying the endothelial damage caused by sFlt-1 in pregnant women with severe preeclampsia [10].

Management

The objective of management in women with gestational hypertension/preeclampsia must always be safety of the mother and then delivery of a mature newborn who will not require intensive and prolonged neonatal care. This can only be achieved with a plan that takes into consideration one or more of the following: the severity of the disease process, fetal gestational age, maternal and fetal status at time of the initial evaluation, presence of labor, and the wishes of the mother [1].

Mild hypertension or preeclampsia

Once the diagnosis of mild gestational hypertension or mild preeclampsia is made, subsequent therapy will depend on the results of maternal and fetal evaluation. (A suggested algorithm for management of mild preeclampsia is described in Figure 35.1.) In general, women with mild disease developing at 37 weeks' gestation or after have a pregnancy outcome similar to that found in normotensive pregnancy. These patients should undergo induction of labor for delivery [11].

All patients with mild preeclampsia at less than 37 weeks should receive maternal and fetal evaluation at the time of their diagnosis. Maternal evaluation includes measurements of blood pressure, weight, and urine protein, and questioning about symptoms of headache, visual disturbances, and epigastric pain.

Laboratory evaluation includes determinations of hematocrit, platelet counts, liver enzyme levels, and a 24-h urine collection once a week. This evaluation is important because patients may develop thrombocytopenia and abnormal liver enzyme levels with minimal BP elevations. Fetal evaluation should include ultrasonography to determine fetal growth and amniotic fluid volume every 3 weeks, daily fetal movement count ("kick count"), and nonstress testing (NST) at least once weekly.

Patients are instructed to take a regular diet with no salt restriction. Diuretics, antihypertensive drugs, and sedatives are not used. Several studies indicate that these

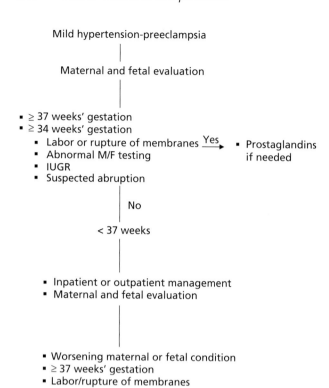

Mild hypertension-preeclampsia

|

Maternal and fetal evaluation

|

- ≥ 37 weeks' gestation
- ≥ 34 weeks' gestation
  - Labor or rupture of membranes <u>Yes</u> → • Prostaglandins if needed
  - Abnormal M/F testing
  - IUGR
  - Suspected abruption

No

|

< 37 weeks

|

- Inpatient or outpatient management
- Maternal and fetal evaluation

|

- Worsening maternal or fetal condition
- ≥ 37 weeks' gestation
- Labor/rupture of membranes

Figure 35.1 Recommended management of mild gestational hypertension or preeclampsia. IUGR, intrauterine growth restriction; M/F, maternal/fetal.

Box 35.1 Indication for delivery in mild preeclampsia

- Gestational age greater than or equal to 37 weeks
- Gestational age greater than or equal to 34 weeks with:
  - Labor
  - Rupture of membranes
  - Vaginal bleeding
  - Persistent headaches or visual symptoms
  - Epigastric pain, nausea, vomiting
- Abnormal biophysical profile
- Criteria for severe preeclampsia met

---

agents do not improve pregnancy outcome, and may increase the incidence of fetal growth restriction [1].

With expectant management, patients are instructed to be on restricted but not complete bedrest, to have BP checked daily and to report symptoms of severe disease.

The women are usually seen twice weekly for evaluation of maternal BP, urine protein, and symptoms of impending eclampsia. Maternal and fetal evaluation is performed once or twice weekly in an ambulatory testing unit. Any evidence of disease progression or development of acute severe hypertension is an indication for prompt hospitalization. Indications for delivery are summarized in Box 35.1.

In women with mild gestational hypertension, fetal evaluation should include an NST and an ultrasound examination of estimated fetal weight and amniotic fluid index. If the results are normal, then there is no need for repeat testing unless there is a change in maternal condition (progression to preeclampsia or severe hypertension) or there is decreased fetal movement or abnormal fundal height growth [1].

Severe preeclampsia

The presence of severe preeclampsia mandates direct admission to labor and delivery. Magnesium sulfate should be administered intravenously to prevent convulsions and antihypertensive medications should be given to lower severe levels of hypertension (systolic pressure greater than 160 mmHg and/or diastolic pressure of at least 110 mmHg). The aim of the antihypertensive therapy is to keep systolic BP at 140–155 mmHg and diastolic BP at 90–105 mmHg and prevent potential cerebrovascular and cardiovascular complications [1–3].

During the observation period, maternal and fetal conditions are assessed and a plan of management formulated regarding the need for delivery. If the patient is less than 34 weeks, betamethasone 12 mg IM is administered × two doses 24 h apart. A suggested algorithm for management of severe preeclampsia is described in Figure 35.2 [12].

Expectant management of severe preeclampsia

There is disagreement about treatment of patients with severe preeclampsia before 34 weeks' gestation where maternal condition is stable and fetal condition is reassuring [12]. In such patients, some authors consider delivery as the definitive treatment regardless of gestational age, whereas others recommend prolonging pregnancy until development of maternal or fetal indications for delivery, achievement of fetal lung maturity or at 34 weeks' gestation. Expectant management is safe in properly selected women with severe disease, although maternal and fetal conditions can deteriorate rapidly. Hospitalization and daily monitoring are required. These pregnancies involve higher rates of maternal morbidity and significant risk of neonatal morbidity. For this reason, expectant management should proceed only in a tertiary care center with adequate maternal and neonatal facilities.

These patients should be advised of the potential risks and benefits of expectant management, which requires daily monitoring of maternal and fetal conditions. It should be explained that the decision to continue expectant management will be revisited on a daily basis and that the median number of days of pregnancy prolongation in these cases is 7 days (range 2–35 days) [12].

A plan for a vaginal delivery should be attempted for all women with mild disease and for the majority of

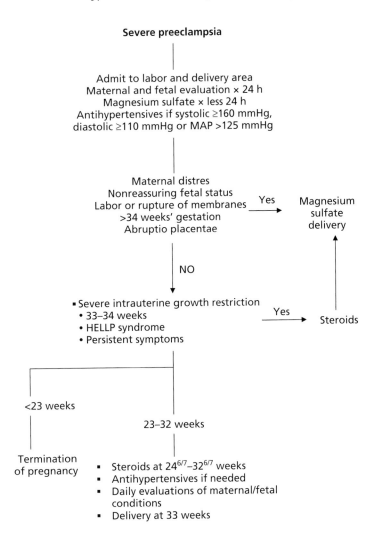

Figure 35.2 Recommended management of severe preeclampsia. MAP, mean arterial pressure; Maternal distress: imminent eclampsia, pulmonary edema, disseminated coagulopathy, eclampsia, acute renal failure. Reproduced from Sibai and Barton [12] with permission from Elsevier.

women with severe disease, particularly those beyond 30 weeks' gestation [2]. Cesarean delivery should be based on fetal gestational age, fetal condition, presence of labor, and cervical Bishop score. The presence of severe pre-eclampsia is not an indication for cesarean delivery. However, elective cesarean section is recommended for women with severe disease below 30 weeks' gestation who are not in labor with a Bishop score of less than 5. Women with severe preeclampsia and fetal growth restriction with unfavorable cervix at less than 32 weeks' gestation are better delivered by cesarean section.

Postpartum management

These women usually receive large amounts of intravenous fluids during labor, as a result of prehydration before the administration of epidural analgesia, and intravenous fluids given during the administration of oxytocin and magnesium sulfate in labor and in the postpartum period. In addition, during the postpartum period there is mobilization of extracellular fluid leading to increased intravascular volume. As a result, women with severe preeclampsia – particularly those with abnormal renal

function, those with capillary leaks, and those with early onset – are at increased risk for pulmonary edema and exacerbation of severe hypertension postpartum. These women should receive frequent evaluation of the amount of intravenous fluids, oral intake, blood products, and urine output as well as monitoring by pulse oximetry and pulmonary auscultation.

In general, in most women with gestational hypertension, the BP becomes normotensive during the first week postpartum. In contrast, in women with preeclampsia, the hypertension takes longer to resolve. In addition, in some women with preeclampsia there is an initial decrease in BP immediately postpartum, followed by development of hypertension again between days 3 and 6. Use of antihypertensive drugs is recommended if the systolic BP is at least 155 mmHg and/or if the diastolic BP is at least 105 mmHg. The drug of choice is oral nifedipine (10 mg every 6 h) or long-acting nifedipine (30–60 mg bid) to keep BP below that level. If BP is well controlled and there are no maternal symptoms, the woman is then discharged home with instructions for daily BP measurements by a home visiting nurse for the first week postpartum or longer, as necessary. Antihypertensive medications are discontinued if the pressure remains below the hypertensive levels for at least 48 h [1].

Hemolysis, elevated liver enzymes, low platelet count syndrome

This term describes preeclamptic patients having hemolysis, elevated liver enzymes, and a low platelet count. The HELLP syndrome has been recognized for many years as a complication of severe preeclampsia/eclampsia [13]. Our criteria for the diagnosis of HELLP syndrome include laboratory findings summarized in Box 35.2.

Approximately 90% of patients with HELLP syndrome are first seen remote from term, complaining of epigastric or right upper quadrant pain. Approximately half have nausea or vomiting, and others have nonspecific viral syndrome-like symptoms. Hypertension or proteinuria may be absent or mild. Thus, some patients may display various signs and symptoms not diagnostic of severe preeclampsia. Consequently, for all pregnant women having any of these symptoms, it is advisable to obtain a complete blood count, platelet count, and liver enzymes [13].

Some patients may first be seen because of jaundice, gastrointestinal bleeding, hematuria, or bleeding from the gums. As a result, these patients are often misdiagnosed as having viral hepatitis, gallbladder disease, peptic ulcer disease, kidney stones, glomerulonephritis, acute fatty liver of pregnancy, idiopathic or thrombotic thrombocytopenia purpura, or hemolytic uremic syndrome [14].

Perinatal outcomes and management

The presence of HELLP syndrome is associated with an increased risk of maternal death (1%) and increased rates of maternal morbidities such as pulmonary edema (8%), acute renal failure (3%), disseminated intravascular coagulopathy (15%), abruptio placentae (9%), liver hemorrhage or failure (1%), adult respiratory distress syndrome,

sepsis, and stroke (less than 1%). Pregnancies complicated by HELLP syndrome are also associated with increased rates of wound hematomas and the need for transfusion of blood and blood products. The development of HELLP syndrome in the postpartum period further increases the risk of renal failure and pulmonary edema [13].

The reported perinatal death rate in recent series is in the range 7.4–20.4%. This high perinatal death rate is mainly experienced at very early gestational age (less than 28 weeks), in association with severe fetal growth restriction or abruptio placentae. Neonatal morbidities are dependent on gestational age at the time of delivery and they are similar to those in preeclamptic pregnancies without the HELLP syndrome. The rate of preterm delivery is approximately 70%, with 15% occurring before 28 weeks' gestation [13].

Patients with the syndrome at less than 37 weeks should be referred to a tertiary care center and managed initially as any patient with severe preeclampsia. The first priority is to assess the mother's condition and stabilize it, particularly if she has coagulation abnormalities. The next step is to investigate fetal well-being with a nonstress test and biophysical profile or Doppler assessment of fetal vessels. Finally, the decision must be made whether or not immediate delivery is indicated. A suggested algorithm for management is summarized in Figure 35.3 [13]. Delivery may be delayed for 24–48 h prior to 34 weeks' gestation to administer corticosteroids if the patient is asymptomatic and the fetus has reassuring testing. High-dose steroids have been shown to improve platelet counts transiently in undelivered women with HELLP. However, these studies did not report improvement in clinically important maternal morbidity such as the need for platelet transfusion, pulmonary, renal, or hepatic complications [15]. In addition, a double-blind, placebo-controlled trial revealed no benefit from high-dose corticosteroids in women with HELLP syndrome [16].

Maternal and fetal conditions are assessed continuously during this period. In some of these patients, there may be transient improvement in maternal laboratory tests but delivery is still indicated despite such improvement.

HELLP syndrome is not an indication for cesarean delivery, although cesarean delivery may be acceptable prior to 32 weeks' gestation with an unfavorable cervix, because of an anticipated long induction time in a clinically deteriorating gravida. Ripening agents as well as oxytocin can be used to initiate labor with a favorable cervix after 30 weeks. If thrombocytopenia is severe, regional anesthesia and pudendal blocks may be contraindicated. In this situation, intravenous narcotics can still be administered for analgesia during labor.

Maintain platelet counts greater than 20,000/μL for vaginal delivery and 40,000/μL for cesarean delivery. If platelets fall below 40,000/μL prior to cesarean delivery, be prepared to administer platelets just prior to surgery

---

Box 35.2 Recommended criteria for HELLP syndrome

- Hemolysis (at least two of these findings):
  - Peripheral smear (schistocytes, burr cells)
  - Serum bilirubin (greater than or equal to 1.2 mg/dL)
  - Low serum haptoglobin
  - Severe anemia, unrelated to blood loss
- Elevated liver enzymes:
  - AST or ALT greater than or equal to twice upper level of normal
  - LDH greater than or equal to twice upper level of normal
- Low platelets (less than 100,000/mm³)

ALT, alanine aminotransferase; AST, aspartate aminotransferase; LDH, lactic dehydrogenase.

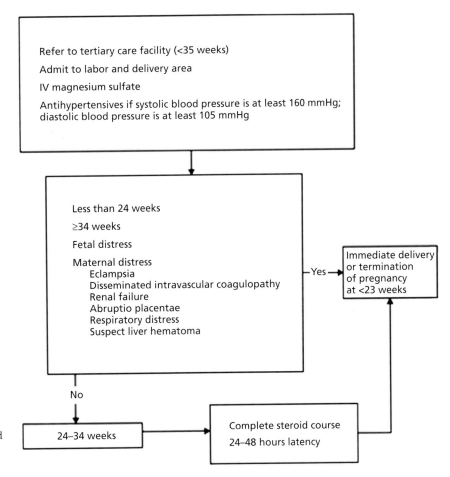

Figure 35.3 Management of HELLP (hemolysis, elevated liver enzymes, and low platelet count) syndrome. Reproduced from Sibai [13] with permission from Lippincott Williams and Wilkins.

and/or intraoperatively. At the time of skin incision, 6–10 units of platelets are usually administered, and an additional 6 units are administered if oozing is noted during surgery. Depending on the platelet count and degree of oozing, leave the bladder flap open and place an intraperitoneal and/or subcutaneous closed suction drain through a separate stab wound in an attempt to prevent wound hematomas. Box 35.3 summarizes the steps taken in cesarean delivery.

After delivery, patients with HELLP syndrome should receive close monitoring of vital signs, fluid intake and output, laboratory values, and pulse oximetry for at least 48h. Intravenous magnesium sulfate prophylaxis should be continued for 48h.

The clinical and laboratory findings of HELLP syndrome may develop for the first time in the postpartum period. In these patients, the time of onset of the manifestations ranges from a few hours to 7 days, with the majority developing within 48h postpartum. Hence, all postpartum women and healthcare providers should be educated as to the signs and symptoms of HELLP syndrome. The treatment of patients with postpartum HELLP syndrome should be similar to that in the antepartum period, including the use of magnesium sulfate [13,15].

Box 35.3 Cesarean delivery in HELLP syndrome

- Epidural anesthesia
  - Platelet count greater than75,000/μL
- General anesthesia
- Platelet transfusion if necessary
  - 6–10 units
  - Platelet count less than 40,000/μL
  - In operating room at time of surgery
- Vesicouterine peritoneum left open
- Subfascial drain if oozing at time of surgery and/or platelet count less than 40,000/μL
- Skin closure
  - Subcutaneous drain (closed system)
  or
  - Secondary closure 3 days later
- Perioperative transfusions as needed
- Intensive monitoring for 48h postpartum

Eclampsia

Eclampsia is defined as the onset of seizures and/or unexplained coma during pregnancy or postpartum in patients with signs and symptoms of preeclampsia. Although most cases (90%) present in the third trimester or within 48 h following delivery, rare cases (1.5%) have been reported at or prior to 20 weeks and as late as 23 days postpartum. The diagnosis of eclampsia is straightforward in the presence of hypertension, proteinuria, generalized edema, and convulsions. However, these patients could present with a broad spectrum of signs, ranging from severe hypertension (20–54%), severe proteinuria and generalized edema (48%), to absent or mild hypertension (30–60%), absent proteinuria (14%), and no edema (26%) [17].

Other symptoms may occur before or after the onset of seizures, including persistent frontal or occipital headaches (50–75%), blurred vision (19–32%), photophobia, epigastric/right upper quadrant pain, and altered mental status. All these symptoms in the presence of the abovementioned risk factors should keep the physician watchful for development of eclampsia [14].

Management

The cardinal steps in the management of eclampsia are as follows. Do not attempt to arrest the first seizure, especially when no intravenous access or skilled personnel for rapid intubation are available. First, support maternal respiratory and cardiovascular functions to prevent hypoxia. Establish airway patency and maternal oxygenation during or immediately after the acute episode. Even if the initial seizure is short, it is important to maintain oxygenation by supplemental oxygen administration via facemask with or without a reservoir at 8–10 L/min because hypoventilation followed by respiratory acidosis often occurs. Pulse oximetry is advisable to monitor oxygenation in these patients. Arterial blood gas analysis is required if the pulse oximetry is abnormal (saturation less than 92%) [17].

Second, prevent maternal injury and aspiration by securing the bed's side rails by elevating them and making sure they are padded. Place the patient in the lateral decubitus position to minimize aspiration of oral secretions and vomitus in the event of emesis.

Third, intravenous magnesium sulfate should be started to treat and prevent further seizures. The recommended regimen is to give a loading dose of 6 g over 15–20 min followed by a continuous infusion of 2 g/h. Ten percent of patients might have a second convulsion after receiving magnesium sulfate. In this case, another 2 g bolus of magnesium sulfate can be given intravenously over 3–5 min. If the patient is still having seizure activity after adequate magnesium sulfate dosing, 250 mg sodium amobarbital may be given intravenously over 3–5 min. Be watchful for magnesium toxicity in women with abnormal renal function. Signs and symptoms and management of magnesium toxicity are given in Box 35.4.

Fourth, it is important to reduce and maintain blood pressure in a safe range. The goal is to keep systolic BP at 140–160 mmHg and diastolic BP at 90–110 mmHg. This

---

Box 35.4 Magnesium toxicity

Manifestations

- Loss of patellar reflex (8–12 mg/dL)
- Feeling of warmth, flushing (9–12 mg/dL)
- Somnolence (10–12 mg/dL)
- Slurred speech (10–12 mg/dL)
- Muscular paralysis (15–17 mg/dL)
- Respiratory difficulty (15–17 mg/dL)
- Cardiac arrest (30–35 mg/dL)

Management

- Discontinue magnesium sulfate
- Obtain magnesium (serum) level
- If magnesium level greater than 15 mg/dL:
  - Give 1 g calcium gluconate IV
  - Intubate
  - Assist ventilation

---

can be achieved with intravenous bolus doses of 5–10 mg hydralazine or 20–40 mg labetalol every 15 min, as needed, or 10–20 mg nifedipine orally every 30 min to a maximum dosage of 50 mg in 1 h. Sodium nitroprusside or nitroglycerine is rarely needed in eclampsia. Diuretics are not used except in the setting of pulmonary edema.

Finally, begin induction of labor within 24 h. It is important to keep in mind that the presence of eclampsia is not an indication for cesarean delivery. The patient should not be rushed to the operating room, especially if maternal condition is not stable. It is to the fetus' advantage to be resuscitated *in utero* first. However, if bradycardia or persistent late decelerations occur despite resuscitative measures then a diagnosis of abruptio placentae or nonreassuring fetal status should be considered. The decision to proceed with cesarean delivery after maternal stabilization is based on the fetal gestational age, fetal condition, presence of labor, and cervical Bishop score. Cesarean delivery is recommended for those with eclampsia before 30 weeks, who are not in labor, and have a Bishop score below 5. Patients in labor or with ruptured membranes are allowed to deliver vaginally in the absence of obstetric complications. Labor can be induced with either oxytocin or prostaglandins in all patients after 30 weeks' gestation irrespective of Bishop score.

During the convulsion there is usually a prolonged deceleration and/or bradycardia. Following the convulsion and as a result of maternal hypoxia and hypercarbia, fetal heart rate monitoring might show compensatory tachycardia, decreased beat-to-beat variability, and transient late decelerations [17]. Additionally, uterine contraction monitors demonstrate increase in both uterine tone and frequency. The duration of the increased uterine activity varies from 2 to 14 min (Box 35.5). Because the fetal heart rate pattern usually returns to normal after a

Box 35.5 Transitory changes associated with eclamptic convulsions

- Uterine hyperactivity
- Increased frequency of contractions
- Increased uterine tone
- Duration of contraction greater than or equal to 2 min
- Fetal heart rate changes
- Bradycardia
- Compensatory tachycardia
- Decreased beat-to-beat variability
- Late decelerations

convulsion, other conditions should be considered if an abnormal pattern persists. It may take longer for the heart rate pattern to return to baseline in an eclamptic woman whose fetus is preterm with growth restriction. Abruptio placentae may occur after the convulsion and should be considered if uterine hyperactivity remains, if there are repetitive late decelerations, or fetal bradycardia persists.

Magnesium sulfate should be continued for at least 24 h after delivery and/or after the last convulsion. In the presence of renal insufficiency, rates of both fluid administration and doses of magnesium sulfate should be reduced. After delivery, oral antihypertensive medication can be used to maintain systolic BP below 155 mmHg and diastolic BP below 105 mmHg. Starting 200 mg labetalol every 8 h (maximum dose 2400 mg/day) or 10 mg nifedipine every 6 h (maximum dose 120 mg/day) is recom-

mended. Oral nifedipine offers a beneficial diuretic effect in the postpartum period. There are no risks from the combined use of magnesium sulfate and oral nifedipine [17].

Prediction and prevention of preeclampsia

Numerous clinical, biophysical, and biochemical tests have been proposed for the prediction or early detection of preeclampsia. Unfortunately, most of these tests suffer from poor sensitivity and poor positive predictive values, and the majority of them are not suitable for routine use in clinical practice. At present, there is no single screening test that is considered reliable and cost-effective for predicting preeclampsia [9].

During the past two decades, numerous clinical reports and randomized trials have described the use of various methods to reduce the rate and/or severity of preeclampsia. Based on the available data, neither calcium supplementation nor low-dose aspirin should be routinely prescribed for preeclampsia prevention in nulliparous women. In addition, zinc, magnesium, fish oil, and vitamins C and E should not be routinely used for this purpose. Even in studies reporting beneficial effects, the results reveal reductions in a "definition of preeclampsia" without concomitant improvement in perinatal outcome [9].

CASE PRESENTATION

A 20-year-old white primigravida at 35w 5d of gestation with an uneventful prenatal course was referred to labor and delivery by ambulance with severe preeclampsia. She had been complaining of headache and visual disturbance for the last 2 days. Her past medical/surgical and social history was completely negative. Upon admission, her BP was 180/110 mmHg. She had 2+ protein on urine dipstick. Bedside ultrasound confirmed a singleton intrauterine pregnancy consistent with 35 weeks' gestation. Fetal heart rate tracing was in the 150 beat/min range with moderate variability. Cervical examination revealed a Bishop score of 7.

Intravenous access was secured and laboratory tests were obtained for complete blood count, including platelet count, liver enzymes, and a metabolic profile. A loading dose of 6 g magnesium sulfate was given intravenously over 20 min which was followed by a maintenance dose of 2 g/h. Because of her severe hypertension, an intravenous 10 mg bolus of hydralazine was administered. Blood pressures were monitored every 5–10 min; after 30 min, BP was 150 mmHg systolic and 105 mmHg diastolic. Maternal urine output and reflexes were moni-

tored every hour. The results of the blood tests revealed a platelet count of 110,000/mm^3, a hematocrit of 38%, and normal liver enzymes. Once maternal and fetal conditions were considered stable, intravenous oxytocin was started to initiate labor.

The patient subsequently underwent a spontaneous vaginal delivery of an infant weighing 2650 g with Apgar scores of 6 and 9 at 1 and 5 min, respectively. Postpartum magnesium sulfate was continued for 24 h. In addition, maternal vital signs, intake, and urine output as well as patellar reflexes were monitored every hour. She was started on 10 mg oral nifedipine every 6 h because of elevated blood pressures. Three days postpartum, she was discharged home to be seen in 1 week at the outpatient clinic.

Because this patient was diagnosed with severe preeclampsia at 35w 5d of gestation, she was not a candidate for steroid injections or expectant management. She was started on magnesium sulfate for seizure prophylaxis and antihypertensive medications to stabilize blood pressure and induction of labor was initiated.

References

1. Sibai BM. Diagnosis and management of gestational hypertension and preeclampsia. Obstet Gynecol 2003;102:181–192.
2. National High Blood Pressure Education Program. Working group report on high blood pressure in pregnancy. Am J Obstet Gynecol 2000;183:S1–S22.
3. American College of Obstetricians and Gynecologists. Diagnosis and management of preeclampsia and eclampsia. Obstet Gynecol 2001;98:159–167.
4. Barton JR, Sibai BM. Prediction and prevention of recurrent preeclampsia. Obstet Gynecol 2008;112(2 Pt 1):359–372.
5. Kyle PM, Fielde JN, Pullar B. Comparison of methods to identify significant proteinuria in pregnancy in the outpatient setting. Br J Obstet Gynaecol 2008;115:523–527.
6. Lindheimer MD, Kanter D. Interpreting abnormal proteinuria in pregnancy. The need for a more pathophysiological approach. Obstet Gynecol 2010;115:365–375.
7. Sibai BM, Stella CA. Diagnosis and management of atypical preeclampsia-eclampsia. Am J Obstet Gynecol 2009;200:481.
8. Buchbinder A, Sibai BM, Caritis S, Macpherson C, Hauth J, Lindheimer MD. Adverse perinatal outcomes are significantly higher in severe gestational hypertension than in mild preeclampsia. Am J Obstet Gynecol 2002;186:66–71.
9. Sibai B, Dekker G, Kupferminc M. Preeclampsia. Lancet 2005;365:785–799.
10. Khankin EV, Royle C, Karumanchi SA. Placental vasculature in health and disease. Semin Thromb Hemost 2010;36:309–320.
11. Koopmans CM, Biglenga D, Groen H et al, for the HYPITAT Study Group. Induction of labour versus expectant monitoring for gestational hypertension or mild pre-eclampsia after 36 weeks' gestation (HYPITAT): a multicentre, open-label randomised controlled trial. Lancet 2009;374:979–988.
12. Sibai BM, Barton JR. Expectant management of severe preeclampsia remote from term: patient selection, treatment and delivery indications. Am J Obstyet Gynecol 2007;196:514.
13. Sibai BM. Diagnosis, controversies, and management of the syndrome of hemolysis, elevated liver enzymes, and low platelet count. Obstet Gynecol 2004;1035:981–991.
14. Sibai BM. Imitators of severe pre-eclampsia. Semin Perinatol 2009;33(3):196–205.
15. Martin JN Jr, Thigpen BD, Rose CH, Cushman J, Moore A, May WL. Maternal benefit of high-dose intravenous corticosteroid therapy for HELLP syndrome. Am J Obstet Gynecol 2003;189:830–834.
16. Fonseca JE, Mendez F, Catano C, Arias F. Dexamethasone treatment does not improve the outcome of women with HELLP syndrome: a double-blind, placebo-controlled, randomized clinical trial. Am J Obstet Gynecol 2005;193:1591–1598.
17. Sibai BM. Diagnosis, prevention, and management of eclampsia. Obstet Gynecol 2005;105:402–410.

Chapter 36
Postpartum Hemorrhage

Michael A. Belfort

Department of Obstetrics and Gynecology, Baylor College of Medicine, Houston, TX, USA

Postpartum hemorrhage (PPH) remains one of the leading causes of maternal death, in both industrialized and non-industrialized nations. Approximately 140,000 women die annually from PPH worldwide, and more than 50% of these mortalities occur within the first 24 h postpartum [1–3]. In the USA, 12% of all maternal mortality is due to obstetric hemorrhage [4].

Recent reports from Europe [5,6] have highlighted the seriousness of the "near miss" and the importance of close monitoring of such cases in any quality assurance program. In most cases substandard care was indentified. The ratio of severe maternal morbidity to maternal mortality is almost 27:1 [5].

Primary (early) PPH refers to excessive blood loss (>500 mL) during the third stage of labor or in the first 24 h after delivery; thereafter, significant bleeding is referred to as secondary (late) PPH. The incidence of significant PPH rises after 30 min in the third stage [7] and active intervention to deliver the placenta between 30 and 60 min into the third stage is advised.

The main causes of PPH include retained placenta/ adherent placenta, uterine atony, placenta accreta/ percreta, upper (uterus, cervix) tract tears and rupture, and lower (vagina, perineum) genital tract trauma, uterine inversion, retained placental tissue, acquired coagulopathy, and disseminated intravascular coagulation (DIC). Major reductions in the frequency and severity of PPH have followed the adoption of routine prophylactic administration of oxytocics in the management of the third stage [8].

Retained and trapped placenta

Retained placenta (more common in preterm deliveries) is diagnosed using a cut off of 1 h [9]. Manual removal occurs in approximately 1–2% of deliveries and is the management of choice when there is active bleeding and a low risk of morbidly adherent placentatation. Clinical endometritis is more common (compared with spontaneous delivery – 7% versus 2%) [9] following manual removal of the placenta, and antibiotic treatment should be instituted. In the absence of active hemorrhage, there is no urgency to resort to manual removal, and potential placenta accreta or percreta should always be considered before any such attempt.

Trapped placenta, as opposed to retained placenta, usually follows rapid contraction of the uterus (oxytocic induced) and the clinical findings include a small, contracted fundus, some vaginal bleeding and cord lengthening indicative of placental separation, and the placental margin often palpable through the closed cervical os. On ultrasound examination, the entire myometrium is thickened and a clear demarcation may be seen between it and the placenta [10]. Delivery of a trapped placenta can usually be achieved using controlled cord traction, which encourages cervical dilation, with or without IV glyceryl trinitrate (100–200 µg) [11]. Releasing the cord clamp, to allow blood trapped in the placenta to drain, may also help.

Adherent placenta

An adherent placenta is not caused by pathologic invasion of the placenta into the uterine muscle, and should not be confused with placenta accreta. On ultrasound, the myometrium appears thick and contracted in all areas (except where the placenta remains attached), and the uterine wall remains less than 2 cm thick [10]. Detachment usually starts in the lower part of the uterus and is associated with bleeding from the placental bed [12]. In the absence of bleeding, a conservative approach can be adopted and manual removal of the placenta can be

Queenan's Management of High-Risk Pregnancy: An Evidence-Based Approach, Sixth Edition. Edited by John T. Queenan, Catherine Y. Spong, Charles J. Lockwood.
© 2012 John Wiley & Sons, Ltd. Published 2012 by John Wiley & Sons, Ltd.

postponed while the problem is investigated (by ultrasound).

When there is heavy bleeding, immediate active management is necessary. Oxytocin is administered via the umbilical vein (first-line recommendation by the WHO) [13], using the Pipingas technique (nasogastric tube in the umbilical vein with prostaglandin $F_{2\alpha}$ (20 mg diluted in 20 mL of normal saline) or oxytocin (30 IU diluted in 20 mL of normal saline) injected through the catheter [14,15].

Uterine atony

Fundal massage and bimanual compression are effective and useful as initial maneuvers for the management of uterine atony. Following vaginal delivery, in cases of life-threatening massive hemorrhage, this may be combined with external aortic compression [16].

Medical treatment of uterine atony

The prophylactic use of uterotonic drugs is an effective means of preventing postpartum hemorrhage from uterine atony [17]. These drugs include oxytocin, methylergonovine and ergot alkaloids, E and F class prostaglandins as well as misoprostol.

Oxytocin

Oxytocin has specific uterine receptors and intravenous administration (dose 5–10 IU) results in immediate onset of action [18]. The mean plasma half-life is 3 min and continuous intravenous infusion is needed to ensure sustained contraction. The usual concentration is 20–40 units per liter of crystalloid, with the infusion rate titrated to response. Steady-state concentration is reached after 30 min. Intramuscular injection has a time to onset of 3–7 min, with a longer clinical effect (30–60 min). Most studies report that oxytocin alone reduces the need for additional medications, and that oxytocin is associated with fewer adverse side-effects [19].

Oxytocin is metabolized by both the liver and kidneys. Because it has approximately 5% of the antidiuretic effect of vasopressin, if given in large volumes of electrolyte-free solution, oxytocin can cause water toxicity (headache, vomiting, drowsiness, and convulsions), symptoms that may be mistakenly attributed to other causes. Rapid administration of an intravenous bolus of oxytocin (5–10 U) results in relaxation of vascular smooth muscle. Hypotension with a reflex tachycardia may occur, followed by a small but sustained increase in blood pressure. In addition, bolus doses have been associated with electrocardiogram (ECG) abnormalities (ST depression) as reduction in cerebral perfusion pressure. Oxytocin is stable at temperatures up to 25°C, but refrigeration may prolong shelf-life.

Methylergonovine/ergometrine

Methylergonovine (methylergometrine) and its parent compound ergometrine result in sustained tonic contraction of uterine smooth muscle by stimulation of α-adrenergic myometrial receptors [18]. The dose of methylergonovine is 0.2 mg, and that of ergometrine is 0.2–0.5 mg. These doses may be repeated in 2–4 h if needed. The onset of action is within 2–5 min when given intramuscularly. These drugs are extensively metabolized in the liver and the mean plasma half-life is approximately 30 min. Plasma levels do not correlate with uterine effect, since the clinical action of ergometrine is sustained for 3 h or more. When oxytocin and ergometrine derivatives are used together, two different mechanisms are in play, oxytocin producing an immediate response and ergometrine a more sustained action. Nausea and vomiting are common side-effects. Vasoconstriction of vascular smooth muscle also occurs as a consequence of their α-adrenergic action. This can result in elevation of central venous pressure and systemic blood pressure and in the risk of pulmonary edema, stroke, and myocardial infarction.

Contraindications include heart disease, autoimmune conditions associated with Raynaud phenomenon, peripheral vascular disease, arteriovenous shunts even if surgically corrected, and hypertension. Women with preeclampsia/eclampsia are particularly at risk of severe and sustained hypertension. These agents should not be used intravenously except perhaps in individualized extreme circumstances (moribund, shocked patient with no other alternative).

Prostaglandins

Prostaglandin $F_{2\alpha}$ results in contraction of smooth muscle cells [18]. Hemabate (carboprost or 15-methyl prostaglandin $F_{2\alpha}$ is an established second-line treatment for postpartum hemorrhage unresponsive to oxytocic agents. It is available in single-dose vials of 0.25 mg and is given by deep intramuscular injection or by direct injection into the myometrium, either under direct vision at cesarean section or transabdominally/transvaginally after vaginal delivery. It is not licensed for the latter route and caution should be exercised to prevent direct injection into a uterine sinus [20]. It may be more effective in shocked patients, when tissue hypoperfusion may compromise absorption following intramuscular injection [21]. A second dose may be given after 90 min or if atony and hemorrhage continue, repeat doses may be given every 15 min to a maximum of 8 doses (2 mg).

F-class prostaglandins cause bronchoconstriction, venoconstriction, and constriction of gastrointestinal smooth muscle. Associated side-effects include nausea, vomiting, diarrhea, pyrexia, and bronchospasm. There are case reports of hypotension and intrapulmonary shunting with arterial oxygen desaturation, and prostaglandin $F_{2\alpha}$

is contraindicated in patients with known cardiac or pulmonary disease.

Prostaglandin E$_2$ (dinoprostone) is generally a vasodilatory prostaglandin; however, it causes contraction of smooth muscle in the pregnant uterus [18]. Dinoprostone is available as an intravaginal pessary (10 mg) and as a vaginal suppository (20 mg) or gel (0.5 mg) for cervical ripening. Rectal administration (2 mg given 2 hourly) has been successful as a treatment for uterine atony. Due to its vasodilatory effect, this drug should be avoided in hypotensive and hypovolemic patients. However, it may be useful in women with heart or lung disease in whom carboprost is contraindicated [22].

Misoprostol

Misoprostol is a synthetic analog of prostaglandin E$_1$ and is metabolized in the liver. The tablet(s) can be given orally, vaginally, or rectally. As prophylaxis for postpartum hemorrhage, an international multicenter randomized trial reported that oral misoprostol is less successful than parenteral oxytocin administration [23]. Misoprostol may, however, be of benefit in treating postpartum hemorrhage. In a recent metaanalysis, oral or sublingual misoprostol at a dose of 600 μg was found to be useful in postpartum hemorrhage but did not demonstrate a benefit over other uterotonics [24].

Mechanical and surgical control of bleeding

If bleeding continues following use of uterotonics and despite adequate uterine contraction, exploration of the genital tract is necessary to detect other causes such as trauma (uterine, cervical, or vaginal tears) or retained placental tissue, particularly in cases where risk factors were present (i.e. obstructed labor, fetal distress, difficult operative delivery, manual removal of placenta). Persisting with the exclusive use of manual uterine compression and oxytocic administration in the face of continuous hemorrhage is not advised. If these measures fail to control bleeding, progressively invasive and sometimes ablative surgical solutions may be required.

Uterine tamponade

Small studies have demonstrated that uterine packing is effective for controlling hemorrhage refractory to other medical treatment [25,26]. Historically, uterine packing was performed using sterile gauze, with up to 5 m of 5–10 cm gauze introduced into the uterus, either using a specific packing instrument or long forceps [27]. Packs are generally left *in situ* for 24–36 h and prophylactic antibiotics are advised. Concerns have been raised about concealed bleeding, infection, trauma, and inadequate packing, but there is a paucity of evidence to support these concerns, and the risks may be overstated [27,28].

Several inflatable mechanical devices are now being used for uterine tamponade. These temporizing devices may allow for correction of coagulopathy in anticipation of, or during, surgical intervention. They may completely control the bleeding and should be considered in cases where future fertility is desired. They may also be lifesaving in low-resource areas. A continuous oxytocin infusion (with or without other uterotonic agents) and prophylactic antibiotic coverage are advised when using these devices. It is possible that balloon tamponade acts by more than one mechanism, including direct pressure on the open venous channels, stretching and compression of the atonic myometrium, increasing intramuscular vascular resistance, and by direct compression of the arteries supplying the uterus [29,30].

Uterine brace sutures

There are a number of uterine brace sutures that are variants of the B-Lynch suture which was designed to vertically compress the uterine body in cases of uterine atony [31–34]. In order to assess whether the suture will be effective, bimanual compression is applied to the uterus. If bleeding stops, compression with a brace suture should be equally successful. Most commonly, a 70 mm round-bodied needle with number 2 chromic catgut suture is used. Normal uterine anatomy has been demonstrated on follow-up [35]. Resumption of normal menses along with uncomplicated pregnancies following the B-Lynch procedure for postpartum hemorrhage have also been described [35]. Unexpected occlusion of the uterine cavity with subsequent development of infection (pyometria) has been reported with the occlusive square-stitch [36]. A summary of studies on brace sutures was published in 2001 [37].

Uterine devascularization

Uterine devascularization has been used for stepwise management of postpartum hemorrhage due to atony, placenta previa, and trauma [38]. These techniques can also be used prophylactically in the operating room (OR) at the time of delivery in pregnancies complicated by placenta accreta. Ligation procedures of the uterine arteries, internal iliac arteries, and ovarian arteries have been described [38,39]. A vaginal route for uterine artery ligation has also been reported, with moderate success [38].

Internal iliac artery ligation has been shown to decrease distal arterial pulse pressure by 85%, with a 24% reduction in mean arterial pressure [40]. In addition, a 48% reduction in blood flow resulted following ipsilateral ligation. It is generally accepted that internal iliac artery ligation controls pelvic hemorrhage mainly by decreasing arterial pulse pressure and by transforming the arterial system into a venous-like circulation. As a result, clot formation is more likely to occur at the site of injury with arrest of the bleeding. Complications of this procedure include damage to the internal iliac vein and to the ureter. Tissue edema, ongoing hemorrhage, and the presence of a large atonic uterus may make identification of anatomy difficult and prolong operating time. The author has found that traction on the postpartum uterus in a caudal direction and adequate exposure of the common iliac bifurcation allows opening of the retroperitoneal space directly over the distended internal iliac artery (as opposed to a more indirect passage from the lateral broad ligament). It should be remembered that in some cases (accreta and percreta), the internal iliac artery may be a larger diameter vessel than the external iliac artery and absolute identification is critical. Incorrect identification of the internal iliac artery may result in accidental ligation of the external or common iliac artery, resulting in lower limb and pelvic ischemia. Femoral or pedal pulses should therefore be checked before and after the procedure. Recanalization of ligated vessels may occur, and successful pregnancy has been reported whether or not recanalization has taken place. Success rates are generally reported to be approximately 40% [41].

Arterial embolization

Uterine devascularization by selective arterial embolization using pledgets of absorbable gelatin sponge can effect a temporary blockade with resorption within approximately 10 days [42]. If the site of bleeding cannot be identified, embolization of the anterior branch of the internal iliac artery or the uterine artery is performed. Uterine atony and pelvic trauma have been indications for embolization, and overall success rates of 85–100% are reported [43,44]. Higher failure rates are associated with placenta accreta and following failed bilateral internal iliac artery ligation. Subsequent successful pregnancies have been documented [38]. Fever, contrast media renal toxicity, and leg ischemia are rare but reported complications of this procedure.

A variation on this theme is the prophylactic placement of inflatable balloon catheters in the internal iliac arteries of patients who are expected to bleed excessively at the time of surgery, for example elective cesarean delivery in a patient with placenta percreta [42]. This practice may result in opening deeper and more inaccessible collateral vessels in the pelvis and may not be as helpful as initially thought.

It should be clearly understood that arterial embolization should not be used in a critically unstable and profusely bleeding patient. This technique is best suited to those patients with persistent bleeding amenable to embolization who are hemodynamically stable and who, it is anticipated, can be maintained that way for at least a few hours with transfusion and drug support. In most cases, these procedures are performed in an interventional radiology suite that is not staffed or equipped for the management of a critical and unstable bleeding patient. There may be significant delays in instituting the embolization, difficult or impossible access depending on the surgery already performed, and an uncertain result.

Severe hemorrhage uncontrolled by medical means and tamponade procedures requires decisive and definitive surgical treatment in an operating room setting. In those operating rooms equipped for intraoperative embolization, combined surgical and radiological procedures may be appropriate.

Hysterectomy

Peripartum hysterectomy is frequently considered the definitive procedure for obstetric hemorrhage, but is not without complications. The procedure can be complicated by ongoing blood loss and grossly distorted pelvic anatomy due to edema, abnormal vascularization and dilated vessels, retroperitoneal and other hematoma formation, and trauma. Adequate hemostasis is not always easily achieved, and further procedures may be necessary. Relook laparotomy may also be required; this has been reported in up to 13% of patients [45]. The incidence of febrile morbidity is high, with rates of 5–85% in different series.

The interval between delivery and successful surgery is a very important prognostic factor, and if a primary procedure (such as brace suture or devascularization) fails, hysterectomy should be undertaken promptly, without attempts at other conservative measures [46]. In severely shocked patients with life-threatening hemorrhage, hysterectomy is in most circumstances the first-line treatment [41].

A subtotal hysterectomy can be performed if bleeding is from the uterine body, and it is generally simpler than a total hysterectomy. The cervix and vaginal angles can be difficult to identify in women who have labored to full dilation, and a subtotal hysterectomy has less risk of injury to the ureters and bladder (13%) compared with total hysterectomy (25%) [47]. If placenta accreta/percreta is suspected, the use of preoperatively placed ureteral stents will help determine the location of the ureters, and can be extremely useful when dealing with difficult dissection planes and distorted anatomy. In addition, intraoperative intentional cystotomy may improve visualization of bladder invasion. If the bleeding is from the lower segment (placenta previa/accreta, trauma) and cervix, the cervical branch of the uterine artery will usually have to be ligated, and a total hysterectomy will usually be necessary.

In almost all cases, general endotracheal anesthesia is best because of prolonged surgical time, need for abdominal packing, extensive surgical dissection and manipulation, and anticipated massive blood transfusion. Prophylaxis for thromboembolism should be initiated before surgery. Compression stockings placed before induction of anesthesia and the use of compression devices during surgery are important [47]. Intraoperative prevention of extreme hypotension, hypothermia, hypoxia, acidosis, and coagulopathy are critical anesthesia-related issues. Postpartum monitoring should in most cases be in an intensive care unit setting. Because of prolonged operative time combined with massive transfusion, there is an increased risk of laryngeal edema, pulmonary edema, delayed extubation, and prolonged ventilation. Continuous vital sign determination (including respiratory rate and pulse oximetry) along with meticulous urine output measurement is warranted after significant hemorrhage and blood product replacement. Patients with periods of prolonged hypotension during surgery should also be followed postoperatively for evidence of the partial or full Sheehan syndrome.

Pelvic pressure pack

The pelvic pressure pack, also known as the "mushroom," "umbrella" or "Logothetopoulos" pack, has been successfully used for control of posthysterectomy hemorrhage in both gynecologic and obstetric patients. The most common method of construction involves the use of a sterile radiology plastic bag filled with gauze bandages tied together (Fig. 36.1). The bag is inserted abdominally and the open end is passed through the vaginal cuff and out of the vagina. It is then placed on traction to fit the pack snugly into the pelvic bowl and compress the pelvic structures. Once bleeding has abated, the bandage can be gradually removed from the bag which is then pulled out of the vagina. Although studies are limited, the success rate of the pelvic pressure pack in the control of posthysterectomy bleeding in obstetrics has approached 86% after other therapies were attempted [49].

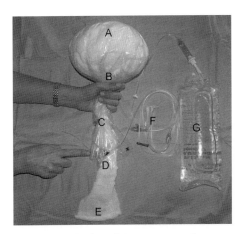

Figure 36.1 Photograph of a pelvic pressure pack, as constructed from an x-ray cassette drape, sterile gauze rolls, and an intravenous infusion setup. A, dome of the pack. B, base of pack located above vaginal cuff. C, neck of pack located in vagina. D, continuous gauze roll exiting neck of pack. E, end of gauze. F, intravenous tubing. G, 1 liter intravenous fluid bag. Reproduced from Dildy *et al* [49] with permission from Wolters Kluwer Health.

Placenta accreta/percreta

Placenta accreta is a condition in which all or part of the placenta is adherent to the uterine wall because of myometrial invasion by chorionic villi. The definition, incidence and risk factors, pathophysiology, and clinical presentation are discussed in Chapter 45. In this chapter specific aspects of management are covered.

Management options

Known placenta percreta

Once the diagnosis is established, the treatment options and potential complications should be clearly discussed with the patient and the discussion should be documented. The delivery is preferably handled using a dedicated and practiced team of clinicians and support staff.

Preoperative consultation with blood bank personnel is essential given the expected intraoperative blood loss of at least 3000–5000 mL and in some cases much more [48,50,51]. These patients frequently will require more blood products than the average hospital blood bank has in stock. It is recommended that adequate amounts of packed red blood cells (PRBCs), fresh frozen plasma (FFP), platelets, and cryoprecipitate should be available to prevent (or treat) coagulopathy [48]. It is also advisable to have recombinant factor VIIa in the operating room at the time of the surgery. When autotransfusion (cell-saver) blood is used, it is recommended that there be double washing of the recovered blood, which should only be suctioned after double irrigation of the abdominal cavity following delivery [52]. Attention should also be paid to the volume of reinfused washed PRBCs to ensure that adequate FFP, cryoprecipitate, and platelets are given along with the cell-saver blood because of the lack of these products in the reconstituted red cells.

Preoperative anesthesia consultation is essential to allow appropriate planning and allocation of personnel. Anesthetic considerations include the need for general endotracheal anesthesia in anticipation of prolonged surgical time, consideration of a lumbothoracic epidural catheter for postpartum pain relief, and readiness for massive blood and blood product transfusion. The anesthesia service will be primarily responsible during the surgery for preventing the deadly triad of hypovolemia, hypothermia, and acidosis that increases the risk for coagulopathy. Shock trauma fluid infusion devices capable of high flow rate transfusion of blood products, adequate central venous access (bilateral central line sheaths with quadruple catheter capability), arterial line placement, and multiple suction devices should all be part of the anesthesia preparation. In addition, thromboembolism prophylaxis should also be initiated before surgery.

Bladder involvement is extremely common in anterior placenta previa with accreta/percreta and in such cases there is frequently hypervascularity and distortion of the ureterovesical junction. In such cases preoperative cystoscopy and placement of ureteric stents allow palpation of the ureters during difficult and often obscured surgery. In those cases where there is obvious penetration of the trophoblast into the bladder wall, it is helpful to create an intentional cystotomy in an uninvolved area of the bladder and directly visualize the area of invasion. This allows for a better appreciation of the extent of the bladder invasion and for protection of the trigone and ureterovesical junction. Another benefit is that it allows the surgeon to simply excise that portion of the bladder involved in the percreta under direct vision without the risk of inadvertently increasing the hemorrhage during blind dissection of percreta tissue.

Preoperative pelvic artery occlusion has been proposed as an adjunct to minimize blood loss at the time of hysterectomy [53]. Others have determined that preoperative placement of balloon catheters in the internal iliac arteries has not proven useful and the inflation of the balloons after delivery may actually complicate the hysterectomy by opening up collateral vessels deeper in the pelvis that are more difficult to control than the immediate branches of the internal iliac artery [54]. The placement of balloon catheters may also add to the complexity of the surgery, and can potentially result in significant complications such as insertion site hematoma, precipitation of unanticipated fetal decompensation, insertion site abscess formation, and tissue infarction and necrosis.

Gynecologic oncology, urology and general and vascular surgery consultants should be recruited as necessary for assistance in cases of placenta accreta/percreta. These specialists are invaluable when major pelvic vessel, lateral pelvic side wall, bladder, or bowel invasion has occurred.

Most planned cases of cesarean hysterectomy for adherent placenta will be performed between 34 and 35 weeks of gestation and neonatal personnel should be present [55].

Specific intraoperative management suggestions include the following.
• Low lithotomy positioning with an assistant placed between the patient's legs.
• Vertical skin incision (median or paramedian) dependent on the site of placental invasion.
• Vertical upper segment uterine incision (fundal or posterior classical).
• Avoid disturbing the placenta during delivery of the baby.
• No attempts should be made to remove the placenta. The umbilical cord should be tied off and replaced within the uterus. The uterus should then be closed in a single layer with a locked suture.

• Minimize the chances of inadvertent partial placental separation or placental disruption before the major supplying vessels are ligated and the uterus is devascularized. Minimize manipulation of the uterus and specifically the lower segment.
• Infiltrate the upper segment and noninvolved myometrium with 15-methyl-prostaglandin $F_{2\alpha}$ (250 μg of carboprost tromethamine (Hemabate) in 20 cc saline) given through a 22 gauge spinal needle in multiple areas to facilitate contraction to prevent loss of a significant amount of blood into the uterine cavity during the surgery. A red rubber catheter can be used as a tourniquet above the level of the placental edge to help compress the uterus [48].
• Large abdominal retractor (Bookwalter or similar) should be optimally placed, the bowel packed away and pelvic visualization optimized before proceeding with definitive surgery.
• The vagina should also be packed with gauze after delivery of the baby since this helps with elevating the cervix and lower uterine segment into the pelvis, and also shows the vaginal fornices more clearly, preventing unnecessary removal of vaginal tissue.
• After delivery of the baby and contraction of the uterus, a reevaluation of the extent of the placental invasion may show that any attempts at surgical removal will be more risky than anticipated. A flexible approach is important. A placenta percreta that has penetrated the lateral wall of the uterus and is deeply invading the lateral pelvic side wall may be deemed impossible to remove without damaging vital structures or causing uncontrollable bleeding. In such cases, as long as the patient is stable and not actively bleeding from the placenta (i.e. partial separation), the safest approach may be to close the abdomen and manage the patient conservatively (see below), or transfer her to another facility that may be in a better position to deal with the problem.
• Hysterectomy using careful systematic stepwise devascularization.
• Avoid making any holes in the peritoneal covering of the placenta which is usually all that covers the highly vascular placental tissue. Caution should be exercised with placement of instruments, positioning of clamps (especially the tip), pressure from finger tips on areas of placental invasion when grasping the uterus during exposure or traction.
• Careful dissection of the retroperitoneal space and modified radical hysterectomy with removal of the uterus along with a significant portion of the broad ligament and lateral structures.
• In anterior percreta into the bladder, an intentional cystotomy should be made to identify the extent of the involved bladder wall [48]. This region can then be excised and left attached to the uterus, as long as it does not involve the trigone. The bladder can then

be reconstituted. This technique avoids unnecessary bleeding that will occur with attempted dissection of adherent bladder. If the trigone and ureters are involved, reimplantation may be needed.

• Avoid supracervical hysterectomy in true placenta previa percreta because of the risk of disruption of the vascular channels supplying the placenta. Collateral blood supply to the uterus and cervix via the bladder, bowel, pelvic side wall or other organs attached to the placenta may still lead to massive hemorrhage from the uterus if a supracervical hysterectomy is attempted too early in the process.

Intraoperative blood product and fluid administration

A full discussion of blood product replacement strategies in massive hemorrhage in pregnancy is beyond the scope of this chapter. In patients with massive hemorrhage from trauma, early and extensive use of FFP and platelets, in a 1:1:1 ratio with PRBCs, is of benefit in terms of reducing mortality [56]. There are no comparable published data for use of this ratio in obstetrics, but the empiric use of early FFP in a 1:1 ratio with PRBCs in massive obstetric hemorrhage is potentially a strategy that could be of benefit, and one deserving of investigation.

The associated potentially acute metabolic effects of massive transfusion should also be kept in mind. These include hypothermia, citrate toxicity, and hyperkalemia.

Activated factor VII

There are many case reports and case series regarding the use of recombinant activated factor VII for control of hemorrhage in massive obstetric bleeding. The data are generally encouraging although caution is still advised since serious adverse events such as thromboembolism and myocardial infarction have been noted [57]. The dose is generally between 60 and 90 μg/kg, and a median dose of 72 μg/kg has been shown to be effective in stopping or reducing bleeding in nearly 90% of reported cases [58].

Persistent hemorrhage

Aortic clamping

Temporary compression of the infrarenal (or infradia-phragmatic) aorta can decrease blood loss and allow time for resuscitation with blood products during resuscitation [48,59].

Pelvic pressure pack

In those cases where there is refractory pelvic bleeding after hysterectomy, placement of a pelvic pressure pack should be considered. This temporizing step has been shown to be effective in allowing hemodynamic stabilization of the patient and correction of coagulopathy [49] (see Fig. 36.1).

Internal iliac artery embolization

There have been a number of reports suggesting that this technique is the preferred method for managing persistent but noncatastrophic bleeding [60]. The author is, however, personally aware of a number of cases of severe morbidity associated with complications from attempted selective embolization under emergency conditions in unstable patients. These patients suffered hepatic, pancreatic, splenic, gluteal, and limb ischemia that required emergency surgery and resulted in permanent injury. As with any salvage procedure, individualization is essential. Embolization (internal iliac or uterine) is not a procedure that should be used in a hemodynamically unstable patient (as discussed above). Rapid control of bleeding is essential in such situations and definitive surgical therapy (or temporizing maneuvers – see below) is generally the best route for management.

Temporizing management in uncontrolled hemorrhage

When uncontrolled massive pelvic bleeding occurs after the hysterectomy, temporary cessation of surgery, infrarenal aortic clamping, pelvic packing, closure of the skin with towel clips, aggressive resuscitation with blood products, reversal of acid–base imbalances, and patient warming can be life saving. Desperate efforts to stop persistent oozing from hidden bleeding points in the face of coagulopathy is time consuming, may worsen the situation and will lead to hypothermia, acidosis, and hemodynamic collapse. It is preferable to slow the blood loss using temporizing methods such that resuscitation becomes effective, the coagulopathy is reversed, and surgery can be resumed under controlled circumstances. Temporizing may involve keeping the patient on the operating room table or, if appropriate, transport to an adjacent intensive care unit until return to the operating room is possible. The placement of wide-bore pelvic drains is important in this situation to warn of persistent significant bleeding.

Postoperative management

Patients who have had prolonged surgery and undergone massive transfusion may be at risk for a number of problems. These include intraabdominal bleeding, pelvic thromboembolism, renal compromise, bowel ischemia, pulmonary edema, myocardial depression, transfusion-related acute lung injury and/or acute respiratory syndrome, Sheehan syndrome, and infection. The postoperative management team should anticipate and be prepared for such complications.

Conservative management

In some cases removal of the placenta and uterus is simply impossible or too dangerous to attempt. There are a number of papers describing successful conservative approaches which have included closure of the uterus with the placenta *in situ*, selective arterial embolization, and expectant management [61,62]. Without adequate randomized controlled trials, there is considerable risk of publication bias (failure to publish bad outcomes) and caution is advised before employing these techniques liberally. There have been some reports of serious morbidity with conservative management, with subsequent massive hemorrhage and septic shock being the most serious of these complications [63]. Methotrexate use is discouraged by this author given the significant maternal risks and questionable value with a large volume of nonactively dividing trophoblast.

Although mortality for placenta accreta is now uncommon, morbidity with conservative management remains high; consequently, peripartum hysterectomy remains the current treatment of choice in most cases.

Unexpected placenta accreta/percreta at the time of delivery

Placenta accreta or percreta may be first discovered after a vaginal delivery when incomplete placental separation and partial manual removal occur. This highlights the rationale behind always considering accreta as the reason for a failed spontaneous third stage before attempting manual removal. In those cases where there is a risk of accreta, it is essential to delay any action that could result in sudden onset of massive hemorrhage until all preparations have been made to take care of such an eventuality.

More commonly, the placenta accreta or percreta is discovered at the time of repeat cesarean section. If at the time of opening the abdomen, the lower uterine segment appears unusually distorted or thinned, as long as there is no active bleeding the uterine incision should be delayed until all preparations have been made. In addition, after delivery of the baby, if there is suspicion of morbid adherence, there should be no attempt to remove the placenta if there is anything more than a small area of focal accreta.

When there has been partial removal of the placenta with bleeding from areas of accreta, hemostasis may be attained using multiple 3 cm square sutures deep into the myometrium over the area of maximal bleeding [33]. Other methods have been attempted, such as inversion of the cervix into the uterine cavity and suturing the inverted cervical tissue over the area of bleeding placental bed or two parallel vertical compression sutures that are used to suture the anterior and posterior walls of the lower segment together to compress the bleeding placental bed [64,65].

The overarching principle in such cases should always be to limit the hemorrhage as quickly as possible and to perform definitive surgery before the patient develops coagulopathy, hypothermia or circulatory instability. A large part of the mortality and morbidity in these situations is related to unnecessary delay compounded by fruitless attempts to preserve the uterus. Recognition of the problem and decisive surgical action, combined with aggressive resuscitation and use of blood products, is required to deal with massive hemorrhage from accreta.

Uterine inversion

Uterine inversion is the folding of the fundus into the uterine cavity in varying degrees:
• first degree – the wall extends as far as, but not through the cervix
• second degree – the fundus is prolapsed through the cervix but not out of the vaginal opening
• third degree – prolapse of the fundus outside the vagina
• fourth degree – complete prolapse of both uterus and vagina.
Acute inversion occurs within the first 24 h after delivery; subacute refers to inversion between 24 h and 30 days after delivery, and chronic inversion is inversion after 30 days.

Predisposing factors include fundal placenta, flaccid myometrium around the placental site, and a dilated cervix. Other associations include use of intrapartum fundal pressure (Credé maneuver), morbidly adherent placenta, short umbilical cord, inappropriate cord traction, chronic endometritis, fetal macrosomia, vaginal birth after cesarean, intrinsic myometrial weakness/damage, uterine sacculation, precipitate labor, acute tocolysis with potent uterine relaxant or anesthetic drug, and idiopathic factors. Mismanagement of the third stage in unlikely to be a factor in most inversions since almost every vaginal delivery is accompanied by postpartum uterine flaccidity and some degree of cord traction. Fundal implantation is very common and inversion so infrequent that for it to occur must require a number of coincident factors all acting simultaneously. In approximately 60–70% of cases, the placenta is still attached at the moment of inversion. The extent of the bleeding is variable and depends on the degree of prolapse. Frequently the degree of shock is reported to be out of proportion to that attributable to the observed blood loss, and this may be neurogenic shock due to a parasympathetic outflow from stretching peritoneum or reproductive organs. The underestimation of blood loss at the time of delivery may, however, be an important confounder. Most cases will respond to prompt uterine replacement and fluid resuscitation.

The physical examination in cases of partial inversion (first degree) can be very misleading. Abdominal or combined abdominopelvic examination often reveals a mass suggestive of a uterine or pelvic tumor. The partially inverted fundus may feel like a poorly contracted 22–24-week sized uterus. The cervix is still palpable and can be visualized (if the bleeding is not too excessive). Often, the only way to make the diagnosis is with ultrasound or if the inversion progresses. In second-degree inversion, the inverted portion of the fundus remains in the vagina, having passed through the cervix, and the examiner is unable to palpate the uterine fundus on abdominal examination, and cannot see or feel the cervix during pelvic examination. Due to the potential complexities of presentation, prompt ultrasound scanning is the most helpful technique in uncertain cases. The correct diagnosis may only be established at laparotomy.

Management

This includes aggressive blood product and fluid replacement, replacement of the uterus, and administration of potent uterotonics to keep the uterus contracted and prevent reinversion. The placenta should not generally be removed before uterine replacement since this can exacerbate blood loss. Replacement can usually be accomplished manually by placing a hand in the vagina with the fingers placed circumferentially around the prolapsed fundus. The last region of the uterus that inverted should be the first to be replaced. Uterine relaxation may be necessary, with β-sympathomimetic agents, magnesium sulfate, or low-dose nitroglycerine [66]. General anesthesia and use of halogenated gases may be needed to provide full uterine relaxation. Intravaginal hydrostatic replacement is an alternative technique that was at one time promulgated but which in the opinion of the author is difficult and impractical [67].

If there is a tightly contracted cervical ring which prohibits vaginal replacement of the fundus, surgical options may be necessary. These include incising the ring via a vaginal approach, and both anterior and posterior vaginal incisions have been described with subsequent repair once the fundus has been replaced [68]. If these measures fail, at least three abdominal procedures have been described at laparotomy: (a) stepwise traction on the funnel of the inverted uterus or the round ligaments, using ring or Allis forceps reapplied progressively as the fundus emerges (Huntington procedure); (b) longitudinal incision posteriorly through the cervix, relieving cervical

constriction and allowing traction on the round ligaments (as in the Huntington procedure) combined with stepwise replacement of the uterus from below with subsequent repair of the incision from inside the abdomen (Haultain procedure); and (c) dissection of the bladder off the cervix and entry into the vagina with a longitudinal incision. Two fingers are advanced through this incision, above the invaginated uterine body, and, exerting counterpressure with the other hand, the inversion can be reversed. Uterotonic drugs are then given immediately to maintain uterine contraction and to prevent reinversion (Tews procedure). Recurrent uterine inversion may be prevented by placement of a balloon catheter [69].

Once the uterus has been replaced, all uterine relaxant drugs should be stopped and manual removal of the placenta should follow. With early diagnosis and prompt replacement of the fundus, laparotomy and hysterectomy can be avoided [70]. In many cases, delay in definitive management is what leads to increased edema, blood loss, and associated morbidities.

Most authorities would recommend antibiotic use after manual replacement although specific evidence of the utility of this is lacking.

Uterine rupture

This subject has been dealt with elsewhere (see Chapter 49) but the general principles addressed above apply in this situation.

Conclusion

Postpartum hemorrhage remains one of the major contributors to maternal mortality, and in many cases, that mortality may have been prevented by the institution of prophylactic and interventional measures. Recognition of risk factors, institution of standard procedures and protocols, and a team approach to this problem will almost certainly result in drastically decreased morbidity and mortality.

CASE PRESENTATION

A 26-year-old gravida 7, para 6 woman with four prior pregnancies complicated by gestational diabetes presented at term with polyhydramnios and a large for gestational age baby. Following a protracted labor course, complicated by chorioamnionitis, she was delivered vaginally with forceps and a third-degree episiotomy that extended into a fourth-degree laceration. The baby weighed 4.3 kg and did well. The placenta was adherent and was removed

manually in pieces. Heavy vaginal bleeding ensued within minutes, and in addition to a routine oxytocin infusion (20 U in 1 L Ringer's lactate at 250 mL/h), because her uterus was felt to be atonic, she was given an intramuscular dose of methylergonovine (0.2 mg). At this time estimated blood loss was 1500 mL. Manual compression of the uterus was initiated and a second intravenous line was started. Because of the piecemeal placental removal, an ultrasound

Continued

unit was brought to the bedside and transabdominal scanning revealed retained placental fragments. Curettage was performed with a wide-diameter curette under US guidance.

The patient continued to bleed heavily and when blood loss was estimated to be in excess of 2000 mL it was noted that her vital signs indicated incipient collapse (decreasing systolic pressure with narrowed pulse pressure, tachycardia, increased respiratory rate, and restlessness). A complete blood count and coagulation profile were obtained. The patient was given an intramuscular injection of carboprost tromethamine (250 μg) and a second obstetric physician and the anesthesiologist were summoned. Four units of PRBCs were ordered along with 4 units of FFP. Both IV lines were opened fully and crystalloid (2 L of Ringer's lactate solution) was rapidly infused while the patient was taken to the operating room.

In the operating room, the patient was placed in lithotomy position and a tamponade balloon was placed through her cervix into the uterus and filled with 500 mL of normal saline. Six hundred micrograms of misoprostol was placed in the patient's rectum. At this point the bleeding slowed dramatically and the patient was resuscitated with the 4 units of PRBCs and 4 units of FFP. A Foley catheter was placed and urine output was measured. The patient was monitored closely in the OR until it was determined that the bleeding was controlled. She was then moved to the ICU where she continued a uneventful recovery. The tamponade balloon was removed after 18 h when her coagulation profile was normal and there was no abnormal bleeding. Three additional units of PRBCs were given in the ICU. The patient was discharged in stable condition 4 days postpartum.

References

1. Chang J, Elam-Evans L, Berg C et al. Pregnancy-related mortality surveillance – United States. 1991–1999. MMWR Surveill Summ 2003;52(2):1–8.

2. Berg C, Chang J, Callaghan W, Whitehead S. Pregnancy related mortality in the United States, 1991–1997. Obstet Gynecol 2003;101(2):289–296.

3. AbouZahr C. Global burden of maternal death and disability. Br Med Bull 2003;67:1–11.

4. Clark S, Belfort M, Dildy G, Herbst M, Meyers J, Hankins G. Maternal death in the 21st century: causes, prevention, and relationship to cesarean delivery. Am J Obstet Gynecol 2008;199(1):36; discussion 91–92.

5. Lynch C, Sheridan C, Breathnach F, Said S, Daly S, Byrne B. Near miss maternal morbidity. Ir Med J 2008; 101:134–136.

6. Zwart J, Richters J, Ory F, Vries J, Bloemenkamp K, Roosmalen J. Severe maternal morbidity during pregnancy, delivery and puerperium in the Netherlands: a nationwide population-based study of 371,000 pregnancies. Br J Obstet Gynaecol 2008;115:842–850.

7. Combs C, Laros R. Prolonged third stage of labor: morbidity and risk factors. Obstet Gynecol 1991;77:863–867.

8. Prendiville W, Elbourne D, Chalmers I. The effects of routine oxytocic administration in the management of the third stage of labor: an overview of the evidence from controlled trials. Br J Obstet Gynaecol 1988;95:3–16.

9. Ely J, Rijhsinghani A, Bowdler N, Dawson J. The association between manual removal of the placenta and postpartum endometritis following vaginal delivery. Obstet Gynecol 1995;86:1002–1006.

10. Herman A, Weinraub Z, Bukovsky I et al. Dynamic ultrasonographic imaging of the third stage of labor: new perspective into third stage mechanism. Am J Obstet Gynecol 1993;168: 1469–1496.

11. Lowenwirt I, Zauk R, Handwerker S. Safety of intravenous glyceryl trinitrate in management of retained placenta. Aust N Z J Obstet Gynaecol 1997;37(1):20–24.

12. Herman A, Zimerman A, Arieli S et al. Down-up sequential separation of the placenta. Ultrasound Obstet Gynecol 2002; 19:278–281.

13. Purwar M. Practical recommendations for umbilical vein injection for management of retained placenta. In: AM Gulmezoglu, J Villar, eds. The WHO Reproductive Health Library, vol. 4. Geneva: World Health Organization, 2001.

14. Bider D, Dulitzky M, Goldenberg M, Lipitz S, Mashiach S. Intraumbilical vein injection of prostaglandin F2α in retained placenta. Eur J Obstet Gynecol Reprod Biol 1996;64: 59–61.

15. Pipingas A, Hofmeyr G, Sesel K. Umbilical vessel oxytocin administration for retained placenta: in vitro study of various infusion techniques. Am J Obstet Gynecol 1993;168: 793–795.

16. Riley D, Burgess R. External abdominal aortic compression: a study of a resuscitation manoeuvre for postpartum haemorrhage. Anaesth Intensive Care 1994;37:237–238.

17. McDonald S, Prendiville W, Elbourne D. Prophylactic syntometrine versus oxytocin for delivery of the placenta. Cochrane Database Syst Rev 2000;2:CD000201. Update in: Cochrane Database Syst Rev 2004;1:CD000201.

18. Chelmow C, O'Brien B. Postpartum haemorrhage: prevention. Clin Evid 2006:1932–1950.

19. McDonald S, Abbott J, Higgins S. Prophylactic ergometrine-oxytocin versus oxytocin for the third stage of labour. Cochrane Database Syst Rev 2007;3:CD000201.

20. Hayashi R, Castillo M, Noah M. Management of severe postpartum hemorrhage with a prostaglandin F2 alpha analogue. Obstet Gynecol 1984;63:806–808.

21. Toppozada M, El-Bossaty M, El-Rahman H, El-Din A. Control of intractable atonic postpartum hemorrhage by 15-methyl prostaglandin F2 alpha. Obstet Gynecol 1981;58:327–330.

22. Barrington J, Roberts A. The use of gemeprost pessaries to arrest postpartum haemorrhage. Br J Obstet Gynaecol 1993;100:691–692.

23. Gülmezoglu A, Villar J, Ngoc N et al. WHO Collaborative Group to Evaluate Misoprostol in the Management of the Third Stage of Labour. WHO multicentre randomised trial of misoprostol in the management of the third stage of labour. Lancet 2001;358:689–695.

24. Gülmezoglu A, Forna F, Villar J, Hofmeyr G. Prostaglandins for preventing postpartum haemorrhage.Cochrane Database Syst Rev 2007;3:CD000494.

25. Naqvi S, Makhdoom K. Conservative management of primary postpartum haemorrhage. J Coll Physicians Surg Pak 2004; 14:296–297.

26. Haq G, Tayyab S. Control of postpartum and post abortal haemorrhage with uterine packing. J Pak Med Assoc 2005;55: 369–371.

27. Katesmark M, Brown R, Raju K. Successful use of a Sengstaken-Blakemore tube to control massive postpartum haemorrhage. Br J Obstet Gynaecol 1994;101(3):259–260.

28. Bagga R, Jain V, Kalra J, Chopra S, Gopalan S. Uterovaginal packing with rolled gauze in postpartum hemorrhage. MedGenMed 2004;6(1):50.

29. Cho Y, Rizvi C, Uppal T, Condous G. Ultrasonographic visualization of balloon placement for uterine tamponade in massive primary postpartum hemorrhage. Ultrasound Obstet Gynecol 2008;32:711–713.

30. Belfort MA, Dildy GA, Garrido J, White GL. Intraluminal pressure in a uterine tamponade balloon is curvilinearly related to the volume of fluid infused. Am J Perinatol 2011;28(8):659–66. Epub 2011 Apr 15.

31. B-Lynch C, Coker A, Lawal A, Abu J, Cowen M. The B-Lynch surgical technique for the control of massive postpartum haemorrhage: an alternative to hysterectomy? Five cases reported. Br J Obstet Gynaecol 1997;104(3):372–375.

32. Hayman R, Arulkumaran S, Steer P. Uterine compression sutures: surgical management of postpartum hemorrhage. Obstet Gynecol 2002;99(3):502–506.

33. Cho J, Jun H, Lee C. Hemostatic suturing technique for uterine bleeding during cesarean delivery. Obstet Gynecol 2000;96(1): 129–131.

34. Smith K, Baskett T. Uterine compression sutures as an alternative to hysterectomy for severe postpartum hemorrhage. J Obstet Gynecol Can 2003;25:197–200.

35. Habek D, Kulas T, Bobi-Vukovi M, Selthofer R, Vuji B, Ugljarevi M. Successful of the B-Lynch compression suture in the management of massive postpartum hemorrhage: case reports and review. Arch Gynecol Obstet 2006;273:307–309.

36. Ochoa M, Allaire A, Stitely M. Pyometria after hemostatic square suture technique. Obstet Gynecol 2002;13:127–131.

37. Tamizian O, Arulkumaran S. The surgical management of postpartum haemorrhage. Curr Opin Obstet Gynecol 2001; 13(2):127–131.

38. AbdRabbo S. Stepwise uterine devascularization: a novel technique for management of uncontrolled postpartum hemorrhage with preservation of the uterus. Am J Obstet Gynecol 1994;171:694–700.

39. Hebisch G, Huch A. Vaginal uterine artery ligation avoids high blood loss and puerperal hysterectomy in postpartum hemorrhage. Obstet Gynecol 2002;100:574–578.

40. Burchell R, Olson G. Internal iliac artery ligation: aortograms. Am J Obstet Gynecol 1966;94:117–124.

41. Dildy G. Postpartum hemorrhage: new management options. Clin Obstet Gynecol 2002;45:330–344.

42. Hansch E, Chitkara U, McAlpine J, El-Sayed Y, Dake M, Razavi M. Pelvic arterial embolization for control of obstetric hemorrhage: a five-year experience. Am J Obstet Gynecol 1999;180: 1454–1460.

43. Pelage J, LeDref O, Mateo J et al. Life-threatening primary postpartum hemorrhage: treatment with emergency selective arterial embolization. Radiology 1998;208:359–362.

44. Soncini E, Pelicelli A, Larini P, Marcato C, Monaco D, Grignaffini A. Uterine artery embolization in the treatment and prevention of postpartum hemorrhage. Int J Gynaecol Obstet 2007;96(3):181–185.

45. Lau W, Fung H, Rogers M. Ten years experience of caesarean and postpartum hysterectomy in a teaching hospital in Hong Kong. Eur J Obstet Gynecol Reprod Biol 1997;74:133–137.

46. Ledee N, Ville Y, Musset D, Mercier F, Frydman R, Fernandez H. Management in intractable obstetric haemorrhage: an audit study on 61 cases. Eur J Obstet Gynecol Reprod Biol 2001; 94(2):189–196.

47. Usta I, Hobeika E, Musa A, Gabriel G, Nassar A. Placenta previa-accreta: risk factors and complications. Am J Obstet Gynecol 2005;193:1045–1049.

48. Hudon L, Belfort M, Broome D. Diagnosis and management of placenta percreta: a review. Obstet Gynecol Surv 1998;53: 509–517.

49. Dildy GA, Scott JR, Saffer CS, Belfort MA. An effective pressure pack for severe pelvic hemorrhage. Obstet Gynecol 2006;108:1222–1226.

50. Clark S, Phelan J, Yeh S, Bruce S, Paul R. Hypogastric artery ligation for obstetric hemorrhage. Obstet Gynecol 1985;66: 353–356.

51. Catanzarite V. Prophylactic intramyometrial carboprost tromethamine does not substantially reduce blood loss relative to intramyometrial oxytocin at routine cesarean section. Am J Perinatol 1990;7:39–42.

52. Sullivan I, Faulds J, Ralph C. Contamination of salvaged maternal blood by amniotic fluid and fetal red cells during elective Caesarean section. Br J Anaesth 2008;101(2): 225–229.

53. Bodner L, Nosher J, Gribbin C, Siegel R, Beale S, Scorza W. Balloon-assisted occlusion of the internal iliac arteries in patients with placenta accreta/percreta. Cardiovasc Intervent Radiol 2006;29:354–361.

54. Mok M, Heidemann B, Dundas K, Gillespie I, Clark V. Interventional radiology in women with suspected placenta accreta undergoing caesarean section. Int J Obstet Anesth 2008;17:255–261.

55. Belfort MA. Indicated preterm birth for placenta accreta. Semin Perinatol 2011;35(5):252–256.

56. Gunter O, Au B, Isbell J, Mowery N, Young P, Cotton B. Optimizing outcomes in damage control resuscitation: identifying blood product ratios associated with improved survival. J Trauma 2008;65:527–534.

57. Franchini M, Franchi M, Bergamini V, Salvagno G, Montagnana M, Lippi G. A critical review on the use of recombinant factor VIIa in life-threatening obstetric postpartum hemorrhage. Semin Thromb Hemost 2008;34:104–112.

58. Welsh A, McLintock C, Gatt S, Somerset D, Popham P, Ogle R. Guidelines for the use of recombinant activated factor VII in massive obstetric haemorrhage. Aust N Z J Obstet Gynaecol 2008;48:12–16.

59. Belfort M, Kofford S, Varner M. Massive obstetric hemorrhage in a Jehovah's Witness: intraoperative strategies and high-dose erythropoietin use. Am J Perinatol 2011;28(3):207–210.

60. Uchiyama D, Koganemaru M, Abe T, Hori D, Hayabuchi N. Arterial catheterization and embolization for management of emergent or anticipated massive obstetrical hemorrhage. Radiat Med 2008;26(4):188–197.

61. Alkazaleh F, Geary M, Kingdom J, Kachura J, Windrim R. Elective non-removal of the placenta and prophylactic uterine artery embolization postpartum as a diagnostic imaging approach for the management of placenta percreta: a case report. J Obstet Gynaecol Can 2004;26(8):743–746.

62. Timmermans S, van Hof A, Duvekot J. Conservative management of abnormally invasive placentation. Obstet Gynecol Surv 2007;62:529–539.

63. Teo S, Kanagalingam D, Tan H, Tan L. Massive postpartum haemorrhage after uterus-conserving surgery in placenta percreta: the danger of the partial placenta percreta. Br J Obstet Gynaecol 2008;115:789–792.

64. Dawlatly B, Wong I, Khan K, Agnihotri S. Using the cervix to stop bleeding in a woman with placenta accreta: a case report. Br J Obstet Gynaecol 2007;114:502–504.

65. Hwu Y, Chen C, Chen H, Su T. Parallel vertical compression sutures: a technique to control bleeding from placenta praevia or accreta during caesarean section. Br J Obstet Gynaecol 2005;112:1420–1423.

66. Dayan S, Schwalbe S. The use of small-dose intravenous nitroglycerin in a case of uterine inversion. Anesth Analg 1996;82:1091–1093.

67. Ogueh O, Ayida G. Acute uterine inversion: a new technique of hydrostatic replacement. Br J Obstet Gynaecol 1997;104: 951–952.

68. Platt L, Druzin M. Acute puerperal inversion of the uterus. Am J Obstet Gynecol 1981;141:187–190.

69. Majd H, Pilsniak A, Reginald P. Recurrent uterine inversion: a novel treatment approach using SOS Bakri balloon. Br J Obstet Gynaecol 2009;116(7):999–1001.

70. Watson P, Besch N, Bowes W. Management of acute and subacute puerperal inversion of the uterus. Obstet Gynecol 1980;55:12–16.

Chapter 37
Emergency Care

Garrett K. Lam[1] *and Michael R. Foley*[2]

[1]Department of Obstetrics and Gynecology, University of Tennessee-Chattanooga, Chattanooga, TN, USA
[2]Department of Obstetrics and Gynecology, University of Arizona, Tucson, AZ, USA

Incidents requiring emergency care of the gravid patient represent some of the most difficult clinical scenarios faced by the practicing clinician. There are multiple causes for maternal collapse, and commonly the clinical situation is so dire that there is no time for a detailed diagnostic work-up. Attempts to resuscitate the mother are the starting point for intervention; however, as the resuscitation progresses, consideration of fetal well-being must be addressed.

It is not the intention of the authors to cover all causes of obstetric emergencies in a single chapter. Instead, we focus on amniotic fluid embolism (AFE), and the management of its sequelae: disseminated intravascular coagulopathy (DIC), blood product replacement, and perimortem cesarean delivery as prototypical examples of obstetric emergent care as their attendant management principles and guidelines are applicable to most obstetric emergencies.

Amniotic fluid embolism

Amniotic fluid embolism is one of the most catastrophic causes of maternal collapse. Published literature, including data from a national registry, have estimated the incidence to be between 1 in 8000 and 1 in 80,000 livebirths worldwide [1,2]. A recent review of over 3 million birth records produced an estimate of 7.7 cases/100,000 livebirths [3]. Illustrative of its severity is its extremely high maternal mortality rate, reported in different sources to be 60–90%. In the US, AFE and pulmonary thromboembolism combine to account for approximately 20% of maternal mortality [4,5].

The diagnosis of AFE requires a high index of suspicion and clinical context. Contributing factors include grand multiparity, precipitous or tumultuous labor, uterine hyperstimulation, rupture of membranes, and use of oxytocin. Episodes usually occur during labor and delivery, or in the immediate postpartum period, although individual cases have occurred around the time of cesarean delivery, dilation and curettage (D&C) for termination of pregnancy, and amniocentesis.

Clinically, the signs of AFE include the triad of hypoxia, cardiovascular collapse, and coagulopathy. Sudden onset of dyspnea and hypoxemia is usually the earliest sign of AFE, with rapid progression to respiratory failure. Indeed, 50% of patients who expire within the first hour of incident have cause of death attributed to profound hypoxemia and bronchospasm [6]. Affected patients may rapidly progress to cardiovascular failure, manifested by dysrhythmias, pulseless electrical activity, and, ultimately, asystole. The events leading to total cardiac collapse are not definitively known, but are thought to be triggered by pulmonary artery vasospasm and right ventricular failure, which causes potentially irreversible hypoxic damage to the left ventricle, producing an estimated 86% mortality rate [1]. While DIC has been reported in over 50% of cases, its specific cause remains unclear, but is believed to be related to leakage of thromboplastin-like material into the maternal circulation [7]. Symptoms of agitation, nausea, mental status changes, and tonic–clonic seizures have also been reported in AFE patients [1].

Patients who weather these initial insults may develop noncardiogenic pulmonary edema (disease worsens even though left ventricular function improves), possibly due to inflammatory damage to the endothelial lining of the alveoli [8]. Affected serum specimens display decreased complement levels and increased cytokine levels, intimating that AFE results from a unique maternal immunologic response to fetal antigens in amniotic fluid introduced into the maternal circulation. Studies have identified elevated serum levels of tryptase, a protein released along with histamine by mast cells in cases of fatal anaphylaxis [9]. Furthermore, a study of registry data revealed that 41% of women with AFE had a history of allergy. Thus, the term "anaphylactoid syndrome of pregnancy" has been suggested in lieu of AFE [1].

No prophylaxis for AFE is available as there are no definitive predisposing factors, nor is there a definitive treatment. The basic tenets of care, as in any case of maternal cardiovascular collapse, emphasize the need to maintain the patient's ABCs (airway, breathing, circulation) to prevent maternal end-organ damage and maintain fetal oxygenation, if applicable, until resuscitation or delivery is accomplished. Continuous monitoring of oxygen saturation, electrocardiogram (ECG) monitoring, and pulmonary artery catheterization are vital to monitoring respiratory status, cardiovascular function, and intravascular volume. Cardiopulmonary resuscitation with consistent ventilation must be initiated quickly to maintain placental perfusion in women who become unresponsive during the antepartum period from AFE, and continued until the woman is fully resuscitated. Rapid intubation should be considered to ensure adequate fetal oxygenation, which requires maternal $PaO_2 > 70\,mmHg$ or an oxyhemoglobin saturation of $> 95\%$ [10].

For those patients who survive the initial cardiopulmonary incident, left ventricular failure eventually develops. In order to ensure organ perfusion, forward flow of circulation must be maintained. Thus, optimizing ventricular preload, even at the potential expense of pulmonary congestion, is imperative. Use of inotropic medications may also be considered, particularly when hypotension persists, despite aggressive volume expansion. It is at this point where the use of Swan–Ganz catheterization is valuable.

Steroid administration has also been suggested as a theoretical treatment based on the putative anaphylactoid reaction previously described. However, not enough evidence exists to show benefit.

Disseminated intravascular coagulopathy

This coagulopathic state is caused by the rapid consumption of clotting factors. Although there are two described clinical forms of DIC, this chapter focuses on acute DIC, not chronic DIC from long-standing disease (e.g. cancer).

Episodes of DIC are triggered when the clotting cascade is rapidly activated via exposure of blood to massive amounts of tissue factor, a natural procoagulant. This generates large amounts of thrombin which ultimately cause extensive clot formation that obstructs the microvasculature of tissues and organs. Patients exhibit thrombocytopenia ($<100,000/\mu L$) and microangiopathic hemolytic anemia can be seen on peripheral smears (Fig. 37.1). Initially, affected women exhibit petechiae and ecchymoses (Fig. 37.2). However, as the quantity of intravascular thrombi builds, tissue necrosis and ischemia of multiple organ systems occur. An early study by Siegal *et al* [11] looked at a series of patients with DIC (unrelated to pregnancy), and found that the most commonly affected organ systems were the kidneys, followed by liver, lungs, heart (cardiogenic shock), and then the central nervous system (CNS).

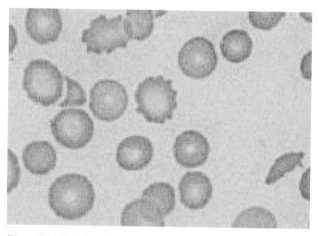

Figure 37.1 Peripheral smear of patient with disseminated intravascular coagulopathy (DIC). Schistocytes and helmet cells are characteristic of microangiopathic hemolytic anemia. Note the lack of platelets seen in the microscopic field. Reproduced from Ramanarayanan and Krishnan [18] with permission from Emedicine.com.

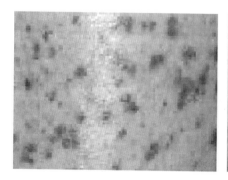
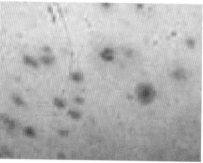

Figure 37.2 Petechiae and purpura seen in DIC. Reproduced from Ramanarayanan and Krishnan [18] with permission from Emedicine.com.

In addition to ischemic sequelae, widespread thrombus formation depletes the patient's intrinsic clotting factors, causing a paradoxical state of anticoagulation illustrated clinically by signs such as "oozing" of blood from intravenous sites, catheters, or friable surfaces such as mucosal membranes. In the pregnant patient, vaginal bleeding is one of the most common signs. The inability to clot can lead to multiorgan failure as a vicious cycle is created whereby continued blood loss consumes more clotting factors, which leads to further blood loss that reduces intravascular volume and oxygen-carrying capacity, worsening chances for successful resuscitation. Given the potential severity of the disease, it is not surprising that DIC itself has a very high mortality rate. In the general literature on DIC, mortality rates are reported in the range 40–80% [12,13]; however, many of those findings were based on trauma and burn cases, rather than pregnancy-related causes. There do not appear to be any data available directly addressing maternal mortality and DIC specifically.

Treatment of DIC is reviewed partly in the following section on blood product replacement; however, a short discussion on the use of heparin to treat DIC is warranted. Given that DIC is based on consumption of clotting factors, use of anticoagulants such as heparin to interrupt the clotting cascade is a theoretically sensible treatment option. However, no controlled trials exist to indicate that heparin is beneficial [6]. Furthermore, there is logical concern that heparinization would exacerbate bleeding, which could create further complications in the patient who is postoperative from delivery. Thus, the mainstay of therapy would appear to be related to replacement therapy with blood products and recombinant factors.

Blood product replacement

In the treatment of DIC from AFE, the cardinal principle is continuing replacement of consumed blood products to maintain perfusion and circulation. This is a temporizing measure until the patient has been resuscitated and the bleeding is stabilized. Thus, it is imperative to understand what comprises each type of blood product in order to choose which to use (Table 37.1).

The basic tenets for blood product replacement are to improve oxygen-carrying capacity, maintain intravascular volume, and treat coagulopathy. Transfusion with packed red blood cells (PRBCs) meets the first two purposes. Each unit of packed cells contains approximately 200 mL of red cells in a total volume of 300 mL. In an adult patient without active bleeding, 1 unit should raise the hematocrit by approximately 3%. In nonacute settings, blood that is specifically typed and crossmatched to the patient is used, and a leukopoor option is requested to decrease the risk of febrile transfusion reaction. In an acute setting of bleeding, where blood group and antibody screens are lacking, use of O negative PRBCs is the safest, quickest, temporizing option until properly matched products are available. In most acute care hospitals, typed and screened blood products that were ordered prior to surgery can be made available within 30 min (Transfusion Services, Banner Good Samaritan Regional Medical Center, personal communication, 2010).

Platelet transfusion is considered when thrombocytopenia becomes severe enough that persistent bleeding becomes problematic. It has been our experience that people have idiosyncratic cut-offs for determining when platelet transfusion is prescribed; however, a general

Table 37.1 Blood products used for replacement

Blood product	Contents	Indications	Volume added (mL)	Effect
Packed RBCs	Red cells, ~50 mL of plasma, WBCs	Increases red cell mass, oxygen-carrying capacity, intravascular volume (secondary)	300	Increases hematocrit on average 3% per unit
Platelets (usually available as 10-pack of single donor platelets)	Platelets, small amount of plasma, RBCs and WBCs	Treats bleeding from thrombocytopenia	50	Increases total platelet count between 7500–10,000/mm^3
Fresh frozen plasma	Plasma and all clotting factors, fibrinogen	Coagulation disorders, increases intravascular volume (secondary effect)	250	Increases fibrinogen levels 10–15 mg/dL per unit
Cryoprecipitate	Fibrinogen, factors V, VIII, XIII, von Willebrand and fibrinogen	Treats specific bleeding disorders (von Willebrand disease, hemophilia) and any fibrinogen disorders	40	Same as FFP; however, does not add as much intravascular volume

FFP, fresh frozen plasma; RBC, red blood cell; WBC, white blood cell.

consensus exists that excessive bleeding from major trauma or surgery follows platelet counts less than 50,000/mm^3, and spontaneous bleeding occurs with platelet counts below 10,000/mm^3 (note that this threshold has been reduced from the previous value of 20,000/mm^3 based on recent evidence [14]. Furthermore, dilutional thrombocytopenia requiring platelet transfusion can occur when a patient receives over 1.5–2 times their normal blood volume. Platelets can be collected from single or random donors, but are more commonly available as a group of 10 units from a single donor. One single donor unit should increase the platelet count 7500–10,000/mm^3 after equilibration, usually occurring within 10 min of transfusion [15]. Thus, in the setting of pathologic processes with massive platelet destruction or consumption, such as HELLP (hemolysis, elevated liver enzymes, and low platelet count) or DIC, platelet transfusions have very limited effect, and are often avoided except in a temporizing capacity (e.g. cesearean delivery in an affected patient). Of note, platelet concentrates also contain RBCs in the approximately 50 mL of serum present in each unit; thus, Rh-negative patients should receive Rh-immune prophylaxis.

The use of plasma products is more germane to the treatment of our AFE patient, as they can replace many of the coagulation products consumed or lost during the course of DIC. Several different preparations of plasma and coagulation products are available. Fresh frozen plasma (FFP) is separated from freshly drawn blood, and is used to correct any factor deficiency in a patient. It needs to be ABO-compatible with the patient, but does not require antibody crossmatching or Rh typing. A typical unit will provide an extra 250 mL of volume, and contains approximately 700 mg of fibrinogen, which should raise a patient's fibrinogen level 10–15 mg/dL per unit. Different recommendations exist for the amount of FFP to be administered, based on the number of PRBC units transfused (i.e. 1 unit FFP per 3–5 units PRBCs). No specific ratio of plasma products:PRBCs has proven optimal; however, when blood products are administered for mass transfusion cases, according to a preexisting, defined protocol, reductions in complications such as organ failure and infection have been observed [16,17].

When specific factors, such as factors VIII, XIII and von Willebrand factor, or fibrinogen are needed, cryoprecipitate is a better choice. Cryoprecipitate is cold-insoluble and is separated from FFP that has been warmed to refrigerator temperatures. Akin to FFP, it raises fibrinogen levels 10–15 mg/dL per unit but only adds 40 mL in volume per unit, making it a logical choice in patients who require fibrinogen but are at risk for fluid overload. Additionally, as cryoprecipitate is collected from a single donor unit of FFP, it carries less risk for hepatitis and HIV transmission.

Recombinant factor VIIa (rVIIa, aka NovoSeven™) has been released for treatment of bleeding diathesis, primarily for hemophilias. This synthesized protein combines with tissue factor to activate factors IX and X, and increase production of thrombin that stimulates platelet recruitment (Fig. 37.3). Thus, it has been used, off-label, for bleeding disorders from extensive surgery, trauma, thrombocytopenia, liver disease, or qualitative platelet dysfunction [18]. Moreover, rVIIa may be useful for patients with coagulopathy as it does not add extensive volume load and has a short half-life (<3 h). It has been selectively used for individual cases of obstetric hemorrhage [19]. One case report describes its successful use for DIC in the setting of AFE [20]. Given its novelty, there is no known optimal or minimal dosing regimen for its use in pregnancy. Case reports have described dosages ranging from 20 to 120 μg/kg for treatment of serious bleeding, and have reported clinically significant hemostasis within 30 min of administration. Although there appears to be great potential for the use of rVIIa in obstetric hemorrhage and DIC, reservation of its use for the most severe cases of hemorrhage seems most prudent.

Perimortem cesarean delivery

The final consideration in all cases of obstetric collapse is timing of delivery to salvage the fetus. Unfortunately, there is a lack of data on this topic for the obvious reason that the opportunity to study this technique is rare and unpredictable. Thus, our knowledge is based on theoretical conclusions drawn from physiologic data and case studies.

According to a paper by Katz *et al* [21], the decision to perform perimortem cesarean delivery must be made quickly and without equivocation. Their paper states that any maternal patient who suffers cardiac arrest in the third trimester should have cesarean delivery initiated within 4 min of the time of arrest, and delivery performed within 5 min of the seminal event. The recommendation for timing of delivery is based on the physiologic principle that irreversible anoxic damage occurs within 4–6 min from cessation of adequate cerebral perfusion. In the pregnant woman, anoxia occurs more quickly given the preexisting reduction in functional residual capacity caused by the gravid uterus. Furthermore, it is maintained that cardiopulmonary resuscitation likely does not produce adequate blood flow in the pregnant patient. In nonpregnant patients, the thoracic compressions of cardiopulmonary resuscitation produce a stroke volume 30% of normal [21]. This stroke volume is reduced another two-thirds in pregnancy because of caval compression by the gravid uterus, such that chest compressions are likely only producing a cardiac output that is 10% of normal [22]. Measures to improve preload and cardiac stroke volume are thus vital to maternal survival. Delivery of the

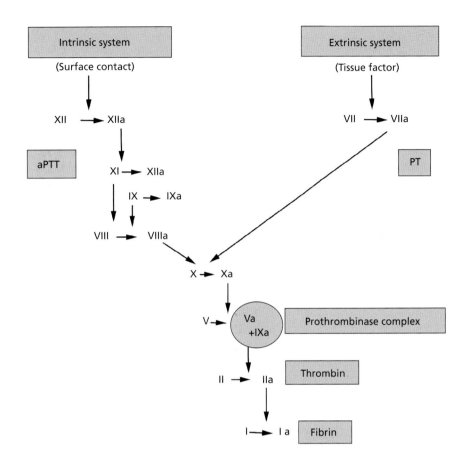

Figure 37.3 The coagulation cascade. Reproduced from Ramanarayanan and Krishnan [18] with permission from Emedicine.com.

near term infant will decrease uterine pressure on the vena cava, thus increasing venous return to the heart. Involution of the uterus also produces an "autotransfusion" of blood from the uterine sinuses into maternal circulation. Both measures have been estimated to improve maternal circulation 30–80% [23] and will improve the likelihood for resuscitation.

The 5-min rule for delivery of the infant also appears to be supported by physiologic studies and case reports in the literature. Physiologic studies in animals show that a normal fetus has an oxygen reserve of around 2 min but compensatory mechanisms and shunting may preserve oxygenation for vital organs for periods of time longer than 5 min. Katz *et al*'s original paper [21] reviewed the available data on fetal survivors from perimortem delivery, and found that most survivors were delivered within 5 min of arrest. Their follow-up paper in 2005 [22] reported seven cases of infants surviving after delivery was accomplished over 15 min from maternal cardiac arrest. Given that full-term infants have sufficient reserve to recover from hypoxic insult, recommendations are for delivery of any fetus exhibiting a heart rate, even if it is past the 5-min period.

Conclusion

Emergency care in pregnancy is a broad topic encompassing myriad causes. We hope that this review of the treatment of AFE and its attendant co-morbidities has provided the reader with guidelines germane to the management of most types of maternal crises. The key principle for treatment of the patient with AFE is devoting full attention to maintaining her circulation and perfusion, which is necessary for support of the fetus in addition to the mother. Awareness of time spent in resuscitation is a critical element in deciding when to perform perimortem cesarean delivery, as the goal for delivery should occur within minutes of complete arrest. Timely delivery may not only salvage a viable infant, but also improves the efforts for maternal resuscitation. Even if resuscitation is successful, vigilance must be maintained towards latent issues, notably DIC and blood product replacement. Correct usage of replacement products will maintain hemostasis and tissue oxygenation, and normalize intravascular volume, and is protective against major sequelae such as organ failure and infection.

CASE PRESENTATION

A 29-year-old African-American female, gravida 2, para 1001, at 38 weeks' gestation, has been on pitocin augmentation for the past 12h. Fetal heart rate is consistently in the 140–150 beat per minute (bpm) range, with good variability and no signs of hypoxia. At 4cm dilation, amniotomy is performed, with light meconium-stained fluid noted. The patient then complains to her labor nurse that she is "feeling strange," with light-headedness and the inability to "think clearly." She then, oddly, begins counting backwards from 10 spontaneously and, before she finishes, loses consciousness.

The labor nurse notes that her oxygen saturations are acutely falling, dropping to the 80s. The resident attempts bedside revival, but no response is obtained. Fetal heart tones become bradycardic to 80bpm within minutes from loss of consciousness. She is rushed to the operating room for resuscitation, and has a grand mal seizure on the operating table. The anesthesiologist notes that the patient's rhythm strip shows asystole. The fetal heart monitor verifies a severe bradycardia.

The decision is made to perform a perimortem cesarean delivery of the fetus. Cardiopulmonary resuscitation is performed concurrently. The infant is successfully delivered by low transverse cesarean section, and requires resuscitation in the operating room by the neonatal team.

Full code resuscitation is carried out on the patient throughout the completion of the cesarean delivery. An inordinately small amount of blood loss is noted from the uterine incision. As the patient's skin is being closed, a watery-bloody discharge begins to ooze between the staples. She is also noted to be bleeding from her intravenous sites, and a large pool of blood is noted on the sheets of the operating table between her legs. The code is carried out for a full 50min from the initiation of the cesarean, but the patient never recovers a consistent heart rhythm. Death is pronounced approximately 50min from membrane rupture.

References

1. Clark SL, Hankins GD, Dudley DA et al. Amniotic fluid embolism: analysis of the national registry. Am J Obstet Gynecol 1995;172:1158–1167.

2. Tuffnell DJ. Amniotic fluid embolism. Curr Opin Obstet Gynecol 2003;15:119–122.

3. Abenheim HA, Azoulay L, Kramer MS et al. Incidence and risk factors of amniotic fluid embolisms: a population based study on 3 million births in the United States. Am J Obstet Gynecol 2008;199:49.

4. Chang J, Elam-Evans LD, Berg CJ et al. Pregnancy-related mortality surveillance, United States, 1991–1999. MMWR Surveill Summ 2003;52:1–8.

5. Kaunitz AM, Hughes JM, Grimes DA. Causes of maternal mortality in the United States. Obstet Gynecol 1985;65:605–612.

6. Baldiserri M. Amniotic fluid embolism. UpToDate.com.

7. Davies S. Amniotic fluid embolism and isolated disseminated intravascular coagulation. Can J Anaesth 1999;46:456–459.

8. Benson MD. A hypothesis regarding complement activation and amniotic fluid embolism. Med Hypotheses 2007;68:101–122.

9. Bradley, JM, Collins KM, Harley RA. Ancillary studies in amniotic fluid embolism: a case report and review of the literature. Am J Forensic Med Pathol 2005;26:92.

10. Cole DE, Taylor TL, McCullough DM et al. Acute respiratory distress syndrome in pregnancy. Crit Care Med 2005;33:S269–272.

11. Siegal T, Seligsohn U, Aghai E, Modan M. Clinical and laboratory aspects of disseminated intravascular coagulation: a study of 118 cases. Thromb Haemost 1978;39:122–134.

12. Stephan F, Hollande J, Richard O et al. Thrombocytopenia in the surgical ICU. Chest 1999;115:1363–1370.

13. Gando S, Nanzaki S, Kemmotsu O. Disseminated intravascular coagulation and sustained systemic inflammatory response syndrome predict organ dysfunctions after trauma. Ann Surg 1999;229:121–127.

14. May AK. Use of blood products in the critically ill. UpToDate.com.

15. Martin SM, Strong TH. Transfusion of blood components and derivatives in the obstetric intensive care patient. In: Foley MR, Strong TH, Garite TJ, eds. Obstetric Intensive Care Manual, 2nd edn. London: McGraw-Hill, 2004.

16. Cotton BA, Au BK, Nunez TC et al. Predefined massive transfusion protocols are associated with a reduction in organ failure and postinjury complications. J Trauma 2009;66:41–48.

17. Gunter OL, Au BK, Isbell JM et al. Optimizing outcomes in damage control resuscitation: identifying blood product rations associated with improved survival. J Trauma 2008;65:527–534.

18. Ramanarayanan J, Krishnan G. Factor VII. Emedicine.com.

19. Bouwmeester FW, Jonkhoff AR, Verheijen RH, van Geijn HP. Successful treatment of life-threatening postpartum hemorrhage with recombinant activated factor VII. Obstet Gynecol 2003;101:1174–1176.

20. Lim Y, Loo CC, Chia V, Fun W. Recombinant factor VIIa after amniotic fluid embolism and disseminated intravascular coagulopathy. Int J Gynecol Obstet 2004;87:178–179.

21. Katz VL, Dotters DJ, Droegemueller W. Perimortem cesarean delivery. Obstet Gynecol 1986;68:571–576.

22. Katz VL, Balderston K, DeFreest M. Perimortem cesarean delivery: were our assumptions correct? Am J Obstet Gynecol 2005;192:1916.

23. DePace NL, Betesh JS, Kotler MN. "Postmortem" cesarean section with recovery of both mother and offspring. JAMA 1982;248:971–973.

Chapter 38
Rh and Other Blood Group Alloimmunizations

Kenneth J. Moise Jr

Department of Obstetrics, Gynecology and Reproductive Sciences, University of Texas School of Medicine at Houston and the Texas Fetal Center of Memorial Hermann Children's Hospital, Houston, TX, USA

The time-honored concept that the placenta is relatively impervious to cell trafficking between the fetus and its mother is no longer accepted. Flow cytometry can detect fetal red cell and red cell precursors in the maternal circulation in virtually all pregnancies [1,2].

In some patients, this exposure to fetal red cell antigens produces an antibody response that can be harmful to future offspring. The process is known as red cell alloimmunization (formerly isoimmunization). Active transplacental transport of these antibodies leads to their attachment to fetal red cells and sequestration in the fetal spleen. The quantity of the maternal antibody (see below), the subclass of immunoglobulin G (IgG), and even the response of the fetal reticuloendothelial system have roles in the development of fetal anemia – a disease state known as hemolytic disease of the fetus and newborn (HDFN). In extreme cases, this severe anemia is associated with the accumulation of extracellular fluid in the form of ascites, pleural effusions, and scalp edema, a condition termed hydrops fetalis.

Prophylaxis

Prevention of maternal alloimmunization is almost uniformly successful in the case of exposure to the RhD or "rhesus" antigen. Prophylactic immunoglobulin (rhesus immunoglobulin; RhIg) is now available in the USA in the form of four commercial preparations – two can only be administered intramuscularly while two can be given either intramuscularly or intravenously. RhIg is not effective once the patient has developed endogenous antibodies. Immunoglobulins to prevent sensitization to other red cell antigens are not available.

All pregnant patients should undergo an antibody screen to red cell antigens at the first prenatal visit. In the case of a negative screen in the RhD-negative patient, further testing is unnecessary until 28 weeks' gestation. Unless the patient's partner is documented to be RhD negative, a 300 µg dose of RhIg should be administered at 28 weeks. In addition, a repeat antibody screen should also be obtained at that time as recommended by the American Association of Blood Banks, although the American Congress of Obstetricians and Gynecologists has left this to the discretion of the clinician [3]. Although this has not been studied for cost-effectiveness, a repeat screen will detect the rare patient who becomes RhD sensitized early in pregnancy. If a repeat screen is obtained, the intramuscular RhIg injection can be administered before the patient is sent for venepuncture. The short time interval between procedures will not affect the results of the antibody screen.

At delivery, a cord blood sample should be tested for neonatal RhD typing. If the neonate is determined to be RhD positive, a second dose of 300 µg RhIg should be administered to the mother within 72 hours of delivery. Approximately 0.1% of deliveries will be associated with a fetomaternal hemorrhage (FMH) in excess of 30 mL. More than the standard dose of RhIg will be required in these cases. Because risk factor assessment will only identify 50% of patients who have an excessive FMH at delivery, the routine screening of all postpartum women is now recommended. Typically, this involves a sheep rosette test which is read qualitatively as positive or negative. If negative, one vial of RhIg (300 µg) is given. If positive, the bleed is quantitated with a Kleihauer–Betke stain or fetal cell stain by flow cytometry. Blood bank consultation should then be undertaken to determine the number of doses of RhIg to administer.

The mechanism by which RhIg prevents sensitization is not well understood. Biochemical studies have revealed

Queenan's Management of High-Risk Pregnancy: An Evidence-Based Approach, Sixth Edition. Edited by John T. Queenan, Catherine Y. Spong, Charles J. Lockwood.

Table 38.1 Indications for administration of Rhesus immunoglobulin

Indication	Level of evidence
Spontaneous abortion	A
Elective abortion	A
Threatened abortion	C
Ectopic pregnancy	A
Hydatidiform mole	B
Genetic amniocentesis	A
Chorion villus biopsy	A
Fetal blood sampling	A
Placenta previa with bleeding	C
Suspected abruption	C
Intrauterine fetal demise	C
Blunt trauma to the abdomen (includes motor vehicle accidents)	C
At 28 weeks' gestation, unless father of fetus is RhD negative	A
Amniocentesis for fetal lung maturity	A
External cephalic version	C
Within 72 h of delivery of an RhD-positive infant	A
After administration of RhD-positive blood components	C

Level A evidence (good and consistent scientific evidence) [3].
Level C evidence (consensus and expert opinion) [3].
Reproduced with permission from Moise KJ. Red cell alloimmunization. In: Gabbe S, Niebyl J, J Simpson *et al* (eds) *Obstetrics: Normal and Abnormal Pregnancies*, 5th edn. Philadelphia: Elsevier Saunders, 2007.

that the standard dose is insufficient to block all of the antigenic sites on the fetal red cells in the maternal circulation [4]. Therefore, if RhIg is inadvertently omitted after delivery, some protection has been proven with administration within 13 days. It should not be withheld as late as 28 days after delivery if the need arises [5].

Additional indications for RhIg are listed in Table 38.1. Although a 50 μg dose of RhIg has been recommended for clinical situations up to 13 weeks' gestation, most hospitals no longer stock this preparation and the cost is comparable to the standard 300 μg dose.

Methods of surveillance

In recent years, techniques for fetal surveillance in cases of RhD alloimmunization have evolved to a more noninvasive approach. Many of these have led to a reduction in the rate of enhanced maternal immunization as a result of invasive procedures as well as a reduction in the rate of perinatal loss. Consultation with a maternal-fetal specialist should be considered in these cases in an effort to offer the patient the latest advancements in the field.

Antibody titer

In the first affected pregnancy, the maternal antibody titer continues to be used as the first level of surveillance in the USA. Once the maternal antibody screen indicates the presence of an anti-D antibody, a titer should be ordered. A critical titer has been defined as the value for a particular institution that is associated with a risk for fetal hydrops. An anti-D titer of 32 in the first affected pregnancy is often used. However, one must be cautious in the interpretation of antibody titers as they are crude estimates of the amount of circulating antibody.

Today titers are performed much the same as they have been for several decades. Preserved human red cells are used as the indicator for the measurement of a biologic endpoint. These cells have a shelf-life of 4 weeks, leading to the likely situation that subsequent titers will be performed using a different batch of indicator cells. In addition, large differences in titer can be seen between laboratories in the same patient, as many commercial facilities use such techniques as enzymatic treatment of the indicator red cells to overestimate the actual value of the titer. Additionally, newer gel technology will often produce titer results that are two or more dilutions higher than expected with older tube technology [6].

Ultrasound

Ultrasound has revolutionized the surveillance of the anemic fetus. An early study is indicated in an affected pregnancy to determine the gestational age accurately. In the past, ultrasound was used to detect fetal hydrops. Unfortunately, this represents an end-stage phase of HDFN with more than two-thirds reduction in the fetal hemoglobin below the norm [7]. The most significant breakthrough in the surveillance of the potentially anemic fetus has been the validation of the peak systolic middle cerebral artery (MCA) Doppler velocity. For many years, alloimmunized women were subjected to repetitive amniocenteses to measure the amount of bilirubin in the amniotic fluid – a surrogate test for the degree of ongoing fetal hemolysis. The test was often referred to as the ΔOD_{450} as it measured the change in optical density at 450 nm for the bilirubin peak using spectrophotometry. Results were plotted on various longitudinal curves named after their authors – the Liley and Queenan curves [8,9]. Recent studies have verified the MCA Doppler to be more sensitive for predicting fetal anemia than the ΔOD_{450} [10]. The

Table 38.2 Peak systolic middle cerebral artery values

Weeks of gestation	1.29 MoM (mild anemia) (cm/s)	1.50 MoM (moderate–severe anemia) (cm/s)
18	29.9	34.8
20	32.8	38.2
22	36.0	41.9
24	39.5	46.0
26	43.3	50.4
28	47.6	55.4
30	52.2	60.7
32	57.3	66.6
34	62.9	73.1
36	69.0	80.2
38	75.7	88.0
40	83.0	96.6

MoM, multiples of the mean.
Source: Mari [11].

MCA can be easily visualized with color flow Doppler. Pulsed Doppler is then used to measure the peak systolic velocity of the MCA just distal to its bifurcation from the internal carotid artery. Enhanced fetal cardiac output and a decrease in blood viscosity contribute to an increased blood flow velocity in fetal anemia. Because the general trend is for the MCA velocity to increase with advancing gestational age, results are reported in multiples of the median (MoM), much like serum α-fetoprotein. The actual value can be plotted on standard curves (Table 38.2) or entered into a website that will calculate the MoM value (www.perinatology.com). A value greater than 1.5 MoM is suggestive of moderate-to-severe fetal anemia and requires further investigation through direct ultrasound-guided fetal blood sampling (cordocentesis) [11].

Middle cerebral artery Dopplers can be initiated as early as 18 weeks' gestation and should be repeated every 1–2 weeks as the clinical situation warrants. After 35 weeks' gestation, the false-positive rate for the prediction of fetal anemia is increased probably as a result of fetal heart rate accelerations [12]. The advantage of serial MCA measurements is a reduction of over 80% in the need for invasive diagnostic procedures such as amniocentesis and cordocentesis.

Fetal blood typing through DNA analysis

Paternal testing should begin early in the evaluation process of the alloimmunized patient. An RhD-negative result with assurance of paternity requires no further maternal testing after proper documentation of the paternity discussion with the patient in the medical record. Because more than 50% of RhD-positive partners are heterozygous, testing in consultation with the blood bank should be employed to determine the paternal zygosity. This is undertaken through DNA analysis for RhD; serologic testing can be used to detect paternal zygosity in the case of other Rh antibodies (C, c, E, e) or other irregular anti-red cell antibodies such as Kell.

An exciting new development in fetal RhD typing involves the isolation of free fetal DNA in maternal serum [13]. In the UK, this technique has virtually replaced amniocentesis for fetal RhD determination in the case of a heterozygous paternal phenotype. This test is now commercially available in the US. In the case of a heterozygous paternal phenotype for other red cell antigens, amniocentesis can be undertaken at 15–17 weeks to obtain fetal DNA from the amniotic fluid to determine the fetal genotype for the involved red cell antigen. Both paternal and maternal blood samples should be sent to the reference laboratory with the amniotic fluid aliquot in order to exclude gene rearrangements that may invalidate the fetal DNA result. If the patient's partner is not available or if there is a question regarding paternity, paired maternal titers can be tested 8–10 weeks apart. If there is an increase in titer of more than fourfold (i.e. 4–32), an antigen-negative fetal genotype by previous amniocentesis or free fetal DNA testing may be erroneous.

Overall clinical management

First sensitized pregnancy

- Follow maternal titers every 4 weeks up to 20 weeks' gestation; repeat every 2 weeks thereafter.
- Assess paternal zygosity for the Rh gene.
- Once a critical value (usually 32) is reached in cases of a heterozygous paternal phenotype, perform free fetal DNA from maternal blood or amniocentesis at 15–17 weeks to determine the fetal RhD status. Send maternal and paternal blood samples (usually in an EDTA tube) with the amniotic fluid.
- If an RhD-negative fetus is found, no further testing is warranted.
- If a there is homozygous paternal phenotype or RhD-positive fetus by DNA analysis, begin serial MCA Dopplers as early as 24 weeks' gestation. Repeat weekly three times and assess trend. If not rising rapidly, consider MCAs every 2 weeks.
- If the MCA Doppler is >1.5 MoM, perform cordocentesis with blood readied for intrauterine transfusion (IUT; see below) for a fetal hematocrit of <30%.
- If repeat MCA velocities remain <1.5 MoM, consider induction by 38 weeks' gestation.
- In the case of an elevated MCA after 35 weeks' gestation, consider repeating the study the following day. If the

value remains elevated, perform amniocentesis for fetal lung maturity and ΔOD_{450}. If immature and the ΔOD_{450} value is not in the upper zone 2 of the Liley curve, consider repeat amniocentesis 1 week later to confirm maturity.

• Induce by 38 weeks' gestation.

Previous severely affected fetus or infant (previous child requiring intrauterine or neonatal transfusion)

• Maternal titers are *not* helpful in predicting the onset of fetal anemia after the first affected gestation.

• In cases of a heterozygous paternal phenotype, analyze free fetal DNA from maternal blood or following amniocentesis at 15–16 weeks' gestation to determine the fetal RhD status. If an RhD-negative fetus is found, no further testing is warranted.

• If fetus is Rh positive, begin MCA Doppler assessments at 18 weeks' gestation. Repeat every week.

• When an MCA Doppler >1.5 MoM is noted, perform cordocentesis with blood readied for IUT for fetal hematocrit of <30%.

• If the MCA Doppler value does not become elevated, follow the same protocol after 35 weeks as for the first affected pregnancy (see above).

Intrauterine transfusion

First introduced in 1963 by Sir William Liley, IUT has withstood the test of time as the most successful fetal therapy [14]. Initially the peritoneal cavity was used as the site of transfusion; however, hydropic fetuses were found to exhibit poor absorption of transfused red blood cells. Today the direct intravascular transfusion (IVT) of donor red blood cells into the fetal umbilical vein at its placental insertion is the most common method of IUT. Variations in the standard IVT approach include the inclusion of additional transfused cells into the peritoneal cavity at the same setting to prolong the interval between procedures [15]. Additionally, the intrahepatic portion of the umbilical vein is used as the access site for IVT in many centers in Europe [16].

Limited visualization of the umbilical cord insertion precludes successful IVT prior to 18 weeks' gestation. Most centers will not perform an IUT after 35 weeks. After the first IVT, the second procedure is usually planned 7–10 days later with an expected decrement in the fetal hematocrit of approximately 1% per day. Subsequent procedures are repeated at 2–3-week intervals based on fetal response and suppression of fetal erythropoiesis.

After the last procedure, the patient is scheduled for induction of labor at 38–39 weeks' gestation to allow for fetal liver maturity. The addition of oral maternal phenobarbital may further enhance the ability of the fetal liver to conjugate bilirubin, thereby preventing the need for neonatal exchange transfusions [17]. Currently, the typical neonatal course for the fetus treated successfully with serial IUTs includes minimal need for phototherapy and discharge to home with the mother at the end of a routine postpartum stay. Postpartum is not contraindicated.

Outcome

In experienced centers, the overall perinatal survival with IUT is 85–90% [18]. Hydropic fetuses fare more poorly, with a 15% decrease in survival over their nonhydropic counterparts [19]. Suppression of fetal erythropoiesis because of serial IUTs can be associated with profound anemia in the first few months of life. Weekly neonatal hematocrit and reticulocyte counts should be followed until there is evidence of renewed production of red cells. Top-up red cell transfusions may be required in as many as 50% of cases [20].

Neurodevelopmental follow-up studies of neonates transfused by IVT are limited in number. Most point to over a 90% chance of intact survival [21]. Hydrops fetalis does not seem to affect this outcome. Sensorineural hearing loss may be slightly increased as a result of prolonged exposure of the fetus to high levels of bilirubin. A hearing screen should be performed during the early neonatal course and repeated by 2 years of life.

Hemolytic disease of the fetus and newborn caused by non-RhD antibodies

Antibodies to the red cell antigens Lewis, I, and P are often encountered through antibody screening during prenatal care. Because these antibodies are typically of the IgM class, they do not cross the placenta and are not associated with HDFN [22].

Antibodies to more than 50 other red cell antigens have been reported to be associated with HDFN (Table 38.3). However, only three of these antibodies cause significant hemolytic disease where treatment with IUT is necessary: anti-RhD, anti-Rhc, and anti-Kell (K1). Most centers use a maternal titer of 32 in cases of non-RhD antibodies to initiate fetal surveillance. Because the Kell antibody affects the fetus both at the level of the bone marrow to suppress erythropoiesis as well as causing the destruction of circulating red cells, a critical titer of 8 is used in the case of Kell antibodies [23].

Table 38.3 Non-RhD antibodies and associated hemolytic disease of the fetus and newborn (HDFN)

Antigen system	Specific antigen	Antigen system	Specific antigen	Antigen system	Specific antigen
Frequently associated with severe disease					
Kell	K (K1)				
Rhesus	c				
Infrequently associated with severe disease					
Colton	Co^a	MNS	Mur	Scianna	Sc2
	Co3		M^V		Rd
Diego	ELO		s	Other Ag	Bi
	Di^a		s^D		Good
	Di^b		S		Heibel
	Wr^a		U		HJK
	Wr^b		Vw		Ht^a
Duffy	Fy^a	Rhesus	Be^a		Jones
Kell	Js^b		C		Joslin
	k (K2)		Ce		Kg
	Kp^a		C^w		Kuhn
	Kp^b		ce		Li^a
	K11		E		MAM
	K22		E^w		Niemetz
	Ku		Evans		REIT
	Ul^a		G		Reiter
Kidd	Jk^a		Go^a		Rd
MNS	En^a		Hr		Sharp
	Far		Hr$_o$		Vel
	Hil		JAL		Zd
	Hut		Rh32		
	M		Rh42		
	Mi^a		Rh46		
	Mt^a		STEM		
	MUT		Tar		
Associated with mild disease					
Duffy	Fy^b	Kidd	Jk^b	Rhesus	Riv
	Fy3		Jk3		RH29
Gerbich	Ge2	MNS	Mit	Other	At^a
	Ge3	Rhesus	C^X		JFV
	Ge4		D^w		Jr^a
	Ls^a		e		Lan
Kell	Js^a		HOFM		
			LOCR		

Reproduced with permission from Moise KJ. Hemolytic disease of the fetus and newborn. In: Creasy RK, Resnik R, Iams J, eds. Maternal-Fetal Medicine, 5th edn. Philadelphia: wb Saunders, 2004.

CASE PRESENTATION 1: SURVEILLANCE OF THE FIRST AFFECTED GESTATION

A 30-year-old gravida 2, para 1001 was noted to have a positive antibody screen for anti-D at her first prenatal visit at 8 weeks' gestation. The patient had not received Rh immunoglobulin after her previous delivery in Mexico 3 years earlier. Her titer was 32 for anti-D. Paternal DNA testing revealed a heterozygous state. The patient was scheduled for amniocentesis at 16 weeks' gestation but elected to undergo free fetal DNA testing instead. Results indicated an RhD-positive fetus. At 24 weeks' gestation the anti-D titer remained stable at 32. Serial MCA Doppler studies were initiated each week. After 3 weeks, these

remained at 1.1–1.2 MoM so the testing interval was lengthened to every 2 weeks. The MCA Dopplers remained normal. Induction of labor was undertaken at 38 weeks' gestation. A healthy 3713 g (8 lb 3 oz) female fetus was born vaginally. Cord blood revealed the child to be A, RhD positive, the direct Coombs was 1+, and the total bilirubin was 2.1 mg/dL. The infant required 3 days of bililight therapy with a peak bilirubin of 10 mg/dL. The infant was discharged on the fourth day of life and required no further treatment.

CASE PRESENTATION 2: SURVEILLANCE OF A SUBSEQUENT AFFECTED GESTATION

The patient in case presentation 1 returned 2 years later with her third pregnancy. The current pregnancy had been fathered by the same partner as her previous gestation. At 10 weeks' gestation, the maternal anti-D titer was 128. An amniocentesis at 15 weeks indicated an RhD-positive fetus. Serial MCA Dopplers were initiated each week starting at 18 weeks' gestation. At 25 weeks, the MCA peak systolic velocity was 1.45 MoM. One week later it had risen to 1.7 MoM. The following day, an IUT was scheduled. Initial fetal blood at the time of cordocentesis revealed blood type O, RhD positive, with a 3+ direct Coombs test. The fetal hematocrit was 25% with 15% reticulocytes. An intravascular transfusion of 45 mL raised the fetal hematocrit to 50%. The patient returned for five additional IUTs, the last one being performed at 35 weeks' gestation. Oral phenobarbital was prescribed to the

patient 10 days prior to her planned induction date in an effort to enhance the neonatal capability to conjugate bilirubin.

She was induced at 38 weeks' gestation and delivered a healthy 3004 g (6 lb 10 oz) male fetus. Cord blood testing revealed a hematocrit of 45% with a Kleihauer–Betke stain consisting of 100% adult hemoglobin-containing red cells, indicating complete suppression of the fetal bone marrow. The infant was discharged on the second day of life and did not require bililight therapy. He was followed with weekly hematocrit and reticulocyte counts by his pediatrician. At 4 weeks of age he was noted to be feeding poorly; the hematocrit had declined to 23%. He was admitted overnight for a "top-up" red cell transfusion. Subsequent testing revealed a rising reticulocyte count. The infant required no further therapy.

References

1. Wataganara T, Chen AY, LeShane ES et al. Cell-free fetal DNA levels in maternal plasma after elective first-trimester termination of pregnancy. Fertil Steril 2004;81:638–644.
2. Medearis AL, Hensleigh PA, Parks DR, Herzenberg LA. Detection of fetal erythrocytes in maternal blood postpartum with the fluorescence-activated cell sorter. Am J Obstet Gynecol 1984;148:290–295.
3. American College of Obstetricians and Gynecologists. Prevention of RhD alloimmunization. Practice Bulletin No. 4. Washington, DC: American College of Obstetricians and Gynecologists, 1999.
4. Kumpel BM. On the mechanism of tolerance to the Rh D antigen mediated by passive anti-D (Rh D prophylaxis). Immunol Lett 2002;82:67–73.
5. Bowman JM. Controversies in Rh prophylaxis. Who needs Rh immune globulin and when should it be given? Am J Obstet Gynecol 1985;151:289–294.
6. Novaretti MC, Jens E, Pagliarini T et al. Comparison of conventional tube test with diamed gel microcolumn assay for anti-D titration. Clin Lab Haematol 2003;25:311–315.
7. Nicolaides KH, Warenski JC, Rodeck CH. The relationship of fetal plasma protein concentration and hemoglobin level to the development of hydrops in rhesus isoimmunization. Am J Obstet Gynecol 1985;152:341–344.
8. Liley AW. Liquor amnii analysis in the management of pregnancy complicated by rhesus sensitization. Am J Obstet Gynecol 1961;82:1359–1370.
9. Queenan JT, Tomai TP, Ural SH, King JC. Deviation in amniotic fluid optical density at a wavelength of 450 nm in Rh-immunized pregnancies from 14 to 40 weeks' gestation: a

proposal for clinical management. Am J Obstet Gynecol 1993;168:1370–1376.

10. Opekes D, Seward G, Vandenbussche F et al. Minimally invasive management of Rh alloimmunization: can amniotic fluid delta OD450 be replaced by Doppler studies? A prospective study multicenter trial. Am J Obstet Gynecol 2004;191:S3.

11. Mari G, for the Collaborative Group for Doppler Assessment of the Blood Velocity in Anemic Fetuses. Noninvasive diagnosis by Doppler ultrasonography of fetal anemia due to maternal red-cell alloimmunization. N Engl J Med 2000;342:9–14.

12. Zimmerman R, Carpenter RJ Jr, Durig P, Mari G. Longitudinal measurement of peak systolic velocity in the fetal middle cerebral artery for monitoring pregnancies complicated by red cell alloimmunisation: a prospective multicentre trial with intention-to-treat. Br J Obstet Gynaecol 2002;109: 746–752.

13. Finning KM, Martin PG, Soothill PW, Avent ND. Prediction of fetal D status from maternal plasma: introduction of a new noninvasive fetal RHD genotyping service. Transfusion 2002;42:1079–1085.

14. Liley AW. Intrauterine transfusion of foetus in haemolytic disease. BMJ 1963;2:1107–1109.

15. Moise KJ Jr, Carpenter RJ Jr, Kirshon B, Deter RL, Sala JD, Cano LE. Comparison of four types of intrauterine transfusion: effect on fetal hematocrit. Fetal Ther 1989;4:126–137.

16. Nicolini U, Nicolaidis P, Fisk NM, Tannirandorn Y, Rodeck CH. Fetal blood sampling from the intrahepatic vein: analysis of safety and clinical experience with 214 procedures. Obstet Gynecol 1990;76:47–53.

17. Trevett T, Dorman K, Lamvu G, Moise KJ. Does antenatal maternal administration of phenobarbital prevent exchange transfusion in neonates with alloimmune hemolytic disease? Am J Obstet Gynecol 2005;192:478–482.

18. Van Kamp IL, Klumper FJ, Oepkes D et al. Complications of intrauterine intravascular transfusion for fetal anemia due to maternal red-cell alloimmunization. Am J Obstet Gynecol 2005;192:171–177.

19. Van Kamp IL, Klumper FJ, Bakkum RS et al. The severity of immune fetal hydrops is predictive of fetal outcome after intrauterine treatment. Am J Obstet Gynecol 2001;185: 668–673.

20. Saade GR, Moise KJ, Belfort MA, Hesketh DE, Carpenter RJ. Fetal and neonatal hematologic parameters in red cell alloimmunization: predicting the need for late neonatal transfusions. Fetal Diagn Ther 1993;8:161–164.

21. Hudon L, Moise KJ Jr, Hegemier SE et al. Long-term neurodevelopmental outcome after intrauterine transfusion for the treatment of fetal hemolytic disease. Am J Obstet Gynecol 1998;179:858–863.

22. Brecher ME. Technical Manual of the American Association of Blood Banks. Bethesda, MD: American Association of Blood Banks, 2002.

23. Bowman JM, Pollock JM, Manning FA, Harman CR, Menticoglou S. Maternal Kell blood group alloimmunization. Obstet Gynecol 1992;79:239–244.

Chapter 39
Multiple Gestations

Karin E. Fuchs and Mary E. D'Alton
Department of Obstetrics and Gynecology, Columbia University Medical Center and Columbia Presbyterian Hospital, New York, NY, USA

An epidemic of multiple gestations has occurred over the past two decades, attributed largely to an older patient population secondary to delayed child bearing and the rise in the use of assisted reproductive technology (ART) and ovulation induction. According to the National Vital Statistics Report for 2007, the twinning rate was 32.2 twin births per 1000 total livebirths with a 70% rise between 1980 and 2004 [1]. More impressive are the numbers of triplets and high-order multiples, which rose over 400% between 1980 and 1998 to a high of 193.5 per 100,000 births before declining again to a rate of 148.9 per 100,000 births in 2007 [1]. Perinatal complications have been strongly affected by the widespread prevalence of multiple gestations as these pregnancies account for a disproportionate share of adverse outcomes.

The most profound implication of this epidemic of multiple gestations is the problem of preterm delivery, which remains the leading cause of hospitalization among pregnant women and the leading cause of infant death [2]. In addition to prematurity, multiple pregnancy is known to be associated with a greater number of other maternal and fetal problems including gestational hypertension, placental abruption, operative delivery, low birthweight, and adverse neurologic outcomes [3]. The overall increased perinatal risks associated with multiple gestations compared with singleton pregnancies are well documented, and these high-risk pregnancies have a profound effect on medical expenditures and public health [1]. This chapter reviews multiple gestations and the current strategies for managing these complex pregnancies.

Impact on perinatal outcomes

The two most important contributors to increased perinatal morbidity and mortality in multiple gestations appear to be increased rates of prematurity and complications of monochorionicity. In 2002 in the USA, the mean age at delivery was 35.3 weeks for twins, 32.2 weeks for triplets, and 29.9 weeks for quadruplets, compared to 38.8 weeks for singletons [4]. Offspring of multiple pregnancies also have lower birthweights than singletons, with the mean birthweight for singletons being 3332 g compared to 2347 g for twins, 1687 g for triplets, and 1309 g for quadruplets [4]. In 2007, 57% of twins were low birthweight (LBW) [1]. In addition, neonates from multiple gestations currently comprise a disproportionate share of neonatal intensive care admissions and recent National Vital Statistics data indicate that nearly 20% of neonatal deaths are from multiple gestations. While the offspring of multiple gestations may be born earlier than singletons, preterm twin and triplet neonates appear to have similar birthweights, morbidities, and mortalities as gestational age-matched singleton controls [5–7], suggesting that the increased risk of perinatal morbidity and mortality among multiples can be explained by the increased rate of preterm delivery in this population.

Besides prematurity, patients with multiples are at increased risk for adverse perinatal outcomes resulting from complications unique to the twinning process. In particular, monochorionic placentation accounts for 20% of all twin pregnancies and carries a worse prognosis than dichorionicity. Complications from monochorionicity such as twin–twin transfusion syndrome (TTTS) continue to place these offspring at higher risk for long-term adverse outcomes. Cases of single intrauterine fetal death (IUFD) in twins sharing a single placenta can be associated with a coincident insult leading to white matter damage in the surviving co-twin. Other unique but rare problems that occur in monochorionic pregnancies include cord entanglement in monoamniotic twins, conjoined twins, and twin reversed arterial perfusion (TRAP) sequence, also known as a cardiac twinning.

Multiple gestation is an independent risk factor for long-term neurologic impairment. In various studies,

Queenan's Management of High-Risk Pregnancy: An Evidence-Based Approach, Sixth Edition. Edited by John T. Queenan, Catherine Y. Spong, Charles J. Lockwood.

children from a multiple pregnancy have a 4–17 times higher risk of developing cerebral palsy compared to their singleton counterparts [3,8–10]. With more investigators finding this correlation to be true at higher birthweights, this suggests that the risk is not simply related to an increased preterm delivery rate [9,10]. One epidemiologic study reported that the risk of producing one child with cerebral palsy in twin, triplet, and quadruplet gestations was 15 per 1000 twins, 80 per 1000 triplets, and 429 per 1000 quadruplets [10]. While many previous studies investigating this association were not optimally designed, the prevalence of cerebral palsy in multiple pregnancies reported in these studies is similar and ranges from 6.7 to 12.6 per 1000 surviving infants [9]. This consistent conclusion suggests an association between multiple birth and cerebral palsy. While a portion of this risk appears to be related to the higher rates of prematurity, there are many other risk factors for cerebral palsy seen with higher frequency in multiples, including maternal hypertensive disease, bleeding in pregnancy, LBW infants, congenital anomalies, and complications specific to monochorionicity [9,11].

Zygosity and chorionicity

Embryology

Zygosity refers to the genetic constitution of a twin pregnancy, while chorionicity indicates the pregnancy's membrane composition. In dizygotic twins, chorionicity is determined by the mechanism of fertilization, while in monozygotic twins it is determined by the timing of embryonic division. The vast majority of dizygotic twins have separate dichorionic diamniotic placentas (each fetus has its own placental disk with a separate amnion and chorion). This is because dizygotic twins result from the fertilization of two different ova by two separate sperm. The type of placenta that develops in a monozygotic pregnancy is determined by the timing of cleavage of the fertilized ovum. If twinning is accomplished during the first 2–3 days, it precedes the separation of cells that eventually become the chorion. In that case, two chorions and two amnions will be formed. After approximately 3 days, twinning cannot split the chorionic cavity and from that time forward, a monochorionic placenta results. If the split occurs between the third and eighth days, a diamniotic monochorionic placenta develops. Between the 8th and 13th days, the amnion has already formed, and the placenta will therefore be monoamniotic and monochorionic. Embryonic cleavage between the 13th and 15th days results in conjoined twins within a single amnion and chorion; beyond that point, the process of twinning does not occur [12]. Interestingly, rare cases of dizygotic monochorionic twins conceived following ART have been reported [13,14].

Ultrasound diagnosis of chorionicity

The determination of chorionicity is important in the management of multiple gestations as monochorionic twins are at increased risk for adverse outcomes. Antenatal knowledge of chorionicity can be critical for determining optimal management of a variety of pregnancy complications, including growth disorders. Precise knowledge of chorionicity is imperative when contemplating the selective termination (ST) of one abnormal twin or when performing elective first-trimester multifetal pregnancy reduction (MPR). If the gestation is monochorionic, a shared placental circulation could result in death or injury to a surviving fetus, depending on the technique utilized for the termination procedure.

Chorionicity is most accurately determined in the first trimester. From 6 to 10 weeks, counting the number of gestational sacs with evaluation of the thickness of the dividing membrane is the optimal method. Two separate gestational sacs, each containing a fetus and a thick dividing membrane, suggests a dichorionic diamniotic pregnancy, while one gestational sac with a thin dividing membrane and two fetuses suggests a monochorionic diamniotic pregnancy [15]. The number of yolk sacs can also be used as an indirect method of determining amnionicity [16]. After 9 weeks, the dividing membranes become progressively thinner in monochorionic pregnancies. In dichorionic pregnancies, they remain thick and easy to identify at their attachment to the placenta as a triangular projection (lambda or twin peak sign) [17–19]. Thus, in the late first trimester, sonographic examination of the base of the intertwin membrane for the presence or absence of the lambda sign provides reliable distinction between dichorionic and monochorionic pregnancies [20].

Later in pregnancy, determination of chorionicity and amnionicity becomes less accurate and requires different techniques. The sonographic prediction of chorionicity and amnionicity should be systematically approached by determining the number of placentas visualized and the sex of each fetus and then by assessing the membranes that divide the sacs. If two separate placental disks are seen, the pregnancy is dichorionic. Likewise, if the twins are different genders, the pregnancy is most likely dichorionic. When a single placenta is present and the twins are of the same sex, careful sonographic examination of the dividing membrane will typically result in a correct diagnosis. Evaluation of three features in the intertwin membrane will provide an almost certain diagnosis about the chorionicity of a twin pregnancy:
- thickness of the intertwin membrane
- number of layers visualized in the membrane
- assessment of the junction of the membrane with the placenta for the "twin peak" sign [21].

It should be mentioned that the absence of the twin peak sign does not guarantee that the pregnancy is monochorionic.

In some pregnancies with monochorionic diamniotic placentation, the dividing membranes may not be sonographically visualized because they are very thin. In other cases, they may not be seen because severe oligohydramnios causes them to be closely apposed to the fetus in that sac. This results in a "stuck twin" appearance, where the trapped fetus remains firmly held against the uterine wall despite changes in maternal position. Diagnosis of this condition confirms the presence of a diamniotic gestation, which should be distinguished from a monoamniotic gestation with an absent dividing membrane. In the latter situation, free movement of both twins, and entanglement of their umbilical cords, can be identified [22].

Fetal complications and multiple gestations

The offspring of a multiple gestation are at risk for many complications *in utero* that may lead to long-term adverse outcomes, including growth abnormalities, fetal loss, and complications unique to the twinning process (Box 39.1).

Intrauterine growth restriction and growth discordance

Birthweight is a function of many factors, including gestational age, rate of fetal growth, ethnicity, and genetic composition. Two important antenatal markers for growth abnormalities are intrauterine growth restriction (IUGR) and growth discordance. IUGR remains a sonographic and statistical diagnosis consisting of either an estimated fetal weight (EFW) less than the 3rd percentile (two standard deviations from the mean) for gestational age or an EFW <10th percentile for gestational age along with evidence of fetal compromise (usually oligohydramnios or

---

Box 39.1 Multiple gestation: fetal and neonatal risks

- Fetal loss
- Chromosomal abnormalities
- Congenital malformations
- Monochorionicity:
  - TTTS
  - Monoamnionicity
  - TRAP
- Growth discordance/IUGR
- Amniotic fluid volume abnormalities
- Prematurity
- Low birthweight
- Perinatal mortality
- Cerebral palsy

IUGR, intrauterine growth restriction; TRAP, twin reversed arterial perfusion; TTTS, twin–twin transfusion syndrome.

---

abnormal umbilical artery Doppler velocimetry) [23]. Growth discordance is generally defined as >20% difference in EFW between fetuses of the same pregnancy expressed as a percentage of the larger EFW [23]. Both growth abnormalities are seen with increased frequency in multiple gestations.

Intrauterine growth restriction has long been known to be associated with adverse perinatal outcomes. Neonatal morbidity (such as meconium aspiration syndrome, hypoglycemia, polycythemia, and pulmonary hemorrhage) may be present in up to 50% of IUGR neonates [23]. Long-term studies show a twofold increased incidence of cerebral dysfunction (ranging from minor learning disabilities to cerebral palsy) in IUGR infants delivered at term and an even higher incidence if the infant was born preterm [9]. Multiple gestations present a dilemma both in diagnosis and management of IUGR. For example, fetuses suspected to be normally grown may be affected by iatrogenic preterm delivery secondary to interventions for a growth-restricted co-twin. Current management of IUGR is aimed at early diagnosis and fetal surveillance to aid in timing delivery.

Like IUGR, growth discordance has been associated with an increased risk for adverse perinatal outcomes [24]. Approximately 15% of twins are diagnosed with this condition [24]. Risk factors include monochorionicity, velamentous cord insertion, antenatal bleeding, uteroplacental insufficiency, and gestational hypertensive disease [24]. Growth discordance has different implications depending on chorionicity and is more concerning in monochorionic twinning. Although IUGR can complicate a pregnancy with growth discordance, the second does not necessarily imply the first. While some studies have demonstrated an increased risk for perinatal morbidity in growth discordant twins, others have not. In approximately two-thirds of discordant twin pairs, the smaller twin has a birthweight of less than 10% [25]. In a study of more than 10,000 discordant twins, the neonatal mortality rates were 29 versus 11 per 1000 livebirths when the smaller twin weighed less than the 10th percentile, compared with those who were above it [25]. Conversely, a recent study suggests that 20% growth discordance may result in an increased risk for some adverse outcomes but not for serious sequelae [26]. After adjusting for chorionicity, antenatal steroids, oligohydramnios, preeclampsia, and gestational age at delivery, discordant twins were at increased risk for low or very low birthweight, neonatal intensive care unit (NICU) admission, neonatal oxygen requirement, and hyperbilirubinemia but did not seem to be at increased risk for serious neonatal morbidity and mortality.

Fetal loss

The incidence of early pregnancy loss in multiple gestations is higher than previously thought. The routine use of ultrasound has shown that early fetal loss is common in multiple gestations. In patients with twin gestations scanned in the first trimester, rates of demise ranged from 13% to 78% [27]. This phenomenon has been termed the *vanishing twin*. Explanations for this occurrence include physiologic resorption, artifact, and sonographic error. Although this condition has been associated with first-trimester bleeding and spotting, it has not been associated with adverse pregnancy outcomes.

During the second and third trimester, IUFD occurs more commonly in multiple gestations than in singletons, with IUFD of one fetus occurring in approximately 2–5% of twin pregnancies. In patients with high-order multiples, however, death of a single fetus may be more common with single IUFD rates up to 17% in triplet pregnancies [28]. Recent literature has suggested that the risk of intrauterine death of one or both twin is higher in monochorionic than dichorionic pregnancies. In a study of 1000 consecutive twin-pairs, monochorionic-diamniotic twins had a higher risk of stillbirth compared with dichorionic-diamniotic twins, both overall and at each gestational age after 24 weeks [29]; this increased risk of fetal loss persisted in "apparently normal" monochorionic-diamniotic twins unaffected by growth abnormalities, congenital anomalies, or TTTS.

Death of one twin in the second or third trimesters can adversely affect the surviving fetus or fetuses in two ways:
- risk for multicystic encephalomalacia and multiorgan damage in monochorionic pregnancies
- preterm labor and delivery in both dichorionic and monochorionic twins resulting in prematurity.

Although the multiorgan damage in surviving monochorionic twins was once thought to be due to disseminated intravascular coagulation in the surviving twin caused by transfer of thromboplastic materials from the dead fetus [30], a more recent and widely accepted theory suggests that the surviving twin may rapidly "back-bleed" into the dead twin through placental anastomoses (a capacitance effect), resulting in profound hypovolemia and anemia in the surviving twin [31]. Decreased circulatory tone in the dead twin causing blood to flow from the viable to the dead twin may be the underlying pathophysiology [32]. If the hypotension is severe enough, the surviving twin is at risk for ischemic damage to vital organs. Most evidence in the literature suggests that "back-bleeding" and subsequent hemodynamic changes are the cause of multiorgan injury in surviving co-twins. As a result, immediate delivery of the co-twin following single IUFD in a monochorionic pregnancy does not improve outcome but rather adds to the additional risk of prematurity. Most cases are managed expectantly with close fetal surveillance. Normal fetal heart rate patterns and biophysical profile scores cannot rule out multicystic encephalomalacia. Normal fetal magnetic resonance imaging, while investigational, may be reassuring [33].

In addition to multiorgan ischemic damage in monochorionic pregnancies, studies have demonstrated that IUFD of one twin can result in preterm delivery. Both dichorionic and monochorionic pregnancies are at risk for preterm delivery. In a study of 17 twin pregnancies complicated by IUFD, 76% of these pregnancies were delivered before 37 weeks. Eighty-six percent of the patients delivering prematurely presented in active labor [34].

When IUFD occurs in a multiple pregnancy, baseline maternal hematologic laboratory investigation is suggested, including prothrombin time (PT), partial thromboplastin time (PTT), fibrinogen level, and platelet count, because of the theoretical risk of maternal consumptive coagulopathy in the setting of a single IUFD. If these values are within normal limits, further surveillance is not indicated. Of note, mothers with IUFD in one twin do not appear to be at increased risk of infection from a retained twin [34]. Dystocia secondary to the dead fetus has been reported infrequently. Cesarean delivery rates appear increased in patients with single IUFD complicating a twin gestation because of higher rates of nonreassuring fetal status in the surviving twin [34].

Discordant anatomic abnormalities

There is general agreement that anomalies occur more frequently in twins than in singletons, but controversy exists regarding the degree of difference [35–38]. The diagnosis of discordance for major genetic disorders or anatomic abnormalities in the second trimester places parents in a difficult position. Management choices include:
- expectant management
- termination of the entire pregnancy
- selective termination of the anomalous fetus.

The term "selective termination" (ST) refers to terminating a specific fetus that is known to be abnormal. In contrast, the term multifetal pregnancy reduction (MPR) refers to reduction in the number of fetuses a woman is carrying in order to reduce her risk of preterm delivery. For dichorionic pregnancies, intracardiac injection with potassium chloride is utilized. Because of the placental anastomoses between monochorionic fetuses, however, cord occlusive procedures are employed in monochorionic pregnancies in order to reduce the risk to the surviving twin [39]. Cord occlusion techniques include suture ligation, bipolar or laser coagulation, or radiofrequency ablation.

Several issues should be considered when counseling patients about the management of a multiple pregnancy complicated by a discordant anomaly.
- Severity of the anomaly
- Chorionicity

• Effect of the anomalous fetus on the remaining fetus or fetuses

• The parents' personal, moral, and ethical beliefs

It is important to counsel patients that conservative management can result in adverse outcomes for the healthy twin. Several studies have demonstrated that the normal fetus in a twin pregnancy discordant for major fetal anomalies may be at increased risk for preterm delivery, low birthweight, and perinatal morbidity and mortality [40–42].

Complications unique to monochorionicity

Monoamnionicity

Less than 1% of monozygotic twins are monoamniotic [43]. Monoamniotic twins have been associated with a high rate of perinatal mortality. Previous studies report a fetal mortality rate of greater than 50% but more recent studies indicate a perinatal mortality rate ranging from 10% to 21% [44–46]. Preterm delivery, IUGR, congenital anomalies, cord entanglement, and cord accidents remain common in monoamniotic pregnancies. The management of these pregnancies is controversial, particularly regarding the optimal protocol for antenatal surveillance and the optimal timing for delivery. Because IUFD can occur at any gestational age, some experts suggest early delivery in the late preterm period [47]. Other studies have suggested that early delivery is not prudent secondary to the risks of prematurity [48]. The nonstress test is generally the preferred method of testing over the biophysical profile, as cord compression may be indicated by variable decelerations. While the optimal management and timing of delivery for monoamniotic twins remain uncertain, our current practice includes routine hospitalization beginning at 24–26 weeks, daily nonstress tests, and, if uncomplicated, delivery at 34 weeks is offered after antenatal corticosteroid administration and thorough counseling of the risks and benefits of elective preterm delivery.

Twin–twin transfusion syndrome

Monochorionic twins occur spontaneously in 0.4% of the general population. However, studies have reported that monozygotic twinning may be greater than 10 times higher in pregnancies following fertility treatment [49,50]. The primary concerns about monochorionic placentation include complications such as TTTS characterized by an unequal distribution of the blood flow across the shared placenta of two fetuses. Although all monochorionic twins share a portion of their vasculature, only approximately 15–20% will develop this condition [43,51]. Left untreated, there is up to 60–100% mortality rate for both twins.

Antenatal diagnosis of TTTS is made sonographically and findings include the presence of a single placenta, same-gender fetuses, weight discordance, and significant amniotic fluid discordance. The recipient twin may have signs of heart failure and hydrops and the donor may demonstrate IUGR and a "stuck" appearance. Umbilical artery Doppler studies can be variable [52]. TTTS may be chronic or acute. A staging system devised by Quintero *et al* [53] is commonly utilized to categorize disease severity and standardize comparison of different therapies. The net effect of this hemodynamic imbalance is a large, plethoric recipient twin and a small, anemic donor twin. While the exact etiology has not been clearly delineated, the mechanism is likely to involve shunting of arteriovenous anastomoses [54].

Treatment depends on gestational age at diagnosis. Patients with early-onset TTTS may opt for selective termination of one twin (usually the donor twin) or voluntary termination of the entire pregnancy. Diagnosis in the middle to late third trimester may be less aggressive, depending on disease severity and the proximity to term. Patients with mild TTTS (Quintero stage I) are generally followed expectantly with serial ultrasound examinations whereas treatments for severe TTTS include serial amnioreduction, septostomy, or selective fetoscopic laser coagulation of the communicating vessels. Compared to amnioreduction, several studies have shown that treatment with laser ablation is associated with a higher likelihood of the survival of at least one twin due to a lower rate of perinatal and neonatal mortality, and a lower likelihood of neurologic morbidity at 6 months [55–59]. Based on the published literature, laser ablation of placental anastomoses is often recommended for Quintero stage II-IV TTTS between 16 and 26 weeks of gestation, whereas amnioreduction remains the preferred treatment for severe TTTS beyond 26 weeks or when laser ablation is not available.

Maternal obstetric complications

Antepartum complications develop in over 80% of multiple pregnancies compared to 25% of singleton gestations [23]. Examples of adverse outcomes that may arise include anemia, urinary tract infections, gestational diabetes, abnormal placentation, thromboembolism, preterm premature rupture of membranes, abruption, and postpartum hemorrhage (Box 39.2) [3,60–62]. Pulmonary embolism, the leading cause of maternal death in the USA and around the world, and thromboembolism are about five times more likely during pregnancy or the puerperium than in the nonpregnant state [63]. Women carrying multiples are believed to be at increased risk for both.

Preeclampsia and its related spectrum of diseases occur in approximately 5–8% of singleton pregnancies but the

---

Box 39.2 Multiple gestation: maternal risks

- Hyperemesis
- Threatened miscarriage
- Anemia
- Gestational hypertension
- Preterm labor/delivery:
  - Tocolysis complications
  - Long-term bedrest
- Placental abnormalities:
  - Abruption
  - Abnormal placentation
- Urinary tract infection
- Gestational diabetes
- Postpartum hemorrhage
- Operative delivery
- Thromboembolism

---

incidence is higher in multiples [64,65]. Hypertensive diseases during pregnancy may manifest as hemolysis, elevated liver enzymes, and low platelet (HELLP) syndrome or eclampsia and can be associated with adverse sequelae including IUGR, placental abruption, disseminated intravascular coagulation, renal failure, and IUFD [64]. Unfortunately, no intervention to date (including aspirin and calcium supplementation) has been shown to prevent or reduce the incidence of preeclampsia in these high-risk pregnancies and delivery remains the only definitive cure [66,67]. Both gestational hypertension and preeclampsia are more common in women carrying multiples, with the rates estimated to be 2–2.6 times higher in twins compared to singletons [65]. Rates of preeclampsia seem to be the same for both monozygotic and dizygotic twins [68]. When preeclampsia occurs in triplets and higher order multiples, it often happens earlier, with more severity, and in an atypical presentation [60,69]. Finally, women carrying multifetal pregnancies may also be prone to developing acute fatty liver of pregnancy, one of the most serious maternal obstetric complications [70]. This disease process is characterized by hepatic dysfunction, severe coagulopathy, hypoglycemia, and hyperammonemia, and can result in fetal and/or maternal death.

Antepartum management of multiple gestations

The antepartum management of multiple pregnancies warrants attention to ensure adequate nutrition, avoidance of strenuous physical activity, and increased frequency of prenatal visits. Patients should be counseled regarding the increased risk of complications associated with multiple gestations. Women with multifetal pregnancies are currently recommended to increase their daily caloric intake approximately 300 kcal more than women with singletons. Iron and folic acid supplementation is also advised. While the optimal weight gain for women with multiples has not been determined, it has been suggested that women with twins gain 15.87–20.41 kg (35–45 lb) [3,71]. Patients with multiples should be followed with serial growth scans because clinical examination is inadequate in assessing growth of individual fetuses and because of the increased risk of fetal growth abnormalities in these pregnanacies.

Multifetal pregnancy reduction

Ovulation induction and ART have greatly contributed to the increasing number of high-order multiples. The purpose of first-trimester MPR is to improve perinatal outcomes by decreasing maternal complications secondary to multiple gestations and by decreasing adverse fetal outcomes associated with preterm delivery. Reducing a high-order multiple gestation to twins lowers the risk of preterm labor and delivery and increases the chances of higher birthweight and gestational age at delivery. In some instances, such as a history of a previous second-trimester loss, reduction from twins to a singleton may be indicated.

Nonetheless, MPR is an ethical dilemma. The starting number of fetuses needed to justify the procedure is controversial. There have been conflicting studies regarding whether or not MPR from triplets to twins results in improved perinatal outcomes compared to expectant management [72]. In addition, while most women do not regret their decision, women undergoing multifetal pregnancy reduction may have feelings of loss, guilt, and sadness.

The procedure is most commonly performed transabdominally under ultrasound guidance between 10 and 13 weeks' gestation. Potassium chloride is injected into the fetal heart until asystole is achieved. If chorionic villus sampling is performed prior to the procedure and one fetus is found to have a genetic anomaly, that fetus is targeted. Otherwise, the fetus with a crown–rump length smaller than expected for gestational age or the fetus most physically accessible is chosen. The fetus over the cervix is usually avoided. This procedure is reserved for dichorionic pregnancies. In monochorionic pregnancies, selectively reducing one fetus utilizing intracardiac potassium chloride is contraindicated because of the presence of communicating placental anastomoses. Selective reduction in these cases involves more technically challenging procedures.

There are several studies documenting pregnancy loss rates associated with MPR. With extensive experience, the current loss rate is approximately 6% [73]. There is little maternal risk associated with the procedure. The terminated fetus is usually resorbed or becomes a small papyraceous fetus. There have been no reports of coagulation disorders following this procedure [74]. Maternal serum α-fetoprotein (MSAFP) is elevated following MPR and ST and therefore cannot be used as a screening tool in these pregnancies.

Prenatal diagnosis

Prenatal diagnosis and genetic counseling are important in the management of patients with a multiple gestation because these pregnancies are at increased risk for both chromosomal and structural anomalies. All women, regardless of age, should be counseled about the option for either screening or diagnostic testing for fetal aneuploidy [75].

Many known chromosomal anomalies have been reported in twins. The maternal age-related risk for chromosomal abnormalities for each twin in dizygotic pregnancies is the same as in singleton pregnancies and, because each fetus has its own independent risk of aneuploidy, the chance of at least one chromosomally abnormal fetus is increased. Reports suggest that the risk of having one fetus with Down syndrome is similar for a woman between the ages of 31 and 33 carrying dizygotic twins and a 35-year-old woman with a singleton [76,77]. In monozygotic twins, the risk for chromosomal abnormalities is the same as in singletons, and in the vast majority of cases both fetuses are affected or both are unaffected [78]. However, there are occasional case reports of monozygotic twins discordant for abnormalities of autosomal or sex chromosomes [79,80].

Screening for fetal aneuploidy

Both first- and second-trimester serum markers are approximately twice as high in twin pregnancies as in singleton pregnancies [81]. Interpretation of abnormal serum screening results is difficult because it is not possible to determine which of the fetuses is responsible for the abnormal analyte concentration. In cases discordant for abnormalities, altered serum levels from the affected fetus will be brought closer to the mean by the unaffected twin.

First-trimester nuchal translucency ultrasound measurement, which assesses each fetus independently, is a promising method for aneuploidy screening in patients with multiples. Because the nuchal translucency distribution does not differ significantly in singletons compared to twins, the Down syndrome detection rate in multiples using nuchal translucency measurement together with maternal age is similar to that of singletons [82]. Nuchal translucency appears to be higher in patients with monochorionic pregnancies and it has been suggested that this may reflect an early manifestation of TTTS in a proportion of cases [83]. Nuchal translucency can also be performed in triplet and higher order multiple pregnancies with similar accuracy as in singletons.

In singletons, first-trimester combined screening, including maternal age and nuchal translucency combined with maternal serum free β-human chorionic gonadotropin (B-hCG) and pregnancy-associated plasma protein A (PAPP-A), has been shown to detect approximately 82% of cases of Down syndrome for a 5% false-positive rate [84]. In a prospective study, Spencer and Nicolaides reported a 75% detection rate of Down syndrome for a 9% false-positive rate using nuchal translucency and first-trimester serum markers in 206 twin pregnancies [85]. The combination of nuchal translucency and biochemistry studies in twins may prove to give detection rates similar to singleton pregnancies, but larger prospective studies on first-trimester combined screening in twins are needed before definitive conclusions and recommendations for practice can be made.

Diagnostic testing for fetal aneuploidy

Diagnostic testing should be performed on one fetus only if monozygosity is certain. Otherwise, diagnostic testing should be done on all fetuses given the individual risk of aneuploidy in each fetus.

Genetic amniocentesis in multiples is usually performed using an ultrasound-guided multiple-needle approach. Indigo carmine dye may be used to confirm proper needle placement. Although pregnancy loss rates after genetic amniocentesis in twins has been considered similar to singletons, recent literature suggests an increased risk of loss after amniocentesis of twin gestations [86]. Chorionic villus sampling (CVS) offers the advantage of earlier diagnosis, and can be performed between 10 and 13 weeks with a loss rate similar to amniocentesis [87].

Screening for neural tube defects in multiples

In singletons, a second-trimester MSAFP of greater than 2.5 multiples of the median (MoM) has been used to screen for neural tube defects. Different MSAFP cut-offs are needed for twin pregnancies because the MSAFP level in a twin pregnancy is approximately double that of a singleton pregnancy. A cut-off of 4.5 MoM is often used for twins because it has a detection rate of 50–85% for a 5% false-positive rate [88]. If an abnormal MSAFP is found, ultrasound is required for further evaluation. It is important to note that similar to maternal serum screening for aneuploidy, maternal serum screening for neural tube defects in a twin pregnancy will always be limited because it is impossible to confirm which fetus is affected without performing an ultrasound examination. As a result, many centers do not offer this type of serum screening for twin pregnancies.

Screening for anatomic abnormalities

The fetuses of multiple gestations seem to be at increased risk for anatomic abnormalities. Careful sonographic, anatomic evaluation of each fetus should be obtained. No large-scale studies of ultrasound for fetal anatomy in multiples have been performed. Small studies have attempted to determine the predictive value of ultrasound in the detection of fetal anomalies in multiples, and found it effective [89]. Recent studies have also demonstrated that monochorionic-diamniotic twins, both with and without TTTS, appear to be at increased risk of congenital heart disease, suggesting that screening fetal echocardiography may be considered in these pregnancies [90].

Prevention of preterm delivery

Patients with multiples are at increased risk for preterm labor and delivery. No therapy has proven to be efficacious in decreasing the adverse outcomes from prematurity except the administration of corticosteroids and surfactant to improve fetal lung maturity and antibiotics to lengthen the latency period for patients with premature rupture of membranes [91–93]. This therapy does not treat the primary problem of preterm labor. Management strategies aimed at reducing the rate of preterm delivery that have not proven beneficial include prophylactic cervical cerclage, routine bedrest, prophylactic tocolytics, progesterone supplementation, or home uterine monitoring [3,94,95].

Prophylactic cervical cerclage in patients with a multiple gestation has not been consistently proven to prevent prematurity. A randomized trial of 128 patients with twins offered elective cerclage at 18–26 weeks did not demonstrate any benefit [96]. Likewise, this intervention has not been shown to significantly improve perinatal outcomes in triplets [97]. A recent metaanalysis of randomized controlled trials examined individual patient-level data to determine whether cerclage prevented preterm birth in women with a short cervical length [98]. In the subgroup analysis of three trials including 49 twins, cerclage was associated with a significantly higher incidence of preterm birth and perinatal mortality. However, this investigation was limited by small sample size. Until a large prospective randomized trial of cerclage in multiples is performed, it remains difficult to refute a potential benefit from this procedure for a select group of women. Because this surgical procedure carries potential risks for both the mother and her fetuses, cerclage placement for multiple gestations is generally reserved for women with either a strong history or objectively documented cervical incompetence.

The idea that prophylactic bedrest may decrease uterine activity makes common sense to both patients and physicians. However, the literature does not support any significant benefit from routine bedrest or hospitalization in multiples [3,99]. A Cochrane database review of six randomized trials involving over 600 multiples demonstrated a trend toward a decrease in LBW infants and a paradoxical increased risk of delivery at less than 34 weeks' gestation with inpatient bedrest [100]. In addition, prophylactic bedrest may be associated with adverse complications such as thromboembolic disease and can be disruptive to families.

Administration of prophylactic tocolytic agents has been attempted but has not been beneficial. Women with multifetal pregnancies appear to be particularly prone to developing pulmonary edema and cardiovascular complications after administration of β-adrenergic agents because of their higher blood volume and lower colloid osmotic pressure [23,101]. As such, it seems prudent to restrict the use of those agents to women who are confirmed to be in preterm labor. Similarly, there is no evidence to suggest that prophylactic supplementation with either vaginal or intramuscular progesterone is effective in reducing the rate of spontaneous preterm delivery in twin gestations [94,95].

Ambulatory home monitoring of uterine contractions with a tocodynamometer in an attempt to predict preterm labor has not been shown to be useful. A metaanalysis of six randomized trials was unable to demonstrate a significant benefit of home uterine activity monitoring to reduce the risk of preterm delivery in patients with twins [102]. Furthermore, a prospective trial of 2422 patients (including 844 twins) randomized women to weekly nurse contact, daily nurse contact, or daily nurse contact in addition to home uterine activity monitoring, and demonstrated no difference in preterm delivery prior to 35 weeks' gestation [103].

Specialized twin clinics and transvaginal cervical length surveillance are two current management strategies utilized in attempts to reduce the risk of adverse outcomes associated with multifetal pregnancies. In these clinics, patients have the opportunity to develop rapport with a small group of dedicated caregivers [104]. Heightened awareness can increase compliance with therapeutic directives and mothers are able to provide psychologic support to one another. Another more commonly utilized strategy in managing multiples is cervical length measurements. Premature cervical shortening and cervical funneling detected by transvaginal ultrasound examination have good predictive capabilities for the development of preterm labor and delivery in women with multiple gestations [105–108]. Studies suggest that a cervical length measurement of >35 mm at 24–26 weeks identifies women with twins who are at low risk for delivery prior to 34 weeks' gestation [106]. On the other hand, a cervical length of 25 mm or less with or without funneling at 24 weeks' gestation predicts a high risk for preterm labor and delivery [105]. One study also found that a positive fetal fibronectin test at 28 weeks is a significant predictor of spontaneous preterm labor prior to 32 weeks' gestation [105].

Antenatal surveillance

Although it is prudent to follow fetal growth with serial ultrasound scans, routine antenatal testing in patients with an uncomplicated multiple gestation has not been demonstrated to improve outcomes. Antenatal testing is suggested in all patients with multiple gestations complicated by IUGR, discordant growth, abnormal amniotic fluid volumes, TTTS, monoamnionicity, fetal anomalies, single IUFD, and other medical or obstetric complications (Box 39.3). For women with twins, options for antenatal testing include the nonstress test, the biophysical profile, and Doppler velocimetry assessment if IUGR is suspected.

When patients with a multiple gestation present for antenatal testing or labor monitoring, each fetal heart rate should be independently identified to ensure precision. Monitoring of triplets and high-order multiples may require frequent sonographic identification of the appropriate fetus.

Box 39.3 Ultrasound management of patients with twins

- Ideally, ultrasound is performed in the first trimester to determine the number of fetuses and amnionicity and chorionicity. Patients are also offered nuchal translucency ultrasound at 10–14 weeks' gestation.
- A detailed ultrasound is scheduled at 18–20 weeks' gestation. This includes standard biometry, assessment of amniotic fluid volume in each sac, and an anatomic survey of each fetus. If the patient did not have a first-trimester ultrasound, an attempt is made to determine chorionicity by examining fetal gender, the number of placentas, the thickness as well as number of layers in the membrane separating the sacs, and the presence or absence of the lambda or twin peak sign.
- If the first two scans are suggestive of a dichorionic pregnancy, fetal growth is performed every 3–4 weeks thereafter as long as fetal growth and amniotic fluid volume in each sac remain normal.
- If the initial scan is suggestive of a monochorionic diamniotic pregnancy, subsequent scans are repeated every 2–3 weeks to follow for signs of TTTS. Fetal echocardiography is offered to patients with monochorionic twins because these pregnancies may be at increased risk for congenital heart defects.
- In either dichorionic or monochorionic pregnancies, if there is evidence of IUGR, discordant fetal growth, or discordant fluid volumes, fetal surveillance is intensified and includes frequent nonstress tests along with biophysical profile and Doppler velocimetry studies.
- Daily nonstress testing starting at approximately 24–26 weeks' gestation is suggested for patients with monoamniotic twins because of their risk for sudden IUFD from cord entanglement. Although cord accidents cannot be predicted, daily fetal heart rate monitoring may reveal increasing frequency of variable decelerations. When variable decelerations are identified, continuous monitoring is recommended and may ultimately require delivery for nonreassuring fetal testing.

IUFD, intrauterine fetal death; IUGR, intrauterine growth restriction; TTTS, twin–twin transfusion syndrome.

Routine Doppler studies have not been found to be helpful in the management of women with multiple gestations [109,110]. However, when IUGR or growth discordance is suspected in one or more fetuses, Doppler velocimetry of the umbilical artery is a useful adjunct in assessing and following these pregnancies. Furthermore, in cases of monochorionic twins with IUGR, discordant growth, or amniotic fluid volume abnormalities, Doppler studies of the ductus venosus may be helpful in identifying the possible overlapping pathologies of uteroplacental insufficiency and cardiac dysfunction.

Intrapartum period

A number of factors must be considered when determining the mode of delivery for patients with multiple gestations. These variables include the gestational age and estimated weights of the fetuses, their positions, the availability of real-time ultrasound on the labor floor and in the delivery room, the capability of monitoring each twin independently during the entire intrapartum period, and the healthcare provider experience. When both twins are vertex, vaginal delivery is possible. During the time period between the delivery of the first and second twin, it is important to demonstrate reassuring status of the undelivered twin as evidenced by continuous fetal heart rate monitoring or by ultrasound. If the presenting twin is nonvertex, cesarean delivery is suggested. Management of vertex/nonvertex twins is variable. Vaginal delivery of a breech second twin with an estimated fetal weight of 1500–3500 g in a woman with an adequate pelvis is reasonable. Cesarean delivery may be the preferred route of delivery if there is significant growth discordance between the twins or if the provider does not have adequate experience with such deliveries. Some obstetricians have had favorable experiences delivering triplets vaginally. Nonetheless, most providers deliver triplets and higher order multiples by cesarean section because continuous fetal heart rate monitoring of triplets and higher order multiples in labor is challenging [3,71].

Conclusion

Advances in fertility treatment and delayed child bearing have resulted in a substantial increase in the incidence of multiple gestations. The high perinatal morbidity and mortality rates associated with multiple gestations are the result of a variety of factors, some of which cannot be altered. Nonetheless, technologic advances in recent years have given us new insights into problems particular to multifetal pregnancies as well as tools with which to detect and treat these problems. Early diagnosis of multiple gestations and serial ultrasound studies are important in the management of these high-risk pregnancies and will hopefully have a beneficial impact on maternal and neonatal outcomes.

CASE PRESENTATION

A 38-year-old gravida 1 with twins in the moderate preterm gestation presented to a routine prenatal care visit and reported an "upset stomach" the previous weekend. Her prenatal course was significant for a history of polycystic ovarian syndrome and an initial quadruplet pregnancy conceived with ovulation induction and intrauterine insemination. She had elected to have chorionic villus sampling and subsequent MPR to a dichorionic twin gestation. During a routine anatomic ultrasound survey at 20 weeks, the patient was noted to have a short cervix measuring 24 mm. Preterm labor precautions were reviewed, light activity was advised, and serial cervical length measurements were scheduled. At 28 weeks' gestation, the patient was diagnosed with gestational diabetes which subsequently required insulin for glycemic control.

At her office visit at 30w 6d gestation, the patient's blood pressure was 150/92 mmHg and a urine dipstick revealed 2+ proteinuria. She was admitted and corticosteroids were administered to assist fetal lung maturation. After 72h of hospitalization, a 24-h urine collection revealed 6 g protein and the patient developed unremitting epigastric pain. Laboratory evaluation revealed a platelet count of 70, liver enzymes of 530 and 478, and a lactic dehydrogenase (LDH) of 990; the findings were consistent with HELLP syndrome. A bedside ultrasound revealed the fetal presentations to be cephalic/breech. The cervix was 3 cm dilated with a Bishop score of 8. However, a 38% twin weight discordance had been estimated during a routine scan at 30 weeks, with a higher estimated fetal weight for twin B.

Immediate delivery was recommended and the risks and benefits of attempted vaginal delivery and cesarean were discussed. The patient underwent an uncomplicated, primary low transverse cesarean delivery. Vigorous male and female infants were born. Although each neonate spent a brief period in the neonatal ICU, they were both discharged home after 2 weeks. There were no postpartum maternal complications and the patient was discharged home on postoperative day 4.

This case highlights many of the common features of multiple pregnancy, including assisted conception, MPR, medical and obstetric complications, and preterm delivery. While the outcome for the majority of multiple gestations is favorable, these high-risk pregnancies can be associated with maternal and neonatal morbidity and mortality and thus warrant increased vigilance.

References

1. Martin JA, Hamilton BE, Sutton PD et al. Births: final data for 2007. Natl Vital Stat Rep 2010;58:1–125.
2. Beato CV. Healthy People 2010 Progress Report: Maternal, Infant, and Child Health. Washington, DC: US Department of Health and Human Services, 2003.
3. American College of Obstetricians and Gynecologists. Multiple gestation: complicated twin, triplet, and high-order multifetal pregnancy. ACOG Practice Bulletin No. 56. Obstet Gynecol 2004;104:869–883.
4. Martin JA, Hamilton BE, Sutton PD, Ventura SJ, Menacker F, Munson ML. Births: final data for 2002. Natl Vital Stat Rep 2002;52:1–113.
5. Martin JA, Hamilton BE, Ventura SJ, Menacker F, Park MM, Sutton PD. Births: final data for 2001. Natl Vital Stat Rep 2001;51:1–102.
6. Nielson HC, Harvey-Wilkes K, MacKinnon B, Hung S. Neonatal outcome of very premature infants from multiple and singleton gestations. Am J Obstet Gynecol 1997;177: 653–659.
7. Kaufman GE, Malone FD, Harvey-Wilkes KB, Chelmow D, Penzias AS, D'Alton ME. Neonatal morbidity and mortality associated with triplet pregnancy. Obstet Gynecol 1998;91: 342–348.
8. Topp M, Huusom LD, Langhoff-Roos J et al. Multiple birth and cerebral palsy in Europe: a multicenter study. Acta Obstet Gynecol Scand 2004;83:548–553.
9. American College of Obstetricians and Gynecologists. Neonatal Encephalopathy and Cerebral Palsy: Defining the Pathogenesis and Pathophysiology. Washington, DC: American College of Obstetricians and Gynecologists, 2003.
10. Yokoyama Y, Shimizu T, Hayakawa K. Prevalence of cerebral palsy in twins, triplets and quadruplets. Int J Epidemiol 1995;24:943–948.
11. Russell EM. Cerebral palsied twins. Arch Dis Child 1961;36:328–336.
12. Benirschke K. The biology of the twinning process: how placentation influences outcome. Semin Perinatol 1995;19: 342–350.
13. Souter VL, Kapur RP, Nyholt DR et al. A report of dizygous monochorionic twins. N Engl J Med 2003;349:154–158.
14. Miura K, Niikawa NJ. Do monochorionic dizygotic twins increase after pregnancy by assisted reproductive technology? Hum Genet 2005;50:1–6.
15. Barth RA, Crowe HC. Ultrasound evaluation of multifetal gestations. In: Callen PW, ed. Ultrasonography in Obstetrics and Gynecology, 4th edn. Philadelphia: WB Saunders, 2000, p.171.
16. Bromley B, Benacerraf B. Using the number of yolk sacs to determine amnionicity in early first trimester monochorionic twins. J Ultrasound Med 1995;14:415–419.
17. Bessis R, Papiernik E. Echographic imagery of amniotic membranes in twin pregnancies. In: Gedda L, Parisi P, eds. Twin Research 3: Twin Biology and Multiple Pregnancy. New York: Alan R. Liss, 1981, p.183.

18. Finberg HJ. The "twin peak" sign: reliable evidence of dichorionic twinning. J Ultrasound Med 1992;11:571–577.

19. Monteagudo A, Timor-Tritsch IE, Sharma S. Early and simple determination of chorionic and amniotic type in multifetal gestations in the first fourteen weeks by high-frequency transvaginal ultrasonography. Am J Obstet Gynecol 1994;170:824–829.

20. Sepulveda W, Seibre NJ, Hughes K et al. The lambda sign at 10–14 weeks of gestation as a predictor of chorionicity in twin pregnancies. Ultrasound Obstet Gynecol 1996;7:421–423.

21. Egan JFX, Borgida AF. Multiple gestations: the importance of ultrasound. Obstet Gynecol Clin North Am 2004;31:141–158.

22. Nyberg DA, Filly RA, Golbus MS et al. Entangled umbilical cords: a sign of monoamniotic twins. J Ultrasound Med 1984;3:29–32.

23. Norwitz ER, Valentine E, Park JS. Maternal physiology and complications of multiple pregnancy. Semin Perinatol 2005;29:338–348.

24. Demissie K, Ananth CV, Martin J et al. Fetal and neonatal mortality among twin gestations in the United States: the role of intrapair birth weight discordance. Obstet Gynecol 2002;100:474–480.

25. Blickstein I, Keith LG. Neonatal mortality rates among growth-discordant twins, classified according to the birth weight of the smaller twin. Am J Obstet Gynecol 2004;190:170–174.

26. Amaru RC, Bush MC, Berkowitz RL, Lapinski RH, Gaddipati S. Is discordant growth in twins an independent risk factor for adverse neonatal outcome? Obstet Gynecol 2004;103:71–76.

27. Landy HJ, Keith L, Keith D. The vanishing twin. Acta Genet Med Gemellol (Roma) 1982;31:179–194.

28. Cleary-Goldman J, D'Alton M. Management of single fetal demise in a multiple gestation. Obstet Gynecol Surv 2004;59:285–298.

29. Lee YM, Wylie BJ, Simpson LL, D'Alton ME. Twin chorionicity and the risk of stillbirth. Obstet Gynecol 2008;111:301–308.

30. Landry HJ, Weingold AB. Management of a multiple gestation complicated by antepartum fetal demise. Obstet Gynecol Surv 1989;44:171–176.

31. Okamura K, Murotsuki J, Tanigawara S, Uehara S, Yajima A. Funipuncture for evaluation of hematologic and coagulation indices in the surviving twin following co-twins death. Obstet Gynecol 1994;83:975–978.

32. Fusi L, McParland P, Fisk N, Wigglesworth J. Acute twin–twin transfusion: a possible mechanism for brain-damaged survivors after intrauterine death of a monochorionic twin. Obstet Gynecol 1991;78:517–520.

33. Weiss JL, Cleary-Goldman J, Budorick N, Tanji K, D'Alton ME. Multicystic encephalomalacia after first trimester intrauterine fetal demise in monochorionic twins. Am J Obstet Gynecol 2004;190:563–565.

34. Carlson N, Towers C. Multiple gestation complicated by the death of one fetus. Obstet Gynecol 1989;73:685–689.

35. Onyskowova A, Dolezal A, Jedlicka V. The frequency and the character of malformations in multiple birth (a preliminary report). Teratology 1971;4:496.

36. Hendricks CH. Twinning in relation to birth weight, mortality, and congenital anomalies. Obstet Gynecol 1966;27:47–53.

37. Kohl SG, Casey G. Twin gestation. Mt Sinai J Med 1975;42:523–539.

38. Benirschke K, Kim CK. Multiple pregnancy [first of two parts]. N Engl J Med 1973;288:1276–1284.

39. Spadola AC, Simpson LL. Selective termination procedures in monochorionic pregnancies. Semin Perinatol 2005;29:330–337.

40. Malone FD, Craigo SD, Chelmow D, D'Alton ME. Outcome of twin gestations complicated by a single anomalous fetus. Obstet Gynecol 1996;88:1–5.

41. Sebire NJ, Sepulveda W, Hughes KS et al. Management of twin pregnancies discordant for anencephaly. Br J Obstet Gynaecol 1997;107:216–219.

42. Gul A, Cebecia A, Aslan H et al. Perinatal outcomes of twin pregnancies discordant for major fetal anomalies. Fetal Diagn Ther 2005;20:244–248.

43. D'Alton ME, Simpson LL. Syndromes in twins. Semin Perinatol 1995;19:375–386.

44. Carr SR, Aronson MP, Coustan DR. Survival rates of monoamniotic twins do not decrease after 30 weeks' gestation. Am J Obstet Gynecol 1990;163:719–722.

45. Rodis JF, McIlveen PF, Egan JF et al. Monoamniotic twins: improved perinatal survival with accurate prenatal diagnosis and antenatal fetal surveillance. Am J Obstet Gynecol 1997;177:1046–1049.

46. Allen VM, Windrim R, Barrett J et al. Management of monoamniotic twin pregnancies: a case series and systematic review of the literature. Br J Obstet Gynaecol 2001;108:931–936.

47. Rogue H, Gillen-Goldstein J, Funai E et al. Perinatal outcomes in monoamniotic gestations. J Mat Fetal Neonatal Med 2003;13:414–421.

48. Tessen JA, Zlatnik FJ. Monoamniotic twins: a retrospective controlled study. Obstet Gynecol 1991;77:832–834.

49. Blickstein I, Verhoeven HC, Keith LG. Zygotic splitting after assisted reproduction. N Engl J Med 1999;340:738–739.

50. Blickstein I. Estimation of iatrogenic monozygotic twinning rate following assisted reproduction: pitfalls and caveats. Am J Obstet Gynecol 2005;192:365–368.

51. Jain V, Fisk NM. The twin–twin transfusion syndrome. Clin Obstet Gynecol 2004;47:181–202.

52. Malone FD, D'Alton ME. Anomalies peculiar to multiple gestations. Clin Perinatol 2000;27:1033–1046.

53. Quintero RA, Morales WJ, Allen MH, Bornick PW, Johnson PK, Kruger M. Staging of twin–twin transfusion syndrome. J Perinatol 1999;19:550–555.

54. Bajoria R, Wigglesworth J, Fisk NM. Angioarchitecture of monochorionic placentas in relation to the twin–twin transfusion syndrome. Am J Obstet Gynecol 1995;172:856–863.

55. De Lia JE, Cruikshank DP, Keye WR Jr. Fetoscopic neodymium:YAG laser occlusion of placental vessels in severe twin-twin transfusion syndrome. Obstet Gynecol 1990;75:1046.

56. Hecher K, Plath H, Bregenzer T, Hansmann M, Hackeloer BJ. Endoscopic laser surgery versus serial amniocenteses in the treatment of severe twin–twin transfusion syndrome. Am J Obstet Gynecol 1999;180:717–724.

57. Quintero RA, Dickinson JE, Morales WJ et al. Stage-based treatment of twin twin transfusion syndrome. Am J Obstet Gynecol 2003;188:1333–1340.

58. Senat MV, Deprest J, Boulvain M, Paupe A, Winer N, Ville Y. Endoscopic laser surgery versus serial amnioreduction for severe twin-to-twin transfusion syndrome. N Engl J Med 2004;351:136–144.

59. Rossi A C, D'Addario V. Laser therapy and serial amnioreduction as treatment for twin-twin transfusion syndrome: a metaanalysis and review of literature. Am J Obstet Gynecol 2008;198:147.

60. Devine PC, Malone FD, Athanassiou A, Harvey-Wilkes K, D'Alton ME. Maternal and neonatal outcome of 100 consecutive triplet pregnancies. Am J Perinatol 2001;18:225–235.

61. Graham G, Simpson LL. Diagnosis and management of obstetrical complications unique to multiple gestations. Clin Obstet Gynecol 2004;47:163–180.

62. Campbell DM, Templeton A. Maternal complications of twin pregnancy. Int J Gynaecol Obstet 2004;84:71–73.

63. American College of Obstetricians and Gynecologists. Thromboembolism in pregnancy. ACOG Practice Bulletin No. 19. Obstet Gynecol 2000;96(2).

64. American College of Obstetricians and Gynecologists. Diagnosis and management of preeclampsia and eclampsia. ACOG Practice Bulletin No. 33. Obstet Gynecol 2002;99: 159–167.

65. Sibai BM, Hauth J, Caritis S et al. Hypertensive disorders in twin versus singleton gestations. National Institute of Child Health and Human Development Network of Maternal-Fetal Medicine Units. Am J Obstet Gynecol 2000;182:938–942.

66. Caritis S, Sibai B, Hauth J et al. Low-dose aspirin to prevent preeclampsia in women at high risk. National Institute of Child Health and Human Development Network of Maternal-Fetal Medicine Units. N Engl J Med 1998;338:701–705.

67. Levine RJ, Hauth JC, Curet LB et al. Trial of calcium to prevent preeclampsia. N Engl J Med 1997;337:69–76.

68. Maxwell CV, Lieberman E, Norton M, Cohen A, Seely EW, Lee-Parritz A. Relationship of twin zygosity and risk of preeclampsia. Am J Obstet Gynecol 2001;185:819–821.

69. Hardardottir H, Kelly K, Bork MD, Cusick W, Campbell WA, Rodis JF. Atypical presentation of preeclampsia in high-order multifetal gestations. Obstet Gynecol 1996;87:370–374.

70. Davidson KM, Simpson LL, Knox TA, D'Alton ME. Acute fatty liver of pregnancy in triplet gestation. Obstet Gynecol 1998;91:806–808.

71. American College of Obstetricians and Gynecologists and the American Academy of Pediatrics. Guidelines for Perinatal Care, 5th edn. Washington DC: American College of Obstetricians and Gynecologists and the American Academy of Pediatrics, 2002.

72. Bush MC, Malone FD. Down syndrome screening in twins. Clin Perinatol 2005;32:373–386.

73. Stone J, Eddleman K, Lynch L, Berkowitz RL. A single center experience with 1000 consecutive cases of multifetal pregnancy reduction. Am J Obstet Gynecol 2002;187:1163–1167.

74. Malone FD, D'Alton ME. Anomalies peculiar to multiple gestations. Clin Perinatol 2000;27:1033–1046.

75. American College of Obstetricians and Gynecologists. Invasive prenatal testing for aneuploidy. ACOG Practice Bulletin No. 88. Obstet Gynecol 2007;110:1459–1467.

76. Meyers C, Adam R, Dungan J, Prenger V. Aneuploidy in twin gestations: when is maternal age advanced? Obstet Gynecol 1997;89:248–251.

77. Odibo AO, Elkousy MH, Ural SH et al. Screening for aneuploidy in twin pregnancies: maternal age- and race-specific risk assessment between 9–14 weeks. Twin Res 2003;6: 251–256.

78. Cleary-Goldman J, D'Alton ME, Berkowitz RL. Prenatal diagnosis and multiple pregnancy. Semin Perinatol 2005;29: 312–320.

79. Rogers JG, Voullaire L, Gold H. Monozygotic twins discordant for trisomy 21. Am J Med Genet 1982;11:143–146.

80. Dallapiccola B, Stomeo C, Ferranti B et al. Discordant sex in one of three monozygotic triplets. J Med Genet 1985;22:6–11.

81. Graham G, Simpson LL. Diagnosis and management of obstetrical complications unique to multiple gestations. Clin Obstet Gynecol 2004;47:163–180.

82. Odibo AO, Lawrence-Cleary K, Macones GA. Screening for aneuploidy in twins and higher-order multiples: is first-trimester nuchal translucency the solution? Obstet Gynecol Surv 2003;58:609–614.

83. Sebire NJ, D'Ercole C, Hughes K, Carvalho M, Nicolaides KH. Increased nuchal translucency thickness at 10–14 weeks of gestation as a predictor of severe twin-to-twin transfusion syndrome. Ultrasound Obstet Gynecol 1997;10:86–89.

84. Malone FD, D'Alton ME, Society for Maternal-Fetal Medicine. First-trimester sonographic screening for Down syndrome. Obstet Gynecol 2003;102:1066–1079.

85. Spencer K, Nicolaides KH. Screening for trisomy 21 in twins using first trimester ultrasound and maternal serum biochemistry in a one stop clinic: a review of three years experience. Br J Obstet Gynaecol 2003;110:276–280.

86. Cahill AG, Macones GA, Stamilio DM, Dicke JM, Crane JP, Odibo AO. Pregnancy loss rate after mid-trimester amniocentesis in twin pregnancies. Am J Obstet Gynecol 2009; 200(3):257.

87. Jenkins TM, Wapner RJ. The challenge of prenatal diagnosis in twin pregnancies. Curr Opin Obstet Gynecol 2000;12: 87–92.

88. Wapner RJ. Genetic diagnosis in multiple pregnancies. Semin Perinatol 1995;19:351–362.

89. Edwards MS, Ellings JM, Newman RB et al. Predictive value of antepartum ultrasound examination for anomalies in twin gestations. Ultrasound Obstet Gynecol 1995;6: 43–49.

90. Bahtiyar MO, Dulay AT, Weeks BP, Friedman AH, Copel JA. Prevalence of congenital heart defects in monochorionic/diamniotic twin gestations: a systematic literature review. J Ultrasound Med 2007;26(11):1491–1498.

91. National Institutes of Health. National Institutes of Health Consensus Development Conference Statement: effect of corticosteroids for fetal maturation on perinatal outcomes, February 28–March 2, 1994. Am J Obstet Gynecol 1995;173: 246–252.

92. Mercer BM, Miodovnik M, Thurnau GR et al. Antibiotic therapy for reduction of infant morbidity after preterm premature rupture of the membranes: a randomized controlled trial. JAMA 1997;278:989–995.

93. Lovett SM, Weiss JD, Diogo MJ, Williams PT, Garite TJ. A prospective double-blind, randomized, controlled clinical trial of ampicillin-sulbactam for preterm premature rupture of membranes in women receiving antenatal corticosteroid therapy. Am J Obstet Gynecol 1997;176:1030–1038.

94. Rouse DJ, Caritis SN, Peaceman AM et al. A trial of 17 alpha-hydroxyprogesterone caproate to prevent prematurity in twins. N Engl J Med 2007;357(5):454–461.

95. Norman JE, Mackenzie F, Owen P et al. Progesterone for the prevention of preterm birth in twin pregnancy (STOPPIT): a randomised, double-blind, placebo-controlled study and meta-analysis. Lancet 2009;373(9680):2034–2040.

96. Newman RB, Krombach RS, Myers MC et al. Effect of cerclage on obstetric outcome in twin gestations with a shortened cervical length. Am J Obstet Gynecol 2002;186:634–640.

97. Elimian A, Figueroa R, Nigam S et al. Perinatal outcome of triplet gestation: does prophylactic cerclage make a difference? J Maternal Fetal Med 1999;8:119–122.

98. Berghella V, Odibo AO, To MS, Rust OA, Althuisius SM. Cerclage for short cervix on ultrasonography: meta-analysis of trials using individual patient-level data. Obstet Gynecol 2005;106:181–189.

99. Saunders MC, Dick JS, Brown IM, McPherson K, Chalmers I. The effects of hospital admission for bed rest on the duration of twin pregnancy: a randomized trial. Lancet 1985;2: 793–795.

100. Crowther CA. Hospitalization and bed rest for multiple pregnancy. Cochrane Database Syst Rev 2001;1:CD000110.

101. Katz M, Robertson PA, Creasy RK. Cardiovascular complications associated with terbutaline treatment for preterm labor. Am J Obstet Gynecol 1981;139:605–608.

102. Colton T, Kayne HL, Zhang Y et al. A meta-analysis of home uterine activity monitoring. Am J Obstet Gynecol 1995; 173:1499–1505.

103. Dyson DC, Danbe KH, Bamber JA et al. Monitoring women at risk for preterm labor. N Engl J Med 1998;338:15–19.

104. Luke B, Brown MB, Misiunas R et al. Specialized prenatal care and maternal and infant outcomes in twin pregnancy. Am J Obstet Gynecol 2003;189:934–938.

105. Goldenberg RL, Iams JD, Miodovnik M et al. The preterm prediction study: risk factors in twin gestations. National Institute of Child Health and Human Development Maternal-Fetal Medicine Units Network. Am J Obstet Gynecol 1996; 175:1047–1053.

106. Imseis HM, Albert TA, Iams JD. Identifying twin gestations at low risk for preterm birth with a transvaginal ultrasonographic cervical measurement at 24 to 26 weeks' gestation. Am J Obstet Gynecol 1997;177:1149–1155.

107. Ramin KD, Ogburn PL Jr, Mulholland TA et al. Ultrasonographic assessment of cervical length in triplet pregnancies. Am J Obstet Gynecol 1999;180:1442–1445.

108. Gibson JL, Macara LM, Owen P, Young D, Maculey J, Mackenzie F. Prediction of preterm delivery in twin pregnancy: a prospective, observational study of cervical length and fetal fibronectin testing. Ultrasound Obstet Gynecol 2004;23:561–566.

109. Geipel A, Berg C, Germer U et al. Doppler assessment in the uterine circulation in the second trimester in twin pregnancies: prediction of pre-eclampsia, fetal growth restriction and birth weight discordance. Ultrasound Obstet Gynecol 2002;20:541–545.

110. Giles W, Bisits A, O'Callahan S, Gill A, DAMP Study Group. The Doppler assessment in multiple pregnancy randomised controlled trial of ultrasound biometry versus umbilical artery Doppler ultrasound and biometry in twin pregnancy. Br J Obstet Gynaecol 2003;110:593–597.

Chapter 40
Polyhydramnios and Oligohydramnios

Ron Beloosesky and Michael G. Ross
Department of Obstetrics, Gynecology and Public Health, UCLA School of Medicine and Public Health and Harbor-UCLA Medical Center, Torrance, CA, USA

All that fluid which is contained in the ovum is called by the general name of the waters. The quantity, in proportion to the size of the different parts of the ovum, is greatest by far in early pregnancy. At the time of parturition, in some cases, it amounts to or exceeds four pints. In others, it is scarcely equal to as many ounces. It is usually in the largest quantity when the child has been some time dead, or is born in a weakly state. (T. Denman, 1815)

In 1815, Denman recognized the great variation in amniotic fluid (AF) volume and associated polyhydramnios with congenital malformations, fetal death, and fetal disease [1]. Although our current knowledge of the intrauterine environment has expanded many fold, we have not overturned any of Denman's concepts (1).

Polyhydramnios and oligohydramnios are pathologic conditions representing excess AF and diminished AF, respectively. Numerous serious clinical conditions are associated with polyhydramnios and oligohydramnios. An understanding of the normal AF parameters and the AF turnover is necessary before embarking on the pathologic considerations.

Normal amniotic fluid composition and volume

During the first trimester, AF is isotonic with maternal plasma [2] but contains minimal protein. It is thought that the fluid arises either from a transudate of fetal plasma through nonkeratinized fetal skin, or maternal plasma across the uterine decidua and/or placenta surface [3]. Thus, fetuses with renal agenesis may demonstrate normal first-trimester AF volumes. With advancing gestation, AF osmolality and sodium concentration decrease, a result of the mixture of dilute fetal urine and isotonic fetal lung liquid production. In comparison with the first half of pregnancy, AF osmolality decreases by 20–30 mOsm/

kg with advancing gestation to levels approximately 85–90% of maternal serum osmolality [4]. AF urea, creatinine, and uric acid increase during the second half of pregnancy, resulting in AF concentrations of the urinary by-products two to three times higher than fetal plasma [4].

Throughout the history of medicine, investigators have been intrigued with the concept of quantitating the volume of AF. In 1972, Queenan *et al*, using dye dilution technique, measured the AF volumes in 187 samples from 115 patients with normal pregnancies [5]. The volumes varied widely for the various weeks of gestation. The mean volumes were 239 mL at 25–26 weeks, 984 mL at 33–34 weeks (the peak volume), 836 mL at term, and 544 mL at 41–42 weeks (Fig. 40.1).

Brace and Wolf analyzed AF volumes in 12 published studies including 705 normal pregnancies at 8–43 weeks' gestation [6]. They found that AF volume rises linearly from early gestation until 32 weeks, whereupon it remains constant until term, ranging between 700 and 800 mL. After 40 weeks, AF volume declines at a rate of 8% a week, to an average of 400 mL at 42 weeks. At 30 weeks' gestation, the 95% confidence intervals about the mean (817 mL) cover the range 18–2100 mL. Thus, a volume less than 318 mL is considered oligohydramnios and more than 2100 mL polyhydramnios. The wide biologic variability in the AF volume with advancing gestational age, especially before 32–35 weeks, makes an absolute volume criterion for oligohydramnios or polyhydramnios inappropriate. Accordingly, AF volume abnormalities are best defined as a volume below the 5th percentile or above the 95th percentile for gestational age.

Dynamics of amniotic fluid turnover

Amniotic fluid is produced and resorbed in a dynamic process with large volumes of water circulated between the AF and fetal compartments. During the latter half of

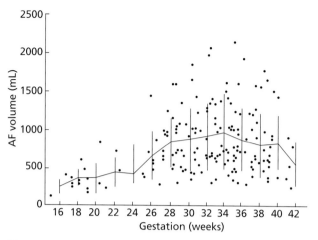

Figure 40.1 Normal amniotic fluid (AF) volumes are plotted against weeks of gestation. The mean values ± 1 SD are calculated for each 2-week period. Reproduced from Queenan *et al* [5] with permission from Elsevier.

gestation, the primary sources of AF include fetal urine excretion and fluid secreted by the fetal lung. The primary pathways for water exit from the AF include removal by fetal swallowing and intramembranous absorption across the fetal membranes into fetal blood. If the balance of fluid exchange is disturbed, polyhydramnios or oligohydramnios develops. For instance, if a pathologic condition increased the AF volume by 1 oz or 30 mL/day, 1 L of excess AF would accumulate in a month.

Fetal urine

Fetal micturition is known to be the major source of AF. Chez *et al* [9] studied fetal urine production with indwelling catheters in rhesus monkeys, and reported the rate to be 5 mL/kg/h, which correlates with the rate of swallowing in Pritchard's studies [7]. In humans, fetal urine production changes with increasing gestation. The amount of urine produced by the human fetus has been estimated by the use of ultrasound assessment of fetal bladder volume [8], although the accuracy of these measurements has been called into question. Exact human fetal urine production rates across gestation are not established but appear to be in the range of 25% of bodyweight per day or nearly 1000 mL/day near term [8,9]. AF is isotonic in early pregnancy, but by term it becomes hypotonic, a result of the increased contribution of hypotonic urine.

Kurjak *et al* studied fetal renal function in 255 normal singleton pregnancies and 133 complicated pregnancies between 22 and 41 weeks' gestation [10]. They evaluated the hourly fetal urine production rate (HFUPR), fetal glomerular filtration rate (GFR), fetal tubular water reabsorption (TWR), and the effect of furosemide on fetal micturition by sonography and biochemical tests. In normal pregnancies, the HFUPR increased from 2.2 mL/h

at 22 weeks to 26.3 mL/h at 40 weeks' gestation. The fetal GFR was 2.66 mL/min at term and the percentage of TWR was 78%. In growth-restricted fetuses, the HFUPR was below the 10th centile in 59% and above normal in only 6%. The diuretic effect of furosemide was the same in growth-restricted and normal fetuses. In diabetic pregnancies, HFUPR values varied considerably and correlated with fetal size. In 90% of pregnancies with polyhydramnios, the HFUPR was normal.

Oligohydramnios is associated with severe malformations of the fetal urinary system (e.g. renal agenesis), which is incompatible with urine production. In a review of 295 fetuses with renal agenesis, Jeffcoate and Scott found sufficient clinical data in 100 to establish a diagnosis of oligohydramnios [11]. From these data, the investigators inferred that conditions affecting fetal urine production would alter the AF volume. On the other hand, they also reported renal agenesis in a fetus with polyhydramnios. Others reported renal agenesis and normal AF volume [12,13].

Fetal lung fluid

All mammalian fetuses normally secrete fluid from their lungs. In the human, AF clearly contains phospholipids, such as lecithin and sphingomyelin derived from type II aveolar cells; thus, at least some of the tracheal fluid contributes to the AF volume. Liley described some 800 mothers who had radiologic contrast media injected into the AF and noted that only four had the medium demonstrated in the fetal or neonatal lungs [14].

The absolute rate of fluid production by the human fetal lungs has not been determined, although animal studies suggest that the respiratory tract has a major role in AF production. Goodlin and Lloyd demonstrated that the fetal lamb produces 50–80 mL/day tracheal fluid [15]. Adamson *et al* reported that the near term lamb has tracheal secretions of 200–400 mL/day [16]. Tracheal ligation in animals leads to overdistension of the lungs, suggesting a relatively large outflow of fluid from the lungs. This knowledge has been utilized in the development of therapeutic approaches to the treatment of diaphragmatic hernia; tracheal occlusion results in pulmonary distension despite the presence of a thoracic mass. Under physiologic conditions, half of the fluid exiting the lungs enters the AF and half is swallowed [17]; therefore, an average of approximately 165 mL/day lung liquid enters the AF near term.

Fetal lung fluid production is affected by physiologic and endocrine factors, but nearly all stimuli have been demonstrated to reduce fetal lung liquid production, with no evidence of stimulated production and nominal changes in fluid composition. Increased arginine vasopressin [18], catecholamines [19], and cortisol [20] decrease lung fluid production. The marked increase in fetal plasma levels of these hormones during labor results in a cessation of lung fluid production, after which lung liquid is resorbed into pulmonary lymphatics to prepare for newborn respiration.

Fetal swallowing

Swallowing is the major pathway for AF removal. Evidence of fetal swallowing of AF was established many years ago by amniography, Studies of near term pregnancies suggest that the human fetus swallows an average of 210–760 mL/day [21], which is considerably less than the volume of urine produced each day. However, fetal swallowing may be reduced beginning a few days before delivery [22], so the rate of human fetal swallowing is probably underestimated. Fetal swallowing is increased during active as compared with quiet sleep states. Furthermore, the near term fetus develops functional ingestive responses such that fetal swallowing may increase in response to thirst or appetite stimulation. Of note, fetal swallowing decreases with acute arterial hypotension [23] or hypoxia [17,24], indicating that oligohydramnios associated with fetal hypoxia is not caused by increased AF resorption via swallowing.

The effect of fetal swallowing can be demonstrated by studying mothers who have delivered babies with tracheo-esophageal fistulas. Of 228 such cases, 25 fetuses had complete obstruction between the mouth and the stomach and 19 (76%) of these had polyhydramnios [25]. In a study of 169 cases of polyhydramnios, 54 (32%) of the fetuses were unable to swallow [11].

Anencephaly is also associated with a high incidence of polyhydramnios. Although swallowing has been demonstrated in some of these fetuses, it is reasonable to believe that the swallowing capability is reduced or absent in many. The exposed meninges in anencephaly have been described as the source of the production of the excess AF [26]. Other authors disagreed [27], noting that the rudimentary and distorted brain is almost always covered with a collagen membrane. They proposed that fetal polyuria may contribute to the polyhydramnios because anencephalic fetuses lack antidiuretic hormone. Naeye *et al* also suggested that polyuria of the anencephalic fetus causes polyhydramnios [28].

The importance of swallowing in controlling AF volume remains undefined. An inability to swallow in the setting of esophageal atresia but not in anencephaly appears to result in polyhydramnios in some cases.

Intramembranous flow

The amount of fluid swallowed by the fetus does not equal the amount of fluid produced by both the kidneys and the lungs in either human or ovine gestation. As the volume of AF does not greatly increase during the last half of pregnancy, another route of fluid absorption is needed. The intramembranous (IM) pathway refers to the route of absorption between the fetal circulation and the amniotic cavity directly across the amnion. Although the contribution of the IM pathway to the overall regulation and maintenance of AF volume and composition has yet to be completely understood, results from *in vivo* and *in vitro* studies of ovine membrane permeability suggest that the permeability of the fetal chorio-amnion is important in determining AF composition and volume [29–31]. This IM flow, recirculating AF water to the fetal compartment, is thought to be driven by the significant osmotic gradient between the hypotonic AF and isotonic fetal plasma [32]. In addition, electrolytes (e.g. Na^+) may diffuse down a concentration gradient from fetal plasma into the AF while peptides (e.g. arginine vasopressin) and other electrolytes (e.g. Cl^-) may be recirculated to the fetal plasma. Recent studies have demonstrated the expression of aquaporins (AQP; 1, 3, 8, and 9), which are cell membrane proteins that serve as water channels, in human chorio-amniotic membranes and placenta. The expression of AQP8 and AQP9 mRNA and protein was significantly increased in the amnion and placenta of patients with polyhydramnios, suggesting that aquaporins may play an important role in the regulation of amniotic fluid resorption via the IM pathway [33–36].

Although never directly measured in humans, indirect evidence supports the presence of IM flow. Studies of intraamniotic ^{51}Cr injection demonstrated appearance of the tracer in the circulation of fetuses with impaired swallowing [37]. Additionally, alterations in IM flow may contribute to AF clinical abnormalities, as membrane ultrastructure changes are noted with polyhydramnios or oligohydramnios [38]. Experimental estimates of the net IM flow average 200–250 mL/day in fetal sheep and likely this balances the flow of urine and lung liquid with fetal swallowing under homeostatic conditions.

Amniotic fluid turnover

The AF is constantly recirculating. When diffusion of water is measured, approximately 500 mL water enters and leaves the amniotic sac each hour, with little effect on the total AF volume. However, estimates of actual bulk flow of water suggest that approximately 1000 mL/day enter and leave the amniotic cavity at term. This results in a turnover of the entire volume of AF each day.

Clinical measurement of amniotic fluid

A few decades ago, AF volume was estimated in crude ways such as measurement of fundal height, roentgenographic, or direct measurement at the time of delivery. The PAH dye dilution technique provides an accurate measurement but is an invasive technique and therefore limited to research settings [39].

Ultrasound examination is the only practical clinical means of assessing the AF volume. Several ultrasound methods have been used to estimate the AF volume; each has limitations in the detection of abnormal AF volumes. These methods can better identify true normal AF volumes than abnormal AF volumes (oligohydramnios and polyhydramnios), which they all detect poorly.

The single deepest pocket (SDP) measurement refers to the vertical dimension of the largest pocket of AF not containing umbilical cord or fetal extremities and measured at a right angle to the uterine contour. The horizontal component of this vertical dimension must be at least 1 cm. A normal SDP measurement is 2.1–8 cm, with oligohydramnios defined as less than 2.0 cm and polyhydramnios as more than 8.0 cm. In a comparison of SDP with dye-determined AF volume, SDP poorly identifies patients with oligohydramnios [40,41].

The Amniotic Fluid Index (AFI) is measured by first dividing the uterus into four quadrants using the linea nigra for the right and left divisions and the umbilicus for the upper and lower quadrants. The maximum vertical AF pocket diameter in each quadrant not containing cord or fetal extremities is measured in centimeters; the sum of these measurements is the AFI. A normal AFI is 5.1 to <25 cm, with oligohydramnios defined as less than 5.0 cm and polyhydramnios as more than 25 cm. Borderline normal values are 5.1–8.0 cm. The accuracy of the AFI has been examined in several studies [40,42–45]. In comparison to dye dilution, the AFI overestimated actual volumes by 89% at low volumes and underestimated actual volumes by 54% at high volumes. Chauhan *et al* demonstrated that the sensitivity, specificity, positive, and negative predictive values of AFI ≤5 for prediction of oligohydramnios were 5%, 98%, 80%, and 49%; these same characteristics for AFI >24 for prediction of polyhydramnios were 30%, 98%, 57%, and 93%, respectively [44]. Notably, AFI standards have been demonstrated using gray-scale ultrasound. When color flow Doppler is utilized for AFI determination, oligohydramnios may be overdiagnosed [46–48].

The two-diameter AF pocket is the product of the vertical depth multiplied by the horizontal diameter of the largest pocket of AF not containing umbilical cord or extremities (with the transducer held at a right angle to the uterine contour). A normal two-dimensional measurement is 15.1–50 cm^2, with oligohydramnios defined as less than 15 cm^2 and polyhydramnios as more than 50 cm^2. Two series that compared the two-diameter pocket and dye-determined AF volume found that the former identified 81–94% of the dye-determined normal volumes and approximately 60% of pregnancies with low volumes [38,43]. Receiver operator curve analysis showed that for any specific two-diameter pocket, the 95% confidence range was so wide that ultrasonographic assessment was not a reasonable reflection of actual AF volume, and thus was not clinically useful [44].

Subjective assessment of AF volume refers to visual interpretation without sonographic measurements [49]. The ultrasonographer scans the uterine contents and subsequently reports the AF volume as oligohydramnios, normal, or polyhydramnios. One study involving 63 pregnancies compared the subjective assessment of AF volume with ultrasound measurement of AFI, the single deepest pocket technique, and the two-diameter pocket method in the identification of dye-determined AF volume [49]. The subjective assessment of AF volume by an experienced examiner had a similar sensitivity to the other techniques for identifying dye-determined AF volumes.

All obstetric ultrasound examinations should include an assessment of AF volume. Although the ultrasonographer may elect to use only a subjective assessment, we recommend use of an objective measure (e.g. AFI) if the subjective assessment is abnormal, in patients at increased risk of pregnancy complications, and in all patients examined in the third trimester.

Polyhydramnios

Definition

Historically, polyhydramnios has been characterized by an excessive accumulation of AF, usually more than 2000 mL. However, this definition does not take account of the normal physiologic changes that occur in the volume of AF as the gestational weeks change. There is a progressive increase in AF volume from a mean of 30 mL at 10 weeks to 190 mL at 16 weeks, peaking at 780 mL at 32–35 weeks' gestation; thereafter, AF volume progressively decreases to approximately 550 mL at 42 weeks [6]. The wide biologic variability in the AF volume with advancing gestational age makes an absolute volume criterion for oligohydramnios or polyhydramnios inappropriate. Accordingly, AF volume abnormalities are best defined as a volume below the 5th percentile or above the 95th percentile for gestational age.

Diagnosis

Polyhydramnios is generally a problem of the late second to early third trimester. The clinician may notice that the uterus is consistently larger than expected for the stage of gestation, or there may be a sudden increase in uterine size. The fetal parts may be difficult to palpate and the fetal heart may be difficult to hear with Doppler ultrasound if the fetus moves about in the large volume of AF.

The diagnosis of polyhydramnios can be confirmed by sonography by quantifying the AF. When one is scanning the pregnant uterus, it is possible to make a qualitative judgment as to the presence or absence of polyhydramnios. At 16 weeks' gestation, when genetic amniocentesis is commonly performed, the fetus and placenta each weigh approximately 100 g and the AF volume is 200 mL. Therefore, at this time the AF volume constitutes approximately 50% of the uterine image. At 28 weeks, when the fetus weighs 1000 g and the placenta weighs 200 g, the AF volume is approximately 1000 mL and comprises approximately 45% of the image of the uterus. At term, when the fetus and placenta weigh 3300 and 500 g respectively, the AF volume is approximately 800 mL and makes up only approximately 17% of the image of the uterus. Keeping these guidelines in mind will facilitate making a judgment about the normalcy of AF volume versus polyhydramnios or oligohydramnios.

In severe cases, the mere image confirms the diagnosis because the findings are dramatic. Nonetheless, it is useful to have a quantifiable value such as the AFI. The diagnosis of polyhydramnios is established by an AFI ≥25 cm.

Polyhydramnios may have both maternal and fetal sequelae. In mild cases, there are minimal maternal symptoms, generally consisting of abdominal discomfort and slight dyspnea. In moderate-to-severe polyhydramnios (AF volume greater than 4000 mL), there may be marked respiratory distress: dyspnea and orthopnea and usually edema of the lower extremities.

The increased AF volume and overstretched myometrium place the patient with polyhydramnios at risk of certain complications. Spontaneous labor with intact membranes usually produces contractions that are of poor quality because of the excessive uterine size. There is an increased incidence of abnormal presentations, and therefore there are more operative deliveries. Spontaneous rupture of the membranes causes a sudden decompression of the uterus, which increases the incidence of abruptio placentae and cord prolapse. There is a marked increase in the incidence of postpartum hemorrhage as a result of uterine overdistension, resulting in uterine atony. Fetal complications include myriad congenital anomalies or abnormalities that result in increased fluid production or reduced fluid resorption.

Associations

Clinically detectable polyhydramnios occurs in 0.4–0.5% of pregnancies. Most cases of mild polyhydramnios (e.g. AFI 25–30 cm) are idiopathic (35–66%), and have a good prognosis, although the risks of preterm labor and fetal malpresentation remain. With increasing degrees of AF volume, the rate of fetal anomalies approaches 50%. It may be associated with diabetes mellitus, structural congenital malformations (usually of the central nervous system or gastrointestinal tract) impairing fetal swallowing, chromosomal abnormalities, multiple pregnancy (especially twin–twin transfusion syndrome or an

Table 40.1 Polyhydramnios: associated conditions

Cause	1970*	1987†	1999‡
Idiopathic (%)	35	66	66
Diabetes mellitus (%)	25	15	28
Congenital malformations (%)	21	13	4
Rh incompatibility (%)	11	1	–
Multiple pregnancy (%)	8	5	–

*Queenan and Gadow [50]; † Hill [51]; ‡ Panting-Kemp [53].

acardiac twin), or blood group incompatibilities. When associated with fetal hydrops, polyhydramnios may be a result of fetal cardiac abnormalities, anemia or hypoproteinemia. Once polyhydramnios is diagnosed, a systematic maternal work-up is necessary to determine the cause. Management is determined by the underlying cause. The clinician should rule out such conditions as diabetes mellitus, erythroblastosis fetalis, and multiple pregnancy (e.g. twin–twin transfusion) by performing a glucose tolerance test, indirect Coombs test, and sonography, respectively.

In Queenan and Gadow's 1970 series of 358 patients with polyhydramnios, the major associated conditions were diabetes mellitus (25%), congenital malformations (20%), and erythroblastosis fetalis (11%) (Table 40.1) [50]. By 1987, the causes had changed considerably, according to Hill *et al* [51]. The representation of diabetes mellitus was lower, reflecting stricter blood glucose control, and the occurrence of polyhydramnios resulting from rhesus (Rh) incompatibility was markedly decreased as a result of Rh immunoglobulin prophylaxis. Idris *et al* recently reported an 18.8% incidence of polyhydramnios among patients with pregestational diabetes, with the AF excess associated with poor diabetes control [52]. Panting-Kemp *et al* reported a 66% incidence of idiopathic polyhydramnios, with 4% of patients demonstrating fetal congenital malformation and 28% with maternal diabetes mellitus [53]. The reduction in the rate of fetal malformations associated with polyhydramnios may represent a higher detection rate of the malformation by second-trimester ultrasound and termination of severe cases before reaching viability.

Management

Treatment of polyhydramnios depends on the etiology and prognosis for effective treatment. Therapeutic amniocentesis is an option for the treatment of twin–twin transfusion syndrome. However, recent studies have indicated that fetoscopic laser ablation of the communicating blood vessels is of greater efficacy in severe cases presenting prior to fetal viability.

Conservative management includes modified bedrest and assessment of uterine activity and fetal well-being.

Diuretics are generally contraindicated because they deplete maternal vascular volume with little effect on the total AF volume. If moderate-to-severe polyhydramnios results in pronounced maternal distress, and sonographic study reveals a normal-appearing fetus, a more aggressive approach becomes necessary. If the fetus is mature, delivery is indicated. If the fetus is too immature for delivery, amniocentesis with drainage to normalize AF volume may be indicated. Complications of rapid removal of AF occur in 2–3% of procedures and include premature separation of the placenta, placental abruption, and premature rupture of membranes [54–56]. Reaccumulation of AF may rapidly occur and the procedure may need to be repeated every 2–3 days. A tocolytic agent should be considered to decrease the occurrence of uterine contractions.

For severe symptomatic polyhydramnios at less than 32 weeks' gestation, we suggest treatment with indomethacin following the amniocentesis to maintain normal AF volume without exposing the fetus to the risks of serial invasive procedures. Prostaglandin synthetase inhibitors may stimulate fetal secretion of arginine vasopressin and facilitate vasopressin-induced renal antidiuretic responses and reduced renal blood flow, thereby reducing fetal urine flow. These agents may also impair production or enhance reabsorption of lung liquid [57]. Indomethacin is started at 25 mg orally four times daily. If there is no reduction in AF volume, then the dosage is gradually increased to 2–3 mg/kg/day [58]. Maternal side-effects, such as nausea, esophageal reflux, gastritis, and emesis, are seen in approximately 4% of patients treated with indomethacin for preterm labor. The primary fetal concern with use of indomethacin is constriction of the ductus arteriosus and recent information suggests an increased risk of intraventricular hemorrhage. During indomethacin therapy, we monitor AF volume 2–3 times per week. The drug is tapered when there is a reduction in AF volume, and stopped when polyhydramnios is no longer severe. We obtain fetal echocardiographic evaluations at intervals to examine ductal flow. If the fetus is found to have major malformations incompatible with life, delivery may be considered.

Future therapies

Future therapeutic approaches for polyhydramnios include the use of intraamniotic pharmacologic agents to reduce fetal fluid production. In ovine pregnancy, intraamniotic administration of either arginine vasopressin or deamino arginine vasopressin results in rapid fetal plasma absorption and a marked decrease in fetal urine flow [59], although there is no effect on fetal swallowing [59].

The recent discovery of the aquaporins and their different expression in hydramnios may facilitate novel therapeutic approaches, targeting those cell membrane proteins that serve as water channels.

Oligohydramnios

Definition

Oligohydramnios is a pathologic condition characterized by a decrease in AF volume. Although it can occur in the first half of pregnancy, it is generally a problem of the second half.

Diagnosis

Oligohydramnios is suspected when the uterus is smaller than the date of gestation would suggest, and the diagnosis is made by sonography. The clinician relies on a quantifying method such as depth of the SDP or, more commonly, the AFI. An AFI of 5.0–8.0 cm indicates borderline AF, whereas an AFI of 5.0 or less indicates oligohydramnios. The time in pregnancy when it develops has a bearing on the prognosis. When oligohydramnios occurs as early as the second trimester, the prognosis is very poor [60].

Moore *et al* demonstrated the reliability and predictive value of a scoring system for oligohydramnios in the second trimester [61]. Sixty-two cases of oligohydramnios were diagnosed sonographically between 13 and 28 weeks' gestation. Three experienced sonographers used a subjective scale to rate the oligohydramnios as mild, moderate, severe, or anhydramniotic. Intraobserver reliability was excellent (intraclass correlation coefficient, 0.81). The overall perinatal mortality was 43% and the incidence of pulmonary hypoplasia was 33%. One-third had lethal congenital anomalies. The frequency of adverse outcomes strongly correlated with the most severe oligohydramnios or anhydramnios; 88% of the fetuses with severe oligohydramnios or anhydramnios had lethal outcomes, compared with 11% in the mild and moderate oligohydramnios group. The presence of an anuric urinary tract anomaly was associated with the most severe grade of oligohydramnios and was uniformly fatal. Pulmonary hypoplasia was diagnosed in 60% of the severe oligohydramnios group versus 6% of the moderate group.

The investigators concluded that subjective grading of oligohydramnios by experienced observers in the second trimester is both reliable and predictive of outcome. The finding of severe oligohydramnios in the second trimester is highly predictive of a poor fetal outcome and should stimulate an extensive search for the etiology and consideration of intervention.

Clinical significance

Oligohydramnios occurring as early as the second trimester is associated with a poor prognosis. Mercer and Brown reported 39 cases of oligohydramnios in the second trimester, diagnosed by sonography [62]. Nine of the pregnancies were associated with fetal malformations: Potter syndrome (5), atrioventricular disassociation (39), congenital absence of the thyroid (1), and multiple anomalies (5). There were 10 unexplained stillbirths, one death resulting from abruptio placentae, eight with perinatal mortality and morbidity after premature labor or abruptio placentae, and six live-born term infants. Although oligohydramnios in the second trimester is associated with a marked increase in perinatal mortality, it is not uniformly associated with a poor outcome.

Although oligohydramnios can be idiopathic, commonly it is associated with a specific clinical condition. The clinical conditions most commonly associated with oligohydramnios are discussed below.

Premature rupture of membranes

Premature rupture of membranes (PROM) occurs in 2–4% of preterm gestations. The clinical implications for oligohydramnios in the setting of PROM are as follows. If PROM occurs before 24 weeks, there is an 80% chance of labor, infection, or both. The rate of perinatal mortality is 54% and the risk of permanent handicap in survivors is 40% [63]. It is not unusual for a pregnancy complicated by PROM to present initially as oligohydramnios with a normally functioning fetal bladder. Further work-up reveals a slow leak of AF resulting from PROM.

The earlier in pregnancy that PROM occurs, the more likely the risk of fetal pulmonary hypoplasia. If the PROM occurs at 16–24 weeks' gestation, the threat of pulmonary hypoplasia is great. A recent review emphasized that the benefits of amnio-infusion for periviable PROM are unproven and the risks remain undetermined [64].

Oligohydramnios occurring secondary to PROM later in pregnancy creates a risk of umbilical cord compression. If compression occurs during labor, variable decelerations may become very problematic. This can be treated with amnio-infusion to create a cushion to relieve the cord compression.

Congenital malformation

When managing oligohydramnios, the clinician should always rule out chromosome abnormalities and structural malformations. Malformations of the urogenital system are the most commonly associated with oligohydramnios. The classic is Potter syndrome, with renal agenesis, low-set ears, and facial pressure deformities. With little or no AF, it is very difficult to image the fetus and adrenal glands may be mistaken for kidneys. Transabdominal amnio-infusion can help in providing fluid contrast for proper imaging. Additional urogenital problems can be encountered in the form of obstructive uropathy, such as posterior urethral valve syndrome, ureteropelvic junction syndrome, or ureterocystic junction

obstruction. The obstructive uropathies can be detected as early as 14–16 weeks' gestation. Bilateral cystic dysplasia of the fetal kidneys may be detected as early as 12 weeks' gestation. If the problem is unilateral, oligohydramnios is not likely. Cystic kidneys and renal pelvis dilation are found with trisomy 21 and trisomy 18, so karyotype should be determined.

Intrauterine growth restriction

Between 3% and 7% of all pregnancies are complicated by intrauterine growth restriction (IUGR). These fetuses have a considerably higher incidence of problems including hypoxia, acidosis, meconium aspiration, and polycythemia. After birth, potential complications include hypoglycemia, necrotizing enterocolitis, and impaired growth and development.

Approximately 60% of fetuses with IUGR have decreased AF volume discernible on sonographic examination. This feature may be very useful in differentiating the pathologically growth-restricted fetus from the one that is merely constitutionally small. Generally, oligohydramnios in the IUGR fetus is a sign of potential fetal jeopardy and a thorough evaluation of fetal well-being is indicated.

Postdate pregnancy

Approximately 3–7% of pregnancies extend beyond 42 completed weeks of gestation, dated from the first day of the last normal menstrual period. These pregnancies have a higher incidence of perinatal mortality, perinatal morbidity, and macrosomia. Postdate pregnancies are a leading cause of obstetric malpractice litigation, with most of the cases involving neurologically impaired babies [65].

The incidence of oligohydramnios increases in postdate pregnancies, in part as a result of normal shifts in the rates of fluid production and resorption (e.g. increased fetal swallowing) as well as a potential response to relative fetal hypoxia or nutrient restriction secondary to placental aging. The significance of oligohydramnios and spontaneous fetal heart rate decelerations during antepartum testing of postdate pregnancies was evaluated by Small *et al* [66]. The occurrence of oligohydramnios or spontaneous decelerations during testing necessitates consideration of prompt delivery. Fetuses with decreased AF volume are at increased risk for umbilical cord compression, meconium aspiration, and fetal compromise.

Twin pregnancy

Seventy-five percent of twin pregnancies are dichorionic and 25% are monochorionic. The fetal loss rate is much higher in monochorionic pregnancies as a result of twin–twin transfusion syndrome. Monochorionic twin pregnancies may be identified by the telltale "T sign" at the base of the intertwin membrane. The first manifestation of twin–twin transfusion syndrome is an increased nuchal translucency in one or both fetuses at 10–14 weeks' gestation. Subsequently, at 15–17 weeks' gestation there is intertwin disparity of AF volume manifested by folding of the intertwin membrane [67].

In multiple pregnancies where polyhydramnios and oligohydramnios occur in separate sacs, there is a serious danger to the fetus with oligohydramnios. Chescheir and Seeds reported on seven such twins with twin–twin transfusion syndrome resulting in a perinatal mortality rate of 71% [68]. The occurrence of the complication before 26 weeks' gestation resulted in death of all fetuses despite a variety of attempted therapies. In twin–twin transfusion syndrome, the donor twin becomes anemic and, over time, growth restricted, and develops oligohydramnios. When the oligohydramnios is severe, the fetus becomes immobilized, generally against the uterine wall because of pressure from the sac with polyhydramnios. The fetus does not move despite changing of maternal position. This has been called the trapped twin syndrome.

Endoscopic laser ablation of the intercommunicating placental vessels is recommended for severe twin–twin transfusion syndrome presenting prior to fetal viability [69]. Following viability, amniodrainage from the twin with polyhydramnios may improve the AF volume of the donor twin with oligohydramnios [67].

Management

Amnio-infusion may be considered in pregnancies complicated by oligohydramnios when the physician feels that augmenting the AF volume will provide diagnostic or therapeutic benefit. Amnio-infusion may be performed therapeutically, prophylactically, or as a diagnostic intervention. Maternal hydration via oral hydration or intravenous hypotonic fluid is a means of transiently increasing amniotic fluid volume, and is less invasive than amnio-infusion [70–72]. Hydration with oral water reduces maternal plasma osmolality and sodium concentration, resulting in an osmotically driven maternal-to-fetal water flux. Increased placental blood flow volume, fetal urine output, and possibly decreased reabsorption of amniotic fluid via swallowing or intramembranous flow increases the amniotic fluid volume [73].

Conclusion

Recent clinical and laboratory studies have provided an ever increasing understanding of the dynamics of amniotic fluid volume, the clinical importance of oligo- and polyhydramnios, and the potential use of the amniotic cavity as a route for the administration of therapeutic agents to the fetus. AF is a dynamic body of water which provides essential functions for appropriate fetal growth and development. The extremes of volume – too much or too little – may be associated with an unfavorable prognosis. Appropriate diagnosis and management of polyhydramnios and oligohydramnios are essential to optimize fetal outcome.

CASE PRESENTATION

A 26-year-old gravida 2, para 1 with a history of one prior term vaginal delivery presented for prenatal care in the first trimester. The patient's fundal height was slightly greater than her dates, and a subsequent ultrasound revealed a twin gestation with a dividing membrane consistent with diamniotic monochorionic placentation. Repeat ultrasounds demonstrated symmetric growth until a 26-week scan revealed a 20% weight discordance. A repeat ultrasound 2 weeks later demonstrated marked oligohydramnios (i.e. stuck twin) in the smaller twin, associated with an absence of bladder filling and polyhydramnios in the larger twin. A diagnosis of twin–twin transfusion syndrome was made. As the gestation was beyond fetal viability, laser ablation of placental anastomoses was not entertained. An amnioreduction procedure was performed with withdrawal of 2 L fluid from the polyhydramnios sac. Subsequent ultrasound confirmed a reduction in amniotic fluid in the polyhydramnios sac, and reaccumulation of fluid in the oligohydramnios sac, although still subjectively reduced. A repeat amnioreduction was performed 1 week later. Shortly thereafter,

the patient progressed into spontaneous labor and was operatively delivered at 29 weeks' gestation. Twins demonstrated a 25% discordancy in weight, with evidence of polycythemia and anemia in the larger and smaller twin, respectively.

This case represents an example of twin–twin transfusion syndrome. The donor twin's anemia, reduced intravascular volume, and mild hypoxemia result in relative oliguria. Continued fetal swallowing, despite reduced amniotic fluid (e.g. urine) production, contributes to the oligohydramnios. Conversely, the recipient twin develops polycythemia, increased intravascular volume, and elevated plasma atrial natriuretic factor levels. Markedly increased urine production contributes to the polyhydramnios state. Amnioreduction reduces intraamniotic pressure, potentiating increased maternal-to-fetal placental water flow, and facilitating intravascular volume repletion and urine output in the donor twin. However, the twin–twin transfusion pathophysiology continues, with continued transfer of plasma and red cells, and polyhydramnios/oligohydramnios recurs.

References

1. Denman T. An Introduction to the Practice of Midwifery. London: Bliss and White, 1825.

2. Campbell J, Wathen N, Macintosh M, Cass P, Chard T, Mainwaring BR. Biochemical composition of amniotic fluid and extraembryonic coelomic fluid in the first trimester of pregnancy. Br J Obstet Gynaecol 1992;99(7):563–565.

3. Faber JJ, Gault CF, Green TJ, Long LR, Thornburg KL. Chloride and the generation of amniotic fluid in the early embryo. J Exp Zool 1973;183(3):343–352.

4. Gillibrand PN. Changes in the electrolytes, urea and osmolality of the amniotic fluid with advancing pregnancy. J Obstet Gynaecol Br Commonw 1969;76(10):898–905.

5. Queenan JT, Thompson W, Whitfield CR, Shah SI. Amniotic fluid volumes in normal pregnancies. Am J Obstet Gynecol 1972;114(1):34–38.

6. Brace RA, Wolf EJ. Normal amniotic fluid volume changes throughout pregnancy. Am J Obstet Gynecol 1989;161(2):382–388.

7. Pritchard JA. Deglutition by normal and anencephalic fetuses. Obstet Gynecol 1965;25:289–297.

8. Rabinowitz R, Peters MT, Vyas S, Campbell S, Nicolaides KH. Measurement of fetal urine production in normal pregnancy by real-time ultrasonography. Am J Obstet Gynecol 1989; 161(5):1264–1266.

9. Chez RA, Smith RG, Hutchinson DL. Renal function in the intrauterine primate fetus. I. Experimental technique: rate of formation and chemical composition of urine. Am J Obstet Gynecol 1964;90:128–131.

10. Kurjak A, Kirkinen P, Latin V, Ivankovic D. Ultrasonic assessment of fetal kidney function in normal and complicated pregnancies. Am J Obstet Gynecol 1981;141(3):266–270.

11. Jeffcoate TN, Scott JS. Polyhydramnios and oligohydramnios. Can Med Assoc J 1959;80(2):77–86.

12. Shiller W, Toll CM. An inquiry into the cause of oligohydramnios. Am J Obstet Gynecol 1927;12:689.

13. Sylvester PE, Hughes DR. Congenital absence of both kidneys; a report of four cases. BMJ 1954;4853:77–79.

14. Liley AW. Disorders of amniotic fluid. In: Assali NS, ed. Pathophysiology of Gestation. New York: Academic Press, 1972.

15. Goodlin R, Lloyd D. Fetal tracheal excretion of bilirubin. Biol Neonat 1968;12(1):1–12.

16. Adamsons TM, Brodecky V, Lambert V et al. The production and composition of lung liquid in the in utero foetal lamb. In: Dawes GS, ed. Foetal and Neonatal Physiology.Cambridge, UK: Cambridge University Press, 1973.

17. Brace RA, Wlodek ME, Cock ML, Harding R. Swallowing of lung liquid and amniotic fluid by the ovine fetus under normoxic and hypoxic conditions. Am J Obstet Gynecol 1994;171(3):764–770.

18. Ross MG, Ervin G, Leake RD, Fu P, Fisher DA. Fetal lung liquid regulation by neuropeptides. Am J Obstet Gynecol 1984; 150(4):421–425.

19. Lawson EE, Brown ER, Torday JS, Madansky DL, Taeusch HW Jr. The effect of epinephrine on tracheal fluid flow and surfactant efflux in fetal sheep. Am Rev Respir Dis 1978;118(6): 1023–1026.

20. Dodic M, Wintour EM. Effects of prolonged (48h) infusion of cortisol on blood pressure, renal function and fetal fluids in the immature ovine foetus. Clin Exp Pharmacol Physiol 1994; 21(12):971–980.

21. Pritchard JA. Fetal swallowing and amniotic fluid volume. Obstet Gynecol 1966;28(5):606–610.

22. Bradley RM, Mistretta CM. Swallowing in fetal sheep. Science 1973;179(77):1016–1017.

23. El-Haddad MA, Ismail Y, Guerra C, Day L, Ross MG. Effect of oral sucrose on ingestive behavior in the near-term ovine fetus. Am J Obstet Gynecol 2002;187(4):898–901.

24. Sherman DJ, Ross MG, Day L, Humme J, Ervin MG. Fetal swallowing: response to graded maternal hypoxemia. J Appl Physiol 1991;71(5):1856–1861.

25. Carter CO. Congenital malformation. Ciba Foundation Symposium 1960;264.

26. Gadd RL. Liquor amnii. In: Phillipp EE, Barnes J, Newton M, eds. Scientific Foundations of Obstetrics and Gynaecology. London: Butterworth Heinemann, 1987, p.254.

27. Benirschke K, McKay DG. The antidiuretic hormone in fetus and infant: histochemical observations with special reference to amniotic fluid formation. Obstet Gynecol 1953;1(6):638–649.

28. Naeye RL, Milic AM, Blanc W. Fetal endocrine and renal disorders: clues to the origin of hydramnios. Am J Obstet Gynecol 1970;108(8):1251–1256.

29. Lingwood BE, Wintour EM. Amniotic fluid volume and in vivo permeability of ovine fetal membranes. Obstet Gynecol 1984;64(3):368–372.

30. Gilbert WM, Newman PS, Eby-Wilkens E, Brace RA. Technetium Tc 99m rapidly crosses the ovine placenta and intramembranous pathway. Am J Obstet Gynecol 1996;175(6): 1557–1562.

31. Lingwood BE, Wintour EM. Permeability of ovine amnion and amniochorion to urea and water. Obstet Gynecol 1983;61(2): 227–232.

32. Gilbert WM, Brace RA. The missing link in amniotic fluid volume regulation: intramembranous absorption. Obstet Gynecol 1989;74(5):748–754.

33. Huang J, Qi HB. [Expression of aquaporin 8 in human fetal membrane and placenta of idiopathic polyhydramnios]. Zhonghua Fu Chan Ke Za Zhi 2009;44(1):19–22.

34. Zhu XQ, Jiang SS, Zou SW, Hu YC, Wang YH. [Expression of aquaporin 3 and aquaporin 9 in placenta and fetal membrane with idiopathic polyhydramnios]. Zhonghua Fu Chan Ke Za Zhi 2009;44(12):920–923.

35. Mann SE, Dvorak N, Gilbert H, Taylor RN. Steady-state levels of aquaporin 1 mRNA expression are increased in idiopathic polyhydramnios. Am J Obstet Gynecol 2006;194(3):884–887.

36. Wang S, Chen J, Huang B, Ross MG. Cloning and cellular expression of aquaporin 9 in ovine fetal membranes. Am J Obstet Gynecol 2005;193(3):841–848.

37. Queenan JT, Allen FH Jr, Fuchs F et al. Studies on the method of intrauterine transfusion. I. Question of erythrocyte absorption from amniotic fluid. Am J Obstet Gynecol 1965;92: 1009–1013.

38. Hebertson RM, Hammond ME, Bryson MJ. Amniotic epithelial ultrastructure in normal, polyhydramnic, and oligohydramnic pregnancies. Obstet Gynecol 1986;68(1):74–79.

39. Charles D, Jacoby HE. Preliminary data on the use of sodium aminohippurate to determine amniotic fluid volumes. Am J Obstet Gynecol 1966;95(2):266–269.

40. Magann EF, Nolan TE, Hess LW, Martin RW, Whitworth NS, Morrison JC. Measurement of amniotic fluid volume: accuracy of ultrasonography techniques. Am J Obstet Gynecol 1992; 167(6):1533–1537.

41. Horsager R, Nathan L, Leveno KJ. Correlation of measured amniotic fluid volume and sonographic predictions of oligohydramnios. Obstet Gynecol 1994;83(6):955–958.

42. Dildy GA III, Lira N, Moise KJ Jr, Riddle GD, Deter RL. Amniotic fluid volume assessment: comparison of ultrasonographic estimates versus direct measurements with a dyedilution technique in human pregnancy. Am J Obstet Gynecol 1992;167(4 Pt 1):986–994.

43. Magann EF, Morton ML, Nolan TE, Martin JN Jr, Whitworth NS, Morrison JC. Comparative efficacy of two sonographic measurements for the detection of aberrations in the amniotic fluid volume and the effect of amniotic fluid volume on pregnancy outcome. Obstet Gynecol 1994;83(6):959–962.

44. Chauhan SP, Magann EF, Morrison JC, Whitworth NS, Hendrix NW, Devoe LD. Ultrasonographic assessment of amniotic fluid does not reflect actual amniotic fluid volume. Am J Obstet Gynecol 1997;177(2):291–296.

45. Magann EF, Doherty DA, Chauhan SP, Busch FW, Mecacci F, Morrison JC. How well do the amniotic fluid index and single deepest pocket indices (below the 3rd and 5th and above the 95th and 97th percentiles) predict oligohydramnios and hydramnios? Am J Obstet Gynecol 2004;190(1):164–169.

46. Magann EF, Chauhan SP, Barrilleaux PS, Whitworth NS, McCurley S, Martin JN. Ultrasound estimate of amniotic fluid volume: color Doppler overdiagnosis of oligohydramnios. Obstet Gynecol 2001;98(1):71–74.

47. Goldkrand JW, Hough TM, Lentz SU, Clements SP, Bryant JL, Hodges JA. Comparison of the amniotic fluid index with grayscale and color Doppler ultrasound. J Matern Fetal Neonatal Med 2003;13(5):318–322.

48. Zlatnik MG, Olson G, Bukowski R, Saade GR. Amniotic fluid index measured with the aid of color flow Doppler. J Matern Fetal Neonatal Med 2003;13(4):242–245.

49. Magann EF, Nevils BG, Chauhan SP, Whitworth NS, Klausen JH, Morrison JC. Low amniotic fluid volume is poorly identified in singleton and twin pregnancies using the 2 x 2cm pocket technique of the biophysical profile. South Med J 1999;92(8):802–805.

50. Queenan JT, Gadow EC. Polyhydramnios: chronic versus acute. Am J Obstet Gynecol 1970;108(3):349–355.

51. Hill LM, Breckle R, Thomas ML, Fries JK. Polyhydramnios: ultrasonically detected prevalence and neonatal outcome. Obstet Gynecol 1987;69(1):21–25.

52. Idris N, Wong SF, Thomae M, Gardener G, McIntyre DH. Influence of polyhydramnios on perinatal outcome in pregestational diabetic pregnancies. Ultrasound Obstet Gynecol 2010;36(3):338–343.

53. Panting-Kemp A, Nguyen T, Chang E, Quillen E, Castro L. Idiopathic polyhydramnios and perinatal outcome. Am J Obstet Gynecol 1999;181(5 Pt 1):1079–1082.

54. Queenan JT. Recurrent acute polyhydramnios. Am J Obstet Gynecol 1970;106(4):625–626.

55. Elliott JP, Sawyer AT, Radin TG, Strong RE. Large-volume therapeutic amniocentesis in the treatment of hydramnios. Obstet Gynecol 1994;84(6):1025–1027.

56. Leung WC, Jouannic JM, Hyett J, Rodeck C, Jauniaux E. Procedure-related complications of rapid amniodrainage in the treatment of polyhydramnios. Ultrasound Obstet Gynecol 2004;23(2):154–158.

57. Kramer WB, van den Veyver, I, Kirshon B. Treatment of polyhydramnios with indomethacin. Clin Perinatol 1994;21(3): 615–630.

58. Cabrol D, Landesman R, Muller J, Uzan M, Sureau C, Saxena BB. Treatment of polyhydramnios with prostaglandin synthetase inhibitor (indomethacin). Am J Obstet Gynecol 1987; 157(2):422–426.

59. Gilbert WM, Cheung CY, Brace RA. Rapid intramembranous absorption into the fetal circulation of arginine vasopressin injected intraamniotically. Am J Obstet Gynecol 1991;164(4): 1013–1018.

60. Moore TR. Oligohydramnios. In: Queenan JT, Hobbins JC, eds. Protocols in High-Risk Pregnancies. Cambridge, MA: Blackwell Science, 1996, p.488.

61. Moore TR, Longo J, Leopold GR, Casola G, Gosink BB. The reliability and predictive value of an amniotic fluid scoring system in severe second-trimester oligohydramnios. Obstet Gynecol 1989;73(5 Pt 1):739–742.

62. Mercer LJ, Brown LG. Fetal outcome with oligohydramnios in the second trimester. Obstet Gynecol 1986;67(6):840–842.

63. Ghidini A, Romero R. Prelabor rupture of the membranes. In: Queenan JT, Hobbins JC, eds. Protocols in High-Risk Pregnancies. Cambridge, MA: Blackwell Science, 1996, p.547.

64. Waters TP, Mercer BM. The management of preterm premature rupture of the membranes near the limit of fetal viability. Am J Obstet Gynecol 2009;201(3):230–240.

65. Quilligan EJ. Postdate pregnancies. In: Queenan JT, Hobbins JC, eds. Protocols in High-Risk Pregnancies. Cambridge, MA: Blackwell Science, 1996, p.633.

66. Small ML, Phelan JP, Smith CV, Paul RH. An active management approach to the postdate fetus with a reactive nonstress test and fetal heart rate decelerations. Obstet Gynecol 1987;70(4):636–640.

67. Nicolaides K, Sebire N, d'Ercole C. Prediction, diagnosis and management of twin-to-twin transfusion syndrome. In: Cockburn F, ed. Advances in Perinatal Medicine. New York: Parthenon Publishing, 1997, p.200.

68. Chescheir NC, Seeds JW. Polyhydramnios and oligohydramnios in twin gestations. Obstet Gynecol 1988;71(6 Pt 1): 882–884.

69. Ville Y, Hecher K, Gagnon A, Sebire N, Hyett J, Nicolaides K. Endoscopic laser coagulation in the management of severe twin-to-twin transfusion syndrome. Br J Obstet Gynaecol 1998;105(4):446–453.

70. Ghafarnejad M, Tehrani MB, Anaraki FB, Mood NI, Nasehi L. Oral hydration therapy in oligohydramnios. J Obstet Gynaecol Res 2009;35(5):895–900.

71. Yan-Rosenberg L, Burt B, Bombard AT et al. A randomized clinical trial comparing the effect of maternal intravenous hydration and placebo on the amniotic fluid index in oligohydramnios. J Matern Fetal Neonatal Med 2007;20(10): 715–718.

72. Doi S, Osada H, Seki K, Sekiya S. Effect of maternal hydration on oligohydramnios: a comparison of three volume expansion methods. Obstet Gynecol 1998;92(4 Pt 1):525–529.

73. Hofmeyr GJ, Gulmezoglu AM. Maternal hydration for increasing amniotic fluid volume in oligohydramnios and normal amniotic fluid volume. Cochrane Database Syst Rev 2002;1:CD000134.

Chapter 41
Prevention of Preterm Birth

Paul J. Meis

Department of Obstetrics and Gynecology, Wake Forest University School of Medicine, Winston-Salem, NC, USA

Preterm birth is defined as a livebirth before 37 completed weeks' gestation. Preterm births can be classified by their apparent etiology as spontaneous preterm labor and delivery, constituting approximately 45% of preterm births; births occurring after spontaneous premature preterm rupture of the fetal membranes (PPROM), approximately 35% of preterm births; and preterm births that result from a medical or obstetric complication of the pregnancy, approximately 20% of preterm births [1]. Based on common risk factors for their occurrence, it may be appropriate to consider those births caused by spontaneous preterm labor and PPROM as a single entity and likely to be caused by similar pathogeneses [2].

The rate of preterm birth has been rising in the USA and in many other countries. The rate reached 12.8% of all livebirths in 2006, but more recently decreased to 12.3% in 2008, the most recent year of available data. This improvement is somewhat encouraging, but the rate of 12.3% remains very high compared to other developed countries. Compared with singleton births (one baby), multiple births in the USA were about six times more likely to be preterm in 2002 [3].

Preterm birth demonstrates a marked racial disparity. The rate of preterm birth for black infants is 17.6%, compared to 10.7% for white infants. However, the rate of preterm birth for white infants in the USA remains high compared to rates of 6–8% for most European countries [4]. Preterm birth is the most common reason for the death of a newborn infant with no birth defects. It is also the leading cause of cerebral palsy in the surviving children and is linked to other long-term developmental problems. In very premature infants, weighing 501–700 g, the mortality rate is approximately 70%, and with neonatal intensive care many of these deaths may occur as late as 100 days of hospitalization. The risk of severe handicap (cerebral palsy, mental retardation, epilepsy, blindness, or deafness) in survivors is approximately 20% [4].

The financial costs of preterm birth are very high. In 2005, prematurity-related infant stays resulted in hospital charges of $26,200,000. The costs of hospital care for infants born at 25–27 weeks' gestation were more than 28 times those of infants born at term: $280,146 versus $9803 [5]. Hospital costs in 2010 are likely to be even higher. These figures do not include the financial costs to the families of handicapped children over their lifespan. In addition to the financial costs of preterm birth, the families of very preterm infants are exposed to considerable stress in dealing with this problem and dysfunctional family patterns are common. For these reasons, preterm birth is recognized as a major public health problem and reduction of the rates of preterm birth as the most important goal in contemporary obstetric practice and research.

Preterm birth as a social phenomenon

Many studies have shown that the risk of preterm birth is related to low socio-economic status. Given this relationship, why does the USA have high rates of preterm birth when it has one of the highest rates of per capita income of all the nations of the world? Several facts may explain this seeming contradiction. Access to healthcare for individuals in the USA may be limited by the lack of health insurance. From 2008 census data, 20.1% of women aged 15–44 were uninsured and women of child-bearing age accounted for 27.1% of uninsured Americans [6].

The racial disparity of insurance coverage is striking. In a study by Families USA, nearly 35% of Hispanics were uninsured, as were 20% of blacks and 12% of whites [7]. While many states have attempted to improve insurance coverage with Medicaid for low-income pregnant women, many gaps in coverage persist, and health problems of the women may not be covered by Medicaid insurance until the time of pregnancy.

Queenan's Management of High-Risk Pregnancy: An Evidence-Based Approach, Sixth Edition. Edited by John T. Queenan, Catherine Y. Spong, Charles J. Lockwood.

Income inequality is greater in the USA than in other major industrialized countries such as Canada, Australia, and European countries. In 2002, a total of 34.6 million Americans, 12.1% of the population, lived in poverty. A monograph by Miller [8] described some of the social support benefits enjoyed by pregnant women in Europe. The countries surveyed were Belgium, Denmark, Germany, France, Ireland, Netherlands, Norway, Spain, Switzerland, and the UK. In all of these countries, prenatal care is available to all regardless to their ability to pay. Many of these countries provide financial incentives to pregnant women for attending prenatal visits. They all provide paid pregnancy leave with job security, and routine home visits by a nurse following the delivery. In The Netherlands, women receive 100% of their salaries during maternity leave, and in Denmark and Sweden 90%. These programs are in contrast to the relative lack of organized social support for pregnant women in the USA.

Tocolytic drugs

Since the 1970s, much of the effort toward preventing preterm birth has been focused on attempts to halt preterm labor through the use of tocolytic drugs. Despite the wide usage of these drugs, the results have been disappointing. Since the time of the introduction of these drugs, no reduction has been observed in the rates of preterm birth in the USA or in other countries. Randomized placebo-controlled trials of these drugs have found that the use of these drugs can be effective in delaying preterm delivery for a matter of days, but that ultimate preterm delivery is not prevented [9]. The short-term delay in delivery, however, can be useful in allowing time for the effective use of antenatal steroid therapy to enhance fetal lung maturity. This lack of effectiveness of tocolytic therapy and the lack of other effective methods to reduce rates of preterm birth have led to the opinion of many that no effective and reproducible method of preventing preterm birth has been demonstrated [9]. Although magnesium sulfate therapy, like other tocolytic drugs, has limited effectiveness in preventing preterm delivery, a large randomized trial found that this treatment was effective in preventing moderate or severe cerebral palsy when measured at 1 year of age [10].

It would appear that once the labor process has begun, which likely occurs earlier than the clinical onset of labor, attempts to halt this process are futile and that effective prevention for preterm labor must rely on programs or interventions that are introduced early in pregnancy. Current evidence suggests that we may be at the threshold of implementing effective and clinically useful methods of preventing preterm birth. It is tempting to speculate that these new therapies are beginning to have an impact on preterm delivery rates.

Prevention of preterm birth in France

The French experience in preterm birth prevention in the 1970s and 1980s is worthy of attention because it represented a formal program to reduce the rate of preterm births and because France was the only European country to experience a significant decrease in the rate of preterm births. The program was under the direction of Dr Emile Papiernik. A full description of this program was published by Papiernik and Goffinet [11]. Papiernik first tested this program in a small district of France containing the city of Hagenau in the region of Alsace. The basic features of the program included the availability of early and equal prenatal care for all women regardless of ability to pay; provision of information that would convince the women to change their lifestyles; recognition, during prenatal care, of risk factors and warning signs of preterm birth; and appropriate use of maternity work leave and reduction of physical activity. The program was directed at all pregnant women, not only those at high risk. The success of this program in Hagenau led to its adoption throughout the entire country. In France, the proportion of deliveries at less than 37 weeks decreased from 8.2% in 1972 to 6.8% in 1976, 5.6% in 1982, and 4.9% in 1988. Of even greater significance, births at less than 34 weeks decreased from 2.4% of deliveries in 1972 to 1.7% in 1976, 1.2% in 1981, and 0.9% in 1988 [11]. Analysis of the preterm births revealed that the reduction occurred for spontaneous preterm births, and no decrease occurred for indicated preterm deliveries [12]. The decrease in preterm deliveries occurred mainly for women at low or moderate risk. Women at high risk for preterm delivery, because of a history of a previous preterm delivery or a previous stillbirth, did not experience a decreased rate of preterm delivery.

Since 1988 a trend has been seen in France for a modest increase in preterm births, to 4.43% in 1995 and 6.27% in 1998. The largest increases were identified in the subgroup of indicated preterm births, from 0.51% in 1972 to 2.31% in 1998 [12]. France has experienced an increased number of births to immigrant women who were born outside continental France. An analysis of births in the Seine–Saint-Denis district in 2000 found that almost half of all births occurred to these women. The only groups who experienced an increased rate of preterm births were women born in the French Caribbean or sub-Saharan Africa, who had rates of preterm birth of 7.9% and 7.2%, respectively [13]. These rates are still low compared with rates of preterm birth in the USA.

Unfortunately, attempts to duplicate the French experience in the USA have not been successful. A multicenter randomized trial of a system of patient education, physician education, and weekly pelvic examination enrolled 2395 women. The results showed no significant reduction in the study group compared to the control group [14].

There are several reasons that can be advanced for this lack of success. The program did not receive the same level of support from the popular media as was present in France in helping to promote healthier lifestyles, and no governmental policy was in place that encouraged liberal pregnancy work leave. Perhaps more importantly, the trial was limited to women who were at high risk for preterm birth. In general, this group of women did not show benefit in the French program.

Likewise, trials of increased social support for women at high risk for preterm delivery have failed to show results in improved birth outcomes [15,16]. A recent trial by Ayman *et al* is an exception to the disappointing results of social support. These investigators provided individually tailored counseling for women who reported environmental smoke exposure. The subjects randomized to this treatment had lower rates of very low birthweight and very preterm births [17].

The results achieved by the French experience are important, but without changes in healthcare policy, they may not be translatable to the current health delivery system in the USA.

Infection and preterm birth

Several lines of evidence link the presence of infection and/or inflammation and preterm birth. These include a strong association between histologic chorioamnionitis and preterm birth [18], particularly early preterm birth, an association of bacterial vaginosis with preterm birth [19], and of periodontitis with preterm birth [20]. In addition, a small percentage of women in preterm labor with intact membranes have demonstrated the presence of bacterial invasion of the amniotic space [21].

These associations have stimulated a number of clinical trials of antibiotic therapy for women in preterm labor, and pregnant women with positive vaginal fetal fibronectin, vaginal infections, or periodontal disease [22–26] and of interconceptional antibiotics for women following an early preterm birth [27]. Unfortunately, the results of these trials have been disappointing, showing a lack of positive prevention of preterm birth or, in some cases, an increase in preterm birth in some groups of women treated with antibiotics [23,25,26]. Similarly, trials of oral treatment of periodontal disease in pregnancy have found that improvement in periodontal health did not improve pregnancy outcome [28,29]. An exception to these disappointing results of trials of antibiotic therapy is the improvement demonstrated by treating women with PPROM with antibiotics such as erythromycin. These treatments resulted in an increased latency period before labor and improved neonatal outcome [30].

Several trials have evaluated omega-3 fatty acid supplementation in pregnancy to prevent preterm birth, presumably through antiinflammatory effects. The results of a trial by Olsen found that the supplementation was effective only in women with low dietary fish intake [31]. A trial by Harper of omega-3 supplementation in addition to treatment with 17α-hydroxyprogesterone caproate (17P) found no additional benefit to the fish oil treatment, but the rate of preterm delivery was noted to be significantly lower in subjects with a history of dietary fish intake [32].

Cervical changes and preterm birth

The concept of weakness in the compliance and passive ability of the uterine cervix to retain the fetus in pregnancy was first advanced more than 50 years ago, but has remained controversial up to the present time.

In 1955, Shirodkar proposed surgical cerclage of the cervix as a treatment for women with a history of habitual abortion [33]. The surgical technique that he reported and other similar procedures have been used frequently since that time with an estimated current frequency of use between 1 in 200 and 1 in 2000 deliveries [34]. The traditional concept of this entity has been to consider the cervix as being competent or incompetent, with the treatment of cervical incompetence (better referred to as insufficiency) requiring surgical cerclage. Despite the relative popularity of this treatment to prevent preterm delivery, controversies have persisted regarding the best means of diagnosis of cervical insufficiency, appropriate indications for the procedure, and the efficacy of the treatment to prevent preterm birth. The classic indications for the procedure using the patient's historical factors include a history of two or more consecutive second-trimester pregnancy losses, a history of painless dilation of the pregnant cervix to 4–6 cm, and a history of diethylstilbestrol (DES) exposure *in utero* of the pregnant women.

The availability of endovaginal ultrasonography to measure cervical length accurately and identify funneling of the internal os has both focused increased attention on the role of the cervix in preterm delivery and provided a potentially better means of evaluating cervical function.

Cervical length remains relatively stable up to the early third trimester of pregnancy at which time progressive shortening begins. The median cervical length is 35–40 mm at 14–22 weeks and falls to approximately 35 mm at 24–28 weeks, and 30 mm after 32 weeks [35]. The cervical length at 22–32 weeks' gestation displays a normal distribution, with the 50th percentile approximately 35 mm and the 10th and 90th at 25 and 45 mm, respectively [36,37]. The studies reported by Iams and other investigators have shown that the likelihood of preterm delivery is inversely related to the length of the cervix when measured at 24–28 weeks' gestation. While the cervical length can now be measured with accuracy and the associated risk of preterm delivery better assessed, it is unclear how best to treat a shortened cervix and what degree of shortening merits treatment.

Perhaps the most common cause of a shortened cervix is inflammation, resulting from local effects of intravaginal and/or intrauterine infection or decidual hemorrhage with consequent biochemically induced change in the cervix. These inflammatory alterations in the cervix are similar to the changes that occur in preparation for labor at term, and are a prelude to preterm labor and delivery. The cervical appearance in these women is currently indistinguishable from a shortened cervix resulting from intrinsic physical causes, but surgical cerclage in this circumstance would be counterproductive and would likely enhance the inflammatory or hemorrhagic process.

The efficacy of cervical cerclage in preventing preterm delivery has been evaluated by a number of randomized trials. Some of these trials enrolled women on the basis of historical pregnancy factors; other more recent trials enrolled patients on the basis of ultrasound measurement of cervical length. Grant reported a metaanalysis of four earlier trials [38]. Enrollment into these trials was essentially by the subject's past pregnancy history. A total of 1509 women were enrolled. The largest trial was conducted by the Medical Research Council and Royal College of Obstetrics and Gynaecology Working Group (MRC/RCOG) and enrolled 905 subjects [39]. The combined odds ratios (OR) of the trials did not find a statistically significant reduction of delivery at less than 33 weeks' gestation or at less than 37 weeks' gestation. The largest single trial (MRC/RCOG) found OR of delivery at less than 33 weeks of 0.67, which barely met statistical significance (95% confidence interval [CI] 0.47–0.97). Subgroup analysis of this trial found that the only group of subjects who benefited was women with a history of combination of three or more preterm births or second-trimester pregnancy losses.

Several randomized trials have reported the results of cervical cerclage for patients with a shortened cervix on ultrasound measurement. Rush *et al* [40] randomly assigned patients with sonographic evidence of cervical shortening (<25 mm) or funneling (>25%) between 16 and 24 weeks' gestation to cerclage (n = 55) versus no cerclage (n = 58). There were no significant differences in preterm birth rate (cerclage 35% versus no cerclage 36%) or other perinatal outcomes between the two groups.

Althuisius *et al* [41] recruited 35 women with a history of preterm birth at less than 34 weeks to the Cervical Incompetence Prevention Randomized Cerclage Trial (CIPRACT). Study subjects were followed with endovaginal sonography and randomized to cerclage versus bedrest if the cervical length fell below 25 mm. Of the 35 women enrolled, 19 were randomly assigned to cerclage

with modified bedrest and 16 were assigned to bedrest alone. A preterm birth rate of 44% (seven of the 16 women) occurred in those women treated with bedrest alone, compared with zero in those treated with cerclage and modified bedrest (0 of the 19 women; P < 0.002).

Berghella *et al* [42] randomized 61 women found to have a shortened cervix to either bedrest or bedrest plus cervical cerclage. Some of the women had singleton pregnancies and had risk factors for preterm delivery, some of the women had a twin gestation, and some were at low risk for preterm delivery but were identified on routine screening to have a shortened cervix. Preterm delivery at less than 35 weeks occurred in 45% of the subjects in the cerclage group and 47% of the women in the bedrest group. No difference existed in any obstetric or neonatal outcome.

In 2004, To *et al* [43] performed the largest randomized multicenter study examining the usefulness of cervical cerclage placement in women with a short cervix. The investigators screened 47,123 women using transvaginal ultrasound at 22–24 weeks' gestation and identified 470 women with a cervical length of 15 mm or less. Two hundred and fifty three patients were randomized to receive either a Shirodkar cervical cerclage (n = 127) or expectant management (n = 126). Study subjects in the cerclage arm received a single dose of intravenous intraoperative antibiotics and all participants were administered prophylactic steroids (two doses) for fetal lung maturity at 26–28 weeks' gestation. There were no significant differences in proportion of preterm birth rate before 33 weeks' gestation (cerclage 22% versus no cerclage 26%; relative risk [RR] 0.84; P = 0.44) or other differences in perinatal or maternal morbidity or mortality. This study is remarkable for the large number of women screened, the strict definition of shortened cervix (<15 mm), the relatively large number of subjects recruited and randomized, and the careful control of the quality of the surgical procedure used. The researchers concluded that, while transvaginal sonographic measurement of the cervical length at 22–24 weeks identifies a group at high risk of preterm delivery, the insertion of a cerclage suture in such women with short cervices does not substantially reduce the risk of prematurity.

Berghella *et al* [44] performed a metaanalysis of these four trials, including some additional subjects in the Rush and Althuisius trials. The total number of subjects was 607. The combined OR for these trials did not reach statistical significance for delivery prior to 35 weeks (OR 0.84, 95% CI 0.67–1.06). Berghella also performed subgroup analysis of these data, which found an increased RR for delivery at less than 35 weeks among women with twins having a short cervix who had a cerclage performed, compared with mothers of twins not so treated (RR 2.15, 95% CI 1.15–4.01). In contrast, subgroup analysis of women with a history of a previous preterm delivery and a shortened cervix had a decreased chance of preterm delivery at less than 35 weeks when cerclage was performed (RR 0.61, 95% CI 0.40–0.92).

Owen *et al* [45] performed a trial of cerclage versus no cerclage for women with a history of prior spontaneous preterm delivery and a cervix found to be less than 25 mm in length. The results of the trial found a significant improvement in delivery at less than 24 weeks' gestation and less than 37 weeks' gestation, although no significant difference in the primary outcome of the trial, delivery at less than 35 weeks' gestation. In subjects found to have a cervix 15 mm or less in length, cerclage demonstrated a clear benefit in prolonging pregnancy.

A subset of the subjects in the Owen trial were offered weekly injections of 17α-hydroxyprogesterone caproate (17P). Berghella *et al* analyzed the pregnancy outcomes for these women and found similar reductions in the rate of preterm delivery in the women treated with 17P or with cervical cerclage [46]. Treatment with both modalities did not significantly improve outcome compared with either treatment.

Fonseca *et al* screened with transvaginal ultrasound a large number of women (24,620) presenting for prenatal care [47]. Of these, 250 women found to have a cervix measuring 15 mm or less were randomly allocated to treatment with daily vaginal micronized progesterone or placebo. The results of the trial found a decrease in the rate of preterm delivery of less than 34 weeks' gestation in the progesterone group. No difference was found in any measure of neonatal morbidity or mortality.

In a subset of subjects in a trial of vaginal progesterone in women with a prior preterm delivery, DeFranco examined results for subjects who were found to have a shortened cervix of less than 28 mm, and found that treatment with progesterone reduced the likelihood of delivery at less than 32 weeks' gestation [48]. These results, however, must be viewed with caution. The overall results of the trial were negative, not all subjects had measurements of their cervix, multiple comparisons were made, and the subset evaluated had uneven distribution between the progesterone and placebo group.

In summary, while the ability to measure the cervix accurately by means of transvaginal ultrasound improves the accuracy of predicting risk for preterm delivery, the use of this method has been disappointing for selecting women who might benefit from cervical cerclage. It seems clear that women with twin gestations who may have a short cervix are poor candidates for a cerclage. Women with a prior preterm delivery and a short cervix may benefit from this procedure and additional randomized trials of treatment of this group of women with cerclage are needed.

Progesterone prophylactic therapy to prevent preterm birth

The use of progesterone to prevent preterm delivery is not new, and the first randomized trial of progesterone for this purpose was by Papiernik [49]. Several other small trials of progesterone therapy were reported over the next two decades. Recently, interest in this therapy has been reinvigorated as evidenced by the recent publication of several review articles and an American College of Obstetricians and Gynecologists (ACOG) Committee Opinion [50]. The origin of this new enthusiasm and interest in progesterone was the publication in 2003 of two randomized trials, one using progesterone vaginal suppositories and the other 17P injections to prevent recurrent preterm delivery [51,52].

The results of the early reported trials of progesterone were evaluated by two metaanalyses. Goldstein *et al*, in 1989, published the results of a metaanalysis of randomized controlled trials involving the use of progesterone or other progestogenic agents for the maintenance of pregnancy [53]. Fifteen trials of variously defined, high-risk subjects were felt to be suitable for analysis. The trials employed six progestational drugs. The pooled OR for these trials showed no statistically significant effect on rates of miscarriage, stillbirth, neonatal death, or preterm birth. The authors concluded that "progestogens should not be used outside of randomized trials at present."

In response to this publication, in 1990 Keirse presented the results of an analysis of a more focused selection of trials [54]. This metaanalysis was restricted to trials that employed 17P, the most fully studied progestational agent, and included all placebo-controlled trials that used this drug. Pooled OR found no significant effect on rates of miscarriage, perinatal death, or neonatal complications. However, in contrast to Goldstein *et al*'s review, the OR for preterm birth was significant at 0.5 (95% CI 0.30–0.85), as was the OR for birthweight less than 2500 g, 0.46 (95% CI 0.27–0.80). Keirse remarked that the results demonstrated by these trials contrasted markedly with the poor effectiveness of other efforts to reduce the occurrence of preterm birth, but that because no effect was demonstrated to result in lower perinatal mortality or morbidity, "further well-controlled research would be necessary before it is recommended for clinical practice."

A large trial of an oral progestogen was reported by Hobel *et al* [55] in 1994. As part of a larger preterm birth prevention program, 823 patients were identified as being at risk for preterm birth by a high-risk pregnancy scoring system. The drug used was Provera (medroxyprogesterone acetate), and 411 patients were assigned to take 20 mg/day orally. The control group of 412 patients was given placebo tablets. The allocation to drug or placebo was on the basis of the particular prenatal clinic that the patient attended. The subjects were enrolled prior to 31 weeks' gestation. The outcome of interest was delivery at less than 37 weeks. The rate of preterm delivery in the treatment group was 11.2%, compared with 7.3% in the placebo group. The rate of compliance for the subjects was low, with only 55% of the patients assigned to the Provera group actually taking the drug. This remains the only large trial of an oral progestational agent to prevent preterm birth.

Two large trials have been reported on the use of progestogens to prevent preterm birth. In 2003, Fonseca *et al* reported the results of a randomized, placebo-controlled trial of vaginal progesterone suppositories in 142 women [51]. The subjects were selected as being at high risk for preterm birth. The risk factor in over 90% of the subjects was that of a previous preterm delivery. The patients were randomly assigned to daily insertion of either a 100 mg progesterone suppository or a placebo suppository. The treatment period was 24–34 weeks' gestation. All patients were monitored for uterine contractions once weekly for 1 h with an external tocodynamometer. Although 81 progesterone and 76 placebo patients were entered into the study, several patients were excluded from analysis because of PPROM or were lost to follow-up, leaving 72 progesterone and 70 placebo subjects. The rate of preterm delivery at less than 37 weeks in the progesterone patients was 13.8%, significantly less than the rate in the placebo patients of 28.5%. The rate of preterm delivery at less than 34 weeks in the treatment group was 2.8% compared to 18.6% in the placebo group. These differences were statistically significant. The rate of uterine contractions measured by the weekly hour-long recording was significantly less at 28–34 weeks in the progesterone patients compared to the placebo patients. Analysis of the results by intent to treat showed smaller differences between the groups but these differences remained statistically significant [56].

Meis *et al* reported the results of a large multicenter trial of 17P conducted by the Maternal Fetal Medicine Units (MFMU) Network of the National Institute of Child Health and Human Development [52]. The study enrolled women with a documented history of a previous spontaneous preterm delivery, which occurred as a consequence of either spontaneous preterm labor or PPROM. After receiving an ultrasound examination to rule out major fetal anomalies and determine gestational age, the subjects were offered the study and given a test dose of the placebo injection to assess compliance. If they chose to continue, they were randomly assigned, using a 2:1 ratio, to weekly injections of 250 mg 17P or a placebo injection. Treatment was begun at 16–20 weeks' gestation and was continued until delivery or 37 weeks' gestation, whichever came first. The study planned to enroll 500 subjects, a sample size estimated to be sufficient to detect a 37%

reduction in the rate of preterm birth. However, enrollment was halted at 463 subjects, 310 in the treatment group and 153 in the placebo group, following a scheduled evaluation by the Data Safety and Monitoring Committee, which found that the evidence of efficacy for the primary outcome was such that further entry of patients was unnecessary.

In this study, delivery at less than 37 weeks was reduced from 54.9% in the placebo group to 36.3% in the treatment group. Similar reductions were seen in delivery at less than 35 weeks, from 30.7% to 20.6%, and in delivery at less than 32 weeks, from 19.6% to 11.4%. All these differences were statistically significant. Rates of birthweight less than 2500 g were significantly reduced, as were rates of intraventricular hemorrhage, necrotizing enterocolitis, and need for supplemental oxygen and ventilatory support. Rates of neonatal death were reduced from 5.9% in the placebo group to 2.6% in the treatment group, although this difference did not reach statistical significance.

The women enrolled in this study had unusually high rates of preterm birth. This could be explained in part by the fact that the mean gestational age of their previous preterm delivery was quite early, at 31 weeks. In addition, one-third of the women had had more than one previous spontaneous preterm delivery. Despite random allocation, more women in the placebo group had had more than one preterm delivery. Adjustment of the analysis controlling for the imbalance found that the treatment effect remained significantly different from that of the placebo. A majority of the women were of African-American ethnicity and the treatment with 17P showed equal efficacy in the African-American women and in the non-African-American subjects.

The results of the MFMU trial of 17P in women with a prior spontaneous preterm delivery stimulated other trials of 17P or vaginal progesterone for women with other high-risk conditions. Several trials of 17P or vaginal progesterone in women with twins or triplets have found disappointing results, with no improvement in any pregnancy outcome [57–60]. Unfortunately, no current treatment has shown any effectiveness in reducing the rate of preterm delivery in women with multiple gestation.

A large multicenter trial of progesterone vaginal gel treatment for women with a prior preterm delivery at less than 35 weeks' gestation was conducted at 53 medical centers [61]. Sponsored by Columbia Labs, 659 subjects were randomly assigned to daily application of progesterone gel or placebo gel. The results were disappointing, as no improvement in rates of preterm birth or neonatal outcome was found in the group treated with the progesterone gel.

In 2005, Sanchez-Ramos *et al* published a meta-analysis of trials of progestational agents to prevent preterm births [62]. They included the two recent trials in a total of 10 trials that met the search criteria. The analysis found that "compared with women randomized to the placebo, those who received progestational agents had lower rates of preterm delivery" (26.2% versus 35.9%, OR 0.45, 95% CI 0.25–0.80). The comparison of rates of perinatal mortality did not reach a statistically significant difference (OR 0.69, 95% CI 0.38–1.26). Petrini *et al* reported an interesting analysis of the potential impact of 17P treatment of women at risk for recurrent preterm delivery [63]. Their calculations assumed a 33% reduction of preterm births (based on the results of the MFMU Network trial). By their calculations, if all women at risk for recurrent preterm delivery in the USA were treated with 17P, 10,000 spontaneous preterm births would be prevented. However, the overall rate of preterm birth in the USA would be reduced only from 12.1% (in 2005) to 11.8%.

Although no evidence has been reported that progesterone treatment during pregnancy could have harmful effects on the fetus and subsequent child, a recent study provides further evidence of the safety of progesterone treatment. Northen *et al* evaluated 278 children born to women in the MFMU 17P trial [64]. The children were evaluated at about age 4 using an Ages to Stages questionnaire, a physical examination and gender-specific play scores. No difference was found in health status between the 17P-treated and placebo-treated children.

In summary, progesterone treatment has been demonstrated to be an effective reproducible treatment to reduce the rate of preterm delivery in a select group of women (those with a prior spontaneous preterm delivery). Whether this treatment is effective for other groups of high-risk pregnant women must await the results of further randomized trials. It is important to realize that most preterm births in the USA occur to women with no identified risk factors. Large reductions in the rate of preterm birth in the USA will likely depend on policies or treatments that can apply to the broad population of pregnant women.

CASE PRESENTATION

The patient was a 25-year-old, gravida 2, para 1, whose previous pregnancy was delivered following spontaneous preterm rupture of the fetal membranes at 25 weeks followed by subsequent labor and delivery of a 625 g infant. The child survived but has been diagnosed with spastic quadriplegia form of cerebral palsy. The patient presented for prenatal care at 12 weeks. Physical examination was unremarkable. At 16 weeks, ultrasonography revealed a 16-week gestation with no obvious fetal anomalies and transvaginal sonography measured the cervix at 3.5 cm.

The patient was started on weekly injections of 250 mg 17P. The prenatal course was unremarkable until 33w 6d when preterm labor contractions began. On admission to labor and delivery, the cervix was fully effaced and 3–4 cm dilated. Tocolysis with magnesium sulfate was started and the patient was given betamethasone, which was repeated at 24 h. At 36 h after admission, uterine contrac-

tions recurred despite the tocolytic treatment and the patient was delivered of a 2300 g infant at 34 weeks' gestation. Apgar scores were 8 and 9 at 1 and 5 min, respectively. The infant required no ventilatory support in the nursery and mother and infant were discharged home on day 3.

Treatment of this patient with 17P was appropriate as the history of delivery following PPROM is included in the criteria of a prior spontaneous preterm delivery. Tocolysis initially halted labor and allowed time for steroid therapy with betamethasone. However, tocolysis was only effective for a short period, and preterm labor resumed. Treatment with 17P was effective in prolonging the pregnancy compared with the previous delivery, and the birth outcome was excellent. Treatment with 17P is especially effective for women with a history of a very early preterm delivery, but the treatment does not guarantee carrying the pregnancy to term in every case.

References

1. Meis PJ. Indicated preterm births: a review. Perinat Neonat Med 1998;3:113–115.
2. Klebanoff M. Conceptualizing categories of preterm birth. Prenat Neonat Med 1998;3:13–15.
3. National Center for Health Statistics, final natality data 2008. http://www.nchs.gov/
4. Paneth NS. The problem of low birth weight. Future Child 1995;5:19–34.
5. Agency for Healthcare Research and Quality. Overview of the HCUP National Inpatient Sample 2005. http://www.ahrq.gov/.
6. National Centre for Health Statistics Final Natality Data. www.marchofdimes.com/peristats.
7. Families USA. How will association health plans affect minority health? www.familiesusa.org.
8. Miller CA. Maternal Health and Infant Survival. Washington, DC: National Center for Clinical Infant Programs, 1987.
9. Creasy RK. Preventing preterm birth. N Engl J Med 1991; 325:727–728.

10. Rouse DJ, Hirtz DG, Thom E et al. A randomized controlled trial of magnesium sulfate for the prevention of cerebral palsy. N Engl J Med 2008;359:895.

11. Papiernik E, Goffinet F. Prevention of preterm births, the French experience. Clin Obstet Gynecol 2004;47:755–767.

12. Breart G, Blondel B, Tuppin P et al. Did preterm deliveries continue to decrease in France in the 1980s? Paediatr Perinat Epidemiol 1995;9:296–356.

13. Zeitlin J, Bucort M, Rivera L et al. Preterm birth and maternal country of birth in a French district with a multiethnic population. Br J Obstet Gynaecol 2004;111:849–855.

14. Collaborative Group on Preterm Birth Prevention. Multi-centered randomized, controlled trial of a preterm birth prevention program. Am J Obstet Gynecol 1993;169:352–366.

15. Moore ML, Meis PJ, Ernest JM et al. A randomized trial of nurse intervention to reduce preterm and low birth weight births. Obset Gynecol 1998;91:656.

16. Villar J, Farnot U, Barros F et al. A randomized trial of psycho-social support during high risk pregnancies. N Engl J Med 1992;327:1266.

17. Ayman AE, El-Mohandes, Kiely M et al. Am intervention to reduce environmental tobacco smoke exposure improves pregnancy outcomes. Pediatrics 2010;175:721.

18. Mueller-Heubach E, Rubinstein DN, Schwarz SS. Histologic chorioamnionitis and preterm delivery in different patient populations. Obstet Gynecol 1990;75:622–626.

19. Meis PJ, Goldenberg RL, Mercer B et al. The preterm prediction study: significance of vaginal infections. Am J Obstet Gynecol 1995;173:1231–1235.

20. Offenbacher S, Katz V, Fertik G et al. Periodontal infection as a possible risk factor for preterm low birthweight. J Periodontal 1996;67(Suppl 10):1103–1113.

21. Romero R, Sirtori M, Oyarzun E et al. Infection and labor. V. Prevalence, microbiology, and clinical significance of intramniotic infection in women with preterm labor and intact membranes. Am J Obstet Gynecol 1989;161:817–824.

22. Romero R, Sibai B, Caritis S et al. Antibiotic treatment of preterm labor with intact membranes: a multicenter, randomized, double-blinded, placebo-controlled trial. Am J Obstet Gynecol 1993;169:764–774.

23. Klebanoff MA, Carey JC, Hauth JC et al. Failure of metronidazole to prevent preterm delivery in women with asymptomatic Trichomonas vaginalis infection. N Engl J Med 2001;345:487–493.

24. Carey JC, Klebanoff MA, Hauth JC et al. Metronidazole to prevent preterm delivery in pregnant women with asymptomatic bacterial vaginosis. N Engl J Med 2000;342:534–540.

25. Jeffcoat MK, Hauth JC, Geurs NC et al. Periodontal disease and preterm birth: results of a pilot intervention study. J Periodontol 2003;74:1214–1218.

26. Andrews WW, Sibai B, Thom EA et al. Randomized clinical trial of metronidazole plus erythromycin to prevent spontaneous preterm delivery in fetal fibronectin-positive women. Obstet Gynecol 2003;101:847–855.

27. Andrews WW, Goldenberg, RL, Hauth JC et al. Interconceptional antibiotics to prevent spontaneous preterm birtrh: a randomized clinical trial. Am J Obstet Gynecol 2006;194:217.

28. Michalowicz BS, Hodges JS, DiAngelis AJ et al. Treatment of periodontal disease and the risk of preterm birth. N Engl J Med 2006;355:1885.

29. Macones GA, Perry S, Nelson DB et al. Treatment of localized periodontal disease in pregnancy does not reduce the occcurence of preterm birth: results from the Periodontal Infections and Premturity Study. Am J Obstet Gynecol 2010;202:147.

30. Mercer BM, Miodovnik M, Thurnau GR et al. Antibiotic therapy for reduction of infant morbidity after preterm premature rupture of the membranes: a randomized controlled trial. National Institute of Child Health and Human Development Maternal-Fetal Medicine Units Network. JAMA 1997;278:989–995.

31. Olsen SF, Osterdal ML, Salvig JD et al. Duration of pregnancy in relation to fish oil supplementation and habitual fish intake: a randomized clinical trial with fish oil. Eur J Clin Nutr 2007;61:976.

32. Harper M, Thom E, Klebanoff MA et al. Omega-3 fatty acid supplementation to prevent recurrent preterm birth, a randomized controlled trial. Obstet Gynecol 2010;115:234L.

33. Shirodkar VN. A new method of operative treatment for habitual abortion in the second trimester of pregnancy. Antiseptic 1955;52:299.

34. American College of Obstetricians and Gynecologists. Cervical insufficiency. Practice Bulletin No. 48. Obstet Gynecol 2003;102:1091–1099.

35. Iams JD. Abnormal cervical competence. In: Creasy RK, Resnick R, Iams JD, eds. Maternal-Fetal Medicine: Principles and Practice, 5th edn. Philadelphia: WB Saunders, 2004, pp.603–622.

36. American College of Radiology. ACR Appropriateness Criteria: Expert Panel on Women's Imaging. Premature Cervical Dilatation. Reston, VA: American College of Radiology, 1999. www.acr.org.

37. American College of Obstetricians and Gynecologists Committee on Quality Assessment. Criteria Set 18. Washington, DC: American College of Obstetricians and Gynecologists, 1996.

38. Grant A. Cervical cerclage to prolong pregnancy. In: Chalmers I, Enkin M, Keirse M, eds. Effective Care in Pregnancy and Childbirth. Oxford: Oxford University Press, 1989, pp.633–644.

39. MRC/RCOG Working Party on Cervical Cerclage. Interim report of the Medical Research Council/Royal College of Obstetricians and Gynaecologist multicentre randomized trial of cervical cerclage. Br J Obstet Gynaecol 1988;95:437–455.

40. Rush RW, Isaacs S, McPherson K et al. A randomized controlled trial of cervical cerclage in women at high risk of spontaneous preterm delivery. Br J Obstet Gynaecol 1984;91:724–730.

41. Althuisius SM, Decker GA, Hummel P et al. Final results of the Cervical Incompetence Prevention Randomized Cerclage Trial (CIPRACT): therapeutic cerclage with bed rest versus bed rest alone. Am J Obstet Gynecol 2001;185:1106–1112.

42. Berghella V, Odibo AO, Tolosa JE. Cerclage for prevention of preterm birth in women with a short cervix found on transvaginal ultrasound examination: a randomized trial. Am J Obstet Gynecol 2004;191:1311–1317.

43. To MS, Alfirevic Z, Heath VCF et al. Cervical cerclage for prevention of preterm delivery in women with short cervix: randomized controlled trial. Lancet 2004;363:1849–1853.

44. Berghella V, Odibo AO, To MS, Rust OA, Althuisius SM. Cerclage for short cervix on untrasonography. Obstet Gynecol 2005;106:181–189.

45. Owen J, Hankins G, Iams JD et al. Muticenter randomized trial of cerclage for preterm birth prevention in high-risk women with shortened midtrimester cervical length. Am J Obstet Gynecol 2009; 201:375.

46. Berghella V, Figueroa D, Szychowski JM et al. 17 alpha hydroxyprogesterone caproate for the prevention of preterm birth in women with prior preterm birth and a short cervical length. Am J Obstet Gynecol 2010;202:351.

47. Fonseca E, Celik E, Parra M et al. Progesterone and the risk of preterm birth among women with a short cervix. N Engl J Med 2007;357:5.

48. DeFranco EA, O'Brien JM, Adair CD et al. Vaginal progesterone is associated with a decrease in risk for early preterm birth and improved neonatal outcome in women with a short cervix: a secondary analysis from a randomized, double-blind, placebo-controlled trial. Ultrasound Obstet Gynecol 2007;30:697.

49. Papiernik E. Double blind study of an agent to prevent preterm delivery among women at increased risk. In: Edition Schering, Serie IV, fiche 3. 1970, pp.65–68.

50. American College of Obstetricians and Gynecologists. Use of progesterone to reduce preterm birth. Committee Opinion No. 419. Obstet Gynecol 2003;112:963.

51. Fonseca EB, Bittar RE, Carvalho MHB et al. Prophylactic administration of progesterone by vaginal suppository to reduce the incidence of spontaneous preterm birth in women at increased risk: a randomized placebo-controlled double-blind study. Am J Obstet Gynecol 2003;188:419–424.

52. Meis PJ, Klebanoff M, Thom E et al. Prevention of recurrent preterm delivery by 17 alpha-hydroxyprogesterone caproate. N Engl J Med 2003;348:2379–2385.

53. Goldstein P, Berrier J, Rosen S et al. A meta-analysis of randomized control trials of progestational agents in pregnancy. Br J Obstet Gynaecol 1989;96:265–274.

54. Keirse MJNC. Progesterone administration in pregnancy may prevent pre-term delivery. Br J Obstet Gynaecol 1990;97: 149–154.

55. Hobel CJ, Ross MG, Bemis RL et al. The West Los Angeles Preterm Birth Prevention Project. I. Program impact on high-risk women. Am J Obstet Gynecol 1994;170:54–62.

56. Fonseca EB. Progesterone and preterm birth [Letter reply]. Am J Obstet Gynecol 2004;190:1803–1804.

57. Hartikainen-Sorri A, Kauppila A, Tuimala R. Inefficacy of 17 alpha-hydroxyprogesterone caproate in the prevention of prematurity in twin pregnancy. Obstet Gynecol 1980;56:692.

58. Caritis S, Rouse D. A randomized trial of 17-hydroxyprogesterone caproate (17OHP) for the prevention of preterm birth in twins. Am J Obstet Gynecol 2006;195:S2.

59. Briery CM, Veillon EW, Klauser CK et al. Progesterone dies not prevent prterm births in women with twins. South Med J 2009;102:900.

60. Rouse DJ, Caritis SN, Peaceman AM et al. A trial of 17 alpha-hydroxyprogesterone caproate to prevent prematurity in twins. N Engl J Med 2007;357:454.

61. O'Brien JM, Adair CD, Lewis DF et al. Progesterone vaginal gel for the reduction of recurrent preterm birth: primary results from a randomized, double-blind, placebo-controlled trial. Ultrasound Obstet Gynecol 2007;30:687.

62. Sanchez-Ramos L, Kaunitz AM, Delke I. Progestational agents to prevent preterm birth: a meta-analysis of randomized controlled trials. Obstet Gynecol 2005;105:273–279.

63. Petrini JR, Callaghan WM, Klebanoff M et al. Estimated effect of 17 alpha-hydroxyprogesterone caproate on preterm birth in the United States. Obstet Gynecol 2005;105:267–272.

64. Northen AT, Norman GS, Anderson K et al. Follow-up of children exposed in utero to 17 alpha-hydroxyprogesterone caproate compared with placebo. Obstet Gynecol 2007;110: 865.

Chapter 42
Pathogenesis and Prediction of Preterm Delivery

Catalin S. Buhimschi and Charles J. Lockwood

Department of Obstetrics, Gynecology and Reproductive Sciences, Yale University School of Medicine, New Haven, CT, USA

Preterm delivery (PTD) is defined as a birth before 37 weeks' gestation. The percentage of births occurring preterm in the US has recently declined after many years of sustained increases, and was 12.3% in 2008 [1]. The decline in preterm births for 2007–2008 was mostly among infants born at 34–36 weeks (late preterm). Specifically, the rate of prematurity for this category decreased from 9.14% in 2006 to 8.77% in 2008. The percentage of infants born at less than 34 weeks also dropped, albeit more modestly, from 3.63% to 3.56%. Declines were registered for almost all age, race, and ethnic categories. Compared to 2007, in 2008 there was a decrease in preterm birth of 4% for non-Hispanic white (11.5% to 11.1%), 6% for non-Hispanic black (18.3% to 17.5%) and 2% for Hispanic infants (12.3% to 12.1%) [1]. Unfortunately, the percentage of infants delivered at very low birthweight (less than 1500 g) has only declined minimally for 2007–2008, from 1.48% to 1.46%, respectively. The medical relevance of this observation is that it is these newborns who are at the highest risk of early death or disability. Moreover, the overall rate of prematurity continues to represent a relative increase of nearly 20% from 1990 levels.

For the last two decades much of the increase in prematurity has been attributed to the epidemic of multifetal gestations and to generally later PTDs deemed necessary due to deteriorating maternal or fetal health [2].

Etiology and pathogenesis of spontaneous preterm delivery

Proximate causes of PTD include medically indicated PTDs (18.7–35.2% of cases) and spontaneous PTDs resulting from either preterm labor (PTL) with intact fetal membranes (23.2–64.1%) or preterm premature rupture of membranes (PPROM) (7.1–51.2%) [3]. There is compelling evidence to suggest that spontaneous PTD involves multiple underlying pathogenic pathways and etiologic factors [4–6]. At least four distinct pathways have been defined: maternal/fetal stress, decidual-amnion-chorion inflammation, decidual hemorrhage, and excessive myometrial stretching [7]. Increasingly inherited variations, primarily in inflammatory cytokine and proteolytic pathway genes, have been described which predispose to PTD [8].

Regrettably, because of the large number of pathways leading to prematurity and complex interactions among putative effectors, no single genetic factor accounts for more than a fraction of PTD cases. However, regardless of the initial pathogenic and etiologic stimulus and genetic predisposition, all spontaneous PTDs utilize a common final biochemical pathway characterized by increased genital tract inflammation, enhanced prostaglandin (PG) and protease production in the cervix, decidua, myometrium, and fetal membranes coupled with alterations in progesterone receptor (PR) levels or the relative expression of PR isoforms in the cervix, decidua, and myometrium that together lead to a functional progesterone withdrawal [9–11]. This final common pathway is employed by each of the main four major pathogenic pathways as well as minor pathways (e.g. allergies).

Maternal and/or fetal stress: premature activation of the placental–fetal hypothalamic–pituitary–adrenal axis

Human parturition involves complex maternal, fetal, and placental interactions. Stress can be a common element activating a series of physiologic adaptive responses in each of these compartments [12]. Periconceptional maternal stress and anxiety are associated with modestly increased rates of spontaneous PTD with odds ratios (ORs) of 1.16 (95% confidence interval [CI]1.05–1.29) [13]. Recent data derived from registry-linked births to mothers with posttraumatic stress disorder noted higher odds of PTD (adjusted OR 2.48, 95% CI 1.05–5.84) [14]. Depression

Queenan's Management of High-Risk Pregnancy: An Evidence-Based Approach, Sixth Edition. Edited by John T. Queenan, Catherine Y. Spong, Charles J. Lockwood.
© 2012 John Wiley & Sons, Ltd. Published 2012 by John Wiley & Sons, Ltd.

among women of African descent is associated with an adjusted OR for PTD of 1.96 (95% CI 1.04–3.72) [15]. What can be concluded from the existing body of literature is that during pregnancy, women with depression are at increased risk for PTD, although the magnitude of the effect varies as a function of the method of ascertainment of depression and socio-economic status [16]. Interestingly, placental pathologic changes consistent with infection and ischemia-induced fetal stress are 3–7 times more common in patients with spontaneous PTD compared with term controls [17,18]. Both elevated maternal stress and aberrant placentation are more common with first pregnancies. In addition, there appears to be a genetic predisposition to both maternal mood disorders [19] and impaired placentation [20].

Corticotropin-releasing hormone (CRH), a 41-amino acid peptide initially discovered in the hypothalamus but also expressed by placental, chorionic, amnionic, and decidual cells, appears to be the mediator of stress-associated PTDs [21]. In uncomplicated (physiologic) pregnancies maternal plasma free CRH concentrations, which are almost entirely placental derived, rise during the second half of pregnancy and peak during labor [22]. The CRH concentration curve across gestation in women with subsequent PTD runs parallel to the CRH curve of normal pregnancy, but the absolute CRH level for a given week of gestation is displaced significantly upward and to the left [23]. In contrast to the hypothalamus, where glucocorticoids inhibit CRH release, cortisol enhances placental production of CRH [24]. This positive feed-forward system is a unique biologic feature causing progressive increases in placental CRH production as pregnancy advances to term. Both maternal and fetal stress (i.e. fetal growth restriction) are associated with elevated maternal and/or fetal cortisol levels [25–27].

Lockwood and colleagues [28] examined paired maternal and fetal hypothalamic–pituitary–adrenal (HPA) axis hormone levels in patients undergoing cordocentesis across the second half of gestation and noted that placental-derived maternal serum CRH values correlated best with fetal cortisol (r = 0.40, P = 0.0002) but also modestly correlated with maternal cortisol levels (r = 0.28, P = 0.01). Thus, rising maternal and/or fetal cortisol levels likely establish a positive feedback loop, i.e. placental-derived CRH stimulates the release of fetal pituitary adrenocorticotropin (ACTH) to enhance fetal adrenal cortisol production which further stimulates placental CRH release [28].

Despite the above evidence, it is unclear whether precocious elevation of plasma CRH levels is an epiphenomenon rather than a trigger for PTD mechanisms [29]. For example, there is evidence for a myometrial relaxing effect of CRH, favoring uterine quiescence, in contrast to its indirect uterotonic effect documented *in vitro* and its increased bio-availability at term [30].

The output of prostaglandins (PGs) $F_{2\alpha}$ and/or E_2 is increased by CRH in cultured amnionic, chorionic, decidual, and placental cells [31,32]. Both $PGF_{2\alpha}$ and/or E_2 bind to uterotonic receptors, F-prostanoid, and EP-1/3, respectively, in the fundus and corpus of the uterus to mediate calcium flux which triggers effective contractions and to increase myometrial expression of oxytocin receptor, connexin 43 (gap junctions), and cyclooxygenase (COX)-2 [33–36]. In turn, the latter generates additional PGs. Together, these data suggest that a functional increase in myometrial CRH signaling may lead to activation of uterine contractility and labor. In addition, CRH-induced PG synthesis can promote preterm premature rupture of the membranes (PROM) and cervical change by enhancing the synthesis of matrix metalloproteinases (MMPs) in the fetal membranes and cervix [34,37]. Moreover, PGs increase cervical expression of interleukin (IL)-8 which recruits and activates neutrophils, releasing additional MMPs and elastases which can promote cervical extracellular matrix (ECM) dissolution and weakening of the fetal membranes [38].

Finally, both PGE_2 and $PGF_{2\alpha}$ have been reported to increase the PR-A isoform and decrease the PR-B isoform in myometrium, cervix, and decidua [39–41]. Because PR-A antagonizes the classic PR-mediated genomic effects of PR-B, PGs appear to induce a functional progesterone withdrawal. Merlino *et al* have reported that in contrast to the intense nuclear PR mRNAs and proteins expression observed in decidual cells, PR expression is barely detectable in amnion and chorion [42]. The authors suggest that decidual cells, and not amnion and chorion cells, are the direct target of progesterone during human pregnancy.

At term, cortisol released into the amniotic fluid can directly stimulate fetal membrane PG production by increasing amnionic COX-2 expression and inhibiting the chorionic PG metabolizing enzyme, 15-hydroxy-prostaglandin dehydrogenase (PGDH) [43,44]. This suggests that a local amniotic fluid positive feedback loop exists to tie fetal HPA axis maturation to parturition which is likely operational in stress-induced PTD.

With the development of the fetal adrenal zone of the fetal adrenal after 28–30 weeks' gestation, stress-associated activation of the placental–fetal HPA axis also mediates PTD by enhancing placental estrogen production. This is because increased fetal adrenal zone production of dehydroepiandrosterone sulfate (DHEAS) accompanies ACTH-induced fetal adrenal cortisol production. In addition, CRH can directly augment fetal adrenal DHEAS production [45]. Placental sulfatases cleave the sulfate conjugates of DHEAS and its 16-hydroxy hepatic derivative, allowing their conversion to estradiol (E2) and estrone (E1), as well as estriol (E3), respectively. These estrogens increase myometrial expression of contraction-associated proteins such as oxytocin receptor and connexion-43 [46,47]. Because reductions in PR-B expression lead to increased expression of the active form of the estrogen receptor-β (ER-β), rising placental estrogen production would be matched to PG-induced increases in myometrial ER-β expression [31,48].

As shown above, compelling data suggest that the fetus actively participates in controlling the timing of labor, via production of adrenal hormonal precursors [49]. This premise is also supported by the evidence that at term, prior to the onset of labor, the weight and volume of the fetal adrenal gland equal those of the adult [50]. Interestingly, a recent study showed that in the setting of intraamniotic inflammation, the fetal cortisol-to-DHEAS ratio was low, with no direct correlation between the adrenal gland volume and either cortisol or DHEAS [51]. This suggests that infection-mediated PTD may act via a different pathway (see below).

Decidual-amnion-chorion inflammation

Inflammation is a highly orchestrated process designed to assure survivability of the host [52]. When properly controlled, the inflammatory response is beneficial but when dysregulated, it becomes harmful [53]. There is consensus that the balance between the expression of pro- and antiinflammatory molecules determines the magnitude of the damage [54].

Systemic inflammation resulting from pneumonia, sepsis, pancreatitis, acute cholecystitis, pyleonephritis, and asymptomatic bacteriuria as well as genital tract inflammatory states such as deciduitis, chorioamnionitis, and intraamniotic infections are all associated with PTD [55–60]. Results of several recent hypothesis-driven studies have indicated that periodontal infection and subsequent systemic inflammation may be implicated in triggering PTD [61,62]. Unfortunately, intervention studies have generally not demonstrated a benefit to treatment [63] although possible beneficial effects of periodontal treatment may be dependent on time of initiation and success of therapy [64].

Genital tract inflammation is recognized as the most common antecedent of very early PTDs, accounting for more than half of cases [58,59]. Bacterial vaginosis (BV) is the most common lower genital tract microbial-related syndrome among women of reproductive age [65]. Studies of the efficacy of screening and treating asymptomatic and symptomatic women at high risk for PTD are conflicting. Specifically, multiple prospective cohort studies have established a modest association between BV and an increased risk of spontaneous PTD (OR 1.4–2.2), with the strongest association noted for BV detected at less than 16 weeks (OR 7.55, 95% CI 1.80–31.65) [66–68]. The occurrence of BV facilitates overgrowth of upper genital tract facultative bacteria such as Mycoplasma species and Gardnerella vaginalis, gram-negative bacteria such as Escherichia coli, and gram-positive cocci [64,69], as well as urinary tract colonization and infections [70].

In turn, several studies report that asymptomatic bacteriuria and vaginal E. coli colonization are linked to a twofold increase in PTD [71–73].

The mechanism by which BV affects PTD risk remains unknown. Experimental studies lend support to the concept that BV is responsible for inflammatory changes in the genital tract, and antibiotic treatment can reverse this trend [74,75]. However, a recent report from the US Preventive Services Task Force concluded that there is no evidence to support screening or treating low-risk pregnant women asymptomatic for BV [76]. A subgroup of high-risk women may still benefit from BV screening and treatment. However, there may also be a subgroup for which BV treatment with metronidazole could increase the occurrence of PTD [77].

In multicellular organisms, two complementary inflammatory networks have been described: the innate and the adaptive immune systems. Innate immunity is an evolutionarily preserved defense mechanism, designed to provide the first line of resistance against exogenous and endogenous pathogens. Genetically programmed "modules" of the innate immune system respond rapidly, nonspecifically and without memory to pathogens [78,79]. The best characterized inflammatory response is that elicited by microbial pathogens which are triggering a vast array of transcriptional events following engagement of Toll-like receptors (TLRs). The TLRs are trans-membrane receptors that participate in host defense mechanisms through engagement of pathogen-associated molecular patterns (PAMPs) [80]. Owing to their strategic positioning at the maternal/fetal interface and cervical mucosa, TLRs are considered key operative agents of the host response to infection. For example, gram-negative bacteria-derived endotoxins bind to cervical and fetal membrane TLR-4 and gram-positive bacteria-derived exotoxins bind to TLR-2 on decidual cells and leukocytes to elicit production of tumor necrosis factor-α (TNF-α) and IL-1β [81–83]. In turn, TNF-α, IL-1β, and/or endotoxins such as lipopolysaccharide (LPS) induce expression of the transcription factor NFκB, which enhances MMP-1, 3, and 9 as well as COX-2 expression while promoting apoptosis in amnion epithelial cells. These chains of events underline the central role of inflammation in promoting ECM remodeling processes linked to PPROM and to early cervical ripening and dilation [84–93].

It was shown that PGDH activity and PGDH mRNA were significantly lower in membranes of women with infection-induced chorioamnionitis compared to women with idiopathic PTD or at term [86]. This NFκB-mediated effect may allow passage of the unmetabolized PG to the decidua and myometrium, and contribute to premature activation of myometrial contractility and PTD. In addition, TNF-α, IL-1β, and endotoxin stimulate IL-6 production in amniochorion and decidua [94,95], which further augments amnionic and decidual PG production [96]. Using specific inhibitors of NFκB activation, Lockwood et al were able to demonstrate that inhibition of IL-1β enhanced IL-6 expression levels in cultured decidual cells [97]. Finally, TNF-α and IL-1β induce IL-8 production in the fetal membranes, decidua, and cervix, effects that are potentiated by IL-6 [93,98]. Given that IL-8 causes recruitment and activation of neutrophils that release additional MMPs and elastases, it further exacerbates the PTD-enhancing effects of genital tract inflammation.

Recently, it was proven that the biologic activity of the TLRs is dependent not only on the presence of bacterial PAMPs but also on a palette of intracellular signaling adaptors (e.g. MyD88) and co-receptor molecules (e.g. CD14) that associate with TLRs in complex supramolecular arrangements [99]. Equally important is that TLR signaling can be elicited by endogenous damage-associated molecular pattern molecules (DAMPs) [100]. Owing to their similarity to cytokines and their release by activated or damaged cells under inflammatory conditions, DAMPs are endogenous proinflammatory molecules. Acting through TLR2, TLR4, and the receptor for advanced glycation end-products (RAGE), DAMPs recruit inflammatory cells, which in turn amplify innate immune responses and enhance levels of cytokine activation [98]. Buhimschi et al reported that the DAMP-RAGE system is present in women with PTD and intraamniotic infection and its activation correlates with the degree of inflammation in amnion epithelial, decidual, and extravillous trophoblast cells [101]. Lastly, the roles of soluble receptor modulators (soluble TLR2, soluble TNF receptor-1, soluble IL-6 receptor, soluble gp130 and soluble RAGE) in fine-tuning human TLR-mediated signaling have just begun to be elucidated [102–105].

Culture-based approaches suggest that the most common microorganisms identified in the fetal membranes and amniotic fluid of patients with inflammation-associated PTD are Ureaplasma urealyticum, Mycoplasma hominis, Gardnerella vaginalis, and Bacteroides species, relatively weak pathogens [106–108]. Moreover, 16S rRNA-based culture-independent methods suggest that the diversity of the amniotic fluid microbiome is far greater than what was once believed [109]. As most cultivated and uncultivated organisms are generally of low virulence, it has been posited that a genetically determined exaggerated maternal and/or fetal inflammatory response rather than the presence of microorganisms per se triggers PTD. Indeed, the 15% recurrence risk of PTD coupled with its predilection for certain families and concordance in twins are consistent with a genetic link [110–113]. The availability of a reference sequence of the genome provides the basis for studying the nature of sequence variation, particularly single nucleotide polymorphisms (SNPs), in human populations [114]. The T2 allele of the TNF-α gene causes increased expression of

TNF-α and confers an increased risk of PPROM in African-American women [115]. Moreover, African-American mothers harboring both this polymorphism and BV are at even greater risk of PTD (OR 6.1, 95% CI 1.9–21.0) [116], suggesting that gene–environment interactions are important contributors to inflammation-associated PTD. Conversely, concurrent carriage of TNF(–308A) and IL-6(–174C) alleles which reduce inflammation may decrease the risk of PTD in women with BV [114,117]. Lorenz et al [118] observed an increased frequency of two (Asp299Gly and Thr399Ile) polymorphisms for TLR-4, the major endotoxin-signaling receptor, in a population of white infants delivering preterm. Other examples of gene–environment interactions in PTD have been observed, including polymorphisms in drug-metabolizing genes, CYP1A1 HincII RFLP and GSTT1, that shorten gestation among Chinese women exposed to benzene [119] and US women exposed to cigarette smoke [120].

Fetal genotypes may also have a role in the genesis of inflammation-associated PTD. The presence of a fetal MMP-1 mutation has been found to increase the risk of PPROM in African-American fetuses, suggesting that genetic influences on fetal membrane structural integrity contribute to PPROM [121]. Similarly, a 14 CA-repeat allele in the MMP-9 gene enhances transcription and is more common in African-American neonates whose mothers had experienced PPROM [122]. Homozygosity for the IL-1β 3953 allele 1 in African-American fetuses is associated with an increased risk of PTD while Hispanic fetuses carrying the IL-1RN allele 2 have an increased risk for PPROM (OR 6.5, 95% CI 1.25–37.7) [123]. These findings help account for disparate ethnic and racial patterns in PTD rates and may also identify subsets of women who would benefit from targeted interventions based on specific genetic markers.

Abruption-associated preterm delivery

Decidual hemorrhage (placental abruption) originates in damaged spiral arteries or arterioles and presents clinically as vaginal bleeding or either a retroplacental or retrochorionic hematoma formation noted on ultrasound. The incidence ranges from 0.5% to 2% depending on the clinical definition and criteria used to characterize abruption intensity [124]. Abruption-associated PTDs are more common in older, white, married, parous, college-educated patients presenting a demographic profile distinct from that associated with patients with stress-induced PTDs (nulliparous, anxious, or depressed patients) or inflammation-associated PTDs (young, minority, poor socio-economic status) [125]. Large prospective studies reported that vaginal bleeding during the first half of pregnancy increases the relative risk of spontaneous PTD (relative risk 1.4, 95% CI 1.2–1.5), PPROM (relative risk 2.1, 95% CI 1.2–2.3) and placental abruption (relative risk

1.1, 95% CI 1.01–1.2) [126]. When vaginal bleeding occurs in more than one trimester, it is associated with a nearly 50% risk of PPROM (OR 7.4, 95% CI 2.2–25.6) [127]. That inherited or acquired thrombophilias are associated with adverse pregnancy outcomes such as placental abruption is controversial [128–130]. Thus, testing for inherited thrombophilias in women who have experienced placental abruption is not recommended [128].

The key histologic finding in placental abruption is hemorrhage in the decidua basalis. Decidual hemosiderin deposition and retrochorionic hematoma formation is present in 38% of patients with PTD between 22 and 32 weeks' gestation resulting from PPROM and 36% of patients experiencing PTD after preterm labor with intact membranes (PTL) compared with only 0.8% following term delivery [131]. Uteroplacental vascular lesions associated with abruption include spiral artery vascular thrombosis and failed physiologic transformation of uteroplacental vessels. Placental abruption is regarded as an acute event. This assertion is supported by the histologic evidence that acute lesions of chorioamnionitis and funisitis are frequently associated with decidual bleeding [122]. Nevertheless, evaluation of the vasculopathy accompanying decidual hemorrhage suggests that the process of placental abruption has chronic histologic features. Chronic deciduitis and villitis, infarcts, necrosis, blood vessels with absent physiologic changes, vascular thrombosis and increased numbers of circulating nucleated erythrocytes are the most frequently encountered histopathologic lesions co-associated with chronic decidual bleeding leading to PTD [129]. Trauma, hypertension, heavy cigarette smoking and cocaine use may induce or exacerbate the acute and chronic vasculopathies attendant upon placental abruption [132]. The association of abruption with increasing maternal age may reflect increased myometrial artery sclerosis present in 11% of spiral arteries at age 17–19 years but in 83% after age 39 [133].

Dysregulation of the molecular mechanisms responsible for vascular and decidual penetration by extravillous trophoblasts increases the risk of hemorrhage leading to abruption [134]. The decidua is a rich source of tissue factor, the primary initiator of clotting through thrombin generation [135]. Thus, decidual hemorrhage results in intense local thrombin generation. Hormonal factors such as progesterone play an important modulator role [136]. The expression of MMP-1 and MMP-3 protein and mRNA output by cultured term decidual cells is significantly enhanced by thrombin binding to the protease-activated receptor (PAR) type-1 [137,138]. Lockwood et al [139] reported that abruption-associated PPROM is accompanied by dense decidual neutrophil infiltration in the absence of infection. Decidual neutrophils co-localized with areas of thrombin-induced fibrin deposition and thrombin–PAR-1 interactions enhance IL-8 mRNA and

protein expression in cultured term decidual cells [137]. Neutrophils are a rich source of elastase and MMP-9 [140] which contribute to PPROM and cervical effacement. Stephenson et al [141] have shown that thrombin also enhances MMP-9 expression in cultured amniochorion. These studies suggest a mechanism linking abruption-associated PPROM to decidual thrombin–PAR interactions. A link between thrombin and PTL has been described by Phillippe and Chien [142] who reported that thrombin–PAR interactions trigger myometrial contractions. In either case, abruption can be accompanied by a robust intraamniotic inflammatory process in the absence of infection [143]. Proteomics-based studies demonstrated that coagulation proteases and free hemoglobin chains control different modules of the innate immunity and a feed-forward mechanism reinforces a "sterile" inflammatory process leading to PPROM, PTL, and PTD [141].

Mechanical stretching of the uterus

Pregnancy transforms the uterus into a thin-walled muscular organ to accommodate the fetus, placenta, and amniotic fluid [144]. These changes facilitate uterine adaptation to stretch such that a state of myometrial contractile quiescence can be maintained. Ultrasonography has opened a new window into the evaluation of the uterus and its physiologic adaptation to pregnancy. Buhimschi et al showed that in singleton gestations there is significant and widespread ultrasonographic thinning of the myometrium during active labor whether this occurs at term or preterm [142,145]. Various mathematical models indicate that wall stress (applied force per unit of cross-sectional area) is directly proportional to intracavitary pressure and radius of the curvature but inversely proportional to the thickness of the muscle [146]. Thus, the thinner the myometrium during contraction, the greater will be the generated uterine wall stress.

There is a decrease in the gestational age at delivery with increasing numbers of fetuses. For example, the average gestational age of delivery with twins is 35.3 weeks compared with 29.9 weeks for quadruplets [147], implicating mechanical stretching directly in the PTD process. Sfakianaki et al investigated whether the higher uterine volume of a multiple gestation could lead to a thinner uterine wall and increased uterine wall stress and therefore potentially explain the tendency for twin gestations to deliver earlier than singletons [148]. Twin pregnancy was characterized by a significant, selective and gradual thinning of the lower uterine segment during gestation. Thinning of the lower uterine segment occurred earlier in twin pregnancies destined to deliver preterm [146].

There has been an increased interest in identifying the role of excessive myometrial stretch and wall stress on gene expression patterns and pathways that orchestrate transition from quiescence to active myometrial contractions. Korita and colleagues examined the effect of labor-like cyclic mechanical stretch on possible upregulation of prostacyclin (PGI_2) synthase expression by examining the PGI_2 production by cultured human myometrial cells [149]. Cyclic mechanical stretch of myometrial cells augmented PGI_2 synthase gene promoter activity, via activation of activator protein-1 (AP-1) sites, and PGI_2 synthase mRNA and protein expression in cultured human myometrial cells. *In vitro*, mechanical stretch increased MMP-1 secretion from cultured human uterine cervical fibroblast cells [37]. Similarly, stretching of the human uterine myocytes induces oxytocin receptor, COX-2, IL-8, and connexin-43 expression [150–153]. *In vivo*, mechanical dilation of the cervix promoted cervical ripening through the induction of endogenous PGs [154] and increased MMP-1 expression [155]. Polyhydramnios and multifetal gestation-induced mechanical stretch increases amnion COX-2 expression and related PG production [156,157]. These data consolidate the argument that mechanical stretch contributes to the massive increase in the expression of procontractile molecules with central roles in premature activation of the myometrial contractile machinery leading to PTD.

Final common pathway of preterm delivery

The generation of PGs, proteases and a large array of proinflammatory cytokines reflects the final common pathway of both term and all spontaneous preterm deliveries. Levels of PGs increase in reproductive tract tissues, maternal plasma, and amniotic fluid immediately before and during parturition [158–161]. Concomitant with rising PG levels is the upregulation of myometrial PG receptors prior to the onset of labor [162,163]. PGs appear to induce functional progesterone withdrawal in the myometrium, enhance sensitivity to estrogens, and increase MMP and IL-8 expression. Moreover, all the pathways of prematurity described above also directly trigger MMP and IL-8 expression to mediate cervical change and fetal membrane rupture. Prior to 20 weeks' gestation, the myometrium is quiescent because of the high PR-B, low ER-β, low circulating estrogen levels, and inhibition of contraction-associated proteins gene expression, causing incompetent cervix to be the *forme fruste* of the PTD process in the first half of gestation. Figure 42.1 presents a schematic of the discrete pathogenic processes leading to prematurity and their final common biochemical pathway.

Prediction of preterm delivery: interpretation of test results

The four PTD pathogenic processes outlined above present unique biochemical or biophysical signatures. Efforts to exploit these "signatures" to identify patients at

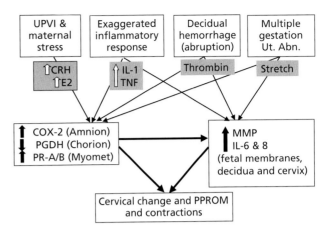

Figure 42.1 Pathogenesis of preterm delivery (PTD). COX-2, cyclooxygenase 2; IL, interleukin; MMP, metalloproteinase; Myomet, myometrium; PGDH, 15-hydroxy-prostaglandin dehydrogenase; PR-A/B progesterone receptor isoform A to B ratio; PPROM, preterm premature rupture of the membranes; TNF, tumor necrosis factor; UPVI, uteroplacental vascular insufficiency; Ut Abn, uterine abnormality.

risk for PTD from a given pathway have met with only modest success. The final common pathway of cervical and fetal membrane proteolysis can be discerned by assessment of cervicovaginal levels of fetal fibronectin (fFN) derived from the chorion or cervical length determination by ultrasound. In addition, high-throughput, high-dimensional proteomics technologies provide early detection of the pathophysiologic conditions leading to PTD. Unfortunately, studies examining the efficacy of various putative biomarkers continue to be marked by heterogeneous patient populations with varying distributions of pathogenic mechanisms and prevalence of PTD, as well as by diverse assay strategies, inconsistent cut-off values, and varying definitions of PTD.

Clinical epidemiology has long focused on sensitivity and specificity in interpreting diagnostic test results. These measures are not absolute and the various limitations of this approach have been described [164,165]. Comparison of markers therefore requires conversion of their predictive estimates to positive and negative likelihood ratios (LR) [166]. The LR is a measure of the predictive accuracy of a diagnostic test, yet independent of disease prevalence. The LR expresses how many more times (LR positive (+)) or fewer times (LR negative (-)) a test result is to be identified in subjects with the outcome of interest compared with those without the outcome. Interpretation of LRs is intuitive. The higher the LR(+) and the lower the LR(−), the better the diagnostic test performance. A LR(+) is calculated by dividing the sensitivity by the false-positive rate. A LR(−) is calculated by dividing the false-negative rate by specificity. A LR of 1.0 indicates no change from pretest probability, suggesting a useless test. As general guidelines, a LR(+) >2 corresponds to the probability of disease of approximately 67% [167,168]. Values of LR(+) >5 argue strongly for presence of the disease, while values of LR(−) <0.2 strongly militate against the presence of a disease.

Pathway-specific markers

Biomarkers and ultrasonographic markers of maternal-fetal stress

Putative markers of maternal-fetal stress include CRH and salivary estriol. Maternal levels of CRH rise in the weeks before labor [22]. However, the largest studies have not found CRH to be predictive of PTD [169,170]. Among those studies finding an association between maternal CRH levels and PTD, the available LRs have been less than robust: 1.8–4.0 for LR(+) and 0.47–0.77 for LR(−) for second-trimester maternal CRH levels predicting PTD among asymptomatic patients [171–174]. The test performs no better among symptomatic patients with LR(+) of 3.9 and LR(−) of 0.67 [175]. The detection of salivary estriol levels >2.1 ng/mL is predictive of PTD within 72 h between 32 and 37 weeks but again with only a modest LR(+) of 2.37 and LR(−) of 0.61 [176,177].

As noted, fetal adrenal activation is a key initiator of physiologic and stress-induced labor [48]. By using volume analysis – VOCAL (Virtual Organ Computerized Aided Analysis) – of three-dimensional (3D) ultrasonographic images, Turan *et al* demonstrated that a birthweight-corrected fetal adrenal gland volume of >422 mm^3/kg was a significant predictor of PTD within 5 days of the measurement with a very robust LR(+) and a LR(−) of 93.5 and 0.08, respectively [178].

Inflammatory biomarkers

Markers of the inflammatory pathway perform modestly better. Although anatomically part of the uterus, the cervix is perhaps best viewed as a separate, complex, and heterogeneous organ [179]. Its biology undergoes major molecular, enzymatic, and biomechanical transformations that may aid with prediction of PTD. Lockwood *et al* [180] conducted a prospective study cohort among 161 high-risk asymptomatic patients sampled every 3–4 weeks between 24 and 36 weeks and noted a 4.2-fold increase in maximal cervical IL-6 concentrations among patients with subsequent PTDs <37 weeks compared with those with subsequent term deliveries [178]. A single cervical IL-6 value >250 pg/mL identified patients with subsequent PTD compared with those having term deliveries with LR(+) of 3.33 and LR(−) of 0.59. Multiple logistic regression indicated that a cervical IL-6 level >250 pg/mL was an independent predictor of spontaneous PTD with an adjusted OR of 4.8 (95% CI 1.7–14.3).

The Maternal Fetal Medicine Units (MFMU) Network conduced a nested case–control study in an asymptomatic high-risk population and noted that while IL-6 concentrations were significantly higher in cases compared with controls (212 ± 339 versus 111 ± 186 pg/mL, P < 0.008), only 20% of cases had IL-6 values >90th percentile [181]. Moreover, regression analysis suggested that after adjusting for other PTD risk factors, including a positive fFN test result, Body Mass Index (BMI) <19.8 kg/m^2, vaginal bleeding in the first or second trimester, previous spontaneous PTD and short cervix, elevated cervical IL-6 levels were not independently associated with spontaneous PTD. Among symptomatic patients, the published LRs for cervical IL-6 for the prediction of PTD were 1.82–3.63 for LR(+) and 0.3–0.8 for LR(−) [96,[182–185].

Holst and associates [98] found higher cervical IL-8 levels among women who subsequently delivered preterm compared with those delivering at term (median 11.3 ng/mL, range 0.15–98.1 ng/mL versus 4.9 ng/mL, range 0.15–41.0 ng/mL, P < 0.002). The presence of cervical IL-8 values >7.7 ng/mL predicted PTD <7 days with LR(+) of 2.38 and LR(−) of 0.51. Kurkinen-Raty *et al* [183] observed LR(+) of 1.4 (95% CI 0.9–2.4) for a cervical IL-8 value >3.74 μg/L among symptomatic patients sampled between 22 and 32 weeks. Rizzo and colleagues [186] observed that cervical IL-8 values >450 pg/mL were comparable with fFN values >50 ng/mL in predicting PTD and that a cervical IL-8 level >860 pg/mL predicted a positive amniotic fluid culture with LR(+) of 2.4 and LR(−) of 0.28. In contrast, Coleman *et al* [184] were not able to confirm any PTD predictive value for cervical IL-8 determinations. Other markers of lower genital tract infection including cervical lactoferrin, sialidase, defensins, follistatin-free activin, serum β2-microglobulin, latex C-reactive protein, intracellular adhesion molecule-1, elevated vaginal pH, and cervical neutrophils do not appear to be predictive of PTD [187–192].

Identification of relevant cervicovaginal protein biomarkers that can lead to early diagnosis and treatment of PTD is theoretically possible through application of proteomics high-throughput technologies that directly interrogate differences in protein biomarkers [193]. Based on previous studies, the cervicovaginal proteome of pregnant women is rich in innate defense proteins [194]. Several of the identified immunoregulatory proteins, such as lactotransferin, neutrophil gelatinase, S100 A8 (calgranulin A), S100A9 (calgranulin B), haptoglobin, defensins, lactoferrin, azurocidin, annexins and transferrin, were previously linked to PTD [195–197]. The presence of these proteins in cervicovaginal secretions does not appear to be necessarily the result of an inflammatory response triggered, for example, by microbial invasion of the amniotic fluid sac, but rather that these proteins are normal components of the cervical innate immune system [198]. The PTD predictive value of the reported cervicovaginal proteomic biomarkers has not been tested prospectively in large population-based studies. Most data were analyzed based on fold-change rather than LRs. Hence, at this time, the true PTD predictive value of most proteomic biomarkers is difficult to determine.

The immunologic separation between maternal, fetal, and amniotic fluid compartments characteristic of human pregnancy may represent an evolutionary mechanism aimed to protect the fetus from its mother and vice versa. This isolation process offers an alternative explanation for the modest ability of several proposed acute-phase reactant inflammatory biomarkers (C-reactive protein, fibrinogen, amyloid protein A, procalcitonin) to predict PTD in asymptomatic women with intraamniotic inflammation [199]. The clinical relevance of this paradigm is that identification of inflammatory specific biomarkers which predispose to PTD is possible for the most part only through direct evaluation of the affected compartment.

The attention of several recent studies has been concentrated on identification of amniotic fluid protein biomarkers which could accurately predict PTD in women with intraamniotic inflammation [200–202]. Buhimschi and associates used surface-enhanced laser desorption ionization time-of-flight (SELDI-TOF) mass spectrometry and named the analysis method mass restricted (MR) scoring. Proteomic identification techniques established that presence of four protein biomarkers (defensin-2, defensin-1, S100A12, S100A8) in the amniotic fluid was diagnostic of intraamniotic inflammation [199]. The MR score was reproducible and maintained its highly accurate signature when tested prospectively in women with intraamniotic fluid inflammation/infection [203]. A key finding of the aforementioned study was that women with "severe amniotic fluid inflammation" (MR score with three or four proteomic biomarkers present) had shorter amniocentesis-to-delivery intervals than women with "no inflammation" (MR 0, all four markers absent) or even "minimal inflammation" (MR score with one or two markers present). Nonetheless, a "minimal" degree of inflammation was associated with PTD regardless of membrane status. This is relevant because in this population, biochemical tests such as amniotic fluid glucose and lactate dehydrogenase levels and white blood cell count traditionally used to diagnose intraamniotic inflammation were reported as normal. These findings suggest that detection of one or two biomarkers in the amniotic fluid of women with symptoms of PTL is associated with an increased risk of PTD even when clinical laboratory results are within normal limits. Interventional trials aimed to prevent activation of the final common pathway leading to premature activation of myometrial contractility, PPROM, and PTD are warranted based on the above results.

Ultrasonographic markers of uterine wall stretch and activation

The prevailing theories surrounding PTD may well overestimate the importance of the cervix, leaving the role played by myometrial activation subsequent to stretch

largely unexplored. As noted, mathematical modeling suggests that wall stress is directly proportional to both the intracavitary pressure and the radius of the curvature, but inversely proportional to the thickness of the myometrium. Thus, the thicker the myometrium at rest, the lower the uterine wall stress. Direct measurement of the uterine wall tension subsequent to stretch is not possible. Thus, sonographic evaluation of myometrial wall thickness may represent an alternative clinical tool for prediction of a short latency interval in women with twins or PPROM [146,143].

Biomarkers of decidual hemorrhage and dysregulation in coagulation pathways

Given the high concentrations of tissue factor in the decidua [133], abruption leads to excess thrombin generation, explaining the consumptive coagulopathy noted in severe cases. Thus, thrombin would appear to be an ideal marker for the detection of abruption-associated PTDs. Rosen *et al* [204] noted that thrombin–antithrombin complexes (TAT) >3.9 μg/L predict subsequent PPROM in asymptomatic patients with LR(+) of 2.75 and LR(−) of 0.18. Among symptomatic patients, TAT complex levels >6.3 μg/L between 24 and 33 weeks predict PTD within 3 weeks with LR(+) of 5.5 and LR(−) of 0.55 [205]. Chaiworapongsa *et al* [206] observed that TAT complex levels >20 μg/L predict PTD <37 weeks with LR(+) of 2.9 and LR(−) of 0.6.

Markers of the final preterm delivery common pathway

Fibronectins are large extracellular matrix and plasma proteins. A heavily glycosylated form, termed fFN, is present in the amniotic fluid, placental, and fetal membranes [207]. The fFN molecule is produced by extravillous cytotrophoblasts in the anchoring villi and cytotrophoblastic shell as well as the chorion; it is released into cervicovaginal secretions when the extracellular matrix of the chorionic–decidual interface is disrupted prior to labor [208]. It is also produced by amnion epithelium and released into amniotic fluid where it attains high concentrations [205]. Thus, fFN is positioned to be deported into the cervicovaginal secretions following occult or overt PPROM [205].

Lockwood and colleagues [207] first described the association between the presence of cervicovaginal fFN (>50 ng/mL) between 22 and 37 weeks' gestation and an increased risk of PTD among symptomatic patients with LR(+) of 4.67 and LR(−) of 0.22. Given evidence that fFN determinations retained their predictive value for only 2–3 weeks, Peaceman *et al* [209] assessed the value of fFN for predicting PTD within 7–14 days in symptomatic patients and noted LR(+) of 4.9 and 4.9, respectively, and LR(−) of 0.15 and 0.21, respectively. Of note, the corresponding negative predictive values in this population-based study were 99.5% and 99.2%, respectively. A metaanalysis of 14 studies examining the accuracy of fFN reported pooled LRs for the prediction of PTD within 7–14 days in symptomatic patients of 5.43 (95% CI 4.36–6.74) for LR(+) and 0.25 (95% CI 0.2–0.31) for LR(−). The comparable values for predicting PTD prior to 34 weeks were 3.64 (95% CI 3.32–5.73) and 0.32 (95% CI 0.16–0.66), respectively, among eight studies [210]. A recent metaanalysis of 32 pooled studies confirmed these results with LRs for a positive and negative fFN test of 4.20 (95% CI 3.53–4.99) and 0.29 (95% CI 0.22–0.38), respectively [211].

Lockwood *et al* [212] also initially assessed the utility of cervicovaginal fFN in the prediction of subsequent PTD amongst high-risk asymptomatic patients sampled every 2–4 weeks between 24 and 37 weeks' gestation. A vaginal fFN value >50 ng/mL predicted PTD with LR(+) of 3.4 and LR(−) of 0.4. Vaginal fFN predicted PTDs resulting from PTL and PPROM with equal efficiency. The MFMU Network subsequently assessed the value of cervicovaginal fFN obtained at 22–24 weeks among nearly 3000 asymptomatic women and found an even more robust LR(+) of 6.3 but less strong LR(−) of 0.84 [213]. A metaanalysis of studies among high-risk asymptomatic patients has demonstrated a pooled LR(+) for the prediction of PTD <34 weeks of 4.01 (95% CI 2.93–5.49) and a LR(−) of 0.78 (95% CI 0.72–0.84) [208].

The fFN test appears equally valid in patients with twins, cervical cerclage, and prior multifetal reduction procedures [214–216]. While the principal utility of the fFN lies in its very high negative predictive value (>99% for delivery within 2 weeks), most studies suggest a positive predictive value for PTD in general of >50%, suggesting that fFN-positive patients beyond 23 completed weeks of gestation should receive corticosteroids. A speculum exam need not be used to obtain a vaginal specimen [217]. At this point fFN remains the cervical biomarker with the greatest clinical usefulness [211,218].

Between 22 and 30 weeks' gestation, the length of the cervix assumes a Gaussian distribution with the 5th percentile at 20 mm, 10th percentile at 25 mm, 50th percentile at 35 mm, and 90th percentile at 45 mm [219]. The relative risk of PTD increases as the length of the cervix decreases. When women with shorter cervixes at 24 weeks were compared with women with values above the 75th percentile, the relative risks of PTD among the women with shorter cervixes were as follows: 1.98 for cervical lengths ≤40 mm, 2.35 for lengths ≤35 mm, 3.79 for lengths ≤30 mm, 6.19 for lengths ≤26 mm, 9.49 for lengths ≤22 mm, and 13.99 for lengths ≤13 mm [217].

Among symptomatic women who go on to deliver preterm, 80–100% have a cervical length ≤30 mm when initially evaluated because of contractions. As a rule, a subsequent PTD is highly unlikely in symptomatic women when the cervix is longer than 30 mm, unless an acute abruption is the cause of their contractions. Conversely, PTD is quite likely when a cervix measures <15 mm [220]. In one study of 216 women, in 173 cases the cervical length was ≥15 mm and only one of these women delivered within 7 days, while in the 43 patients with cervical lengths <15 mm, delivery within 7 days occurred in 37% [221]. Venditelli and Volumenie [222] conducted a metaanalysis of the utility of cervical sonographic length determination for the prediction of PTD among symptomatic patients. Nine articles met their inclusion criteria, the optimal predictive cut-off varied from 18 to 30 mm, and the prevalence of PTD was 37.3%. The authors found that relative risk for the occurrence of PTD when the cervical length was ≤18 mm was 3.9 (95% CI 1.8–8.5) and that sensitivities for predicting PTD ranged from 68% to 100%, while the specificity ranged from 30% to 78%.

In asymptomatic women with a history of PTD, the gestational age at PTD in the previous pregnancy correlates with the cervical length in the subsequent gestation [223]. Cervical length measurements in the second trimester in asymptomatic women with a history of prior spontaneous PTD predict recurrent spontaneous PTD. The MFMU Network examined the value of cervical ultrasound in predicting PTD <35 weeks among high-risk asymptomatic patients [224]. Patients underwent cervical sonography every 2 weeks and lengths <25 mm noted at any time were associated with a relative risk for spontaneous PTD of 4.5 (95% CI 2.7–7.6) but LR(+) of only 1.5 and LR(−) of 0.39. The efficacy of cervical length in predicting PTD in asymptomatic low-risk women is quite low. In a series of 3694 unselected Finnish women scanned at 18–24 weeks, a 25 mm cut-off yielded insignificant LR(+) and LR(−) [225]. Similar results were found in a large US cohort [226].

The optimal PTD diagnostic accuracy occurs when combining vaginal fFN with cervical length determinations. Hincz *et al* [227] prospectively evaluated 82 symptomatic patients with cervical sonography and fFN if the cervical length was between 2.0 and 3.1 cm. Defining positive patients as those with either a cervical length <2.1 cm or a positive fFN, they predicted delivery within 28 days with LR(+) of 8.6 and LR(−) of 0.16. The sensitivity of this two-step method was 86%, with a specificity of 90%, positive predictive value of 63%, and negative predictive value of 97%. Interestingly, among patients with a cervical length of 2.0–3.1 mm, 71.4% of those with a positive fFN delivered within 28 days while only 7.4% of those with negative fFN delivered within 28 days. Figure 42.2 describes this algorithm for evaluating symptomatic patients with both fFN and cervical sonography. It represents the most sensitive, specific, and accurate diagnostic paradigm available. Patients found to be at risk would qualify for a course of antenatal steroids when ≥24 weeks,

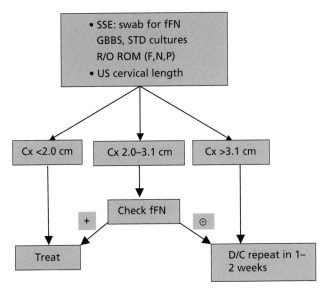

Figure 42.2 Algorithm for using fetal fibronectin (fFN) and/or cervical ultrasound in symptomatic patients. Cx, cervix; D/C, discharge patient; GBBS, group B β-streptococcus; R/O ROM, rule out rupture of fetal membranes; SSE, sterile speculum exam; STD, sexually transmitted disease; US, ultrasound.

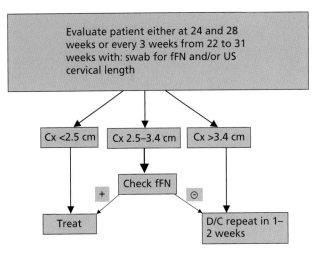

Figure 42.3 Algorithm for using fFN and/or cervical ultrasound (US) in high-risk asymptomatic patients. Cx, cervix; D/C, discharge patient.

as well as short-term tocolysis, and antibiotic therapy for urinary tract infections, or group B β-streptococcus if present or while cultures are pending.

The MFMU Network examined high-risk asymptomatic women between 24 and 28 weeks with fFN and cervical sonography and observed that patients with both a positive fFN and a short cervix on transvaginal ultrasound were at relatively high risk of spontaneous PTD (33.3%) while the absence of either marker placed them at very low risk of PTD <34 weeks (1.3%) [228]. Based on expert opinion and these data, we employ the algorithm outlined in Figure 42.3 for evaluating high-risk asymptomatic patients. Patients are evaluated every 3 weeks from 22 to 32 weeks. Again, patients found to be at risk can be treated with a course of antenatal corticosteroids and may benefit from decreased work and more intense surveillance.

Conclusion

Substantial strides have been made in our understanding of the pathogenesis of PTD. However, evaluation of the utility of biochemical and biophysical mediators of the major pathogenic markers has not produced efficient and noninvasive predictors of PTD (i.e. markers with high LR(+) and low LR(−) values). Identification of cervicovaginal fFN and cervical shortening on transvaginal sonography is the most accurate and efficient marker of PTD. Both are indicators of the final common pathway of genital tract ECM breakdown. High-risk asymptomatic patients found with either a short cervix or positive fFN are eligible for antenatal corticosteroids. However, most physicians rely on the high negative predictive value of a long cervix and/or negative fFN to avoid introduction of costly and potentially dangerous interventions of unproven efficacy. Future methods of risk assessment will likely rely on assessment of multiple markers. Opportunities presented by the advances of genomics and proteomics are expected to translate into useful clinical diagnostic tools and therapies which can target specific biologic processes leading to PTD.

CASE PRESENTATION 1

A 37-year-old primigravida at 31 weeks notes sudden onset of intermittent abdominal tightening and back pain. She contacts the on-call obstetrician who instructs her to go to the hospital. At presentation, she is noted to have a category I fetal heart rate tracing and contractions occurring three times every 10 min for 30 minu. Intravenous fluids are administered. An ultrasonographic cervical length of 2.2 cm is noted. A vaginal swab was obtained prior to the ultrasound and was sent for fFN determination. The fFN returns positive. The patient is admitted, tocolysis commenced, penicillin given for group B β-streptococcus prophylaxis after rectovaginal cultures were obtained and steroids given. After 72 h of observation, uterine contractions subside. She is discharged home with specific instructions including reduced physical effort. At 36 weeks she enters into spontaneous labor and delivers a healthy infant.

CASE PRESENTATION 2

A 38-year-old gravida 1, para 0, at 32 weeks, presents to labor and delivery with sudden onset of abdominal pain and vaginal bleeding. The pregnancy had been complicated by vaginal bleeding of uncertain etiology in the first trimester and at 20 weeks. The fetal heart rate tracing remains category 1 with rare contractions, her fibrinogen level is stable at 345 and 338 mg/dL over 4h and she is observed for 24h without cervical change or increasing contractions. Vaginal spotting continues intermittently for 1 week and she re-presents 7 days later with frank PPROM. The patient is admitted, given intravenous fluids, antibiotics, and two doses of corticosteroids. After 72h of observation, she develops sudden onset of heavy vaginal bleeding, fetal bradycardia and uterine hypertonus, prompting intensive resuscitation with blood and crystalloids and an emergency cesarean delivery. A Couvelaire uterus and a large retroplacental hematoma are noted.

References

1. Hamilton BE, Martin JA, Ventura SJ. Births: Preliminary Data for 2008. Health E-stats. Hyattsville, MD: National Center for Health Statistics, 2010.

2. Ananth CV, Vintzileos AM. Medically indicated preterm birth: recognizing the importance of the problem. Clin Perinatol 2008;35:53–67.

3. Moutquin JM. Classification and heterogeneity of preterm birth. Br J Obstet Gynaecol 2003;10(Suppl 20):30–33.

4. Muglia LJ, Katz M. The enigma of spontaneous preterm birth. N Engl J Med 2010;362:529–535.

5. Mendelson CR. Minireview: fetal-maternal hormonal signaling in pregnancy and labor. Mol Endocrinol 2009;23: 947–954.

6. Buhimschi CS, Rosenberg VA, Dulay AT et al. Multidimensional system biology: genetic markers and proteomic biomarkers of adverse pregnancy outcome in preterm birth. Am J Perinatol 2008;25:175–187.

7. Lockwood CJ, Kuczynski E. Risk stratification and pathological mechanisms in preterm delivery. Paediatr Perinat Epidemiol 2001;2:78–89.

8. Anum EA, Springel EH, Shriver MD, Strauss JF 3rd. Genetic contributions to disparities in preterm birth. Pediatr Res 2009;65:1–9.

9. Challis JR, Lockwood CJ, Myatt L, Norman JE, Strauss JF 3rd, Petraglia F. Inflammation and pregnancy. Reprod Sci 2009;16: 206–215.

10. Zakar T, Hertelendy F. Progesterone withdrawal: key to parturition. Am J Obstet Gynecol 2007;196:289–296.

11. Lockwood CJ, Stocco C, Murk W, Kayisli UA, Funai EF, Schatz F. Human labor is associated with reduced decidual cell expression of progesterone, but not glucocorticoid, receptors. J Clin Endocrinol Metab 2010;95:2271–2275.

12. Petraglia F, Imperatore A, Challis JR. Neuroendocrine mechanisms in pregnancy and parturition. Endocr Rev 2010;31(6):783–816.

13. Copper RL, Goldenberg RL, Das A et al. The preterm prediction study: maternal stress is associated with spontaneous preterm birth at less than thirty-five weeks' gestation. National Institute of Child Health and Human Development Maternal-Fetal Medicine Units Network. Am J Obstet Gynecol 1996;175:1286–1292.

14. Lipkind HS, Curry AE, Huynh M, Thorpe LE, Matte T. Birth outcomes among offspring of women exposed to the September 11, 2001, terrorist attacks. Obstet Gynecol 2010;116:917–925.

15. Orr ST, James SA, Blackmore Prince C. Maternal prenatal depressive symptoms and spontaneous preterm births among African-American women in Baltimore, Maryland. Am J Epidemiol 2002;156:797–802.

16. Grote NK, Bridge JA, Gavin AR, Melville JL, Iyengar S, Katon WJ. A meta-analysis of depression during pregnancy and the risk of preterm birth, low birth weight, and intrauterine growth restriction. Arch Gen Psychiatry 2010;67: 1012–1024.

17. Germain AM, Carvajal J, Sanchez M, Valenzuela GJ, Tsunekawa H, Chuaqui B. Preterm labor: placental pathology and clinical correlation. Obstet Gynecol 1999;94:284–289.

18. Arias F, Rodriquez L, Rayne SC, Kraus FT. Maternal placental vasculopathy and infection: two distinct subgroups among patients with preterm labor and preterm ruptured membranes. Am J Obstet Gynecol 1993;168:585–591.

19. Craddock N, Forty L. Genetics of affective (mood) disorders. Eur J Hum Genet 2006;14:660–668.

20. Svensson AC, Pawitan Y, Cnattingius S, Reilly M, Lichtenstein P. Familial aggregation of small-for-gestational-age births: the importance of fetal genetic effects. Am J Obstet Gynecol 2006;194:475–479.

21. Challis JR, Lye SJ, Gibb W, Whittle W, Patel F, Alfaidy N. Understanding preterm labor. Ann N Y Acad Sci 2001;943: 225–234.

22. McLean M, Bisits A, Davies J, Woods R, Lowry P, Smith R. A placental clock controlling the length of human pregnancy. Nat Med 1995;1:460–463.

23. Wolfe CD, Patel SP, Linton EA et al. Plasma corticotrophin-releasing factor (CRF) in abnormal pregnancy. Br J Obstet Gynaecol 1988;95:1003–1006.

24. Jones SA, Brooks AN, Challis JR. Steroids modulate corticotropin-releasing hormone production in human fetal membranes and placenta. J Clin Endocrinol Metab 1989;68: 825–830.

25. Sandman CA, Glynn L, Schetter CD et al. Elevated maternal cortisol early in pregnancy predicts third trimester levels of placental corticotropin releasing hormone (CRH): priming the placental clock. Peptides 2006;27:1457–1463.

26. Economides DL, Nicolaides KH, Linton EA, Perry LA, Chard T. Plasma cortisol and adrenocorticotropin in appropriate and small for gestational age fetuses. Fetal Ther 1988;3:158–164.

27. Amiel-Tison C, Cabrol D, Denver R, Jarreau PH, Papiernik E, Piazza PV. Fetal adaptation to stress. Part I: acceleration of fetal maturation and earlier birth triggered by placental insufficiency in humans. Early Hum Dev 2004;78:15–27.

28. Lockwood CJ, Radunovic N, Nastic D, Petkovic S, Aigner S, Berkowitz GS. Corticotropin-releasing hormone and related pituitary-adrenal axis hormones in fetal and maternal blood during the second half of pregnancy. J Perinat Med 1996; 24:243–251.

29. Florio P, Zatelli MC, Reis FM, degli Uberti EC, Petraglia F. Corticotropin releasing hormone: a diagnostic marker for behavioral and reproductive disorders? Front Biosci 2007; 12:551–560.

30. Challis JRG, Matthews SG, Gibb W, Lye SJ. Endocrine and paracrine regulation of birth at term and preterm. Endocr Rev 2000;21:514–50.

31. Jones SA, Challis JR. Effects of corticotropin-releasing hormone and adrenocorticotropin on prostaglandin output by human placenta and fetal membranes. Gynecol Obstet Invest 1990;29:165–168.

32. Jones SA, Challis JR. Steroid, corticotrophin-releasing hormone, ACTH and prostaglandin interactions in the amnion and placenta of early pregnancy in man. J Endocrinol 1990;125:153–159.

33. Myatt L, Lye SJ. Expression, localization and function of prostaglandin receptors in myometrium. Prostaglandins Leukot Essent Fatty Acids 2004;70:137–148.

34. Garfield RE, Sims S, Daniel EE. Gap junctions: their presence and necessity in myometrium during parturition. Science 1977;198:958–960.

35. Olson DM. The role of prostaglandins in the initiation of parturition. Best Pract Res Clin Obstet Gynaecol 2003;17: 717–730.

36. Cook JL, Zaragoza DB, Sung DH, Olson DM. Expression of myometrial activation and stimulation genes in a mouse model of preterm labor: myometrial activation, stimulation, and preterm labor. Endocrinology 2000;141:1718–1728.

37. Yoshida M, Sagawa N, Itoh H et al. Prostaglandin F(2alpha), cytokines and cyclic mechanical stretch augment matrix metalloproteinase-1 secretion from cultured human uterine cervical fibroblast cells. Mol Hum Reprod 2002;8:681–687.

38. Denison FC, Calder AA, Kelly RW. The action of prostaglandin E2 on the human cervix: stimulation of interleukin 8 and inhibition of secretory leukocyte protease inhibitor. Am J Obstet Gynecol 1999;180:614–620.

39. Madsen G, Zakar T, Ku CY, Sanborn BM, Smith R, Mesiano S. Prostaglandins differentially modulate progesterone receptor-A and -B expression in human myometrial cells: evidence for prostaglandin-induced functional progesterone withdrawal. J Clin Endocrinol Metab 2004;89:1010–1013.

40. Stjernholm-Vladic Y, Wang H, Stygar D, Ekman G, Sahlin L. Differential regulation of the progesterone receptor A and B in the human uterine cervix at parturition. Gynecol Endocrinol 2004;18:41–46.

41. Oh SY, Kim CJ, Park I et al. Progesterone receptor isoform (A/B) ratio of human fetal membranes increases during term parturition. Am J Obstet Gynecol 2005;193:1156–1160.

42. Merlino A, Welsh T, Erdonmez T et al. Nuclear progesterone receptor expression in the human fetal membranes and decidua at term before and after labor. Reprod Sci 2009; 16:357–363.

43. Zakar T, Hirst JJ, Mijovic JE, Olson DM. Glucocorticoids stimulate the expression of prostaglandin endoperoxide H synthase-2 in amnion cells. Endocrinology 1995;136: 1610–1619.

44. Patel FA, Clifton VL, Chwalisz K, Challis JR. Steroid regulation of prostaglandin dehydrogenase activity and expression in human term placenta and chorio-decidua in relation to labor. J Clin Endocrinol Metab 1999;84:291–299.

45. Parker CR Jr, Stankovic AM, Goland RS. Corticotropin-releasing hormone stimulates steroidogenesis in cultured human adrenal cells. Mol Cell Endocrinol 1999;155:19–25.

46. Di WL, Lachelin GC, McGarrigle HH, Thomas NS, Becker DL. Oestriol and oestradiol increase cell to cell communication and connexin43 protein expression in human myometrium. Mol Hum Reprod 2001;7:671–679.

47. Richter ON, Kubler K, Schmolling J et al. Oxytocin receptor gene expression of estrogen-stimulated human myometrium in extracorporeally perfused non-pregnant uteri. Mol Hum Reprod 2004;10:339–346.

48. Mesiano S, Chan EC, Fitter JT, Kwek K, Yeo G, Smith R. Progesterone withdrawal and estrogen activation in human parturition are coordinated by progesterone receptor A expression in the myometrium. J Clin Endocrinol Metab 2002;87:2924–2930.

49. Challis JR. CRH, a placental clock and preterm labour. Nat Med 1995;1:416.

50. Langlois D, Li JY, Saez JM. Development and function of the human fetal adrenal cortex. J Pediatr Endocrinol 2002;15(Suppl 5):1311–1322.

51. Buhimschi CS, Turan OM, Funai EF et al. Fetal adrenal gland volume and cortisol/dehydroepiandrosterone sulfate ratio in inflammation-associated preterm birth. Obstet Gynecol 2008;111:715–722.

52. Martinon F, Mayor A, Tschopp J. The inflammasomes: guardians of the body. Annu Rev Immunol 2009;27:229–265.

53. Stutz A, Golenbock DT, Latz E. Inflammasomes: too big to miss. J Clin Invest 2009;119:3502–3511.

54. Reddy RC, Chen GH, Tekchandani PK, Standiford TJ. Sepsis-induced immunosuppression: from bad to worse. Immunol Res 2001;24:273–287.

55. Offenbacher S, Boggess KA, Murtha AP et al. Progressive periodontal disease and risk of very preterm delivery. Obstet Gynecol 2006;107:29–36.

56. Locksmith G, Duff P. Infection, antibiotics, and preterm delivery. Semin Perinatol 2001;25:295–309.

57. Richey SD, Roberts SW, Ramin KD, Ramin SM, Cunningham FG. Pneumonia complicating pregnancy. Obstet Gynecol 1994;84:525–528.

58. Goldenberg RL, Hauth JC, Andrews WW. Intrauterine infection and preterm delivery. N Engl J Med 2000;342: 1500–1507.

59. Mueller-Heubach E, Rubinstein DN, Schwarz SS. Histologic chorioamnionitis and preterm delivery in different patient populations. Obstet Gynecol 1990;75:622–626.

60. Andrews WW, Hauth JC, Goldenberg RL, Gomez R, Romero R, Cassell GH. Amniotic fluid interleukin-6: correlation with

upper genital tract microbial colonization and gestational age in women delivered after spontaneous labor versus indicated delivery. Am J Obstet Gynecol 1995;173:606–612.

61. Han YW. Oral health and adverse pregnancy outcomes – what's next? J Dent Res 2011;90(3):289–293.

62. Polyzos NP, Polyzos IP, Mauri D et al. Effect of periodontal disease treatment during pregnancy on preterm birth incidence: a metaanalysis of randomized trials. Am J Obstet Gynecol 2009;200:225–232.

63. Macones GA, Parry S, Nelson DB et al. Treatment of localized periodontal disease in pregnancy does not reduce the occurrence of preterm birth: results from the Periodontal Infections and Prematurity Study (PIPS). Am J Obstet Gynecol 2010; 202:147.

64. Jeffcoat M, Parry S, Sammel M, Clothier B, Catlin A, Macones G. Periodontal infection and preterm birth: successful periodontal therapy reduces the risk of preterm birth. Br J Obstet Gynaecol 2011;118(2):250–256.

65. Pirotta M, Fethers KA, Bradshaw CS. Bacterial vaginosis – more questions than answers. Aust Fam Physician 2009;38: 394–397.

66. Meis PJ, Goldenberg RL, Mercer B et al. The preterm prediction study: significance of vaginal infections. National Institute of Child Health and Human Development Maternal-Fetal Medicine Units Network. Am J Obstet Gynecol 1995; 173:1231–1235.

67. Hillier SL, Nugent RP, Eschenbach DA et al. Association between bacterial vaginosis and preterm delivery of a low-birth-weight infant. The Vaginal Infections and Prematurity Study Group. N Engl J Med 1995;333:1737–1742.

68. Leitich H, Bodner-Adler B, Brunbauer M, Kaider A, Egarter C, Husslein P. Bacterial vaginosis as a risk factor for preterm delivery: a meta-analysis. Am J Obstet Gynecol 2003;189: 139–147.

69. Hillier SL. The complexity of microbial diversity in bacterial vaginosis. N Engl J Med 2005;353:1886–1887.

70. Hillebrand L, Harmanli OH, Whiteman V, Khandelwal M. Urinary tract infections in pregnant women with bacterial vaginosis. Am J Obstet Gynecol 2002;186:916–917.

71. Romero R, Oyarzun E, Mazor M, Sirtori M, Hobbins JC, Bracken M. Meta-analysis of the relationship between asymptomatic bacteriuria and preterm delivery/low birth weight. Obstet Gynecol 1989;73:576–578.

72. Villar J, Gulmezoglu AM, de Onis M. Nutritional and antimicrobial interventions to prevent preterm birth: an overview of randomized controlled trials. Obstet Gynecol Surv 1998; 53:575–585.

73. Krohn MA, Thwin SS, Rabe LK, Brown Z, Hillier SL. Vaginal colonization by Escherichia coli as a risk factor for very low birth weight delivery and other perinatal complications. J Infect Dis 1997;175:606–610.

74. Diaz-Cueto L, Dominguez-Lopez P, Tena-Alavez G, Cuica-Flores A, Rosales-Ortiz S, Arechavaleta-Velasco F. Effect of clindamycin treatment on vaginal inflammatory markers in pregnant women with bacterial vaginosis and a positive fetal fibronectin test. Int J Gynaecol Obstet 2009;107:143–146.

75. Mitchell C, Balkus J, Agnew K, Lawler R, Hitti J. Changes in the vaginal microenvironment with metronidazole treatment for bacterial vaginosis in early pregnancy. J Womens Health (Larchmt) 2009;18:1817–1824.

76. Nygren P, Fu R, Freeman M, Bougatsos C, Guise JM. Screening and Treatment for Bacterial Vaginosis in Pregnancy: Systematic Review to Update the 2001 U.S. Preventive Services Task Force Recommendation [Internet]. Rockville, MD: Agency for Healthcare Research and Quality, 2008.

77. Shennan A, Crawshaw S, Briley A et al. A randomised controlled trial of metronidazole for the prevention of preterm birth in women positive for cervicovaginal fetal fibronectin: the PREMET Study. Br J Obstet Gynaecol 2006;113:65–74.

78. Kapetanovic R, Cavaillon JM. Early events in innate immunity in the recognition of microbial pathogens. Expert Opin Biol Ther 2007;7:907–918.

79. Medzhitov R. Inflammation 2010: new adventures of an old flame. Cell 2010;140:771–776.

80. Brodsky IE, Medzhitov R. Targeting of immune signalling networks by bacterial pathogens. Nat Cell Biol 2009;11: 521–526.

81. Pioli PA, Amiel E, Schaefer TM, Connolly JE, Wira CR, Guyre PM. Differential expression of Toll-like receptors 2 and 4 in tissues of the human female reproductive tract. Infect Immunol 2004;72:5799–5806.

82. Kim YM, Romero R, Chaiworapongsa T et al. Toll-like receptor-2 and -4 in the chorioamniotic membranes in spontaneous labor at term and in preterm parturition that are associated with chorioamnionitis. Am J Obstet Gynecol 2004;191:1346–1345.

83. Holmlund U, Cebers G, Dahlfors AR et al. Expression and regulation of the pattern recognition receptors Toll-like receptor-2 and Toll-like receptor-4 in the human placenta. Immunology 2002;107:145–151.

84. Belt AR, Baldassare JJ, Molnar M, Romero R, Hertelendy F. The nuclear transcription factor NF-κB mediates interleukin-1β-induced expression of cyclooxygenase-2 in human myometrial cells. Am J Obstet Gynecol 1999;181:359–366.

85. Yan X, Wu Xiao C, Sun M, Tsang BK, Gibb W. Nuclear factor κB activation and regulation of cyclooxygenase type-2 expression in human amnion mesenchymal cells by interleukin-1β. Biol Reprod 2002;66:1667–1671.

86. Lee Y, Allport V, Sykes A, Lindstrom T, Slater D, Bennett P. The effects of labour and of interleukin 1 beta upon the expression of nuclear factor κB related proteins in human amnion. Mol Hum Reprod 2003;9:213–218.

87. Arechavaleta-Velasco F, Ogando D, Parry S, Vadillo-Ortega F. Production of matrix metalloproteinase-9 in lipopolysaccharide-stimulated human amnion occurs through an autocrine and paracrine proinflammatory cytokine-dependent system. Biol Reprod 2002;67:1952–1958.

88. Van Meir CA, Sangha RK, Walton JC, Mathews SG, Keirse MJ, Challis JR. Immunoreactive 15-hydroxyprosta-glandin dehydrogenase (PGDH) is reduced in fetal membranes from patients at preterm delivery in the presence of infection. Placenta 1996;17:291–297.

89. McLaren J, Taylor DJ, Bell SC. Prostaglandin E(2)-dependent production of latent matrix metalloproteinase-9 in cultures of human fetal membranes. Mol Hum Reprod 2000;6: 1033–1040.

90. Ito A, Nakamura T, Uchiyama T et al. Stimulation of the biosynthesis of interleukin 8 by interleukin 1 and tumor necrosis factor alpha in cultured human chorionic cells. Biol Pharm Bull 1994;17:1463–1467.

91. So T, Ito A, Sato T, Mori Y, Hirakawa S. Tumor necrosis factor-alpha stimulates the biosynthesis of matrix metalloproteinases and plasminogen activator in cultured human chorionic cells. Biol Reprod 1992;46:772–778.

92. Fortunato SJ, Menon R, Lombardi SJ. Role of tumor necrosis factor-alpha in the premature rupture of membranes and preterm labor pathways. Am J Obstet Gynecol 2002;187: 1159–1162.

93. Lei H, Furth EE, Kalluri R et al. A program of cell death and extracellular matrix degradation is activated in the amnion before the onset of labor. J Clin Invest 1996;98: 1971–1978.

94. Dudley DJ, Trautman MS, Araneo BA, Edwin SS, Mitchell MD. Decidual cell biosynthesis of interleukin-6: regulation by inflammatory cytokines. J Clin Endocrinol Metab 1992;74: 884–889.

95. Fortunato SJ, Menon RP, Swan KF, Menon R. Inflammatory cytokine (interleukins 1, 6 and 8 and tumor necrosis factor-alpha) release from cultured human fetal membranes in response to endotoxic lipopolysaccharide mirrors amniotic fluid concentrations. Am J Obstet Gynecol 1996;174: 1855–1861.

96. Mitchell MD, Dudley DJ, Edwin SS, Schiller SL. Interleukin-6 stimulates prostaglandin production by human amnion and decidual cells. Eur J Pharmacol 1991;192:189–191.

97. Lockwood CJ, Murk WK, Kayisli UA et al. Regulation of interleukin-6 expression in human decidual cells and its potential role in chorioamnionitis. Am J Pathol 2010;177: 1755–1764.

98. Holst RM, Mattsby-Baltzer I, Wennerholm UB, Hagberg H, Jacobsson B. Interleukin-6 and interleukin-8 in cervical fluid in a population of Swedish women in preterm labor: relationship to microbial invasion of the amniotic fluid, intra-amniotic inflammation, and preterm delivery. Acta Obstet Gynecol Scand 2005;84:551–557.

99. Miyake K. Innate immune sensing of pathogens and danger signals by cell surface Toll-like receptors. Sem Immunol 2007;19:3–10.

100. Lotze MT, Zeh HJ, Rubartelli A et al. The grateful dead: damage-associated molecular pattern molecules and reduction/oxidation regulate immunity. Immunol Rev 2007;220:60–81.

101. Buhimschi IA, Zhao G, Pettker CM et al. The receptor for advanced glycation end products (RAGE) system in women with intraamniotic infection and inflammation. Am J Obstet Gynecol 2007;196:181.

102. Dulay AT, Buhimschi CS, Zhao G et al. Soluble TLR2 is present in human amniotic fluid and modulates the intraamniotic inflammatory response to infection. J Immunol 2009;182:7244–7253.

103. Menon R, Velez DR, Morgan N, Lombardi SJ, Fortunato SJ, Williams SM. Genetic regulation of amniotic fluid TNF-alpha and soluble TNF receptor concentrations affected by race and preterm birth. Hum Genet 2008;124:243–253.

104. Buhimschi CS, Baumbusch MA, Dulay AT et al. Characterization of RAGE, HMGB1, and S100beta in inflammation-induced preterm birth and fetal tissue injury. Am J Pathol 2009;175:958–975.

105. Lee S, Buhimschi IA, Zhao G et al. The interleukin-6 (IL-6) Trans-signaling system: evidence for presence and activation in pregnancies complicated by intra-amniotic infection. Am J Obstet Gynecol 2008;199:S141.

106. Hillier SL, Martins J, Krohn M, Kiviat N, Holmes KK, Eschenbach DA. A case–control study of chorioamnionic infection and histologic chorioamnionitis in prematurity. N Engl J Med 1988;319:972–978.

107. Andrews WW, Goldenberg RL, Hauth JC. Preterm labor: emerging role of genital tract infections. Infect Agents Dis 1995;4:196–211.

108. Pettker CM, Buhimschi IA, Magloire LK, Sfakianaki AK, Hamar BD, Buhimschi CS. Value of placental microbial evaluation in diagnosing intra-amniotic infection. Obstet Gynecol 2007;109:739–749.

109. Han YW, Shen T, Chung P, Buhimschi IA, Buhimschi CS. Uncultivated bacteria as etiologic agents of intra-amniotic inflammation leading to preterm birth. J Clin Microbiol 2009;47:38–47.

110. Porter TF, Fraser A, Hunter CY, Ward R, Varner MW. The intergenerational predisposition to preterm birth. Obstet Gynecol 1997;90:63–67.

111. Winkvist A, Mogren I, Hogberg U. Familial patterns in birth characteristics: impact on individual and population risks. Int J Epidemiol 1998;27:248–254.

112. Treloar SA, Macones GA, Mitchell LE, Martin NG. Genetic influences on premature parturition in an Australian twin sample. Twin Res 2000;3:80–82.

113. Clausson B, Lichtenstein P, Cnattingius S. Genetic influence on birthweight and gestational length determined by studies in offspring of twins. Br J Obstet Gynaecol 2000;107: 375–381.

114. International HapMap Consortium. The International HapMap Project. Nature 2003;426:789–796.

115. Roberts AK, Monzon-Bordonaba F, van Deerlin PG et al. Association of polymorphism within the promoter of the tumor necrosis factor alpha gene with increased risk of preterm premature rupture of the fetal membranes. Am J Obstet Gynecol 1999;180:1297–1302.

116. Macones GA, Parry S, Elkousy M, Clothier B, Ural S, Strauss JF III. A polymorphism in the promoter region of TNF and bacterial vaginosis: preliminary evidence of gene-environment interaction in the etiology of spontaneous preterm birth. Am J Obstet Gynecol 2004;190:1504–1508.

117. Simhan HN, Krohn MA, Roberts JM, Zeevi A, Caritis SN. Interleukin-6 promoter-174 polymorphism and spontaneous preterm birth. Am J Obstet Gynecol 2003;189:915–918.

118. Lorenz E, Hallman M, Marttila R, Haataha R, Schwartz D. Association between the Asp299Gly polymorphisms in the toll-like receptor 4 and premature births in the Finnish population. Pediatr Res 2002;52:373–376.

119. Wang X, Chen D, Niu T et al. Genetic susceptibility to benzene and shortened gestation: evidence of gene–environment interaction. Am J Epidemiol 2000;152:693–700.

120. Wang X, Zuckerman B, Pearson C et al. Maternal cigarette smoking, metabolic gene polymorphism, and infant birth weight. JAMA 2002;287:195–202.

121. Fujimoto T, Parry S, Urbanek M et al. A single nucleotide polymorphism in the matrix metalloproteinase-1 (MMP-1) promoter influences amnion cell MMP-1 expression and risk for preterm premature rupture of the fetal membranes. J Biol Chem 2002;277:6296–6302.

122. Ferrand PE, Parry S, Sammel M et al. A polymorphism in the matrix metalloproteinase-9 promoter is associated with increased risk of preterm premature rupture of membranes in African Americans. Mol Hum Reprod 2002;8:494–501.

123. Genc MR, Gerber S, Nesin M, Witkin SS. Polymorphism in the interleukin-1 gene complex and spontaneous preterm delivery. Am J Obstet Gynecol 2002;187:157–163.

124. Elsasser DA, Ananth CV, Prasad V, Vintzileos AM, New Jersey-Placental Abruption Study Investigators. Diagnosis of placental abruption: relationship between clinical and histopathological findings. Eur J Obstet Gynecol Reprod Biol 2010;148:125–130.

125. Strobino B, Pantel-Silverman J. Gestational vaginal bleeding and pregnancy outcome. Am J Epidemiol 1989;129:806–815.

126. Dadkhah F, Kashanian M, Eliasi G. A comparison between the pregnancy outcome in women both with or without threatened abortion. Early Hum Dev 2010;86:193–196.

127. Harger JH, Hsing AW, Tuomala RE et al. Risk factors for preterm premature rupture of fetal membranes: a multicenter case–control study. Am J Obstet Gynecol 1990;163:130–137.

128. Roque H, Paidas MJ, Funai EF, Kuczynski E, Lockwood CJ. Maternal thrombophilias are not associated with early pregnancy loss. Thromb Haemost 2004;91:290–295.

129. Nurk E, Tell GS, Refsum H, Ueland PM, Vollset SE. Associations between maternal methylenetetrahydrofolate reductase polymorphisms and adverse outcomes of pregnancy: the Hordaland Homocysteine Study. Am J Med 2004;117:26–31.

130. American College of Obstetricians and Gynecologists. Inherited thrombophilias in pregnancy. Practice Bulletin No. 113. Obstet Gynecol 2010;116:212–222.

131. Salafia CM, Lopez-Zeno JA, Sherer DM et al. Histologic evidence of old intrauterine bleeding is more frequent in prematurity. Am J Obstet Gynecol 1995;173:1065–1070.

132. Misra DP, Ananth CV. Risk factor profiles of placental abruption in first and second pregnancies: heterogeneous etiologies. J Clin Epidemiol 1999;52:453–461.

133. Naeye RL. Maternal age, obstetric complications, and the outcome of pregnancy. Obstet Gynecol 1983;61:210–216.

134. Buhimschi CS, Schatz F, Krikun G, Buhimschi IA, Lockwood CJ. Novel insights into molecular mechanisms of abruption-induced preterm birth. Expert Rev Mol Med 2010;12:e35.

135. Lockwood C, Krikun G, Schatz F. The decidua regulates hemostasis in the human endometrium. Semin Reprod Endocrinol 1999;17:45–51.

136. Lockwood CJ, Murk W, Kayisli UA et al. Progestin and thrombin regulate tissue factor expression in human term decidual cells. J Clin Endocrinol Metab 2009;94:2164–2170.

137. Mackenzie AP, Schatz F, Krikun G, Funai EF, Kadner S, Lockwood CJ. Mechanisms of abruption-induced premature rupture of the fetal membranes: thrombin enhanced decidual matrix metalloproteinase-3 (stromelysin-1) expression. Am J Obstet Gynecol 2004;191:1996–2001.

138. Rosen T, Schatz F, Kuczynski E, Lam H, Koo AB, Lockwood CJ. Thrombin-enhanced matrix metalloproteinase-1 expression: a mechanism linking placental abruption with premature rupture of the membranes. J Matern Fetal Neonatal Med 2002;11:11–17.

139. Lockwood CJ, Toti P, Arcuri F et al. Mechanisms of abruption-induced premature rupture of the fetal membranes: thrombin-enhanced interleukin-8 expression in term decidua. Am J Pathol 2005;167:1443–1449.

140. Lathbury LJ, Salamonsen LA. In vitro studies of the potential role of neutrophils in the process of menstruation. Mol Hum Reprod 2000;6:899–906.

141. Stephenson CD, Lockwood CJ, Ma Y, Guller S. Thrombin-dependent regulation of matrix metalloproteinase (MMP)-9 levels in human fetal membranes. J Matern Fetal Neonatal Med 2005;18:17–22.

142. Phillippe M, Chien EK. Intracellular signaling and phasic myometrial contractions. J Soc Gynecol Invest 1998;5:169–177.

143. Buhimschi IA, Zhao G, Rosenberg VA, Abdel-Razeq S, Thung S, Buhimschi CS. Multidimensional proteomics analysis of amniotic fluid to provide insight into the mechanisms of idiopathic preterm birth. PLoS One 2008;3:e2049.

144. Buhimschi CS, Buhimschi IA, Malinow AM, Weiner CP. Myometrial thickness during human labor and immediately postpartum. Am J Obstet Gynecol 2003;188:553–559.

145. Buhimschi CS, Buhimschi IA, Norwitz ER et al. Sonographic myometrial thickness predicts the latency interval of women with preterm premature rupture of the membranes and oligohydramnios. Am J Obstet Gynecol 2005;193:762–770.

146. Veille JC, Hosenpud JD, Morton MJ, Welch JE. Cardiac size and function in pregnancy induced hypertension. Am J Obstet Gynecol 1984;150:443–449.

147. Centers for Disease Control and Prevention. National Vital Statistic Reports. Births: Final data for 2002. Vol 52:1–118. Released December 17, 2003.

148. Sfakianaki AK, Buhimschi IA, Pettker CM et al. Ultrasonographic evaluation of myometrial thickness in twin pregnancies. Am J Obstet Gynecol 2008;198:530.

149. Korita D, Sagawa N, Itoh H. Cyclic mechanical stretch augments prostacyclin production in cultured human uterine myometrial cells from pregnant women: possible involvement of up-regulation of prostacyclin synthase expression. J Clin Endocrinol Metab 2002;87:5209–5219.

150. Terzidou V, Sooranna SR, Kim LU, Thornton S, Bennett PR, Johnson MR. Mechanical stretch up-regulates the human oxytocin receptor in primary human uterine myocytes. J Clin Endocrinol Metab 2005;90:237–246.

151. Sooranna SR, Engineer N, Loudon JA, Terzidou V, Bennett PR, Johnson MR. The mitogen-activated protein kinase dependent expression of prostaglandin H synthase-2 and interleukin-8 messenger ribonucleic acid by myometrial cells: the differential effect of stretch and interleukin-1β. J Clin Endocrinol Metab 2005;90:3517–3527.

152. Loudon JA, Sooranna SR, Bennett PR, Johnson MR. Mechanical stretch of human uterine smooth muscle cells increases IL-8 mRNA expression and peptide synthesis. Mol Hum Reprod 2004;10:895–899.

153. Ou CW, Orsino A, Lye SJ. Expression of connexin-43 and connexin-26 in the rat myometrium during pregnancy and labor is differentially regulated by mechanical and hormonal signals. Endocrinology 1997;138:5398–5407.

154. Levy R, Kanengiser B, Furman B, Ben Arie A, Brown D, Hagay ZJ. A randomized trial comparing a 30-mL and an 80-mL Foley catheter balloon for preinduction cervical ripening. Am J Obstet Gynecol 2004;191:1632–1636.

155. Olund A, Jonasson A, Kindahl H, Fianu S, Larsson B. The effect of cervical dilatation by laminaria on the plasma levels of 15-keto-13,14-dihydro-PGF2 alpha. Contraception 1984;30: 23–27.

156. Leguizamon G, Smith J, Younis H, Nelson DM, Sadovsky Y. Enhancement of amniotic cyclooxygenase type 2 activity in women with preterm delivery associated with twins or poly-hydramnios. Am J Obstet Gynecol 2001;184:117–122.

157. Terakawa K, Itoh H, Sagawa N et al. Site-specific augmenta-tion of amnion cyclooxygenase-2 and decidua vera phospholipase-A2 expression in labor: possible contribution of mechanical stretch and interleukin-1 to amnion prostaglan-din synthesis. J Soc Gynecol Invest 2002;9:68–74.

158. Husslein P, Sinzinger H. Concentration of 13,14-dihydro-15-keto-prostaglandin E2 in the maternal peripheral plasma during labour of spontaneous onset. Br J Obstet Gynaecol 1984;91:228–231.

159. Sellers SM, Hodgson HT, Mitchell MD, Anderson AB, Turnbull AC. Raised prostaglandin levels in the third stage of labor. Am J Obstet Gynecol 1982;144:209–212.

160. Keirse MJNC, Turnbull AC. Prostaglandins in amniotic fluid during late pregnancy and labour. J Obstet Gynaecol Br Commonw 1973:80:970–973.

161. Casey ML, MacDonald PC. Biomolecular processes in the initiation of parturition: decidual activation. Clin Obstet Gynecol 1988;31:533–552.

162. Matsumoto T, Sagawa N, Yoshida M et al. The prostaglandin E2 and F2 alpha receptor genes are expressed in human myo-metrium and are down-regulated during pregnancy. Biochem Biophys Res Commun 1997;238:838–841.

163. Brodt-Eppley J, Myatt L. Prostaglandin receptors in lower uterine segment myometrium during gestation and labor. Obstet Gynecol 1999;93:89–93.

164. Hawass NE. Comparing the sensitivities and specificities of two diagnostic procedures performed on the same group of patients. Br J Radiol 1997;70:360–366.

165. Biggerstaff BJ. Comparing diagnostic tests: a simple graphic using likelihood ratios. Stat Med 2000;19:649–663.

166. Attia J. Moving beyond sensitivity and specificity: using like-lihood ratios to help interpret diagnostic tests. Aust Prescr 2003; 26:111–113.

167. Foy R, Warner P. About time: diagnostic guidelines that help clinicians. Qual Saf Health Care 2003;12:205–209.

168. Wang ST, Pizzolato S, Demshar HP. Receiver operating char-acteristic plots to evaluate Guthrie, Wallac, and Isolab pheny-lalanine kit performance for newborn phenylketonuria screening. Clin Chem 1997;43:1838–1842.

169. Sibai B, Meis PJ, Klebanoff M et al, Maternal Fetal Medicine Units Network of the National Institute of Child Health and Human Development. Plasma CRH measurement at 16 to 20 weeks' gestation does not predict preterm delivery in women at high-risk for preterm delivery. Am J Obstet Gynecol 2005;193:1181–1186.

170. Berkowitz GS, Lapinski RH, Lockwood CJ, Florio P, Blackmore-Prince C, Petraglia F. Corticotropin-releasing factor and its binding protein: maternal serum levels in term and preterm deliveries. Am J Obstet Gynecol 1996;174: 1477–1483.

171. Holzman C, Jetton J, Siler-Khodr T, Fisher R, Rip T. Second trimester corticotropin-releasing hormone levels in relation to preterm delivery and ethnicity. Obstet Gynecol 2001;97: 657–663.

172. McLean M, Bisits A, Davies J et al. Predicting risk of preterm delivery by second-trimester measurement of maternal plasma corticotropin-releasing hormone and alpha-fetoprotein concentrations. Am J Obstet Gynecol 1999; 181:207–215.

173. Leung TN, Chung TK, Madsen G, McLean M, Chang AM, Smith R. Elevated mid-trimester maternal corticotrophin-releasing hormone levels in pregnancies that delivered before 34 weeks. Br J Obstet Gynaecol 1999;106:1041–1046.

174. Inder WJ, Prickett TC, Ellis MJ et al. The utility of plasma CRH as a predictor of preterm delivery. J Clin Endocrinol Metab 2001;86:5706–5710.

175. Coleman MA, France JT, Schellenberg JC et al. Corticotropin-releasing hormone, corticotropin-releasing hormone-binding protein, and activin A in maternal serum: prediction of preterm delivery and response to glucocorticoids in women with symptoms of preterm labor. Am J Obstet Gynecol 2000;183:643–648.

176. Heine RP, McGregor JA, Goodwin TM et al. Serial salivary estriol to detect an increased risk of preterm birth. Obstet Gynecol 2000;96:490–497.

177. McGregor JA, Jackson GM, Lachelin GC et al. Salivary estriol as risk assessment for preterm labor: a prospective trial. Am J Obstet Gynecol 1995;173:1337–1342.

178. Turan OM, Turan S, Funai EF, Buhimschi IA, Copel JA, Buhimschi CS. Fetal adrenal gland volume: a novel method to identify women at risk for impending preterm birth. Obstet Gynecol 2007;109:855–862.

179. Garfield RE, Saade G, Buhimschi CS et al. Control and assess-ment of the uterus and cervix during pregnancy and labour. Hum Reprod Update 1998;4:673–695.

180. Lockwood CJ, Ghidini A, Wein R, Lapinski R, Casal D, Berkowitz RL. Increased interleukin-6 concentrations in cer-vical secretions are associated with preterm delivery. Am J Obstet Gynecol 1994;171:1097–1010.

181. Goepfert AR, Goldenberg RL, Andrews WW et al, National Institute of Child Health and Human Development Maternal-Fetal Medicine Units Network. The Preterm Prediction Study: association between cervical interleukin 6 concentration and spontaneous preterm birth. National Institute of Child Health and Human Development Maternal-Fetal Medicine Units Network. Am J Obstet Gynecol 2001;184:483–488.

182. Trebeden H, Goffinet F, Kayem G et al. Strip test for bedside detection of interleukin-6 in cervical secretions is predictive for impending preterm delivery. Eur Cytokine Netw 2001;12:359–360.

183. Kurkinen-Raty M, Ruokonen A, Vuopala S et al. Combination of cervical interleukin-6 and -8, phosphorylated insulin-like growth factor-binding protein-1 and transvaginal cervical ultrasonography in assessment of the risk of preterm birth. Br J Obstet Gynaecol 2001;108:875–881.

184. Coleman MA, Keelan JA, McCowan LM, Townend KM, Mitchell MD. Predicting preterm delivery: comparison of cer-vicovaginal interleukin (IL)-1β, IL-6 and IL-8 with fetal fibronectin and cervical dilatation. Eur J Obstet Gynecol Reprod Biol 2001;95:154–158.

185. Lange M, Chen FK, Wessel J, Buscher U, Dudenhausen JW. Elevation of interleukin-6 levels in cervical secretions as a

predictor of preterm delivery. Acta Obstet Gynecol Scand 2003;82:326–329.

186. Rizzo G, Capponi A, Vlachopoulou A, Angelini E, Grassi C, Romanini C. The diagnostic value of interleukin-8 and fetal fibronectin concentrations in cervical secretions in patients with preterm labor and intact membranes. J Perinat Med 1997;25:461–468.

187. Goldenberg RL, Andrews WW, Guerrant RL et al. The Preterm Prediction Study: cervical lactoferrin concentration, other markers of lower genital tract infection, and preterm birth. National Institute of Child Health and Human Development Maternal-Fetal Medicine Units Network. Am J Obstet Gynecol 2000;182:631–635.

188. Andrews WW, Tsao J, Goldenberg RL et al. The Preterm Prediction Study: failure of midtrimester cervical sialidase level elevation to predict subsequent spontaneous preterm birth. Am J Obstet Gynecol 1999;180:1151–1154.

189. Wang EY, Woodruff TK, Moawad A. Follistatin-free activin A is not associated with preterm birth. Am J Obstet Gynecol 2002;186:464–469.

190. Moawad AH, Goldenberg RL, Mercer B et al. The Preterm Prediction Study: the value of serum alkaline phosphatase, alpha-fetoprotein, plasma corticotropin-releasing hormone, and other serum markers for the prediction of spontaneous preterm birth. Am J Obstet Gynecol 2002;186:990–996.

191. Simhan HN, Caritis SN, Krohn MA, Hillier SL. Elevated vaginal pH and neutrophils are associated strongly with early spontaneous preterm birth. Am J Obstet Gynecol 2003; 189:1150–1154.

192. Simhan HN, Caritis SN, Krohn MA, Hillier SL. The vaginal inflammatory milieu and the risk of early premature preterm rupture of membranes. Am J Obstet Gynecol 2005;192: 213–218.

193. Buhimschi CS, Baumbusch MA, Campbell KH, Dulay AT, Buhimschi IA. Insight into innate immunity of the uterine cervix as a host defense mechanism against infection and preterm birth. Expert Rev Obstet Gynecol 2009;4:9–15.

194. Klein LL, Jonscher KR, Heerwagen MJ, Gibbs RS, McManaman JL. Shotgun proteomic analysis of vaginal fluid from women in late pregnancy. Reprod Sci 2008;15:263–273.

195. Shaw JL, Smith CR, Diamandis EP. Proteomic analysis of human cervico-vaginal fluid. J Proteome Res 2007;6: 2859–2865.

196. Pereira L, Reddy AP, Jacob T et al. Identification of novel protein biomarkers of preterm birth in human cervical-vaginal fluid. J Proteome Res 2007;6:1269–1276.

197. Hitti J, Lapidus JA, Lu X et al. Noninvasive diagnosis of intraamniotic infection: proteomic biomarkers in vaginal fluid. Am J Obstet Gynecol 2010;203:32.

198. Buhimschi IA, Buhimschi CS, Weiner CP et al. Proteomic but not enzyme-linked immunosorbent assay technology detects amniotic fluid monomeric calgranulins from their complexed calprotectin form. Clin Diagn Lab Immunol 2005;12: 837–844.

199. Gabay C, Kushner I. Acute-phase proteins and other systemic responses to inflammation. N Engl J Med 1999;340:448–454.

200. Rüetschi U, Rosén A, Karlsson G et al. Proteomic analysis using protein chips to detect biomarkers in cervical and amniotic fluid in women with intra-amniotic inflammation. J Proteome Res 2005;4:2236–2242.

201. Buhimschi IA, Christner R, Buhimschi CS. Proteomic bio-marker analysis of amniotic fluid for identification of intra-amniotic inflammation. Br J Obstet Gynaecol 2005; 112:173–181.

202. Gravett MG, Novy MJ, Rosenfeld RG et al. Diagnosis of intra-amniotic infection by proteomic profiling and identification of novel biomarkers. JAMA 2004;292:462–469.

203. Buhimschi CS, Bhandari V, Hamar BD et al. Proteomic profiling of the amniotic fluid to detect inflammation, infection, and neonatal sepsis. PLoS Med 2007;4:e18.

204. Rosen T, Kuczynski E, O'Neill LM, Funai EF, Lockwood CJ. Plasma levels of thrombin–antithrombin complexes predict preterm premature rupture of the fetal membranes. J Matern Fetal Med 2001;10:297–300.

205. Elovitz MA, Baron J, Phillippe M. The role of thrombin in preterm parturition. Am J Obstet Gynecol 2001;185: 1059–1063.

206. Chaiworapongsa T, Espinoza J, Yoshimatsu J et al. Activation of coagulation system in preterm labor and preterm premature rupture of membranes. J Matern Fetal Neonatal Med 2002;11:368–373.

207. Lockwood CJ, Senyei AE, Dische MR et al. Fetal fibronectin in cervical and vaginal secretions as a predictor of preterm delivery. N Engl J Med 1991;325:669–674.

208. Feinberg RF, Kliman HJ, Lockwood CJ. Is oncofetal fibronectin a trophoblast glue for human implantation? Am J Pathol 1991;138:537–543.

209. Peaceman AM, Andrews WW, Thorp JM et al. Fetal fibronectin as a predictor of preterm birth in patients with symptoms: a multicenter trial. Am J Obstet Gynecol 1997;177:13–18.

210. Honest H, Bachmann LM, Gupta JK, Kleijnen J, Khan KS. Accuracy of cervicovaginal fetal fibronectin test in predicting risk of spontaneous preterm birth: systematic review. BMJ 2002;325:301–304.

211. Sanchez-Ramos L, Delke I, Zamora J, Kaunitz AM. Fetal fibronectin as a short-term predictor of preterm birth in symptomatic patients: a meta-analysis. Obstet Gynecol 2009;114:631–640.

212. Lockwood CJ, Wein R, Lapinski R et al. The presence of cervical and vaginal fetal fibronectin predicts preterm delivery in an inner-city obstetric population. Am J Obstet Gynecol 1993;169:798–804.

213. Goldenberg RL, Mercer BM, Meis PJ, Copper RL, Das A, McNellis D. The Preterm Prediction Study: fetal fibronectin testing and spontaneous preterm birth. NICHD Maternal Fetal Medicine Units Network. Obstet Gynecol 1996;87: 643–648.

214. Goldenberg RL, Iams JD, Miodovnik M et al. The Preterm Prediction Study: risk factors in twin gestations. National Institute of Child Health and Human Development Maternal-Fetal Medicine Units Network. Am J Obstet Gynecol 1996;175:1047–1053.

215. Roman AS, Rebarber A, Sfakianaki AK et al. Vaginal fetal fibronectin as a predictor of spontaneous preterm delivery in the patient with cervical cerclage. Am J Obstet Gynecol 2003;189:1368–1373.

216. Roman AS, Rebarber A, Lipkind H, Mulholland J, Minior V, Roshan D. Vaginal fetal fibronectin as a predictor of spontaneous preterm delivery after multifetal pregnancy reduction. Am J Obstet Gynecol 2004;190:142–146.

217. Roman AS, Koklanaris N, Paidas MJ, Mulholland J, Levitz M, Rebarber A. "Blind" vaginal fetal fibronectin as a predictor of spontaneous preterm delivery. Obstet Gynecol 2005;105: 285–289.

218. Audibert F, Fortin S, Delvin E et al. Contingent use of fetal fibronectin testing and cervical length measurement in women with preterm labour. J Obstet Gynaecol Can 2010;32:307–312.

219. Iams JD, Goldenberg RL, Meis PJ et al. The length of the cervix and the risk of spontaneous premature delivery. National Institute of Child Health and Human Development Maternal Fetal Medicine Unit Network. N Engl J Med 1996;334:567–572.

220. Iams JD. Prediction and early detection of preterm labor. Obstet Gynecol 2003;10:402–412.

221. Tsoi E, Akmal S, Rane S, Otigbah C, Nicolaides KH. Ultrasound assessment of cervical length in threatened preterm labor. Ultrasound Obstet Gynecol 2003;21:552–555.

222. Vendittelli F, Volumenie J. Transvaginal ultrasonography examination of the uterine cervix in hospitalised women undergoing preterm labour. Eur J Obstet Gynecol Reprod Biol 2000;90:3–11.

223. Iams JD, Johnson FF, Sonek J, Sachs L, Gebauer C, Samuels P. Cervical competence as a continuum: a study of ultrasonographic cervical length and obstetric performance. Am J Obstet Gynecol 1995;172:1097–1103.

224. Owen J, Yost N, Berghella V et al. National Institute of Child Health and Human Development, Maternal-Fetal Medicine Units Network. Mid-trimester endovaginal sonography in women at high risk for spontaneous preterm birth. JAMA 2001;286:1340–1348.

225. Taipale P, Hiilesmaa V. Sonographic measurement of uterine cervix at 18–22 weeks' gestation and the risk of preterm delivery. Obstet Gynecol 1998;92:902–907.

226. Iams JD, Goldenberg RL, Mercer BM et al. The Preterm Prediction Study: can low-risk women destined for spontaneous preterm birth be identified? Am J Obstet Gynecol 2001;184:652–655.

227. Hincz P, Wilczynski J, Kozarzewski M, Szaflik K. Two-step test: the combined use of fetal fibronectin and sonographic examination of the uterine cervix for prediction of preterm delivery in symptomatic patients. Acta Obstet Gynecol Scand 2002;81:58–63.

228. Goldenberg RL, Iams JD, Das A et al. The Preterm Prediction Study: sequential cervical length and fetal fibronectin testing for the prediction of spontaneous preterm birth. National Institute of Child Health and Human Development Maternal-Fetal Medicine Units Network. Am J Obstet Gynecol 2000;182:636–643.

Chapter 43
Preterm Premature Rupture of Membranes

Brian M. Mercer

Department of Reproductive Biology, Case Western Reserve University and MetroHealth Medical Center, Cleveland, OH, USA

Rupture of fetal membranes before the onset of labor (premature rupture of membranes, PROM) complicates 8–10% of pregnancies, and is responsible for nearly one-third of preterm births. PROM, especially preterm PROM (PPROM), has been associated with brief latency from membrane rupture to delivery, an increased risk of chorioamnionitis, and umbilical cord compression. As such, PPROM is associated with increased risk of perinatal complications. An understanding of gestational age-dependent risks of delivery, the risks and potential benefits of conservative management, and opportunities to reduce complications of preterm birth will help clinicians improve outcomes after this frequent pregnancy complication.

Mechanisms

Spontaneous membrane rupture at term results from progressive weakening of the membranes because of collagen remodeling and cellular apoptosis, and from increased intrauterine pressure with uterine contractions when membrane rupture occurs subsequent to the onset of labor. While PPROM near term likely results in many cases from these same physiologic processes, PPROM remote from term has been associated with several pathologic processes, especially infection and inflammation. Reported clinical risk factors predisposing to intrauterine infection, inflammation, membrane stretch, and local tissue hypoxia have included low socio-economic status, maternal undernutrition, cigarette smoking, uterine bleeding and work in pregnancy, cervical cerclage, prior preterm labor and acute pulmonary disease in the current pregnancy, and bacterial vaginosis in addition to other urogenital infections [1–6]. It has been proposed that there could be a genetic predisposition to PPROM in some women, either through inheritance of polymorphisms for proinflammatory cytokines and matrix metalloproteinases [7,8] or through heritable connective tissue disorders of collagen metabolism.

Among the strongest risk factors for PPROM is a history of preterm birth in a previous gestation, particularly one resulting from PPROM (odds ratio [OR] 3.3–6.3) [6]. The role of ascending infection in the pathogenesis of PPROM is particularly plausible as bacterial proteases (collagenases and phospholipases) can cause membrane weakening. Ascending bacterial colonization can also cause a maternal inflammatory response including production of cytokines, prostaglandins, and metalloproteinases locally which cause membrane degradation and weakening. Preterm contractions can lead to separation of the amnion and choriodecidua with an overall reduction in membrane tensile strength [9] while cervical dilation can result in exposure of the membranes to vaginal microorganisms and reduce underlying tissue support.

Prediction and prevention

Although the above-mentioned clinical risk factors have been associated with PPROM, most women with these characteristics do not develop PPROM and the majority of women with PPROM lack these risk factors. This has led to interest in ancillary testing for prediction of PPROM. Both short cervical length on transvaginal ultrasound (less than 25 mm; relative risk [RR] 3.2) and the presence of fetal fibronectin (fFN) in cervicovaginal secretions (RR 2.5) in the later second trimester are associated with an increased risk of preterm birth resulting from PPROM [6]. However, like clinical risk factors, these modalities also fail to identify the majority of women destined to have PPROM and are not recommended as routine screening tests for low-risk women.

Women suffering PPROM are at increased risk for recurrence in a future pregnancy. While general guidance directed against factors associated with spontaneous

Queenan's Management of High-Risk Pregnancy: An Evidence-Based Approach, Sixth Edition. Edited by John T. Queenan, Catherine Y. Spong, Charles J. Lockwood.

preterm birth (e.g. adequate nutrition, smoking cessation, avoidance of heavy lifting and prolonged standing without breaks, early treatment of urogenital infections) may reduce the risk of PPROM, direct benefit from these has not been demonstrated. Identification and treatment of sexually transmitted urogenital infections such as *Chlamydia trachomatis* and *Neisseria gonorrhoeae* can reduce the risks of PROM and preterm birth. While treatment of symptomatic bacterial vaginosis and *Trichomonas vaginalis* infection is appropriate, treatment of women with asymptomatic vaginal infections is controversial and may even promote preterm birth [10,11].

Antenatal treatment with 17-hydroxyprogesterone caproate therapy has been demonstrated to be effective in reducing the risk of recurrent spontaneous preterm birth due to preterm labor or PPROM [12]. In this multicenter trial, authors found 17-hydroxyprogesterone caproate treatment (250 mg given intramuscularly each week through 36 weeks of gestation) to reduce the risk of recurrent preterm birth (RR 0.66, 95% confidence interval [95% CI] 0.54–0.81) and spontaneous preterm birth (RR 0.65, 95% CI 0.51–0.83), potentially resulting in fewer newborn complications. Nightly vaginal progesterone suppository (100 mg) treatment has also been shown to prevent preterm birth in women with incidentally discovered short cervices but treatment with progesterone gel is apparently not effective in other high-risk women [13,14]. Alternatively, though vitamin C deficiency has been linked to PPROM, data are conflicting regarding the potential risks and benefits of treatment with vitamin C supplementation and this treatment is not recommended to prevent recurrent PPROM [15–17].

Diagnosis

Diagnosis of membrane rupture is best made by sterile speculum examination of women presenting with a suspicious clinical history or who are found to have oligohydramnios on ultrasonography. Evident fluid passing through the cervical os is diagnostic. An alkaline vaginal pH (>6.0–6.5) with Nitrazine paper and the presence of a "ferning" pattern on microscopic examination of dried secretions obtained from the vaginal side wall are supportive when visual inspection is equivocal. These tests are subject to false-positive findings because of the presence of cervical mucus, blood, semen, alkaline antiseptics, or bacterial vaginosis, and can be falsely negative with prolonged leakage and oligohydramnios. Repeat speculum examination after prolonged bedrest may provide needed diagnostic information if initial testing is negative despite a suspicious history. In the absence of fetal growth restriction or urogenital abnormalities, ultrasound evidence of oligohydramnios is suggestive but not diagnostic of membrane rupture. The diagnosis can be confirmed

unequivocally by indigo carmine amnio-infusion with observation for passage of dye *per vaginam*.

Although a variety of substances, including fFN, α-fetoprotein, total T4 and free T4, prolactin, human chorionic gonadotropin, interleukin-6, placental α-microglobulin (PAMG)-1, and insulin-like growth factor-binding protein (IGFBP)-1, among others, have been evaluated for their ability to assist in the diagnosis of membrane rupture, these have not generally been studied for their diagnostic ability among women in whom the diagnosis of membrane rupture remains unclear after clinical examination. Further, some of these markers do not require membrane rupture to be found in cervico-vaginal secretions [18–20]. In a comparative study of two rapid tests, PAMG-1 identified lower concentrations of amniotic fluid than IGFBP-1 [21]. PAMG-1 in cervicovaginal secretions can confirm PROM in nearly 99% of cases where the diagnosis is evident on traditional testing [18]. But it has also been found to be positive among 30.9% of laboring women and in 4.8% of nonlaboring women without suspected membrane rupture, raising questions regarding its utility when membrane rupture is not clinically evident [22]. For these reasons, routine testing with these markers is not recommended until their clinical value is clarified.

Clinical course

Brief latency from membrane rupture to delivery, increased risk of intrauterine and neonatal infection, and oligohydramnios have been considered hallmarks of PPROM. Each can affect pregnancy outcomes, and each has implications regarding clinical management of women with PPROM.

While it is true that mean and median latency from membrane rupture to delivery increase with decreasing gestational age at membrane rupture, the clinical importance of this finding is overstated. The likelihood that a conservatively managed woman with PPROM at 24–31 weeks will deliver within 1 week is approximately 50%.[23]. Approximately one-quarter of those with membrane rupture near the limit of viability will remain pregnant for 1 month or more. Alternatively, those with PROM at or near term are rarely given the opportunity to remain pregnant for an extended time and the natural labor process can be anticipated to occur in over 90% of women within about 24 h. Benefits of conservative management include additional time for induction of fetal pulmonary maturity and prevention of intraventricular hemorrhage through administration of antenatal corticosteroids (24–48 h latency required), and reduction of gestational age-dependent morbidity through extended latency (more than approximately 1 week latency required).

Chorioamnionitis complicates 13–60% of pregnancies with PROM, and is increasingly common with decreasing gestational age at membrane rupture [24]. Abruptio placentae, amnionitis, and endometritis complicate 4–12%, 13–60%, and 2–13% of pregnancies, respectively, when membrane rupture occurs remote from term [24–28]. Amniotic fluid cultures from amniocentesis specimens are positive in 25–35% of asymptomatic women after PPROM [29]. Maternal sepsis is uncommon (approximately 1%) but is a serious complication of PROM remote from term. Conservative management of PROM at any gestational age increases the risk of chorioamnionitis. Fetal demise after PPROM is believed to result in most cases from umbilical cord compression. Fetal infection, placental abruption, and umbilical cord prolapse can also lead to fetal death. Overall, fetal death complicates approximately 1–2% of pregnancies conservatively managed after PPROM. This risk increases in the face of chorioamnionitis, and when PROM occurs near the limit of potential viability (periviable).

Therefore, expeditious delivery should be considered if the fetus is considered to be at low risk for gestational age-dependent morbidity, if antenatal corticosteroids are not going to be administered when only brief pregnancy prolongation is anticipated, or after antenatal corticosteroid treatment has been completed if continued attempts to extend latency more than approximately 1 week are not planned.

Evaluation

In general, women with PROM at term do not require additional specific evaluations unless additional complications occur. Initial evaluation of the woman presenting with PPROM includes (Box 43.1):
• maternal uterine activity and fetal heart rate monitoring for labor, umbilical cord compression, and for fetal well-being if the limit of potential viability has been reached
• clinical assessment for chorioamnionitis (fever ≥38.0°C [100.4°F] with uterine tenderness, maternal or fetal tachycardia, vaginal discharge)
• ultrasound to confirm gestational age and to identify fetal malformations associated with PROM and oligohydramnios if not previously performed, to determine fetal presentation, and to estimate fetal weight and amniotic fluid volume.
Digital cervical examination should be avoided if possible until the diagnosis of PPROM has been excluded or a decision to deliver has been made. Digital examination in this setting shortens latency and increases the risk of chorioamnionitis while adding little information over that obtained by visual examination [30]. Cervical cultures for *Neisseria gonorrhoeae* and *Chlamydia trachomatis*,

---

Box 43.1 Considerations for initial evaluation of the woman with preterm premature rupture of membranes

• Maternal uterine activity monitoring for labor
• Fetal heart rate monitoring for umbilical cord compression (and fetal well-being if the limit of viability has been reached)
• Clinical assessment for chorioamnionitis
• Ultrasound to confirm gestational age, estimate fetal growth, and amniotic fluid volume, identify fetal malformations associated with PROM/oligohydramnios if not previously carried out, and to determine fetal presentation
• Visual inspection of cervical dilation and effacement if not in active labor
• Cervical cultures for *Neisseria gonorrhoeae* and *Chlamydia trachomatis* if not recently performed
• Anovaginal culture for group B streptococcus if not recently performed
• Urinalysis with urine culture if not recently performed
• Baseline maternal blood white blood cell
• Vaginal pool or ultrasound-guided amniocentesis sampling for fetal pulmonary maturity at 32–33 weeks' gestation

PROM, premature rupture of membranes.

Box 43.2 Adjuncts to the evaluation of the woman with equivocal findings of intraamniotic infection

• Maternal blood white blood cell count: rising values and a value above 16,000/mm³ are supportive of the diagnosis if antenatal corticosteroids not administered within 5–7 days
• Ultrasound-guided amniocentesis: positive culture considered abnormal
• Positive gram stain supportive but may be falsely positive as a result of contamination
• White blood cell count ≥30 cells/μL considered abnormal
• Glucose concentration <16–20 mg/dL considered abnormal

---

anovaginal culture for group B β-hemolytic streptococci (GBS), and urinalysis with urine culture should be considered if not recently performed.

If the diagnosis of chorioamnionitis is suspected but not clear, maternal blood white blood cell (WBC) count and ultrasound-guided amniocentesis can sometimes be helpful (Box 43.2). A maternal blood WBC count above 16,000/mm³ is supportive of suspicious clinical findings. It is helpful to obtain a baseline blood WBC count on presentation after PPROM to be used during initial assessment and for subsequent comparison if needed during conservative management. It is important to remember that there is significant variation in WBC count between patients, and that the WBC count is elevated in pregnancy and for 5–7 days after administration of antenatal corticosteroids. As such, this test should not be used in isolation. Amniotic fluid gram stain, WBC count (≥30 cells/µL considered abnormal), and glucose concentration (less than 16–20 mg/dL considered abnormal) can also provide rapid supportive information regarding the presence of intraamniotic infection [31,32]. Elevated amniotic fluid and vaginal fluid cytokine levels have also been associated with intrauterine infection after PPROM; however, tests for these markers are not generally available for clinical use. Amniotic fluid culture for aerobic and anaerobic bacteria and for mycoplasma can be helpful, but results are generally not available before a management decision is needed.

Management

Delivery after PPROM is mandated by the presence of clinical chorioamnionitis, nonreassuring fetal testing, significant vaginal bleeding, and advanced labor (Box 43.3). In the absence of these conditions, conservative management may be appropriate. If conservative management of the patient with PPROM is being considered, initial extended monitoring followed by intermittent monitoring at least daily is appropriate if testing remains reassuring. Biophysical profile testing can be helpful if fetal heart rate testing is nonreactive. A nonreactive fetal heart rate or a nonreassuring biophysical profile score can be a sign of intrauterine infection, particularly if testing had previously been reassuring [33,34]. In the stable patient, gestational age is important in determining whether conservative management or expeditious delivery should be pursued [29].

Intrapartum GBS prophylaxis should be given to women with a recent (less than 6 weeks) positive anovaginal GBS culture regardless of intervening antibiotic treatments [35]. Intrapartum GBS prophylaxis should also be given to women delivering preterm without a recent anovaginal recent culture result, to all women with GBS bacteriuria at any time in the current pregnancy, and to all women with a previously affected infant regardless of culture results in the current pregnancy.

Preterm premature rupture of membranes near term (34–36w 6d)

Infants born after PROM near term (34–36w 6d) have a relatively low risk of serious morbidity and antenatal corticosteroids are not generally recommended for fetal maturation at this gestation. Although there are risks of neonatal morbidity at this gestation, these risks are not likely to be reduced with the relatively brief latency anticipated at this gestation, and the risks related to intrauterine infection and umbilical cord compression outweigh the potential benefits of conservative management [36,37]. Because of these factors, women with PPROM at 34–36w 6d are best treated by delivery.

Premature rupture of membranes near term (32–33w 6d)

When PROM occurs at 32–33w 6d gestation, fetal pulmonary maturity should be assessed from amniotic fluid collected from the vaginal pool or by amniocentesis if feasible. From either site, a Foam Stability Index ≥47, phosphatidyl glycerol positive, lecithin:sphingomyelin (L:S) ratio ≥2:1, or uncentrifuged lamellar body count (LBC) ≥50,000/µL can be considered indicative of fetal pulmonary maturity [38–42]. The L:S ratio results may be falsely immature in the presence of blood or meconium contamination, although the presence of a mature ratio should lead to consideration of delivery. Unfortunately, the L:S ratio is difficult to perform. The LBC can be altered by either blood or meconium contamination and should not be relied upon if either is present. Vaginal pool specimens should not be analyzed if there is evident mucus as it can obstruct counter channels. Should centrifugation be performed, an LBC cut-off of 30,000/µL has been suggested to be predictive of pulmonary maturity [43,44]. If a mature fetal pulmonary profile is obtained, expeditious delivery should be considered in accordance with the recommendations for PROM at 34–36w 6d as these infants are at low risk for complications of prematurity and conservative management increases the risk of infectious morbidity [37]. If testing reveals an immature pulmonary profile or if fluid cannot be obtained, in the absence of chorioamnionitis, induction of fetal pulmonary maturation with antenatal corticosteroids followed by delivery at 24–48h or at 34 weeks' gestation is recommended. If after antenatal corticosteroid administration the patient is ≥33 weeks' gestation, it is unlikely that further delay of delivery to 34 weeks will result in substantial reduction in infant morbidities. Delivery is recommended before complications ensue. If conservative management is pursued, evaluation and treatment should be as described below for PROM at 23–31w 6d.

Premature rupture of membranes remote from term (23–31w 6d)

Delivery at 23–31w 6d gestation is associated with significant risks of neonatal morbidity and mortality resulting from prematurity. These women are generally best served by conservative inpatient management after PPROM to prolong pregnancy and reduce gestational age-dependent morbidity in the absence of chorioamnionitis, placental abruption, advanced labor, or nonreassuring fetal testing. Because the latency is frequently brief and clinical findings can change over a short period of time, transfer to a tertiary care facility before acute complications occur should be considered if adequate facilities are not available at the initial institution.

During conservative management, patients should have at least daily assessment for evidence of labor,

Box 43.3 Options for management of the woman with preterm premature rupture of membranes according to gestational age at membrane rupture

PROM near term (34–36w 6d)*

- Expeditious delivery, by labor induction or cesarean delivery as indicated
- Intrapartum GBS prophylaxis **
- Broad-spectrum intrapartum antibiotics for suspected chorioamnionitis

PROM near term (32–33w 6d)*

- Expeditious delivery, by labor induction or cesarean delivery as indicated, if fetal pulmonary maturity evident on sampling from the vaginal pool or by amniocentesis
- Antenatal corticosteroids for fetal maturation if amniotic fluid testing reveals an immature profile or if fluid unavailable, followed by:
  - delivery 24–48h after antenatal corticosteroids if ≥33 weeks' gestation
  or
  - delivery 24–48 hours after antenatal corticosteroids or at 34 weeks if <33 weeks' gestation (if conservatively managed, treat as described for PROM at 23–31w 6d)
- Intrapartum GBS prophylaxis **
- Broad-spectrum intrapartum antibiotics for suspected chorioamnionitis

PROM remote from term (23–31w 6d)*

- Conservative inpatient management
- Antenatal corticosteroids for fetal maturation if not previously administered
- Broad-spectrum antibiotics to prolong pregnancy and reduce neonatal morbidity
- Transfer to a tertiary care facility if adequate facilities for neonatal care not available
- At least daily assessment for labor, amnionitis, placental abruption, and fetal well-being
- Leg exercises, antiembolic stockings, and/or prophylactic heparin

- Fetal growth assessment by ultrasound every 3–4 weeks
- Tocolytic therapy for labor can be given but should not be administered if there is suspicion of intrauterine infection, fetal compromise, or placental abruption
- Consider elective delivery at 34 weeks' gestation if remains pregnant to this time
- Intrapartum GBS prophylaxis **
- Broad-spectrum intrapartum antibiotics for suspected chorioamnionitis

Previable PROM (<23 weeks)

- Counsel regarding:
  - potential for previable, periviable, and preterm birth
  - impact of oligohydramnios on pulmonary development and risk of lethal pulmonary hypoplasia and restriction deformities
  - risks of adverse fetal, neonatal, and long-term infant outcomes with early preterm birth
  - risks of maternal morbidities with conservative management
- Deliver by labor induction or dilation and evacuation according to individual circumstances
  or
- Manage conservatively with:
  - initial evaluation for intrauterine infection, labor, fetal death, or placental abruption
  - strict pelvic rest and modified bed/couch rest
  - serial ultrasound for fetal pulmonary growth and amniotic fluid volume with additional counseling as appropriate for persistent oligohydramnios or suspected pulmonary hypoplasia
  - serial ultrasound for fetal weight and pulmonary growth, and amniotic fluid volume
  - broad-spectrum antibiotics to prolong pregnancy and reduce neonatal morbidity may be helpful but no specific data are available for this gestational age
  - treat as for PROM at 23–31w 6d once the limit of viability has been reached

GBS, group B streptococcus; PROM, premature rupture of membranes.
*Delivery is mandated by the presence of chorioamnionitis, nonreassuring fetal testing/fetal death, significant vaginal bleeding, and for advanced labor.
**Once the limit of viability has been reached, intrapartum GBS prophylaxis should be given to women with a recent positive anovaginal GBS culture regardless of intervening antibiotic treatments. Intrapartum GBS prophylaxis should also be given to women delivering preterm without a recent anovaginal culture result, to all women with GBS bacteriuria at any time in the current pregnancy, and to all women with a previously affected infant regardless of culture results in the current pregnancy.

chorioamnionitis, placental abruption, and fetal well-being. Leg exercises, antiembolic stockings, and/or prophylactic doses of subcutaneous heparin may be of value in preventing thromboembolic complications. Fetal growth should be assessed with ultrasound every 3–4 weeks. Although the extent of oligohydramnios is inversely related to latency, low amniotic fluid volume is an inaccurate predictor of latency and neonatal outcome,

and should not be used to determine clinical management other than as a tool to confirm resealing of the membranes with restoration of a normal Amniotic Fluid Index. The patient who remains stable is generally delivered at 34 weeks' gestation because of the ongoing but low risk of fetal loss with conservative management and the high likelihood of survival without long-term complications after delivery at this gestational age.

Several adjunctive therapies have been proposed during conservative management of PROM remote from term. A single course of antenatal corticosteroids for fetal maturation is recommended to reduce the risks of neonatal respiratory distress and intraventricular hemorrhage, without increasing the risk of neonatal infection [45,46]. Either 12 mg betamethasone IM every 24 h for two doses, or 6 mg dexamethasone IM every 12 h for four doses is appropriate. Broad-spectrum antibiotic therapy should be administered to treat or prevent ascending subclinical decidual infection in order to prolong pregnancy, and to reduce neonatal infectious and gestational age-dependent morbidity [46–48]. Intravenous therapy (48 h) with ampicillin (2 g IV every 6 h) and erythromycin (250 mg IV every 6 h) followed by limited-duration oral therapy (5 days) with amoxicillin (250 mg PO every 8 h) and enteric-coated erythromycin base (333 mg PO every 8 h) has been recommended by the National Institute of Child Health and Human Development and the Maternal Fetal Medicine Units (NICHD-MFMU) Network. Therapy for shorter periods has not been studied with adequate numbers, has not been shown to offer equivalent neonatal benefits [49,50], and is not recommended.

Recent shortages have led to the need for substitution of alternative antibiotic agents. Oral ampicillin, erythromycin, and azithromycin are likely appropriate substitutions for the above agents, as needed. The optimal broad-spectrum therapy for women who are penicillin allergic has not been determined. The Oracle trial [51] has suggested that single-agent erythromycin may be appropriate, and has also raised concern that broad-spectrum amoxicillin-clavulanate therapy might increase the risk of necrotizing enterocolitis. This latter finding is not consistent with the NICHD-MFMU trial in which broad-spectrum antibiotic therapy in a higher risk population reduced the risk of stage 2–3 necrotizing enterocolitis [47]. Of note, despite conflicting results from a concurrent study of antibiotics for preterm labor with intact membranes, the Oracle trial for women with PPROM revealed no increases or decreases in long-term morbidities at 7 years for infants exposed to antepartum antibiotics [52].

Management of GBS carriers after the initial 7 days of antibiotic therapy has not been well studied. Options include:
- subsequent intrapartum prophylaxis only
- continued narrow-spectrum GBS prophylaxis from completion of the initial 7-day course through delivery, or
- follow-up anovaginal culture after completion of the 7-day course, with continued narrow-spectrum therapy against GBS until delivery for those with persistently positive cultures.

Regardless of antepartum antibiotic treatments, intrapartum prophylaxis should be given to all known GBS carriers.

Tocolytic therapy for women with PPROM has been shown to reduce the likelihood of delivery at 24–48 h in some studies [53–56]. However, such treatment has not been shown to improve neonatal outcomes. Tocolytic therapy should not be administered after PPROM if there is suspicion of intrauterine infection, fetal compromise, or placental abruption. Further study is needed regarding tocolytic therapy after PPROM.

Previable premature rupture of membranes (less than 23 weeks)

Preterm premature rupture of membranes before the limit of viability (currently 23 weeks' gestation) is particularly concerning as it can lead to previable delivery with no potential for survival, periviable delivery near the limit of viability where the majority of survivors are at risk for acute and long-term complications, or to delivery after extended latency with pulmonary hypoplasia and restriction deformities resulting from severe oligohydramnios at the time of critical pulmonary and skeletal development. Alternatively, some conservatively managed patients will have extended latency with survival of a healthy infant, and some may have spontaneous resealing of the membranes with reaccumulation of amniotic fluid.

Gestational age should be estimated based on the earliest available ultrasound and menstrual history. These patients should be counseled realistically regarding potential fetal and neonatal outcomes after early preterm birth [29]. The risk of stillbirth during conservative management and delivery is approximately 15%. Most of these pregnancies will deliver before or near the limit of viability, where neonatal death is either assured or common. The risk of long-term sequelae will depend on the gestational age at delivery. Persistent oligohydramnios is a prognostic indicator of poor outcomes after PROM before 20 weeks, with a high risk of lethal pulmonary hypoplasia regardless of extended latency. Conservative management is also associated with frequent chorioamnionitis (39%), endometritis (14%), retained placenta/postpartum hemorrhage necessitating curettage (12%), and placental abruption (3%).

Should the patient desire delivery after counseling, options for labor induction include high-dose intravenous oxytocin, intravaginal prostaglandin E_2, and oral or intravaginal prostaglandin E_1 (misoprostol) according to clinical circumstances. Dilation and evacuation can be an option for caregivers with experience in this technique. Placement of intracervical laminaria before labor induction or dilation and evacuation may be helpful. Women undergoing conservative management should be initially evaluated for evidence of intrauterine infection, labor, or placental abruption. Although supportive data are lacking, it is prudent to advise the patient managed in an ambulatory setting to pursue strict pelvic rest to reduce the potential for ascending infection and it may be helpful to maintain modified bed or couch rest to enhance the potential for membrane resealing. In the absence of data supporting either approach, inpatient or outpatient monitoring after initial evaluation may be considered appropriate with consideration given to individual clinical circumstances. Serial ultrasound can be helpful to evaluate for persistent oligohydramnios and to estimate fetal pulmonary growth (e.g. measurement of thoracic/abdominal circumference ratio or chest circumference) [57–59]. Information from such testing is useful in counseling and ongoing care of the patient with PROM before the limit of viability.

A number of small studies have evaluated the potential to reseal the fetal membranes after previable PROM. Some techniques have included transabdominal/transcervical amnio-infusion, and Gelfoam or fibrin-platelet-cryoprecipitate instillation [60–62]. Data regarding efficacy and safety of these techniques are too limited at this time to warrant their incorporation into clinical practice.

Once the limit of viability has been reached, many clinicians will admit the patient with PPROM for ongoing bedrest in order to allow early diagnosis and intervention for infection, abruption, labor, and nonreassuring fetal heart rate patterns (see management of PROM at 23–31w 6d above). Administration of antenatal corticosteroids for fetal maturation is appropriate at this time. Women with PROM before the limit of viability have been included in some studies of broad-spectrum antibiotic therapy after PPROM. However, the numbers of these women are too small to know if treatment is effective for this subgroup. It is also unknown if antibiotic administration at the time of readmission at viability will improve pregnancy outcomes for women who have already had a prolonged latency without evident infection.

Special circumstances

Cerclage

Cerclage is a well-described risk factor for PROM [63,64]. When the cerclage is removed after PROM occurs, the risk of perinatal complications is comparable to patients with PROM who had no cerclage [64,65]. Although no individual study has achieved statistical significance, reviews of studies comparing cerclage retention or removal after PPROM suggest a trend towards increased maternal infection with retained cerclage [66–68]. Perhaps more important is that no study has found cerclage retention after PPROM to significantly reduce infant morbidity, and

one study has found increased infection-related neonatal death with cerclage retention. As such, cerclage should generally be removed when PROM occurs. If the cerclage is retained concurrent to antenatal corticosteroid treatment for fetal maturation, broad-spectrum antibiotic administration should be given to reduce the risk of infection and the cerclage should generally be removed after steroid benefit has been achieved (24–48 h).

Herpes simplex virus

Typically, women with active primary or secondary herpes simplex virus (HSV) infection should be delivered expeditiously by cesarean delivery when PROM occurs at or near term. Alternatively, when PROM complicates HSV infection before 32 weeks' gestation and the mother shows no evidence of systemic infection, conservative management may be appropriate [69]. During conservative management, treatment with acyclovir (200 mg PO five times a day or 500 mg IV every 6 h) would be appropriate to reduce viral shedding and the likelihood of recurrences before delivery.

Human immunodeficiency virus

There are not adequate data to make evidence-based recommendations for treatment of the HIV-infected woman with PPROM. Given the poor prognosis of perinatally acquired HIV infection and increasing risk of vertical transmission with increasing duration of membrane rupture, expeditious cesarean delivery is generally recommended when PROM occurs after the limit of fetal viability. Conservative management to prolong pregnancy may be appropriate for selected women with an undetectable titer at the time of PPROM remote from term, but the gestational age limit, risks, and benefits or this approach have not been studied. If conservative management is undertaken, multiagent antiretroviral therapy with serial monitoring of maternal viral load and CD4 counts should be initiated.

Resealing of the membranes

A small number of women will have cessation of leakage with resealing of the membranes, particularly those with PROM after amniocentesis [70,71]. In the absence of data in this regard, we empirically continue inpatient observation for approximately 1 week after cessation of leakage and normalization of the Amniotic Fluid Index to encourage healing of the membrane rupture site. These women are subsequently discharged with instructions for modified bedrest and pelvic rest, and are advised to return should labor, vaginal bleeding, abdominal tenderness or fever, or recurrent membrane rupture ensue.

CASE PRESENTATION

A 23-year-old, gravida 2, para 0101, with singleton gestation, presented at 28 weeks with perineal wetness for approximately 2 h. She denied contractions, abdominal pain, vaginal bleeding, fever, or chills. She had a prior 32-week preterm birth resulting from preterm labor, but no other pregnancy complications. Past medical and allergy histories were negative. Specific clinical findings included temperature 37.2°C, pulse 92 beats/min, respiratory rate 18/min, symphysis-fundal height 27 cm, with no fundal tenderness. A catheterized urine specimen revealed no leukocytes and culture was subsequently negative. Sterile speculum examination revealed moist vaginal side walls but no fluid pool in the posterior fornix. A sterile swab of the vaginal side walls revealed a complex arborized ferning pattern and Nitrazine paper applied to this site turned blue, confirming the clinical suspicion of membrane rupture. Visual inspection suggested a cervix 2 cm dilated and approximately 1.5 cm long. Endocervical swabs for *Neisseria gonorrhoeae* and *Chlamydia trachomatis*, and distal vagina/anal swabs for GBS were obtained. Ultrasound revealed appropriate fetal growth, a longitudinal cephalic lie, and oligohydramnios (Amniotic Fluid Index = 36 mm). The fetal bladder was normal in size and position. There was no evident hydronephrosis. Monitoring revealed a fetal heart rate of 140–150 beats/min with moderate variability, and with intermittent accelerations and no decelerations or contractions. Maternal WBC count was 12,000/mm³.

After counseling regarding the risks of preterm birth at 28 weeks and of conservative management, and the potential benefits of conservative management, antibiotics (NICHD-MFMU protocol) and corticosteroid treatment (12 mg betamethasone IM every 24 h for two doses) were initiated, and neonatology consultation was obtained. The patient was transferred to the antepartum unit after 6 h of reassuring continuous fetal/contraction monitoring, for continued bedrest with bathroom privileges. Daily assessments revealed no clinically evident chorioamnionitis, abruption, or contractions. Fetal testing remained reassuring. Cultures were negative.

On hospital day 23, at 31 weeks' gestation, the patient reported mild lower abdominal cramping. External monitoring revealed irregular brief contractions with moderate variable-type decelerations. Speculum examination revealed umbilical cord at the external os. With the patient in knee–chest position and a vaginal hand elevating the presenting part, the patient was taken for immediate cesarean delivery, resulting in a liveborn infant with Apgar scores of 4 and 7 at 1 and 5 min. Newborn resuscitation and intubation were performed before transfer to the neonatal ICU. Cord blood pH was within normal limits and placental evaluation revealed no chorioamnionitis. The mother was discharged home on postoperative day 4 for outpatient postoperative evaluation and for counseling regarding her risk of recurrent preterm birth. The infant suffered mild respiratory distress syndrome and hyperbilirubinemia requiring phototherapy, but no sepsis or intraventricular hemorrhage, and is gaining weight at 2 weeks of life.

References

1. Skinner SJM, Campos GA, Liggins GC. Collagen content of human amniotic membranes: effect of gestation length and premature rupture. Obstet Gynecol 1981;57:487–489.
2. Lavery JP, Miller CE, Knight RD. The effect of labor on the rheologic response of chorioamniotic membranes. Obstet Gynecol 1982;60:87–92.
3. Taylor J, Garite T. Premature rupture of the membranes before fetal viability. Obstet Gynecol 1984;64:615–620.
4. Naeye RL. Factors that predispose to premature rupture of the fetal membranes. Obstet Gynecol 1992;60:93.
5. Harger JH, Hsing AW, Tuomala RE et al. Risk factors for preterm premature rupture of fetal membranes: a multicenter case–control study. Am J Obstet Gynecol 1990;163:130.
6. Mercer BM, Goldenberg RL, Meis PJ et al. NICHD-MFMU Network. The Preterm Prediction Study: prediction of preterm premature rupture of the membranes using clinical findings and ancillary testing. Am J Obstet Gynecol 2000;183: 738–745.
7. Roberts AK, Monzon-Bordonaba F, van Deerlin PG et al. Association of polymorphism within the promoter of the tumor necrosis factor alpha gene with increased risk of preterm premature rupture of the fetal membranes. Am J Obstet Gynecol 1999;180:1297–1302.
8. Ferrand PE, Parry S, Sammel M et al. A polymorphism in the matrix metalloproteinase-9 promoter is associated with increased risk of preterm premature rupture of membranes in African Americans. Mol Hum Reprod 2002;8:494–501.
9. Strohl A, Kumar D, Novince R et al. Decreased adherence and spontaneous separation of fetal membrane layers – amnion and choriodecidua – a possible part of the normal weakening process. Placenta 2010;31(1):18–24.
10. Klebanoff MA, Carey JC, Hauth JC et al, National Institute of Child Health and Human Development Maternal-Fetal Medicine Units Network. Failure of metronidazole to prevent preterm delivery among pregnant women with asymptomatic Trichomonas vaginalis infection. N Engl J Med 2001;345: 487–493.
11. Carey JC, Klebanoff MA, Hauth JC et al, National Institute of Child Health and Human Development Maternal-Fetal Medicine Units Network. Metronidazole to prevent preterm delivery in pregnant women with asymptomatic bacterial vaginosis. N Engl J Med 2000;342:534–540.

12. Meis PJ, Klebanoff M, Thom E et al, National Institute of Child Health and Human Development Maternal-Fetal Medicine Units Network. Prevention of recurrent preterm delivery by 17 alpha-hydroxyprogesterone caproate. N Engl J Med 2003;348:2379–2385. Erratum in: N Engl J Med 2003;349:1299.

13. Da Fonseca EB, Bittar RE, Carvalho MH, Zugaib M. Prophylactic administration of progesterone by vaginal suppository to reduce the incidence of spontaneous preterm birth in women at increased risk: a randomized placebo-controlled double-blind study. Am J Obstet Gynecol 2003;188:419–424.

14. O'Brien JM, Adair CD, Lewis DF et al. Progesterone vaginal gel for the reduction of recurrent preterm birth: primary results from a randomized, double-blind, placebo-controlled trial. Ultrasound Obstet Gynecol 2007;30:687–696.

15. Spinnato JA, Freire S, Pinto e Silva JL et al. Antioxidant supplementation and premature rupture of the membranes: a planned secondary analysis. Am J Obstet Gynecol 2008;199:433.

16. Mercer BM, Abdelrahim A, Moore RM et al. The impact of vitamin C supplementation in pregnancy and in vitro upon fetal membrane strength and remodeling. Reprod Sci 2010;17:685–695.

17. Casanueva E, Ripoll C, Tolentino M et al. Vitamin C supplementation to prevent premature rupture of the chorioamniotic membranes: a randomized trial. Am J Clin Nutr 2005;81:859–863.

18. Lee SE, Park JS, Norwitz ER et al. Measurement of placental alpha-microglobulin-1 in cervicovaginal discharge to diagnose rupture of membranes. Obstet Gynecol 2007;109:634–640.

19. Lockwood CJ, Wein R, Chien D et al. Fetal membrane rupture is associated with the presence of insulin-like growth factor-binding protein-1 in vaginal secretions. Am J Obstet Gynecol 1994;171:146–150.

20. Gaucherand P, Guibaud S, Awada A, Rudigoz RC. Comparative study of three amniotic fluid markers in premature rupture of membranes: fetal fibronectin, alpha-fetoprotein, diamino-oxydase. Acta Obstet Gynecol Scand 1995;74:118–121.

21. Chen FC, Dudenhausen JW. Comparison of two rapid strip tests based on IGFBP-1 and PAMG-1 for the detection of amniotic fluid. Am J Perinatol 2008;25:243–246.

22. Lee SM, Lee J, Seong HS et al. The clinical significance of a positive Amnisure test in women with term labor with intact membranes. J Matern Fetal Neonatal Med 2009;22:305–310.

23. Mercer BM, Goldenberg RL, Das AF et al, National Institute of Child Health and Human Development Maternal-Fetal Medicine Units Network. What have we learned regarding antibiotic therapy for the reduction of infant morbidity? Semin Perinatol 2003;27:217–230.

24. Hillier SL, Martius J, Krohn M, Kiviat N, Holmes KK, Eschenbach DA. A case–control study of chorioamnionic infection and histologic chorioamnionitis in prematurity. N Engl J Med 1988;319:972–978.

25. Gunn GC, Mishell DR, Morton DG. Premature rupture of the fetal membranes: a review. Am J Obstet Gynecol 1970;106:469–482.

26. Garite TJ, Freeman RK. Chorioamnionitis in the preterm gestation. Obstet Gynecol 1982;59:539–545.

27. Vintzileos AM, Campbell WA, Nochimson DJ, Weinbaum PJ. Preterm premature rupture of the membranes: a risk factor for the development of abruptio placentae. Am J Obstet Gynecol 1987;156:1235–1238.

28. Mercer BM, Moretti ML, Prevost RR, Sibai BM. Erythromycin therapy in preterm premature rupture of the membranes: a prospective, randomized trial of 220 patients. Am J Obstet Gynecol 1992;166:794–802.

29. Mercer BM. Preterm premature rupture of the membranes. Obstet Gynecol 2003;101:178–193.

30. Alexander JM, Mercer BM, Miodovnik M et al. The impact of digital cervical examination on expectantly managed preterm rupture of membranes. Am J Obstet Gynecol 2000;183:1003–1007.

31. Broekhuizen FF, Gilman M, Hamilton PR. Amniocentesis for gram stain and culture in preterm premature rupture of the membranes. Obstet Gynecol 1985;66:316–321.

32. Romero R, Yoon BH, Mazor M et al. A comparative study of the diagnostic performance of amniotic fluid glucose, white blood cell count, interleukin-6, and Gram stain in the detection of microbial invasion in patients with preterm premature rupture of membranes. Am J Obstet Gynecol 1993;169:839–851.

33. Vintzileos AM, Campbell WA, Nochimson DJ, Weinbaum PJ. Fetal breathing as a predictor of infection in premature rupture of the membranes. Obstet Gynecol 1986;67:813–817.

34. Vintzileos AM, Campbell WA, Nochimson DJ, Connolly ME, Fuenfer MM, Hoehn GJ. The fetal biophysical profile in patients with premature rupture of the membranes: an early predictor of fetal infection. Am J Obstet Gynecol 1985;152:510–516.

35. Centers for Disease Control. Prevention of perinatal group B streptococcal disease. Revised guidelines. MMWR 2010;59:1–36.

36. Naef RW 3rd, Allbert JR, Ross EL, Weber BM, Martin RW, Morrison JC. Premature rupture of membranes at 34 to 37 weeks' gestation: aggressive versus conservative management. Am J Obstet Gynecol 1998;178:126–130.

37. Mercer BM, Crocker L, Boe N, Sibai B. Induction versus expectant management in PROM with mature amniotic fluid at 32–36 weeks: a randomized trial. Am J Obstet Gynecol 1993;82:775–782.

38. Shaver DC, Spinnato JA, Whybrew D, Williams WK, Anderson GD. Comparison of phospholipids in vaginal and amniocentesis specimens of patients with premature rupture of membranes. Am J Obstet Gynecol 1987;156:454.

39. Estol PC, Poseiro JJ, Schwarcz R. Phosphatidylglycerol determination in the amniotic fluid from a pad placed over the vulva: a method for diagnosis of fetal lung maturity in cases of premature ruptured membranes. J Perinatol Med 1992;20:65.

40. Edwards RK, Duff P, Ross KC. Amniotic fluid indices of fetal pulmonary maturity with preterm premature rupture of membranes. Obstet Gynecol 2000;96:102.

41. Neerhof MG, Haney EI, Silver RK et al. Lamellar body counts compared with traditional phospholipid analysis as an assay for evaluating fetal lung maturity. Obstet Gynecol 2001;97:305.

42. Neerhof MG, Dohnal JC, Ashwood ER. Lamellar body counts: a consensus on protocol. Obstet Gynecol 2001;97:318.

43. Fakhoury G, Daikoku NH, Benser J et al. Lamellar body concentrations and the prediction of fetal pulmonary maturity. Am J Obstet Gynecol 1994;170:72.

44. Dalence CR, Bowie LJ, Dohnal JC et al. Amniotic fluid lamellar body count: a rapid and reliable fetal lung maturity test. Obstet Gynecol 1995;86:235.

45. Harding JE, Pang J, Knight DB, Liggins GC. Do antenatal corticosteroids help in the setting of preterm rupture of membranes? Am J Obstet Gynecol 2001;184:131–139.

46. American College of Obstetricians and Gynecologists. Antenatal corticosteroid therapy for fetal maturation. Committee Opinion 210. Obstet Gynecol 2002;99:871–873.

47. Mercer B, Miodovnik M, Thurnau G et al, National Institute of Child Health and Human Development Maternal-Fetal Medicine Units Network. Antibiotic therapy for reduction of infant morbidity after preterm premature rupture of the membranes: a randomized controlled trial. JAMA 1997;278: 989–995.

48. Kenyon S, Boulvain M, Neilson J. Antibiotics for preterm rupture of the membranes: a systematic review. Obstet Gynecol 2004;104:1051–1057.

49. Lewis DF, Adair CD, Robichaux AG et al. Antibiotic therapy in preterm premature rupture of membranes: are seven days necessary? A preliminary, randomized clinical trial. Am J Obstet Gynecol 2003;188:1413–1416; discussion 1416–1417.

50. Segel SY, Miles AM, Clothier B, Parry S, Macones GA. Duration of antibiotic therapy after preterm premature rupture of fetal membranes. Am J Obstet Gynecol 2003;189:799–802.

51. Kenyon SL, Taylor DJ, Tarnow-Mordi W, Oracle Collaborative Group. Broad spectrum antibiotics for preterm, prelabor rupture of fetal membranes: the Oracle I randomized trial. Lancet 2001;357:979–988.

52. Kenyon S, Pike K, Jones DR et al. Childhood outcomes after prescription of antibiotics to pregnant women with preterm rupture of the membranes: 7-year follow-up of the ORACLE I trial. Lancet 2008;372:1310–1318.

53. Christensen KK, Ingemarsson I, Leideman T, Solum T, Svenningsen N. Effect of Ritodrine on labor after premature rupture of the membranes. Obstet Gynecol 1980;55:187–190.

54. Weiner CP, Renk K, Klugman M. The therapeutic efficacy and cost-effectiveness of aggressive tocolysis for premature labor associated with premature rupture of the membranes. Am J Obstet Gynecol 1988;159:216–222.

55. Garite TJ, Keegan KA, Freeman RK, Nageotte MP. A randomized trial of Ritodrine tocolysis versus expectant management in patients with premature rupture of membranes at 25 to 30 weeks of gestation. Am J Obstet Gynecol 1987;157: 388–393.

56. How HY, Cook CR, Cook VD, Miles DE, Spinnato JA. Preterm premature rupture of membranes: aggressive tocolysis versus expectant management. J Matern Fetal Med 1998;7:8–12.

57. Lauria MR, Gonik B, Romero R. Pulmonary hypoplasia: pathogenesis, diagnosis, and antenatal prediction. Obstet Gynecol 1995;86:466–475.

58. D'Alton M, Mercer B, Riddick E, Dudley D. Serial thoracic versus abdominal circumference ratios for the prediction of pulmonary hypoplasia in premature rupture of the membranes remote from term. Am J Obstet Gynecol 1992;166: 658–663.

59. Vintzileos AM, Campbell WA, Rodis JF, Nochimson DJ, Pinette MG, Petrikovsky BM. Comparison of six different ultrasonographic methods for predicting lethal fetal pulmonary hypoplasia. Am J Obstet Gynecol 1989;161:606–612.

60. Sciscione AC, Manley JS, Pollock M et al. Intracervical fibrin sealants: a potential treatment for early preterm premature rupture of the membranes. Am J Obstet Gynecol 2001; 184:368–373.

61. Quintero RA, Morales WJ, Bornick PW, Allen M, Garabelis N. Surgical treatment of spontaneous rupture of membranes: the amniograft–first experience. Am J Obstet Gynecol 2002; 186:155–157.

62. O'Brien JM, Barton JR, Milligan DA. An aggressive interventional protocol for early midtrimester premature rupture of the membranes using gelatin sponge for cervical plugging. Am J Obstet Gynecol 2002;187:1143–1146.

63. Treadwell MC, Bronsteen RA, Bottoms SF. Prognostic factors and complication rates for cervical cerclage: a review of 482 cases. Am J Obstet Gynecol 1991;165:555–558.

64. Blickstein I, Katz Z, Lancet M, Molgilner BM. The outcome of pregnancies complicated by preterm rupture of the membranes with and without cerclage. Int J Gynaecol Obstet 1989;28:237–242.

65. Yeast JD, Garite TR. The role of cervical cerclage in the management of preterm rupture of the membranes. Am J Obstet Gynecol 1988;158:106–110.

66. Ludmir J, Bader T, Chen L, Lindenbaum C, Wong G. Poor perinatal outcome associated with retained cerclage in patients with premature rupture of membranes. Obstet Gynecol 1994;84:823–826.

67. Jenkins TM, Berghella V, Shlossman PA et al. Timing of cerclage removal after preterm premature rupture of membranes: maternal and neonatal outcomes. Am J Obstet Gynecol 2000;183:847–852.

68. McElrath TF, Norwitz ER, Lieberman ES, Heffner LJ. Perinatal outcome after preterm premature rupture of membranes with in situ cervical cerclage. Am J Obstet Gynecol 2002;187: 1147–1152.

69. Major CA, Towers CV, Lewis DF, Garite TJ. Expectant management of preterm premature rupture of membranes complicated by active recurrent genital herpes. Am J Obstet Gynecol 2003;188:1551–1554.

70. Johnson JWC, Egerman RS, Moorhead J. Cases with ruptured membranes that "reseal." Am J Obstet Gynecol 1990;163: 1024–1032.

71. Gold RB, Goyer GL, Schwartz, Evans MI, Seabolt LA. Conservative management of second trimester post-amniocentesis fluid leakage. Obstet Gynecol 1989;74: 745–747.

Chapter 44
Management of Preterm Labor

Vincenzo Berghella

Department of Obstetrics and Gynecology, Thomas Jefferson University, Philadelphia, PA, USA

Major advances in reducing the incidence of prematurity will only come from a better understanding of the pathophysiology leading to preterm birth (PTB). Prevention efforts in asymptomatic women are more beneficial than treatment of symptomatic women. Despite massive research efforts in primary or secondary prevention, millions of women in the USA present with symptoms of preterm labor (PTL) every year, and over 500,000 deliver before 37 weeks. Given the dire consequences of PTB, especially very early PTB (<32 weeks), proven interventions should be performed to avoid it even when it is most difficult (i.e. the woman has manifest symptoms of PTL).

Management of the woman with symptoms of PTL starts with initial assessment of history, physical exam, and specific laboratory and other screening tests to establish diagnosis and prognosis, in order to obtain an accurate initial assessment and to decide the correct interventions.

Evaluation: history, physical exam, and screening tests

As a minimum, the history should include a review of specific symptoms, such as cramps, abdominal "tightenings," low backache, pelvic pressure, increased vaginal discharge, or spotting. It is paramount to obtain the exact determination of gestational age. To assess prognosis, specific risk factors for PTB should be carefully reviewed. These are listed in Box 44.1.

The physical exam should include an assessment of vital signs, fetal heart and toco-monitoring, an abdominal exam for uterine tenderness and contractions, cervical exam by speculum for pooling, Nitrazine, ferning, visual examination of cervix (especially if preterm premature rupture of membranes [PPROM] is suspected), collection

for fetal fibronectin (fFN) and group B streptococci (GBS), and *Chlamydia* and gonorrhea DNA tests. If PPROM is ruled out, a manual cervical exam can be performed for dilation, cervical length and/or effacement, station, and presentation.

Laboratory tests that should be considered include rapid plasma reagin (RPR) or Venereal Disease Research Laboratory (VDRL) to rule out syphilis in high-risk women, rapid HIV (if status unknown), cervicovaginal fFN, vaginorectal GBS, urinary drug screen (UDS), urinalysis, and urine culture. In women without specific symptoms of these infections, there is no evidence that screening for bacterial vaginosis (BV), *Trichomonas*, *Mycoplasma* or *Ureaplasma* is beneficial.

In addition, there are other important screening tests that are suggested. An ultrasound should assess for fetal demise, major anomaly, polyhydramnios, placenta previa, placental abruption, fetal presentation, and estimated fetal weight. A transvaginal ultrasound (TVU) can be performed for cervical length (CL) evaluation. Amniocentesis may be considered to check for intraamniotic infection (IAI) (incidence approximately 5–15%) if equivocal signs of chorioamnionitis are present, and/or for fetal lung maturity (FLM) (the latter especially if between 33 and 37 weeks). If the diagnosis of IAI is made clinically (≥2 of uterine tenderness, maternal fever ≥38°C (≥100.4°F), maternal tachycardia, fetal tachycardia, in the absence of other infection), delivery is recommended even without amniocentesis. The rates of IAI (documented by amniotic fluid culture) by pregnancy status at <37 weeks are approximately 5–15% for PTL (intact membranes), 20–30% for PPROM (no labor), 30–40% for PPROM (labor), and 50% if cervix ≥2cm/80% in second trimester. The rates of infection are indirectly proportional to gestational age, as well as CL. There is insufficient evidence to recommend amniocentesis in all cases of PTL.

Queenan's Management of High-Risk Pregnancy: An Evidence-Based Approach, Sixth Edition. Edited by John T. Queenan, Catherine Y. Spong, Charles J. Lockwood.

Initial assessment

Diagnosis of preterm labor

The vast majority of women who present with symptoms of PTL do not deliver preterm even without intervention. Therefore, it is important to establish the diagnosis of PTL before any treatment is ever considered. One of the most commonly used PTL diagnoses is the presence of uterine contractions (≥4/20 min or ≥8/h) *and* documented cervical change with intact membranes at 20–36w 6d. In fact, 70–80% of women even with this diagnosis of PTL do not deliver preterm. Women without manual cervical change do not have PTL and should not receive tocolysis.

Fetal fibronectin and cervical length

Because so many women with a diagnosis of PTL do not deliver preterm, two predictive tests, fFN and TVU CL, can be used, where available, in the initial assessment of the chance of delivering preterm. Women with PTL but TVU CL ≥30 mm have a less than 2% chance of delivering within 1 week, and a more than 95% chance of delivering ≥35 weeks without therapy [1], and should therefore not

receive any treatment. Women with TVU CL 20–29 mm and positive fFN, or especially those with TVU CL less than 20 mm, are at highest risk of PTB and should receive treatment interventions. This management (Fig. 44.1) has been associated with a significant reduction in PTB <37 weeks in a randomized controlled trial [2].

Management

The main interventions for the woman with PTL at high risk for delivering preterm are aimed at increasing fetal maturation and stopping uterine contractions to avoid PTB. In addition, it is important to consider referral to a tertiary care center if the neonatal intensive care unit (NICU) is not adequate for the gestational age. The woman and her family members should be counseled regarding morbidity and mortality for the possible preterm infant. Current (2011) survival is 0% at 21 weeks, 75% at 25 weeks, and more than 95% at 29 weeks, while intact survival at 18 months is over 50% after 25 weeks. Disabilities in mental and psychomotor development, neuromotor function (including cerebral palsy), or sensory and communication function are present in at least 50% of fetuses born ≤25 weeks' gestation [3]. A neonatology consult at 22–34 weeks should always be obtained to discuss neonatal prognosis and management. Obstetric counseling should review the principles and progress of management of PTL. Specific interventions should aim to treat any positive tests or infections, such as urinary tract infections, sexually transmitted diseases (STDs), GBS, and HIV.

Women with multiple gestations should not be treated differently from those with singletons, except for caution in that their risk of pulmonary edema is greater when exposed to β-mimetics or magnesium sulfate [4]. There is insufficient evidence to justify the use of steroids for FLM and tocolysis before 23 weeks and after 33w 6d.

Prophylaxis to prevent neonatal morbidity/mortality from preterm birth (fetal maturation)

Betamethasone and dexamethasone are the only two corticosteroids that cross the placenta reliably and have been shown to benefit the fetus. The regimen for one course of betamethasone is 12 mg IM every 24 h for two doses and for dexamethasone is 6 mg IM every 6 h for four doses. Betamethasone, if available, is preferred to dexamethasone [5]. Corticosteroids given prior to PTB (either spontaneous or indicated) are effective in preventing respiratory distress syndrome (RDS), intraventricular hemorrhage (IVH), and neonatal mortality [6]. Antenatal administration of 24 mg of betamethasone or dexamethasone to women expected to give birth preterm is associated with a 40% reduction in neonatal mortality, 47%

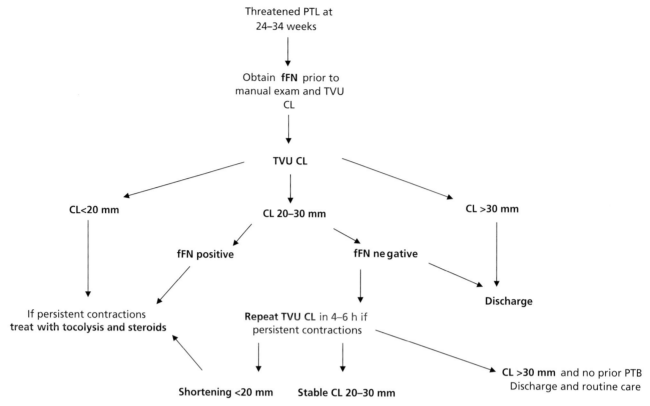

Figure 44.1 Preterm labor management algorithm. Reproduced from Ness *et al* [2] with permission from Elsevier. CL, cervical length; fFN, fetal fibronectin; PTB, preterm birth; PTL, preterm labor; TVU CL, transvaginal ultrasound cervical length.

reduction in RDS, and 52% reduction in IVH in preterm infants. There is a trend for a 41% reduction in necrotizing enterocolitis (NEC). These benefits apply to at least 24–33w 6d and are not limited by gender or race. The effects are significant mostly at 48 h to 7 days from the first dose, but treatment should not be withheld even if delivery appears imminent, and effects even for babies delivered more than 7 days later have been reported. Such steroids should therefore be administered to any woman at these gestational ages at significant PTB risk upon identification of that risk. The results are mostly from singleton gestations, with fewer data on multiple gestations. There is no increase in maternal or fetal/neonatal infection. There are no contraindications. When used for only one course, no significant side-effects have been reported. No adverse consequences of prophylactic corticosteroids for PTB in either the mothers or, most importantly, the infants, even at 10 years follow-up, have been identified.

One single additional rescue course of betamethasone has been associated with a 36% decrease in RDS with no other additional benefits or detriments in women who remain undelivered more than 14 days after the first course, but who are at continued risk of PTB before 30 weeks in a randomized trial [7]. More than two repeated courses of steroids for FLM should NOT be administered [8]. While repeated courses have been associated with

fewer infants with severe lung disease compared with infants in the placebo group [8], if repeated courses, especially four courses or more, are used, there is a possible association with birthweight <10th percentile and small neonatal head circumference (<10th percentile), with evidence of some later "catch-up" growth.

Thyrotropin-releasing hormone, phenobarbital, and vitamin K have not been shown to be beneficial for fetal maturation and PTL management.

Neuroprotection
Antenatal magnesium sulfate given to women at immediate risk for PTB because of PTL or PPROM at around 24–33 weeks is associated with a 32% decrease in the incidence of cerebral palsy, with no other significant benefits or detriments. This is based on data from five randomized trials, establishing the neuroprotective effect of magnesium [9]. Dose, timing, exact patient population, and other long-term outcomes will require further trials.

Nontocolytic interventions
Activity restriction (e.g. bedrest), hydration, and sedation have not been shown to be beneficial in the management of PTL. Bedrest has never been tested by itself in singleton gestations complicated by PTL or PPROM. In twin

pregnancies, bedrest in hospital has not been shown to decrease PTB [10].

Hydration

Intravenous hydration does not seem to be beneficial, even during the period of evaluation soon after admission, in the management of women with PTL. Compared with bedrest alone, hydration is associated with similar incidence of PTB at <37, <34, or <32 weeks [9]. Admission to the neonatal ICU occurs with similar frequency in both groups. Cost of treatment is obviously higher in the hydration group. No studies have evaluated oral hydration in women with evidence of dehydration [11].

Prophylactic antibiotics

There is no clear overall benefit from prophylactic antibiotic treatment for women with PTL with intact membranes on neonatal outcomes, and there are concerns about a trend for increased neonatal mortality for those who received antibiotics (relative risk [RR] 1.52, 95% confidence interval [CI] 0.99–2.34) [12]. Rates of PTB at less than 36–37 weeks are similar in antibiotics and placebo groups, as is perinatal mortality. In the largest trial, with the longest (7 years) follow-up, co-amoxiclav or erythromycin was associated with significant increase in cerebral palsy, and erythromycin with an increase in functional impairment [13]. Therefore antibiotics should not be used for prophylaxis in women with PTL.

Group B streptococcus prophylaxis

As antibiotics can be detrimental, they should be used for GBS prophylaxis only in those pregnancies deemed at high risk to deliver preterm within 2–3 days, such as those with TVL CL less than 20 mm. Until GBS maternal status is known, these women should receive penicillin (or ampicillin if penicillin is not available) to prevent GBS neonatal infections, unless allergic [14].

Progesterone

Progesterone has been associated with prevention of PTB in certain asymptomatic women, i.e. those with prior PTB and/or with short CL before 28 weeks. In women symptomatic with PTL, progestational agents instead cannot be advocated for prevention of PTB when used in addition to tocolytics or solely for this purpose [15].

Tocolysis

The principles of tocolytic therapy are listed in Box 44.2, and contraindications are listed in Box 44.3.

Primary tocolysis – single agent

β-Mimetics

Ritodrine and terbutaline have been the more commonly studied agents.

Box 44.2 Principles of tocolytic therapy

- At 24–33w 6d, steroids for fetal maturation should always be given if tocolysis is initiated. Tocolytics should not be used without concomitant use of steroids for fetal maturation
- Tocolysis is typically used for 48h to allow steroid effect. Given side-effects, stop tocolytic therapy at 48h after steroids given if PTL under control
- No tocolytic agent has been shown to improve perinatal mortality
- There is no tocolytic agent that is more safe and efficacious. COX inhibitors are the only class of primary tocolytics shown to decrease PTB <37 weeks compared with placebo, while COX inhibitors, β-mimetics and ORA have been shown to significantly prolong pregnancy at 48h and 7 days compared with placebo. COX inhibitors, CCB, and ORA, properly used, have significantly fewer side-effects than β-mimetics
- There is no *maintenance* tocolytic agent that has been proven to prevent PTB or perinatal morbidity/mortality. There is insufficient evidence to evaluate multiple tocolytic agents for primary tocolysis, refractory (primary agent is failing, so another is started) tocolysis, or repeated tocolysis (after successful primary tocolysis)

CCB, calcium channel blocker; COX, cyclooxygenase; ORA, oxytocin receptor antagonist; PTB, preterm birth; PTL, preterm labor.

Box 44.3 Contraindications to tocolytic therapy

Maternal

- Chorioamnionitis
- Severe vaginal bleeding/abruption
- Preeclampsia
- Medical contraindications to specific tocolytic agent (see text)
- Other maternal medical condition that makes continuing the pregnancy inadvisable

Fetal

- Intrauterine fetal death
- Major (especially if lethal) fetal anomaly or chromosome abnormality
- Other fetal conditions in which prolongation of pregnancy is inadvisable
- Documented fetal maturity

Dose. Ritodrine: 50–100 µg/min IV initial dose, increase 50 µg/min every 10 min (max 350 µg/min) (PO 1–20 mg every 2–4 h). Terbutaline: 25 mg SQ every 20 min at first, then 2–3 h, or 5–10 µg/min IV, max 80 µg/min; or 2.5–5 mg PO every 2–4 h (hold if maternal heart rate over 120/min).

Mechanism of action. Stimulate B_2 receptor through cyclic adenosine monophosphate, so no free calcium for myometrial contraction.

Evidence for effectiveness. β-Mimetics decrease by 37% the number of women in PTL giving birth within 48h compared with placebo, but are associated with no significant decrease in births within 7 days or prior to 37 weeks [15]. No benefit is demonstrated for β-mimetics on RDS or perinatal death. A few trials reported no difference detected in cerebral palsy, infant death, and NEC. Ritodrine has been the agent studied usually, with insufficient evidence to evaluate effectiveness of other β-mimetics [16].

Comparison with other tocolytics. See below.

Specific contraindications. Cardiac arrhythmia or other significant cardiac disease; diabetes mellitus (DM); poorly controlled thyroid disease (for ritodrine).

Side-effects. Maternal: hyperglycemia (140–200 mg/dL glucose in 20–50%. Mechanism: decreased peripheral insulin sensitivity and increased endogenous glucose production). Hyperinsulinemia; hypokalemia (K <3 mEq/L in 50%); tremors, nervousness, dyspnea (10%), chest pain (5–10%), tachycardia/palpitations, arrhythmia (3%); ECG changes (2–3%); hypotension (2–3%); pulmonary edema (<1–5%; mechanism: reduced sodium excretion, leading to sodium and therefore fluid retention); headaches; nausea/vomiting; and nasal stuffiness. Ritodrine specific: altered thyroid function, antidiuresis. Fetal/neonatal: ritodrine: tachycardia, hypoglycemia, hypocalcemia, hyperbilirubinemia, hypotension, IVH. Terbutaline: tachycardia, hyperinsulinemia, hyperglycemia, myocardial and septal hypertrophy, myocardial ischemia.

Calcium-channel blockers

Nifedipine (most commonly) and nicardipine have been the calcium channel blocker (CCB) agents studied.

Dose. Nifedipine 20–30 mg for one dose, then 10–20 mg every 4–8 h (max. 90 mg/day) (nicardipine dose similar).

Mechanism of action. Impair calcium channels, so inhibit influx of calcium into cell, and therefore myometrial contraction.

Evidence for effectiveness. There are no studies of CCB compared with placebo for PTB prevention. When compared with any other tocolytic agent (mainly β-mimetics), CCB reduce the number of women giving birth within 7 days of receiving treatment by 24% and PTB at less than 34 weeks' gestation by 17% [17]. CCB show a trend to reduce PTB within 48 h of initiation of treatment (RR 0.80, 95% CI 0.61–1.05), and PTB at less than 37 weeks' gestation (RR 0.95, 95% CI 0.83–1.09). CCB also reduces the frequency of neonatal RDS by 37%, NEC by 79%, IVH by 41%, and neonatal jaundice by 27%. CCB also reduce the requirement for women to have treatment stopped for adverse drug reaction by 86%. There are insufficient data regarding the effects of different dosage regimens and formulations of CCB on maternal and neonatal outcomes; the most studied is nifedipine, at the dosage shown above. CCB should therefore be preferred to β-mimetics for tocolysis [17].

Specific contraindications. Cardiac disease; hypotension (<90/50 mmHg); concomitant use of magnesium; caution in renal disease.

Side-effects. Maternal: flushing, headache, dizziness, nausea, transient hypotension. Caution in women with hypotension and renal disease, as well as those on magnesium (cardiovascular collapse). Fetal/neonatal: None.

Cyclooxygenase inhibitors

Nonselective cyclooxygenase (COX) inhibitors: indomethacin (Indocin). Selective COX inhibitors (preferential COX-2 inhibitors): sulindac (Clinoril); rofecoxib (Vioxx); celecoxib (Celebrex); ketorolac (Toradol); nimesulide.

Dose. Indomethacin: 50–100 mg loading dose (rectal or vaginal route preferred, oral otherwise), then 25–50 mg every 6 h for 48 h max, and always <32 weeks. Sulindac: 200 mg PO every 12 h for 48 h. Ketorolac: 60 mg IM, then 30 mg IM every 6 h for 48 h.

Mechanism of action. COX inhibitors, so inhibit prostaglandin synthesis, therefore inhibit myometrial contraction.

Evidence for effectiveness. The nonselective COX inhibitor indomethacin was used in 10/13 trials.

When compared with placebo, COX inhibition (indomethacin only studied) results in a 79% reduction in PTB at less than 37 weeks, an increase in gestational age of 3.5 weeks, and an increase in birthweight of approximately 700 g in two small trials [18–20]. There is a trend towards a reduction in delivery within 48 h of initiation of treatment (RR 0.20, 95% CI 0.03–1.28) and within 7 days (RR 0.41, 95% CI 0.10–1.66) [18]. No differences are detected in any other reported outcomes including perinatal mortality and RDS.

Used for 48 h only, the intravaginal route (100 mg every 12 h) decreases delivery at 48 h (3/23 versus 8/23) and at less than 7 days (5/23 versus 13/23) compared with rectal/oral (100 mg rectally, followed by 25 mg PO every 6 h), with some improvement in neonatal morbidities [21].

Compared with β-mimetics, COX inhibitors significantly reduce by 63% the number of women delivering within 48 h of initiation of treatment. Compared with magnesium sulfate, COX inhibitors have a trend for a lower number of women delivering within 48 h of initiation of treatment (RR 0.75, 95% CI 0.40–1.40) and lower PTB at less than 37 weeks (RR 0.55, 95% CI 0.17–1.73).

A comparison of nonselective (indomethacin and sulindac) versus selective (rofecoxib and nimesulide) COX-2 inhibitor [22,23] does not demonstrate any differences in maternal or neonatal outcomes. Because of the small numbers, all estimates of effect are imprecise and need to be interpreted with caution.

Specific contraindications. Renal or hepatic disease, active peptic ulcer disease, poorly controlled hypertension (HTN), nonsteroidal antiinflammatory drug

(NSAID)-sensitive asthma, coagulation disorders/thrombocytopenia.

Side-effects. When used for only 48h, no serious maternal or fetal/neonatal side-effects occur, and fetal surveillance is not indicated. Usually COX inhibitors are better tolerated by the mother than other tocolytics such as magnesium and betamimetics. Maternal: as with any NSAID, mild gastrointestinal upset – nausea, heartburn (take with some food/milk) (COX-1). Gastrointestinal bleeding (COX-1), coagulation and platelet abnormalities (COX-1), asthma if aspirin sensitive. NSAIDs may obscure elevation in temperature. Long-term rofecoxib (Vioxx) use in adults has been associated with stroke, so this drug is now not available in many countries. Fetal/neonatal: in randomized controlled trials (RCTs), 403 women received short-term tocolysis (up to 48h) with COX inhibitors (mainly indomethacin) and there was only one case of antenatal closure of the ductus arteriosus (incidence <0.3%). There was no increase in the incidence of patent ductus arteriosus postnatally [18]. No difference in incidences of IVH, bronchopulmonary dysplasia, patent ductus arteriosus, NEC, or perinatal mortality was noted in a review of RCTs aimed at evaluating safety [24]. Use for more than 48h, especially ≥32 weeks, is associated with significant fetal effects such as constriction of the ductus arteriosus, which can lead to hydrops, pulmonary hypertension, and death, and renal insufficiency, manifested *in utero* by oligohydramnios. Other effects with prolonged use such as hyperbilirubinemia, NEC, and IVH have not been shown with less than 72-h use. Selective COX-2 inhibitors have not been shown consistently to be any safer for the fetus/neonate than nonselective COX inhibitors such as indomethacin. Therefore, continuous use of COX inhibitors for more than 48 hours and ≥32 weeks is contraindicated.

Magnesium sulfate (MgSO$_4$)

Dose. 40 g MgSO$_4$ in 1 L d51/2NS. Initial: 4–6 g/30 min, then 2–4 g/h. A dose of 5 g/h has not been shown to be beneficial in perinatal outcome compared with a dose of 2 g/h, and is associated with significant side-effects [25]. Weaning MgSO$_4$ tocolysis has no benefits and a few harmful side-effects compared with stopping MgSO$_4$ abruptly [26].

Mechanism of action. Intracellular calcium antagonist.

Evidence for effectiveness. Compared with placebo, there is insufficient evidence to show if magnesium sulfate reduces the incidence of PTB or perinatal morbidity and mortality [27–29]. Compared with all controls (including other tocolytics), magnesium sulfate did not prevent PTB at 48h, PTB at less than 37 weeks or PTB at less than 32 weeks. Perinatal death was higher but very rare, while perinatal morbidities were similar [27]. Dosage of magnesium did not affect efficacy.

Specific contraindications. Myasthenia gravis.

Management. Aim for 4–7 MgSO$_4$ level. Monitor urinary output. Follow deep tendon reflexes: ↓ at ≥8, absent ≥10. ≥10: respiratory depression; ≥15 risk of cardiac arrest.

Side-effects. Maternal: flushing, lethargy, headache, muscle weakness, diplopia, dry mouth, pulmonary edema (1%; Mechanism: intravenous overhydration), cardiac arrest. Fetal/neonatal: lethargy, hypotonia, hypocalcemia, respiratory depression. Prolonged use: demineralization.

Oxytocin receptor antagonists

Atosiban (Tractocile in Europe) is not Food and Drug Administration (FDA) approved, and therefore not available in the USA.

Dose. Atosiban 6.75 mg bolus, then 300 μg/min IV for 3h, then 100 μg/min (max. 45 h).

Mechanism of action. Competitive inhibitor of oxytocin via blockade of oxytocin receptor.

Evidence for effectiveness. Compared with placebo, atosiban did not reduce incidence of preterm birth or improve neonatal outcome. In one trial, atosiban was associated with an increase in infant deaths at 12 months of age compared with placebo [30]. However, this trial randomized significantly more women to atosiban before 26 weeks' gestation. Use of atosiban resulted in lower infant birthweight and more maternal adverse drug reactions. Compared with β-mimetics, atosiban had similar incidences of PTB or perinatal morbidity/mortality. Atosiban was associated with fewer maternal drug reactions requiring treatment cessation [31].

Side-effects. Minimal to none.

There is currently insufficient evidence to support the administration of nitric oxide donors [32], progesterone, or alcohol for prevention of PTB in women with PTL.

Primary tocolysis – multiple agents simultaneously

Indomethacin and ampicillin-sulbactam do not prevent PTB compared with placebo in women in PTL already receiving MgSO$_4$ tocolysis [33].

Refractory tocolysis – primary agent is failing

Indomethacin is similar to sulindac in prevention of PTB in women failing primary MgSO$_4$ tocolysis [34].

Maintenance tocolysis – after successful primary tocolysis

There is evidence that all agents used so far for maintenance tocolysis do not prevent PTB, recurrent PTL, recurrent hospitalizations, or perinatal morbidity and mortality. These include oral β-mimetics [35], terbutaline pump [36], CCB [37], COX inhibitors [38,39], magnesium [40], or atosiban [41].

Mode of delivery

There is insufficient evidence to evaluate the use of a policy for uniform planned cesarean delivery (CD) compared with expectant management and selective CD for preterm babies (approximately 24–36 weeks) [42]. Mothers in the planned CD group have higher morbidity, while babies in the planned CD group show no statistical differences compared with expectant management, except a more frequent low cord pH. The numbers so far are too small for definite conclusions, including for differentiating by fetal presentation [42].

CASE PRESENTATION

A 25-year-old, African-American, gravida 6, para 0141 calls her obstetrician at 28w 6d with complaints of vaginal pressure. Upon questioning, she states that she might have intermittent cramps. Based on this history, the attending physician asks her to come to labor and delivery to be evaluated.

Her past obstetric history is significant for two spontaneous abortions, two induced abortions, and one PTB at 30 weeks the year before. This PTB had been preceded by PTL, unsuccessfully treated with magnesium sulfate. She received steroids for fetal maturation, and her 1484 g (3 lb 4 oz) baby is currently doing well. She denies any other risk factors for PTB. Her prenatal course has been uneventful. Her expected date of confinement has been confirmed by an 18-week ultrasound. Her prenatal laboratory tests were within normal limits, including a negative HIV test.

On physical exam, her blood pressure is 110/74 mmHg, pulse 86 beats/min, temperature 36.9°C (98.4°F), respiratory rate 20. No tenderness or contractions are identified. On speculum exam, pooling, ferning, and nitrazine are negative, and so rupture of membranes is ruled out. Tests for fFN, GBS, gonorrhea and *Chlamydia* are collected. Her cervical exam is 2 cm dilated, 1 cm long, -2 station. The clinical impression is vertex presentation and size less than dates. Fetal heart and tocomonitoring are initiated.

Twenty minutes after arrival, the fetal heart appears reassuring and appropriate for gestational age. On toco-

monitoring, she is contracting every 4 min. An ultrasound is performed and reveals an appropriate for gestational age estimated fetal weight (1498 g), vertex presentation, no placenta previa, and Amniotic Fluid Index of 10. TVU reveals a cervical length of 19 mm.

Based on contraction frequency and cervical exam findings, especially the short CL <20 mm, a diagnosis of PTL is made. Betamethasone 12 mg IM is given with a plan to give a second dose at 24 h. 100 mg indomethacin is given *per rectum*, with a plan for continuing this drug 50 mg every 6 h for 48 h. Extensive counseling is given regarding safety and effectiveness of all interventions, prognosis, and possible complications. A neonatal consult is ordered. The NICU is level III, and there is availability for care in case of a 28-week PTB.

An hour later, contractions are diminishing in frequency and intensity. Regular nutrition is allowed. Later, the contractions resolve, the fFN result returns as positive, while GBS, gonorrhea, *Chlamydia*, and urine culture are negative. Antibiotics for GBS prophylaxis are discontinued. Hospitalization is continued as planned for a total of 48 h, with tocomonitoring for 1 h every shift and at the patient's request if she feels symptoms of PTL.

Forty-eight hours after initial assessment, she is discharged home with PTL precautions and close follow-up, aware of her high chance of PTB at less than 35 weeks and its consequences.

References

1. Berghella V, Ness A, Bega G, Berghella M. Cervical sonography in women with symptoms of preterm labor. Obstet Gynecol Clin North Am 2005;32:383–396.
2. Ness A, Visintine J, Ricci E, Berghella V. Does knowledge of cervical length and fetal fibronectin affect management of women with threatened preterm labor? A randomized trial. Am J Obstet Gynecol 2007;197(4):426.
3. Larson JE, Desai SA, McNett W. Perinatal care and long-term implications. In: Berghella V, ed. Preterm Birth. Oxford: Blackwell Publishing, 2010.
4. American College of Obstetrics and Gynecology. Management of preterm labor. Obstet Gynecol 2003;82:127–135.
5. Jobe AH, Soll RF. Choice and dose of corticosteroid for antenatal treatments. Am J Obstet Gynecol 2004;190: 878–881.
6. Crowley P. Prophylactic corticosteroids for preterm birth. Cochrane Database Syst Rev 2000;2:CD000065.
7. Garite TJ, Kurtzman J, Maurel K, Clark R. Impact of a 'rescue course' of antenatal corticosteroids: a multicenter randomized placebo-controlled trial. Am J Obstet Gynecol 2009;248.
8. Crowther CA, Harding, JE. Repeat doses of prenatal corticosteroids for women at risk of preterm birth for preventing neonatal respiratory disease. Cochrane Database Syst Rev 2007;3:CD003935.
9. Doyle LW, Crowther CA, Middleton P, Marret S, Rouse D. Magnesium sulphate for women at risk of preterm birth for

neuroprotection of the fetus. Cochrane Database Syst Rev 2009;1:CD004661.

10. Crowther CA, Neilson JP, Verkuyl DAA, Bannerman C, Ashurst HM. Preterm labour in twin pregnancies: can it be prevented by hospital admission? Br J Obstet Gynaecol 1989;96:850–853.

11. Stan C, Boulvain M, Pfister R, Hirsbrunner-Amagbaly P. Hydration for treatment of preterm labour. Cochrane Database Syst Rev 2002;2:CD003096.

12. King J, Flenady V, Murray L. Prophylactic antibiotics for inhibiting preterm labour with intact membranes. Cochrane Database Syst Rev 2002;4:CD000246.

13. Kenyon S, Pike K, Jones DR et al. Childhood outcomes after prescription of antibiotics to pregnant women with spontaneous preterm labor: 7-year follow-up of the ORACLE II trial. Lancet 2008;372:1319–1327.

14. Gibbs RS, Schrag S, Schuchat A. Perinatal infections due to group B streptococci. Obstet Gynecol 2004;104: 1062–1076.

15. Su LL, Samuel M, Chong YS. Progestational agents for treating threatened or established preterm labour. Cochrane Database Syst Rev 2010;1:CD006770.

16. Anotayanonth S, Subhedar NV, Neilson JP, Harigopal S. Betamimetics for inhibiting preterm labour. Cochrane Database Syst Rev 2004;4:CD004352.

17. King JF, Flenady VJ, Papatsonis DNM, Dekker GA, Carbonne B. Calcium channel blockers for inhibiting preterm labour. Cochrane Database Syst Rev 2003;1:CD002255.

18. King J, Flenady V, Cole S, Thornton S. Cyclooxygenase (COX) inhibitors for treating preterm labour. Cochrane Database Syst Rev 2005;2:CD001992.

19. Niebyl JR, Blake DA, White RD et al. The inhibition of premature labor with indomethacin. Am J Obstet Gynecol 1980;136: 1014–1019.

20. Zuckerman H, Shalev E, Gilad G, Katzuni E. Further study of the inhibition of premature labor by indomethacin. Part II. Double-blind study. J Perinatal Med 1984;12:25–29.

21. Abramov Y, Nadjari M, Weinstein D, Ben-Shachar I, Plotkin V, Ezra Y. Indomethacin for preterm labor: a randomized comparison of vaginal and rectal routes. Obstet Gynecol 2000; 95:482–486.

22. Sawdy RJ, Lye S, Fisk NM, Bennett PR. A double-blind randomized study of fetal side effects during and after the short-term maternal administration of indomethacin, sulindac, and nimesulide for the treatment of preterm labor. Am J Obstet Gynecol 2003;188:1046–1051.

23. Stika CS, Gross GA, Leguizamon G et al. A prospective randomized safety trial of celecoxib for treatment of preterm labor. Am J Obstet Gynecol 2002;187:653–660.

24. Loe SM, Sanchez-Ramos L, Kaunitz A. Assessing the neonatal safety of indomethacin tocolysis: a systematic review with meta-analysis. Obstet Gynecol 2005;106:173–179.

25. Terrone DA, Rinehart BK, Kimmel ES, May WL, Larmon JE, Morrison JC. A prospective randomized controlled trial of high and low maintenance doses of magnesium sulfate for acute tocolysis. Am J Obstet Gynecol 2000;182:1477–1482.

26. Lewis DF, Bergstedt S, Edwards MS et al. Successful magnesium sulfate tocolysis: is "weaning" the drug necessary? Am J Obstet Gynecol 1997;177:742–745.

27. Crowther CA, Hiller JE, Doyle LW. Magnesium sulfate for preventing preterm birth in threatened preterm labour. Cochrane Database Syst Rev 2002;4:CD001060.

28. Cotton DB, Strassner HT, Hill LM, Schifrin BS, Paul RH. Comparison of magnesium sulfate, terbutaline and a placebo for inhibition of preterm labor: a randomized study. J Reprod Med 1984;29:92–97.

29. Cox SM, Sherman ML, Leveno KJ. Randomized investigation of magnesium sulfate for prevention of preterm birth. Am J Obstet Gynecol 1990;163:767–772.

30. Romero R, Sibai BM, Sanchez-Ramos L et al. An oxytocin receptor antagonist (atosiban) in the treatment of preterm labor: a randomized, double-blind, placebo-controlled trial with tocolytic rescue. Am J Obstet Gynecol 2000;182: 1173–1183.

31. Papatsonis D, Flenady V, Cole S, Liley H. Oxytocin receptor antagonists for inhibiting preterm labour. Cochrane Database Syst Rev 2005;3:CD004452.

32. Duckitt K, Thornton S. Nitric oxide donors for the treatment of preterm labour. Cochrane Database Syst Rev 2002;3:CD002860.

33. Newton ER, Shields L, Rigway LE, Berkus MD, Elliott BD. Combination antibiotics and indomethacin in idiopathic preterm labor: a randomized double-blind study. Am J Obstet Gynecol 1991;165:1753–1759.

34. Carlan S, O'Brien WF, O'Leary TD, Mastrogiannis D. Randomized comparative trial of indomethacin and sulindac for the treatment of refractory preterm labor. Obstet Gynecol 1992;79:223–228.

35. Dodd JM, Crowther AD, Dare MR, Middleton P. Oral betamimetics for maintenance therapy after threatened preterm labour. Cochrane Database Syst Rev 2006;1:CD003927.

36. Nanda K, Cook LA, Gallo MF, Grimes DA. Terbutaline pump maintenance therapy after threatened preterm labour for preventing preterm birth. Cochrane Database Syst Rev 2002;4:CD003933.

37. Carr DB, Clark AL, Kernek K, Spinnato JA. Maintenance oral nifedipine for preterm labor: a randomized clinical trial. Am J Obstet Gynecol 1999;181:822–827.

38. Carlan SJ, O'Brien WF, Jones MH, O'Leary TD, Roth L. Outpatient oral sulindac to prevent recurrence of preterm labor. Obstet Gynecol 1995;85:769–774.

39. Humprey RG, Bartfield MC, Carlan SJ, O'Brien WF, O'Leary TD, Triana T. Sulindac to prevent recurrent preterm labor: a randomized controlled trial. Obstet Gynecol 2001;98:555–562.

40. Crowther CA, Moore V. Magnesium maintenance therapy for preventing preterm birth after threatened preterm labor. Cochrane Database Syst Rev 2000;2:CD000940.

41. Valenzuela GJ, Sanchez-Ramos L, Romero R et al. Maintenance treatment of preterm labor with the oxytocin antagonist atosiban. Am J Obstet Gynecol 2000;182:1184–1190.

42. Grant A, Glazener CMA. Elective caesarean section versus expectant management for delivery of the small baby. Cochrane Database Syst Rev 2001;2:CD000078.

Chapter 45
Placenta Previa and Related Placental Disorders

Yinka Oyelese

Department of Obstetrics and Gynecology, Jersey Shore University Medical Center, Neptune and UMDNJ-Robert Wood Johnson Medical School, New Brunswick, NJ, USA

The placenta usually implants in the upper uterine segment. However, in some cases, it implants in the lower uterine segment, either covering the internal cervical os or lying in close proximity to it. This abnormal implantation into the lower segment, called placenta previa, is one of the most important causes of bleeding in the second half of pregnancy and during labor, and is associated with significant maternal and perinatal morbidity and occasionally mortality. Placenta previa may also be associated with two other clinically important conditions, placenta accreta and vasa previa, which are also discussed in this chapter.

Placenta previa

Placenta previa has traditionally been classified into four types (Figs 45.1 and 45.2).
1. *Complete placenta previa*, where the placenta completely overlies the internal os (see Fig. 45.2).
2. *Partial placenta previa*, where the placenta partially overlies the internal os.
3. *Marginal placenta previa*, where the placental edge just reaches to the internal os, but does not cover it (Fig. 45.3).
4. *Low-lying placenta*, which reaches into the lower uterine segment but does not reach the internal os.

Incidence and risk factors
Placenta previa complicates approximately 1 in 200 pregnancies (0.5%) [1,2]. Studies have identified several risk factors for placenta previa. These include prior cesarean delivery [3], prior uterine surgery, smoking [2], multifetal gestation [4], cocaine use, increasing parity, and increasing maternal age [1,2,5]. The risk of placenta previa increases with the number of prior cesarean deliveries in a dose–response manner. It is not clear why the placenta implants in the lower uterine segment in some

pregnancies. However, it has been established that scarring of the endometrium as a consequence of cesarean delivery or intrauterine surgery significantly increases the risk of placenta previa.

Clinical presentation
Patients with placenta previa typically present with painless bleeding in the early third trimester. The initial bleed is usually not very heavy and typically does not lead to delivery, but is frequently sufficient to cause significant alarm. However, approximately one-third of cases of placenta previa will experience no bleeding prior to the onset of labor [6]. Not infrequently, there is a fetal malpresentation or unstable lie. This is because the placenta lies in the lower uterine segment, preventing engagement of the fetal head.

Diagnosis
The diagnosis of placenta previa is usually made by sonography. This typically occurs in one of two scenarios. In the first, the diagnosis is made in asymptomatic women on routine sonography, and the second is when sonography is performed in women who present with vaginal bleeding in the late second or early third trimester. Transabominal sonography will detect the majority of cases of placenta previa. However, transabdominal sonography will produce false-positive or false-negative diagnoses of placenta previa in 10–20% of cases [7]. A common reason for false-positive diagnoses is the approximation of the anterior and posterior walls of the lower uterine segment that occurs with the bladder filling that is necessary for transabdominal sonography; this may give a false impression of a placenta previa [8]. Crucial landmarks such as the internal os and the lower placental edge are frequently not adequately visualized using transabdominal sonography, producing a false-negative diagnosis [7]. In addition, the fetal head may prevent adequate visualization of the region over the cervix [8].

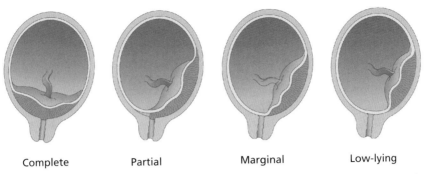

Complete   Partial   Marginal   Low-lying

Figure 45.1 Types of placenta previa. *Complete:* placental tissue completely overlies the internal os (can be central or noncentral, depending on whether or not the center of the placenta is directly over the os). *Partial:* placental tissue is situated over part of the os but does not completely overlie it. *Marginal:* placental tissue approaches the edge of the os but does not overlie any part of it. *Low-lying:* placental tissue is implanted in the lower uterine segment but does not reach the edge of the os. Reproduced from Oyelese and Smulian [39] with permission from Lippincott, Williams and Wilkins.

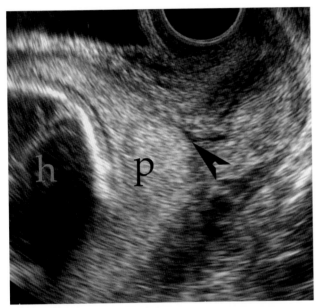

Figure 45.2 Transvaginal sonogram of a complete placenta previa (placenta marked "p"). The placenta can be seen completely overlying the internal os (indicated by the arrow). The fetal head is marked "h".

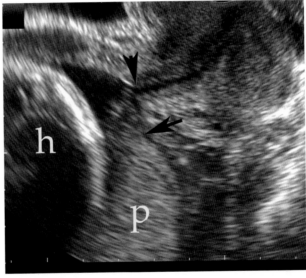

Figure 45.3 Transvaginal sonogram demonstrating a marginal placenta previa (p). The internal os is again clearly shown (*short arrow*). There is a prominent sinus at the placental edge. The actual placental edge is indicated by the long arrow. Because this placenta was less than 2 cm from the internal os, the patient required a cesarean delivery. The fetal head is marked "h".

Finally, a posterior placenta may be difficult to image transabdominally. Transvaginal sonography places the transducer closer to the region of interest, and because of the higher frequencies produced by transvaginal transducers, produces images of superior resolution to those obtained by transabdominal sonography [8]. In virtually all cases, the internal os and the placenta can be adequately visualized using this technique (see Figs 45.2 and 45.3). Numerous studies have consistently demonstrated that transvaginal sonography is more accurate in the diagnosis of placenta previa than transabdominal sonography [8,9]. Furthermore, the technique is

safe and does not lead to an increase in vaginal bleeding [9,10]. When transvaginal sonography is used, false-positive diagnoses of placenta previa are avoided; thus, the reported incidence of placenta previa using transvaginal sonography is considerably lower than that obtained by transabdominal sonography. This has several potential benefits, the main one being that women who do not actually have a placenta previa do not have unnecessary lifestyle restrictions and interventions. Translabial or transperineal sonography and magnetic resonance imaging (MRI) have also been used for placental location. However, these techniques have no benefits over the more readily available transvaginal sonogram.

Placental migration

It has been well documented that the majority of women in whom a placenta previa is detected in the second trimester will no longer have a placenta previa by the third trimester. It is not clear why this occurs. Studies using transvaginal sonography have shown that the incidence of second-trimester placenta previa is 1.1–4.9% [11]. Approximately 90% of these will resolve before term [11]. The apparent movement of the placenta away from the cervix is most likely the consequence of the development of the lower uterine segment, leading to a stationary lower placental edge appearing to move away from the cervix. Another proposed mechanism is preferential growth of the placenta towards the better vascularized fundus.

The likelihood that a second-trimester placenta previa will persist until term can be determined by the degree by which the placenta overlies the internal os in the second trimester. Placentas that do not cover the internal os in the second trimester are unlikely to be placenta previas at term. Conversely, placentas that overlie the internal os by 1.5 cm or more are less likely to resolve by term [11].

Management

Women who present with vaginal bleeding in the late second or third trimester should be considered to have a placenta previa until proven otherwise. However, it must be emphasized that even though this bleeding is classically described as painless, there may be pain, probably the consequence of contractions or placental separation. A digital vaginal examination is contraindicated; this may provoke torrential vaginal bleeding. At least one (and preferably two) wide-bore intravenous cannulae should be inserted and intravenous fluids should be started. Blood should be taken for a complete blood count, blood type, and screen, and at least 2 units of blood should be crossmatched. Sonography, preferably by the transvaginal route, should be performed to confirm or rule out the diagnosis of placenta previa. The patient should be admitted and, initially at least, placed on bedrest. Blood pressure, pulse, and urine output should be monitored closely. Fetal sonography should be performed to rule out fetal anomalies, evaluate fetal growth and amniotic fluid volume. Continuous fetal heart rate monitoring should be commenced. Steroids should be administered to promote fetal lung maturation if the gestational age is between 24 and 32 weeks.

In women who are having contractions, cautious use of tocolytics is reasonable [12]. Frequently, the contractions cause further placental separation, which causes further bleeding, which in turn causes more contractions, and

thus a vicious cycle is set up. It was traditionally taught that tocolytics should not be used in the presence of vaginal bleeding. However, studies of tocolytic usage in women with placenta previa have demonstrated that they may safely be used with caution, and are associated with significant prolongation of gestation and increased birthweight [12,13].

The subsequent management depends on gestational age, fetal and maternal status, and the presence of any other co-existing conditions. At a gestational age of less than 36 weeks, conservative management, rather than immediate delivery, is desirable, because prematurity is the cause of most of the perinatal mortality associated with placenta previa. Blood transfusions may be given as required. Cotton *et al* [14] found that delivery could be deferred with conservative management in two-thirds of patients with symptomatic placenta previa, and that half of patients with an initial hemorrhagic episode exceeding 500 mL did not require immediate delivery. These authors achieved a mean prolongation of pregnancy of 16.8 days in women with symptomatic previas. Similarly, Silver *et al* [15], with conservative aggressive management, prolonged gestation by at least 4 weeks in 50% of patients with a symptomatic previa.

If the mother and fetus are stable, hospitalization for at least 48 h is justified. When there has been no bleeding for at least 24–48 h, the patient may be discharged and subsequently managed as an outpatient [16]. However, it is essential that women who are considered for outpatient management live in close proximity to the hospital, have a responsible adult at home, and have access to telephone services and transportation. Outpatient management has been compared with inpatient management in a few studies [16,17]. A randomized controlled study found that stable patients with placenta previa could be safely managed as outpatients with substantial savings in hospital costs and no worse outcomes (assessed by gestational age at delivery, birthweights, blood transfusions, and neonatal outcomes) than women managed as inpatients [17]. A recent study found that the cervical length was predictive of bleeding; patients with a cervical length of less than 3 cm were at increased risk for bleeding [18]. In another study, cervical lengths were not associated with bleeding, but women with shorter cervices had higher rates of emergency cesarean delivery at <34 weeks. Thus cervical lengths may play a role in the management of women with placenta previa [19].

Complications

Fetal

Placenta previa is associated with increased perinatal mortality as well as an excess in neonatal deaths after live births [19,20]. There is a higher risk of preterm birth, and prematurity is the reason for most of the perinatal deaths

[18]. Placenta previa is also associated with an increased risk of congenital malformations, respiratory distress syndrome, and intrauterine growth restriction [20]. The perinatal mortality rate associated with placenta previa is approximately three times that of controls [20,21].

Maternal

Women with complete or partial placenta previa require cesarean delivery. In addition, the condition is a major cause of obstetric hemorrhage [22]. Frequently, blood transfusions are necessary. While in almost all cases of placenta previa there is some degree of placental separation, women with placenta previa are also at increased risk of concurrent placental abruption. Prolonged bedrest may put women at greater risk of thromboembolic disease [22]. Morbid adherence of the placenta occurs more frequently in women with placenta previa, and frequently these women will go on to have a hysterectomy [22].

Timing of delivery

Women with a placenta previa should be delivered by cesarean at a time when fetal lung maturation is likely and before catastrophic bleeding occurs. Doubtless, these patients are better delivered in a controlled scheduled setting, rather than as an emergency for bleeding. A 2003 study demonstrated that the perinatal mortality for pregnancies complicated by placenta previa started to rise after approximately 37 weeks [21]. For these reasons, scheduled cesarean delivery at 36–37 weeks after documentation of fetal lung maturity by amniocentesis appears reasonable.

Mode of delivery and uterine incisions

There is consensus that women with complete or partial placenta previa require cesarean delivery. What is more controversial is the mode of delivery of women with placentas that lie in close proximity to the internal os but do not cover it. A few studies have addressed the mode of delivery in these patients [23–27]. In an early study, Oppenheimer *et al* [23] found that a lower placental edge to internal os distance of 2 cm or greater on transvaginal sonography was likely to result in a successful trial of labor. Similar findings were noted by Bhide *et al* [24]. Women who had a placental edge to os distance in excess of 2 cm did not require cesarean delivery for bleeding, whereas when the distance was less, the patients invariably required cesarean delivery. However, a more recent study by Vergani and co-workers found that more than two-thirds of women delivered vaginally if the distance between the placental edge and the internal cervical os was 11 mm or greater [26]. When this distance was between 0 and 10 mm, 75% of women required a cesarean delivery and 29% experienced bleeding before labor. In another retrospective study, Bronsteen and colleagues found that 76.5% of women with a placental

edge-to-internal os distance of 1–2 cm successfully delivered vaginally, compared with only 27.3% when this distance was 0–1 cm [27]. It must be pointed out that in several of these studies, the delivering obstetricians were not blinded to the ultrasound results, and thus these results may be significantly biased. Nonetheless, based on newer data, it does appear reasonable to offer a trial of labor to women with a placental edge-to-os distance of 11 mm or greater by transvaginal sonography, who have no other contraindications to vaginal delivery.

In women with an anterior placenta previa, the surgeon generally has to either incise through the placenta and separate the placenta prior to delivery of the fetus or make an incision that avoids the placenta, such as a vertical fundal incision. Generally, a lower segment transverse incision can be used, but it is useful to determine placental location by sonography prior to the operation, and preferably to avoid the placenta.

Vasa previa

The term "vasa previa" refers to fetal blood vessels running through the membranes over the cervix, unprotected by umbilical cord or placental tissue (Fig. 45.4) [28]. Consequently, when the membranes rupture, these vessels frequently rupture also, often resulting in fetal exsanguination [28]. Undiagnosed prenatally, this condition carries a perinatal mortality of approximately 56%

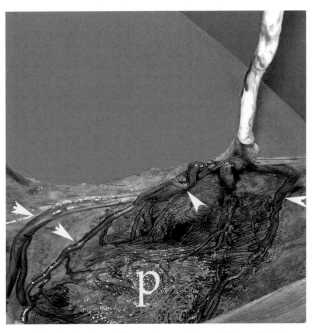

Figure 45.4 Vasa previa shown after cesarean delivery. In this case, the diagnosis had been made prenatally. Prominent velamentous vessels traverse the membranes (*arrows*). "p" marks the placenta.

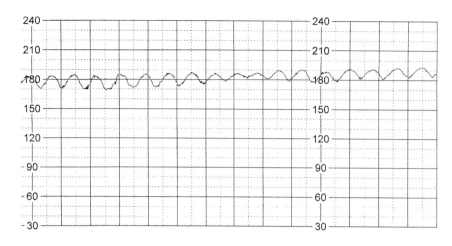

Figure 45.5 Sinusoidal fetal heart rate tracing in a patient with a ruptured vasa previa. The patient, in labor, ruptured her membranes and had bleeding at the same time. Emergency cesarean delivery was performed. The infant was born extremely pale, was immediately transfused, and did well.

[29]. Vasa previa can result from velamentous insertion of the umbilical cord into the placenta or from vessels running between lobes of a placenta with accessory lobes [28].

Incidence and risk factors

The diagnosis of vasa previa is often missed, and thus accurate estimates of the frequency of this condition are difficult to make. Nonetheless, studies suggest that the incidence of clinically recognized vasa previa is approximately 1 in 2500 deliveries [28]. Major risk factors for vasa previa include second-trimester low-lying placentas or placenta previa [28–31]. This risk exists even when the placenta previa is no longer low-lying by the time of delivery [29,31]. Other risk factors include pregnancies resulting from *in vitro* fertilization [28,32], multifetal gestations, and pregnancies where the placenta has one or more succenturiate lobes [28,29].

Pathophysiology

While the exact reason for developing vasa previa remains unknown, two main hypotheses exist as to the condition's pathogenesis. In the first, it is thought that the portion of the placenta that overlies the cervix early in pregnancy undergoes atrophy because of poor vascularity in that region, leaving blood vessels running exposed through the membranes. The second hypothesis suggests that the placenta grows preferentially toward the better vascularized upper segment, again leaving blood vessels exposed during its differential growth.

Clinical presentation

The classic presentation of vasa previa is of vaginal bleeding at the time of rupture of the membranes followed by fetal death or distress. A sinusoidal fetal heart rate tracing in this scenario is virtually pathognomonic of vasa previa (Fig. 45.5). Pressure on the exposed vessels by the presenting part may lead to recurrent variable decelerations, even in cases with intact membranes. Rarely, fetal vessels may be palpated in the unruptured membranes during a cervical examination [24]. More recently, vasa previa has been diagnosed during routine second-trimester sonography or during sonography in patients presenting with bleeding in the second half of pregnancy or patients having sonography for low-lying placentas [29–33].

Diagnosis

The diagnosis of vasa previa may be made based on a history of fetal death or distress associated with bleeding when the membranes rupture. The delivery of an extremely pale, exsanguinated infant and the finding of ruptured velamentous vessels on placental examination after delivery confirm the diagnosis. The diagnosis of vasa previa may be made in asymptomatic women during second-trimester obstetric sonography. Vasa previa has the appearance of linear or tubular structures overlying the cervix. Color Doppler should be employed to demonstrate flow through these vessels, and if pulsed Doppler demonstrates a fetal umbilical or venous waveform, the diagnosis is confirmed (Fig. 45.6). Care must be taken to distinguish a vasa previa from a funic presentation. In a funic presentation, the vessels will move away from the cervix with changes in maternal position, while the position will remain constant.

Several studies have examined the utility of routine screening for vasa previa in asymptomatic patients during the second-trimester obstetric sonogram [33–36]. These studies have consistently demonstrated that vasa previa can be diagnosed with accuracy and without excessive extra time over that required for the obstetric examination [33–36]. The strategy for screening for vasa previa consists of identifying the placental cord insertion during the sonographic examination. This essentially excludes a vasa previa unless there is a multilobed placenta. In women with multilobed placentas, those with second-trimester low-lying placentas, and those with multifetal gestations, transvaginal sonography with a color Doppler sweep of the region over the cervix should be performed.

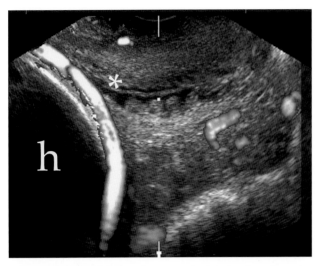

Figure 45.6 Color Doppler of vasa previa showing flow through a vessel running over the internal os (marked by the asterisk). The fetal head is marked "h".

The diagnosis of vasa previa has been made in women presenting with third-trimester bleeding by testing the vaginal blood for fetal blood cells using a test such as the Apt test or Kleihauer–Betke test. However, these tests are rarely used for this purpose, and diagnosis by ultrasound is preferable.

Management
Asymptomatic women with a second-trimester diagnosis of vasa previa should be informed about the diagnosis and about the severity of the condition. These women should report to hospital immediately should they experience contractions, bleeding, or loss of fluid. Coitus should be avoided. Consideration should be given to admission to the hospital at approximately 32 weeks' gestation. The major purpose for admission is to ensure quick access to immediate cesarean delivery should the membranes rupture. In selected cases in which the cervical length is >3cm on transvaginal sonography, and in which the fetal fibronectin test is negative and there are no symptoms, outpatient management may be an option. Because the majority of these women will be delivered preterm, steroids should be administered to promote fetal lung maturation. The patient should be seen by a neonatologist, and facilities for immediate neonatal blood transfusion in the delivery room should be available. Delivery should be by cesarean at 35–36 weeks or after documentation of fetal lung maturation, or if in the third trimester, should significant bleeding, labor, or rupture of the membranes occur. This is earlier than the 39 weeks which is generally recommended for elective deliveries. However, the risk of prematurity may be less than that of fetal exsanguination should the membranes rupture. When the membranes have ruptured, immediate cesar-

ean delivery and neonatal blood transfusion may be lifesaving [37].

Recently, we have used three-dimensional sonography to map out the course of the vessels prior to surgery in order to plan our incision to avoid transecting the vessels. At cesarean delivery, a transverse uterine incision may be made, but it is important to avoid incising or rupturing the membranes after the uterine incision. Every attempt should be made to deliver the fetus *en caul*, with intact membranes.

Outcomes
Perinatal deaths from vasa previa are for the most part preventable; good outcomes depend on prenatal diagnosis and delivery by cesarean before the membranes rupture [28]. Because the fetal blood volume is only approximately 100mL/kg at term, relatively small amounts of blood loss may prove catastrophic to the fetus, and thus everything must be done to ensure delivery before fetal hemorrhage occurs [28]. A study of 155 cases of vasa previa demonstrated that the most important factor in assuring a good perinatal outcome was prenatal diagnosis; the perinatal mortality in pregnancies in which the prenatal diagnosis had been made was 56% [29]. Furthermore, in survivors in cases where the prenatal diagnosis had not been made, the median Apgar scores were 1 at 1min and 4 at 5minu [29]. In addition, over half of these survivors required neonatal blood transfusions [29]. Conversely, when the diagnosis was made prenatally, less than 3% of fetuses/neonates died (over 97% survived), and the median Apgar scores were 7 and 9 at 1 and 5min, respectively [29]. In these patients, neonatal blood transfusions were rarely required [29].

Placenta accreta

Placenta accreta refers to a placenta that is abnormally adherent. This condition is caused by a deficiency of the decidua basalis. Invasion into the myometrium is called placenta increta, while invasion through the serosa is termed placenta percreta. In placenta percreta, the placenta may invade adjacent structures such as the bladder, ureters, bowel, and omentum. In all these entities, the placenta does not separate after delivery and the condition is associated with massive blood loss and high maternal morbidity and mortality.

Incidence and risk factors
The incidence of placenta accreta is estimated at 1 in 500–2500 pregnancies [38,39]. The most important risk factors for placenta accreta are a prior cesarean delivery and a placenta previa in the current pregnancy [38–42]. Clark *et al* [41] showed that the incidence of placenta accreta increased with the number of prior cesarean deliveries,

rising from 25% in women with one prior cesarean to 68% in women with a low-lying placenta and three prior cesarean deliveries. Consequently, as a result of increasing cesarean rates, the incidence of placenta accreta is rising.

Pathophysiology

Recently, it has become clear that prior cesarean deliveries are a risk factor for placenta accreta. In a retrospective study of first-trimester ultrasound images of patients who later ended up with placenta accreta, Comstock and colleagues found that the gestational sac was implanted abnormally low and in the anterior part of the uterus [43]. Observations such as these have led to the hypothesis that placenta accreta generally starts off as pregnancy implantation in the deficient scar of a prior cesarean. Thus, it is possible that the placenta does not actually invade the myometrium but rather, there is abnormal pregnancy implantation in the deficient myometrium at the scar site rather than in the decidua.

Clinical presentation and diagnosis

Placenta accreta should be suspected, particularly in women with a history of prior cesarean or intrauterine surgery, when the placenta fails to separate after delivery. However, the diagnosis may be made prenatally using sonography [42,44,45]. Placenta accreta should be suspected in women with a prior cesarean delivery who have a placenta previa in the current pregnancy [42,44,45]. These women should have a targeted sonographic examination for evidence of placenta accreta [44,45]. Comstock reviewed the antenatal sonographic diagnosis of placenta accreta and found that the most reliable sign of placenta accreta is the presence of prominent vascular spaces or lacunae in the placenta [44,45]. This may give the placenta a "moth-eaten" appearance (Fig. 45.7). Other sonographic signs of placenta accreta include absence of the retroplacental clear space, the presence of a highly vascular myometrial–bladder interface, and invasion into the bladder [44,45]. These authors found a sensitivity of 93%

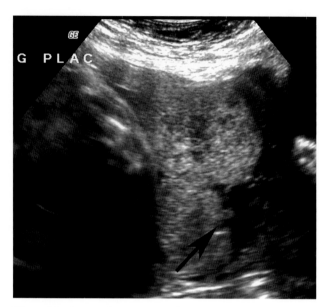

Figure 45.7 Gray-scale sonogram of placenta accreta. Note the prominent lacunae in the placenta, giving a "moth-eaten" appearance (*arrow*).

and a positive predictive value of 92% using gray-scale ultrasound for placenta accreta.

Color Doppler imaging has been used in the diagnosis of placenta accreta, with the main finding being turbulent lacunar blood flow extending from the placenta into the surrounding tissues. MRI is useful and accurate in diagnosing placenta accreta, but does not appear to offer any advantages over sonography, except in cases where there is a posterior placenta. Elevated maternal serum α-fetoprotein (MSAFP) levels may be found in women with placenta accreta [46], and therefore women with unexplained elevated MSAFP levels should have targeted sonography to rule out placenta accreta. The management of placenta accreta is covered elsewhere in this book (see Chapter 36).

CASE PRESENTATION

A 46-year-old gravida 1, para 0 woman became pregnant with twins following *in vitro* fertilization with donor eggs due to infertility. An early sonogram showed that the twins were dichorionic diamniotic. Transabdominal sonography at 20 weeks showed a complete placenta previa. Transvaginal sonography confirmed this. At 30 weeks' gestation she experienced painless vaginal bleeding. Transabdominal and transvaginal sonography showed that there was a vasa previa of twin A. She was admitted to hospital at 32 weeks and steroids were administered. At 35 weeks, the patient was delivered by elective cesarean delivery. Examination of the placenta after delivery confirmed the presence of velamentous vessels, consistent with the diagnosis of a vasa previa.

Management points

The patient conceived by *in vitro* fertilization, was expecting twins, and had a second-trimester complete placenta previa. These are all risk factors for vasa previa. In these patients, it is especially important to screen for vasa previa using transvaginal sonography with color Doppler. Good outcomes depend on a high degree of suspicion and elective delivery by cesarean prior to membrane rupture.

The patient was admitted to hospital at 32 weeks. While admission is not mandatory, it allows quick access to the operating room for emergency cesarean delivery should the membranes rupture. In cases in which the cervix is >3 cm long on transvaginal sonography, closed with no funneling or dynamic changes, and the patient does not have any contractions, outpatient management may be a reasonable option. However, it must be emphasized that not all cases of membrane rupture can be predicted accurately. Steroids should be administered, since these fetuses are at high risk of preterm delivery.

The patient was managed conservatively until 35 weeks. Earlier cesarean delivery would have been performed if she had experienced rupture of the membranes, significant bleeding or had gone into labor.

The patient was delivered electively at 35 weeks. This is earlier than the 39 weeks generally recommended for elective delivery. The risks of fetal exsanguinations should the membranes rupture may exceed those of prematurity at 35 weeks. Amniocentesis for fetal lung maturity studies may be considered prior to delivery.

These babies should be delivered in centers with neonatal units and the neonatologists should be informed prior to delivery.

References

1. Iyasu S, Saftlas AK, Rowley DL, Koonin LM, Lawson HW, Atrash HK. The epidemiology of placenta previa in the United States, 1979 through 1987. Am J Obstet Gynecol 1993;168:1424–1429.

2. Faiz AS, Ananth CV. Etiology and risk factors for placenta previa: an overview and meta-analysis of observational studies. J Matern Fetal Neonatal Med 2003;13:175–190.

3. Ananth CV, Smulian JC, Vintzileos AM. The association of placenta previa with history of cesarean delivery and abortion: a metaanalysis. Am J Obstet Gynecol 1997;177:1071–1078.

4. Ananth CV, Demissie K, Smulian JC, Vintzileos AM. Placenta previa in singleton and twin births in the United States, 1989 through 1998: a comparison of risk factor profiles and associated conditions. Am J Obstet Gynecol 2003;188:275–281.

5. Zhang J, Savitz DA. Maternal age and placenta previa: a population-based, case–control study. Am J Obstet Gynecol 1993;168:641–645.

6. Hill DJ, Beischer NA. Placenta praevia without antepartum haemorrhage. Aust N Z J Obstet Gynaecol 1980;20:21–23.

7. Smith RS, Lauria MR, Comstock CH et al. Transvaginal ultrasonography for all placentas that appear to be low-lying or over the internal cervical os. Ultrasound Obstet Gynecol 1997;9:22–24.

8. Timor-Tritsch IE, Monteagudo A. Diagnosis of placenta previa by transvaginal sonography. Ann Med 1993;25:279–283.

9. Leerentveld RA, Gilberts EC, Arnold MJ, Wladimiroff JW. Accuracy and safety of transvaginal sonographic placental localization. Obstet Gynecol 1990;76:759–762.

10. Timor-Tritsch IE, Yunis RA. Confirming the safety of transvaginal sonography in patients suspected of placenta previa. Obstet Gynecol 1993;81:742–744.

11. Taipale P, Hiilesmaa V, Ylostalo P. Transvaginal ultrasonography at 18–23 weeks in predicting placenta previa at delivery. Ultrasound Obstet Gynecol 1998;12:422–425.

12. Sharma A, Suri V, Gupta I. Tocolytic therapy in conservative management of symptomatic placenta previa. Int J Gynaecol Obstet 2004;84:109–113.

13. Besinger RE, Moniak CW, Paskiewicz LS, Fisher SG, Tomich PG. The effect of tocolytic use in the management of symptomatic placenta previa. Am J Obstet Gynecol 1995;172:1770–1775; discussion 1775–1778.

14. Cotton DB, Read JA, Paul RH, Quilligan EJ. The conservative aggressive management of placenta previa. Am J Obstet Gynecol 1980;137:687–695.

15. Silver R, Depp R, Sabbagha RE, Dooley SL, Socol ML, Tamura RK. Placenta previa: aggressive expectant management. Am J Obstet Gynecol 1984;150:15–22.

16. Mouer JR. Placenta previa: antepartum conservative management, inpatient versus outpatient. Am J Obstet Gynecol 1994;170:1683–1685; discussion 1685–1686.

17. Wing DA, Paul RH, Millar LK. Management of the symptomatic placenta previa: a randomized, controlled trial of inpatient versus outpatient expectant management. Am J Obstet Gynecol 1996;175:806–811.

18. Stafford IA, Dashe JS, Shivvers SA, Alexander JM, McIntire DD, Leveno KJ. Ultrasonographic cervical length and risk of hemorrhage in pregnancies with placenta previa. Obstet Gynecol 2010;116:595–600.

19. Ghi T, Contro E, Martina T et al. Cervical length and risk of antepartum bleeding in women with complete placenta previa. Ultrasound Obstet Gynecol 2009;33(2):209–212.

20. Crane JM, van den Hof MC, Dodds L, Armson BA, Liston R. Neonatal outcomes with placenta previa. Obstet Gynecol 1999;93:541–544.

21. Ananth CV, Smulian JC, Vintzileos AM. The effect of placenta previa on neonatal mortality: a population-based study in the United States, 1989 through 1997. Am J Obstet Gynecol 2003;188:1299–1304.

22. Crane JM, van den Hof MC, Dodds L, Armson BA, Liston R. Maternal complications with placenta previa. Am J Perinatol 2000;17:101–105.

23. Oppenheimer LW, Farine D, Ritchie JW, Lewinsky RM, Telford J, Fairbanks LA. What is a low-lying placenta? Am J Obstet Gynecol 1991;165:1036–1038.

24. Bhide A, Prefumo F, Moore J, Hollis B, Thilaganathan B. Placental edge to internal os distance in the late third trimester and mode of delivery in placenta praevia. Br J Obstet Gynaecol 2003;110:860–864.

25. Dawson WB, Dumas MD, Romano WM, Gagnon R, Gratton RJ, Mowbray RD. Translabial ultrasonography and placenta

previa: does measurement of the os–placenta distance predict outcome? J Ultrasound Med 1996;15:441–446.

26. Vergani P, Ornaghi S, Pozzi I et al. Placenta previa: distance to internal os and mode of delivery. Am J Obstet Gynecol 2009;201(3):266.

27. Bronsteen R, Valice R, Lee W, Blackwell S, Balasubramaniam M, Comstock C. Effect of a low-lying placenta on delivery outcome. Ultrasound Obstet Gynecol 2009;33(2):204–208.

28. Oyelese KO, Turner M, Lees C, Campbell S. Vasa previa: an avoidable obstetric tragedy. Obstet Gynecol Surv 1999;54:138–145.

29. Oyelese Y, Catanzarite V, Prefumo F et al. Vasa previa: the impact of prenatal diagnosis on outcomes. Obstet Gynecol 2004;103:937–942.

30. Oyelese Y, Spong C, Fernandez MA, McLaren RA. Second trimester low-lying placenta and in vitro fertilization? Exclude vasa previa. J Matern Fetal Med 2000;9:370–372.

31. Francois K, Mayer S, Harris C, Perlow JH. Association of vasa previa at delivery with a history of second-trimester placenta previa. J Reprod Med 2003;48:771–774.

32. Schachter M, Tovbin Y, Arieli S, Friedler S, Ron-El R, Sherman D. In vitro fertilization is a risk factor for vasa previa. Fertil Steril 2002;78:642–643.

33. Lee W, Lee VL, Kirk JS, Sloan CT, Smith RS, Comstock CH. Vasa previa: prenatal diagnosis, natural evolution, and clinical outcome. Obstet Gynecol 2000;95:572–576.

34. Catanzarite V, Maida C, Thomas W, Mendoza A, Stanco L, Piacquadio KM. Prenatal sonographic diagnosis of vasa previa: ultrasound findings and obstetric outcome in ten cases. Ultrasound Obstet Gynecol 2001;18:109–115.

35. Nomiyama M, Toyota Y, Kawano H. Antenatal diagnosis of velamentous umbilical cord insertion and vasa previa with color Doppler imaging. Ultrasound Obstet Gynecol 1998;12:426–429.

36. Sepulveda W, Rojas I, Robert JA, Schnapp C, Alcalde JL. Prenatal detection of velamentous insertion of the umbilical cord: a prospective color Doppler ultrasound study. Ultrasound Obstet Gynecol 2003;21:564–569.

37. Schellpfeffer MA. Improved neonatal outcome of vasa previa with aggressive intrapartum management: a report of two cases. J Reprod Med 1995;40:327–332.

38. Miller DA, Chollet JA, Goodwin TM. Clinical risk factors for placenta previa–placenta accreta. Am J Obstet Gynecol 1997;177:210–214.

39. Oyelese Y, Smulian JC. Placenta previa, accreta, and vasa previa. Obstet Gynecol 2006;107:927–941.

40. Wu S, Kocherginsky M, Hibbard JU. Abnormal placentation: twenty-year analysis. Am J Obstet Gynecol 2005;192:1458–1461.

41. Clark SL, Koonings PP, Phelan JP. Placenta previa/accreta and prior cesarean section. Obstet Gynecol 1985;66:89–92.

42. Hudon L, Belfort MA, Broome DR. Diagnosis and management of placenta percreta: a review. Obstet Gynecol Surv 1998;53:509–517.

43. Comstock CH, Lee W, Vettraino IM, Bronsteen RA. The early sonographic appearance of placenta accreta. J Ultrasound Med. 2003;22:19–23.

44. Comstock CH. Antenatal diagnosis of placenta accreta: a review. Ultrasound Obstet Gynecol 2005;26:89–96.

45. Comstock CH, Love JJ Jr, Bronsteen RA et al. Sonographic detection of placenta accreta in the second and third trimesters of pregnancy. Am J Obstet Gynecol 2004;190:1135–1140.

46. Zelop C, Nadel A, Frigoletto FD Jr, Pauker S, MacMillan M, Benacerraf BR. Placenta accreta/percreta/increta: a cause of elevated maternal serum alpha-fetoprotein. Obstet Gynecol 1992;80:693–694.

Chapter 46
Prolonged Pregnancy

Teresa Marino and Errol R. Norwitz
Department of Obstetrics and Gynecology, Tufts Medical Center and Tufts University School of Medicine, Boston, MA, USA

The timely onset of labor and delivery is an important determinant of perinatal outcome. Both preterm births (defined as delivery prior to 37 weeks' gestation) and postterm births (defined as delivery after 42 weeks' gestation) are associated with increased neonatal morbidity and mortality. Much attention has been paid to the problem of preterm birth. Despite the observation that antepartum stillbirths account for more perinatal deaths than either complications of prematurity or sudden infant death syndrome and the fact that the risks of postterm pregnancy can be easily avoided by earlier induction of labor, the issue of postterm pregnancy has received little attention. This chapter reviews in detail the risks of continuing pregnancy beyond the due date, the option of induction of labor, and the management of low-risk postterm pregnancies.

Definitions

Prolonged or postterm pregnancy is defined as one that continues to or beyond 42 weeks 0 days (294 days) from the first day of the last normal menstrual period or 14 days beyond the best obstetric estimate of the date of delivery (EDD) [1]. The term "postdates" is not well defined and, as such, is best avoided. Accurate pregnancy dating is critical to the diagnosis.

Prevalence

The prevalence of postterm pregnancy depends on the patient population, including such factors as the percentage of primigravid women, women with pregnancy complications, and the frequency of preterm birth. Local practice patterns such as the rates of scheduled cesarean delivery and routine labor induction will also affect the overall prevalence of postterm birth. In the USA, approximately 18% of all singleton pregnancies continue beyond 41 weeks, 10% (range 3–14%) continue beyond 42 weeks and are therefore post term, and 4% (2–7%) continue beyond 43 completed weeks in the absence of obstetric intervention [1].

Etiology

The most common cause of prolonged pregnancy is an error in gestational age dating. Reliance on clinical criteria alone (Box 46.1) tends to overestimate gestational age [2–4]. Uncertainty in dating parameters should prompt an ultrasound examination. Most cases of "true" postterm pregnancy have no known cause. Risk factors include nulliparity and a prior postterm pregnancy. Rarer causes include placental sulfatase deficiency (an X-linked recessive disorder characterized by low circulating estriol levels), fetal adrenal insufficiency or hypoplasia, and fetal anencephaly without polyhydramnios. Genetic factors may also have a role in prolonging pregnancy [1,5]. There is no consistent association between postterm pregnancy and maternal age, parity, or ethnicity.

Complications of postterm pregnancy

Recent studies have shown that the fetal [6–14] and maternal risks [11,15–18] of continuing the pregnancy beyond the EDD are greater than originally appreciated.

Fetal risks
Antepartum stillbirths account for more perinatal deaths than either complications of prematurity or sudden infant death syndrome [10]. Perinatal mortality (defined as stillbirths plus early neonatal deaths) at 42 weeks' gestation is twice that at 40 weeks (4–7 versus 2–3 per 1000 deliveries, respectively) and increases fourfold at 43 weeks and 5–7-fold at 44 weeks [8–11]. Additionally,

Queenan's Management of High-Risk Pregnancy: An Evidence-Based Approach, Sixth Edition. Edited by John T. Queenan, Catherine Y. Spong, Charles J. Lockwood.

recent epidemiologic studies suggest that these calculations may actually underestimate the risk of stillbirth and early neonatal death. This is because these data used all pregnancies rather than ongoing (undelivered) pregnancies as the denominator (Figs 46.1 and 46.2); however, once a fetus is delivered, it is no longer at risk of stillbirth. For example, in one retrospective study of over 170,000 singleton births, Hilder *et al* [9] demonstrated that, when calculated per 1000 ongoing pregnancies, fetal and neonatal mortality rates increase sharply after 40 weeks (see Fig. 46.1). Cotzias *et al* [10] used the same database to calculate the *absolute risk* of stillbirth in ongoing pregnancies for each gestational age from 35 to 43 weeks. The risk of stillbirth was 1 in 926 ongoing pregnancies at 40 weeks' gestation, 1 in 826 at 41 weeks, 1 in 769 at 42 weeks, and 1 in 633 at 43 weeks. Uteroplacental insufficiency, asphyxia, and intrauterine infection all contribute to the excess perinatal deaths.

Postterm infants are larger than term infants with a higher incidence of fetal macrosomia (2.5–10% versus 0.8–1%, respectively), such that twice as many postterm infants weigh over 4000 g at birth [19]. Complications associated with fetal macrosomia include prolonged labor, cephalopelvic disproportion, and shoulder dystocia. Approximately 20% of postterm fetuses have "fetal dysmaturity (postmaturity) syndrome," which describes infants with characteristics of chronic intrauterine growth restriction from uteroplacental insufficiency. These pregnancies are at increased risk of oligohydramnios, nonreassuring fetal testing, intrauterine passage of meconium, and short-term neonatal complications (e.g. hypoglycemia, seizures, and respiratory insufficiency).

Meconium aspiration syndrome refers to respiratory compromise with tachypnea, cyanosis, and reduced pulmonary compliance in newborn infants exposed to meconium *in utero*. It is primarily a disease of postterm infants. The fourfold decrease in the incidence of the meconium aspiration syndrome in the USA from 1990 to 1998 has been attributed primarily to a reduction in the postterm delivery rate [20], with very little contribution from conventional interventions designed to protect the lungs from the chemical pneumonitis caused by chronic meconium exposure, such as amnio-infusion and routine nasopharyngeal suctioning of meconium-stained neonates.

Postterm pregnancy is also an independent risk factor for neonatal encephalopathy [21] and for death in the first year of life [9–11].

Maternal risks

The maternal risks of prolonged pregnancy are often underappreciated. These include an increase in labor dystocia, third- and fourth-degree perineal lacerations, and cesarean delivery [11,15–18]. The latter is associated with higher risks of complications such as endometritis, hemorrhage, and thromboembolic disease. In addition to the medical risks, the emotional impact (anxiety and frustration) of carrying a pregnancy 2 weeks beyond the EDD should not be underestimated.

Prevention and management of postterm pregnancy

Appropriate management of postterm pregnancy includes accurate gestational age assessment in early pregnancy, antenatal fetal surveillance, and the timely initiation of delivery if spontaneous labor does not occur.

Accurate gestational age assessment

An accurate EDD should be calculated early in pregnancy. Although often based upon standard clinical criteria (see Box 46.1), any uncertainty in dating parameters should prompt an ultrasound examination. *Routine* early ultrasound examination has been shown to reduce the rate of false-positive diagnoses and thereby the overall rate of postterm pregnancy from 10% to 1–3%, thereby minimizing unnecessary interventions [1–4,22]. However, the practice of ultrasound for pregnancy dating has not been recommended as a standard of care in the USA [23].

Antenatal fetal surveillance

Postterm pregnancy is a universally accepted indication for antenatal fetal monitoring [1,23,24]. The efficacy of this approach has not been validated by prospective

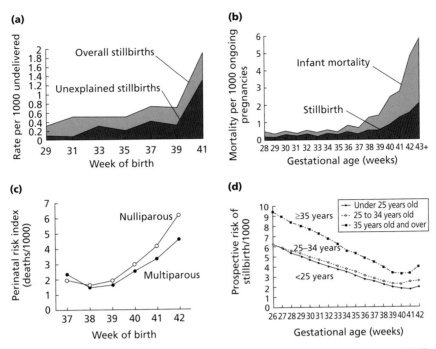

Figure 46.1 Multiple studies have reported that antepartum stillbirths increase after 38–39 weeks' gestation. (a) This was first demonstrated in 1987 (Yudkin *et al* [6]). (b) Subsequent studies showed that this was true not only of antepartum stillbirth, but also of mortality within the first year of life (e.g. Rand *et al* [11]). (c) Further studies have shown that the same relationship exists in both nulliparous and multiparous women (Smith [12]) and (d) in women of advanced maternal age (Feldman [8]).

randomized trials. Indeed, because of ethical and medicolegal concerns, there are no studies of postterm pregnancies that include a nonmonitored control group, and it is highly unlikely that such a trial will ever be performed. Options for evaluating fetal well-being include nonstress testing (NST) with or without amniotic fluid volume assessment, the biophysical profile (BPP), the oxytocin challenge test, or a combination of these modalities. There is no consensus in the literature as to which of these modalities is preferred, and no single method has been shown to be superior [1,23,24].

The American College of Obstetricians and Gynecologists has recommended that antepartum fetal surveillance be initiated by 42 weeks (EDD+14 days) without a specific recommendation regarding the type of test or frequency [1,23]. Many investigators would advise twice-weekly testing with some evaluation of amniotic fluid volume [24]. There is insufficient evidence to show that initiating antenatal surveillance at 40–42 weeks' gestation improves pregnancy outcome [1,24].

Timing of delivery

Delivery is typically recommended when the risks to the fetus from continuing the pregnancy are greater than those faced by the neonate after birth. The pregnancies of high-risk patients (Box 46.2) should not be allowed to progress into the postterm period because, in these pregnancies, the balance often shifts in favor of delivery at around 38–39 weeks' gestation. Management of low-risk pregnancies is more controversial. Because delivery cannot always be expedited, maternal risks and considerations are more likely to confound this decision. Factors that need to be considered include results of antepartum fetal assessment, favorability of the cervix for induction, gestational age, and maternal preference. These factors will guide discussion of the risks, benefits, and alternatives to expectant management with antepartum monitoring versus immediate labor induction.

Antepartum fetal assessment

Delivery should be effected immediately if there is evidence of fetal compromise or oligohydramnios [1]. Oligohydramnios may result from uteroplacental insufficiency or increased renal artery resistance and may predispose to umbilical cord compression, thus leading to intermittent fetal hypoxemia, meconium passage, or meconium aspiration. Adverse pregnancy outcomes (i.e. nonreassuring fetal heart rate tracing, neonatal intensive care unit (ICU) admission, and low Apgar scores) are more common when oligohydramnios is present [1]. Twice-weekly screening of postterm patients for oligohydramnios is important because amniotic fluid can become drastically reduced within 24–48 h. However, a consistent definition of low amniotic fluid volume in the postterm

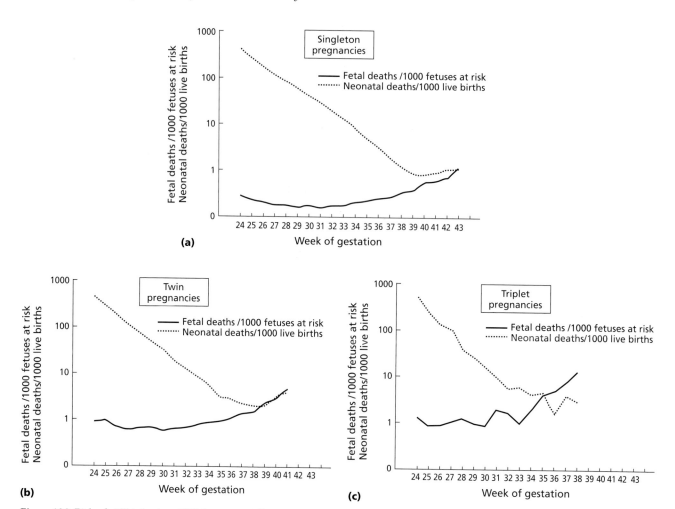

Figure 46.2 Risk of stillbirths (per 1000 fetuses at risk) and neonatal deaths (per 1000 livebirths) in singleton (n = 11,061,599), twin (n = 297,622), and triplet (n = 15,375) gestations drawn from the 1995–1998 National Center for Health Statistics linked birth and death files. Reproduced from Kahn *et al* [14] with permission from Lippincott Williams and Wilkins.

Box 46.2 High-risk pregnancies

Maternal factors

- Preeclampsia (gestational proteinuric hypertension)
- Chronic hypertension
- Diabetes mellitus (including gestational diabetes)
- Maternal cardiac disease
- Chronic renal disease
- Chronic pulmonary disease
- Active thromboembolic disease

Fetal factors

- Nonreassuring fetal testing ("fetal distress")
- Intrauterine growth restriction
- Isoimmunization

- Intraamniotic infection
- Known fetal structural anomaly
- Prior unexplained stillbirth
- Multiple pregnancy

Uteroplacental factors

- Premature rupture of fetal membranes
- Unexplained oligohydramnios
- Prior classic (high vertical) hysterotomy
- Placenta previa
- Abruptio placentae
- Vasa previa

pregnancy has not been established. Options include largest vertical fluid pocket <2 cm or Amniotic Fluid Index (AFI) <5 cm.

Favorability of the cervix

There is insufficient evidence to determine whether expectant management or labor induction in postterm pregnancies with a *favorable* cervical examination yields a better outcome. A favorable cervical examination is defined as a Bishop score >6. This has been shown to be superior to transvaginal ultrasound assessment of cervical length to predict the time interval from induction to delivery [25,26]. One of the reasons for the lack of data is that the majority of studies comparing induction to expectant management excluded this group of patients or initiated induction at the time the cervix became favorable. In studies that did examine this subgroup, there was no apparent increased risk associated with expectant management [1]. When the ongoing risk of stillbirth (albeit small) is weighed against the very low risk (both in absolute and relative terms) of failed induction leading to cesarean delivery with a *favorable* cervical examination, common sense suggests that routine induction of labor is a reasonable option for such women at or after 41 weeks' gestation.

In the setting of an *unfavorable* cervical examination, both expectant management and labor induction are associated with low complication rates in low-risk, postterm gravidae. However, there appears to be a slight advantage to labor induction at 41 weeks' gestation using cervical ripening agents, when indicated, regardless of parity or method of induction. The introduction of preinduction cervical maturation has resulted in fewer failed and serial inductions, lower fetal and maternal morbidity, a shorter hospital stay, lower medical cost, and possibly a lower rate of cesarean delivery in the general obstetric population [1].

The largest trial of routine postterm induction compared with expectant management randomly assigned 3407 low-risk women with uncomplicated singleton pregnancies at 41 weeks' gestation to either induction of labor (with or without cervical ripening agents) within 4 days of randomization or expectant management until 44 weeks [27]. Elective induction resulted in a modestly lower cesarean delivery rate (21.2% versus 24.5%), primarily because of fewer surgeries for nonreassuring fetal tracings. A subsequent cost analysis of these data reported that a policy of routine labor induction resulted in lower costs compared with expectant management [28]. In addition, a metaanalysis of 19 trials of routine versus selective induction of labor in postterm patients found that routine induction after 41 weeks was associated with a lower rate of perinatal mortality (odds ratio [OR] 0.2, 95% confidence interval [CI] 0.06–0.70) and no increase in the cesarean delivery rate (OR 1.02, 95% CI 0.75–1.38) [29]. The actual risk of stillbirth during the 41st week (41 weeks 0 days to 41 weeks 6 days) was 1.04–1.27 per 1000 undelivered women compared with 1.55–3.10 at or beyond 42 weeks [30].

These findings, similar to those of other metaanalyses [31], suggest that routine induction at 41 weeks' gestation has fetal benefit without incurring additional maternal risks because of a higher rate of cesarean delivery [11]. An improved ability to identify women who will have a successful induction of labor would allow obstetric care providers to better individualize their recommendations.

In patients with a prior cesarean delivery who desire a trial of labor (i.e. decline elective repeat cesarean at 39 weeks' gestation), failure to go into labor spontaneously by 41 weeks should prompt further discussion about elective repeat cesarean. An effort should be made to avoid induction of labor in such patients, because of the increased risk of uterine rupture [32].

Gestational age

The American College of Obstetricians and Gynecologists no longer defines any specific upper limit of gestational age for expectantly managed pregnancies [1]. Although postterm pregnancy is defined as a pregnancy >42 weeks' gestation, the two large multicenter randomized studies of management of prolonged pregnancy reported favorable outcomes with routine induction as early as 41 weeks' gestation [27,33]. Many physicians now induce labor between weeks 41 and 42, and virtually all do not allow pregnancy to extend beyond 43 weeks' gestation (EDD + 3 weeks). This practice is supported by recent studies suggesting that the rate of fetal demise is significantly higher than the rate of neonatal death at any time after 283 days' gestation (40 weeks 3 days) [12,34,35].

What is post term for multiples?

The definition of term (and hence post term) in multifetal gestations should incorporate not only the natural history of such pregnancies but also the effect of gestational age on perinatal mortality. The average length of gestation is 40 weeks in singletons, 36 weeks in twins, 33 weeks in triplets, and 29 weeks in quadruplets [36]. To investigate the effect of gestational age on perinatal mortality, Minakami and Sato [37] compared the outcome of 88,936 infants born of multiple pregnancies (96% of which were twins) with that of 6,020,542 infants born of singleton pregnancies after 26 weeks' gestation between 1989 and 1993. In this cohort, the lowest perinatal mortality rate was seen at 38 weeks in multiple pregnancies compared with 40 weeks in singleton pregnancies (10.5 versus 9.7 deaths per 1000 deliveries, respectively). Thereafter, the perinatal mortality rate increased for both groups, but was more exaggerated in multiple pregnancies. Indeed, the risk of perinatal death was sixfold higher for fetuses of multiple pregnancies born after 37 weeks compared with singleton fetuses born at or after 40 weeks (relative risk [RR] 6.6, 95% CI 6.1–7.1) [37]. Although no consensus has been reached, these data suggest that the normal length of gestation for twins should be regarded as 38 rather than 40 weeks. As such, every effort should be made to deliver uncomplicated twins by 40 weeks' gestation (post term for twins).

Intrapartum management

The postterm fetus is at high risk of intrapartum fetal heart rate abnormalities. For this reason, most authors recommend continuous electronic fetal monitoring in labor for these pregnancies. Intrapartum spontaneous or induced fetal heart rate accelerations coupled with moderate fetal heart rate variability (category 1 tracings) are reliable signs of a nonacidotic fetus.

Prognosis

At 1 and 2 years of age, the general intelligence quotient, physical milestones, and frequency of intercurrent illnesses are the same for normal term infants and those from prolonged pregnancies [38].

Conclusion

The risks of routine induction of labor (specifically failed induction leading to cesarean delivery) in the era of cervical ripening agents is lower than previously reported. The risk of fetal death is also low, but not zero, with expectantly managed, carefully monitored postterm pregnancies. For these reasons, the authors favor a policy of routine induction of labor for low-risk singleton pregnancies at 41 weeks' gestation.

CASE PRESENTATION

A 33-year-old Asian woman, gravida 3, para 0, presents for routine prenatal care at 41 weeks 0 days gestation. Her prior pregnancies included a first-trimester spontaneous abortion and a 20-week previable delivery as a result of cervical insufficiency. Dating criteria include a firm last menstrual period, confirmed by a 6-week ultrasound. An elective cervical cerclage was placed at 14 weeks and removed without incident at 37 weeks. Level II ultrasound at 18 weeks' gestation confirmed a structurally normal male fetus and a fundal placenta.

The woman perceives good fetal movements but reports only irregular uterine contractions and no leakage of fluid. A rectovaginal culture taken at 37 weeks confirms that she is not a group B streptococcus carrier. Abdominal examination confirms a singleton fetus with an estimated fetal weight of 3500 g. The presentation is cephalic and the vertex is engaged in the maternal pelvis. Pelvic examination confirms a gynecoid pelvis with adequate clinical pelvimetry. The cervix is posterior, firm, and closed. Fetal well-being is confirmed with a baseline fetal heart rate of 140 beats/min and a reactive NST. The patient strongly desires a vaginal delivery and understands that obstetric intervention in the setting of an unfavorable cervical examination may increase her risk of cesarean delivery. You review symptoms and signs of labor, and discharge the woman home to follow up in 1 week.

The patient returns at 42 weeks 0 days gestation. She again reports good fetal movements and rare contractions. Estimated fetal weight is 4200 g. Pelvic examination shows the cervix to be 1 cm dilated, 50% effaced, –2 station, and posterior. You offer the patient cervical ripening and induction for postterm pregnancy, but she declines. Fetal NST is reactive and Amniotic Fluid Index is 12.2 cm. You again discharge the woman home after reviewing symptoms and signs of labor. A follow-up visit is planned in 2 days.

The woman presents the next day to labor and delivery with regular contractions every 3–4 min. Initial cervical examination is 4 cm dilated, 90% effaced, with the vertex at 0 station and membranes bulging. Position is noted to be occiput posterior. Fetal heart rate tracing is reactive with a baseline of 140–145 beats/min and moderate variability. Intermittent variable decelerations are noted. Over the next 2 h, the patient's contractions become milder and less frequent and there is no further cervical change or descent of the presenting part. Fetal well-being remains reassuring. After counseling, you rupture the fetal membranes and note moderate meconium staining of the amniotic fluid. You start oxytocin augmentation. Because of a difficulty in tracing the fetal heart rate, you place a fetal scalp electrode. Over the next 4 h, the contractions are noted to be adequate (>200 Montevideo units), but there is no further cervical dilation or descent of the presenting part. Moreover, you note increasing caput succedaneum, more exaggerated molding of the fetal skull bones, and repetitive severe variable decelerations on cardiotocography. You make a diagnosis of cephalopelvic disproportion and recommend cesarean delivery which is performed under spinal anesthesia. A viable male infant is delivered in the occiput posterior position without difficulty. Moderate meconium staining of the amniotic fluid is confirmed. The baby is vigorous at birth. Apgar scores are assigned as 8 at 1 min and 9 at 5 min. No cord gases are sent. The birth weight is 4890 g. The baby is discharged home on day 4 of life along with the mother.

References

1. American College of Obstetricians and Gynecologists Committee on Practice Bulletins-Obstetrics. Management of postterm pregnancy. ACOG Practice Bulletin No. 55. Obstet Gynecol 2004;104:639–646.

2. Neilson JP. Ultrasound for fetal assessment in early pregnancy. Cochrane Database Syst Rev 2000;2:CD000182.

3. Taipale P, Hiilermaa V. Predicting delivery date by ultrasound and last menstrual period on early gestation. Obstet Gynecol 2001;97:189–194.

4. Caughey AB, Nicholson JM, Washington AE. First- vs second-trimester ultrasound: the effect on pregnancy dating and perinatal outcomes. Am J Obstet Gynecol 2008;198:703.

5. Laursen M, Bille C, Olesen AW, Hjelmborg J, Skytthe A, Christensen K. Genetic influence on prolonged gestation: a population-based Danish twin study. Am J Obstet Gynecol 2004;190:489–494.

6. Yudkin PL, Wood L, Redman CW. Risk of unexplained stillbirth at different gestational ages. Lancet 1987;1:1192–1194.

7. Herabutya Y, Prasertsawat PO, Tongyai T, Isarangura NA, Ayudthya N. Prolonged pregnancy: the management dilemma. Int J Gynecol Obstet 1992;37:253–258.

8. Feldman GB. Prospective risk of stillbirth. Obstet Gynecol 1992;79:547–553.

9. Hilder L, Costeloe K, Thilaganathan B. Prolonged pregnancy: evaluating gestation-specific risks of fetal and infant mortality. Br J Obstet Gynaecol 1998;105:169–173.

10. Cotzias CS, Paterson-Brown S, Fisk NM. Prospective risk of unexplained stillbirth in singleton pregnancies at term: population based analysis. BMJ 1999;319:287–288.

11. Rand L, Robinson JN, Economy KE, Norwitz ER. Post-term induction of labor revisited. Obstet Gynecol 2000;96:779–783.

12. Smith GC. Life-table analysis of the risk of perinatal death at term and post term in singleton pregnancies. Am J Obstet Gynecol 2001;184:489–496.

13. Froen JF, Arnestad M, Frey K, Vege A, Saugstad OD, Stray-Pedersen B. Risk factors for sudden intrauterine unexplained death: epidemiologic characteristics of singleton cases in Oslo, Norway, 1986–1995. Am J Obstet Gynecol 2001;184:694–702.

14. Kahn B, Lumey LH, Zybert PA et al. Prospective risk of fetal death in singleton, twin, and triplet gestations: implications for practice. Obstet Gynecol 2003;102:685–692.

15. Campbell MK, Ostbye T, Irgens LM. Post-term birth: risk factors and outcomes in a 10-year cohort of Norwegian births. Obstet Gynecol 1997;89:543–548.

16. Alexander JM, McIntire DD, Leveno KJ. Forty weeks and beyond: pregnancy outcomes by week of gestation. Obstet Gynecol 2000;96:291–294.

17. Treger M, Hallak M, Silberstein T, Friger M, Katz M, Mazor M. Post-term pregnancy: should induction of labor be considered before 42 weeks? J Matern Fetal Neonatal Med 2002;11:50–53.

18. Caughey AB, Stotland NE, Washington AE, Escobar GJ. Maternal and obstetric complications of pregnancy are associated with increasing gestational age at term. Am J Obstet Gynecol 2007;196:155.

19. Spellacy WN, Miller S, Winegar A, Peterson PQ. Macrosomia: maternal characteristics and infant complications. Obstet Gynecol 1985;66:158–161.

20. Yoder BA, Kirsch EA, Barth WH, Gordon MC. Changing obstetric practices associated with decreasing incidence of meconium aspiration syndrome. Obstet Gynecol 2002;99:731.

21. Badawi N, Kurinczuk JJ, Keogh JM et al. Antepartum risk factors for newborn encephalopathy: the Western Australian case–control study. BMJ 1998;317:1549–1553.

22. Bennett KA, Crane JM, O'Shea P, Lacelle J, Hutchens D, Copel JA. First trimester ultrasound screening is effective in reducing postterm labor induction rates: a randomized controlled trial. Am J Obstet Gynecol 2004;190:1077–1081.

23. American Academy of Pediatrics and American College of Obstetricians and Gynecologists. Guidelines for Perinatal Care, 6th edn. Washington, DC: AAP and ACOG, 2007.

24. American College of Obstetricians and Gynecologists. Antepartum fetal surveillance. ACOG Practice Bulletin No. 9. Obstet Gynecol 1999;94(4).

25. Roman H, Verspyck E, Vercoustre L et al. The role of ultrasound and fetal fibronectin in predicting the length of induced labor when the cervix is unfavorable. Ultrasound Obstet Gynecol 2004;23:567–573.

26. Rozenberg P, Chevret S, Ville Y. Comparison of pre-induction ultrasonographic cervical length and Bishop score in predicting risk of cesarean section after labor induction with prostaglandins. Gynecol Obstet Fertil 2005;33:17–22.

27. Hannah ME, Hannah WJ, Hellmann J, Hewson S, Milner R, Willan A. Induction of labor as compared with serial antenatal monitoring in post-term pregnancy: a randomized controlled trial. The Canadian Multicenter Post-Term Pregnancy Trial Group. N Engl J Med 1992;326:1587–1592.

28. Goeree R, Hannah M, Hewson S. Cost-effectiveness of induction of labour versus serial antenatal monitoring in the Canadian Multicentre Postterm Pregnancy Trial. CMAJ 1995;152:1445–1450.

29. Crowley P. Interventions for preventing or improving the outcome of delivery at or beyond term. Cochrane Database Syst Rev 2000;2:CD000170.

30. Menticoglou SM, Hall PF. Routine induction of labour at 41 weeks gestation: nonsensus consensus. Br J Obstet Gynaecol 2002;109:485–491.

31. Sanchez-Ramos L, Olivier F, Delke I, Kaunitz AM. Labor induction versus expectant management for postterm pregnancies: a systematic review with meta-analysis. Obstet Gynecol 2003;101:1312–1318.

32. Lydon-Rochelle M, Holt VL, Easterling TR, Martin DP. Risk of uterine rupture during labor among women with a prior cesarean delivery. N Engl J Med 2001;345:3–35.

33. National Institute of Child Health and Human Development Network of Maternal-Fetal Medicine Units. A clinical trial of induction of labor versus expectant management in postterm pregnancy. Am J Obstet Gynecol 1994;170:716–723.

34. Caughey AB, Stotland NE, Escobar GJ. What is the best measure of maternal complications of term pregnancy: ongoing pregnancies or pregnancies delivered? Am J Obstet Gynecol 2003;189:1047–1052.

35. Divon MY, Ferber A, Sanderson M, Nisell H, Westgren M. A functional definition of prolonged pregnancy based on daily fetal and neonatal mortality rates. Ultrasound Obstet Gynecol 2004;23:423–426.

36. Kahn B, Lumey LH, Zybert PA et al. Prospective risk of fetal death in singleton, twin, and triplet gestations: implications for practice. Obstet Gynecol 2003;102:685–692.

37. Minakami H, Sato I. Reestimating date of delivery in multifetal pregnancies. JAMA 1996;275:1432–1434.

38. Shime J, Librach CL, Gare DJ, Cook CJ. The influence of prolonged pregnancy on infant development at one and two years of age: a prospective controlled study. Am J Obstet Gynecol 1986;154:341–345.

Chapter 47
Induction of Labor

Nicole M. Petrossi and Deborah A. Wing
Department of Obstetrics and Gynecology, University of California, Irvine, CA, USA

One of the most routinely performed obstetric procedures in the United States is induction of labor. This procedure involves iatrogenic stimulation of uterine contractions prior to the onset of spontaneous labor to accomplish vaginal delivery. Increasing the frequency and improving the intensity of existing uterine contractions in a patient who is in labor and not progressing sufficiently is referred to as augmentation of labor. From 1990 to 2007, there was a sharp increase in the frequency of labor induction, from 9.5% to 22.8% [1]. The principal reason for this increase is the availability of superior cervical ripening agents and an increase in *bona fide* indications for induction of labor (e.g. preterm premature rupture of the membranes at term and postdates pregnancies), as well as a more relaxed attitude toward marginal indications for induction, and clinician's and/or patient's desire to arrange an opportune time of delivery [2].

Indications and contraindications

Indications for induction of labor can be classified as either maternal or fetal in nature. In most cases, when the benefits of expeditious delivery to the mother or fetus outweigh the risk of continuing the pregnancy, induction of labor should take place [3]. There are several relative indications for labor induction and many accepted medical and obstetric indications (Box 47.1). The degree of maternal and/or fetal risk for morbidities such as cesarean delivery or neonatal respiratory compromise is contingent upon factors such as cervical status, severity of the clinical condition, the presence or absence of fetal lung maturity, and gestational age.

A few examples of common obstetric and medical conditions for which induction may be indicated include preeclampsia/eclampsia, intrauterine fetal growth restriction, rupture of membranes, postterm pregnancy, and fetal demise. Fetal and/or maternal outcome is thought to be improved through appropriately timed induction of women with these pregnancy complications [4]. Unfortunately, there is only limited high-quality evidence showing any benefits for specific medical and obstetric indications for induction, with the recent exception of gestational hypertension beyond 36 weeks in which induction was associated with improved maternal outcomes [5].

Contraindications include all those which proscribe vaginal delivery (Box 47.2), and other clinical scenarios that require a cautious approach when induction is considered, including nonreactive nonstress testing, multifetal pregnancy, and previous low transverse cesarean delivery. These latter scenarios may be associated with an increased risk of maternal or fetal morbidity during induction. Close monitoring during induction is required in these cases, along with a low threshold for intervention if labor is not progressing or there are no reassuring signs of fetal well-being.

Elective induction of labor

The initiation of labor for convenience in a mother with a term pregnancy with no medical or obstetric indication is referred to as elective induction of labor, and should be differentiated from those inductions that are undertaken for indications but without the presence of endogenous labor. Major concerns associated with elective induction include iatrogenic prematurity, increased rates of cesarean delivery, and cost. A further concern is that putative maternal-fetal medical benefits, such as reduction in stillbirth, have not been proven. Nevertheless, scheduled induction of labor has many potential advantages, such as avoiding the risk of delivery *en route* to the hospital if labor is rapid or the healthcare facility is remotely located.

Queenan's Management of High-Risk Pregnancy: An Evidence-Based Approach, Sixth Edition. Edited by John T. Queenan, Catherine Y. Spong, Charles J. Lockwood.
© 2012 John Wiley & Sons, Ltd. Published 2012 by John Wiley & Sons, Ltd.

Box 47.1 Indications for labor induction

Accepted absolute indications

- Hypertensive disorders
  - Preeclampsia/eclampsia
- Maternal medical conditions
  - Diabetes mellitus
  - Renal disease
  - Chronic pulmonary disease
- Prelabor rupture of membranes
- Chorioamnionitis
- Fetal compromise
  - Fetal growth restriction
  - Isoimmunization
  - Nonreassuring antepartum fetal testing
- Fetal demise
- Postdates pregnancy (>42 weeks)

Relative indications

- Hypertensive disorders
  - Chronic hypertension
- Maternal medical conditions
  - Systemic lupus erythematosus
  - Gestational diabetes
- Logistic factors
  - Risk of rapid labor
  - Distance from hospital
  - Psychosocial indications
- Previous stillbirth

Box 47.2 Contraindications to labor induction

Accepted absolute contraindications

- Prior classic uterine incision or transfundal uterine surgery
- Active genital herpes infection
- Placenta or vasa previa
- Umbilical cord prolapse
- Transverse or oblique fetal lie
- Absolute cephalopelvic disproportion (as in women with pelvic deformities)

Relative contraindications

- Cervical carcinoma
- Funic presentation
- Malpresentation (breech)

Data to support a policy of routine elective induction of labor at term are lacking. Large, randomized trials with emphasis on maternal and neonatal safety, cost-effectiveness/cost-benefit analyses, and determination of neonatal benefit as a reflection of reduced unexplained fetal death are needed.

Failed induction cesarean delivery rates by parity

Nulliparas

The risk of cesarean delivery following an elective induction attempt, especially for the nullipara with an unfavorable cervix, is clearly established in literature. Cammu *et al* performed the largest trial to date in Flanders, Belgium, examining outcomes after elective labor induction in nulliparous women [6]. A matched cohort study was performed, which included 7683 nulliparas undergoing elective labor induction and 7683 nulliparas who developed spontaneous labor. The results showed that cesarean delivery was considerably more frequent in the elective induction group, occurring in 9.9% of patients compared with 6.5% of the spontaneous labor group (relative risk [RR] 1.52 95% confidence interval [CI] 1.37–1.70). The majority of these cesarean deliveries were a result of an elevated incidence of first-stage labor disorders. In addition, babies who were born after induced labor were more often transferred to the neonatal ward.

Multiparas

By comparison, most studies in multiparous women have not shown an increased risk of cesarean delivery with induction of labor [7,8]. In one retrospective cohort study, the rates of cesarean delivery in multiparas in spontaneous labor (n = 7208), induced with oxytocin (n = 2190), and induced with cervical ripening agents (n = 239) were 4.2%, 6.3%, and 14.2%, respectively. Oxytocin-induced multiparas were 37% more likely to require cesarean delivery than those with spontaneous labor (odds ratio [OR] 1.37, 95% CI 1.10–1.71) and nearly three times more likely to undergo cesarean when cervical ripening agents were used (OR 2.82, 95% CI 1.84–4.53).

Pediatric issues and maternal risks

The foremost pediatric concern associated with induced labor and delivery is neonatal respiratory compromise. These issues can result from inadvertent delivery of a premature infant or transient tachypnea associated with cesarean delivery after failed induction. This risk is somewhat counterbalanced by observations that fewer induced infants have meconium passage when compared to spontaneously labored infants. In addition, macrosomia also may be reduced. Guidelines to help guarantee that gestational age is at least 39 weeks before elective delivery are listed in Table 47.1.

A retrospective review attempted to quantify the risk of respiratory morbidity defined as infants with transient tachypnea or respiratory distress of the newborn admitted to the neonatal intensive care unit following induced labor and delivery at term [9]. The data were stratified by

Table 47.1 Criteria for confirmation of gestational age and/or fetal pulmonary maturity [3]

	Parameters
Clinical criteria	**1.** ≥39 weeks' gestation have elapsed since the first day of the last menstrual period in a woman with a regular menstrual cycle
	2. Fetal heart tones have been documented for ≥20 weeks' gestation by nonelectronic fetoscope or for ≥30 weeks by Doppler ultrasound
Laboratory determination	**1.** ≥36 weeks' gestation have elapsed since a positive serum human chorionic gonadotropin pregnancy test
	2. Ultrasound estimation of gestational age is considered accurate if it is based on crown–rump measurements obtained at 6–11 weeks' gestation or on biparietal diameter measurements obtained before 20 weeks' gestation
Fetal pulmonary maturity	According to the Guidelines for Perinatal Care, term gestation can be confirmed if two or more of the above obstetric clinical or laboratory criteria are present. If term gestation cannot be confirmed, amniotic fluid analyses can be used to provide evidence of fetal lung maturity. A variety of tests is available. The parameters for evidence of fetal pulmonary maturity are listed below:
	1. Lecithin:sphingomyelin (L:S) ratio >2.1
	2. Presence of phosphatidylglycerol (PG)
	3. Presence of saturated phosphatidylcholine (SPC) ≥500 ng/mL in nondiabetic patients (≥1000 ng/mL for pregestational diabetic patients)

gestational age and route of delivery. Baseline incidence of respiratory distress syndrome and transient tachypnea at term were 2.2/1000 deliveries (95% CI 1.7–2.7/1000) and 5.7/1000 deliveries (95% CI 4.9–6.5/1000), respectively. The frequencies of respiratory morbidity following vaginal delivery were reduced proportionally with advancing gestational age by week, and cesareans following labor were significantly reduced compared to cesareans without labor. For example, respiratory morbidity at 39 weeks occurred following vaginal delivery with a frequency of 3.2 (1.8–4.5)/1000 deliveries (OR 0.6, 95% CI 0.4–1.0) compared to cesarean following labor at 16.2 (5.9–35.0)/1000 deliveries (OR 3.2, 95% CI 1.4–7.4) and to cesarean without labor at 17.8 (8.0–33.5)/1000 deliveries (OR 3.5, 95% CI 1.7–7.1).

Preinduction assessment

Prior to undergoing labor induction, careful examination of the maternal and fetal condition is essential to ensure that there are no contradictions to labor or vaginal delivery and to evaluate the likelihood of successful induction. Indications and contraindications for induction should be reviewed, and risks and benefits of labor induction should be discussed with the patient, including the risk of cesarean delivery. Verification of gestational age and evaluation of fetal lung maturity status should be performed if necessary (see Table 47.1). If time allows, steroids should be permitted in preterm gestations when delivery is indicated. Other prerequisites include evaluation of fetal presentation and cervical examination, along with an estimate of fetal weight, and clinical pelvimetry, all of which should be documented. In addition, the timing and

location of labor induction should be contingent upon the availability of personnel who are familiar with the process and its potential complications in nonemergency settings. Electronic fetal monitoring (EFM) and uterine activity are recommended for any gravida receiving uterotonic drugs.

Predicting a successful induction

There are many clinical and a few biochemical assays [10,11] which could assist in prediction of successful labor induction. The strongest available tool for predicting the likelihood that induction will lead to vaginal delivery is the Bishop score. This conclusion is backed by systematic reviews of controlled studies that found the Bishop score was as, or more, predictive of the outcome of labor induction as cervicovaginal fetal fibronectin (fFN) determination [12] or sonographic measurement of cervical length [12,13], and that dilation was the most vital element of the Bishop score [12]. The modified Bishop score system formulates a score based upon the station of the presenting part and four characteristics of the cervix: consistency, effacement, dilation, and position. If the Bishop score is high (approximately defined as ≥5 or ≥8), the probability of vaginal delivery is comparable whether labor is spontaneous or induced [14]. In contrast, a low Bishop score is predictive that induction will fail and result in vaginal delivery. These relationships are particularly strong in nulliparous women who undergo induction [15,16]. For example, a large retrospective review from a university setting revealed that for women with a Bishop score of less than 5 who undertook labor induction, the relative risk of cesarean was 3.00 (2.38–3.73) compared to those women who entered in spontaneous labor [16]. The relationship between a low Bishop score and failed induction, prolonged labor, and a high cesarean birth rate was first reported prior to widespread use of cervical ripening agents [17].

Sonographically measured cervical length

In pregnant women, the risk of preterm birth increases as cervical length decreases. Cervical length is also predictive of the probability of unprompted onset of labor post term [18]. Many studies have assessed the sonographic assessment of cervical length for predicting the outcome of labor induction. A systematic review of 20 prospective studies found that cervical length was predictive of successful induction (likelihood ratio of a positive test 1.66, 95% CI 1.20–2.31) and failed induction (likelihood ratio of a negative test 0.51, 95% CI 0.39–0.67) [19]. Importantly, though sonographic cervical length did not perform well for prediction of vaginal delivery within 24 h (sensitivity 59%, specificity 65%), vaginal delivery (sensitivity 67%, specificity 58%), achieving active labor (sensitivity 57%, specificity 60%), and delivery within 24 h (sensitivity 56%, specificity 47%), and did not perform considerably better than the Bishop score for predicting a successful induction. Further, in a subanalysis of seven of the 20 included investigations in which a cervical length of 30 mm was used as the discriminator, this value effectively predicted neither vaginal delivery nor cesarean birth, with a likelihood ratio for a positive test of 1.22 (95% CI 0.67–2.22) for the former and likelihood ratio for a negative test of 0.62 (95% CI 0.35–1.10) for the latter. Considerable heterogeneity among the studies limits the data. As with fFN, the role of ultrasound examination as a tool for selecting women likely to have a successful induction is uncertain. More data, including cost-benefit analysis, are necessary before this test can be recommended in choosing candidates for semielective induction.

Complications of induction of labor

All methods of labor induction carry risks.

Uterine overactivity

Uterine overactivity is the most regularly encountered complication of oxytocin or prostaglandin administration. The terms most commonly used to describe uterine overactivity are tachysystole, hypertonus, and hyperstimulation. Previously, there was inconsistent usage and varying definitions for these terms in the obstetric literature. However, a 2008 Eunice Kennedy Shriver National Institutes of Child Health and Human Development (NICHD) workshop issued revised standardized definitions for fetal heart rate and uterine contraction patterns that have the potential for reducing miscommunication

among obstetric care providers [20]. Tachysystole is now the preferred term and defined as more than five contractions in 10 min, averaged over a 30-min window. Any co-existent fetal heart rate abnormality is described separately. Indeed, increased uterine activity is associated with a considerably higher incidence of an umbilical artery pH of 7.05 or less, more nonreassuring fetal heart rate patterns, and decreased fetal oxygen saturation [21,22]. Tachysystole may also cause uterine rupture of unscarred uteri on rare occasions, a phenomenon more common in multigravidas than primigravidas [23]. Various prostaglandin E2 (PGE$_2$) preparations have up to a 5% rate of uterine tachysystole, which is typically well tolerated and not associated with an unfavorable outcome. The reported risk of tachysystole with oxytocin varies widely, and tachysystole occurs more frequently when higher doses of oxytocin, PGE$_2$, or misoprostol are used [24,25].

Hyponatremia

Oxytocin has a comparable structure to vasopressin (antidiuretic hormone) and can crossreact with the renal vasopressin receptor. If high doses (e.g. 40 mU/min) of oxytocin are administered in large quantities (e.g. over 3 L) of hypotonic solutions (e.g. dextrose in water, D5W) for extended periods of time, excessive water retention can occur and result in severe, symptomatic hyponatremia which is similar to the syndrome of inappropriate antidiuretic hormone secretion. Symptoms of severe acute hyponatremia include abdominal pain, headache, nausea, unconsciousness, vomiting, lethargy, anorexia, drowsiness, grand mal type seizures, and potentially irreversible neurologic injury. Oxytocin and any hypotonic solutions should be halted if water intoxication occurs. Careful correction of hyponatremia must be performed and includes restricting water intake and, if the patient is symptomatic, hypertonic saline should be cautiously administered.

Hypotension

Rapid intravenous injection of oxytocin can result in hypotension; however, studies demonstrating this result were performed in men, nonpregnant women, and first-trimester women under general anesthesia. A randomized trial of oxytocin bolus versus slow infusion in women at delivery of the anterior shoulder did not find clinically significant differences in hemodynamic responses [26]. Nonetheless, oxytocin should be administered by infusion pump or slow drip, since bolus injections of oxytocin can cause tachysystole.

Failed induction

Inducing labor usually results in vaginal delivery, though this occurs less often than among women who experience spontaneous labor. A low Bishop score, even after administration of prostaglandins, carries a poor prognosis for successful induction. Women whose induction of labor does not result in delivery are generally offered cesarean birth. There are no standards for what constitutes a failed induction. In one large prospective study, the mean duration of the latent phase of labor (defined as the interval from initiation of induction with either prostaglandins or oxytocin to a cervical dilation of 4 cm) in women with a Bishop score of 0–3 was 12 h in multiparas and 16 h in nulliparas [14]. In another study, a minimum of 12 h of oxytocin administration after membrane rupture was required prior to permitting a diagnosis of failed induction [27]. This led to vaginal deliveries in 75% of nulliparas and eliminated failed labor induction as an indication for cesarean birth in parous women [27]. A third series reported that 73% of women who ultimately delivered vaginally had a latent phase of up to 18 h [28]. Latent phase was defined as the interval from initiation of oxytocin/amniotomy to the start of the active phase (i.e. cervical dilation of 4 cm with 80% effacement or 5 cm dilation). New studies challenge these historic definitions for the duration of the phases of labor [29].

Amniotic fluid embolism

A population-based retrospective cohort study including 3 million deliveries found that medical induction of labor was associated with an increased risk of amniotic fluid embolism (adjusted OR 1.8, 95% CI 1.2–2.7) [30]. However, the absolute risk was small, 10.3 per 100,000 births with medical induction versus 5.2 per 100,000 births without medical induction. Furthermore, failure to induce labor could potentially result in greater maternal-fetal morbidity/mortality than inducing labor, given that these women were induced for serious medical indications.

Uterine rupture

Induction of labor is a risk factor for uterine rupture, though the incidence of rupture is small, with most cases occurring in women with a previously scarred uterus. As noted, uterine rupture in an unscarred uterus has been found to occur with the use of oxytocin, PGE_2, and misoprostol (PGE_1). In 2006, a study reported that of 41 true uterine ruptures occurring in a hospital system, 27 occurred in women with prior uterine surgery (cesarean delivery or other uterine surgery) and 12 of the remaining 14 ruptures occurred in patients who received uterotonic drugs. Additionally, two of these 14 women were nulliparous [31].

Management considerations

Unfavorable cervix

In women with unfavorable cervices who are scheduled for labor induction, prostaglandins are recommended for cervical ripening. Data from randomized trials show that prostaglandins are more effective than placebo, while evidence regarding the efficacy of other drugs and techniques is limited. Misoprostol, in a dose of 25 µg intravaginally every 3–6 h, is generally considered superior when compared with other prostaglandins. If oxytocin is required, the dosage can be started 4 h after the last dose of misoprostol. Uterine tachysystole with fetal heart rate changes appears to be more common with misoprostol than with other prostaglandins.

Favorable cervix

Most inductions are successful in women with favorable cervices (Bishop score >6), and cervical ripening is unnecessary.

Induction of labor in women with prior cesarean delivery

In 2007, the cesarean delivery rate climbed to 31.8% of all births, another all-time high [1]. A trial of labor, whether spontaneous or induced, in women after a previous cesarean delivery (TOLAC, formerly called vaginal birth after a previous cesarean [VBAC]) carries increased risk because of the enhanced potential for uterine rupture. Assessments of the efficacy and safety of cervical ripening and/or labor induction in these women are derived largely from retrospective studies of limited quality [32].

Success rate of induction in women with prior cesarean births

A systematic review identified 14 fair-quality studies and no good-quality studies, on the benefits and risks of inducing labor in patients with prior cesarean delivery [33]. The authors found that induction was more likely to result in cesarean delivery than spontaneous labor, which is not unexpected given that this has been consistently shown in women without a scarred uterus. The cesarean rates for women with prior cesarean delivery undergoing spontaneous labor and oxytocin induction averaged 20% (range 11–35%) and 32% (range 18–44%), respectively.

Risk of uterine rupture in women undergoing labor induction with prior cesarean births

In women with a prior cesarean delivery, induced labor appears to be associated with a higher rate of uterine rupture than spontaneous labor. A systematic review of pooled data from controlled studies of women with prior cesarean delivery reported an OR for uterine rupture of 6.15 (95% CI 0.74–51.4) for induction compared to spontaneous labor [33]. All but one study had a point estimate indicating increased risk of rupture, but confidence intervals were wide. A large, well-designed prospective study, not included in the pooled estimate, reported an OR of 2.86 (95% CI 1.75–4.67) (absolute risk of rupture with induction was 1% versus 0.4% with spontaneous labor) [34].

Approach to management of women with prior cesarean births and labor induction

At 38 weeks of gestation in an uncomplicated pregnancy with a live fetus, stripping the membranes to hasten the onset of spontaneous labor and thereby reducing the likelihood of postterm pregnancy is a reasonable option. If expedited delivery is indicated for maternal and fetal indications, counseling the patient about the risks and benefits of induction versus repeat cesarean delivery, as well as the risks associated with awaiting spontaneous labor, if permissible, should occur. Women who wish to minimize the risk of uterine rupture can reasonably choose repeat cesarean delivery rather than induction.

Administration of low-dose oxytocin for cervical ripening followed by amniotomy and continued oxytocin infusion for augmentation is another option. However, this approach has the potential for serial induction over several days and delaying delivery for this length of time may not be advisable. Use of intracervically applied or intravaginally applied dinsoprostone may be appropriate following informed consent of the risk of uterine rupture with these agents, as described above. Because of the possible increase in the rate of uterine rupture associated with misoprostol use, particularly from intravaginal administration, it should not be administered to women with prior cesarean deliveries.

Conclusion

Induction of labor is performed frequently for a variety of medical and obstetric indications. The best predictor of labor induction success is cervical dilation at the time of initiation. A variety of methods exist for cervical ripening; augmentation of labor is usually accomplished with intravenous oxytocin.

CASE PRESENTATION

A 22-year-old primigravida presents to your office for a routine prenatal care visit at 40 2/7 weeks' gestation. You have seen her since 8 weeks and her antepartum course has been uncomplicated. She is anxious because she has gone beyond her due date, and wishes to discuss with you induction of labor. At this visit, you find that she is in good health, normotensive, and has an unfavorable cervix that is long and closed. The fetus is in vertex presentation.

You engage the patient in a discussion about expectant management with fetal surveillance that would require twice-weekly nonstress or modified biophysical profile testing, and compare outcomes to an elective induction of labor. Concerns regarding a protracted induction and the possibility of a failed induction leading to cesarean delivery are sufficiently deterring to the patient. You discuss the importance of cervical ripening or priming before beginning an induction. You also discuss how, despite advances in the various mechanical and pharmacologic methods by which to prepare the cervix prior to labor induction, no method has been proven to be universally effective in culminating in vaginal delivery for all women in which they are used. She understands that even with optimal cervical ripening, there will be no guarantee that she will achieve a vaginal delivery, although the likelihood that she will enter active labor will be higher. She understands that one of her officemates also recently underwent a labor induction, and inquires about the possibility of beginning the process of cervical ripening at home with a pill to be taken by mouth known as misoprostol. You explain that while there are anecdotal reports of using this prescription medication to induce labor, there is insufficient evidence to support its use in the way she has requested.

References

1. Martin JA, Hamilton BE, Sutton PD et al. Births: Final data for 2007. Natl Vital Stat Rep 2010;58(24):1–86.
2. Rayburn WF, Zhang J. Rising rates of labor induction: present concerns and future strategies. Obstet Gynecol 2002;100:164.
3. American College of Obstetricians and Gynecologists. Induction of labor. Practice Bulletin No. 107. Obstet Gynecol 2009;114:386.
4. Nicholson JM, Parry S, Caughey AB et al. The impact of the active management of risk in pregnancy at term on birth outcomes: a randomized clinical trial. Am J Obstet Gynecol 2008;198:511.
5. Koopmans CM, Bijlenga D, Groen H et al, HYPITAT Study Group. Induction of labour versus expectant monitoring for gestational hypertension or mild pre-eclampsia after 36 weeks' gestation (HYPITAT): a multicentre, open-label randomised controlled trial. Lancet 2009;374(9694):979–988.
6. Cammu H, Martens G, Ruyssinck G, Amy JJ. Outcome after elective labor induction in nulliparous women: a matched cohort study. Am J Obstet Gynecol 2002;186:240.
7. Nielsen PE, Howard BC, Hill CC et al. Comparison of elective induction of labor with favorable Bishop scores versus expectant management: a randomized clinical trial. J Matern Fetal Neonatal Med 2005;18:59.

8. Dublin S, Lydon-Rochelle M, Kaplan RC et al. Maternal and neonatal outcomes after induction of labor without an identified indication. Am J Obstet Gynecol 2000;183:986.

9. Morrison JJ, Rennie JM, Milton PJ. Neonatal respiratory morbidity and mode of delivery at term: influence of timing of elective caesarean section. Br J Obstet Gynaecol 1995;102:101.

10. Chandra S, Crane JM, Hutchens D, Young DC. Transvaginal ultrasound and digital examination in predicting successful labor induction. Obstet Gynecol 2001;98:2.

11. Kiss H, Ahner R, Hohlagschwandtner M et al. Fetal fibronectin as a predictor of term labor: a literature review. Acta Obstet Gynecol Scand 2000;79:3.

12. Crane JM. Factors predicting labor induction success: a critical analysis. Clin Obstet Gynecol 2006;49:573.

13. Hatfield AS, Sanchez-Ramos L, Kaunitz AM. Sonographic cervical assessment to predict the success of labor induction: a systematic review with metaanalysis. Am J Obstet Gynecol 2007;197:186.

14. Xenakis EM, Piper JM, Conway DL, Langer O. Induction of labor in the nineties: conquering the unfavorable cervix. Obstet Gynecol 1197;90:235.

15. Vrouenraets FP, Roumen FJ, Dehing CJ et al. Bishop score and the risk of cesarean delivery after induction of labor in nulliparous women. Obstet Gynecol 2005;105:690.

16. Johnson DP, Davis NR, Brown AJ. Risk of cesarean delivery after induction at term in nulliparous women with an unfavorable cervix. Am J Obstet Gynecol 2003;188:1565.

17. Arulkumaran S, Gibb DM, TambyRaja RL et al. Failed induction of labour. Aust N Z J Obstet Gynaecol 1985;25:190.

18. Vankayalapati P, Sethna F, Roberts N et al. Ultrasound assessment of cervical length in prolonged pregnancy: prediction of spontaneous onset of labor and successful vaginal delivery. Ultrasound Obstet Gynecol 2008;31:328.

19. Hatfield AS, Sanchez-Ramos L, Kaunitz AM. Sonographic cervical assessment to predict the success of labor induction: a systemic review with metaanalysis. Am J Obstet Gynecol 2007;197:186.

20. Macones GA, Hankins GD, Spong CY, Hauth J, Moore T. The 2008 National Institute of Child Health and Human Development Research Workshop Report on electronic fetal heart rate monitoring. Obstet Gynecol 2008;112:661–666.

21. Jonsson M, Norden-Lindeberg S, Ostlund I, Hanson U. Acidemia at birth, related to obstetric characteristics and to oxytocin use, during the last two hours of labor. Acta Obstet Gynecol Scand 2008;87:745.

22. Simpson KR, James DC. Effects of oxytocin-induced uterine hyperstimulation during labor on fetal oxygen status and fetal heart rate patterns. Am J Obstet Gynecol 2008;199:34.

23. Catanzarite V, Cousins L, Dowling D, Daneshmand S. Oxytocin-associated rupture of an unscarred uterus in a primigravida. Obstet Gynecol 2006;108:723.

24. Smith JG, Merrill DC. Oxytocin for induction of labor. Clin Obstet Gynecol 2006;49:594.

25. Wing DA, Ortiz-Omphroy G, Paul RH. A comparison of intermittent vaginal administration of misoprostol with continuous dinoprostone for cervical ripening and labor induction. Am J Obstet Gynecol 1997;177:612.

26. Davies GA, Tessier JL, Woodman MC et al. Maternal hemodynamics after oxytocin bolus compared with infusion in the third stage of labor: A randomized controlled trial. Obstet Gynecol 2005;105:294.

27. Rouse DJ, Owen J, Hauth JC. Criteria for failed labor induction: prospective evaluation of a standardized protocol. Obstet Gynecol 2000;96:671.

28. Simon CE, Grobman WA. When has an induction failed? Obstet Gynecol. 2005;105:705.

29. Zhang J, Yancey MK, Henderson CE. U.S. national trends in labor induction, 1989–1998. J Reprod Med 2002;47:120.

30. Kramer MS, Rouleau J, Baskett TF, Joseph KS. Amniotic-fluid embolism and medical induction of labour: a retrospective, population-based cohort study. Lancet 2006;368:1444.

31. Porreco RP, Clark SL, Belfort MA et al. The changing specter of uterine rupture. Am J Obstet Gynecol 2009;200:269.

32. American College of Obstetricians and Gynecologists. Vaginal birth after prior cesarean delivery. Practice Bulletin No. 115. Obstet Gynecol 2010;116(2 Pt 1):450–463.

33. McDonagh MS, Osterweil P, Guise JM. The benefits and risks of inducing labour in patients with prior caesarean delivery: a systematic review. Br J Obstet Gynaecol 2005;112:1007.

34. Landon MB, Hauth JC, Leveno KJ et al. Maternal and perinatal outcomes associated with a trial of labor after prior cesarean delivery. N Engl J Med 2004;351:2581.

Chapter 48
Cesarean Delivery

Michael W. Varner

Department of Obstetrics and Gynecology, University of Utah Health Sciences Center, Salt Lake City, UT, USA

By the mid-20th century, cesarean delivery (CD) was firmly established in Western obstetric practice, primarily as a procedure to improve maternal outcomes in labor. With the evolution of neonatal medicine through the latter half of the century, CD has been increasingly performed for fetal indications.

The 15-year interval from 1970 through 1985 saw an unparalleled increase in the CD rate, both in the USA [1] and elsewhere [2], with the cesarean rate in the USA temporarily peaking at 24.4% in 1987. The ensuing 15-year interval saw a stabilization of this rate (down to 20.6% in 1996), in large part as a result of efforts to encourage vaginal birth following previous CD [3,4], widely abbreviated as VBAC (vaginal birth after cesarean).

The first decade of the 21st century has again witnessed a progressive increase in the CD rate, primarily as a result of evolving pressures against VBAC in community hospitals and an increasing frequency of CD for failure to make adequate progress in labor [5]. An additional factor, the performance of CD on demand, has become more widespread since its endorsement by the American College of Obstetricians and Gynecologists (ACOG) [6]. The most recent US CD rate available at the time of writing is 32%, a 53% increase from 1996 [7] (Fig. 48.1).

Maternal and perinatal morbidity and mortality

For the past several decades the maternal mortality ratios in the USA have remained essentially unchanged [8]. However, within that relatively constant prevalence, there has been a gradual shift in etiologies. The historic HIT (hemorrhage, infection, toxemia) maternal mortality triad is being replaced by the TEC (trauma, embolism, cardiac) triad. While one might argue that increasing CD rates are decreasing maternal deaths from some of the HIT triad (particularly hemorrhage), one might equally argue that the increasing CD rate is associated with an increased risk of maternal death from some of the TEC triad, particularly thromboembolic disease. What does seem clear, however, is that the dramatic increase in CD rates seen over the past two decades has not been associated with a corresponding decrease in maternal mortality.

Fortunately, maternal mortality is a relatively rare event in the USA. However, a recent report by Clark and associates suggests that CD *per se* increases the maternal mortality ratio by approximately 2 per 100,000 livebirths [9]. "Near-miss" maternal morbidity, on the other hand, is a more common entity, occurring in 0.4–1.0% of pregnancies in developed countries [10]. Geller *et al* [11] have described a useful set of clinical criteria for this definition: organ failure (≥1 organ system), extended intubation (>12 h), intensive care unit (ICU) admission, surgical intervention, and transfusion (>3 units). Several of these conditions are more likely associated with CD but the extent to which CD *per se* increases the risk of near-miss mortality to a previously healthy woman remains unclear.

However, neonatal mortality rates continue to decrease, primarily as a result of continuing advances in neonatal medicine. Peripartum deaths resulting from birth asphyxia are very uncommon in contemporary US obstetric practice. However, the contribution to these ongoing perinatal improvements has as yet not been proven to be a result of the increasing CD rates. In fact, there is evidence that babies delivered by scheduled elective repeat CD at term are at increased risk of developing respiratory problems (adjusted odds ratio [OR] 2.3, 95% confidence interval [CI] 1.4–3.8) [12].

Evidence-based operative considerations

While debate about indications for CD is ongoing, there has been a substantial body of evidence-based

Queenan's Management of High-Risk Pregnancy: An Evidence-Based Approach, Sixth Edition. Edited by John T. Queenan, Catherine Y. Spong, Charles J. Lockwood.

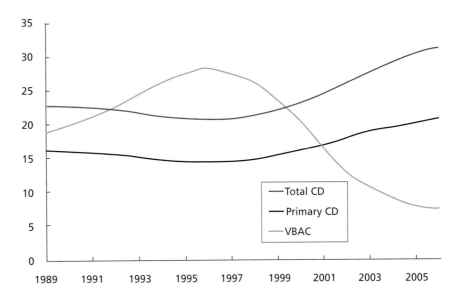

Figure 48.1 Change in vaginal birth after cesarean (VBAC), total cesarean, and primary cesarean delivery rates, USA, 1989–2006. Reproduced from www.cdc.gov/nchs/births.htm with permission from CDC.

recommendations that address various aspects of the surgical technique.

Abdominal surgical incision

The Joel-Cohen incision has advantages compared to the Pfannenstiel incision. A 2007 Cochrane review documented less fever, pain and analgesic requirements, less blood loss and shorter duration of surgery and hospital stay with the Joel-Cohen incision [13].

Antibiotic prophylaxis

It is clear that women who are delivered abdominally are at increased risk of endometritis and/or wound infection. The Cochrane review of 86 clinical trials confirms that it is beneficial for these women to receive antibiotics immediately before, during, or immediately after their CD, whether or not they have clinical evidence of infection. Women who receive antibiotic prophylaxis at the time of CD have lower rates of endometritis (relative risk [RR] 0.38, 95% CI 0.3–0.42) [11]. The risk of wound infection was also reduced in women receiving antibiotic prophylaxis at the time of CD (RR 0.39, 95% CI 0.32–0.48), as was the incidence of febrile morbidity (RR 0.45, 95% CI 0.39–0.51) [14]. More recent reviews suggest that antibiotic administration prior to surgical incision may reduce postcesarean maternal infection by up to 50% [15].

Vaginal antiseptic prophylaxis

Vaginal preparation immediately before CD with povidone-iodine significantly reduces the incidence of postcesarean endometritis from 9.4% in control groups to 5.2% in vaginal cleansing groups (RR 0.57, 95% CI 0.38–0.87) [16]. The risk reduction was particularly strong for women with ruptured membranes (1.4% in the vaginal cleansing group versus 15.4% in the control group; RR 0.13, 95% CI 0.02–0.66). No other outcomes realized statistically significant differences between the vaginal cleansing and control groups and no adverse effects were reported with the povidone-iodine vaginal cleansing.

Manual removal of the placenta

Manual removal of the placenta is associated with a clinically relevant and statistically significant increase in maternal blood loss (weighted mean difference 94 mL; 95% CI 17–172 mL) [17]. Manual removal was also associated with increased postpartum endometritis (OR 1.64, 95% CI 1.42–1.90) and lower hematocrit after delivery (weighted mean difference –1.55%, 95% CI –3.09 to –0.01).

Extraabdominal versus intraabdominal repair of the uterine incision

Six randomized clinical trials, consisting of 1221 participating women, compared uterine exteriorization with intraabdominal repair. There were no significant differences between the groups in most of the outcomes examined, with the exceptions of febrile morbidity and length of hospital stay. Febrile morbidity was lower (RR 0.41, 95% CI 0.17–0.97) and length of hospital stay was longer (weighted mean difference 0.24 days, 95% CI 0.08–0.39) with extraabdominal closure of the hysterotomy [18].

Single-layer versus two-layer hysterotomy closure

In a 2008 Cochrane review, single-layer closure compared with double-layer closure was associated with a statistically significant reduction in mean blood loss (three studies, 527 women, MD –70.11, 95% CI –101.61 to –38.60), duration of the operative procedure (four studies, 645 women, MD –7.43, 95% CI –8.41 to –6.46), and presence of postoperative pain (one study, 158 women, RR 0.69,

95% CI 0.52–0.91) [19]. There are insufficient long-term follow-up data to make any conclusions regarding risks for subsequent pregnancies.

Peritoneal closure

Previous metaanalyses have demonstrated that nonclosure of the visceral and parietal peritoneum decreased operative time (RR −7.33 min, 95% CI −8.43 to −6.24 min), decreased postoperative fever, and reduced postoperative hospital stay [20]. At the time of this analysis, published in 2005, only one study had evaluated long-term adhesion formation and demonstrated no differences. However, a 2009 metaanalysis of five studies demonstrated a significantly increased likelihood of adhesion formation with nonclosure (OR 2.60, 95% CI 1.48–4.56) [21]. Particularly in women planning additional cesarean deliveries, it may therefore be prudent to consider peritoneal closure.

Abdominal wall closure techniques

In a metaanalysis of seven studies involving over 2000 women, Anderson and Gates [22] concluded that the risk of hematoma or seroma was reduced with closure of the subcutaneous tissue compared with nonclosure (RR 0.52, 95% CI 0.33–0.82). The risk of wound complications (defined as hematoma, seroma, wound infection, or wound separation) was also reduced with subcutaneous tissue closure (RR 0.68 95% CI 0.52–0.88). There are no data to address questions of either suture techniques or materials for closure of the rectus sheath.

Thromboprophylaxis

In the developed world, thromboembolic disease is now the most common cause of direct obstetric death. Thromboembolic disease is at least two times more likely following CD [23]. The ACOG does not have a specific policy statement regarding thromboprophylaxis following CD and there are inadequate randomized controlled trial data on which to make firm recommendations. The National Collaborating Center for Women's and Children's Health does have a policy statement on this issue: "Women having a CD should be offered thromboprophylaxis, as they are at increased risk of venous thromboembolism. The choice of method of prophylaxis (e.g. graduated stockings, hydration, early mobilization, low molecular weight heparin) should take into account risk of thromboembolic disease and following existing guidelines [24]." It is important to note that thromboprophylaxis is optimally effective when initiated preoperatively. Because of concerns about procedure-related bleeding at the time of neuraxial anesthesia administration when heparin has been administered, pneumatic compression devices have been recommended by several expert opinions. Thus, while the optimum regimen(s) have yet to be clearly delineated, it is clear that

consideration should be given to the possibility of thromboembolic complications after any CD.

Treatment of postoperative endometritis

In a review of 15 clinical trials, the Cochrane review also confirmed that the combination of gentamicin and clindamycin has fewer treatment failures than other regimens (treatment failure with other regimens RR 1.44, 95% CI 1.15–1.80) [25]. Drug regimens with poor activity against penicillin-resistant anaerobes were particularly likely to be unsuccessful (RR 1.94, 95% CI 1.38–2.72) [17]. Three studies that compared continued oral antibiotic therapy after intravenous therapy with no oral therapy found no differences in recurrent infection or any other adverse outcomes [25].

Potential risks of repeat cesarean delivery

One major contributor to the current increase in the overall CD rate is the dramatic decline in VBAC. A modest decline in VBAC rates had started in 1998 but this was accelerated by a 1999 Technical Bulletin from the ACOG [26] that cautioned against VBAC unless the facilities and staff to perform emergency repeat CD were "immediately available." A recent revision of this Technical Bulletin has emphasized informed consent discussions between pregnant women and their providers and has acknowledged that "immediately available," while ideal, may not always be possible [27]. As of this writing, it remains to be seen whether this change in perspective will lead to a change in practice patterns.

The VBAC rate in 2006 was only 8% [28], a 35% decline from 2002. Overall, the VBAC rate in 2006 was less than half that reported in 1996, while the primary cesarean section rate has climbed 53% during this same interval. At the time of this writing, the definitive statements on risks associated with VBAC are the papers produced by the Eunice Kennedy Shriver National Institute of Child Health and Human Development (NICHD) funded Maternal-Fetal Medicine Units Network Cesarean Registry [29]. These results are outlined in more detail in Chapter 49. While the magnitude of these risks is small, physician practice patterns and medicolegal concerns will undoubtedly keep interest in VBAC low in the near future.

While substantial attention has been paid to the risks of VBAC, rather less attention has been directed to the risks of repeat CD. In the largest series to address this issue, Silver [30] reviewed the outcomes of 30,132 CDs performed without labor. He found that the risk of accreta, hysterectomy, blood transfusion, cystotomy, bowel injury, ureteric injury, previa, ileus, postoperative ventilation, ICU admission, operative time, and hospital days significantly increased with increasing numbers of CDs. Accreta was present in 15 (0.24%), 49 (0.31%), 36 (0.57%), 31 (2.13%), six (2.31%), and six (6.74%) women undergoing their first, second, third, fourth, fifth, and sixth or more cesareans. Hysterectomy was required in 40 (0.65%) first, 67 (0.42%) second, 57 (0.90%) third, 35 (2.40%) fourth, nine (3.46%) fifth, and eight (8.99%) sixth or more cesareans. In the 723 women with previa, the risk for accreta was 3%, 11%, 40%, 61%, and 67% for first, second, third, fourth, and fifth or more repeat cesareans, respectively. Silver confirmed that serious maternal morbidity increases with increasing numbers of CD and suggested that the number of intended pregnancies should be factored into consideration of elective repeat CD versus trial of labor in women with prior CD. He also noted that in 2003 over 80,000 women in the USA had their fourth or more cesarean delivery, making his recommendations more widely applicable than might often be expected.

Influence of different patient populations on cesarean delivery rates

Cesarean delivery rates vary substantially between geographic areas in the USA [28] and often between hospitals in the same community. Numerous factors contribute to these differences, including the availability of ancillary staff (e.g. anesthesia, pediatrics), training and experience of the surgeon(s), and characteristics of particular patient populations. The latter observation has been frequently cited as an explanation for these observed differences.

Although not widely utilized in the USA, the Robson CD classification system [31] allows comparison of cesarean rates within specific subsets of an obstetric population and thereby obviates many of the historic arguments that have arisen when comparing overall cesarean rates between different populations. In this system, any CD can be placed in one, but only one, of 10 mutually exclusive patient population categories (Box 48.1). This classification system could be of value for defining and comparing optimum CD rates for different patient populations. Fischer *et al* [32] demonstrated significant practice pattern differences in Robson group 1 women (term primigravidas, vertex presentation, spontaneous labor; see Box 48.1) between hospitals in the same geographic area with high (16.3%) and low (7.8%) CD rates. Although women delivering in the low CD rate hospital were not more likely to receive oxytocin augmentation, their mean maximum oxytocin dosage was higher (14.5 versus 11.5 units; P < 0.001) and they were more likely to receive both fetal scalp electrodes (60.9% versus 37.3%; P < 0.001) and intrauterine pressure catheters (63.8% versus 26.0%; P < 0.001) compared with an equivalent population in a high CD rate hospital with a similar patient population. They

---

Box 48.1 Robson cesarean classification [31]

1 Nullipara, >37 weeks, single, cephalic presentation, spontaneous labor
2 Nullipara, >37 weeks, single, cephalic presentation, induced labor or CD before labor
3 Multipara, no previous CD, >37 weeks, single, cephalic presentation, spontaneous labor
4 Multipara, no previous CD, >37 weeks, single, cephalic presentation, induced labor
5 Multipara, previous CD, >37 weeks, single, cephalic presentation
6 Nullipara, single breech presentation
7 Multipara, single breech presentation
8 Multiple gestation (with or without previous CD)
9 Singleton pregnancy, oblique or transverse lie (excluding breech, with or without previous CD)
10 Single, cephalic pregnancy, <37 weeks (including previous CD)

---

concluded that such benchmarking practices could be considered in obstetric practices interested in long-term reductions of their CD rates.

Current indications for cesarean delivery

Failure to progress in labor

The most common indication for primary CD is failure to progress in labor. Although the reports of Friedman [33,34] have defined the expectations of normal labor progress for the past generation of obstetric practitioners in the USA, more recent data from the Consortium for Safe Labor suggest that these historic expectations do not reflect normal labor in contemporary American women, particularly prior to 6 cm dilation [35].

In the 1980s, there was hope that the active management of labor, as initially championed by the National Maternity Hospital in Dublin [36], might reverse the increasing CD rates. Unfortunately, this management approach has ultimately failed to stop a rising CD rate in the developed world, including in Ireland [37].

There has been no suggestion that maternal pelves or uterine activity have changed appreciably in the USA over the past several decades. Likewise, mean birthweight has not increased in recent years (1990, 3365 g; 2003, 3325 g) [38]. However, the frequency of CD for the diagnosis of failure to progress in labor has continued to increase during the same interval.

Researchers at the University of Alabama at Birmingham have put forth convincing data that extending the minimum period of oxytocin augmentation for active-phase labor arrest from 2 to at least 4h is effective and safe [39]. Following the diagnosis of a 2-h active-phase arrest, oxytocin was initiated with an intent to achieve a sustained uterine contraction pattern of greater than 200 Montevideo units. CD was not performed for labor arrest until at least 4 h of a sustained uterine contraction pattern of greater than 200 Montevideo units, or a minimum of 6 h of oxytocin augmentation if this contraction pattern could not be achieved. A total of 542 women were managed by this protocol and 92% delivered vaginally. These researchers have subsequently demonstrated that oxytocin-augmented labor proceeds at a slower rate than spontaneous labor [40]. During oxytocin augmentation, nulliparas who were delivered vaginally dilated at a median rate of 1.4 cm/h versus 1.8 cm/h for parous women. In both groups, the 5th percentile of cervical dilatation rate was 0.5 cm/h.

Another contributor to the increased rate of CD because of failure to progress in labor is the epidemic increase in obesity seen in the USA over the past two decades. This diagnosis is most commonly made in the first stage of labor, consistent with observations that leptin inhibits uterine contractility [41]. LaCoursiere *et al* [42] have shown that a 40% increase in prepregnancy overweight (Body Mass Index [BMI] 25.0–29.9) and obesity (BMI ≥30) over a recent 10-year interval in Utah (1991–2001) was accompanied by an attributable fraction of CD of 0.388 (0.369–0.407). Put differently, among all women undergoing CD at the end of this interval, 1 in 7 was attributable to overweight and/or obesity.

Fetal distress

The Cochrane systematic review demonstrated that women followed in labor with electronic fetal heart rate monitoring were more likely to be delivered abdominally and their babies were less likely to suffer neonatal asphyxial seizure (RR 0.52, 95% CI 0.32–0.82) [43]. However, the majority of babies delivered abdominally for "nonreassuring fetal heart rate patterns" or "fetal distress" suffered no perinatal complications, and long-term follow-up of the Dublin population revealed no difference in any neuropsychiatric or developmental landmarks by age 5 years [44].

Earlier attempts to reduce false-positive interventions focused on fetal scalp blood sampling for fetal pH determination and did demonstrate a reduced CD rate for this indication [45]. However, the difficulties of maintaining this equipment, as well as the invasive nature of the procedure, precluded its widescale use, particularly in the community sector. More recently, fetal pulse oximetry has been evaluated as a less invasive technique for assessment of fetal oxygenation during labor, with convincing animal and human data to suggest that a fetal oxygen saturation of greater than 30% was almost never associated with a pH of <7.15 [46–48]. An initial evaluation demonstrated a convincing reduction in CD rates for the diagnosis of "fetal distress" but interestingly demonstrated that those fetuses with nonreassuring fetal heart rates plus reassuring pulse oximetry were more likely to require CD eventually for the diagnosis of failure to progress in labor [49]. More recently, a large randomized controlled trial failed to show any benefit of fetal pulse oximetry when applied prospectively to primigravidas at term in labor [50].

Also recently, the addition of ST waveform analysis to fetal heart rate monitoring has been demonstrated in some, but not all, studies to reduce intrapartum fetal acidosis and/or operative delivery rates [51]. The available data are almost exclusively from European centers, where most intrapartum management protocols are different from North American centers.

Malpresentation

In 3–4% of laboring patients, the fetus is in breech presentation. Current practice calls for CD, except in unusual circumstances. The only ways to lower this figure would be to reduce the frequency of CD for breech presentation (not likely in early 21st-century Western obstetrics in view of the Term Breech Trial results [52]) or to reduce the incidence of breech presentation, which can be accomplished by external cephalic version (ECV). Because breech presentation is more common in primigravidas and because ECV is less likely to be successful near term in this same group, several studies have confirmed that ECV is more likely to be effective if performed at 34–36 weeks in primigravidas. ECV can be deferred to 37–38 weeks in multiparous women. Although historic concerns about complications such as cord entanglement, placental abruption, fetomaternal transfusion, and ruptured uterus have limited the use of ECV in some areas, these problems seem to be more theoretical than real [53]. Nonetheless, ECV should only be performed in a hospital setting where emergency CD is "immediately available."

Repeat cesarean

Safe reduction in CD rates for primigravidas will proportionately reduce the number of repeat CDs required. In view of the aforementioned dominant indications for primary CD, a modern definition of failure to progress in labor, a critical distinction between "fetal distress" versus "fetal stress" and/or "provider distress," and timely identification and correction of breech presentation can all contribute to a lower rate of repeat CD. Higher order repeat CDs are clearly associated with increased maternal morbidity. While it is less clear that a single repeat CD is associated with significant maternal risk, the admonition that "today's primigravidas are tomorrow's multigravidas" is still germane inasmuch as the subgroup of women with the lowest risk of peripartum complications are multiparous women undergoing normal vaginal delivery with a surgically intact uterus.

CASE PRESENTATION 1

A 33-year-old primigravida is admitted at 41w 2d gestation for induction of labor with the diagnosis of postdates pregnancy. Her Bishop score is 3 and she initially receives 25 µg misoprostol *per vaginam* every 4h for a total of three doses, at which time her Bishop score has improved to 7. She is begun on oxytocin and her contractions increase in frequency and intensity. She declines an offer of epidural anesthesia. The fetal heart rate tracing remains reassuring. After 6h her cervix is 4cm dilated and completely effaced, with the vertex estimated at –2 station. An amniotomy is performed for augmentation of labor with return of a large amount of clear fluid. With the next contraction sustained fetal bradycardia is noted on the fetal monitor. A sterile vaginal examination is performed and reveals umbilical cord prolapsing through the cervix. The presenting part is elevated, the oxytocin discontinued, and she is urgently transferred to the operating room where

she initially receives 0.25mg terbutaline subcutaneously for uterine relaxation. Following induction of general anesthesia, an emergency CD is performed via a transverse suprapubic abdominal incision.

She is delivered of a 3600g female whose Apgar scores are 4 and 8 and whose cord artery pH is 7.07 and who thereafter does well. The mother receives 1g cefazolin intravenously following delivery of the baby. She remains afebrile after delivery and is nursing her baby on the third postpartum day when she develops shortness of breath and left-sided chest pain. A chest spiral CT reveals a pulmonary embolism in the lower lobe of the right lung. She is begun on intravenous heparin and oral coumadin. After 2 days her symptoms are greatly improved and the heparin is discontinued. She is discharged on the sixth postpartum day on oral coumadin. She is advised to use condoms and foam for contraception.

CASE PRESENTATION 2

An 18-year-old primigravida who is 1.68m (5 feet 6 inches) tall and whose late-pregnancy BMI is 28.6, presents at 39w 4d gestation for evaluation of labor. She is found to be 3cm dilatated and completely effaced and is contracting painfully every 3 min. She is admitted with the diagnosis of spontaneous labor. After 2h there has been no change in her cervix yet she remains quite uncomfortable. The decision is made to provide an epidural for pain relief and to proceed thereafter with amniotomy. Both are accomplished uneventfully, the latter revealing clear amniotic fluid. The fetal heart rate pattern remains reactive.

After another 2h there has still been no change in her cervical examination. Internal heart rate and pressure catheters are placed, revealing a reactive fetal heart rate with a baseline of 130–140 beats/min and contractions whose total Montevideo units average 140. Oxytocin aug-

mentation is begun with resultant increase of her average Montevideo units to 210.

She progresses to 6cm dilation but thereafter fails to make any further change in either cervical dilation or station of the vertex in the ensuing 2h. As a result, she is taken to the operating room where a primary CD is performed for the diagnosis of failure to progress in labor. A male infant weighing 3280g is delivered whose Apgar scores are 8 and 9 at 1 and 5min, respectively.

Her intraoperative course is complicated by uterine atony that responds to 250mg carboprost given intramuscularly. The estimated blood loss is 1200mL. She has a single temperature elevation to 38.6°C in the recovery room, is started on broad-spectrum antibiotics, and remains afebrile thereafter. Her postoperative course is thereafter uncomplicated and she is discharged with her baby on postoperative day 3.

CASE PRESENTATION 3

A 34-year-old gravida 3, para 2002 is admitted at 39w 0d gestation for scheduled repeat CD. Her first cesarean was performed because of breech presentation diagnosed at the time of labor. Her second delivery was a repeat cesarean at term and she is admitted now for scheduled repeat cesarean and tubal ligation. She is known to be Rh negative and received 300µg RhoGAM intramuscularly at 28 weeks in all three pregnancies and had also received

RhoGAM following delivery of her first child. Her second baby was Rh negative and RhoGAM had not been administered following delivery.

A repeat cesarean is performed following induction of adequate spinal anesthesia. At the time of surgery, multiple dense adhesions are encountered between the omentum and the lower uterine section. After these are removed, further difficulty is encountered dissecting the

Continued

bladder from the anterior lower uterine segment. Because she has requested permanent sterilization, the decision is made to perform a transverse hysterotomy in the lower contractile portion of the uterus. This is performed and a 3760 g male is delivered with some difficulty. The placenta is delivered spontaneously and subsequent inspection reveals a 4 cm extension of the hysterotomy inferiorly on the left side. This is repaired with running, locking, absorbable sutures and the hysterotomy repaired in two layers with similar suture materials. A Pomeroy tubal ligation is performed and segments of fallopian tube are submitted for histologic confirmation.

Prior to closure of the abdomen, the bladder is distended with sterile milk and none is seen intra-abdominally. The remainder of the procedure is accomplished uneventfully. The estimated blood loss is 1000 mL.

Analysis of a cord blood sample reveals the baby to be Rh positive. Although a tubal ligation had been performed, she receives 300 μg RhoGAM intramuscularly.

References

1. Sachs BP. Is the rising rate of cesarean sections a result of more defensive medicine? In: Rostow VP, Bulger RJ, eds. Medical Professional Liability and the Delivery of Obstetrical Care. Vol. II, An Interdisciplinary Review. Washington, DC: National Academies Press, 1989, pp.27–40.
2. Fauendes A, Cecatti JG. Which policy for caesarean sections in Brazil? An analysis of trends and consequences. Health Policy Plan 1993;8:33–42.
3. Menard MK. Cesarean delivery rates in the United States: the 1990s. Obstet Gynecol Clin North Am 1999;26:275–286.
4. Clarke SC, Taffel S. Changes in cesarean delivery in the United States, 1988 and 1993. Birth 1995;22:63–67.
5. Sheiner E, Levy A, Feinstein U, Hallak M, Mazor M. Risk factors and outcome of failure to progress during the first stage of labor: a population-based study. Acta Obstet Gynecol Scand 2002;81:222–226.
6. American College of Obstetricians and Gynecologists. Surgery and patient choice: ethics of decision making. Committee Opinion No. 289. Obstet Gynecol 2003;102:1101–1106.
7. Menacker F, Hamilton BE. Recent trends in caesarean delivery in the United States. NCHS Data Brief No. 35. Hyattsville, MD: National Center for Health Statistics, 2010.
8. Berg CJ, Chang J, Callaghan WM, Whitehead SM. Pregnancy-related mortality in the United States, 1991–1997. Obstet Gynecol 2003;101:289–296.
9. Clark SL, Belfort MA, Dildy GA, Herbst MA, Meyers JA, Hankins GD. Maternal death in the 21st century: causes, prevention and relationship to cesarean delivery. Am J Obstet Gynecol 2008;199:36..
10. Say L, Pattinson RC, Gulmezoglu AM. WHO systematic review of maternal morbidity and mortality: the prevalence of severe acute maternal morbidity (near miss). Reprod Health 2004;1:3.
11. Geller SE, Rosenberg D, Cox S, Brown M, Simonson L, Kilpatrick S. A scoring system identified near-miss maternal morbidity during pregnancy. J Clin Epidemiol 2004;57:716–720.
12. Hook B, Kiwi R, Amini SB, Fanaroff A, Hack M. Neonatal morbidity after elective repeat cesarean section and trial of labor. Pediatrics 1997;100:348–353.
13. Mathai M, Hofmeyr GJ. Abdominal surgical incisions for caesarean section. Cochrane Database Syst Rev 2007;1:CD004453.
14. Smaill FM, Gyte GM. Antibiotic prophylaxis versus no prophylaxis for preventin infection after cesarean section. Cochrane Database Syst Rev 2010;1:CD007482.
15. Tita ATN, Rouse DJ, Blackwell S, Saade GR, Spong CY, Andrews WW. Evolving concepts in antibiotic prophylaxis for cesarean delivery: a systematic review. Obstet Gynecol 2009;113:675–682.
16. Haas DM, Morgain AI, Darei S, Contreras K. Vaginal preparation with antiseptic solution before cesarean section for preventing post-operative infections. Cochrane Database Syst Rev 2010;3:CD007892.
17. Anorlu RI, Maholwana B, Hofmeyr GJ. Methods of delivering the placenta at caesarean section. Cochrane Database Syst Rev 2008;3:CD004737.
18. Jacobs-Jokhan D, Hofmeyr GJ. Extra-abdominal versus intra-abdominal repair of the uterine incision at caesarean section. Cochrane Database Syst Rev 2004;4:CD000085.
19. Dodd JM, Anderson ER, Gates S. Surgical techniques for uterine incision and uterine closure at the time of caesarean section. Cochrane Database Syst Rev 2008;3:CD004732.
20. Berghella V, Baxter JK, Chauhan SP. Evidence-based surgery for cesarean delivery. Am J Obstet Gynecol 2005;193:1607–1617.
21. Cheong YC, Premkumar G, Metwally M, Peacock JL, Li TC. To close or not to close? A systematic review and a meta-analysis of peritoneal non-closure and adhesion formation after caesarean section. Eur J Obstet Gynecol Reprod Biol 2009;147:3–8.
22. Anderson ER, Gates S. Techniques and materials for closure of the abdominal wall at caesarean section. Cochrane Database Syst Rev 2004;18:CD004663.
23. James AH, Jamison MG, Brancazio LR, Myers ER. Venous thromboembolism during pregnancy and the postpartum period: incidence, risk factors, and mortality. Am J Obstet Gynecol 2006;194:1311–1315.
24. National Collaborating Center for Women's and Children's Health. Caesarean Section. London: RCOG Press, 2004, pp.71–72.
25. French LM, Smaill FM. Antibiotic regimens for endometritis after delivery. Cochrane Database Syst Rev 2004;4:CD001067.
26. American College of Obstetricians and Gynecologists. Vaginal birth after previous cesarean delivery. Practice Bulletin No. 5. Washington, DC: American College of Obstetricians and Gynecologists, 1999.
27. American College of Obstetricians and Gynecologists. Vaginal birth after previous cesarean delivery. Practice Bulletin No.

115. Washington, DC: American College of Obstetricians and Gynecologists, 2010.

28. Martin JA, Hamilton BE, Sutton PD et al. Births: Final Data for 2006. National Vital Statistics Reports, vol 57 no 7. Hyattsville, MD: National Center for Health Statistics, 2009.

29. Landon MB, Hauth JC, Leveno KJ et al. The MFMU Cesarean Registry: maternal and perinatal outcome in women undergoing trial of labor after cesarean delivery. N Engl J Med 2004;351:2581–2589.

30. Silver RM, For the NICHD Maternal-Fetal Medicine Units Network. Morbidity associated with multiple repeat cesarean deliveries. Am J Obstet Gynecol 2004;191:S17.

31. Robson MS. Classification of caesarean sections. Fetal Matern Rev 2001;12:123–129.

32. Fischer A, LaCoursiere DY, Barnard P, Bloebaum L, Varner M. Differences in cesarean rates and indications between hospitals for term primigravidas with vertex presentation. Obstet Gynecol 2005;105:816–821.

33. Friedman EA. Primigravid labor: a graphicostatistical analysis. Obstet Gynecol 1955;6:567–589.

34. Friedman EA. Labor in multiparas: a graphicostatistical analysis. Obstet Gynecol 1956;8:691–703.

35. Zhang J, Vanveldhuisen P, Troendel J et al. Normal labor patterns in US women. Am J Obstet Gynecol 2008;199:S36.

36. O'Driscoll K, Foley M, MacDonald D. Active management of labor as an alternative to cesarean section for dystocia. Obstet Gynecol 1984;63:485–490.

37. Farah N, Geary M, Connolly G, McKenna P. The caesarean section rate in the Republic of Ireland in 1998. Ir Med J 2003;96:242–243.

38. Martin JA, Hamilton BE, Sutton PD, Ventura SJ, Menacker F, Munson ML. Births: final data for 2003. Natl Vital Stat Rep 2005;54:85.

39. Rouse DJ, Owen J, Hauth JC. Active-phase labor arrest: oxytocin augmentation for at least 4 hours. Obstet Gynecol 1999;93:323–328.

40. Rouse DJ, Owen J, Savage KG, Hauth JC. Active phase labor arrest: revisiting the 2-hour minimum. Obstet Gynecol 2001; 98:550–554.

41. Moynihan AT, Hehir MP, Glavey SV, Smith TJ, Morrison JJ. Inhibitory effect of leptin on human uterine contractility in vitro. Am J Obstet Gynecol 2006;195:504–509.

42. LaCoursiere DY, Bloebaum L, Duncan JD, Varner MW. Population-based trends and correlates in maternal overweight and obesity, Utah, 1991–2001. Am J Obstet Gynecol 2005;192:832–839.

43. Thacker SB, Stroup D, Chang M. Continuous electronic heart rate monitoring for fetal assessment during labor. Cochrane Database Syst Rev 2001;2:CD000063.

44. MacDonald D, Grant A, Sheridan-Pereira M, Boylan P, Chalmers I. The Dublin randomized controlled trial of intrapartum fetal heart rate monitoring. Am J Obstet Gynecol 1985;152:524–539.

45. Zalar RW Jr, Quilligan EJ. The influence of scalp sampling on the cesarean section rate for fetal distress. Am J Obstet Gynecol 1979;135:239–246.

46. Luttkus AK, Friedmann W, Homm-Luttkus C, Dudenhausen JW. Correlation of fetal oxygen saturation to fetal heart rate patterns: evaluation of fetal pulse oximetry with two different oxisensors. Acta Obstet Gynecol Scand 1998;77:307–312.

47. Carbonne B, Langer B, Goffinet F et al. Multicenter study on the clinical value of fetal pulse oximetry. II. Compared predictive values of pulse oximetry and fetal blood analysis. Am J Obstet Gynecol 1997;177;593–598.

48. Dildy GA, Thorp JA, Yeast JD, Clark SL. The relationship between oxygen saturation and pH in umbilical blood: implications for intrapartum fetal oxygen saturation monitoring. Am J Obstet Gynecol 1996;175:682–687.

49. Garite TJ, Dildy GA, McNamara H et al. A multicenter controlled trial of fetal pulse oximetry in the intrapartum management of nonreassuring fetal heart rate patterns. Am J Obstet Gynecol 2000;183:1049–1058.

50. Bloom SL, Spong CY, Thom E et al. Fetal pulse oximetry and caesarean delivery. N Engl J Med 2006;355:2195–2202.

51. Neilson JP. Fetal electrocardiogram (ECG) for fetal monitoring during labour. Cochrane Database Syst Rev 2006;3: CD000116.

52. Hannah ME, Hannah WJ, Hewson SA, Hodnett ED, Saigal S, Willan AR. Planned caesarean section versus planned vaginal birth for breech presentation at term: a randomized multicenter trial. Term Breech Trial Collaborative Group. Lancet 2000;356:1375–1383.

53. Ranney B. The gentle art of external cephalic version. Am J Obstet Gynecol 1973;116:239–251.

Chapter 49
Vaginal Birth after Cesarean Delivery

Mark B. Landon

Department of Obstetrics and Gynecology, Ohio State University, Columbus, OH, USA

Trends in vaginal birth after cesarean-trial of labor

A recent review of contemporary caesarean delivery in the United States concluded that primary emphasis should be placed on reducing cesarean deliveries for dystocia and repeat operations as these two indications have contributed most to the rise in the overall caesarean rate [1]. A modest decline in cesarean delivery occurred in the USA from 1988 to 1996, which fell to 21% and was largely the result of an increased trial of labor (TOL) rate in women with prior cesareans. However, at present, only 8.5% of women with prior cesarean undergo TOL in the USA [2]. Remarkably, nearly two-thirds of women with a prior cesarean are actually candidates for a TOL [3]. Thus, the majority of repeat operations can be considered elective and are clearly influenced by physician discretion [4]. TOL rates are consistently lower in the USA when compared with European nations, suggesting significant underutilization of TOL in the USA. As 8–10% of the obstetric population has had previous cesarean delivery, more widespread use of TOL could substantially decrease the overall cesarean delivery rate [5].

The evolution in management of the woman with prior cesarean delivery is apparent through review of several American College of Obstetricians and Gynecologists (ACOG) documents and key studies over the last 15 years. In 1988, the ACOG published "Guidelines for vaginal delivery after a previous cesarean birth," recommending VBAC-TOL (vaginal birth after cesarean delivery–trial of labor), as it became clear that this procedure was safe and did not appear to be associated with excess perinatal morbidity compared with elective cesarean delivery. The guidelines recommended that each hospital develop its own protocol for the management of VBAC-TOL patients and that a woman with one prior low transverse cesarean delivery should be counseled and encouraged to attempt labor in the absence of a contraindication such as a prior classic incision. This recommendation was supported by several large case series attesting to the safety and effectiveness of TOL [6–10]. Driven by this encouraging information, VBAC rates reached a peak of 28.3% by 1996. Third-party payers and managed care organizations embraced these data and began to encourage TOL for women with prior cesarean delivery by tracking provider and institutional VBAC rates. Physicians, feeling pressure to lower cesarean delivery rates, began to offer TOL liberally and may have included less than optimal candidates.

With greater utilization of VBAC-TOLs, reports surfaced suggesting a possibly greater than previously appreciated risk for uterine rupture and its maternal and fetal consequences [11–15]. Descriptions of uterine rupture with maternal hemorrhage, hysterectomy, and adverse perinatal outcomes including death and brain injury set the stage for the precipitous decline in VBAC witnessed during the last decade [16–19].

Eventually, the ACOG acknowledged the apparent statistically small but significant risks of uterine rupture with poor outcomes for both women and their infants during TOL [20]. It was also recognized that such adverse events during a TOL might precipitate malpractice litigation. A more conservative approach to TOL has thus been adopted by even ardent supporters of VBAC. Nonetheless, in the 2004 bulletin, the ACOG stated clearly that most women with one previous cesarean delivery with a low transverse incision are candidates for VBAC and should be counseled about VBAC and offered TOL [21].

In response to a growing body of evidence indicating restriction of a woman's access to TOL-VBAC, despite two recent large-scale contemporary multicenter studies [23,53] attesting to the relative safety of VBAC-TOL, the National Institutes of Health (NIH) held a consensus development conference concerning VBAC in 2010. The panel concluded that trial of labor is a reasonable birth

Queenan's Management of High-Risk Pregnancy: An Evidence-Based Approach, Sixth Edition. Edited by John T. Queenan, Catherine Y. Spong, Charles J. Lockwood.

option for many women with previous caesarean delivery. The panel also found that existing practice guidelines and the medical liability climate were restricting access to VBAC-TOL and that these factors need to be addressed [24]. A specific concern raised was the low level of evidence for the requirement for "immediately available" surgical and anesthesia personnel in existing guidelines and the need to reassess this recommendation with reference to other obstetric complications of comparable risk given limited physician and nursing resources.

Several months later, the ACOG issued an updated practice bulletin concerning VBAC [25]. The ACOG acknowledged a background of limited access to TOL-VBAC evolving over time as well as recommendation by the NIH panel to facilitate access. In doing so, while again recommending that TOL-VBAC be undertaken in facilities with staff immediately available to provide emergency care, the ACOG recognized that resources for immediate cesarean may not be available in smaller institutions. In such cases, the decision to offer and pursue TOL-VBAC should be carefully considered by patients and their healthcare providers. It was recommended that the best alternative may be to refer patients to a facility with available resources.

Candidates for trial of labor

Women who have had low transverse uterine incision with prior cesarean delivery and have no contraindications to vaginal birth can be considered candidates for TOL. The following are criteria suggested by the ACOG [25] for identifying candidates for VBAC.
- One or two previous low transverse cesarean deliveries.
- Clinically adequate pelvis.
- No other uterine scars or previous rupture.
- Physicians immediately available throughout active labor capable of monitoring labor and performing an emergency cesarean delivery.

Additionally, several retrospective studies would indicate that it may be reasonable to offer TOL to women in other clinical situations. These would include: more than two prior low transverse cesarean deliveries, gestation beyond 40 weeks, previous low vertical incision, unknown uterine scar type, and twin gestation [25].

Trial of labor is contraindicated in women at high risk for uterine rupture and should not be attempted in the following circumstances.
- Previous classic or T-shaped incision or extensive transfundal uterine surgery.
- Previous uterine rupture.
- Medical or obstetric complications that preclude vaginal delivery.

Table 49.1 Success rates for trial of labor

	VBAC success (%)
Prior indication	
CPD/FTP	63.5
NRFWB	72.6
Malpresentation	83.8
Prior vaginal delivery	
Yes	86.6
No	60.9
Labor type	
Induction	67.4
Augmented	73.9
Spontaneous	80.6

CPD, cephalopelvic disproportion; FTP, failure to progress; NRFWB, nonreassuring fetal well-being; VBAC, vaginal birth after cesarean delivery.
Adapted from Landon *et al* [22].

- Inability to perform emergency cesarean delivery because of unavailable surgeon, anesthesia, sufficient staff or faculty.

Success rates for trial of labor

The overall success rate for VBAC appears to be in the 70–80% range according to published reports [26–28]. In published series with the highest TOL rates, success was only present in 60% of cases [29]. More recently, selective criteria resulting in TOL rates in the 30% range have been associated with a higher number of vaginal births, 70–75% [30,31]. Several predictors of successful TOL have been well described (Table 49.1). The prior indication for the cesarean delivery clearly affects the likelihood of successful VBAC. A history of prior vaginal birth or a nonrecurring condition such as breech or fetal distress is associated with the highest success rates for VBAC. Grobman and colleagues [32] have developed a nomogram for predicting VBAC. The prediction model is based on a multivariable logistic regression, including the variables of maternal age, Body Mass Index, ethnicity, prior vaginal delivery, the occurrences of a VBAC, and a potential recurrent indication for the cesarean delivery. After analysis of the model with crossvalidation techniques, it was found to be accurate and discriminating. Although there is no reliable method to predict success of TOL for an individual woman, a number of factors have been studied which influence success and these are summarized in the following sections.

Maternal demographics

Race, age, Body Mass Index, and insurance status have all been demonstrated to affect the success of TOL [22]. In a multicenter study of 14,529 term pregnancies undergoing TOL, Caucasian women had an overall 78% success rate compared with 70% in non-Caucasian women [22]. Obese women are more likely to fail TOL as are women older than age 40 [22]. Conflicting data exist with regard to payer status (uninsured versus private patients).

Prior indication for cesarean delivery

Success rates for women whose first cesarean delivery was performed for a nonrecurring indication (breech, nonreassuring fetal well-being) are similar to vaginal delivery rates among nulliparous women [31]. Prior cesarean for breech presentation is associated with the highest reported success rate of 89% [22,31]. In contrast, prior operative delivery for cephalopelvic disproportion or failure to progress is associated with success rates in the range 50–67% [32–34]. If dystocia was diagnosed between 5 and 9 cm in a prior labor, 67–73% of VBAC attempts are successful compared with only 13% if prior cesarean delivery was performed during the second stage of labor [35].

Prior vaginal delivery

Prior vaginal delivery including prior successful VBAC is apparently the best predictor for a successful TOL [22]. In one series, a prior vaginal delivery was associated with an 87% success rate compared with 61% success in women without prior vaginal delivery [28]. Caughey *et al* [36] reported that patients with a previous VBAC had a 93% success rate compared with 85% for women with a vaginal delivery prior to their cesarean birth that were without prior VBAC. Mercer and colleagues [37] have reported that success rate increases from 98.6% with one prior vaginal delivery to 90.0% with two prior successful attempts.

Birthweight

Large for gestational age or fetal macrosomia is associated with a lower likelihood of VBAC success [30]. Birthweight greater than 4000 g in particular is associated with a significantly higher risk of failed TOL [28]. Nonetheless, Flamm and Goings [38] reported that 60–70% of women who attempt VBAC with a macrocosmic fetus are successful. Peaceman and colleagues [39] reported only a 34% success rate when the second pregnancy birthweight exceeded the first by 500 g and the prior indication was dystocia, compared with a 64% success rate with other prior indications.

Labor status and cervical examination

Both labor status and cervical examination upon admission influence VBAC success [40]. An 86% VBAC success rate has been reported in women presenting with cervical dilation greater than or equal to 4 cm [41]. Conversely, the success rate drops to 67% if the cervical examination is less than 4 cm upon admission.

Women who undergo induction of labor are at higher risk for a failed TOL or repeat cesarean delivery compared with those who enter spontaneous labor [22,41]. Landon *et al* [22] reported a 67.4% successful VBAC rate in women undergoing induction versus 80.6% in those entering spontaneous labor. Remarkably, Grinstead and Grobman [42] reported a surprisingly high success rate (78%) in 429 women undergoing induction with prior cesarean delivery. These authors noted several factors in addition to past obstetric history, including indication for induction and need for cervical ripening as determinants of VBAC success [42]. Grobman and colleagues [43] have also reported a VBAC success rate of 83% in 1208 women with a prior cesarean and prior vaginal delivery undergoing induction of labor.

Previous incision type

Previous incision type may be unknown in certain patients. It appears that women with unknown scar have VBAC success rates similar to those of women with documented prior low transverse incisions [22]. Similarly, women with previous low vertical incisions do not appear to have lower VBAC success rates [44].

Multiple prior cesarean deliveries

Women with more than one prior cesarean have been demonstrated to consistently have a lower likelihood of achieving VBAC [45–47]. Caughey *et al* [45] reported a 75% success rate for women with one prior cesarean compared with 62% in women with two prior operations. In contrast, Macones *et al*'s [48] large multicenter study of 13,617 women undergoing TOL revealed a 75.5% success rate for women with two prior cesareans, which was not statistically different from the 75% success rate in women with one prior operation (Table 49.2).

Risks of vaginal birth after cesarean-trial of labor

Uterine rupture

The principal risk associated with VBAC-TOL is uterine rupture. This complication is directly attributable to

Table 49.2 Success rates for trial of labor with two prior cesarean deliveries

Author	n	Success rate (%)
Miller *et al* [46]	2936	75.3
Caughey *et al* [45]	134	62.0
Macones *et al* [48]	1082	74.6
Landon *et al* [47]	876	67.0

Table 49.3 Risk of uterine rupture with trial of labor

Prior incision type	Rupture rate (%)
Low transverse	0.5–1.0
Low vertical	0.8–1.1
Classic or T-shaped	4–9

attempted VBAC, as symptomatic rupture is a rare observation at the time of elective repeat operations [49,50]. An important distinction exists between uterine rupture and uterine scar dehiscence. This difference is clinically relevant as dehiscence most often represents an occult scar separation observed at laparotomy in women with a prior cesarean delivery. The serosa of the uterus is intact with most cases of dehiscence and hemorrhage is absent. In contrast, uterine rupture is a thorough disruption of all uterine layers with consequences of hemorrhage, cord compression, potential abruption, fetal compromise, and significant maternal morbidity. The VBAC literature varies with respect to terminology, definitions, and ascertainment for uterine rupture [51]. A review of 10 observational studies providing the best evidence on the occurrence of symptomatic rupture with TOL revealed rupture rates ranging from 0 in 1000 in a small study to 7.8 in 1000 in the largest study, with a pooled rate of 3.8 per 1000 TOL [51,52]. The large, multicenter, prospective, observational Maternal Fetal Medicine Units (MFMU) Network study reported a 0.69% incidence with 124 symptomatic ruptures occurring in 17,898 women undergoing TOL [53].

The rate of uterine rupture depends on both the type and location of the previous uterine incision (Table 49.3). Uterine rupture rates are highest with previous classic or T-shaped incisions, with a reported range of 4–9% [50]. The risk for rupture with a previous low vertical incision is difficult to determine. Distinguishing this incision type from classic incision can be arbitrary and low vertical incision is relatively uncommon. Two reports suggest a rupture rate of 0.8–1.1% for prior low vertical scar [54,55].

Women with unknown scar type may not be at increased risk for uterine rupture. This may simply be because most cases are undocumented prior low transverse incisions. Among 3206 women with unknown scar in the MFMU Network report, uterine rupture occurred in 0.5% of TOL [53].

The most serious sequelae of uterine rupture include perinatal death, fetal hypoxic brain injury, and hysterectomy. Guise *et al* [52] calculated a rate of 0.14 additional perinatal deaths per 1000 TOL related to uterine rupture. This figure is similar to the NICHD-MFMU Network study in which there were two neonatal deaths among 124 ruptures, for an overall rate of rupture-related perinatal death of 0.11 per 1000 TOL [53]. Chauhan *et al* [56], in reviewing 880 maternal uterine ruptures during a

20-year period, calculated 40 perinatal deaths in 91,039 TOL for a rate of 0.4 per 1000.

In most studies, perinatal hypoxic brain injury has been an underreported adverse outcome related to uterine rupture. Landon *et al* [53] found a significant increase in the rate of hypoxic ischemic encephalopathy (HIE) related to uterine rupture among the offspring of women who underwent TOL at term, compared with the children of women who underwent elective repeat cesarean delivery (0.46 per 1000 TOL versus no cases, respectively). In 114 cases of uterine rupture at term, seven infants (6.2%) sustained HIE and two of these infants died in the neonatal period.

Maternal hysterectomy may be a complication of uterine rupture, particularly if the defect is unrepairable or is associated with uncontrollable hemorrhage. In five studies reporting on hysterectomies related to rupture, seven cases occurred in 60 symptomatic ruptures (13%; range 4–27%), indicating that 3.4 per 10,000 women choosing TOL sustain a rupture that necessitates hysterectomy [51]. The NICHD-MFMU Network study included 5/124 (4%) rupture cases requiring hysterectomy in which the uterus could not be repaired [53].

Risk factors for uterine rupture
Rates of uterine rupture vary significantly depending on a variety of associated risk factors. In addition to uterine scar type, obstetric history characteristics including number of prior cesareans, prior vaginal delivery, interdelivery interval, and uterine closure technique have all been reported to affect the risk of uterine rupture. Similarly, factors related to labor management including induction and the use of oxytocin augmentation have all been studied.

Number of prior cesarean deliveries
Miller *et al* [46] reported uterine rupture in 1.7% of women with two or more previous cesarean deliveries compared with a frequency of 0.6% in those with one prior operation (odds ratio [OR] 3.06, 95% confidence interval [CI] 1.95–4.79). Interestingly, the risk for uterine rupture was not increased further for women with three prior cesareans. Caughey *et al* [45] conducted a smaller study of 134 women with two prior cesareans and controlled for labor characteristics as well as obstetric history. These authors reported a rate of uterine rupture of 3.7% among these 134 women compared with 0.8% in the 3757 women with one previous scar (OR 4.5, 95% CI 1.18–11.5). This information led the ACOG, in 2004, to recommend that TOL for women with two prior cesarean deliveries be limited to those with a history of prior vaginal delivery [21]. Macones *et al* [48] reported a uterine rupture rate of 20/1082 (1.8%) in women with two prior cesareans compared with 113/12,535 (0.9%) in women with one prior operation (adjusted OR 2.3, 95% CI 1.37–3.85). In contrast, an analysis from the MFMU Network Cesarean Registry

found no significant difference in rupture rates in women with one prior cesarean. 115/16,916 (0.7%). versus multiple prior cesareans, 9/982 (0.9%) [47]. Therefore, it appears that if multiple prior cesarean section is associated with an increased risk for uterine rupture, the magnitude of any additional risk is fairly small. Thus, the most current ACOG document considers it reasonable to offer TOL to women with two prior cesareans and to counsel such women on the basis of a combination of factors affecting their probability of achieving a successful TOL [25].

Prior vaginal delivery

Prior vaginal delivery is protective against uterine rupture following TOL. Zelop *et al* [57] noted the rate of uterine rupture among women with prior vaginal birth to be 0.2% (2/1021) compared with 1.1% (30/2762) among women with no prior vaginal deliveries. A similar protective effect of prior vaginal birth has been reported in two large multicenter studies [47,58]. There is currently no information as to whether a history of successful VBAC is also protective against uterine rupture.

Uterine closure technique

Single-layer uterine closure technique continues to be widely employed as it may be associated with shorter operating time with similar short-term complications compared with the traditional two-layer technique. A retrospective study of 292 women undergoing TOL found similar rates of uterine rupture for women with one- and two-layer closures [58]. Chapman *et al* [59] conducted a randomized trial that compared the incidence of uterine rupture in 145 women who received either one- or two-layer closure at their primary cesarean delivery. No cases of uterine rupture were found in either group; however, the study is of insufficient size to detect a potential difference. A large observational cohort study identified an approximate fourfold increased rate of rupture following single-layer closure technique when compared with previous double-layer closure [59,60]. These authors conducted a detailed review of operative reports in which the rate of rupture was 15/1489 (3.1%) with single-layer closure versus 8/1491 (0.5%) with previous double-layer closure. A recent case–control study [61] suggested an increased risk of uterine rupture with single-layer closure (OR 2.69, CI 1.57–5.28) compared to two larger closures. In the absence of randomized controlled studies, it remains unclear whether single-layer closure technique increases the risk for rupture.

Interpregnancy interval

Short interpregnancy intervals have been studied as a risk factor for uterine rupture during TOL [62–64]. Shipp *et al* [62] reported an incidence of rupture of 2.3% (7/311) in women with an interdelivery interval less than 18 months compared with 1.1% (22/2098) with a longer interdelivery interval. In contrast, Huang *et al* [63] found no increased risk for uterine rupture with an interdelivery interval of less than 18 months. Bujold *et al* [64] have reported that an interdelivery interval of less than 24 months is independently associated with an almost three-fold increased risk for uterine rupture. These authors reported a rate of rupture of 2.8% in women with a short interval versus 0.9% in women with more than 2 years since the prior cesarean birth.

Labor induction

Induction of labor appears to be associated with an increased risk of uterine rupture [49,54,61]. Lydon-Rochelle *et al* [65] reported a uterine rupture rate of 24/2326 (1.0%) for women undergoing induction compared with 56/10,789 (1.5%) women with spontaneous onset of labor. In the prospective MFMU Network cohort analysis, Landon *et al* [53] noted the risk for uterine rupture to be elevated nearly threefold (OR 2.86, 95% CI 1.75–4.67), with uterine rupture occurring after 48/4708 (1.0%) of induced TOL versus 24/6685 (0.4%) of spontaneous labors. After controlling for various potential confounders, the risk of uterine rupture in women undergoing oxytocin labor induction has been reported to be increased 4.6-fold compared with spontaneous labor (rupture rate of 2.0% versus 0.7%) [57]. Despite these analyses, it remains unclear whether induction causes uterine rupture or whether an associated risk factor such as cervical status is the ultimate cause.

Conflicting data also exist on whether various induction methods increase the risk for uterine rupture [66]. Lydon-Rochelle *et al*'s [65] study suggested an increased risk for uterine rupture with use of prostaglandins for labor induction. Uterine rupture was noted in 15/1960 (0.8%) of women induced without prostaglandin use compared with 9/366 (2.5%) induced with prostaglandin use. Two recent large studies have failed to confirm the findings of Lydon-Rochelle *et al* of an increased risk of rupture associated with the use of prostaglandin agents alone for induction [23,53]. Macones *et al* [23] did report an increased risk for rupture in women undergoing induction only if they received a combination of prostaglandins and oxytocin. In the MFMU Network study, there were no cases of uterine rupture when prostaglandin alone was used for induction, including 52 cases of misoprostol use [53]. The safety of this medication, which is popular for cervical ripening and labor induction, has been challenged for women attempting VBAC.

In the largest report of women receiving prostaglandins for labor induction attempting VBAC, Smith and colleagues [67] reported a 0.87% risk for uterine rupture among 4475 women receiving unspecified prostaglandins compared to 0.29 in 4429 cases not receiving this class of medication. Although the relative risk associated with prostaglandin use was elevated, clearly the absolute risk for rupture was impressively low in this series. At present, based on limited data, the ACOG suggests avoiding sequential use of prostaglandin E_2 and oxytocin in women undergoing TOL.

Labor augmentation

Excessive use of oxytocin may be associated with uterine rupture such that careful labor augmentation should be practiced in women attempting TOL [18]. In a case–control study, Leung *et al* [18] reported an odds ratio of 2.7 for uterine rupture in women receiving oxytocin augmentation. In contrast, a metaanalysis concluded that oxytocin does not increase the risk for uterine rupture [8]. Dysfunctional labor including arrest disorders actually increased the risk sevenfold and thus may actually be the primary factor responsible for rupture. In support of this concept, Zelop *et al* [57] found that labor augmentation with oxytocin did not significantly increase the risk for rupture. In the MFMU Network study, the rate of uterine rupture with oxytocin augmentation was 52/6009 (0.9%) compared with 24/6685 (0.4%) without oxytocin use [53]. Cahill and colleagues [68] have reported that a dose–response relationship exists between maximal oxytocin dose and the risk for rupture compared with women who attempt VBAC with no oxytocin exposure. At the maximal dose of oxytocin (>20 mg/min), these authors noted the risk of uterine rupture to be only 2.07%.

In summary, oxytocin augmentation may marginally increase the risk for uterine rupture in women undergoing TOL. It follows that judicious use of oxytocin should be employed in this population.

Sonographic evaluation of the uterine scar

To better identify women at risk for uterine rupture undergoing TOL, the thickness of the lower uterine segment (LUS) has been evaluated with ultrasound. Bujold and colleagues [69] conducted a prospective study of 125 women with previous cesarean undergoing TOL who received sonographic measurement of the LUS before labor. There were only three cases of uterine rupture; however, receiver operation curve analysis showed that full thickness of less than 2.3 mm was the optimal cut-off for the prediction of uterine rupture (3/33 versus 0/92; P = 0.02). The rate of uterine rupture reported (9.1%) is significantly greater than previously cited risk factors and thus, if confirmed in additional studies, may identify a subgroup of women at sufficiently high risk to advise against TOL.

Management of vaginal birth after cesarean-trial of labor

Because uterine rupture may be catastrophic, it is recommended that TOL after prior cesarean delivery should only be attempted in institutions equipped to respond to emergencies, with physicians immediately available to provide emergency care [25]. Thus, an obstetrician and anesthesia personnel must both be available to comply with this recommendation.

Recommendations for management of women undergoing a TOL after prior cesarean delivery are primarily based upon expert opinion. Women attempting VBAC should be encouraged to contact their healthcare provider promptly when labor or ruptured membranes occur. Continuous electronic fetal heart rate (FHR) monitoring is prudent, although the need for intrauterine pressure catheter monitoring is debatable. Studies that have examined FHR patterns prior to uterine rupture consistently report that nonreassuring signs, particularly significant variable decelerations or bradycardia, are the most common findings accompanying uterine rupture [70,71]. Despite the presence of adequate personnel to proceed with emergency cesarean delivery, prompt intervention does not always prevent fetal neurologic injury or death [52,72]. In one study, significant neonatal morbidity occurred when 18 min or longer elapsed between the onset of FHR deceleration and delivery [18]. If prolonged deceleration is preceded by variable or late decelerations, fetal injury may occur as early as 10 min from the onset of the terminal deceleration.

Trial of labor is not a contraindication to the use of epidural analgesia. Moreover, epidural use does not appear to affect success rates [22]. Epidural analgesia also does not mask the signs and symptoms of uterine rupture. Oxytocin augmentation is employed as necessary, understanding that hyperstimulation should be avoided. In a case–control study, Goetzl *et al* [73] reported no association between uterine rupture and oxytocin dosing intervals, total dose utilized, and the mean duration of oxytocin administration.

Vaginal delivery is conducted as in cases without a history of prior cesarean. Most individuals do not routinely explore the uterus in order to detect asymptomatic scar dehiscences because these generally heal well. However, excessive vaginal bleeding or maternal hypotension should be promptly evaluated, including assessment for possible uterine rupture. Of 124 cases of uterine rupture accompanying TOL, 14 (11%) were identified following vaginal delivery [53].

Counseling for vaginal birth after cesarean-trial of labor

A pregnant woman with prior cesarean delivery is at risk for both maternal and perinatal complications whether undergoing TOL or choosing elective repeat operation (Table 49.4). Complications of both procedures should be discussed and an attempt should be made to individualize risk for both uterine rupture and the likelihood of successful VBAC (Box 49.1; see Table 49.1). For example,

Table 49.4 Comparison of maternal complications in trial of labor versus elective repeat cesarean delivery

Complication	Trial of labor (n = 17,898)	Elective repeated cesarean delivery (n = 15,801)	Odds ratio (98% CI)
Uterine rupture	124 (0.7)	0	–
Hysterectomy	41 (0.2)	47 (0.3)	0.77 (0.51–1.17)
Thromboembolic disease	7 (0.04)	10 (0.1)	0.62 (0.24–1.62)
Transfusion	304 (1.7)	158 (1.0)	1.71 (1.41–2.08)
Endometritis	517 (2.9)	285 (1.8)	1.62 (1.40–1.87)
Maternal death	3 (0.02)	7 (0.04)	0.38 (1.10–1.46)
One or more of the above	978 (5.5)	563 (3.6)	1.56 (1.41–1.74)

Adapted from Landon *et al* [53].

a woman who might require induction of labor may be at slight increased risk for uterine rupture and is also less likely to achieve vaginal delivery. Future child bearing and the risks of multiple cesarean deliveries including risks of placenta previa and accreta should also be considered.

It is important to make every possible effort to obtain the operative records of a prior cesarean delivery in order to determine previous uterine incision type. This is particularly relevant to cases of prior preterm breech delivery in which vertical uterine incision or a low transverse incision in an undeveloped lower uterine segment might preclude TOL. There may be an increased rate of subsequent uterine rupture in women with a prior preterm cesarean attempting TOL [74]. If previous uterine incision type is unknown, the implications of this missing information should also be discussed.

Following complete informed consent detailing the risks and benefits for the individual woman, the delivery plan should be formulated by both the patient and physician. Documentation of counseling is advisable and some practitioners prefer to use a specific VBAC consent form. Many women will choose repeat operation after thorough counseling. However, VBAC-TOL should continue to remain an option for most women with prior cesarean delivery (Box 49.2; see also Box 49.1). The magnitude of risks accompanying TOL must be conveyed to the woman undergoing counseling. The attributable risk for a serious adverse perinatal outcome (perinatal death or HIE) at term appears to be approximately 1 in 2000 TOL [53]. Combining an independent risk for hysterectomy attributable to uterine rupture at term with the risk for newborn HIE indicates that the chance of one of these adverse events occurring is approximately 1 in 1250 cases [53].

The decision to choose TOL may also increase the risk for perinatal death and HIE unrelated to uterine rupture. For women awaiting spontaneous labor beyond 39

Box 49.1 Risks associated with trial of labor (TOL)

- Uterine rupture and related morbidity
- Uterine rupture (0.5–1.0/100 TOL)
- Perinatal death and/or encephalopathy (0.5/1000 TOL)
- Hysterectomy (0.3/1000 TOL)
- Increased maternal morbidity with failed trial of labor
- Transfusion
- Endometritis
- Length of stay
- Potential risk for perinatal asphyxia with labor (cord prolapse, abruption)
- Potential risk for antepartum stillbirth beyond 39 weeks' gestation

---

Box 49.2 Risks associated with elective repeat cesarean delivery

- Increased maternal morbidity compared with successful trial of labor
- Increased length of stay and recovery
- Increased risks for abnormal placentation and hemorrhage with successive cesarean operations

---

weeks, there is a small possibility of unexplained stillbirth which might be avoidable with scheduled repeat operation. A risk for fetal hypoxia and its sequelae may also accompany labor events unrelated to the uterine scar. In the MFMU Network study, five cases of nonrupture-related HIE occurred in term infants in the TOL group compared with none in the elective repeat cesarean population [53].

CASE PRESENTATION

A 31-year-old gravida 3, para 2 at 36 weeks' gestation is considering her options for delivery. This woman underwent a low transverse cesarean delivery for breech presentation 4 years previously followed by an elective repeat operation 2 years previously. She would like to avoid a third operation. Her cervical examination is 1 cm dilated and 50% effaced. She will require complete counseling regarding benefits and risks of TOL. The counseling should include a detailed discussion of risks of TOL including potential uterine rupture and its sequelae. The benefits of VBAC including faster recovery and shorter hospital stay will be reviewed. The option of scheduled repeat cesarean delivery should also be presented. If the patient is considering several future pregnancies, multiple repeat operations may pose additional risk for her of accreta and hysterectomy.

As this woman has a history of two prior cesareans, her overall chance for successful TOL may be as high as 75%. A history of two prior cesareans may be associated with a slight increased risk of uterine rupture compared to that in women with one prior operation. This information should be shared in planning the mode of delivery. If the woman desires TOL, expectant management until 41 weeks is advised. If the cervix ripens further, induction may be planned or alternatively, a repeat cesarean could be scheduled.

References

1. Zhang T, Troendle J, Reddy UM et al, for the Consortium on Safe Labor. Contemporary cesarean delivery practice in the United States. Am J Obstet Gynecol 2010;203(4):326.

2. Menacker F, Hamilton BE. Recent Trends in Cesarean Delivery in the United States. Hyattsville, MD: Centers for Disease Control and Prevention, National Center for Health Statistics, 2010.

3. Flamm BL. Vaginal birth after cesarean section: controversies old and new. Clin Obstet Gynecol 1985;28:735–744.

4. Korst LM, Gregory KD, Fridman MO, Phelan JP. Nonclinical factors affecting women's access to trial of labor after cesarean delivery. Clin Perinatol 2011;38:193–216.

5. Landon MB. Vaginal birth after cesarean delivery. Clin Perinatol 2008;35:491–504.

6. Flamm BL, Newman LA, Thomas SJ et al. Vaginal birth after cesarean delivery: results of a 5-year multicenter collaborative study. Obstet Gynecol 1990;76:750–754.

7. Flamm B, Goings J, Liu Y, Wolde-Tsadik G. Elective repeat cesarean section delivery versus trial of labor: a prospective multicenter study. Obstet Gynecol 1994;83:927–932.

8. Rosen MG, Dickinson JC, Westhoff CL. Vaginal birth after cesarean: a meta-analysis of morbidity and mortality. Obstet Gynecol 1991;77:465–470.

9. Paul RH, Phelan JP, Yeh S. Trial of labor in the patient with a prior cesarean birth. Am J Obstet Gynecol 1985;151:297–304.

10. Martin JN Jr, Harris BA Jr, Huddleston JF et al. Vaginal delivery following previous cesarean birth. Am J Obstet Gynecol 1983;146:255–263.

11. Beall M, Eglinton GS, Clark SL et al. Vaginal delivery after cesarean section in women with unknown types of uterine scars. J Reprod Med 1984;29:31–35.

12. Pruett K, Kirshon B, Cotton D. Unknown uterine scar in trial of labor. Am J Obstet Gynecol 1988;159:807–810.

13. Scott J. Mandatory trial of labor after cesarean delivery: an alternative viewpoint. Obstet Gynecol 1991;77:811–814.

14. Pitkin RM. Once a cesarean? Obstet Gynecol 1991;77:939.

15. Sachs BP, Kobelin C, Castro MA, Frigoletto F. The risks of lowering the cesarean-delivery rate. N Engl J Med 1990;340;54–57.

16. Farmer RM, Kirschbaum T, Potter D, Strong TH, Medaris AL. Uterine rupture during a trial of labor after previous cesarean section. Am J Obstet Gynecol 1991;165:996–1001.

17. Boucher M, Tahilramaney MP, Eglinton GS et al. Maternal morbidity as related to trial of labor after previous cesarean delivery: a quantitative analysis. J Reprod Med 1984;29:12–16.

18. Leung AS, Farmer RM, Leung EK et al. Risk factors associated with uterine rupture during trial of labor after cesarean delivery: a case controlled study. Am J Obstet Gynecol 1993;168:1358–1363.

19. Arulkumaran S, Chua S, Ratnam SS. Symptoms and signs with scar rupture: value of uterine activity measurements. Aust N Z J Obstet Gynaecol 1992;32:208–212.

20. American College of Obstetricians and Gynecologists. Vaginal birth after previous cesarean delivery: clinical management guidelines for obstetricians-gynecologists. ACOG Practice Bulletin No. 5. Washington, DC: American College of Obstetricians and Gynecologists, 1999.

21. American College of Obstetricians and Gynecologists. Vaginal birth after previous cesarean delivery: clinical management guidelines for obstetrician-gynecologists. ACOG Practice Bulletin No. 54. Washington, DC: American College of Obstetricians and Gynecologists, 2004.

22. Landon MB, Leindecker S, Spong CY, for the National Institute of Child Health and Human Development Maternal-Fetal Medicine Units Network. The MFMU Cesarean Registry. Factors affecting the success and trial of labor following prior cesarean delivery. Am J Obstet Gynecol 2005;193:1016–1023.

23. Macones G, Peipert J, Nelson D et al. Maternal complications with vaginal birth after cesarean delivery: a multicenter study. Am J Obstet Gynecol 2005;193:1656–1662.

24. National Institutes of Health Consensus Development Conference Statement. Vaginal birth after cesarean: new insights, March 8–10, 2010. Obstet Gynecol 2010; 115(6):1279–1295.

25. American College of Obstetricians and Gynecologists. Vaginal birth after previous cesarean delivery. Practice Bulletin No. 115. Washington, DC: American College of Obstetricians and Gynecologists, 2010.

26. Whiteside DC, Mahan CS, Cook JC. Factors associated with successful vaginal delivery after cesarean section. J Reprod Med 1983;28:785–788.

27. Silver RK, Gibbs RS. Prediction of vaginal delivery in patients with a previous cesarean section who require oxytocin. Am J Obstet Gynecol 1987;156:57–60.

28. Flamm BL. Vaginal birth after cesarean section. In: Flamm BL, Quilligan EJ, eds. Cesarean Section: Guidelines for Appropriate Utilization. New York: Springer-Verlag, 1995, pp.51–64.

29. Gregory KD, Korst LM, Cane P, Platt LD, Kahn K. Vaginal birth after cesarean and uterine rupture rates in California. Obstet Gynecol 1999;93:985–989.

30. Elkousky MA, Samuel M, Stevens E, Peipert JF, Macones G. The effect of birthweight on vaginal birth after cesarean delivery success rates. Am J Obstet Gynecol 2003;188:824–830.

31. Coughlan C, Kearney R, Turner MJ. What are the implications for the next delivery in primigravidae who have an elective cesarean section for breech presentation? Br J Obstet Gynaecol 2002;109:624–626.

32. Grobman WA, Lai Y, Landon MB et al, for the National Institute of Child Health and Human Development (NICHD) Maternal-Fetal Medicine Units Network (MFMU). Development of a nomogram for prediction of vaginal birth after cesarean delivery. Obstet Gynecol 2007;109(4):806–812.

33. Ollendorff DA, Goldberg JM, Minoque JP, Socol ML. Vaginal birth after cesarean section for arrest of labor: is success determined by maximum cervical dilatation during the prior labor? Am J Obstet Gynecol 1988;159:636–639.

34. Jongen VHWM, Halfwerk MGC, Brouwer WK. Vaginal delivery after previous cesarean section for failure of second stage of labour. Br J Obstet Gynaecol 1998;195:1079.

35. Hoskins IA, Gomez JL. Correlation between maximum cervical dilation at cesarean delivery and subsequent vaginal birth after cesarean delivery. Obstet Gynecol 1997;89:591–593.

36. Caughey AB, Shipp TD, Repke JT et al. Trial of labor after cesarean delivery: the effects of previous vaginal delivery. Am J Obstet Gynecol 1998;179:938–941.

37. Mercer BM, Gilbert S, Landon MB et al, for the National Institute of Child Health and Human Development (NICHD) Maternal-Fetal Medicine Units Network (MFMU). Labor outcomes with increasing number of prior vaginal births after cesarean delivery. Obstet Gynecol 2008;111:285–291.

38. Flamm BL, Goings JR. Vaginal birth after cesarean section: is suspected fetal macrosomia a contraindication? Obstet Gynecol 1989;74:694–697.

39. Peaceman AM, Gersnoviez R, Landon MB et al, for the NICHD Maternal-Fetal Medicine Units Network. The MFMU Cesarean Registry: impact of fetal size on trial of labor successes for patients with prior cesarean for dystocia. Am J Obstet Gynecol 2005;195(4):1127–1131.

40. Weinstein D, Benshushan A, Tanos V et al. Predictive score for vaginal birth after cesarean section. Am J Obstet Gynecol 1996;174:192–198.

41. Shipp TD, Zelop CM, Repke JT, Cohen A, Caughey AB, Lieberman E. Labor after previous cesarean: influence of prior indication and parity. Obstet Gynecol 2000;95:913–916.

42. Grinstead J, Grobman WA. Induction of labor after one prior cesarean: predictors of vaginal delivery. Obstet Gynecol 2004; 103:534–538.

43. Grobman WA, Gilbert S, Landon MB et al. Outcomes of induction of labor after one prior cesarean. Obstet Gynecol 2007;109(2 Pt 1):262–269.

44. Rosen MG, Dickinson JC. Vaginal birth after cesarean: a meta-analysis of indicators for success. Obstet Gynecol 1990;76: 865–869.

45. Caughey AB, Shipp TD, Repke JT et al. Rate of uterine rupture during a trial of labor in women with one or two prior cesarean deliveries. Am J Obstet Gynecol 1999;181:872–876.

46. Miller DA, Diaz FG, Paul RH. Vaginal birth after cesarean: a 10 year experience. Obstet Gynecol 1994;84:255–258.

47. Landon MB, Spong CY, Thom E, for the National Institute of Child Health and Human Development Maternal-Fetal Medicine Units Network. Maternal morbidity associated with multiple repeat cesarean deliveries. Obstet Gynecol 2006;107: 1226–1232.

48. Macones GA, Cahill A, Para E et al. Obstetric outcomes in women with two prior cesarean deliveries: is vaginal birth after cesarean delivery a viable option? Am J Obstet Gynecol 2005;192:1223–1229.

49. Kieser KE, Baskett TF. A 10-year population-based study of uterine rupture. Obstet Gynecol 2002;100:749–753.

50. Mozurkewich EL, Hutton EK. Elective repeat cesarean delivery versus trial of labor: a meta-analysis of the literature from 1989 to 1999. Am J Obstet Gynecol 2000;183:1187–1197.

51. Agency for Health Care Research and Quality. Vaginal Birth After Cesarean (VBAC). AHRQ Publication No. 03-E018. Rockville, MD: Agency for Health Care Research and Quality, 2003.

52. Guise JM, McDonagh MS, Osterweil P et al. Systematic review of the incidence and consequences of uterine rupture in women with previous cesarean section. BMJ 2004;329:19–25.

53. Landon MB, Hauth JC, Leveno KJ et al, for the National Institute of Child Health and Human Development Maternal-Fetal Medicine Units Network. Maternal and perinatal outcomes associated with a trial of labor after prior cesarean delivery. N Engl J Med 2004;351:2581–2589.

54. Naif RW 3rd, Ray MA, Chauhan SP et al. Trial of labor after cesarean delivery with a lower-segment, vertical uterine incision: is it safe? Am J Obstet Gynecol 1995;172:1666–16673.

55. Shipp TD, Zelop CM, Repke TJ et al. Intrapartum uterine rupture and dehiscence in patients with prior lower uterine segment vertical and transverse incisions. Obstet Gynecol 1999;94:735–740.

56. Chauhan SP, Martin JN Jr, Henrichs CE, Morrison JC, Magann EF. Maternal and perinatal complications with uterine rupture in 142,075 patients who attempted vaginal birth after cesarean delivery: a review of the literature. Am J Obstet Gynecol 2003; 189:408–417.

57. Zelop CM, Shipp TD, Repke JT et al. Uterine rupture during induced or augmented labor in gravid women with one prior cesarean delivery. Am J Obstet Gynecol 1999; 181:882–886.

58. Tucker JM, Hauth JC, Hodgkins P et al. Trial of labor after a one- or two-layer closure of a low transverse uterine incision. Obstet Gynecol 1993;168:545–546.

59. Chapman SJ, Owen J, Hauth JC. One-versus two-layer closure of a low transverse cesarean: the next pregnancy. Obstet Gynecol 1997;89:16–18.

60. Bujold E, Bujold C, Hamilton EF et al. The impact of a single-layer or double-layer closure on uterine rupture. Am J Obstet Gynecol 2002;186:1326–1330.

61. Bujold E, Goyet M, Marcoux S et al. The role of uterine closure in the risk of uterine rupture. Obstet Gynecol 2010;116(1): L43–50.

62. Shipp TD, Zelop CM, Repke JT et al. Interdelivery interval and risk of symptomatic uterine rupture. Obstet Gynecol 2001;97: 175–177.

63. Huang WH, Nakashima DK, Rummey PJ et al. Interdelivery interval and the success of vaginal birth after cesarean delivery. Obstet Gynecol 2002;99:41–44.

64. Bujold E, Mehta SH, Bujold C, Gauthier RJ. Interdelivery interval and uterine rupture. Am J Obstet Gynecol 2002;187: 199–202.

65. Lydon-Rochelle M, Holt V, Easterling TR, Martin DP. Risk of uterine rupture during labor among women with a prior cesarean delivery. N Engl J Med 2001;345:36–38.

66. Stone JL, Lockwood CJ, Berkowitz G et al. Use of cervical prostaglandin E2 gel in patients with previous cesarean section. Am J Perinatol 1994;11:309–312.

67. Smith GC, Peil JP, Pasupathy D et al. Factors predisposing to perinatal death related to uterine rupture during attempted vaginal birth after cesarean section: retrospective cohort study. BMJ 2004;329:359–360.

68. Cahill AG, Waterman BM, Stamilio DM et al. Higher maximum doses of oxytocin are associated with an unacceptably high risk for uterine patients attempting vaginal birth after cesarean delivery. Am J Obstet Gynecol 2008;199(1):32.

69. Bujold E, Jastrow N, Simoneau J et al. Prediction of complete uterine rupture by sonographic evaluation of the lower uterine segment. Obstet Gynecol 2009;201:320.

70. Jones R, Nagashima A, Hartnett-Goodman M, Goodlin R. Rupture of low transverse cesarean scars during trial of labor. Obstet Gynecol 1991;77:815–817.

71. Rodriguez M, Masaki D, Phelan J, Diaz F. Uterine rupture: are intrauterine pressure catheters useful in the diagnosis? Am J Obstet Gynecol 1989;161:666–669.

72. Clark SL, Scott JR, Porter TF et al. Is vaginal birth after cesarean less expensive than repeat cesarean delivery? Am J Obstet Gynecol 2000;182:599–602.

73. Goetzl L, Shipp TD, Cohen A, Zelop CM, Repke JT, Lieberman E. Oxytocin dose and the risk of uterine rupture in trial of labor after cesarean. Obstet Gynecol 2001;97:381–384.

74. Scissione AC, Landon MB, Leveno KJ et al, for the NICHD Maternal-Fetal Medicine Units Network. Previous preterm cesarean delivery and risk of subsequent uterine rupture Am J Obstet Gynecol 2008;111(3):648–653.

Chapter 50
Breech Delivery

Edward R. Yeomans[1] and Larry C. Gilstrap[2]

[1] Department of Obstetrics and Gynecology, Texas Tech University Health Sciences Center, Lubbock, TX, USA
[2] American Board of Obstetrics and Gynecology, Dallas, TX, USA

In the US, the rate of cesarean delivery for infants in breech presentation has been equal to or greater than 80% for the last 30 years [1]. The results of the Term Breech Trial published in 2000 [2] supported a policy of planned cesarean delivery for breech presentation and a Committee Opinion [3] from the American College of Obstetricians and Gynecologists (ACOG) initially upheld the conclusions of the Term Breech Trial. However, we presented evidence in the previous edition of this textbook [1] that supported an attempt at vaginal breech delivery in carefully selected and consenting women. Shortly afterwards, the ACOG issued a revised Committee Opinion [4] recommending that the decision regarding mode of delivery should depend on the experience of the healthcare provider and informed maternal preference. In June 2009, the Society of Obstetricians and Gynaecologists of Canada (SOGC) published a practice guideline on vaginal delivery of breech presentation [5]. That document incorporates many of the principles that we advocated in our previous work [1].

The objectives of this revised chapter are to present up-to-date guidance on selection criteria for attempted vaginal breech delivery, review the management of labor in women with breech presentation at term, and highlight important technical aspects of vaginal breech delivery. Many of these techniques are equally applicable to cesarean delivery of the breech fetus since even for obstetric units with considerable expertise in vaginal breech delivery, it is highly likely that more than half of breech deliveries will be conducted via cesarean section [6].

Epidemiology

The incidence of term breech presentation is approximately 3–4%. Accurate determination of breech presentation during prenatal care, followed by referral for and successful completion of external cephalic version (ECV), may lower that incidence somewhat. The approximate frequencies of the various breech presentations at term are frank (65–70%), complete (5–10%), and footling (20–30%). In 2005, 87% of breech presentations underwent cesarean delivery [7]. It is not possible to determine how many of the vaginal deliveries were planned, nor to analyze the cesarean delivery rate by type of breech.

Maternal/perinatal outcomes following vaginal breech delivery (2000–2006)

The Term Breech Trial [2] compared planned cesarean delivery with planned vaginal delivery for breech presentation at term. The salient and highly publicized conclusion of this trial was that planned cesarean delivery reduced perinatal mortality and serious neonatal morbidity by one-third. However, many of the deaths in the vaginal delivery arm were unrelated to the mode of delivery. Moreover, the definitions used for "serious neonatal morbidity" are at least debatable. Maternal morbidity and mortality was not found to be different between groups. However, the impact of a uterine scar in a subsequent pregnancy, such as uterine rupture, placenta accreta, and the need for repeat cesarean delivery, was not considered. Investigators from the Netherlands reported four (0.47/1000 operations) maternal deaths related to elective cesarean delivery for breech presentation [8]. Clearly, this must be weighed carefully against reduced perinatal morbidity or mortality.

Multiple letters to the editor and editorials have been written that take issue with either the conduct of the Term Breech Trial or the interpretation of the results [9]. Such *post hoc* discussion is interesting but not germane to the readers of this textbook. The cesarean delivery rate prior to the publication of the Term Breech Trial was already high and it was predicted that more cesarean breech deliveries would occur after the trial. However, this has not been the case in all centers. Shown in Table 50.1 are

Queenan's Management of High-Risk Pregnancy: An Evidence-Based Approach, Sixth Edition. Edited by John T. Queenan, Catherine Y. Spong, Charles J. Lockwood.

Table 50.1 Summary of method of breech delivery and perinatal outcomes from reports published after the Term Breech Trial from centers outside the US

Reference	Total breech (n)	Elective C/S	Allowed TOL	Successful TOL	Perinatal morbidity		Perinatal mortality	
					Vag	C/S	Vag	C/S
[10]	841	349 (41.5%)	492 (58.5%)	254 (52%)	–	–	2	0
[11]†	809	427 (52.8%)	382 (47.2%)	284 (74.3%)	0.5%	0%	0	0
[12]	1433	552 (38.5%)	881 (61.5%)	416 (47.2%)	5.9%	0.9%	3	1
[13]	986	396 (40.2%)	590 (59.8%)	455 (77.1%)	1.2%	0.5%	1	1
[14]	699	218 (31.2%)	481 (68.8%)	352 (71%)	2.3%	0.5%	0	0
[15]	641	343 (53.5%)	298 (46.5%)	146 (49%)	0.7%	0%	3	0
[6]*	8105	5579 (68.8%)	2526 (31.2%)	1796 (71%)	1.6%	1.4%	2	8

C/S, cesarean section; TOL, trial of labor; Vag, vaginal.
†73 cases were excluded from the 882 breeches reported by the authors.
*This was a multicenter study from France and Belgium.

data that have accumulated since the Term Breech Trial [6,10–15], demonstrating that vaginal breech delivery is still being conducted at multiple centers. In addition, the success rate for attempted vaginal delivery at these centers is greater than or equal to that in the Term Breech Trial and perinatal morbidity and mortality in the vaginal breech group are significantly less than those reported in the trial though generally higher in the trial of labor/vaginal delivery than elective cesarean delivery groups. For each of the studies cited, the elective cesarean delivery rate was well below that in the US proper. However, as noted in Table 50.1, none of the data came from US centers. Importantly, relatively few reports of vaginal breech delivery after the Term Breech Trial are expected to come from the US, given the excessive litigation burden faced by US providers, and those that do will have very small numbers. A report from the University of Texas (UT) illustrates this point [16].

One exception to the small numbers is a population-based study from California where approximately 5000 vaginal breech deliveries were compared with 60,000 prelabor cesarean breech deliveries [17]. Neonatal mortality was lower than that reported in the Term Breech Trial, though perinatal morbidity was still increased for vaginal breech deliveries compared to elective cesarean deliveries. However, this report was based on birth certificate and maternal and neonatal hospital discharge data. Such methodology imposes significant limitations on the conclusions drawn: selection criteria for vaginal breech delivery were not reported, skill of the operator could not be assessed, and even the type of breech presentation could not be verified. The following sections review selection criteria, labor management, and delivery technique because they dramatically affect outcome.

Selection criteria for attempted vaginal breech delivery

The success rate for vaginal breech delivery (VBD) is defined as the number delivering vaginally divided by the number attempting vaginal delivery. This rate varies between centers, but for the series of articles referenced in Table 50.1, it ranged between 47% and 77%. However, to compute the overall vaginal breech delivery rate, the success rate has to be multiplied by a "first term" which reflects the proportion of term breeches offered an attempt at vaginal breech delivery (see the equation below). This "first term," which we call an "offer rate," is also variable. In Table 50.1, this variability is in the range of 31–69%, but the reader should recall that these reports all came from centers with a strong interest in vaginal breech delivery. In the US, the variability of the "offer rate" is undoubtedly greater, because the low end of the range is lower (near zero in some centers). In other words, the fact that 87% of breeches are delivered abdominally in the US implies that only a small minority of women actually attempt vaginal breech delivery. Of the two terms, it is the "offer rate" that is most affected by selection criteria. It should be apparent to the reader that it is also the one most influenced by the informed consent process.

$$\text{VBD rate} = \frac{\text{Attempted VBD}}{\text{No. term breeches}} \times \frac{\text{Successful VBD}}{\text{Attempted VBD}}$$

In general, selection criteria for vaginal breech delivery can be considered lax or stringent. The more stringent the criteria, the smaller the proportion of term breech presentations allowed a trial of labor. So what are considered reasonable selection criteria? Those cited in Box 50.1

Box 50.1 Selection criteria for vaginal breech delivery

- Estimated fetal weight 2000–4000 g*
- Complete or frank breech presentation
- Fetal head flexed or military†
- Adequate maternal pelvis‡
- Normal fetal morphology
- Experienced operator
- Informed consent

*By either clinical or ultrasound estimation. Others have suggested 2500–3800 g [15] or 2500–4000 g [5].
†Ultrasound or radiographic determination, not clinical.
‡As determined by an experienced examiner or radiographically.

Box 50.2 Neonatal morbidity associated with breech delivery

- Intracranial hemorrhage
- Cervical spine injury
- Injury to liver, adrenal glands or spleen
- Bladder rupture
- Pharyngeal diverticulum
- Brachial plexus palsy
- Scrotal/testicular/labial trauma
- Skull fracture
- Long bone fracture

are open to criticism but they do provide a framework for clinicians to adapt to their local practice environments. These criteria are the ones currently being used at one of the authors' institutions (ERY). Two of the listed criteria deserving special emphasis are the need for an experienced operator and a consenting patient. In much of the literature pertaining to vaginal breech delivery, the concept of an "experienced operator" is frequently encountered [2,5]. Operator experience will eventually diminish without training during residency, and experience affects other selection criteria (e.g. clinical pelvimetry), management of labor, and conduct of vaginal breech delivery. One of the editors of this textbook, Dr Queenan, has suggested that maternal-fetal specialists as well as skilled generalists should be involved in this important training [18]. He also suggested, as have others [19], that simulation training may be valuable in the teaching of such infrequently used skills as vaginal breech delivery. A concern has been expressed from Australia that few of the next generation of specialist obstetricians plan to offer vaginal breech delivery to their patients [20].

Regarding the closely related topic of breech delivery of the second twin, D'Alton [21] urged that those with the requisite skills make "every effort" to train the next generation of obstetricians. Clearly, this message must be disseminated to and acted upon by all those charged with the training of residents.

Finally, the manner in which consent is obtained, the discussion of risks and benefits, along with alternatives, is often biased by the perception of medicolegal risk to the person obtaining the consent and caring for the patient.

Labor management

Once an appropriate candidate for vaginal breech delivery is identified, careful management of labor is essential

to achieve an optimal outcome. All studies report a 20–50% incidence of intrapartum cesarean delivery, commonly attributed to either nonreassuring fetal status or failure to progress. With regard to the former, electronic fetal heart rate monitoring (EFM) is recommended, although it has not been shown to be a clear benefit for either vertex or breech presentations. If the fetal heart rate tracing is concerning enough to consider fetal blood sampling, prompt cesarean delivery is appropriate. The use of oxytocin for induction or augmentation has long been a point of contention in vaginal breech delivery. Alarab *et al* [15] did not allow oxytocin for either indication, but still achieved a respectable rate of vaginal breech delivery. At the junior author's institution, use of oxytocin for either induction or augmentation is permitted, but is individualized and used sparingly. In contrast, the Term Breech Trial [2] had a combined rate of induction and augmentation of more than 60%.

The management of labor in breech presentations is more complex than simply interpreting fetal heart rate information and monitoring the progress of labor. Attention must be paid to position of the patient, timing and type of anesthesia, and emotional support and encouragement. Whether to divide the second stage of labor to include a passive descent phase and an active pushing phase has not been adequately evaluated. Timing and type of episiotomy may also be important factors. Episiotomy is not necessary in all cases.

Technique of vaginal breech delivery

Once careful selection of candidates and astute labor management have allowed for the possibility of vaginal breech delivery, proper conduct of the delivery will minimize trauma and optimize overall outcome. Listed in Box 50.2 are a number of complications associated with, but not unique to, vaginal breech delivery. While not guaranteed to eliminate complications, the suggestions that appear in Box 50.3 should produce the best possible results. Despite the time-honored use of the

Box 50.3 Suggestions for vaginal breech delivery

Do	Do not
Await spontaneous delivery to the umbilicus*	Pull on the fetus prematurely
Perform episiotomy as indicated	Grasp the fetal abdomen
Grasp the fetal pelvis over bony prominences (sacrum and iliac crests)	Put transverse pressure on long bones (risk of fracture)
Apply finger pressure parallel to long bones	Allow the fetus to rotate ventrally
Use forceps for the aftercoming head	Attempt vaginal delivery through an incompletely dilated cervix
If forceps not available, maintain flexion of aftercoming head with suprapubic pressure	Panic

*Except under unusual circumstances.

Mauriceau–Smellie–Veit maneuver, the authors favor the routine application of either Piper or Laufe–Piper forceps to the aftercoming head. Both Laufe–Piper and Piper forceps have a reverse pelvic curve to facilitate application to the aftercoming head from below. The low neonatal morbidity and mortality associated with properly selected candidates for vaginal breech delivery that we and others (see Table 50.1) have reported make it feasible to continue to teach this technique to residents in training.

Cesarean delivery for term breech presentation

Most of the suggestions for vaginal breech delivery listed in Box 50.3 apply equally to cesarean delivery of a breech.

Proper placement of the hands of the operator on the bony pelvis of the infant can prevent some of the abdominal trauma listed in Box 50.2. Given that the current cesarean to vaginal delivery ratio for breech presentation is nearly 9:1, residents can be trained in the application of Laufe–Piper forceps to the aftercoming head at cesarean delivery [22]. Almost all cesarean deliveries for breech presentation are performed for fetal indications; that is, to prevent either birth injury or hypoxia/acidemia that are, albeit infrequently, associated with vaginal breech delivery. With that purpose in mind, it is very important that the uterine incision be adequate to deliver the infant atraumatically.

Conclusion

Some women will still want to attempt a vaginal delivery of a breech fetus. Other women whose fetuses are in a breech presentation will be seen for the first time in either advanced labor or with imminent delivery. Physicians will still be called upon to manage labor and vaginal delivery in these circumstances. Additionally, some physicians remain unconvinced by the evidence against planned vaginal delivery and prefer to offer selected women a trial of labor and vaginal breech delivery. At some centers, additional experience with vaginal breech delivery can be gained via delivery of the second twin, but there are important distinctions between breech singletons and breech second twins. Total breech extraction is permissible for a second twin but is rarely performed for a singleton. Continuing to train the next generation of obstetricians in the principles and conduct of vaginal breech delivery is imperative. Finally, the ACOG should strongly consider publishing a practice guideline similar to that from the SOGC [5] to better inform US practice.

CASE PRESENTATION

A 30-year-old gravida 3, para 2 was admitted in active labor at 39 weeks' gestation. On pelvic examination, her cervix was completely effaced and 5 cm dilated. She had a frank breech presentation confirmed by ultrasound. The fetal head was noted to be flexed and the ultrasound-estimated fetal weight of 3150 g was consistent with a clinical estimate of 3400 g. Ultrasound examination revealed a morphologically normal fetus. Clinical pelvimetry was performed by two residents and an attending and the pelvis was deemed to be adequate for breech delivery. Radiographic pelvimetry was not obtained. The patient had received prenatal care from a midwife and was highly motivated to avoid cesarean delivery. She consented to vaginal breech delivery and requested and received epidural analgesia. She reached complete cervical dilation in 4 h and her second stage lasted 45 min. Assisted vaginal breech delivery was performed by a second-year resident, and a fourth-year resident placed Piper forceps to deliver the aftercoming head. A faculty with 25 years of experience supervised the labor and delivery. Apgar scores were 7 at 1 min and 9 at 5 min. Mother and infant were discharged home on postpartum day 2, doing well.

References

1. Yeomans ER, Gilstrap LC. Breech delivery: In: Queenan JT, Spong CY, Lockwood CJ, eds. Management of High Risk Pregnancy, 5th edn. Oxford: Blackwell Science, 2007, pp.397–400.

2. Hannah ME, Hannah WJ, Hewson SA, Hodnett ED, Saigal S, Willan AR, for the Term Breech Trial Collaborative Group. Planned caesarean section versus planned vaginal birth for breech presentation at term: a randomized multicentre trial. Lancet 2000;356:1375–1383.

3. American College of Obstetricians and Gynecologists. Mode of term singleton breech delivery. Committee Opinion No. 265. Washington, DC: American College of Obstetricians and Gynecologists, 2001.

4. American College of Obstetricians and Gynecologists. Mode of term singleton breech delivery. Committee Opinion No. 340. Washington, DC: American College of Obstetricians and Gynecologists, 2006.

5. Society of Obstetricians and Gynaecologists of Canada. Vaginal delivery of breech presentation. Clinical Practice Guideline No. 226. Ottawa: Society of Obstetricians and Gynaecologists of Canada, 2009.

6. Goffinet F, Carayol M, Foidart JM et al. Is planned vaginal delivery for breech presentation at term still an option? Results of an observational prospective survey in France and Belgium. Am J Gynecol Obstet 2006;194:1002–1011.

7. Martin JA, Hamilton BE, Sutton PD et al. Births: final data for 2005. Natl Vital Stat Rep 2007;56:1–103.

8. Schutte JM, Steegers EAP, Santema JG, Schuitemaker N, van Roosmalen J. Maternal deaths after elective cesarean section for breech presentation in the Netherlands. Acta Obstet Gynecol 2007;86:240–243.

9. Glezerman M. Five years to the term breech trial: the rise and fall of a randomized controlled trial. Am J Obstet Gynecol 2006:194:20–25.

10. Lashen H, Fear K, Strudee D. Trends in the management of the breech presentation at term; experience in a District General hospital over a 10-year period. Acta Obstet Gynecol Scand 2002;81:1116–122.

11. Krupitz H, Arzt W, Ebner T, Sommergruber M, Steininger E, Tews G. Assisted vaginal delivery versus caesarean section in breech presentation. Acta Obstet Gynecol Scand 2005;84: 588–592.

12. Pradhan P, Mohajer M, Deshpande S. Outcome of term breech births: 10-year experience at a district general hospital. Br J Obstet Gynaecol 2005;112:218–222.

13. Uotila J, Tuimala R, Kirkinen P. Good perinatal outcome in selective vaginal breech delivery at term. Acta Obstet Gynecol Scand 2005;84:578–583.

14. Giuliani A, Scholl WMJ, Basver A, Tamussino KF. Mode of delivery and outcome of 699 term singleton breech deliveries at a single center. Am J Obstet Gynecol 2002;187: 1694–1698.

15. Alarab M, Regan C, O'Connell MP, Keane DP, O'Herlihy C, Foley ME. Singleton vaginal breech delivery at term: still a safe option. Obstet Gynecol 2004;103:407–412.

16. Doyle NM, Riggs JW, Ramin SM, Sosa MA, Gilstrap LC. Outcomes of term vaginal breech delivery. Am J Perinatol 2005;22:325–328.

17. Gilbert WM, Hicks SM, Boe NM, Danielson B. Vaginal versus cesarean delivery for breech presentation in California: a population-based study. Obstet Gynecol 2003;102:911–917.

18. Queenan JT. Teaching infrequently used skills: vaginal breech delivery (editorial). Obstet Gynecol 2004;103:405–406.

19. Deering S, Brown J, Hodor J, Satin AJ. Simulation training and resident performance of singleton vaginal breech delivery. Obstet Gynecol 2006;107:86–89.

20. Chinnock M, Robson S. Obstetric trainees' experience in vaginal breech delivery. Obstet Gynecol 2007;110:900–903.

21. D'Alton ME. Delivery of the second twin. Obstet Gynecol 2010;115:221–222.

22. Locksmith GJ, Gei AF, Rowe TF, Yeomans ER, Hankins GD. Teaching the Laufe–Piper forceps technique at cesarean delivery. J Reprod Med 2001;46:457–461.

Chapter 51
Operative Vaginal Delivery

Edward R. Yeomans

Department of Obstetrics and Gynecology, Texas Tech University Health Sciences Center, Lubbock, TX, USA

For women who progress to the second stage of labor, there are three options for delivery: spontaneous vaginal, operative vaginal and cesarean. Between 1996 and 2006 cesarean delivery increased by 50%, while both spontaneous and operative vaginal births declined [1]. Recent literature confirms that operative vaginal delivery remains a valid option when problems arise in the second stage of labor [2,3]. However, training and practice are required to maintain that option. The American College of Obstetricians and Gynecologists (ACOG), the Royal College of Obstetricians and Gynaecologists (RCOG), and the Society of Obstetricians and Gynaecologists of Canada (SOGC) have each published guidelines [4–6] pertaining to operative vaginal delivery and exhort residency programs to teach the necessary skills. In order to optimize maternal and neonatal outcomes from operative vaginal delivery, trainees should receive instruction in both technical and nontechnical skills [7]. Related skills including clinical pelvimetry [8], accurate interpretation of fetal heart rate patterns, and correct assessment of fetal head position are also very important and affect outcomes.

Emphasizing contemporary data, the purpose of this chapter is to illustrate that it is possible to achieve equal neonatal and better maternal outcomes when operative vaginal delivery is compared to cesarean delivery in the second stage. Although the trend to choose vacuum extraction over forceps is undeniable, the evidence supporting that trend is unconvincing. A strong case will be made to preserve the option of forceps delivery for tomorrow's obstetricians.

Prerequisites and indications

Operative vaginal delivery is not an option unless the cervix is fully dilated, i.e. the woman has reached the second stage of labor. The fetal head must at least be engaged (leading bony point at zero station) and, except in unusual circumstances, preferably at +2 cm station or lower. The position of the head must be known and the senior person responsible for the delivery must be experienced. The maternal pelvis should be clinically evaluated and the relationship of the fetus to the pelvis assessed. Operative vaginal delivery may be attempted for evidence of fetal compromise or jeopardy, or it may be tried for failure to progress. The latter indication includes cases of maternal exhaustion, dense epidural anesthesia, soft tissue dystocia, malposition, asynclitism, and relative cephalopelvic disproportion.

Instrument selection

The choice between forceps and vacuum extractor depends mainly on operator preference. However, in a few well-defined instances, forceps are the only option: prematurity (<34 weeks), face presentation, and the aftercoming head of the breech. Shown in Figure 51.1 is the range of instrument preference of 20 obstetricians [9]. Those who preferred forceps (by definition, those who chose forceps for more than 90% of operative vaginal delivery attempts) had a lower rate of deep perineal lacerations than those who used any instrument. The conclusion to be drawn is that most complications of operative vaginal delivery may be related to the skill and experience of the operator, not simply to the instrument selected.

Another important point with regard to instrument selection is that there are choices *within* each category for both forceps and vacuum. This fact is underemphasized in randomized controlled trials and the literature in general. Forceps with a long tapered cephalic curve should be used for a molded head, and forceps with a

Queenan's Management of High-Risk Pregnancy: An Evidence-Based Approach, Sixth Edition. Edited by John T. Queenan, Catherine Y. Spong, Charles J. Lockwood.

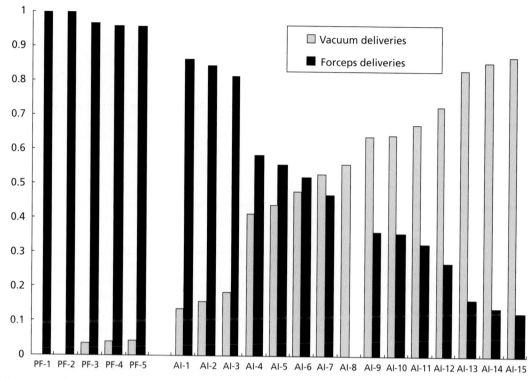

Figure 51.1 Proportion of instrumental deliveries performed using forceps and vacuum between study obstetrician. PF, preferential forceps; AI, any instrument. Reproduced from Abenhaim *et al* [9] with permission from Elsevier.

sliding lock can correct asynclitism. An occiput posterior that is instrumentally rotated to anterior can reduce the risk of deep perineal laceration during delivery. For vacuum extractors, the construction, shape, and size of the cup may be selected to fit a particular clinical situation. The process of instrument selection requires more insight than the old adage "learn to use one instrument well."

Classification

The current three-level classification system (Box 51.1) has been in use for more than 20 years in the United States. It appears in ACOG Practice Bulletin No. 17 from the year 2000 [4] and is only slightly different in the RCOG scheme [5]. The classification highlights the importance of station and rotation in operative vaginal delivery. Application of an instrument to a fetal head in the mid-pelvis in occiput transverse position is much more difficult than a "lift-out" delivery from the pelvic floor. The direction of traction must change continually as the fetal head descends through the maternal pelvis (Fig. 51.2). Importantly, the classification system is the same for both forceps and vacuum deliveries.

Box 51.1 Criteria for types of forceps deliveries

Outlet forceps

1. Scalp is visible at the introitus without separating labia.
2. Fetal skull has reached pelvic floor.
3. Sagittal suture is an anteroposterior diameter or right or left occiput anterior or posterior position.
4. Fetal head is at or on perineum.
5. Rotation does not exceed 45°.

Low forceps

Leading point of fetal skull is at station +2 cm or more (-5 cm to +5 cm scale) and not on the pelvic floor.
 Rotation is 45° or less (left or right occiput anterior to occiput anterior, or left or right occiput posterior to occiput posterior).
 Rotation is greater than 45°.

Mid forceps

Station is above +2 cm but head is engaged.

High forceps

Not included in classification.

Skill

Operative vaginal delivery is a surgical procedure. Various technical skills are required to produce optimal results. An operator's skill set must include the ability to properly apply a given instrument, because experience has shown that, for both forceps and vacuum extraction, misapplication can contribute to fetal injury. With forceps delivery, the goal is a biparietal, bimalar symmetric application. The undesirable brow–mastoid application can lead to unequal pressure and cause injury to the fetal head. With vacuum extraction, failure to center the cup over the sagittal suture 3 cm anterior to the posterior fontanel, referred to as a median flexing application, can increase the risk of cup detachment and fetal injury. Any necessary rotation with forceps involves swinging the handles in an arc, with the notable exception of Kielland forceps. Kielland forceps can be used to rotate heads from the occiput transverse and occiput posterior positions to

occiput anterior. Such rotation can allow delivery of the fetal head in a more favorable diameter, reducing the risk of maternal injury. Appropriate use of Kielland forceps continues to be reported with a "very low rate of adverse maternal and neonatal outcomes" [10]. Although autorotation is sometimes observed with vacuum extraction, no attempt should be made by the operator to manually rotate the vacuum cup once it is applied.

Arguably, the most important technical skill with either type of instrument is traction in the correct axis. Pulling too anteriorly will result in wasted force against the pubic symphysis, whereas pulling too posteriorly will subject the external anal sphincter to injury. In everyday clinical work, experience is the best guide to the amount of traction that can be safely applied. Methods of measuring the force applied are currently being investigated. The central concept in instrumental delivery is that proper traction should produce visible descent of the fetal head. Failure to observe descent should prompt reconsideration and possibly abandonment of the procedure.

Recently, attention has been called to nontechnical surgical skills (NOTSS) for operative vaginal delivery [7]. The authors identified a total of seven NOTSS, shown in Box 51.2. Skill 6 from that box is expanded in Table 51.1

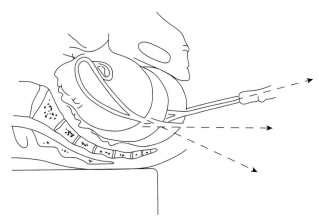

Figure 51.2 Lines of axis traction at different planes of the pelvis. Reproduced from ACOG Technical Bulletin No. 196, August 1994, with permission from the American College of Obstetricians and Gynecologists.

Box 51.2 Categories of nontechnical skills for operative vaginal delivery

1. Situation awareness
2. Decision making
3. Task management
4. Team work and communication
5. Professional relationship with the woman
6. Maintaining professional behavior
7. Crossmonitoring of performance

Adapted from Bahl *et al* [7].

Table 51.1 Maintaining professional behavior

Element	Good behavior	Poor behavior
Calm	Stays calm in an emergency situation Does not appear stressed	Panics in an emergency situation Appears anxious and rushed in a stressful situation
Confident/assertive	Creates a confident atmosphere Clear firm instructions Takes the lead	Does not appear confident Instructions not firm
Able	Knows his/her limitations Open and honest about his/her ability and reflects on the experience Gentle and shows empathy	Does not know his/her limitations Not reflective of his/her practice after an adverse event Rough and lacks empathy

Adapted from Bahl *et al* [7].

and is clearly applicable to obstetricians performing these procedures. An element that might be considered under Skill 3 is choosing the site for the planned delivery. RCOG guidelines specify that operative vaginal births that have a higher rate of failure should be considered a trial and conducted in a place, i.e. "in theater" or in the operating room, where immediate cesarean delivery can be performed if necessary. The concept of a labor-delivery-recovery (LDR) or LDR-postpartum room was not adopted with operative vaginal delivery in mind. Labor beds have thick mattresses and nonadjustable stirrups; labor rooms have suboptimal lighting and no capability for immediate cesarean delivery. If the attempt to deliver with forceps or vacuum extraction fails, time will be lost moving a woman from the labor room to the operating room. The argument is not that all operative vaginal deliveries should be conducted in an operating room. Rather, it is that some such deliveries are ill-suited to being performed in a labor room.

Outcomes

One potential cause of the steady decline in the rate of operative vaginal delivery over the last 30 or more years is concern regarding adverse maternal or neonatal outcomes associated with these procedures. The obstetrician's perception of the threat of litigation if an adverse outcome does occur may be as much or more of a factor than the outcome itself.

On the maternal side, vaginal delivery is less likely to result in hemorrhage, transfusion, infection, pulmonary embolism, or death than cesarean delivery. On the neonatal side, three recent reports provide evidence that neonatal outcomes from either forceps delivery or vacuum extraction are no worse compared to cesarean delivery. In a secondary analysis of data from a randomized clinical trial of fetal pulse oximetry conducted by the Maternal-Fetal Medicine Units Network, Contag and colleagues reported that the occurrence of significant fetal acidemia was not different among the three delivery methods irrespective of indication [11]. Towner reported that the incidence of intracranial hemorrhage in neonates was also no different among the three methods [12]. Alexander and colleagues [13], also in a secondary analysis, reported that cesarean delivery *after* failed attempt at operative vaginal delivery was not associated with adverse neonatal outcomes. This lends credence to the practice of a trial of operative vaginal delivery before resorting to cesarean section. Spencer and co-authors have appropriately called

attention to the maternal morbidity associated with second-stage cesareans [14]. The existing data confirm that operative vaginal delivery in well-selected cases managed by experienced operators lowers maternal risk without increasing neonatal risk.

Training

"Whoever conducts the delivery, high-quality training is crucial" [15]. The written word (this chapter, for example) can affect an operator's skill to only a limited degree [16]. Contemporary training programs face some serious limitations: a shortage of skilled faculty, reluctance of faculty to teach, the threat of litigation, husbands and other observers in the delivery room, nursing bias against the procedures, and uninterested residents. The high cesarean delivery rate means fewer potential cases. It is more difficult to teach and learn forceps skills than vacuum extraction, a fact which contributes to the current 4:1 ratio of vacuum extraction to forceps in the United States. Still, forceps have a lower failure rate than vacuum extractors and vacuum extraction is associated with increased risk to the neonate, particularly the risk for bleeding into the subgaleal space [2].

Simulation training can help. The ACOG has recognized the need for training in operative vaginal delivery and has incorporated simulation training into the curriculum of the Annual Clinical Meeting. Dupuis and colleagues reported on the benefits of simulation training for forceps blade placement using a highly sophisticated simulator [17]. However, after obtaining a working knowledge of mechanical principles, trainees must ultimately participate in a reasonable volume of work involving real patients to attain proficiency. To insure patient safety, such work must be closely supervised [2].

Conclusion

Skillful performance of operative vaginal delivery was once considered to be one of the hallmarks of an obstetrician. There are now fewer such deliveries than at any time in the last century. The risks of a high cesarean delivery rate are just now coming to light. Several prominent organizations [4–6] have called for continued training in operative vaginal procedures to allow women in the second stage of labor to avoid an unnecessary and potentially morbid cesarean delivery.

CASE PRESENTATION

A 25-year-old gravida 1, para 0 has been pushing in the second stage for 3h with a working epidural. Over the last hour, with coached pushing, she moved the fetal head from +2 to +3cm, left occiput anterior at 30° from OA. The pelvis is gynecoid and the estimated fetal weight is 7½ pounds. What are the key points involved in managing this clinical problem?

The case presented would be classified as a low forceps or low vacuum, depending on the instrument selected. The managing obstetrician must assess his/her ability and confidence that operative vaginal delivery is indicated and can be safely performed. Perhaps the patient can be delivered in the labor room, but if the operator is not 100% sure of success, it may be prudent to transport the woman to an operating room and attempt a trial of forceps or vacuum. Such a decision would allow for immediate cesarean if operative vaginal delivery fails. If either forceps or vacuum extraction is attempted, an accurate application is mandatory, followed by traction in the correct axis. In the scenario presented, an experienced operator should be able to successfully deliver a healthy infant to a healthy mother without the need for cesarean section.

References

1. BirthStats. Rates of cesarean delivery, and unassisted and assisted vaginal delivery, United States, 1996, 2000, and 2006. Birth 2009;36:167.
2. Yeomans ER. Operative vaginal delivery. Obstet Gynecol 2010;115:645–653.
3. Goetzinger KR, Macones GA. Operative vaginal delivery: current trends in obstetrics. Women's Health 2008;4:281–290.
4. American College of Obstetricians and Gynecologists. Operative vaginal delivery. Practice Bulletin No. 17. Washington, DC: American College of Obstetricians and Gynecologists, 2000.
5. Royal College of Obstetricians and Gynaecologists. Operative vaginal delivery. RCOG Guideline No. 26. London: Royal College of Obstetricians and Gynaecologists, 2011.
6. Society of Obstetricians and Gynaecologists of Canada. Guidelines for operative vaginal birth. Clinical Practice Guideline No. 148. Ottawa: Society of Obstetricians and Gynaecologists of Canada, 2004.
7. Bahl R, Murphy DJ, Strachan B. Non-technical skills for obstetricians conducting forceps and vacuum deliveries: qualitative analysis by interviews and video recordings. Eur J Obstet Gynecol Reprod Biol 2010;150:147–151.
8. Yeomans ER. Clinical pelvimetry. Clin Obstet Gynecol 2006;49:140–146.
9. Abenhaim HA, Morin L, Benjamin A, Kinch RA. Effect of instrument preference for operative deliveries on obstetrical and neonatal outcomes. Eur J Obstet Gynecol Reprod Biol 2007;134:164–168.
10. Al-Suhel R, Gill S, Robson S, Shadbolt B. Kjelland's forceps in the new millennium. Maternal and neonatal outcomes of attempted rotational forceps delivery. Aust N Z J Obstet Gynecol 2009;49:510–514.
11. Contag SA, Clifton RG, Bloom SL et al. Neonatal outcomes and operative vaginal delivery versus cesarean delivery. Am J Perinatol 2010;27:493–499.
12. Towner D, Castro MA, Eby-Wilkens E, Gilbert WM. Effect of mode of delivery in nulliparous women on neonatal intracranial injury. N Engl J Med 1999;341:1709–1714.
13. Alexander JM, Leveno KJ, Hauth JC et al. Failed operative vaginal delivery. Obstet Gynecol 2009;114:1017–1022.
14. Spencer C, Murphy D, Bewley S. Caesarean delivery in the second stage of labor. BMJ 2006;333:613–614.
15. Ameh CA, Weeks AD. The role of instrumental vaginal delivery in low resource settings. Br J Obstet Gynaecol 2009;116(Suppl 1):22–25.
16. Yeomans ER. Operative vaginal delivery. In: Reece EA, Hobbins JC, eds. Clinical Obstetrics: The Fetus and Mother. Massachusetts: Blackwell Publishing, 2007, pp. 1077–1084.
17. Dupuis O, Moreau R, Pham MT, Redacre T. Assessment of forceps blade orientations during their placement using an instrumented childbirth simulator. Br J Obstet Gynaecol 2009;116:327–332.

Chapter 52
Obstetric Analgesia and Anesthesia

Gilbert J. Grant

Department of Anesthesiology, New York University School of Medicine, New York, NY, USA

Obstetric pain relief has progressed considerably since 1847, when Dr James Young Simpson administered ether to facilitate vaginal delivery for a woman with a deformed pelvis. Analgesics administered by systemic routes (inhalation, intravenous, intramuscular) have been largely supplanted by regional administration of analgesics using the spinal and epidural routes. A distinct advantage of regional analgesia and anesthesia is that profound pain relief may be achieved with relatively low doses of analgesics, preserving maternal alertness and decreasing fetal exposure. Although systemic analgesics remain an option, in the US the regional route is used for the majority of parturients. This chapter describes current practices in obstetric anesthesia.

Labor and vaginal delivery

Consequences of unrelieved pain

The pain of childbirth has untoward effects on the mother and fetus [1]. The hyperventilation that accompanies labor pain causes profound hypocarbia, which may suppress the ventilatory drive between contractions and produce maternal hypoxemia and loss of consciousness [2]. The accompanying respiratory alkalosis interferes with fetal oxygenation by shifting the oxyhemoglobin dissociation curve in favor of the mother and by producing uteroplacental vasoconstriction [3]. The maternal neurohumoral responses to stress and pain also impair placental perfusion and fetal oxygenation, as increased levels of circulating catecholamines produce vasoconstriction and decrease uterine blood flow [4]. Neuraxial (spinal and epidural) analgesia lowers circulating maternal epinephrine and effectively inhibits the respiratory [5] and neurohumoral [6] responses to pain, with a resultant increase in oxygen tension in the parturient and fetus [7]. Accumulating evidence suggests that unrelieved pain

during labor and delivery and even in the immediate postpartum period may contribute to the development of postpartum psychiatric disorders including postpartum depression [8,9] and posttraumatic stress disorder (PTSD) [10].

Multimodal regional analgesia

The current approach to achieving pain relief for labor and vaginal delivery is based on the principle of combining relatively small doses of different classes of analgesics, such as a local anesthetic and an opioid, a concept known as multimodal analgesia [11]. The advantage of this approach is that it is possible to achieve excellent pain relief while minimizing the incidence of unwanted side-effects as the agents used all produce analgesia, but have distinctly different untoward effects. For example, whereas local anesthetics indiscriminately block conduction in all nerves with which they come in contact, at high concentrations they produce hypotension and motor block. Hypotension may decrease fetal oxygen delivery by reducing placental perfusion. Motor block may cause profound lower extremity weakness, which can be distressing for the parturient. Moreover, profound motor and sensory block may interfere with effective pushing during the second stage, particularly if the parturient is unable to perceive rectal or vaginal pressure, as the presence of this pressure facilitates expulsive efforts.

Unlike local anesthetics, opioids administered into the neuraxis (with the exception of meperidine) do not block nerve conduction, but inhibit pain by binding to specific spinal opioid receptors in the spinal cord. In high doses opioids may cause pruritus and nausea, irritating side-effects for a laboring woman. By combining relatively low doses of local anesthetics with opioids, it is possible to achieve reliable analgesia while minimizing the incidence of unwanted side-effects. Some clinicians also combine other classes of analgesics such as those that stimulate spinal adrenergic (e.g. epinephrine, clonidine) and cholinergic (e.g. neostigmine) receptors to further potentiate analgesia.

For parturients, relief of their labor pain and preservation of their lower extremity muscle strength are the most noticeable effects of multimodal analgesia. Although commonly described as a "walking epidural," this term is actually a poor descriptor, as few women walk much during labor after their pain is relieved. Furthermore, the lack of motor block is not a result of the epidural approach *per se*, but may also be achieved with a spinal approach, or a combined spinal–epidural (CSE) approach. The primary determinant of motor block intensity is the concentration of local anesthetic, not its site of administration.

Epidural, spinal, and combined spinal–epidural analgesia

Safe and effective analgesia for labor and delivery may be achieved by using an epidural, spinal or CSE technique. An advantage of the epidural approach is that a catheter may be inserted into the epidural space to facilitate continuous and/or intermittent analgesic dosing to prolong the duration of pain relief. With spinal techniques, the duration of analgesia is limited to the duration of action of a single dose; catheterization of the intrathecal space is infrequently performed. The onset of analgesia is more rapid with the spinal approach (3–5 min) than it is with the epidural approach (approximately 10 min). The CSE approach offers the advantages of both the spinal and epidural techniques: rapid onset of analgesia and prolonged duration if needed.

However, the CSE technique is not without drawbacks. A distressing side-effect sometimes seen after intrathecal injection of opioid is fetal bradycardia or late decelerations of the fetal heart rate, as a result of uterine hyperactivity [12]. This effect is twice as likely to occur after intrathecal administration of opioid alone than after epidural administration of local anesthetic and opioid (24% versus 11%) [13]. The fetal bradycardia may be reversed by administration of a tocolytic, such as terbutaline or nitroglycerine. Whether an epidural or CSE is used to provide labor analgesia, there is no difference with regard to maternal satisfaction, ability to ambulate, or maternal or neonatal outcomes [14].

The particular type of regional analgesia chosen for a parturient depends on many factors. One of the most important determinants is the anticipated duration of labor. In early labor, catheterization of the epidural space is indicated (epidural or CSE technique) to establish a conduit for administering continuous and/or multiple doses of analgesics. Epidural analgesics are typically administered using an infusion pump, perhaps with patient-controlled epidural analgesia (PCEA; see below). For a CSE technique, a dose of analgesic is administered intrathecally and then a catheter is inserted into the epidural space. The epidural analgesics may be administered either immediately after the intrathecal injection or when the pain relief from the initial intrathecal dose begins to wane.

Epidural catheterization is a sensible approach at any time during labor for parturients who have a high likelihood of an instrumental or operative delivery, for example, a woman attempting a vaginal birth after cesarean (VBAC), as it enables rapid administration of additional anesthetics, should they be needed. If delivery is imminent, a single-shot spinal is a reasonable choice, because analgesia onset is rapid. However, these patients may benefit more from a CSE technique, as it requires little additional time compared to a spinal technique, and an indwelling epidural catheter confers considerable versatility. The epidural catheter may be used to administer additional analgesics if delivery does not occur as quickly as anticipated, if the intrathecal medication does not produce adequate analgesia, or if an instrumental or operative delivery is required.

Patient-controlled epidural analgesia

Programmable infusion pumps facilitate precise administration of analgesics into the epidural space. Continuous infusion of analgesics avoids the peaks and valleys of pain and relief that were commonplace with intermittent bolus dosing. PCEA is a further refinement of this technology, enabling the parturient to "fine-tune" her pain relief. PCEA may be administered using intermittent boluses exclusively, or intermittent boluses superimposed on a background infusion, which appears to be a superior strategy [15]. PCEA has many advantages over non-PCEA techniques, including better analgesia and decreased anesthetic requirement, as well as improved patient satisfaction [16], because the patient feels empowered by having some control over her pain relief.

Ideally, PCEA is used to provide analgesia for the duration of labor and delivery. For some women, the low dose delivered from the infusion pump may not be adequate for the late first stage and second stage of labor, when a somatic pain component is superimposed on the visceral pain input. Breakthrough pain that occurs during continuous epidural infusion is treated by increasing the rate of the infusion and/or by administration of a more concentrated dose of anesthetic as a "rescue dose." Ideally, with PCEA, the parturient titrates the analgesia to experience a sensation of pressure during the second stage of labor, while maintaining motor strength. PCEA may be continued to provide analgesia through delivery. However, many practitioners prefer to decrease or halt the epidural administration of analgesics during the second stage of labor, believing that curtailing epidural analgesia will increase the likelihood of spontaneous vaginal delivery. Although conclusive data are not yet available, a metaanalysis showed that discontinuing epidural analgesia during the second stage did not decrease the incidence of instrumental deliveries, but did significantly increase pain intensity [17].

Timing of regional pain relief

The optimal timing for administering regional analgesia for labor has been an issue plagued by misunderstanding and controversy for decades. Those opposed to "early" administration of epidural analgesia have claimed that it would interfere with the progress and outcome of labor. Proponents of "early" administration of regional analgesia have maintained that there is no proven deleterious effect on labor's progress or outcome, and moreover, that parturients should not be denied the right to have their pain relieved at any time.

The four most recent prospective randomized studies of this issue have shown that administration of regional analgesia prior to 4cm cervical dilation in nulliparous women did not affect the outcome of labor. Wong *et al* [18] compared the effect of CSE analgesia administered prior to 4cm cervical dilation to epidural analgesia initiated after 4cm dilation. The women randomized to receive epidural analgesia had their initial pain managed with intravenous opioids. The rate of cesarean delivery was not statistically different whether the women received CSE analgesia prior to 4cm (18%) or epidural analgesia after 4cm dilation (21%). Interestingly, labor progressed more rapidly in the women who received early regional analgesia; the time from initiation of analgesia to full dilation was 90min shorter in the early analgesia group. In a follow-up study, the same investigators studied the effect of early and late administration of CSE in induced labors. The results were very similar, with no difference in the cesarean or forceps rates, and again, a shorter duration of labor among women who received early CSE [19]. In a study of epidural analgesia alone administered either prior to 3 or after 4cm dilation, Ohel *et al* [20] found no difference in the rate of forceps or cesarean delivery. The time to full dilation was approximately one half-hour less in women given early epidurals. In another large study of epidural analgesia alone (nearly 13,000 parturients), Wang *et al* [21] found no difference between the early (1–4cm dilation) or late (greater than 4cm) groups with regard to forceps or cesarean delivery; the duration of labor was not different between the groups.

These studies demonstrate that administering epidurals or spinals early in labor does not increase the likelihood of cesarean or forceps delivery, and does not slow labor; on the contrary, the studies suggest that early administration of regional analgesia may hasten delivery. These studies support the principle of allowing women to have pain relief whenever they choose, as the American College of Obstetricians and Gynecologists has noted: "In the absence of a medical contraindication, maternal request is a sufficient medical indication for pain relief during labor" [22].

Cesarean delivery

Most planned cesarean deliveries in the USA are performed under spinal anesthesia, although epidural anesthesia and CSE anesthesia are also used. If the decision to perform a cesarean delivery is reached after labor has commenced, and the parturient is receiving epidural analgesia, surgical anesthesia is readily achieved by injecting a more concentrated dose of local anesthetic through the epidural catheter. Currently, in the USA, general anesthesia is used for 3–5% of planned and 15–30% of emergency cesarean deliveries [23]. The unconsciousness that accompanies general anesthesia increases the risk of pulmonary aspiration of gastric contents. A large survey found that maternal mortality associated with general and regional anesthesia was 32 and 2 per million cases, respectively [24], reinforcing the belief that regional anesthesia is inherently safer. In addition to the potential safety issues, general anesthesia-induced unconsciousness prevents the mother from experiencing the moment of birth. However, regional anesthesia is associated with its own unique side-effects, such as postspinal headache and, rarely, spinal hematoma, epidural abscess, meningitis, or nerve damage.

The status of the fetus is an important factor in determining the anesthetic choice. If urgent delivery of the fetus is indicated, and if there is no indwelling epidural catheter, general anesthesia is preferred. However, in some circumstances there may be sufficient time to induce spinal anesthesia. Epidural anesthesia is the least desirable choice if time is of the essence because of the prolonged latency of block onset compared to the spinal approach. Ultimately, the choice of anesthetic technique is influenced by a variety of factors including the urgency of the procedure, maternal and fetal status, and physician and patient preference.

Compared to labor analgesia, a more intense block is needed to inhibit the perception of surgical stimulation during caesarean. This is achieved by administering a relatively high concentration of local anesthetic, up to 10-fold greater than the concentration used to provide labor analgesia. This dose predictably produces a profound motor block. In addition, cesarean delivery necessitates a higher dermatomal anesthetic level than does labor analgesia. Whereas sensory block to the 10th thoracic dermatome is sufficient to provide labor analgesia, the anesthetic level must reach the 4th thoracic dermatome at a minimum for cesarean delivery, lest the parturient perceive surgical pain.

Physiologic changes of pregnancy have important clinical implications for providing anesthesia for cesarean delivery. The gastroesophageal sphincter is relatively incompetent, increasing the risk of pulmonary aspiration of gastric contents when upper airway reflexes are compromised during induction of general anesthesia. Pain, anxiety, sedatives, and opioids contribute by prolonging intestinal transit time, increasing the risk of aspiration of gastric contents. Edema of upper airway tissues, especially in preeclamptic parturients, may render tracheal intubation more difficult. The parturient's increased basal metabolic rate and reduced pulmonary functional residual capacity predispose to the development of hypoxemia during the apneic interval that accompanies the induction of general anesthesia. Compression of the aorta and vena cava by the gravid uterus decreases venous return, cardiac output, and blood pressure. Thus, when the parturient is in the supine position, the uterus must be displaced off the great vessels by placing a wedge under the right hip (left uterine displacement).

Left uterine displacement does not eliminate the occurrence of maternal hypotension during induction of anesthesia. In contrast to the low concentrations of local anesthetic used for labor analgesia, which are unlikely to cause maternal hypotension, the higher concentrations used for cesarean delivery often produce hypotension. The reduction in blood pressure is caused by sympathetic block-mediated vasodilation, which causes pooling of blood in capacitance vessels. Hypotension is particularly likely to occur with spinal anesthesia (55–71% of women) [25]. Interestingly, spinal anesthesia is also associated with relatively greater fetal acidemia than epidural or general anesthesia [26]. Strategies to mitigate regional anesthesia-induced hypotension include prophylactic volume expansion with intravenous fluids and administration of vasopressors. Although prophylactic intravenous fluid administration does not prevent maternal hypotension resulting from regional anesthesia, it does reduce its incidence. Vasopressors are administered intravenously to reverse the regional anesthesia-induced hypotension. Mixed α- and β-agonists such as ephedrine produce a greater degree of fetal acidosis than a pure α-agonist such as phenylephrine [27].

Postoperative analgesia

The pain that accompanies cesarean delivery has pathophysiologic consequences that may result in postoperative medical complications. For example, discomfort induced by moving about may limit ambulation and lead to the formation of venous thrombi. Remaining on bedrest promotes atelectasis, makes clearing of pulmonary secretions more difficult, and predisposes to pneumonia. Good pain relief may help to prevent these effects.

Systemically administered opiates have been the mainstay of postoperative pain relief regimens. On-demand intramuscular techniques have been largely replaced by intravenous patient-controlled analgesia (PCA). In comparison with intramuscular administration, intravenous PCA results in more reliable plasma levels and a more rapid onset of analgesia. Various opioids may be used for intravenous PCA, including morphine, fentanyl, and its congeners. For patients receiving regional anesthesia for cesarean delivery, postoperative analgesia is often provided by administration of opioids into the intrathecal or epidural space. Morphine (0.2–0.4 mg intrathecal, 2–4 mg epidural) is the most popular opioid for this application because of its relatively prolonged duration of action. A single morphine dose in the neuraxis provides analgesia for up to 24 h. Bothersome side-effects, including pruritus and nausea, are best treated with specific opioid antagonists, such as naloxone or naltrexone. Respiratory depression, a feared side-effect of neuraxial opioids, is not likely to occur during the postpartum period, because of the persistence of pregnancy-associated increases in ventilatory drive. Another option to provide excellent postoperative analgesia is PCEA. Whether an intravenous or neuraxial approach is used after cesarean delivery, administration of a nonsteroidal antiinflammatory drug (NSAID) such as ketorolac is helpful in potentiating the analgesia [28]. Furthermore, NSAIDs are particularly effective in relieving the cramping pain of postpartum uterine involution.

CASE PRESENTATION

A 31-year-old gravida 2, para 0 presents to the labor and delivery suite at 38 weeks' gestation with presumed rupture of membranes. She says she is experiencing severe pain in her lower abdomen with each uterine contraction. A pelvic examination confirms rupture of membranes and finds cervical dilation to be 2 cm, fetal head not engaged. The patient indicates her desire for pain relief. Her obstetrician and the anesthesiologist on duty are consulted. They agree that the patient is a candidate for regional analgesia, as rupture of membranes and a diagnosis of labor have committed the patient to delivery. The patient is offered and accepts epidural analgesia. An epidural catheter is inserted at the L3–L4 interspace and analgesia is initiated with 20 mL 0.06% bupivacaine and 0.4 μg/mL sufentanil. Analgesia is maintained with an infusion of the same solution at 6 mL/h. PCEA is instituted, giving the parturient the option of self-dosing 5 mL every 10 min.

When her cervical dilation reaches 8 cm, she states that her self-administered doses are no longer sufficient to relieve her pain, so the anesthesiologist administers a rescue dose of 5 mL 0.125% bupivacaine. Within 10 min, this provides relief of her pain, and afterwards she only senses rectal pressure with each contraction. After reaching full dilation, she delivers a 3130 g baby boy over an intact perineum after a 67-min second stage. Although she sensed pressure while she was pushing, she denied experiencing pain.

References

1. Brownridge P. The nature and consequences of childbirth pain. Eur J Obstet Gynecol Reprod Biol 1995;59(Suppl):S9–15.

2. Burden RJ, Janke EL, Brighouse D. Hyperventilation-induced unconsciousness during labour. Br J Anaesth 1994;73:838–839.

3. Ralston DH, Shnider SM, DeLorimier AA. Uterine blood flow and fetal acid–base changes after bicarbonate administration to the pregnant ewe. Anesthesiology 1974;40:348–353.

4. Shnider SM, Wright RG, Levinson G et al. Uterine blood flow and plasma norepinephrine changes during maternal stress in the pregnant ewe. Anesthesiology 1979;50:524–527.

5. Reynolds F, Sharma SK, Seed PT. Analgesia in labour and fetal acid–base balance: a meta-analysis comparing epidural with systemic opioid analgesia. Br J Obstet Gynaecol 2002;109:1344–1353.

6. Shnider SM, Abboud TK, Artal R et al. Maternal catecholamines decrease during labor after lumbar epidural anesthesia. Am J Obstet Gynecol 1983;147:13–15.

7. Bergmans MG, van Geijn HP, Hasaart TH et al. Fetal and maternal transcutaneous PCO_2 levels during labour and the influence of epidural analgesia. Eur J Obstet Gynecol Reprod Biol 1996;67:127–132.

8. Hiltunen P, Raudaskoski T, Ebeling H, Moilanen I. Does pain relief during delivery decrease the risk of postnatal depression? Acta Obstet Gynecol Scand 2004;83:257–261.

9. Eisenach JC, Pan PH, Smiley R, Lavand'homme P, Landau R, Houle TT. Severity of acute pain after childbirth, but not type of delivery, predicts persistent pin and postpartum depression. Pain 2008;140:87–94.

10. Soet JE, Brack GA, DiIorio C. Prevalence and predictors of women's experience of psychological trauma during childbirth. Birth 2003;30:36–46.

11. Kehlet H, Dahl JB. The value of "multimodal" or "balanced analgesia" in postoperative pain treatment. Anesth Analg 1993;77:1048–1056.

12. Abrao KC, Francisco RC, Miyadahira S, Cicarelli DD, Zugaib M. Evaluation of uterine tone and fetal heart rate abnormalities after labor analgesia: a randomized controlled trial. Obstet Gynecol 2009;113:41–47.

13. Van de Velde M, Teunkens A, Hanssens M, Vandermeersch E, Verhaeghe J. Intrathecal sufentanil and fetal heart rate abnormalities: a double-blind, double placebo-controlled trial comparing two forms of combined spinal epidural analgesia with epidural analgesia in labor. Anesth Analg 2004;98:1153–1159.

14. Simmons SW, Cyna AM, Dennis AT, Hughes D. Combined spinal-epidural versus epidural analgesia in labor. Cochrane Database Syst Rev 2007;3:CD003401.

15. Bremerich DH, Waibel HJ, Mierdl S et al. Comparison of continuous background infusion plus demand dose and demand-only parturient-controlled epidural analgesia (PCEA) using ropivacaine combined with sufentanil for labor and delivery. Int J Obstet Anesth 2005;14:114–120.

16. Saito M, Okutomi T, Kanai Y et al. Patient-controlled epidural analgesia during labor using ropivacaine and fentanyl provides better maternal satisfaction with less local anesthetic requirement. J Anesth 2005;19:208–212.

17. Torvaldsen S, Roberts CL, Bell JC, Raynes-Greenow CH. Discontinuation of epidural analgesia late in labour for reducing the adverse delivery outcomes associated with epidural analgesia. Cochrane Database Syst Rev 2009;4:CD004457.

18. Wong CA, Scavone BM, Peaceman AM et al. The risk of cesarean delivery with neuraxial analgesia given early versus late in labor. N Engl J Med 2005;352:655–665.

19. Wong CA, McCarthy RJ, Sullivan JT, Scavone BM, Gerber SE, Yaghmour EA. Early compared with late neuraxial analgesia in nulliparous labor induction: a randomized controlled trial. Obstet Gynecol 2009;113:1066–1074.

20. Ohel G, Gonen R, Vaida S, Barak S, Gaitini L. Early versus late initiation of epidural analgesia in labor: does it increase the risk of cesarean section? A randomized trial. Am J Obstet Gynecol 2006;194:600–605.

21. Wang F, Shen X, Guo X, Peng Y, Gu X. Epidural analgesia in the latent phase of labor and the risk of cesarean delivery: a five-year randomized controlled trial. Anesthesiology 2009;111:871–880.

22. American College of Obstetricians and Gynecologists Committee on Obstetric Practice. Analgesia and cesarean delivery rates. Committee Opinion No. 339. Obstet Gynecol 2006;107:1487–1488.

23. Bucklin BA, Hawkins JL, Anderson JR, Ullrich FA. Obstetric anesthesia workforce survey: twenty-year update. Anesthesiology 2005;103:645–653.

24. Hawkins JL, Koonin LM, Palmer SK, Gibbs CP. Anesthesia-related deaths during obstetric delivery in the United States, 1979–1990. Anesthesiology 1997;86:277–284.

25. Rout CC, Rocke DA, Levin J, Gouws E, Reddy D. A reevaluation of the role of crystalloid preload in the prevention of hypotension associated with spinal anesthesia for elective cesarean section. Anesthesiology 1993;79:262–269.

26. Reynolds F, Seed PT. Anaesthesia for Caesarean section and neonatal acid–base status: a meta-analysis. Anaesthesia 2005;60:636–653.

27. Ngan Kee WD, Lee A, Khaw KS, Ng FF, Karmakar MK, Gin T. A randomized double-blinded comparison of phenylephrine and ephedrine infusion combinations to maintain blood pressure during spinal anesthesia for cesarean delivery: the effects on fetal acid-base status and hemodynamic control. Anesth Analg 2008;107:1295–1302.

28. Pavy TJ, Paech MJ, Evans SF. The effect of intravenous ketorolac on opioid requirement and pain after cesarean delivery. Anesth Analg 2001;92:1010–1014.

Chapter 53
Patient Safety

Christian M. Pettker

Department of Obstetrics, Gynecology and Reproductive Sciences, Yale University School of Medicine, New Haven, CT, USA

Safely providing the most effective care has always been a priority in medicine. However, increasing consumer and provider interest coupled with recent progress in the patient safety movement has now made this a primary concern. The past 50 years have witnessed an evolution in healthcare into a complex environment, requiring integration of advanced technologies and diverse and specialized teams. Thus, opportunities for failure have become more prominent and the costs of errors never greater. In 1999 the Institute of Medicine (IOM) estimated that approximately 44,000–98,000 patients die each year due to medical errors, with a majority of these incidents due to preventable errors and correctable faults [1]. Realizing that this would make medical errors the eighth leading cause of death in the United States, greater than those from motor vehicle collisions, breast cancer, and AIDS, puts the burden of this reality into perspective.

The foundation of the patient safety movement is that fallible individuals and teams working in an increasingly complicated system create substantial opportunities for inadvertent adverse outcomes. Healthcare leaders have responded with improving safety and quality standards, developing better communication and teamwork techniques, and building more robust fail-safes. Today, the science of medicine has renewed a commitment to its ancient credo of "first, do no harm." This chapter discusses the major concepts in patient safety as applied to obstetrics.

Patient safety in obstetrics

The patient safety movement has shown great progress in fields such as cardiology, critical care, and anesthesia, though progress has been slower in obstetrics. This is surprising given that obstetrics is a logical target for safety and quality improvements. Obstetrics is a significant component of US healthcare; childbirth accounts for over 4 million hospitalizations each year, ranking second only to cardiovascular disease [2]. Obstetrics is also unique in that an adverse outcome can often affect two patients (mother and infant) and a neonatal injury may result in significant long-term consequences for the family and society. It is also no secret that perinatal care is in a crisis of professional insurance and medical liability. While obstetricians and gynecologists represent only 5% of the physicians in the US, they are responsible for 15% of liability claims and 36% of total payments [3], with payments for obstetric liability claims averaging $500,000 to $1,900,000 [4]. These latter factors have greatly affected the way obstetrics is practiced in the United States, with more obstetricians practicing defensive medicine and others simply dropping out of obstetric practice altogether [5].

How to measure safety

In general terms, safety efforts can be tracked in three ways, using outcome measures, process measures, and culture measures.

Outcome measures

Patient safety outcome measures track how often patients are harmed or how well the organization is providing favorable (expected) outcomes [6,7]. Most patient safety initiatives focus on adverse outcome measures, as the prevention of these events is often the primary goal of such efforts. Mann and colleagues have proposed one set of measures referred to as the obstetric Adverse Outcome Index (AOI), which is based on measures defined by the Joint Commission, the American College of Obstetricians and Gynecologists (ACOG), and the National Perinatal Information Center [8]. The AOI is calculated as the percentage of mothers with at least one adverse outcome indicator (Box 53.1). This rate can be tracked on a monthly

Queenan's Management of High-Risk Pregnancy: An Evidence-Based Approach, Sixth Edition. Edited by John T. Queenan, Catherine Y. Spong, Charles J. Lockwood.
© 2012 John Wiley & Sons, Ltd. Published 2012 by John Wiley & Sons, Ltd.

Box 53.1 Adverse Outcome Index indicators

- Apgar <7 at 5 min
- Blood transfusion
- Fetal traumatic birth injury
- Intrapartum or neonatal death >2500 g
- Maternal death
- Maternal ICU admission
- Maternal return to operating room or Labor and Delivery
- Unexpected admission to neonatal ICU >2500 g and for >24 h
- Uterine rupture

ICU, intensive care unit.

or quarterly basis and analyzed for trends, and has been used to track the work of various quality improvement programs [8–11]. Units may track these indicators individually, but the critical measure of success is an improvement in overall AOI over time. While the AOI can be compared across units, it is expected that the unique environments, patient demographics, and acuity levels will contribute to high unit-to-unit variability.

Process measures

Process measures analyze the adherence to common or evidence-based standards and practices [12], with the assumption that adherence to these performance measures improves outcomes. The Surgical Care Improvement Project (SCIP), which proposes to measure processes like appropriate antibiotic administration and thromboembolism prophylaxis, is one example of a set of process measures. Whether this, in turn, produces better outcomes is controversial, though one can argue that adherence to good practices in one segment of care produces better compliance across the spectrum of healthcare provisions [13].

Culture measures

Safety culture is the integration of safety thinking and practices into clinical activities. Improving patient safety depends on changing the attitude of an organization, including shifting from a culture of blame to a culture of safety. Safety climate, the quantitative description of the safety culture, can be measured by calibrating a healthcare team's attitudes about issues related to safety through workforce or staff attitude surveys [14]. Many patient safety climate surveys are available. The Agency for Healthcare Research and Quality's Hospital Survey on Patient Safety Culture is a publicly available tool with a centralized comparative database that allows organizations to benchmark survey results [15]. The Safety Attitude Questionnaire (SAQ) is a tool adapted from the aviation industry and subsequently validated in healthcare that can be given to the various staff members of an obstetric

unit [14,16]. Respondents answer a series of statements in agreement or disagreement (on a five-point Likert scale); differences of 10% or more, over time or between groups, are considered clinically significant and overall scores showing 80% agreement with a favorable teamwork climate statement are a target goal. One systematic review has identified the SAQ as the only safety climate survey that has been used to explore the relationship between safety perceptions and patient outcomes [17].

The National Quality Forum (NQF) has suggested 18 consensus standards for assessing quality in perinatal care that combine both outcome and process measures [18]. Those applying to antepartum and intrapartum care include elective delivery prior to 39 completed weeks gestation, incidence of episiotomy, cesarean rate for low-risk first birth women, prophylactic antibiotics in cesarean delivery, appropriate deep vein thrombosis prophylaxis at cesarean delivery, birth trauma rate, and appropriate use of antenatal steroids. These have also been emphasized by the Joint Commission under the Perinatal Care Core Measures.

Tools to improve patient safety

Many strategies have been suggested to improve safety and quality in an obstetric service. Most center on principles of evidence-based practice, the benefits of standardization, and improving communication.

1. *Outside expert review.* Bringing in unbiased and experienced observers to review an obstetrics service for one or several days is often a first step for quality improvement. The review team may consist of any combination of nurses, physicians, or administrators, but should be a group with experience in safety and quality practices. Using a triangulation process to resolve differences in perspectives, the team can interview staff from the various professional domains within the healthcare system to assess the culture of safety. Hospital policies and protocols should be reviewed. The result is usually a written review, with specific recommendations for improvement based on local and national standards, focusing on core principles of safety, and informed by the evidence.

2. *Protocols, guidelines, and checklists.* The initial push for guidelines and protocols can meet high resistance from providers claiming the superiority of experience and intuition over evidence and standardization. A common fear is that guidelines and protocols may dictate all aspects and levels of care, to a level of detail that does not account for individualizing care according to variations in locale, culture, preferences, and experience. In truth, protocols and guidelines merely serve as a common foundation for approaching the aspects of care relative to specific diseases or processes. Variable approaches to similar clinical scenarios, particularly when there is little evidence to demonstrate any as superior, can contribute to confusion and error. Protocols and guidelines create common knowledge structures or shared mental models, improving performance in times of pressure and uncertainty. Higher-risk practices, such as the use of oxytocin, prostaglandins, and magnesium sulfate, are particularly aided by standardized protocols. Checklists, furthermore, aim to implement these protocols and guidelines by distilling and delineating, in real time, the important events and activities required to perform or respond successfully to particular clinical scenarios. The use of checklists, in fact, has demonstrated remarkable reductions in catheter-related bloodstream infections [7] and surgical complications [6] in large-scale trials. The key to developing and implementing these measures is to rely on standards set by the industry or evidence in the literature, and build on these through consensus among staff, preferably through working groups and sufficient comment periods.

3. *Computerized order entry "order sets."* Computerized order entry can potentially contribute to improvements in patient safety by reducing the rates of medication errors. It should also be viewed as a mode of decision support, providing "protocolized" order sets that direct providers to a preferred and uniform management strategy, such as oxytocin administration, antibiotics and steroids for preterm premature rupture of membranes, or preeclampsia management. Converting the relevant aspects of a particular protocol into a formalized order set can direct providers to the institutionally preferred management strategy.

4. *Perinatal patient safety nurse.* The perinatal patient safety nurse is often the crux of a patient safety program, acting as the educator and administrator for most of the subinitiatives. This role is usually filled by a nurse with experience in clinical and administrative systems, in particular relative to obstetrics and/or risk management [19]. Specifically, our patient safety nurse administrated our anonymous event reporting system, safety attitude questionnaire, and electronic fetal monitoring (EFM) certification testing, instructed our staff in crew resource management training, and performed audits of our adverse outcomes data.

5. *Anonymous event reporting system.* Computer-based reporting tools are available that allow for the discrete and anonymous reporting of adverse events, near-misses, and unsafe conditions. In addition to allowing for surveillance of existing and potential unsafe situations, it also empowers staff to participate in the quality improvement process. The patient safety nurse can educate staff on the use of the system, track the data reported for trends, and investigate new or important issues as they arise.

6. *Obstetric hospitalist.* Hospitalist coverage of inpatient services, where a dedicated provider covers the care of inpatients from a variety of primary outpatient caregivers, has become an increasingly utilized service in other fields. The goal of using a hospitalist is to rely on providers with skill sets specific to a particular work environment, improve clinical efficiency, and improve outcomes. The concept of the "laborist" extends this to obstetric units, providing the continuity and availability of a caregiver who does not have responsibilities beyond the unit. While continuity of care is reduced in this model, potential gains come from developing a team that is focused on and has mastered the efficient provision of inpatient obstetric care. Currently, while data suggest superior outcomes in hospitals that employ hospitalists, there are no data available specific to obstetrics [20].

7. *Obstetric patient safety committee.* Forming an obstetric patient safety committee allows representatives of the major stakeholders (e.g. nurses, midwives, obstetricians, pediatricians, anesthesiologists, pharmacists, administration, etc.) to meet on a regular basis to review current practices and important adverse events, and strategize on quality improvement efforts. This multidisciplinary approach fosters change in the organizational culture and allows for an efficient process of developing policies and protocols that have the interests of everyone in mind.

8. *Safety attitude questionnaire (SAQ).* Also discussed above, the SAQ is both an intervention and an assessment tool. As an intervention, a survey demonstrates the interest of the organization in calibrating (and improving) the safety culture. As an assessment tool, the SAQ can be used to track improvements or areas for attention. This feedback is essential for management and administration to respond to the conditions on the front lines of care.

9. *Team training.* Communication failure is overall the dominant root cause of adverse events and near-misses. Crew resource management (CRM), a strategy to improve team functioning derived from civil and defense aviation work, is an important strategy for improving communication and teamwork. Team training aims to reduce the barriers between disciplines (e.g. nurses versus physicians) that arise from these groups training in separate silos. Team training also attempts to combat traditional hierarchies that are common in medicine. Specific concepts that are usually taught are structured handoff techniques (e.g. Situation-Background-Assessment-Recommendation [SBAR]), conflict resolution techniques (concerned, uncomfortable, scared [CUS]; the "two challenge" rule, the chain-of-command), and structured debriefing techniques that are performed after events. Team training has proven helpful in improving teamwork and outcomes in surgical units [21], though a trial to implement CRM in obstetrics units showed no benefit in outcomes as measured by the AOI [9].

10. *Standardization of EFM assessment.* Objective fetal heart rate interpretation relies on a standard set of definitions and descriptions. Indeed, inconsistencies in practice are largely due to obfuscations in the language and terms used to describe particular tracings. The Joint Commission Sentinel Event Alert No. 30 recognized that "inadequate fetal monitoring" was a root cause in 34% of adverse events, recommending units to "develop clear guidelines for fetal monitoring of potential high-risk patients, including nursing protocols for the interpretation of fetal heart rate tracings" and to "educate nurses, residents, nurse midwives, and physicians to use standardized terminology to communicate abnormal fetal heart rate tracings"[22]. Shortly thereafter, in 2005, the ACOG and Association of Women's Health, Obstetric and Neonatal Nurses (AWOHNN) advocated universal implementation of the NIH/NICHD Workshop guidelines on electronic fetal monitoring [23], which were subsequently revised in 2008 [24]. Adoption of such guidelines by a unit is important, and usually relies on formalized programs for training and testing. One example of this is offered by the National Certification Corporation (NCC; www.nccnet.org), a nonprofit group that offers training and testing of fetal monitoring standards based on the NICHD criteria.

11. *Simulation.* The aviation industry has taught us that recreating workplace scenarios in simulations can contribute to acquisition of new skills, particularly for situations that occur infrequently, such as emergencies. Given that obstetrics is characterized mostly by routine labor and delivery, punctuated by low-frequency yet high-severity events (e.g. shoulder dystocia, hemorrhage, and eclampsia), obstetrics is a particular discipline that has rightly incorporated simulation into training. Simulation scenarios are usually focused on either knowledge/skills training or teamwork training, and often units will choose one or the other as the primary objective of particular simulation sessions. High-fidelity simulation technologies that involve sophisticated mannequins and equipment can provide a realistic experience, but require substantial preparation and resources. *In situ* simulation scenarios that take place in the actual patient care units, usually during times of low acuity and census, can provide equally important lessons on teamwork/communication and skills. A recent systematic review of team training for acute obstetric emergencies reports improvements in some clinical outcomes (5-min Apgars and hypoxic-ischemic encephalopathy) as well as in knowledge, skills, communication, and team performance [25].

Evidence to support improvement tools

With the emerging focus on quality and safety in healthcare, research evaluating various tools has increased over the past 5 years. Two of the more notable efforts have involved the implementation of checklists. In Michigan, a statewide effort to implement five evidence-based procedures for the insertion and care of catheters reduced catheter-related bloodstream infections by up to 66% [7]. The World Health Organization international project on a 19-item surgical checklist aiming to improve teamwork, communication, and consistency of care reduced death by nearly 50% (1.5% to 0.8%, $P = 0.003$) and inpatient complications from 11% to 7% ($P = 0.001$) [6].

Obstetrics research has lagged, but is gaining ground. A long-term comprehensive safety effort at Yale-New Haven Hospital, incorporating most of the strategies discussed previously in this chapter, demonstrated significant improvements [10]. Over a 3-year period, comprising over 13,000 deliveries, the AOI declined significantly over time ($P = 0.01$) (Fig. 53.1). The mean quarterly AOI for the second half of the initiative ($2.09 \pm 0.57\%$) was significantly lower than that for the first half ($2.90 \pm 0.64\%$) ($P = 0.04$). A group from the HCA healthcare system, which involves more than 200 hospitals across the United States, implemented a comprehensive effort that included a protocol for oxytocin administration, checklist-based protocols for misoprostol and magnesium, and a standardized shoulder dystocia delivery note. Over time, they witnessed a reduction in annual malpractice claims from 10–13 per 100,000 deliveries to 6–7.5 per 100,000 births ($P < 0.001$) [26].

Demonstrating the power of protocols and guidelines specifically, hospital policies to review and prevent unnecessary elective early term births have been shown to reduce the number of risky and unnecessary inductions as well as the rates of term neonatal admissions [27]. A statewide initiative in Ohio demonstrated a greater than fivefold reduction in inductions without a documented medical indication (25% to 5%, $P < 0.05$) [28]. A randomized trial describing the multifaceted implementation of guidelines for postpartum oxytocin administration and episiotomy repair showed improvements in postpartum hemorrhage rates and episiotomy utilization [29].

Beyond safety and quality

The primary motivations that drive patient safety efforts are providing quality care and eliminating harm, though secondary benefits accrue as well. Eliminating the costs of adverse events provides economic savings, which in turn guides investment in patient safety programs by governments and healthcare institutions [30–32]. Improvements in safety culture can provide more satisfying work environments, improving work efficiency and reducing workforce turnover.

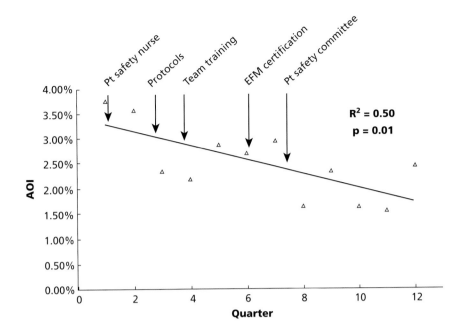

Figure 53.1 Yale-New Haven Hospital quarterly obstetric Adverse Outcome Index.
Reproduced from Pettker *et al* [10] with permission from Elsevier.

CASE PRESENTATION

A 35-year-old gravida 1, para 0 at 39 weeks' gestation is being induced for preeclampsia. She has presented at the end of the day, right before the change of shift, and the physician has ordered both intravenous magnesium sulfate, for seizure prophylaxis, and oxytocin. Before going off her shift, the nurse prepares the magnesium sulfate and oxytocin infusions, but does not start them. The next nurse coming on starts the infusions. Within minutes the patient is noted to have tetanic contractions and a prolonged fetal heart rate deceleration; despite discontinuation of the intravenous infusions and intrauterine resuscitative measures, the team proceeds to a stat cesarean delivery for a fetal bradycardia. A healthy infant is born with Apgars of 5 and 9. After the cesarean is over, the nurse discovers that she confused the magnesium and the oxytocin lines and accidentally gave a large dose of oxytocin thinking it was the magnesium sulfate bolus. Understanding the importance of the team learning from the error, she enters a computerized anonymous event report for the patient safety nurse to review the next morning.

In response to this event, a root cause analysis (RCA) is organized and directed by an outside party experienced in event review. In the spirit of a culture of safety, rather than a culture of blame, the team is able to identify critical areas for potential improvement. Specific system improvements are suggested, such as an appropriate "SBAR" nursing handoff in the patient room, and improved labeling systems for intravenous lines for oxytocin and magnesium sulfate so that they are not confused. The RCA also recognizes that communication during the emergency delivery was suboptimal. The RCA report is reviewed by the Patient Safety Committee, which discusses further enhancements over a longer timeframe, such as creating a computerized SBAR handoff template. The Committee also suggests organizing monthly simulations on Labor and Delivery to train staff on how to perform an efficient and organized emergency cesarean delivery. These ideas create an action plan, which is taken to the staff and administration for implementation.

References

1. Kohn L, Corrigan J, Donaldson M, eds. To Err is Human: Building a Safer Health System. Washington, DC: National Academies Press, 2000.
2. DeFrances C, Cullen K, Kozak L. National Hospital Discharge Survey: 2005 annual summary with detailed diagnosis and procedure data. National Center for Health Statistics. Vital Health Stat 2007;13(165).
3. Sanfilippo J, Robinson C. The Risk Management Handbook for Healthcare Professionals. Pearl River, NY: Parthenon Publishing, 2002.
4. Barbieri RL. Professional liability payments in obstetrics and gynecology. Obstet Gynecol 2006;107(3):578–581.

5. American College of Obstetricians and Gynecologists. 2009 ACOG survey on professional liability results. www.acog.org/departments/dept_notice.cfm?recno=4&bulletin=4309.

6. Haynes AB, Weiser TG, Berry WR et al. A surgical safety checklist to reduce morbidity and mortality in a global population. N Engl J Med 2009;360(5):491–499.

7. Pronovost P, Needham D, Berenholtz S et al. An intervention to decrease catheter-related bloodstream infections in the ICU. N Engl J Med 2006;355(26):2725–2732.

8. Mann S, Pratt S, Gluck P, Nielsen P et al. Assessing quality in obstetrical care: development of standardized measures. Jt Comm J Qual Patient Saf 2006;32:497–505.

9. Nielsen PE, Goldman MB, Mann S et al. Effects of teamwork training on adverse outcomes and process of care in labor and delivery: a randomized controlled trial. Obstet Gynecol 2007;109(1):48–55.

10. Pettker CM, Thung SF, Norwitz ER et al. Impact of a comprehensive patient safety strategy on obstetric adverse events. Am J Obstet Gynecol 2009;200(5):492.

11. Walker S, Strandjord TP, Benedetti TJ. In search of perinatal quality outcome measures: 1 hospital's in-depth analysis of the Adverse Outcomes Index. Am J Obstet Gynecol 2010;203(4):336.

12. Williams SC, Schmaltz SP, Morton DJ, Koss RG, Loeb JM. Quality of care in U.S. hospitals as reflected by standardized measures, 2002–2004. N Engl J Med 2005;353(3):255–264.

13. Hawn MT. Surgical care improvement: should performance measures have performance measures? JAMA 2010;303(24):2527–2528.

14. Sexton JB, Helmreich RL, Neilands TB et al. The Safety Attitudes Questionnaire: psychometric properties, benchmarking data, and emerging research. BMC Health Serv Res 2006;6:44.

15. Agency for Healthcare Research and Quality. Surveys on Patient Safety Culture. www.ahrq.gov/qual/patientsafetyculture/.

16. Sexton JB, Holzmueller CG, Pronovost PJ et al. Variation in caregiver perceptions of teamwork climate in labor and delivery units. J Perinatol 2006;26(8):463–470.

17. Colla JB, Bracken AC, Kinney LM, Weeks WB. Measuring patient safety climate: a review of surveys. Qual Saf Health Care 2005;14(5):364–366.

18. Simpson KR. Quality measures for perinatal care. MCN 2010;35(1):64.

19. Will SB, Hennicke KP, Jacobs LS, O'Neill LM, Raab CA. The perinatal patient safety nurse: a new role to promote safe care for mothers and babies. J Obstet Gynecol Neonatal Nurs 2006;35(3):417–423.

20. Lopez L, Hicks LS, Cohen AP, McKean S, Weissman JS. Hospitalists and the quality of care in hospitals. Arch Intern Med 2009;169(15):1389–1394.

21. Neily J, Mills PD, Young-Xu Y et al. Association between implementation of a medical team training program and surgical mortality. JAMA 2010;304(15):1693–1700.

22. JCAHO. Sentinel Event Alert #30. www.jointcommission.org/SentinelEvents/SentinelEventAlert/sea_30.htm.

23. National Institute of Child Health and Human Development Research Planning Workshop. Electronic fetal heart rate monitoring: research guidelines for interpretation. Am J Obstet Gynecol 1997;177(6):1385–1390.

24. Macones GA, Odibo A, Gross G et al. Standardized multidisciplinary EFM training for the entire obstetric team. Am J Obstet Gynecol 2009;199(6):S211.

25. Merien AE, van de Ven J, Mol BW, Houterman S, Oei SG. Multidisciplinary team training in a simulation setting for acute obstetric emergencies: a systematic review. Obstet Gynecol 2010;115(5):1021–1031.

26. Clark SL, Belfort MA, Byrum SL, Meyers JA, Perlin JB. Improved outcomes, fewer cesarean deliveries, and reduced litigation: results of a new paradigm in patient safety. Am J Obstet Gynecol 2008;199(2):105.

27. Clark SL, Frye DR, Meyers JA et al. Reduction in elective delivery at <39 weeks of gestation: comparative effectiveness of 3 approaches to change and the impact on neonatal intensive care admission and stillbirth. Am J Obstet Gynecol 2010;203(5):449.

28. Donovan EF, Lannon C, Bailit J, Rose B, Iams JD, Byczkowski T. A statewide initiative to reduce inappropriate scheduled births at 36(0/7)-38(6/7) weeks' gestation. Am J Obstet Gynecol 2010;202(3):243.

29. Althabe F, Buekens P, Bergel E et al. A behavioral intervention to improve obstetrical care. N Engl J Med 2008;358(18):1929–1940.

30. Paradis AR, Stewart VT, Bayley KB, Brown A, Bennett AJ. Excess cost and length of stay associated with voluntary patient safety event reports in hospitals. Am J Med Qual 2009;24(1):53–60.

31. Schmidek JM, Weeks WB. What do we know about financial returns on investments in patient safety? A literature review. Jt Comm J Qual Patient Saf 2005;31(12):690–699.

32. Zhan C, Miller MR. Excess length of stay, charges, and mortality attributable to medical injuries during hospitalization. JAMA 2003;290(14):1868–1874.

Chapter 54
Neonatal Encephalopathy and Cerebral Palsy

Maged M. Costantine[1], Mary E. D'Alton[2], and Gary D.V. Hankins[1]

[1]Department of Obstetrics and Gynecology, University of Texas Medical Branch, Galveston, TX, USA
[2]Department of Obstetrics and Gynecology, Columbia University Medical Center and Columbia Presbyterian Hospital, New York, NY, USA

The incidence of cerebral palsy is 1–2 per 1000 births and has remained unchanged over the last 40 years. The occurrence of cerebral palsy is independent of either geographic or economic boundaries. It has also been remarkably resistant to eradication by the introduction of technology such as electronic fetal heart rate monitoring or the increase in cesarean delivery rates. Indeed, the great hope of electronic fetal heart rate monitoring was that intrapartum asphyxia would be promptly identified, delivery rapidly achieved, and neurologic injury of the infant averted. This would in fact parallel the thought processes advanced by the orthopedic surgeon Little [1], over a century ago, who taught that virtually all cerebral palsy was caused by intrapartum events, whether deprivation of oxygen, trauma, or the combination of the two. Unfortunately, despite an escalation of the cesarean delivery rate from approximately 6% in 1970 to a rate of more than 31% nationally today [2], the incidence of cerebral palsy in the USA has remained constant [3].

These facts then would seem to support the evolving concept that cerebral palsy results from the combination of the genetic make-up of the individual and the subsequent interaction of that individual during development with the environment that they are exposed to, both intrauterine as well as extrauterine for the first several days, months, or years of life. As examples, the South Australian Cerebral Palsy Research Group has reported that inheritance of MTHFR C677T approximately doubles the risk of cerebral palsy in preterm infants [4]. A combination of homozygous MTHFR C677T and heterozygous prothrombin gene mutation increased the risk of quadriplegia fivefold in all gestational ages. This is clearly an example of genetic inheritance leading to cerebral palsy. The same group also demonstrated that perinatal exposure to the neurotropic herpes group B viruses nearly doubled the risk of cerebral palsy relative to the control group [5].

Neonatal encephalopathy

Neonatal encephalopathy is a condition defined in and described for term (more than 37 completed weeks' gestation) and near term (more than 34 completed weeks' gestation) infants. It is a clinically defined syndrome of disturbed neurologic function manifest by difficulty with initiating and maintaining respiration, depression of tone and reflexes, altered level of consciousness, and often seizures. Additionally, it must manifest within the first week of life. The differential diagnosis and antecedants for neonatal encephalopathy is shown in Box 54.1.

Hypoxia sufficient to result in hypoxic ischemic encephalopathy (HIE) is only one subset of the larger category of neonatal encephalopathy. If there has been intrapartum asphyxia sufficient to result in long-term neurologic injury manifest as cerebral palsy, then the neonate will manifest the injury as encephalopathy within the first week of life. It is biologically implausible to suggest that one can have sufficient intrapartum asphyxia to result in cerebral palsy, yet the newborn would have a completely normal newborn course void of encephalopathy.

Cerebral palsy

Cerebral palsy is defined as a chronic neuromuscular disability characterized by abnormal control of movement or posture appearing early in life and not the result of recognized progressive disease [6]. The causes of cerebral palsy are in large part the same as the antecedents of neonatal encephalopathy (see Box 54.1). In a sentinel publication, MacLennan [7] notes that epidemiologic studies suggest that in approximately 90% of cases of cerebral palsy, intrapartum hypoxia could not be the cause and in the remaining 10%, intrapartum signs compatible with

---

Queenan's Management of High-Risk Pregnancy: An Evidence-Based Approach, Sixth Edition. Edited by John T. Queenan, Catherine Y. Spong, Charles J. Lockwood.
© 2012 John Wiley & Sons, Ltd. Published 2012 by John Wiley & Sons, Ltd.

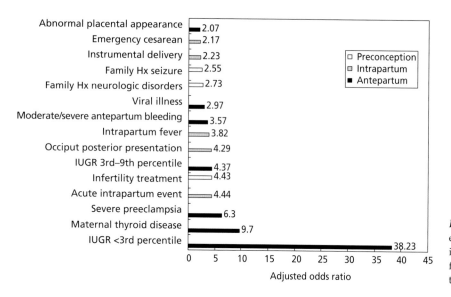

Figure 54.1 Risk factors for newborn encephalopathy. Hx, history; IUGR, intrauterine growth restriction. Reproduced from Badawi *et al* [8] with permission from the *British Medical Journal*.

Box 54.1 Differential diagnosis and antecedants of neonatal encephalopathy

- Developmental abnormalities
- Metabolic abnormalities
- Autoimmune disorders
- Coagulation disorders
- Infections
- Trauma
- Hypoxia
- Intrauterine growth restriction
- Multiple gestations
- Antepartum hemorrhage
- Chromosomal abnormalities
- Persistent breech/transverse lie

---

damaging hypoxia may have had antenatal or intrapartum origins.

A group of investigators led by Badawi [8] reported on the antecedents of moderate-to-severe neonatal encephalopathy from their patient population in metropolitan Western Australia. This study involved 164 term infants with moderate or severe neonatal encephalopathy and 400 randomly selected appropriate controls. Within their population, the prevalence of moderate or severe newborn encephalopathy was 3.8 in 1000 term livebirths. The diagnosis of either moderate or severe newborn encephalopathy was associated with a neonatal fatality rate of 9.1%. In Figure 54.1, the risk factors for newborn encephalopathy in their population that achieved statistical significance are shown and substratified according to whether they occurred preconceptionally, intrapartum, or in the antepartum period. Data shown are the increase in adjusted odds ratio.

Badawi *et al*'s data are striking inasmuch as the traditional risk factors, including abnormal histopathology of the placenta, the need for emergency cesarean section, or the use of vacuum or forceps to achieve vaginal delivery, were among the lowest, although statistically significant, risk factors identified. In contrast, family history of seizure disorder or neurologic disorder and maternal thyroid disease was much more highly associated with moderate-to-severe encephalopathy than the traditional risk factors. This again emphasizes the potential role of genetics in causing both encephalopathy as well as cerebral palsy. The role of environment is also demonstrated from Badawi *et al*'s data, with factors such as viral illness during the index pregnancy, moderate or severe antepartum bleeding, intrapartum fever, and severe preeclampsia being significantly increased risk factors for development of these disorders. Thus, we return to the role of genetics and the impact of environment on causation of this neurologic injury. This is repeatedly being affirmed by clinical studies employing a variety of rapidly advancing technologies [4,5].

When Badawi *et al* analyzed their data with regard to the distribution of risk factors for newborn encephalopathy, they concluded that in 69% of the population there were only antepartum risk factors. In 25%, there were antepartum risk factors and potential impact of intrapartum hypoxia, but in only 4% did intrapartum hypoxia seem to be the logical cause (Fig. 54.2). This team of investigators' overall conclusions were that the causes of newborn encephalopathy are heterogeneous and that many of the causal pathways start before birth. A much earlier study by Blair and Stanley [9] had similarly concluded that in only 8% of all children with spastic cerebral palsy was intrapartum asphyxia the possible cause of their brain damage.

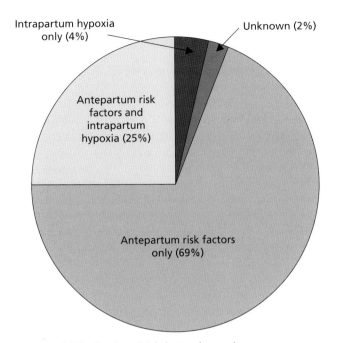

Intrapartum hypoxia only (4%)

Unknown (2%)

Antepartum risk factors and intrapartum hypoxia (25%)

Antepartum risk factors only (69%)

Figure 54.2 Distribution of risk factors for newborn encephalopathy. Reproduced from Badawi *et al* [8] with permission from the *British Medical Journal*.

Box 54.2 Essential criteria to define an acute intrapartum event sufficient to cause cerebral palsy (must meet all four)

- Evidence of a metabolic acidosis in fetal umbilical cord arterial blood obtained at delivery (pH < 7 and base deficit of ≥12 mmol/L)
- Early onset of severe or moderate neonatal encephalopathy in infants born at ≥34 weeks' gestation
- Cerebral palsy of the spastic quadriplegic or dyskinetic type
- Exclusion of other identifiable etiologies, such as trauma, coagulation disorders, infectious conditions, or genetic disorders

The importance of intrauterine growth restriction (IUGR) as a risk factor for newborn encephalopathy deserves special emphasis. In Badawi *et al*'s study, growth restriction between the 3rd and 9th percentile carried an adjusted odds ratio of 4.37 for moderate or severe neonatal encephalopathy. When the growth restriction was severe, defined as less than the 3rd percentile, the adjusted odds ratio increased to a staggering 38.23. In a series reported by Cowan *et al* [10], 11–15% of the population with encephalopathy were at the 3–10th percentile, compared with 13–16% when the growth restriction was less than the 3rd percentile. Their study population was recruited from the Wilhelmina Children's Hospital, Utrecht, The Netherlands, and Hammersmith and Queen Charlotte's Hospitals, London, UK. Substantially similar results were reported from the University of California, San Francisco, and Loma Linda Children's Hospital, where newborns with either a watershed predominant or a total brain/basal ganglia/thalamus predominant injury had a higher incidence of IUGR than did those infants having a normal scan [11].

The clinician is thus cautioned that while all growth-restricted babies are at increased risk for newborn encephalopathy, the risk is extraordinarily high for those infants with growth restriction at less than the 3rd percentile. Accordingly, great care in the timing and route of delivery of these fetuses is encouraged so that they might be delivered in an optimal metabolic condition. It would also seem prudent to have a neonatologist present at the birth to provide immediate care of the newborn. Induction of anesthesia may be a very high-risk period, as many of these fetuses are marginally compensated and will be poorly tolerant of epidural (or spinal)-induced hypotension. Fetal monitoring is necessary in the operating and/or delivery room. In cases of cesarean delivery, the interval from discontinuation of fetal monitoring to delivery should be as short as possible.

Task force on neonatal encephalopathy and cerebral palsy

In January 2003, a monograph summarizing the state of the science on neonatal encephalopathy and cerebral palsy was co-published by the American College of Obstetricians and Gynecologists and the American Academy of Pediatrics. At the time of publication, it was recognized that the topic would require updating as the scientific database and knowledge on the topic expanded and a task force is currently being assembled. In that monograph, the criteria to define an acute event sufficient to cause cerebral palsy were listed, as modified by the task force from the template provided by the International Cerebral Palsy Task Force (Box 54.2). It was emphasized that all four criteria must be met in order to make this association. Additionally, criteria were also listed that collectively suggest an intrapartum timing, defined as within close proximity to labor and delivery (e.g. 0–48h), but which were nonspecific to asphyxia insults (Box 54.3). Among the criteria for elucidating timing were early imaging studies showing evidence of acute nonfocal cerebral abnormalities.

Subsequent to the publication of this monograph, three important papers on neuroimaging have been published. The first of these, by Graham *et al* [12], dealt with an earlier gestation than covered by the task force, which was restricted to the term and near term infant. In contrast, Graham *et al*'s study was of the preterm infant of 23–34 weeks' gestation. The significant findings by these authors included that in this specific population, intrapartum hypoxia ischemia as manifested by metabolic acidosis was rarely associated with white matter injury, and was not different from that seen in premature neonates without injury.

The second study was by Cowan *et al* [10], who divided their population into two groups. Group 1 was defined as those with neonatal encephalopathy with or without seizures, and evidence of perinatal asphyxia. This group consisted of infants with neonatal encephalopathy, defined by abnormal tone pattern, feeding difficulties, altered alertness, and at least three of the following criteria:

- late decelerations on fetal monitoring or meconium staining
- delayed onset of respiration
- arterial cord blood pH <7.14
- Apgar score <7 at 5 min
- multiorgan failure.

Their second group consisted of infants who had seizures within 72 h of birth but who did not meet the criteria for neonatal encephalopathy.

In the first group, brain imaging studies showed evidence of an acute insult without established injury or atrophy in 80% of infants. Magnetic resonance imaging (MRI) showed evidence of established injury in only two infants (<1%), although tiny foci of established white matter gliosis, in addition to acute injury, were seen in 3/21 on postmortem examination. In group 2, acute focal damage was noted in 62 (69%) infants. Two (3%) also had evidence of antenatal injury. Cowan *et al* [10] concluded that although their results could not exclude the possibility that antenatal or genetic factors might predispose some infants to perinatal brain injury, their data strongly suggested that events in the immediate perinatal period were most important in neonatal brain injury. A valid criticism of this study is the criteria selected for inclusion into their group 1. Either late decelerations on fetal monitoring or meconium staining are notoriously poor predictors of intrapartum asphyxia. Delayed onset of respirations can occur for numerous reasons, and a large number of

babies will be born with blood pH <7.1 and almost all will be neurologically intact. What these authors fail to tell us is how many of their total population would have met at least three of the five criteria that they listed for inclusion in the acute injury group.

The study by Miller *et al* [11] reported that the watershed pattern of injury was seen in 78 newborns (45%), the basal ganglia/thalamus pattern was seen in 44 newborns (25%), and normal MRI studies were seen in 51 newborns (30%). Antenatal conditions such as maternal substance abuse, gestational diabetes, premature ruptured membranes, preeclampsia, and IUGR did not differ between the injury patterns. The basal ganglia/thalamus pattern was associated with more severe neonatal signs, including more intensive resuscitation at birth, more severe encephalopathy, and more severe seizures. The basal ganglia/thalamus pattern was most highly associated with impaired motor and cognitive outcome at 30 months. These authors concluded that the patterns of brain injury in term neonatal encephalopathy are associated with different clinical presentation and different neurodevelopmental outcomes. Further, and contrary to prior epidemiologic studies, they noted that measured prenatal factors did not predict the pattern of brain injury. Like Cowan *et al*, they noted that the MRI findings in their cohort were consistent with the recent, rather than chronic brain injury in the majority of patients and the antenatal conditions measured were remarkably similar between newborns with normal and abnormal MRI scan results. They felt that these observations highlighted the potential of interventions to ameliorate brain injury in the newborn. They remarked that the dissociation of antenatal risk factors from the severity of the clinical presentations supports the hypothesis that the etiology of brain injury in neonatal encephalopathy is distinct from these antenatal risk factors. They further noted that the watershed pattern had predominantly cognitive impairments at 30 months that were not detected at 12 months of age. The cognitive deficits in this group often occurred without functional motor deficits. They hypothesized that abnormal outcome after neonatal encephalopathy may not be limited to cerebral palsy and often requires follow-up beyond 12 months of age to be detected.

Cerebral palsy prevention strategies

Magnesium sulfate for neuroprotection for prevention of cerebral palsy

Kuban [13] was the first to report that prenatal magnesium sulfate was associated with a reduction of intraventricular hemorrhage (IVH) in babies with a birthweight of less than 1500 g from 18.9% to 4.4%. In a case–control study of singleton infants weighing less than 1500 g, Nelson [14] reported that administration of magnesium

sulfate to the mother during labor was associated with a marked reduction in the risk of cerebral palsy (odds ratio [OR] 0.14, 95% confidence interval [CI] 0.05–0.51). Different mechanisms of neuroprotection of magnesium sulfate are proposed and include:
- hemodynamic stability by stabilizing the blood pressure and improving cerebral perfusion
- prevention of excitatory injury and neuronal protection by blocking *N*-methyl-D-aspartate (NMDA) receptors and preventing glutamate-induced intracellular calcium influx, which is known to be cytotoxic [15]. Both fetal and newborn brains appear to be more susceptible to glutamate-mediated injury
- prevention of oxidative and inflammatory insults.

While other observational studies also reported a reduction in cerebral palsy and/or IVH, to change clinical practice requires evidence often best gathered by large randomized clinical trials.

Multiple randomized controlled trials have examined the long-term neurologic outcomes of infants exposed antenatally to magnesium sulfate [16–21]. Magnesium sulfate was used for fetal neuroprotection in four trials (Beneficial Effects of Antenatal Magnesium Sulfate (BEAM) [18], the Australasian Collaborative Trial of Magnesium Sulphate (ACTOMgSO4) [16], and PREMAG [19,21]) and in the neuroprotection arm of MagNET [20]. It was used for prevention of eclampsia in the Magnesium Sulphate for the Prevention of Eclampsia (Magpie) trial [17] and for tocolysis in the tocolytic arm of MagNET [20]. Although none of these trials demonstrated significant improvements in their primary outcome with the use of magnesium sulfate, most found benefit in some of their prespecified secondary outcomes. Reduction of "substantial gross motor dysfunction" (3.4% versus 6.6%, relative risk [RR] 0.51, 95% CI 0.29–0.91) and "death or substantial motor gross motor dysfunction" (17.0% versus 22.7%, RR 0.75, 95% CI 0.59–0.96) in ACTOMgSO4, as well as in PREMAG with reduction in death or gross motor dysfunction (25.6% versus 30.8%, OR 0.62, 95% CI 0.41–0.93) and death or motor or cognitive dysfunction (34.9% versus 40.5%, OR 0.68, 95% CI 0.47–0.99). Additionally, the BEAM trial demonstrated reduction in "moderate or severe cerebral palsy" (1.9% compared with 3.5%, RR 0.55, 95% CI 0.32–0.95) and overall cerebral palsy (4.2% compared with 7.3%, P = 0.004) with magnesium sulfate treatment compared to placebo.

Several metaanalyses [22–24] pooled data from all of the five previously mentioned studies and similarly did not show a reduction in the composite outcome of death or cerebral palsy (CP). However, antenatal exposure to magnesium sulfate was found to reduce the rate of CP by ≈30% (RR 0.68, 95% CI 0.54–0.87) and moderate/severe CP by ≈40%, without increasing the rate of death in 6145 infants (RR 1.04, 95% CI 0.92–1.17). Moreover, when only studies designed for neuroprotection (MagNET

preventive arm, ACTOMgSO4, PREMAG, and BEAM) were pooled together (n = 4446 fetuses/infants), the benefit of antenatal exposure to magnesium sulfate was more evident as it additionally showed a reduction in the composite outcomes of combined death or CP (RR 0.85, 95% CI 0.74–0.98), death or moderate-to-severe CP, as well as CP (RR 0.71, 95% CI 0.55–0.91) and moderate-to-severe CP (RR 0.60, 95% CI 0.43–0.84) without increasing the risk of perinatal or infant death (RR 0.95, 95% CI 0.80–1.13) or any other maternal or pediatric adverse events [22,23]. It is important to note that no significant effect of magnesium sulfate therapy was evident for other neurologic impairments such as developmental delay, intellectual impairment, blindness, deafness, or other major neurologic disabilities.

The studies and metaanalyses previously described led the American College of Obstetricians and Gynecologists and Society for Maternal-Fetal Medicine to publish a Committee Opinion stating:

. . . none of the individual studies found a benefit with regard to their primary outcome. However, the available evidence suggests that magnesium sulfate given before anticipated early preterm birth reduces the risk of cerebral palsy in surviving infants. Physicians electing to use magnesium sulfate for fetal neuroprotection should develop specific guidelines regarding inclusion criteria, treatment regimens, concurrent tocolytics, and monitoring in accordance with one of the larger trials [25].

In the Cochrane review, the number of women requiring treatment to prevent one case of cerebral palsy was 63 (95% CI 43–87) if one assumes a CP rate of 5% in the no magnesium group. This number appears justifiable and comparable (or better) to those for eclampsia prevention. Given the relative safety of magnesium sulfate for the mother, the lack of evident risk regarding infant mortality, and the gravity of cerebral palsy, magnesium sulfate should be considered for use as a neuroprotectant in the setting of anticipated preterm birth [25,26].

Key points for implementation of neuroprotection
After discussing the risks and benefits of magnesium sulfate in the setting of anticipated preterm delivery with the patient and obtaining her consent, a protocol similar to one of the large trials should be followed.

There was a reduction in cerebral palsy in the metaanalysis of studies that recruited women at less than 32–34 weeks (RR 0.70, 95% CI 0.55–0.89, n = 5225 infants). Thus, treatment is indicated in women at high risk for delivery at less than 32 weeks' gestation.

Magnesium sulfate regimens
- BEAM: 6 g loading infusion over 20–30 min then 2 g/h for 12 h or delivery, whichever was first. The maintenance was stopped if delivery had not occurred in 12 h and was

no longer considered imminent. Retreatment allowed when delivery was deemed imminent again; if ≥6 h from last infusion, another loading dose given.

• ACTOMgSO4: 4 g loading infusion over 20 min, followed by a maintenance infusion of 1 g/h for 24 h or until birth, whichever was first. No retreatment.

• PREMAG: 4 g infusion bolus. No maintenance. No retreatment.

Hypothermia for perinatal hypoxic ischaemic encephalopathy

Edwards and colleagues [27] performed a metaanalysis using a fixed effect model to determine whether moderate hypothermia after HIE improves survival and neurologic outcomes at 18 months of age. They identified three trials, encompassing 767 infants, that included information on deaths and major neurodevelopmental disability after at least 18 months follow-up. Also identified were seven trials with mortality information but no appropriate neurodevelopmental data. Therapeutic hypothermia reduced the combined rate of death and severe disability in the three trials with 18 month follow-up (RR 0.81, 95% CI 0.71–0.93, P = 0.002) with a number needed to treat of 9 (95% CI 5–25). Hypothermia increased survival with normal neurologic function (RR 1.53, 95% CI 1.22–1.93, P < 0.001) with a number needed to treat of 8 (95% CI 5–17), and in survivors reduced the rates of severe disability (P = 0.006), cerebral palsy (P = 0.004), and mental and psychomotor developmental index of less than 70 (P = 0.01 and P = 0.02, respectively). Mortality was significantly reduced when they assessed all 10 trials (RR 0.78, 95% CI 0.66–0.93). They concluded that in infants with HIE, moderate hypothermia was associated with a consistent reduction in death and neurologic impairment at 18 months of age.

Conclusions

How are we to resolve the epidemiologic studies with the more recent conclusions from imaging studies? Because newborns with severe encephalopathy are more likely to be identified for research studies in the intensive care nursery and these newborns are more likely to have the basal ganglia/thalamus injury pattern, it is possible that the prospective MRI studies of neonatal encephalopathy will overrepresent perinatally acquired injury compared with population-based epidemiologic surveys. Because population-based retrospective studies identify a preponderance of antenatal risk factors and smaller prospective cohort studies identify the perinatal occurrence of brain injury, there is a pressing need to establish the mechanistic link between prenatal risk factors and etiology of brain injury. This is critical to the prevention of acquired neonatal brain injury and may be achieved with the development and application of more accurate *in utero* measures of brain injury, such as fetal MRI.

Both the American College of Obstetricians and Gynecologists and the American Academy of Pediatrics acknowledged that their 2003 summary would require updating as the scientific database and knowledge on the topic expanded. They went on to state that only with more complete understanding of the precise origins of the pathophysiology of neonatal encephalopathy and cerebral palsy could logical hypotheses be designed and tested to reduce this occurrence. Finally, they recommended several important areas of research and for research funding. We would again emphasize the need for funding and studies to address this very important issue in neurodevelopment, neuroimaging, and potential improvements in outcomes for populations worldwide.

CASE PRESENTATION

A 27-year-old gravida 2, para 0100 was accepted for maternal transport with diagnoses of 28 weeks' estimated gestational age and severe preeclampsia. Her past medical history was significant for a prior intrauterine fetal demise at 31 weeks' gestation; that pregnancy was also complicated by severe preeclampsia.

Following successful aeromedical transport, she was received in Labor and Delivery where standard treatment for severe preeclampsia was instituted, including magnesium sulfate for prevention of eclamptic seizures and betamethasone for fetal lung maturation. Because of the severity of her disease process, labor induction with oxytocin was also instituted. Hydralazine was given in 5 mg incremental doses to control and reduce systolic blood pressure to less than 180 mmHg and diastolic blood pres-

sure to less than 110 mmHg. Ten hours into the labor induction, a series of eight repetitive late decelerations was noted. The oxytocin was discontinued, the woman placed in left lateral position, and oxygen was administered at 10 L/min by facemask. The fetal heart rate promptly normalized; however, beat-to-beat variability was judged to be reduced consistent with the estimated gestational age as well as the administration of magnesium sulfate.

As vaginal delivery was remote, the alternative of cesarean section was discussed because of fetal intolerance of labor. Following informed consent, the patient was taken to the operating room for cesarean delivery. General endotracheal anesthesia was necessitated by maternal thrombocytopenia. A low vertical uterine incision was employed as the lower uterine segment was poorly developed and thick and a vertical incision would allow the most atraumatic delivery. A 970 g infant was delivered and passed to a neonatologist who assigned Apgar scores of 1/0/0/0/0. The fetus/infant was pronounced dead at 20 min of age.

The admission cover sheet for this infant produced by the pediatricians recorded a 26–29 weeks' estimated gestational age, male infant with severe birth asphyxia. In the diagnostic codes listed for discharge was included acute respiratory failure with inability to resuscitate the infant in the delivery room and birth asphyxia. The autopsy report also returned findings consistent with chronic intrauterine anoxia, as well as possible acute anoxia secondary to prolonged labor and difficult delivery. These diagnoses were rendered by the pathologist despite the fact that "gross and microscopic examinations were normal." Cord gases were obtained at delivery and showed for the umbilical arterial blood a pH of 7.273, PCO_2 of 57.6, PO_2 of 17.4, HCO_3 of 25.9, and base excess of -4.0. A cord venous blood gas showed a pH of 7.30, PCO_2 of 50.0, PO_2 of 18.6, HCO_3 of 24.1, and base excess of -1.6. Conclusively, then, the cord gases rule out "birth asphyxia" and the fetus was additionally delivered in an atraumatic fashion. Fortunately, when neuropathology results were finalized, they demonstrated lesions within the brain that dated to at least 96 h of age, placing the injury well before the woman presented to the outlying hospital or before transport to the medical center.

This case demonstrates several critical points. Perhaps the most important is the need to be precise in the terminology that we employ and to diagnose birth asphyxia on objective rather than subjective criteria. Secondly, the value of cord blood studies obtained at delivery and of continuous electronic monitoring to exclude intrapartum asphyxia is well demonstrated. Finally, while the pathologist initially listed several erroneous diagnoses, largely based upon erroneous diagnoses contained in the pediatric chart, the record was eventually corrected with the neuropathology results. This would then point out the importance of a pathologic diagnosis of the intrauterine fetal demise and additionally also supplying the pathologist with accurate information upon which to base their conclusions. This case would beg for the establishment of set criteria for the evaluation of a newborn with suspected intrapartum asphyxia to include set times for neuroimaging studies as well as evaluation of the newborn for multiorgan system injury or insult.

References

1. Little WJ. On the influence of abnormal parturition, difficult labours, premature births, and asphyxia neonatorum, on the mental and physical condition of the child, especially in relation to deformities. Trans Obstet Soc Lond 1862;3:293–344.

2. Martin JA, Hamilton BE, Sutton PD, Ventura SJ, Mathews TJ, Kirmeyer S, Osterman MJ. Births: final data for 2007, Natl Vital Stat Rep 2010;58:1–86.

3. Clark SL, Hankins GDV. Temporal and demographic trends in cerebral palsy: fact and fiction. Am J Obstet Gynecol 2003;188:628–633.

4. Gibson CS, MacLennan AH, Hague WM et al. Associations between inherited thrombophilias, gestational age, and cerebral palsy. Am J Obstet Gynecol 2005;193:1437.

5. Gibson CS, MacLennan AH, Goldwater PN et al. Neurotropic viruses and cerebral palsy: population based case–control study. BMJ 2006;332:76–80.

6. Ruth VJ, Raivio KO. Perinatal brain damage: predictive value of metabolic acidosis in the Apgar score. BMJ 1988; 297:24–27.

7. MacLennan A. A template for defining a causal relation between acute intrapartum events and cerebral palsy: international consensus statement. BMJ 1999;319:1054–1059.

8. Badawi N, Kurinczuk JJ, Keogh JM et al. Intrapartum risk factors for newborn encephalopathy: the Western Australian case–control study. BMJ 1998;317:1554–1558.

9. Blair E, Stanley FJ. Intrapartum asphyxia: a rare cause of cerebral palsy. J Pediatr 1988;112:515–519.

10. Cowan FM, Rutherford M, Groenendaal F et al. Origin and timing of brain lesions in term infants with neonatal encephalopathy. Lancet 2003;361:736–742.

11. Miller SP, Ramaswamy V, Michelson D et al. Patterns of brain injury in term neonatal encephalopathy. J Pediatr 2005;146: 453–460.

12. Graham E, Holcroft CJ, Rai KK, Donohue PK, Allen MC. Neonatal cerebral white matter injury in preterm infants is associated with culture positive infections and only rarely with metabolic acidosis. Am J Obstet Gynecol 2004;191:1305–1310.

13. Kuban KCK, Leviton A, Pagano M, Fenton T, Strassfeld R, Wolff M. Maternal toxemia is associated with reduced incidence of germinal matrix hemorrhage in premature babies. J Child Neurol 1992;7:70–76.

14. Nelson KB, Grether JK. Can magnesium sulfate reduce the risk of cerebral palsy in very low birthweight infants? Pediatrics 1995;95:263–269.

15. McDonald JW, Silverstein FS, Johnston MV. Magnesium reduces N-methyl-D-aspartate (NMDA)-mediated brain injury in perinatal rats. Neurosci Lett 1990;109:234–238.

16. Crowther CA, Hiller JE, Doyle LW, Haslam RR, Australasian Collaborative Trial of Magnesium Sulphate (ACTOMgSO4) Collaborative Group. Effect of magnesium sulfate given for neuroprotection before preterm birth: a randomized controlled trial. JAMA 2003;209:2669–2676.

17. Magpie Trial Follow-Up Study Collaborative Group. The Magpie Trial: a randomised trial comparing magnesium sulphate with placebo for pre-eclampsia. Outcome for children at 18 months. Br J Obstet Gynaecol 2007;114:289–299.

18. Rouse DJ, Hirtz DG, Thom E et al, for the Eunice Kennedy Shriver National Institute of Child Health and Human Development Maternal-Fetal Medicine Units Network. A randomized, controlled trial of magnesium sulfate for the prevention of cerebral palsy. N Engl J Med 2008;359:895–905.

19. Marret S, Marpeau L, Zupan-Simunek V et al, on behalf of the PREMAG Trial Group. Magnesium sulphate given before very-preterm birth to protect infant brain: the randomised controlled PREMAG trial. Br J Obstet Gynaecol 2007;114: 310–318.

20. Mittendorf R, Dambrosia J, Pryde PG et al. Association between the use of antenatal magnesium sulfate in preterm labor and adverse health outcomes in infants. Am J Obstet Gynecol 2002;186:1111–1118.

21. Marret S, Marpeau L, Follet-Bouhamed C, Cambonie G, Astruc D, Delaporte B, PREMAG Trial Group. Effect of magnesium sulphate on mortality and neurologic morbidity of the very-preterm newborn with two-year neurologic outcome: results of the prospective PREMAG trial. Gynecol Obstet Fertil 2008;36:278–288.

22. Costantine MM, Weiner SJ, for the Eunice Kennedy Shriver National Institute of Child Health and Human Development Maternal-Fetal Medicine Units Network. Effects of antenatal exposure to magnesium sulfate on neuroprotection and mortality in preterm infants. Obstet Gynecol 2009;114:354–364.

23. Doyle LD, Crowther CA, Middleton P, Marret S, Rouse D. Magnesium sulphate for women at risk of preterm birth for neuroprotection of the fetus. Cochrane Database Syst Rev 2009;1:CD004661.

24. Conde-Agudelo A, Romero R. Antenatal magnesium sulfate for the prevention of cerebral palsy in preterm infants less than 34 weeks' gestation: a systematic review and metaanalysis. Am J Obstet Gynecol 2009;200:595–609.

25. American College of Obstetricians and Gynecologists. Magnesium sulfate before anticipated preterm birth for neuroprotection. Committee Opinion No. 455. Obstet Gynecol 2010;115:669–671.

26. Scott JR. Magnesium sulfate for neuroprotection. What do we do now? Obstet Gynecol 2009;114:500–501.

27. Edwards AD, Brocklehurst P, Gunn AJ et al. Neurological outcomes at 18 months of age after moderate hypothermia for perinatal hypoxic ischaemic encephalopathy: synthesis and meta-analysis of trial data. BMJ 2010;340:363.

Chapter 55
Genetic Amniocentesis and Chorionic Villus Sampling

Ronald J. Wapner

Department of Obstetrics and Gynecology, Columbia University Medical Center, New York, NY, USA

The prenatal diagnosis of genetic disorders is an important component of modern obstetrics. The most common techniques used for obtaining fetal tissues for genetic testing are amniocentesis and chorionic villus sampling (CVS). In this chapter we review the most frequent indications for amniocentesis and CVS, and consider the techniques, safety, and diagnostic aspects of these procedures.

Indications for prenatal diagnosis

Cytogenetic indications include:
• positive screening results for trisomy 21 or 18 [1,2], including increased nuchal translucency
• previous offspring with a chromosome abnormality
• balanced structural chromosome rearrangement in a parent
• risks of fetal mendelian disorder [3]
• fetal structural anomaly on ultrasound
• patient request.

Advanced maternal age is no longer an independent indication for invasive testing [4]. Aneuploid risk assessment has improved to such an extent that women 35 years and older should consider initial risk modification using biochemistry and ultrasound (nuchal translucency) prior to choosing invasive testing.

The indications for the prenatal diagnosis of mendelian disorders have increased rapidly over the past decade. Couples are recognized to be at increased risk by:
• a history of a previously affected child or relative with a mendelian disorder, or
• identification by population screening of a couple in whom both parents are carriers.

Cystic fibrosis, α- or β-thalassemia, sickle cell anemia, hemophilia, Tay–Sachs disease, spinal muscular atrophy, and Duchenne or Becker muscular dystrophy are among the most common conditions. DNA analysis is the primary diagnostic test but enzyme analysis may be required, depending on the specific disorder [3].

Almost all cytogenetic and mendelian diagnoses can be made from either amniotic fluid or chorionic villi. Patients at increased risk for fetal neural tube defects, in which amniotic fluid levels of α-fetoprotein (AFP) are determined, are not candidates for CVS. In many centers, ultrasound is now used as the primary test to evaluate for neural tube defects.

Amniocentesis

Traditional amniocentesis (≥15 weeks' gestation)

Technique

Amniocentesis for genetic evaluation is usually performed at 15–17 weeks' gestation based on the beginning of the last menstrual period but can be performed at any gestational age after 14 weeks. At this stage of gestation, the volume of amniotic fluid is approximately 200 mL and the ratio of viable to nonviable cells in the amniotic fluid is relatively high. Also, the interval prior to fetal viability is adequate to allow the option of pregnancy termination should an abnormality be detected.

An ultrasound examination is performed immediately before the procedure to evaluate fetal number and viability, confirm gestational age by fetal biometric measurements, establish placental location, and estimate amniotic fluid volume. A fetal anatomic survey to screen for major anomalies is routinely performed. In addition, ultrasonography may be useful in discovering maternal gynaecologic conditions (e.g. leiomyoma) that could influence the technique or timing of the amniocentesis.

Ultrasound imaging determines the optimal needle insertion path. An approach is chosen that avoids passage through maternal bowel or bladder and places the needle

Queenan's Management of High-Risk Pregnancy: An Evidence-Based Approach, Sixth Edition. Edited by John T. Queenan, Catherine Y. Spong, Charles J. Lockwood.
© 2012 John Wiley & Sons, Ltd. Published 2012 by John Wiley & Sons, Ltd.

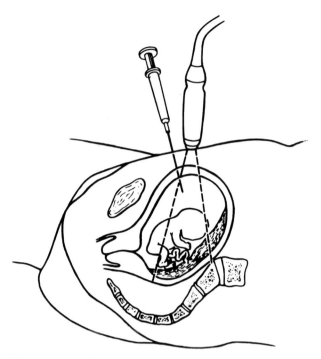

Figure 55.1 Amniocentesis performed concurrently with ultrasound. Reproduced from Simpson and Elias [62] with permission from Elsevier.

into a large pocket of fluid away from the fetus. The placenta should be avoided but on some occasions this is not possible. Use of Doppler color flow imaging is helpful in these situations in avoiding penetration of large placental vessels or the umbilical cord. When traversing the placenta is necessary, select the thinnest portion possible.

The maternal skin is cleaned with an antiseptic solution and sterile drapes may be placed around the needle insertion site. A local anesthetic (e.g. 2–3 mL 1% lidocaine) may be used, but in most cases this is not necessary. We use a 22 gauge spinal needle and recommend a needle no larger than 20 gauge. During the entire procedure, ultrasonographic monitoring with continuous visualization of the needle tip should be performed. Needle insertion should be performed with one smooth continuous motion until the tip is within the amniotic cavity (Fig. 55.1). After the tip is satisfactorily positioned in the amniotic cavity, the stylet is removed and the first 1–2 mL which theoretically contain maternal cells from blood vessels, the abdominal wall, or the myometrium is usually discarded.

Twenty to 30 mL amniotic fluid is aspirated into sterile, disposable plastic syringes. It is preferable to use 10 or 20 mL syringes because only gentle traction on the barrel of the syringe is desirable or necessary. Overly vigorous traction in search of fluid, especially with a 30–50 mL syringe, can result in the amniotic membranes being drawn into the needle, obstructing flow. Once the

amniotic fluid is obtained, the syringe is detached from the needle prior to its removal to minimize contamination. The fluid is either left in the labeled syringes or transferred into labeled tubes that are transported at ambient temperature directly to the laboratory or are prepared for shipping.

Fetal heart activity should be documented post procedure. Patients should be alerted that occasional cramping and vaginal leakage of a small amount of amniotic fluid may occur shortly after the procedure. Instructions to report excessive vaginal fluid loss, bleeding, or fever should be given. We recommend that strenuous exercise (e.g. jogging or aerobic exercises) and coitus be avoided for a day. Most other normal activities may be resumed immediately following the procedure.

Fetomaternal transfusion caused by disruption of the fetoplacental circulation might occur and have an immunizing effect in Rh-negative woman carrying an Rh-positive fetus. While the magnitude of the risk has not been determined, the American College of Obstetricians and Gynecologists recommends that 300 μg Rh-immunoglobulin (RhIG) be administered to all Rh-negative women. This should be carried out irrespective of whether the needle has traversed the placenta [5].

Multiple gestations

Amniocentesis can be performed on each fetus in a multiple gestation, provided the amniotic fluid volume is adequate [6]. In addition to the ultrasound evaluation performed for singletons, the location of the placentas and identification of the dividing membrane is observed and documented. Aspiration of amniotic fluid from the first sac is performed as for a singleton. Prior to removing the needle, 2–3 mL indigo carmine or Evans blue dye is injected. After the membrane separating the two sacs has been revisualized, a second amniocentesis is performed into the sac of the second fetus. Aspiration of clear fluid confirms that the second sac has truly been entered (Fig. 55.2). Methylene blue should never be used as an indicator because it has been associated with fetal jejunoileal atresia or death following intraamniotic injection [7]. Amniocentesis can be performed successfully in almost all twin pregnancies with apparently no increased risks over that of amniocentesis in singletons [6,8].

Triplets (and presumably gestations of greater multiplicity) can be managed by sequentially injecting dye into successive sacs following withdrawal of clear amniotic fluid from each sac. The number of aspirations of clear amniotic fluid should equal the number of fetuses. As long as clear fluid can be aspirated, one can be reassured that a new amniotic sac has been entered.

Safety

Risks of midtrimester amniocentesis can be divided into those affecting the mother and those affecting the fetus.

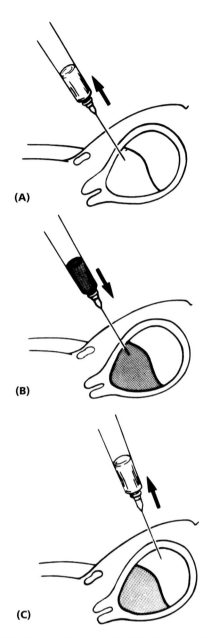

Figure 55.2 Technique of amniocentesis in twin gestations, performed under concurrent ultrasound guidance. (A) Fluid aspirated from the first amniotic sac. (B) Indigo carmine injected into the first amniotic sac. (C) Second tap in the ultrasonographically determined location of the second fetus. Clear fluid confirms that the second amniotic sac was successfully aspirated. Reproduced from Elias *et al* [6] with permission from Elsevier.

Maternal risks are quite low, with amnionitis occurring only rarely. However, cases of maternal sepsis, some of which have led to maternal death, have been reported [9]. These are usually associated with bowel flora such as *Escherichia coli* and underscore the importance of avoiding inadvertent bowel penetration during the procedure. Minor maternal complications such as transient vaginal

spotting and minimal amniotic fluid leakage occur after 1% or less of procedures and almost always are self-limited. Even significant fluid leakage will usually spontaneously resolve with bedrest [10]. Other very rare complications include intraabdominal viscous injury and hemorrhage.

The most concerning complication of amniocentesis is the risk of procedure-induced miscarriage. Only one study has evaluated this in a prospective randomized fashion, comparing women having amniocentesis with those having no procedure. This trial involved 4606 women aged 25–34 years who were without known risk factors for fetal genetic abnormalities who agreed to be randomized to have an amniocentesis or no procedure [11]. Amniocentesis was performed under real-time ultrasound guidance with a 20 gauge needle by experienced operators. The total spontaneous abortion rate after 16 weeks was 1.7% in the amniocentesis patients compared with 0.7% in control subjects (P = 0.01, 95% confidence interval [CI] 0.3–1.5, relative risk [RR] 2.3). Respiratory distress syndrome was diagnosed more often (RR 2.1) in the study group and more infants were treated for pneumonia (RR 2.5).

Seeds [12] has performed a metaanalysis of studies evaluating the pregnancy loss risk associated with second-trimester amniocentesis. Overall, 68,119 amniocenteses from both controlled and uncontrolled studies were included and provided a substantive basis for several conclusions.

• Contemporary amniocentesis with concurrent ultrasound guidance in controlled studies appears to be associated with a procedure-related rate of excess pregnancy loss of 0.6% (95% CI 0.31–0.90).

• The use of concurrent ultrasound guidance appears to reduce the number of punctures and the incidence of bloody fluid.

• Direct fetal needle trauma is rare, but may occur more frequently than is reported because of a failure to diagnose and a failure of consistent production of sequelae.

• There is no additional risk of pregnancy loss if placental puncture is required.

While the above metaanalysis confirmed the safety of second-trimester amniocentesis, in experienced hands the procedure-related loss may even be lower [13–15]. The most recent American College of Obstetricians and Gynecologists practice bulletin suggests that a risk of procedure induced of less than 1 in 300 to 1 in 500 should be used for counseling [4].

Early amniocentesis (<14 weeks' gestation)

Performing amniocentesis at <14 weeks' gestation was once considered an alternative to CVS for patients who desired prenatal diagnosis. However, recent randomized controlled studies have shown that these earlier procedures have an increased procedure-induced pregnancy loss rate and a 10-fold increased risk of club foot [16–23]. Accordingly, amniocentesis should not be performed prior to 14 weeks' gestation and preferably should be deferred until 15 weeks or later.

Chorionic villus sampling

Chorionic villus sampling involves suction aspiration of individual villi from the site of the developing placenta (chorion frondosum). The procedure can be performed by either a transcervical approach using a catheter or transabdominally using a needle. Studies have shown that the sampling routes are equally safe and effective [24], with the best results coming from centers skilled in both procedures. This assures sampling of any placental location and allows the operator to choose the safest approach on an individual basis.

Transcervical chorionic villus sampling

The optimal time to perform transcervical sampling is between 11 and 14 weeks' gestation. Prior to CVS, fetal viability and normal fetal anatomy and growth are confirmed by ultrasound. In addition, ultrasound is used to identify the location of the placenta, evaluate uterine position, assure appropriate bladder filling, eliminate the possibility of additional demised gestational sacs that could contaminate the sample, locate uterine contractions that may distort the sampling path, and image the cervix as it enters into the uterine cavity.

The procedure is performed with a plastic catheter (1.5 mm external diameter) which encloses a metal obturator ending in a blunt tip which extends just distal to the tip of the cannula. Absolute contraindications include maternal blood group sensitization and active cervical infection with gonorrhea or herpes.

The patient is placed in the lithotomy position. The vagina is cleansed with povidone-iodine solution, a speculum inserted in a sterile fashion and the cervix and vagina further cleansed. The catheter and obturator are curved slightly, introduced transcervically under concurrent ultrasonographic visualization, and directed into the placenta, parallel to its long axis (Fig. 55.3). It is important that the catheter is inserted into the plane of the chorion frondosum and avoids injury to the membranes or decidua. Once the catheter is well within the placenta, the obturator is withdrawn and the catheter connected to a 20 or 30 mL syringe containing approximately 5 mL tissue culture medium and a small amount of heparin. Chorionic villi are obtained by slowly removing the catheter as negative pressure is created by retracting the syringe plunger. An adequate sample is at least 5 mg (approximately five moderate-sized villi), but 10–25 mg is preferred.

Adequacy of the sample should be confirmed immediately after retrieval by direct visualization of the villi

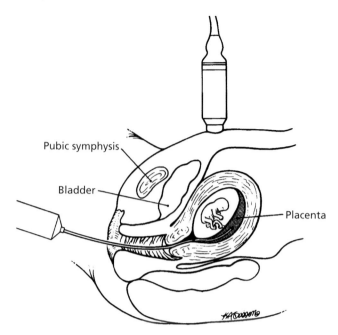

Pubic symphysis

Bladder

Placenta

Figure 55.3 Transcervical chorionic villus sampling.

floating in the syringe. It is important to differentiate villi from the small amount of decidua that is usually also present. Villi have a branching frond-like appearance whereas decidua is amorphous. If necessary, a dissecting microscope can be used to confirm the adequacy of the sample. If additional villi are required, a second attempt is performed with a new catheter. In general, two aspirations can be safely performed. On rare occasions, three attempts may be required but the risk of pregnancy loss is slightly increased when this is necessary.

Villi are retained in a transport medium and transferred to the laboratory, where they are dissected free of decidua and blood clots using fine forceps. Cytogenetic studies are performed either by direct harvest (cytotrophoblast cells) after an overnight incubation or after establishment of *in situ* cultures (mesenchymal core cells) that are harvested at 5–8 days. Chorionic villi are an excellent source for DNA for enzymatic analyses.

Following CVS, fetal heart activity is verified by ultrasonography and the patient discharged. Patients are informed that a small amount of bleeding or spotting is not unusual and is without consequence. They should notify the physician of heavy bleeding, leakage of fluid, or fever. Unsensitized Rh-negative patients are given RhIG. Maternal serum AFP screening for fetal neural tube defects or a detailed ultrasound is necessary at 15–18 weeks' gestation; AFP assay results are not affected by the prior invasive procedure.

Transabdominal chorionic villus sampling

Transabdominal CVS is now widely used as a complement to transcervical sampling. Placentas especially

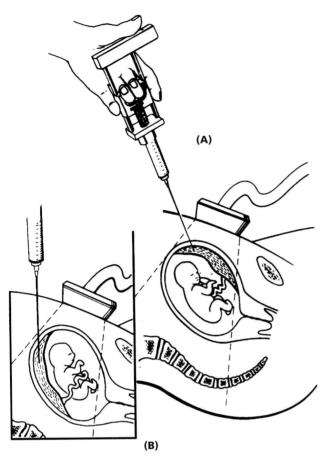

Figure 55.4 Transabdominal chorionic villus sampling performed (A) in an anterior placenta and (B) in a posterior placenta.

amenable to this approach include those located in the fundus or on the anterior uterine wall.

With the patient in the supine position, an insertion path that avoids the bowel and bladder and allows the needle to be placed within the placenta, parallel to the chorionic membrane, is chosen by ultrasonographic examination. The abdominal skin is cleansed with povidone-iodine solution and the area draped in a fashion similar to amniocentesis. The skin may be infiltrated with local anesthetic but this is usually not necessary because any discomfort usually occurs secondary to uterine puncture. A standard 20 gauge spinal needle with stylet is inserted percutaneously through the maternal abdominal wall and myometrium. The tip is advanced into the long axis of the placenta under concurrent ultrasound monitoring (Fig. 55.4). Once in place, the stylet is withdrawn and a 20 mL syringe containing approximately 5 mL of media with heparin is attached to the needle and the plunger pulled back until moderate pressure is felt. Some centers will attach a biopsy aspiration device (Cook Ob/Gyn, Spencer, IN) to the syringe to facilitate one-handed retrieval. We have found this to be unnecessary. Chorionic villi are obtained by moving the needle through approximately 3–7 passes through the placenta, remaining

parallel to the membrane. With each of these passes the needle is slightly redirected to sample different sites. The needle is then withdrawn under continuous negative pressure. The amount of villi obtained by transabdominal CVS is about half that usually obtained by transcervical aspiration [25]. However, such smaller amounts are still adequate for diagnostic testing. If a repeat sampling is required, a new needle is used.

Variations in technique for transabdominal CVS have been proposed in addition to the "freehand technique" described above. Other approaches use small forceps with cutting abilities or double-needle systems. We find that a biopsy guide is quite helpful in defining the exact site and angle for needle insertion.

Transabdominal CVS may be used throughout the late second and third trimesters to obtain late placental biopsies for rapid fetal karyotype analysis, thus offering an alternative to cordocentesis and late amniocentesis. This is particularly helpful in cases of oligohydramnios. Transcervical CVS cannot be used beyond 14–15 weeks' gestation.

Safety comparisons

Pregnancy loss after chorionic villus sampling

Although post-CVS loss rates (calculated from the time of the procedure until 28 weeks' gestation) are approximately 1% greater than those after amniocentesis (2.5% versus 1.5%), this comparison fails to take into consideration that the background miscarriage rate at 11–13 weeks is approximately 1% greater than at 15–16 weeks. To compare the two procedures appropriately, studies must enroll all patients in the first trimester, assign them to either approach, and then calculate the frequency of all subsequent losses, including spontaneous and induced abortions. In 1989, the Canadian Collaborative CVS/Amniocentesis Clinical Trial Group [26] reported such a prospective randomized trial and demonstrated equivalent safety of CVS and second-trimester amniocentesis. In over 2650 patients assigned to either procedure, there was a 7.6% loss rate in the CVS group and a 7.0% loss rate in the amniocentesis group (95% CI 0.92–1.30, RR 1.10). No significant differences were noted in the incidence of preterm birth, low birthweight, or rate of maternal complication. The investigators concluded that these data "may reassure women on the safety of first trimester CVS" [26].

A multicenter, prospective, nonrandomized study has been performed in the USA and enrolled 2235 women in the first trimester who chose either transcervical CVS or second-trimester amniocentesis [27]. An excess pregnancy loss rate of 0.8% in the CVS group over the amniocentesis group was calculated, which was not statistically significant. Repeated catheter insertions were significantly associated with pregnancy loss, with cases requiring three or more passes having a 10.8% spontaneous abortion rate, compared with 2.9% in cases that required only one pass.

Eight US centers later participated in a second National Institute of Child Health and Human Development (NICHD)-sponsored collaborative study to address the relative safety of transcervical and transabdominal CVS [24]. Subjects in whom either procedure was technically feasible were randomized into transabdominal and transcervical arms. Loss rates were nearly identical in the two groups. With availability of both transcervical and transabdominal CVS, total loss rates decreased over the rate seen in the initial trial described above, which only included transcervical CVS, obliterating even the nonsignificant arithmetic difference between amniocentesis and CVS loss rates.

Further information comes from a Danish randomized trial [28] which assigned 1068 patients to transcervical CVS, 1078 to transabdominal CVS, and 1158 to second-trimester amniocentesis. Overall, there was a slight increased risk of pregnancy loss following CVS (95% CI 1.01–1.67, RR 1.30) compared with amniocentesis which was completely accounted for by an excess of losses in the group sampled transcervically (95% CI 1.30–2.22, RR 1.70), the technique with which this group of investigators had the least experience. Excess loss following transcervical CVS has not been replicated in four other direct comparisons [24,29–31,63]. There was no difference in loss rates between transabdominal CVS and amniocentesis (95% CI 0.66–1.23, RR 0.9).

A prospective, randomized, collaborative comparison of more than 3200 pregnancies, sponsored by the European Medical Research Council, reported that CVS had a 4.6% greater pregnancy loss rate than amniocentesis (95% CI 1.24–1.84, RR 1.51) [32]. The present consensus is that operator inexperience with CVS accounts for the discrepancy between this trial in which operators were only required to perform 30 "practice procedures" and the other major studies performed by physicians already performing CVS in clinical practice. The US trial consisted of seven experienced centers and the Canadian trial 11, whereas the Medical Research Council trial used 31. There were, on average, 325 cases per center in the US study, 106 in the Canadian study, and 52 in the European trial.

Chorionic villus sampling, particularly the transcervical approach, has a relatively prolonged learning curve. Saura *et al* [33] suggested that over 400 cases may be required before safety is maximized. The role of experience as demonstrated by three sequential NICHD sponsored trials is of interest. In three sequential studies in which the majority of operators remained relatively constant, the postprocedure loss rate following CVS fell from 3.2% in the initial trial performed 1985–87 [27] to 2.4% for the trial performed 1987–89 [24] to only 1.3% in their most recent experience of 1997–2001 [21]. These data strongly suggest the value of operator experience.

Limb reduction defects

As with amniocentesis, a risk of fetal damage appears to exist if CVS is performed too early in gestation. For CVS this, gestational age "period of vulnerability" exists when procedures are performed under 9 weeks' gestation.

Firth *et al* [34,35] reported five occurrences of severe limb abnormalities out of 289 pregnancies sampled by CVS between 56 and 66 days. Four of these cases had the unusual but severe oromandibular-limb hypogenesis syndrome, which occurs in the general population at a rate of 1 in 175,000 births [36]. Burton *et al* [37] then reported on 14 more post-CVS cases of limb reduction defects (LRD) ranging from mild to severe, only two of which occurred when sampling was performed beyond 9.5 weeks. The infrequent occurrence of LRD after CVS was echoed by the American College of Obstetricians and Gynecologists, who stated that a risk for LRD of 1 in 3000 would be a prudent upper limit for counseling patients [4].

The WHO experience has been expanded and now contains information on 216,381 procedures [38]. These data have been used to analyze the frequency of limb anomalies, their pattern, and their associated gestational age at sampling. No overall increased risk of LRD or any difference in the pattern of defects was identified when compared with the general population. The WHO also investigated a possible temporal relationship between CVS and LRD [38].They evaluated 106,383 cases stratified by the week at which the procedure was performed. The incidence of LRD was 11.7, 4.9, 3.8, 3.4, and 2.3 per 10,000 CVS procedures in weeks 8, 9, 10, 11, and more than 12, respectively. Only the rate at week 8 exceeded the background risk of 6.0 per 10,000 births. The association of LRD and early gestational age sampling has been further supported in reports by Brambati *et al* [39] and Wapner *et al* [40]. Brambati *et al* [39] had a LRD incidence of 1.6% for procedures performed in weeks 6 and 7, 0.1% in week 8, and 0.059% (population frequency) in week 9.

Patients can be reassured that performing CVS beyond 10 weeks' gestation does not increase the risk of any type of fetal anomaly. CVS sampling before 10 weeks is not recommended, except in very unusual circumstances, such as when a patient's religious beliefs may preclude a pregnancy termination beyond a specific gestational age [3]. However, these patients must be informed that the incidence of severe LRD could be as high as 1–2%

Overall safety of chorionic villus sampling

The Committee on Genetics of the American College of Obstetricians and Gynecologists [4] considered all the above data and rendered the following conclusions and recommendations.

- Transcervical and transabdominal CVS, when performed at 10–12 weeks' gestation, are relatively safe and accurate procedures and may be considered acceptable alternatives to mid-trimester genetic amniocentesis.
- Until further information is available, CVS for clinical application should not be performed before 10 weeks' gestation.
- CVS requires appropriate genetic counseling before the procedure is performed, an operator experienced in performing the technique, and a laboratory experienced in processing the villus specimen and interpreting the results. Counseling should include comparing and contrasting the risks and benefits of amniocentesis and CVS.
- Although further studies are needed to determine whether there is an increased risk of transverse digital deficiency following CVS performed at 10–12 weeks' gestation, it is prudent to counsel patients that such an outcome is possible and that the estimated risk may be in the order of 1 in 3000 births.

Diagnostic studies

Cytogenetics

Analysis of either chorionic villi or amniotic fluid cells has certain pitfalls that should be recognized by the obstetrician [41–43]. First, cells may not grow, or growth may be insufficient to perform analyses. Although now uncommon, failure of amniotic cell cultures still occurs. Chorionic villus cultures are likewise usually successful and in fact, may require fewer days for growth than amniotic fluid cell cultures.

A second potential laboratory problem is that *in vitro* chromosome aberrations may arise in amniotic fluid or villus cultures. In fact, cells containing at least one additional structurally abnormal chromosome are detected in 1–3% of all amniotic cell cultures [43]. If such cells are confined to a single culture flask or clone, the phenomenon is termed pseudomosaicism and is not considered clinically important. If a chromosome abnormality is detected in more than one flask or clone, true mosaicism is said to exist, and is considered clinically significant.

While amniocentesis has been available for over three decades, CVS is a relatively new procedure and although almost 10 years was required to learn the unique aspects of evaluating placental tissue, this is now well understood. As opposed to cells retrieved by amniocentesis, which are predominantly extravasated fetal cells, chorionic villi have three major components: an outer layer of hormonally active syncytiotrophoblast, a middle layer of cytotrophoblast from which syncytiotrophoblast cells are derived, and an inner mesodermal core containing fetal blood capillaries. The cytotrophoblast has a high mitotic index, with many spontaneous mitoses available for immediate chromosome analysis, whereas the mesenchymal core requires culture. Because these multiple tissue sources arise from slightly different lineages, the reliability of CVS results needed to be confirmed.

We now know with certainty that genetic evaluation of chorionic villi provides a high degree of accuracy, particularly in regard to the diagnosis of common trisomies. The US collaborative study revealed a 99.7% rate of successful cytogenetic diagnosis, with only 1.1% of the patients requiring a second diagnostic test, such as amniocentesis or fetal blood analysis, to further interpret the results [42,44]. In most cases, the additional testing was required to delineate the clinical significance of mosaic or other ambiguous results (76%), whereas laboratory failure (21%) and maternal cell contamination (3%) also required follow-up testing. As laboratories have become more familiar with handling and interpreting villus material and operators have become more skilled in obtaining adequately sized samples, the need for additional evaluation has continued to decrease.

Array comparative genomic hybridization

Currently prenatal genetic evaluation using banded metaphase karyotypes can identify fetal aneuploidy and other genomic imbalances that are 5 Mb (million base pairs) or larger. Smaller imbalances such as the common deletion leading to DiGeorge syndrome (22q11.2) are also pathologic but will not be routinely identified. However, new technologies using molecular approaches can identify these smaller microdeletions and duplications and are now available for clinical use.

Array comparative genomic hybridization (Fig. 55.5) [45] can identify imbalances as small as 100 Kb (kilobases) by hybridizing patient DNA fragments to arrays having up to a million or more probes. Two types of arrays are presently in clinical use: targeted arrays in which only probes in areas of known pathogenicity are used and whole genome arrays using representative probes throughout the whole genome. Each type of array has advantages. Targeted arrays make counseling abnormal results easier since only known disorders with well-described phenotypes are identified but will miss potentially novel imbalances that may be disease causing. Whole genome arrays will also identify more findings of uncertain clinical significance, making counseling complex.

The value of array technology in prenatal diagnosis has been demonstrated for pregnancies complicated by fetal structural anomalies [46–48]. Arrays may reveal significant findings in 5% or more of these cases with normal karyotypes. The use of arrays in pregnancies without identified anomalies is still being investigated but will probably add additional information since many microdeletion/duplication syndromes will not have

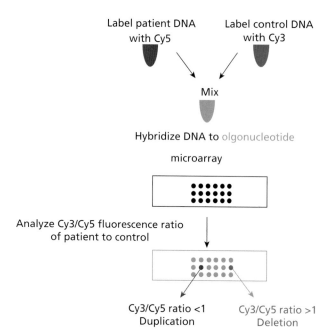

Label patient DNA with Cy5   Label control DNA with Cy3

Mix

Hybridize DNA to olgonucleotide microarray

Analyze Cy3/Cy5 fluorescence ratio of patient to control

Cy3/Cy5 ratio <1   Cy3/Cy5 ratio >1
Duplication   Deletion

Figure 55.5 This figure illustrates the general principle underlying comparative genomic hybridization which is used to identify DNA deletions or duplications. In this technique, fluorescently labeled DNA from a normal control sample is mixed with a test sample which is labeled with a different colored dye. The mixture is then hybridized to an array containing hundreds of thousands of small, well-defined, DNA probes. Regional differences in the fluorescence ratio of gains/losses can be detected and used for identifying abnormal regions in the genome. Courtesy of Dr Ronald Wapner. Modified from Reddy *et al* [45] with permission from Lippincott Williams and Wilkins.

easily identifiable *in utero* anomalies. However, this enthusiasm must be tempered by the anticipated findings of uncertain clinical significance which, depending on the type of array chosen, may exceed 2%.

Maternal cell contamination

Chorionic villus samples typically contain a mixture of placental villi and maternally derived decidua. Although specimens are thoroughly cleaned and separated under a microscope, some maternal cells may occasionally remain and grow in culture. As a result, two cell lines, one fetal and the other maternal, may be identified. In other cases, the maternal cell line may completely overgrow the culture, thereby leading to diagnostic errors, including incorrect sex determination [42,44], and potentially to false-negative diagnoses, although there are no published reports of the latter.

Direct preparations of chorionic villi are generally thought to prevent maternal cell contamination, whereas long-term culture has a rate varying from 1.8% to 4%. Fortunately, when this occurs, the contaminating cells are easily identified as maternal and should not lead to clinical errors. Contamination of samples with significant

amounts of maternal decidual tissue occurs more frequently with a small sample size, making selection of appropriate tissue by the laboratory difficult. In experienced centers in which adequate quantities of villi are available and laboratory personnel are skilled in villus preparation, this problem has disappeared [44,49]. Choosing only whole, clearly typical villus material and discarding any atypical fragments, small pieces, or fragments with adherent decidua will avoid confusion. Therefore, if at the time of sampling the initial aspiration is small, a second pass should be performed rather than risk inaccurate results. When proper care is taken and good cooperation and communication exist between the sampler and the laboratory, prevention of even small amounts of contaminating maternal tissue can be accomplished.

Confined placental mosaicism

Another potential associated with CVS is mosaicism confined to the placenta [50]. Although the fetus and placenta have a common ancestry, chorionic villus tissue will not always reflect fetal genotype [44]. Although initially there was concern that this might invalidate CVS as a prenatal diagnostic tool, subsequent investigations have led to a clearer understanding of villus biology, so that accurate clinical interpretation is now possible and may in some cases add clinically relevant information. It should be recalled that mosaicism also occurs in 0.25% of amniotic cell cultures and is only confirmed in 70–80% of abortuses or livebirths [43,64].

Discrepancies between the cytogenetics of the placenta and fetus can occur because early in development the cells contributing to the chorionic villi become separate and distinct from those forming the embryo. Specifically, at approximately the 32–64-cell stage, only 3–4 cells become the inner cell mass and form the embryo, whereas the remainder become precursors of the extraembryonic tissues. Mosaicism can then occur through two possible mechanisms [51].

An initial meiotic error in one of the gametes can lead to a trisomic conceptus that normally would spontaneously abort. However, if during subsequent mitotic divisions one or more of the early aneuploid cells loses one of the trisomic chromosomes through anaphase lag, the embryo can be "rescued" by reduction of a portion of its cells to disomy. This will result in a mosaic morula with the percentage of normal cells dependent on the cell division at which rescue occurred. Because only a small proportion of cells is incorporated into the inner cell mass and perhaps because the embryo is less tolerant of aneuploid cells than the placenta, the abnormal cells are frequently isolated in the extrafetal tissues, resulting in "confined placental mosaicism."

In the second mechanism, mitotic postzygotic errors produce a mosaic morula or blastocyst with the distribution and percent of aneuploid cells dependent on the timing of nondisjunction. If mitotic errors occur early in the development of the morula, they may segregate to the inner cell mass and have the same potential to produce an affected fetus as do meiotic errors. Mitotic errors occurring after primary cell differentiation and compartmentalization has been completed lead to cytogenetic abnormalities in only one lineage.

The mechanism of meiotic (trisomy) rescue can lead to uniparental disomy (UPD). This occurs when the original trisomic cell containing two chromosomes from one parent and one from the other expels the unmatched chromosome, resulting in progenitor cells containing a pair of chromosomes from a single parent. UPD has clinical consequences when the chromosome pair involved carries imprinted genes in which expression is based on the parent of origin. For example, Prader–Willi syndrome may result from uniparental maternal disomy for chromosome 15. Therefore, a CVS diagnosis of confined placental mosaicism for trisomy 15 may be the initial clue that UPD may be present. Because of this, when trisomy 15 (either complete or mosaic) is confined to the placenta, evaluation for UPD by amniotic fluid analysis is required [52,53]. In addition, chromosomes 7, 11, 14, and 22 are believed to be imprinted and require similar follow-up [54].

Confined placental mosaicism not associated with UPD has been shown to alter placental function and lead to fetal growth failure or perinatal death [55–57]. Although the effect is limited to specific chromosomes, the exact mechanism by which the presence of an abnormal cell line within the placenta alters function is unknown. The most striking example of the clinical impact of confined placental mosaicism occurs with trisomy 16. Confined placental mosaicism for chromosome 16 most often leads to severe intrauterine growth restriction, prematurity, or perinatal death, with less than 35% of pregnancies resulting in normal, appropriate-for-gestational-age, full-term infants [56,58–60].

Enzymatic and DNA analyses

Most biochemical diagnoses that can be made from amniotic fluid or cultured amniocytes can also be made from chorionic villi [3]. In many cases, the results are available more rapidly and efficiently when villi are used because sufficient enzyme or DNA is present to allow direct analysis rather than requiring tissue culture. However, for certain rare biochemical diagnoses, villi will not be an appropriate or reliable diagnostic source [61]. To ensure that appropriate testing is possible, the laboratory should be consulted before sampling.

Because many of these disorders are autosomal recessive or X-linked and have a 25% or greater risk of resulting in an affected pregnancy, performing prenatal diagnosis by amniocentesis is not recommended because:
- the procedure is usually not carried out until 15 weeks' gestation or later, compared to 10–12 weeks' gestation for CVS, and
- amniocentesis does not yield sufficient DNA for many analyses without additional weeks of cell culture [41].

There are potential laboratory pitfalls of CVS biochemical analysis, including maternal cell contamination, failure to optimize laboratory conditions for chorionic villi analyses (e.g. appropriate controls matched for gestational age), or investigator inexperience with a particular assay.

CASE PRESENTATION

Mrs Smith is a 29-year-old gravida 1, para 0 presenting for genetic counseling at 12 weeks' gestation because of a first-trimester combined screen giving her a 1 in 100 risk of fetal Down syndrome.

After a complete pedigree is performed and no other genetic risks are identified, the patient is informed that because of her increased risk of aneuploidy she may wish to consider undergoing invasive prenatal diagnosis. At 12 weeks' gestation the preferred procedure is CVS. She is informed that although there is approximately a 2.5% risk of pregnancy loss following the procedure, most of these miscarriages are unrelated to the sampling. The procedure-induced risk of loss is approximately 1 in 200. This is a similar risk compared to amniocentesis so there is no advantage to waiting until 16 weeks to have an amniocentesis performed. She is also informed that previous concerns that CVS may cause fetal LRD do not apply because this does not occur if the procedure is performed after the 10th week.

Other potential risks include a small chance of bleeding and spotting. Rare complications include leakage of fluid and maternal infections. She is informed that the results of the CVS karyotype are very accurate but in approximately 1% of cases an extra cell line may be present in the placenta which may require further evaluation, including amniocentesis.

The patient decides to undergo the CVS procedure. Prior to the procedure, her physician performs a cervical culture for gonococcus, which is negative. Her blood type is checked and she is found to be A negative with a negative antibody screen. She has a transcervical CVS procedure without difficulty and receives 300 µg RhIG immediately following the CVS. In 7 days, she receives a call from the genetic counselor telling her that she is having a chromosomally normal son. She is advised that CVS does not test for spina bifida so that at 16 weeks she should have a maternal serum AFP drawn and an ultrasound to evaluate fetal anatomy.

References

1. Wapner R et al. First-trimester screening for trisomies 21 and 18. N Engl J Med 2003;349(15):1405–1413.

2. Malone FD et al. First-trimester or second-trimester screening, or both, for Down's syndrome. N Engl J Med 2005;353(19): 2001–2011.

3. Poenaru L. First trimester prenatal diagnosis of metabolic diseases: a survey in countries from the European community. Prenat Diagn 1987;7(5):333–341.

4. American College of Obstetricians and Gynecologists. Invasive prenatal testing for aneuploidy. Practice Bulletin No. 88. Obstet Gynecol 2007;110(6):1459–1467.

5. American College of Obstetricians and Gynecologists. Prevention of D isoimmunization. Technical Bulletin No. 147. Int J Gynaecol Obstet 1992;37(1):53–56.

6. Elias S et al. Genetic amniocentesis in twin gestations. Am J Obstet Gynecol 1980;138(2):169–174.

7. Wapner RJ. Genetic diagnosis in multiple pregnancies. Semin Perinatol 1995;19(5):351–362.

8. Anderson RL, Goldberg JD, Golbus MS. Prenatal diagnosis in multiple gestation: 20 years' experience with amniocentesis. Prenat Diagn 1991;11(4):263–270.

9. Thorp JA et al. Maternal death after second-trimester genetic amniocentesis. Obstet Gynecol 2005;105(5 Pt 2):1213–1215.

10. Crane JP, Rohland BM. Clinical significance of persistent amniotic fluid leakage after genetic amniocentesis. Prenat Diagn 1986;6(1):25–31.

11. Tabor A et al. Randomised controlled trial of genetic amniocentesis in 4606 low-risk women. Lancet 1986;1(8493): 1287–1293.

12. Seeds JW. Diagnostic mid trimester amniocentesis: how safe? Am J Obstet Gynecol 2004;191(2):607–615.

13. Mazza V et al. Age-specific risk of fetal loss post second trimester amniocentesis: analysis of 5043 cases. Prenat Diagn 2007;27(2):180–183.

14. Eddleman KA et al. Pregnancy loss rates after midtrimester amniocentesis. Obstet Gynecol 2006;108(5):1067–1072.

15. Odibo AO et al. Revisiting the fetal loss rate after second-trimester genetic amniocentesis: a single center's 16-year experience. Obstet Gynecol 2008;111(3):589–595.

16. Johnson JM et al. The early amniocentesis study: a randomized clinical trial of early amniocentesis versus midtrimester amniocentesis. Fetal Diagn Ther 1996;11(2):85–93.

17. Canadian Early and Mid-trimester Amniocentesis Trial (CEMAT) Group. Randomised trial to assess safety and fetal outcome of early and midtrimester amniocentesis. Lancet 1998;351(9098):242–247.

18. Vandenbussche FP, Kanhai HH, Keirse MJ. Safety of early amniocentesis. Lancet 1994;344(8928):1032.

19. Brumfield CG et al. Pregnancy outcome following genetic amniocentesis at 11–14 versus 16–19 weeks' gestation. Obstet Gynecol 1996;88(1):114–118.

20. Cederholm M, Axelsson O. A prospective comparative study on transabdominal chorionic villus sampling and amniocentesis performed at 10–13 week's gestation. Prenat Diagn 1997;17(4):311–317.

21. Philip J et al. Late first-trimester invasive prenatal diagnosis: results of an international randomized trial. Obstet Gynecol 2004;103(6):1164–1173.

22. Nicolaides K et al. Comparison of chorionic villus sampling and amniocentesis for fetal karyotyping at 10–13 weeks' gestation. Lancet 1994;344(8920):435–439.

23. Sundberg K et al. Randomised study of risk of fetal loss related to early amniocentesis versus chorionic villus sampling. Lancet 1997;350(9079):697–703.

24. Jackson LG et al. A randomized comparison of transcervical and transabdominal chorionic-villus sampling. The U.S. National Institute of Child Health and Human Development Chorionic-Villus Sampling and Amniocentesis Study Group. N Engl J Med 1992;327(9):594–598.

25. Elias S et al. Transabdominal chorionic villus sampling for first-trimester prenatal diagnosis. Am J Obstet Gynecol 1989;160(4):879–884; discussion 884–886.

26. Canadian Collaborative CVS-Amniocentesis Clinical Trial Group. Multicentre randomised clinical trial of chorion villus sampling and amniocentesis. First report. Lancet 1989;1(8628):1–6.

27. Rhoads GG et al. The safety and efficacy of chorionic villus sampling for early prenatal diagnosis of cytogenetic abnormalities. N Engl J Med 1989;320(10):609–617.

28. Smidt-Jensen S et al. Randomised comparison of amniocentesis and transabdominal and transcervical chorionic villus sampling. Lancet 1992;340(8830):1237–1244.

29. Bovicelli L et al. Transabdominal versus transcervical routes for chorionic villus sampling. Lancet 1986;2(8501): 290.

30. Brambati B, Terzian E, Tognoni G. Randomized clinical trial of transabdominal versus transcervical chorionic villus sampling methods. Prenat Diagn 1991;11(5):285–293.

31. Brambati B et al. First-trimester genetic diagnosis in multiple pregnancy: principles and potential pitfalls. Prenat Diagn 1991;11(10):767–774.

32. MRC Working Party on the Evaluation of Chorion Villus Sampling. Medical Research Council European trial of chorion villus sampling. Lancet 1991;337(8756):1491–1499.

33. Saura R et al. Operator experience and fetal loss rate in transabdominal CVS. Prenat Diagn 1994;14(1):70–71.

34. Firth HV et al. Severe limb abnormalities after chorion villus sampling at 56–66 days' gestation. Lancet 1991;337(8744): 762–763.

35. Firth HV et al. Limb abnormalities and chorion villus sampling. Lancet 1991;338(8758):51.

36. Froster UG, Jackson L. Limb defects and chorionic villus sampling: results from an international registry, 1992–94. Lancet 1996;347(9000):489–494.

37. Burton BK, Schulz CJ, Burd LI. Limb anomalies associated with chorionic villus sampling. Obstet Gynecol 1992;79(5 Pt 1): 726–730.

38. Evaluation of chorionic villus sampling safety: WHO/PAHO consultation on CVS. Prenat Diagn 1999;19(2):97–99.

39. Brambati B et al. Genetic diagnosis by chorionic villus sampling before 8 gestational weeks: efficiency, reliability, and risks on 317 completed pregnancies. Prenat Diagn 1992;12(10):789–799.

40. Wapner RJ et al. Procedural risks versus theology: chorionic villus sampling for Orthodox Jews at less than 8 weeks' gestation. Am J Obstet Gynecol 2002;186(6):1133–1136.

41. Tharapel AT et al. Resorbed co-twin as an explanation for discrepant chorionic villus results: non-mosaic 47,XX,+16 in

villi (direct and culture) with normal (46,XX) amniotic fluid and neonatal blood. Prenat Diagn 1989;9(7):467–472.

42. Ledbetter DH et al. Cytogenetic results from the U.S. Collaborative Study on CVS. Prenat Diagn 1992;12(5): 317–345.

43. Hsu LY, Perlis TE. United States survey on chromosome mosaicism and pseudomosaicism in prenatal diagnosis. Prenat Diagn 1984;4(Spec No):97–130.

44. Ledbetter DH et al. Cytogenetic results of chorionic villus sampling: high success rate and diagnostic accuracy in the United States collaborative study. Am J Obstet Gynecol 1990;162(2):495–501.

45. Reddy UM et al. Stillbirth classification – developing an international consensus for research: executive summary of a National Institute of Child Health and Human Development workshop. Obstet Gynecol 2009;114(4):901–914.

46. American College of Obstetricians and Gynecologists. Array comparative genomic hybridization in prenatal diagnosis. Committee Opinion No. 446. Obstet Gynecol 2009;114(5): 1161–1163.

47. Le Caignec C et al. Detection of genomic imbalances by array based comparative genomic hybridisation in fetuses with multiple malformations. J Med Genet 2005;42(2):121–128.

48. Van den Veyver IB et al. Clinical use of array comparative genomic hybridization (aCGH) for prenatal diagnosis in 300 cases. Prenat Diagn 2009;29(1):29–39.

49. Elles RG et al. Absence of maternal contamination of chorionic villi used for fetal-gene analysis. N Engl J Med 1983;308(24): 1433–1435.

50. Kalousek DK et al. Confined chorionic mosaicism in prenatal diagnosis. Hum Genet 1987;77(2):163–167.

51. Wolstenholme J. Confined placental mosaicism for trisomies 2, 3, 7, 8, 9, 16, and 22: their incidence, likely origins, and mechanisms for cell lineage compartmentalization. Prenat Diagn 1996;16(6):511–524.

52. Cassidy SB et al. Trisomy 15 with loss of the paternal 15 as a cause of Prader–Willi syndrome due to maternal disomy. Am J Hum Genet 1992;51(4):701–708.

53. Purvis-Smith SG et al. Uniparental disomy 15 resulting from "correction" of an initial trisomy 15. Am J Hum Genet 1992;50(6):1348–1350.

54. Ledbetter DH, Engel E. Uniparental disomy in humans: development of an imprinting map and its implications for prenatal diagnosis. Hum Mol Genet 1995;4(Spec No): 1757–1764.

55. Johnson A et al. Mosaicism in chorionic villus sampling: an association with poor perinatal outcome. Obstet Gynecol 1990;75(4):573–577.

56. Breed AS et al. Follow-up and pregnancy outcome after a diagnosis of mosaicism in CVS. Prenat Diagn 1991;11(8): 577–580.

57. Wapner RJ et al. Chorionic mosaicism: association with fetal loss but not with adverse perinatal outcome. Prenat Diagn 1992;12(5):347–355.

58. Post JG, Nijhuis JG. Trisomy 16 confined to the placenta. Prenat Diagn 1992;12(12):1001–1007.

59. Kalousek DK et al. Uniparental disomy for chromosome 16 in humans. Am J Hum Genet 1993;52(1):8–16.

60. Benn P. Trisomy 16 and trisomy 16 mosaicism: a review. Am J Med Genet 1998;79(2):121–133.

61. Gray RG et al. A misdiagnosis of X-linked adrenoleukodystrophy in cultured chorionic villus cells by the measurement of very long chain fatty acids. Prenat Diagn 1995;15(5): 486–490.

62. Simpson JL, Elias S. Prenatal diagnosis of genetic disorders. In: Creasy RK, Resnik R, eds. Maternal-Fetal Medicine: Principles and Practice, 3rd edn. Philadelphia: WB Saunders, 1994, pp.61–88.

63. Tomassini A, Campagna G, Paolucci M et al. Transvaginal CVS vs. transabdominal CVS (our randomized cases). XI European Congress of Prenatal Medicine 1988;1104.

64. Karkut I, Zakrzewski S, Sperling K. Mixed karyotypes obtained by chorionic villi analysis: mosaicism and maternal contamination. In: Fraccaro M et al, eds. First Trimester Fetal Diagnosis. Heidelberg: Springer-Verlag, 1985.

Chapter 56
Fetal Surgery

Robert H. Ball[1] and Hanmin Lee[2]
[1] Department of Obstetrics, Gynecology and Reproductive Sciences
[2] Department of Surgery, University of California, San Francisco, CA, USA

The first open maternal-fetal operation was performed nearly 30 years ago. The indications for intervention have remained largely constant from the first decade of fetal surgery to the start of the fourth decade and the basic tenets of fetal surgery also have remained consistent. The three basic tenets are: (1) the pregnant woman should undergo minimal risk to her health; (2) the fetal disease should be severe and progressive; and (3) fetal intervention should have a high likelihood for reversing fetal disease. While the diseases treated have remained the same, the approach to fetal interventions has changed dramatically. Initial fetal surgical procedures depended on maternal laparotomy and hysterotomy. This approach evolved into maternal laparotomy with uterine endoscopy and most recently into percutaneous approaches. It appears that the less invasive approaches are associated with a less complicated postoperative recovery for the mother, but morbidity is not eliminated [1].

As the proposed indications for fetal surgical interventions and the number of procedures performed have expanded, so too have the centers at which they are performed and the number of physicians performing them. Nevertheless, the availability and proven utility of these procedures remain very limited when compared with the number of fetuses with malformations. One of the responsibilities of physicians with an interest in prenatal diagnosis and intervention is to determine training needs and oversight for operators and centers involved in this field. It is unclear how many centers would be needed given the rarity of these malformations in which a fetal surgical approach may be effective and the even smaller proportion of those with malformations that may need fetal intervention. We must achieve a delicate balance between the ease of accessibility and surgical experience. International fetal surgery consortiums such as Eurofetus and the North American Fetal Therapy Network (NAFTNet) are leading efforts to study and guide fetal surgery through multicenter registries and trials.

Open fetal surgery (hysterotomy)

The feasibility of performing a hysterotomy with subsequent closure of the gravid human uterus was tested in the primate. The maternal safety in this series of primate fetal surgeries was reassuring, including subsequent fertility [2]. The human experience is now quite extensive, both from our own center and others [1,3,4], and has been primarily associated with the large numbers of fetal spina bifida repairs. We currently reserve hysterotomies for repair of spina bifida and resection of fetal tumors causing hydrops fetalis.

Risks and benefits

We recently reviewed our experience at the University of California, San Francisco (UCSF), with maternal hysterotomy (Table 56.1) [1]. Eighty-seven hysterotomies were performed between 1989 and 2003. There were significant postoperative complications. In the early experience, pulmonary edema related to multiple tocolytic use, particularly nitroglycerin, and aggressive fluid management were significant problems [5]. Transfusion for intraoperative blood loss was not uncommon. Pregnancy outcomes were also adversely affected by high rates of premature rupture of membrane and preterm labor. The mean time from hysterotomy to delivery was 4.9 weeks (range 0–16 weeks). The mean gestational age at the time of delivery was 30.1 weeks (range 21.6–36.7 weeks). Others have had similar experiences with respect to an increased risk of preterm delivery following hysterotomy [6,7]. Most of the morbidity associated with hysterotomy has decreased with experience. Significant pulmonary edema or blood loss is now rare, and the mean gestational age at the time of delivery following *in utero* repair of myelomeningocele (MMC) is now around 34 weeks.

The practical aspects of hysterotomy and postoperative management have evolved since the early years of experience. The following is a description of our current

---

Queenan's Management of High-Risk Pregnancy: An Evidence-Based Approach, Sixth Edition. Edited by John T. Queenan, Catherine Y. Spong, Charles J. Lockwood.

Table 56.1 Maternal morbidity and mortality for 178 interventions at UCSF with postoperative continuing pregnancy and divided into operative subgroups

Operative technique	Open hysterotomy	Endoscopy FETENDO/ Lap-FETENDO	Percutaneous FIGS/Lap-FIGS	All interventions
Patients with postop continuing pregnancy	79	68	31	178
Gestational age at surgery (weeks)	25.1	24.5	21.1	24.2
Range (weeks)	17.6–30.4	17.9–32.1	17.0–26.6	17.0–32.1
Gestational age at delivery (weeks)	30.1	30.4	32.7	30.7
Range (weeks)	21.6–36.7	19.6–39.3	21.7–40.4	19.6–40.4
Interval surgery to delivery (weeks)	4.9	6.0	11.6	6.5
Range (weeks)	0–16	0–19	0.3–21.4	0–21.4
Pulmonary edema	22/79 (27.8%)	17/68 (25.0%)	0/31 (0.0%)	39/178 (21.9%)
Bleeding requiring blood transfusion	11/87 (12.6%)	2/69 (2.9%)	0/31 (0.0%)	13/187 (7.0%)
PTL leading to delivery	26/79 (32.9%)	18/68 (26.5%)	4/31 (12.9%)	48/178 (27.0%)
Premature rupture of membranes	41/79 (51.9%)	30/68 (44.1%)	8/31 (25.8%)	79/178 (44.4%)
Chorioamnionitis	7/79 (8.9%)	1/68 (1.5%)	0/31 (0.0%)	8/178 (4.5%)

FETENDO, fetal endoscopic surgery; FIGS, fetal intervention guided by sonography; PTL, preterm labor.

approach. Lengthy discussions regarding the risks, benefits, and alternatives of the procedure are important, including the experimental nature of the surgery. We generally differentiate the risks to the mother, the fetus, and the pregnancy in our counseling. The risks to the mother are similar to other major abdominal surgery, although in this case there is no direct physical benefit to her. In addition, there are the risks associated with aggressive tocolytic therapy and bedrest in a hypercoagulable state. The risks to the fetus are primarily vascular instability and hypoperfusion intraoperatively, leading to injury or death, and prematurity resulting from postoperative complications. The risks to the pregnancy are primarily preterm labor, premature rupture of membranes, and preterm delivery. Infectious complications are rare, except when premature rupture of membranes leads to chorioamnionitis. An important additional counseling point is that all subsequent deliveries, including the index pregnancy, must be by cesarean section. Data regarding future fertility are reassuring, with no increased incidence of infertility in the UCSF experience in those patients subsequently attempting pregnancy [8]. Experience from the Children's Hospital of Philadelphia (CHOP) suggests a substantial risk of uterine rupture in subsequent pregnancies that may be as high as 17%. This is higher than the risk after previous low transverse cesarean delivery (1% or less) or classical cesarean delivery (4–5%). Another potential risk in subsequent pregnancies is placenta accreta. The reason for this is that the uterine location of the hysterotomy incision performed in the second trimester is not in the same area as a cesarean delivery uterine entry site. There is an increased risk of placenta accreta in any setting where implantation occurs in an area of uterine scarring. Multiple incisions will increase the likelihood of implantation in such an area. To our knowledge, there has not been a case of placenta accreta in a fetal surgical patient of ours in a subsequent pregnancy (approximately 80 patients and 40 subsequent pregnancies).

Technique

Prior to surgery, the patients are premedicated with indomethacin and a cephalosporin. Compression stockings and pneumatic antithrombotic boots are placed on the lower extremities. General anesthesia is initiated, with high levels of a halogenated inhalational agent to maximize uterine relaxation. A Foley catheter is placed to drain the bladder. An epidural catheter is placed for postoperative pain control. Following prepping and draping, ultrasound transducers with sterile covers are used to identify fetal lie and placental location. The latter will determine the need for exteriorization of the uterus to allow access to the posterior aspect in cases of an anterior placenta. The transverse skin incision is generally a third of the way between the pubic symphysis and the umbilicus, lower with an anterior placenta, so that the uterus can more easily be exteriorized. Usually, the rectus muscles need to be at least partially transected to allow appropriate exposure.

Once the peritoneal cavity is entered, the ultrasound transducer is placed directly on the uterine serosa and the edge of the placenta is identified and marked. The general strategy is to place the hysterotomy as far from the placenta as possible, with the direction of the incision parallel to its edge. This will minimize the risk of extension towards the placenta, as placental bed bleeding cannot generally be controlled. The additional determinant for the site of the hysterotomy is the fetal surgical site and fetal position. Frequently, transuterine (hands on serosal surface of uterus) fetal manipulation will achieve successful position.

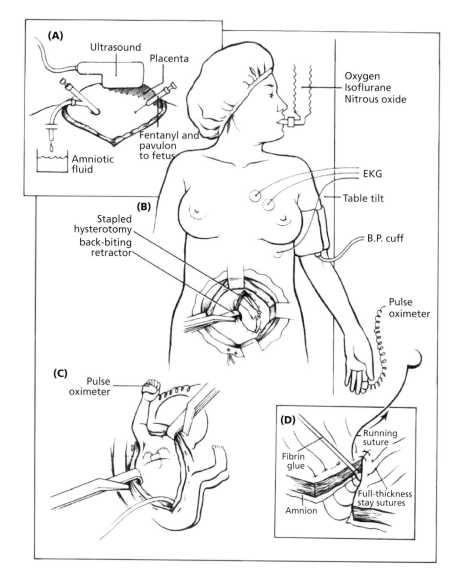

Figure 56.1 Summary of open fetal surgery techniques. (A) The uterus is exposed through a low transverse abdominal incision. Ultrasonography is used to localize the placenta, inject the fetus with narcotic and muscle relaxant, and aspirate amniotic fluid. (B) The uterus is opened with staples that provide hemostasis and seal the membranes. Maternal anesthesia and monitoring are shown. (C) Absorbable staples and backbiting clamps facilitate hysterotomy exposure of the pertinent fetal part. A miniaturized pulse oximeter records pulse rate and oxygen saturation intraoperatively. (D) After fetal repair the uterine incision is closed with absorbable sutures and fibrin glue. Amniotic fluid is restored with warm lactated Ringer solution.

Initial uterine entry can be performed either using the Bruner–Tulipan trocar or direct cutdown. The initial entry is then extended using the Harrison uterine stapler. Use of ultrasound is critical to confirm that the stapler compresses no fetal part or loop of cord, and is definitively intraamniotic. The stapler fires a line of dissolvable staples 8 cm long and cuts in between them. This produces a hemostatic myometrial incision with the membranes tacked to the myometrium, minimizing the risk of dissection. Occasionally, bleeding from the myometrial edge, particularly at the apices, requires placement of atraumatic clamps or a figure-of-eight stitch. Specially designed Harrison–Moran backbiting retractors provide further hemostasis and exposure (Figs 56.1 and 56.2).

Once the hysterotomy incision is appropriately hemostatic, attention can be turned to the fetus. Only that part of the fetus needed to perform the procedure should be exteriorized. This is important for fetal temperature control, and to avoid tissue desiccation and abruption secondary to uterine decompression. The fetus can be monitored using either a pulse oximeter and/or sonographic surveillance of the fetal heart. During the surgery, continued relaxation of the uterus is monitored by palpation, and the serosal surfaces are irrigated with warm saline. If the uterus begins to contract, options include increasing inhalational agents, use of nitroglycerin or loading with magnesium sulfate, or a combination of the above.

Following the procedure on the fetus, the uterine closure begins. This is usually the time we initiate the bolus of magnesium sulfate, followed by a maintenance dose. The uterus is closed in two layers of No. 0 polyglycolic monofilament suture. Full-thickness interrupted stay sutures are placed first but not tied, then the continuous suture is placed. Prior to tying the continuous suture, a catheter is used to refill the amniotic cavity under

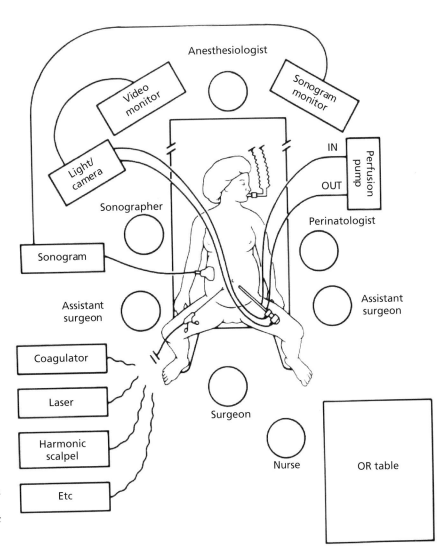

Figure 56.2 Drawing of the operating room set-up. Note that there are two monitors at the head of the table, one for the fetoscopic picture and the other for the real-time ultrasound image.

ultrasound guidance with lactated Ringer solution. The fluid is replenished to a level of low normal fluid, then the stay sutures are tied. When it is assured that the suture line is hemostatic and hydrostatic, the abdominal wall is closed in layers in the usual fashion.

Postoperative recovery in our unit is accomplished in the labor and delivery suite. For pain control, the preoperatively placed epidural catheter is used for the first 48h. Intravenous magnesium sulfate is continued for 24h and oral nifedipine then initiated. Indomethacin is continued for a total of 48h, with ductal constriction surveillance performed by fetal echocardiography daily. The nifedipine is continued long term. Activity is limited to bedrest for the first 48h postoperatively and then liberalized. Upon discharge, patients are still encouraged to limit activity. Close outpatient follow-up with weekly visits and ultrasounds is our routine.

Indications for open fetal surgery

Myelomeningocele

The most common indication for hysterotomy-based fetal intervention currently in our center is MMC. This is a birth defect with sequelae that affect both the central and peripheral nervous systems. A change in cerebrospinal fluid (CSF) dynamics results in the Arnold–Chiari II malformation and hydrocephalus. The abnormally exposed spinal cord results in lifelong lower extremity neurologic deficiency, fecal and urinary incontinence, sexual dysfunction, and skeletal deformities. This defect carries enormous personal, familial, and societal costs, as the near normal lifespan of the affected child is characterized by hospitalization, multiple operations, disability, and, occasionally, institutionalization. Although it has been assumed that the spinal cord itself is intrinsically malformed in children with this defect, recent work suggests that the neurologic impairment after birth may be caused by exposure and trauma to the spinal cord *in utero*, and that covering the exposed cord may prevent the development of the Chiari malformation [9].

Since 1997, more than 200 fetuses have had *in utero* closure of MMC by open fetal surgery. Preliminary clinical evidence suggests this procedure reduces the incidence of shunt-dependent hydrocephalus and restores the cerebellum and brainstem to a more normal configuration. However, clinical results of fetal surgery for MMC are based on comparisons with historical controls, examine only efficacy, not safety, and lack long-term follow-up. The National Institutes of Health (NIH)'s Management of Myelomeningocele Study (MOMS) recently published that prenatal surgery results in a reduction in death or the need for a shunt at 12 months of age and improves motor outcomes at 30 months but is associated with maternal and fetal risks [10]. Prenatal surgery is associated with other favourable secondary outcomes including reducing hindbrain herniation at 12 months (no evidence of herniation in 36% of prenatal versus 4% of postnatal cases), doubling the ability to walk without orthotics (42% in prenatal versus 21% in postnatal cases), and increasing function by two or more levels than that expected based on the anatomic level of the defect (32% versus 12% in postnatal cases). Prenatal surgery was also associated with maternal and fetal risks including preterm birth (80% of prenatal versus 15% of postnatal cases), uterine thinning or dehiscence at the surgical site in (35% in prenatal cases), and higher rates of fetal bradycardia, oligohydramnios, placental abruption, and the need for transfusion at delivery [10].

Congenital pulmonary airway malformation

Congenital pulmonary airway malformation (CPAM), previously termed congenital cystic adenomatoid malformation (CCAM), leading to hydrops is another indication for hysterotomy. Although CPAM often presents as a benign pulmonary mass in infants and children, some fetuses with large lesions die *in utero* or at birth from hydrops and pulmonary hypoplasia [11]. The pathophysiology of hydrops and the feasibility of resecting the fetal lung have been studied in animals [11,12]. Experience managing more than 200 cases suggests that most lesions can be successfully treated after birth, and that some lesions resolve before birth [13]. Although only a few fetuses with very large lesions develop hydrops before 26 weeks' gestation, these lesions may progress rapidly and the fetuses die *in utero*. Careful sonographic surveillance of large lesions is necessary to detect the first signs of hydrops, because fetuses developing hydrops can be successfully treated by emergency resection of the abnormal lobe *in utero*. Fetal pulmonary lobectomy has proven to be surprisingly simple and quite successful at UCSF and

CHOP. For lesions with single large cysts, thoracoamniotic shunting has also been successful [14].

Our group pioneered the use of maternal steroids for treatment of large microcystic or solid appearing CPAMs [15]. The hypothesis is that steroids would cause maturation of the microcystic CPAM and slow growth. We and others have shown successful resolution of hydrops in 80% of fetuses with large microcystic CPAMs and hydrops [16]. What is unclear is the benefit of maternal steroids for large nonhydropic microcystic CPAMs. Others have administered steroids for large macrocystic CPAMs without success.

Sacrococcygeal teratoma

Hysterotomy is the most common fetal surgical approach to treat fetuses in high-output failure and hydrops with large sacrococcygeal teratomas (SCT). Most neonates with SCT survive, and malignant invasion is unusual. However, the prognosis of patients with SCT diagnosed prenatally (by sonogram or elevated α-fetoprotein [AFP]) may be less favorable. There is a subset of fetuses (fewer than 20%) with large tumors who develop hydrops from high-output failure secondary to extremely high blood flow through the tumor. Because hydrops may progress quite rapidly to fetal death, close sonographic follow-up is critical. Attempts to interrupt the vascular steal phenomenon by sonographically guided or fetoscopic techniques have not yet been successful. Excision of the tumor reverses the pathophysiology if it is performed before "mirror syndrome" (maternal preeclampsia) develops in the mother. Hysterotomies in these cases may involve quite large incisions because of the size of the masses.

Fetoscopic surgery

With advances in technology and familiarity with endoscopic techniques, application of this technique to fetal surgery (FETENDO) was natural. Common sense would suggest that the smaller the incision in the uterus, the lower the risk of subsequent pregnancy complications. At UCSF, endoscopic approaches (Lap-FETENDO) were first applied to pregnancies complicated by diaphragmatic hernia, urinary tract obstruction, and twin–twin transfusion.

The initial pioneering approach involved maternal minilaparotomies, with direct exposure of the uterus. Ultrasound is used to determine the point of entry and the laparotomy site, depending on placental location and fetal lie. Once the uterus has been exposed, stay sutures are placed and a 3–5 mm step trocar advanced into the amniotic cavity under direct ultrasound visualization. Initially, several trocars were required for *in utero* dissections, placement of staples, etc. Later, many procedures could be performed through a single trocar using an endoscope with an operating channel. Initial caution regarding this approach led to similar perioperative management compared with hysterotomy cases. This included general anesthesia, use of multiple tocolytics, and prolonged hospitalization. One important difference even initially was that patients could labor following FETENDO procedures.

Since these initial cases, endoscopic procedures have become less invasive with smaller instruments passed through 3 mm ports. This may explain why pregnancy outcomes and pulmonary edema rates were initially similar comparing the hysterotomy and endoscopy groups, although transfusions were required less frequently in the latter cases (see Table 56.1) [1]. The interval from procedure to delivery was also little changed, as was the gestational age at delivery. In our experience, many of the deliveries still required cesarean section to accommodate EXIT procedures [1,17]. This is highly specialized delivery with hysterotomy in which the cord is not clamped until airway management is secure. It involves strategies similar to those used for open surgery, including uterine relaxation with general anesthesia, myometrial incision hemostasis with staples, and fetal monitoring. The endoscopic procedures that necessitated EXITs were balloon tracheal occlusions for congenital diaphragmatic hernias. This was also amongst the most frequent indication for an endoscopic fetal surgical approach at UCSF.

Percutaneous fetoscopic surgery

Currently, we rarely use the more invasive Lap-FETENDO and have since progressed towards a percutaneous approach using a smaller 2–3 mm endoscope with an operating channel. We have used this technique for balloon tracheal occlusions, fetal cystoscopies, and laser ablation in monochorionic twin gestations complicated by severe twin–twin transfusion. Based on our early experience and that of others [13], we anticipate that the risks with percutaneous microendoscopy will be similar to percutaneous sonography-guided procedures (see below). The perioperative management is very different compared to the more invasive procedures. Although patients are treated with prophylactic indomethacin and antibiotics, uterine relaxation from inhalational agents is not required and may in fact be detrimental. Therefore, we generally use regional anesthesia. Ultrasound is again critical for safe uterine access to determine the best entry point. This is based on fetal position, placental location, membrane position in multiple gestations, and uterine vascularity. Postoperative tocolytic therapy is usually based on contraction activity. A 24–48-h course of indomethacin or nifedipine is often all that is required. In cases where there are significant postoperative changes in uterine size, such as with interventions for twin–twin transfusion syndrome (TTTS), prophylactic intravenous magnesium sulfate may be helpful.

Indications for fetoscopic surgery

Congenital diaphragmatic hernia

The fundamental problem in babies born with a congenital diaphragmatic hernia (CDH) is pulmonary hypoplasia. Research in experimental animal models and later in human patients over two decades has aimed to improve growth of the hypoplastic lungs before they are needed for gas exchange at birth. Anatomic repair of the hernia by open hysterotomy proved feasible but did not decrease mortality and was abandoned. Fetal tracheal occlusion was developed as an alternative strategy to promote fetal lung growth by preventing normal egress of lung fluid. Occlusion of the fetal trachea was shown to stimulate fetal lung growth in a variety of animal models. Techniques to achieve reversible fetal tracheal occlusion were explored in animal models and then applied clinically, evolving from external metal clips placed on the trachea by open hysterotomy or fetoscopic neck dissection, to internal tracheal occlusion with a detachable silicone balloon placed by fetal bronchoscopy through a single 5 mm uterine port, as described above.

Our initial experience suggested that fetal endoscopic tracheal occlusion improved survival in human fetuses with severe CDH. To evaluate this novel therapy, we conducted a randomized controlled trial comparing tracheal occlusion with standard care. Survival with fetal endoscopic tracheal occlusion (73%) met expectations (predicted 75%) and appeared better than that of historic controls (37%), but proved no better than that of concurrent randomized controls. The higher than expected survival in the standard care group may be because the study design mandated that patients in both treatment groups be delivered, resuscitated, and intensively managed in a unit experienced in caring for critically ill newborns with suspected pulmonary hypoplasia.

Attempts to improve outcome for severe CDH by treatments either before or after birth have proven to be double-edged swords. Intensive care after birth has improved survival but has increased long-term sequelae in survivors, and is expensive. Intervention before birth may increase lung size, but prematurity caused by the intervention itself can be detrimental. In our study, babies with severe CDH who had tracheal occlusion before birth were born on average at 31 weeks, as a consequence of the intervention. The observation that their rates of survival and respiratory outcomes (including duration of oxygen requirement) were comparable to infants without tracheal occlusion who were born at 37 weeks suggests that tracheal occlusion improved pulmonary hypoplasia, but the improvement in lung growth was adversely affected by pulmonary immaturity related to earlier delivery.

The current results underscore the role of randomized trials in evaluating promising new therapies. This is the second NIH-sponsored trial comparing a new prenatal intervention for severe fetal CDH. The first trial showed that complete surgical repair of the anatomic defect (which required hysterotomy), although feasible, was no better than postnatal repair in improving survival and was ineffective when the liver as well as the bowel was herniated [18]. That trial led to the abandonment of open complete repair at our institution and subsequently around the world. Information derived from that trial regarding measures of severity of pulmonary hypoplasia (including liver herniation and the development of the lung:head ratio [LHR] – the area of contralateral lung in the axial plane at the level of a four-chamber view of the heart, normalized to head circumference) led to the development of an alternative physiologic strategy to enlarge the hypoplastic fetal lung by temporary tracheal occlusion and to the development of less invasive fetal endoscopic techniques that did not require hysterotomy to achieve temporary, reversible tracheal occlusion [19,20].

Our ability to accurately diagnose and assess severity of CDH before birth has improved dramatically. Fetuses with CDH who have associated anomalies do poorly, whereas fetuses with isolated CDH, no liver herniation, and an LHR above 1.4 have an excellent prognosis (100% in our experience). In this study, fetuses with an LHR between 0.9 and 1.4 had a chance of survival greater than 80% when delivered at a tertiary care center. The small number of fetuses with LHR below 0.9 had a poor prognosis in both treatment groups, and should be the focus of further studies [21].

Because tracheal occlusion does work in enlarging hypoplastic lungs, approaches to tracheal occlusion other than that used here might be beneficial. Although the duration of occlusion in this study (36.2 ± 14.7 days) is comparable with that studied in animal models [22,23], the optimal timing and duration of occlusion are not known in humans. Short-term occlusion later in gestation and earlier occlusion (with possible reversal *in utero*) were initially studied in animal models with the potential benefit of improved type II pneumocyte function[24,25]. The group in Leuven, Belgium, has led the effort to study the benefit of percutaneous, reversible balloon tracheal occlusion in human fetuses with severe CDH. The balloon is placed percutanaeously with fetoscopic guidance around 28 weeks and then is removed with percutaneous fetoscopic guidance approximately 4 weeks later [26]. Survival has been shown to be improved compared to a cohort that had standard postnatal care. This technique allows for vaginal delivery, potentially closer to the family's home. Our group has also adopted this approach and is studying this technique under the guidance of the Food and Drug Administration (FDA).

Twin–twin transfusion syndrome

Twin–twin transfusion syndrome (TTTS) is a complication of monochorionic multiple gestations resulting from an imbalance in blood flow through vascular communications. Both twins are compromised, albeit in different ways. The recipient twin is generally the larger twin and receives an excess of blood and can develop high-output cardiac failure. The donor twin is generally the smaller twin and shunts blood to the recipient twin and can develop renal failure from a low-output state.

Twin–twin transfusion syndrome is the most common serious complication of monochorionic twin gestations, affecting between 4% and 35% of monochorionic twin pregnancies, or approximately 0.1–0.9 per 1000 births each year in the USA. Yet despite the relatively low incidence, TTTS disproportionately accounts for 17% of all perinatal mortality associated with twin gestations [27]. Staging for TTTS was pioneered by Quintero based on sonographic measurements. The diagnosis is made by a combination of polyhydramnios in the recipient twin and oligohydramnios for the donor twin. Standard therapy has been limited to serial amnioreduction, which appears to improve the overall outcome but has little impact on the more severe end of the spectrum in TTTS. In addition, survivors of TTTS treated by serial amnioreduction have an 18–26% incidence of significant neurologic and cardiac morbidity. Selective fetoscopic laser photocoagulation of communicating vessels, pioneered by de Lia [28], has emerged as the generally accepted best treatment for advanced stage TTTS, as demonstrated in a randomized trial in Europe [29]. Fetoscopic laser of intertwin vessels for TTTS is now the most common indication for fetoscopic surgery worldwide. Some centers, including ours, routinely use advanced fetal echocardiogram data to further stratify the severity of TTTS.

Urinary tract obstruction

As a group at UCSF we are particularly enthusiastic about the potential of fetal intervention in bladder outlet obstruction by percutaneous fetal cystoscopy. Fetal urethral obstruction produces pulmonary hypoplasia and renal dysplasia, and these often fatal consequences can be ameliorated by urinary tract decompression before birth. The natural history of untreated fetal urinary tract obstruction is well documented, and selection criteria based on fetal urine electrolyte and β2-microglobulin levels and the sonographic appearance of fetal kidneys have proven reliable [30–33]. The vast majority of fetuses with urinary tract dilation do not require intervention. However, fetuses with bilateral hydronephrosis and bladder distension resulting from urethral obstruction subsequently developing oligohydramnios require treatment. Depending on the gestational age, the fetus can be delivered early for postnatal decompression. Alternatively, the bladder can be decompressed *in utero* by a catheter vesicoamniotic shunt placed percutaneously under sonographic guidance [34,35]. Treatment with shunting has been relatively disappointing, as shunts often migrate or do not remain patent. Even when adequately decompressed, the obstructed bladder may not cycle correctly, resulting in a severe bladder dysfunction requiring surgery after birth. We have now developed a percutaneous fetal cystoscopic technique to disrupt posterior urethral valves through a single 3 mm port. This technique would allow the bladder to continue to cycle normally [36].

Fetal intervention guided by sonography

The first fetal procedure, developed in the early 1980s, was percutaneous sonographically guided placement of fetal bladder catheter shunt. Many other catheter-shunt procedures have been developed and described [37]. More recently, we have developed percutaneous sonographically guided radiofrequency ablation procedures for management of anomalous multiple gestations. All these procedures we now group as "fetal intervention guided by sonography" (FIGS).

Fetal intervention guided by sonography is used to sample or drain fetal blood, urine, and fluid collection, to sample fetal tissue, to place catheter shunts in the fetal bladder, chest, abdomen, or ventricles, and to perform radiofrequency ablation (RFA). The most common indication at UCSF is RFA for acardiac twins/twin reversed arterial perfusion (TRAP) sequence or monochorionic twins for selective reduction. Other operators have used bipolar coagulation or umbilical cord ligation for similar indications. Compared with the 17-gauge RFA needles we use, these techniques are more invasive, using at least 3 mm trochars. Additionally, the length of the cord or its position may preclude use of these instruments. The perioperative management of these patients is similar to the current percutaneous FETENDO patients.

The procedures are performed under spinal anesthesia, with prophylactic antibiotics and indomethacin. Postoperative tocolysis is rarely necessary and the patients are frequently discharged within hours of the procedure. Ultrasound is critical for both the planning and execution of the procedure. We attempt to avoid entry into the sac of a normal twin if at all possible. The RFA needle is guided into the abdominal cord insertion of the abnormal twin under ultrasound guidance. The tines (thin wires protruding out of the needle like hooks) are then deployed and energy delivered to the device to create thermal injury to the tissue. The device we currently use measures the temperature at the tines. This allows us to use an energy level to provide the quickest possible obliteration of the vascular communications. This is of benefit as there are theoretical concerns regarding the differential obliteration of arterial and venous vessels, which might place the normal twin at risk for exsanguination. Ultrasound is also used to monitor the procedure and welfare of the normal twin. Thermal injury can be monitored by watching for the characteristic out-gassing in the tissue. Once active energy delivery to the device has ceased, color flow Doppler can be used to detect any residual flow, in both the cord and the abnormal fetus. Once absence of blood flow is confirmed, the tines are retracted and the device then withdrawn.

We have not found an increased frequency of adverse outcomes with a transplacental approach. We have had good success with this approach with a survival rate over 90% and a mean gestational age at delivery of over 35 weeks and an average time from procedure of over 11 weeks. There has been no maternal pulmonary edema or blood loss [38].

There are a few complicated FIGS procedures that may require maternal laparotomy to allow fetal positioning and sonography directly on the uterus (Lap-FIGS). A few simple structural cardiac defects that interfere with development may benefit from prenatal correction. For example, if obstruction of blood flow across the pulmonary or aortic valve interferes with development of the ventricles or pulmonary or systemic vasculature, relief of the anatomic obstruction may allow normal development with an improved outcome. Alternatively, congenital aortic stenosis may lead to hypoplastic left heart syndrome [39]. Stenotic aortic valves have been dilated by a balloon catheter placed using both FIGS and Lap-FIGS in order to prevent the evolution of hypoplastic left heart syndrome. Led by the group in Boston, results have been promising but not proven [40].

Conclusion

In summary, fetal surgery has evolved considerably since its birth at UCSF two decades ago. The indications remain quite limited, but numerically have the potential to expand as patients and providers become increasingly informed. Recent advances in the development of less invasive fetal endoscopic (FETENDO) and sonography-guided techniques (FIGS) have extended the indications for fetal intervention.

CASE PRESENTATION

The patient is a 36-year-old gravida 3, para 2 at 18 weeks' gestation. She is referred to a perinatologist for evaluation because an ultrasound is suspicious for a twin pregnancy with demise of an anomalous fetus with a cystic hygroma.

The perinatologist performs a detailed ultrasound and identifies a monochorionic diamnionic twin pregnancy. One twin is morphologically normal and the other has a torso with edematous skin and no heart and is of similar size to the normal twin. The blood flow in the cord is reversed with flow in the single artery towards the anomalous twin. This therefore is an acardiac twin and the situation represents TRAP. The perinatologist discusses with the patient and her partner that in cases of TRAP, the normal or pump twin is at risk of cardiac failure, hydrops, and stillbirth. They discuss the management options, including observation or intervention with bipolar cord coagulation or RFA.

The family is seen for evaluation. Ultrasound documents the previous findings and also identifies polyhydramnios and an enlarged intraabdominal umbilical vein in the pump twin sac, and significant blood flow into the acardiac twin. Fetal echocardiography shows increased biventricular output in the pump twin with some increased pulsatility in the ductus venosus. The multidisciplinary team meets with the patient and her family and discusses the management options and risks and benefits of each. They decide to proceed with RFA.

The procedure is performed the next day, under spinal anesthesia in the operating room. The RFA device is deployed percutaneously under ultrasound guidance into the abdomen of the acardiac twin at the level of the cord insertion. The device is energized and the tissue is heated acutely. After cooldown, ultrasound documents cessation of blood flow based on color flow and pulse Doppler. The patient stays hospitalized overnight. The next day a repeat ultrasound confirms no acute changes in the pump twin without residual flow into the acardiac twin. The patient is discharged home to return to the care of her referring perinatologist and primary obstetrician. Several months later she delivers a healthy infant at term by induced vaginal delivery.

References

1. Golombeck K, Ball RH, Lee H et al. Maternal morbidity after fetal surgery. Am J Obstet Gynecol 2006;194:834–839.

2. Adzick NS, Harrison MR, Glick PL et al. Fetal surgery in the primate. III. Maternal outcome after fetal surgery. J Pediatr Surg 1986;21:477–480.

3. Bruner JP, Tulipan N, Reed G et al. Intrauterine repair of spina bifida: preoperative predictors of shunt-dependent hydrocephalus. Am J Obstet Gynecol 2004;190:1305–1312.

4. Johnson MP, Sutton LN, Rintoul N et al. Fetal myelomeningocele repair: short-term clinical outcomes. Am J Obstet Gynecol 2003;189:482–487.

5. DiFederico EM, Burlingame JM, Kilpatrick SJ, Harrison MR, Matthay MA. Pulmonary edema in obstetric patients is rapidly resolved except in the presence of infection or of nitroglycerin tocolysis after open fetal surgery. Am J Obstet Gynecol 1998;179:925–933.

6. Wilson RD, Johnson MP, Crombleholme TM et al. Chorioamniotic membrane separation following open fetal surgery: pregnancy outcome. Fetal Diagn Ther 2003;18:314–320.

7. Bruner JP, Tulipan NB, Richards WO, Walsh WF, Boehm FH, Vrabcak EK. In utero repair of myelomeningocele: a comparison of endoscopy and hysterotomy. Fetal Diagn Ther 2000;15:83–88.

8. Farrell JA, Albanese CT, Jennings RW, Kilpatrick SJ, Bratton BJ, Harrison MR. Maternal fertility is not affected by fetal surgery. Fetal Diagn Ther 1999;14:190–192.

9. Bouchard S, Davey MG, Rintoul NE, Walsh DS, Rorke LB, Adzick NS. Correction of hindbrain herniation and anatomy of the vermis after in utero repair of myelomeningocele in sheep. J Pediatr Surg 2003;38:451–458.

10. Adzick NS, Thom EA, Spong CY et al. A randomized trial of prenatal versus postnatal repair of myelomeningocele. N Engl J Med 2011;364(11):993–1004.

11. Adzick NS, Harrison MR, Glick PL et al. Fetal cystic adenomatoid malformation: prenatal diagnosis and natural history. J Pediatr Surg 1985;20:483–488.

12. Adzick NS, Glick PL, Harrison MR et al. Compensatory lung growth after pneumonectomy in the fetus. Surg Forum 1986;37:648–649.

13. MacGillivray TE, Harrison MR, Goldstein RB, Adzick NS. Disappearing fetal lung lesions. J Pediatr Surg 1993;28:1321–1324.

14. Blott M, Nicolaides KH, Greenough A. Postnatal respiratory function after chronic drainage of fetal pulmonary cyst. Am J Obstet Gynecol 1988;159:858–865.

15. Tsao K, Hawgood S, Vu L et al. Resolution of hydrops fetalis in congenital cystic adenomatoid malformation after prenatal steroid therapy. J Pediatr Surg 2003;38:508–510.

16. Curran PF, Jelin EB, Rand L et al. Prenatal steroids for microcystic congenital cystic adenomatoid malformations. J Pediatr Surg 2010;45:145–150.

17. Hirose S, Farmer DL, Lee H, Nobuhara KK, Harrison MR. The ex utero intrapartum treatment procedure: looking back at the EXIT. J Pediatr Surg 2003;39:375–380.

18. Harrison MR, Adzick NS, Bullard KM et al. Correction of congenital diaphragmatic hernia in utero VII: a prospective trial. J Pediatr Surg 1997;32:1637–1642.

19. Harrison MR, Adzick NS, Flake AW et al. Correction of congenital diaphragmatic hernia in utero VIII: response of the

hypoplastic lung to tracheal occlusion. J Pediatr Surg 1996; 31:1339–1348.

20. Skarsgard ED, Meuli M, VanderWall KJ, Bealer JF, Adzick NS, Harrison MR. Fetal endoscopic tracheal occlusion ("Fetendo-PLUG") for congenital diaphragmatic hernia. J Pediatr Surg 1996;31:1335–1338.

21. Lipshutz GS, Albanese CT, Feldstein VA et al. Prospective analysis of lung-to-head ratio predicts survival for patients with prenatally diagnosed congenital diaphragmatic hernia. J Pediatr Surg 1997;32:1634–1636.

22. Papadakis K, de Paepe ME, Tackett LD, Piasecki GJ, Luks FI. Temporary tracheal occlusion causes catch-up lung maturation in a fetal model of diaphragmatic hernia. J Pediatr Surg 1998;33:1030–1037.

23. VanderWall KJ, Bruch SW, Meuli M et al. Fetal endoscopic ("Fetendo") tracheal clip. J Pediatr Surg 1996;31:1101–1103.

24. Luks FI, Wild YK, Piasecki GJ, de Paepe ME. Short-term tracheal occlusion corrects pulmonary vascular anomalies in the fetal lamb with diaphragmatic hernia. Surgery 2000;128: 266–272.

25. Flageole H, Evrard VA, Piedboeuf B, Laberge JM, Lerut TE, Deprest JA. The plug–unplug sequence: an important step to achieve type II pneumocyte maturation in the fetal lamb model. J Pediatr Surg 1998;33:299–303.

26. Deprest J, Jani J, Graticos E et al. Fetal intervention for congenital diaphragmatic hernia. The European experience. Semin Perinatol 2005;29(2):94–103.

27. Quintero RA. Twin–twin transfusion syndrome. Clin Perinatol 2003;30:591–600.

28. De Lia JE, Cruikshank DP, Keye WR Jr. Fetoscopic neodymium:Yag laser occlusion of placental vessels in severe twin-twin transfusion syndrome. Obstet Gynecol 1990;75(6): 1046–1053.

29. Senat MV, Deprest J, Boulvain M, Paupe A, Winer N, Ville Y. Endoscopic laser surgery versus serial amnioreduction for severe twin-to-twin transfusion syndrome. N Engl J Med 2004;351:136–144.

30. Adzick NS, Harrison MR, Glick PL, Flake AW. Fetal urinary tract obstruction: experimental pathophysiology. Semin Perinatol 1985;9:79–90.

31. Crombleholme TM, Harrison MR, Golbus MS et al. Fetal intervention in obstructive uropathy: prognostic indicators and efficacy of intervention. Am J Obstet Gynecol 1990;162: 1239–1244.

32. Nicolaides KH, Cheng HH, Snijders RJ, Moniz CF. Fetal urine biochemistry in the assessment of obstructive uropathy. Am J Obstet Gynecol 1992;166:932–937.

33. Glick PL, Harrison MR, Adzick NS, Noall RA, Villa RL. Correction of congenital hydronephrosis in utero IV: in utero decompression prevents renal dysplasia. J Pediatr Surg 1984;19:649–645.

34. Manning FA, Harrison MR, Rodeck C. Catheter shunts for fetal hydronephrosis and hydrocephalus. Report of the International Fetal Surgery Registry. N Engl J Med 1986;315:336–340.

35. Johnson MP, Bukowski TP, Reitleman C, Isada NB, Pryde PG, Evans MI. In utero surgical treatment of fetal obstructive uropathy: a new comprehensive approach to identify appropriate candidates for vesicoamniotic shunt therapy. Am J Obstet Gynecol 1994;170:1770–1776.

36. Clifton MS, Harrison MR, Ball R, Lee H. Fetoscopic transuterine release of posterior urethral valves: a new technique. Fetal Diagn Ther 2008;23(2):89–94.

37. Wilson RD, Baxter JK, Johnson MP et al. Thoracoamniotic shunts: fetal treatment of pleural effusions and congenital cystic adenomatoid malformations. Fetal Diagn Ther 2004;19:413–412.

38. Lee H, Wagner AJ, Sy E, Ball R, Feldstein VA, Goldstein RB, Farmer DL. Efficacy of radiofrequency ablation for twin-reversed arterial perfusion sequence. Am J Obstet Gynecol 2007;196(5):459.

39. Allan LD, Maxwell D, Tynan M. Progressive obstructive lesions of the heart: an opportunity for fetal therapy. Fetal Ther 1991;6:173–176.

40. Tworetzky W, Wilkins-Haug L, Jennings RW et al. Balloon dilation of severe aortic stenosis in the fetus: potential for prevention of hypoplastic left heart syndrome: candidate selection, technique, and results of successful intervention. Circulation 2004;110(15):2125–2131.

Index

Note: page numbers in *italics* refer to figures; those in **bold** refer to tables and boxes.

abdominal circumference 5, 63–4
  fetal growth restriction 64
abdominal surgical incision, cesarean delivery 407
  vaginal birth after cesarean delivery 416
abdominal wall closure, cesarean delivery 408
abortion
  antiphospholipid antibodies 115
  inherited thrombophilias 116
  recurrent spontaneous 260–6
    aneuploidy 260–1
    antiphospholipid antibody syndrome 264–5, 266
    celiac disease 262
    depression 266
    endocrinopathies 262–3
    evidence-based evaluation 266
    genetic factors **266**
    immunologic causes 265–6
    infections 262
    karyotyping 266
    maternal age 260
    thrombophilias 263–5
    trophoblast inclusions **266**
    uterine abnormalities 263, 266
  see also miscarriage
abruptio placentae *see* placental abruption
acamprosate 27
activated factor VIII, postpartum hemorrhage 295
activated protein C (APC) 123
acute myocardial infarction (AMI), maternal 143–4
acute-phase reactant inflammatory biomarkers, preterm delivery 353
acyclovir
  herpes simplex virus 225
  varicella zoster virus 228
Adverse Outcome Index (AOI) 439–40, 442, *443*
adverse outcomes, incidence 6, **7**
age, maternal and sporadic miscarriage 260
airway obstruction
  asthma 183
  reversible 185
alcohol abuse 23–4, **25**, 26–7, **28–9**, 29–30
  breastfeeding 30
  comprehensive prenatal care 27, **28–9**, 29
  contraception 30
  development effects 26
  education 27
  fetal anomalies 24
  fetal effects 23–4, **25**, 26
  follow-up 30

hospital care 29–30
  pharmacotherapy 26–7
  postpartum care 29–30
  psychiatric disorders 26
  psychosocial interventions 26
  screening for 23, **24**
  therapy during pregnancy 26–7
allergy
  amniotic fluid embolism 301–2
  mite **190**
  penicillin 235, **236**
alloimmune thrombocytopenia 104
  neonatal 104–5, **106**
alpha fetoprotein (AFP) 55
  Down syndrome screening 59
  elevated maternal serum **71**
  maternal serum for neural tube defects 60–1
  placenta accreta 388
amnio-infusion
  normal saline **91**
  oligohydramnios 334
amniocentesis 45, 75, 453–6
  array comparative genomic hybridization 459–60
  complications 454
  congenital malformation risk 456
  cytogenetic diagnosis 459
  diagnostic studies 459–61
  DNA analysis 461
  early 455–6
  enzymatic analysis 461
  fetal platelet antigen typing **106**
  fetomaternal transfusion 454
  genetic evaluation 453–5
    fetal aneuploidy 320
  intraamniotic infection 374
  limb abnormalities 456
  multiple gestations 454
  patient safety 454–5
  procedure-induced miscarriage 455–6
  risks 454–5
  sickle cell disease 96
  twin pregnancy 76
  ultrasound prior to 453–4
  uniparental disomy 461
amnionicity determination 315–16
  monoamnionicity 318
amniotic fluid
  bacterial colonization 274
  bilirubin analysis 387.121
  clinical measurement 329–30
  composition 327, 329
  fetal swallowing 329
  fetal urine 328
  intramembranous flow 329
  osmolality 327

protein biomarkers in preterm delivery 353
  removal 329
  single deepest pocket measurement 330
  techniques for obtaining 75
  turnover 329
    dynamics 327–9
  two-diameter pocket 330
  volume 327, *328*, 329, 331
    assessment 329–30
  see also oligohydramnios; polyhydramnios
amniotic fluid embolism 301–2
  blood product replacement 303–4
  labor induction 403
  plasma preparations 304
Amniotic Fluid Index (AFI) 79, **86**, 330
  biophysical profile 81
  polyhydramnios 331
ampicillin 234
analgesia, obstetric 434–6
  combined spinal-epidural approach 435, 436
  epidural 435
  labor 434–6
  multimodal regional 434–5
  postoperative for cesarean delivery 437
  spinal approach 435
  timing 436
  vaginal delivery 434–6
  see also epidural analgesia
anaphylactoid syndrome of pregnancy 302
anatomic abnormalities *see* congenital malformations; fetal anomalies
anemia 98–100
  consequences 98
  definition 98
  diagnostic work-up 98–100
  macrocytic 98–9
  maternal complications with multiple gestations 318, **319**
  maternal renal disease 157
  microangiopathic hemolytic 302
  microcytic 99
  normocytic 99, **100**
  reticulocyte count 99, **100**
  treatment 98–100
anencephaly
  polyhydramnios 329
  screening 60
anesthesia
  cesarean delivery 436–7
  neonatal encephalopathy risk 447
  physiologic changes of pregnancy 436–7
  see also epidural anesthesia
aneuploidy, fetal
  counseling 58–9
  diagnostic testing 320

Queenan's Management of High-Risk Pregnancy: An Evidence-Based Approach, Sixth Edition. Edited by John T. Queenan, Catherine Y. Spong, Charles J. Lockwood.
© 2012 John Wiley & Sons, Ltd. Published 2012 by John Wiley & Sons, Ltd.

aneuploidy, fetal (*cont.*)
  minor markers 58
  recurrent spontaneous abortion 260–1
  screening 55–60, **61**
    combined first-trimester serum and
      sonographic screening 57
    first-trimester 55–7
    maternal serum with renal disease 157
    multiple gestations 60, 320
    second-trimester serum 59
    second-trimester sonographic 58–9
angiogenesis, preeclampsia 281
angiotensin-converting enzyme (ACE)
      inhibitors, contraindications
  periconceptual period 204–5
  pregnancy 142, 155, 163, 204–5, 206–7
angiotensin receptor blockers,
      contraindications
  periconceptual period 204–5
  pregnancy 142, 155, 204–5, 206–7
anhydramnios 332
anonymous event reporting system 441,
      443
antepartum fetal monitoring 79–84, **84–6**
  Amniotic Fluid Index 79, 81, **86**
  biophysical profile 79, 81–2
    modified 81
  contraction stress test 79, 82–3
  Doppler velocimetry 79, 83, **86**
  indications 84
  nonstress test 79, 80, 81, **86**
  onset of testing 84
anti-β₂-glycoprotein I (β₂GPI) antibodies 214,
      264
anti-D antibody 308, **312**
anti-D immunoglobulin, idiopathic
      thrombocytopenic purpura 103
anti-double-stranded DNA (anti-dsDNA) 205,
      210
  systemic lupus erythematosus 209, 213
anti-La/SSB antibodies 209, 210, 212, 213
anti-ribonucleoprotein (anti-RNP) antibodies
      209, 210
anti-Ro/SSA antibodies 209, 210, 212, 213
anti-Smith (anti-Sm) antibodies 209, 210
antiarrhythmic agents **145–6**
antibiotic prophylaxis
  cervical insufficiency 277
  cesarean delivery 407
  group B streptococcal infection 234–5
  PPROM 339, 369, **371**
  preterm birth 339
  preterm labor 377
anticardiolipin antibodies 264
anticoagulants, endogenous 122–3
anticonvulsants *see* antiepileptic drugs
antidepressants, alcohol abuse withdrawal
      27
antiepileptic drugs 193
  breastfeeding 199
  congenital malformations 194, 195, **200**
  contraception 193, **194**
  embryopathy mechanisms 196
  fetal anticonvulsant syndrome 193–5
  folic acid supplementation 196
  management 197–8
  monotherapy during pregnancy
      194–5
  neural tube defects 194, 195
  neurodevelopmental outcome 196
  postpartum care 199
  vitamin K transport inhibition 198
antigliadin antibodies 262
antihypertensive therapy 206–7, **208**
antimicrosomal antibodies 179
antinuclear antibodies 205, 209–10
antioxidants, maternal nutrition 17
antiphospholipid antibodies
  acquired thrombophilia 114–15
  systemic lupus erythematosus 210,
      213–15

antiphospholipid antibody syndrome (APAS)
      108, 114, 210, 213–15
  clinical complications 214
  diagnosis 214, **215**
  obstetric complications 265
  pathogenesis 265
  recurrent spontaneous abortion 264–5, 266
  treatment 108, 116, 215, 265, 266
antiplatelet therapy, antiphospholipid antibody
      syndrome 108
antiretroviral drugs 245, **246–9**, 250
antithrombin deficiency 108
  inherited thrombophilia 111
antithyroglobulin antibodies 179
antitransglutaminase antibodies 262
aortic aneurysm rupture, risk 139
aortic arch, fetal echocardiography Plate 6.1
aortic clamping, postpartum hemorrhage 295
aortic coarctation, maternal 139, **146**
aortic dissection risk 139
aortic outflow tract 50
aortic regurgitation 136
aortic stenosis 136–7
aortic valve, bicuspid **146**
aquaporins (AQP) 329, 332
arginine vasopressin 332
Arnold-Chiari II malformation 467–8
array comparative genomic hybridization
      459–60
arrhythmias, maternal 144
Arskog syndrome **66**
artemisinin-based combination therapy (ACT)
      232, **233**
arterial embolization, postpartum hemorrhage
      292, 295
arthrogryposis 261
Asherman syndrome 263
Ashkenazi Jews, carrier screening 44–5
asphyxia, intrapartum 446, 448
aspirin
  antiphospholipid antibody syndrome 116,
      215, 265, 266
  factor V Leiden mutation 264
assisted reproductive technologies (ART)
  monozygosity incidence 318
  multiple gestations 314
asthma, maternal 183–90
  acute 189
  assessment 185–7
  chronic 187–8, **189**
  clinical course 183, 184
  controller therapy 187–8
  definition 183
  delivery management 189–90
  diagnosis 185
  effects on pregnancy 184–5
  exacerbations in pregnancy 183
  fetal monitoring 189
  infections 184
  labor management 189–90
  management 189–90
  mechanisms in pregnancy 184–5
  monitoring 185–7
  patient education 187, **190**
  pharmacologic therapy 187–9
  pregnancy effects 183–4
  risk association 183
  severity 184, 187
  symptoms in pregnancy 183
ataxia-telangiectasia syndrome, IUGR **66**
atrial septal defect, maternal 139
atrioventricular node blocking agents **146**
atrioventricular valves, fetal echocardiography
      Plate 6.2
autoimmune thrombocytopenia 102–3, 104
autoimmune thyroiditis 178
  transient 181
autoimmune thyrotoxicosis 179
autonomic dysreflexia, women with physical
      disabilities 256, **257–8**
autosomal dominant inheritance 41–2

autosomal recessive inheritance 41, 42
azathioprine 146, 161–2
  systemic lupus erythematosus 213, **214**

β-blockers **145**, 181, 206
β-mimetics 377–8
bacterial vaginosis 262
  decidual-amnion-chorion inflammation 348
  PPROM risk 365
bacteriuria
  group B streptococcal 234, 236
  renal transplantation patients 161
  sickle cell disease 94
Bacteroides 349
banana sign 61
basiliximab 162
behavioral disorders, family history 41
benzodiazepines, alcohol abuse withdrawal
      27
betamethasone
  preterm birth prevention **342**
  preterm labor prevention 375–6, **380**
bilirubin analysis, amniotic fluid 387.121
biophysical profile (BPP) 79, 81–2
  chronic hypertension 207
  gestational diabetes 171
  modified 81
  prolonged labor prevention 393
  scoring **81–2**
biparietal diameter 63
  neural tube defects 61
birth defects
  folate deficiency 16
  see also congenital malformations; fetal
      anomalies; neural tube defects
birthweight
  large for gestational age infants 416
  low birthweight infants 184
  maternal/paternal 65
  vaginal birth after cesarean delivery 416
  see also macrosomia; small for gestational
      age (SGA) infants
bisphenol A, toxicity 36
bladder
  dysfunction in women with physical
      disability 253
  fetal outlet obstruction 470
  placenta accreta/percreta 294
blocking antibodies, activity in spontaneous
      abortion 265
blood gases, asthma in pregnancy 189
blood pressure
  diastolic 131
  eclampsia 286
  home monitoring 205
  hypotension in labor induction 402
  systolic 131
  see also gestational hypertension;
      hypertension, maternal
blood products
  postpartum hemorrhage 295, 297, **298**
  replacement 301, 303–4
blood transfusion, iron deficiency anemia
      100
blood volume, pregnancy 131
Bloom syndrome
  carrier screening 45
  IUGR **66**
body-length ratio 5
body mass index (BMI)
  adverse pregnancy outcomes 7–9
  prepregnancy
    dietary recommendations **10**, 18–19
    weight retention 13
  preterm delivery incidence 8
  small for gestational age infants 8, 9
brain-sparing reflex 68
breast milk 18
breastfeeding
  alcohol abuse 30
  antiepileptic drug use 199

hepatitis infection **241**
herpes simplex virus 225
HIV infection recommendations 250
maternal nutrition 18
substance abuse 30
breech delivery 424–8
cesarean delivery 416, 427
criteria for attempted delivery 425–6
epidemiology 424
labor management 426
maternal outcome 424–5
neonatal mortality 425
perinatal outcome 424–5
preterm 420
technique 426–7
vaginal 424–7
bronchodilators, congenital malformations 185
bupivacaine **437**
buprenorphine 26, 27

calcitonin 15
calcium
maternal nutrition 15
therapy for lead toxicity 34
calcium *channel* blockers **145**
hypertension treatment 155, 206
renal transplant patients 163
preterm labor prevention 378
calcium supplementation, antiphospholipid
antibody syndrome 215
calf pain **128**
Canavan disease, carrier screening 44, **45**, **46**
carbamazepine 195
neural tube defects 194
induced 16
neurodevelopmental outcome 196
carboprost tromethamine **298**
cardiac anomalies, fetal, Down syndrome/
trisomy 18 58
cardiac anomalies, maternal 139–41
risk 134
cardiac arrest, maternal, perimortem cesarean
delivery 304–5
cardiac disease 131–44, **145–6**, 146, **146–7**
acute myocardial infarction 143–4
aortic regurgitation 136
aortic stenosis 136–7
arrhythmias 144
cardiovascular drugs **145–6**
counseling 131–4
maternal complications 133
mitral stenosis 135–6
mitral valve prolapse 136
peripartum cardiomyopathy 141–3
pulmonary valve stenosis 135
rheumatic heart disease 134
risk factors 133
tricuspid lesions 135
valvular lesions 134, **135**
see also congenital heart disease
cardiac output, pregnancy 131
cardiac screening 47–53
benefits 47
technique 48–51
cardiac transplantation 164–5, **166**
graft rejection 165
pregnancy after 144, 146
cardiomyopathy, peripartum 141–3
cardiopulmonary resuscitation 304, **306**
cardiotocography 66–7
cardiovascular collapse, amniotic fluid
embolism 301
cardiovascular drugs, fetal and uterine blood
flow effects **145–6**
C4b-binding protein 123
CD4 count 244, 245, **251**
celiac disease, recurrent spontaneous abortion
262
cephalopelvic disproportion
cesarean delivery 416
prolonged pregnancy 392

cerebral palsy, infant 445–50
brain imaging 448
genetic inheritance 445, 446
incidence 445
magnesium sulfate prophylaxis 376, 448–50
MTHFR C677T gene 445
multiple gestations 315
neuroprotection in preterm labor 376
preterm birth 337
prevention strategies 448–50
risk factors 446
task force 447–8
watershed injury pattern 448
women with physical disabilities 257
cerebral palsy, maternal 253
cervical cerclage
cervical insufficiency 272, 273–4, 275, **278**
complications 276
history-indicated 272, 273, 275–6
ultrasound-indicated 275–6
vaginal pessary comparison 277
emergency 274
McDonald procedure 273–4, **278**
PPROM 276, 370
preterm birth prevention 339–41
prophylactic in multiple gestations 321
Shirodkar technique 273
cervical competence, biologic continuum
271–2
cervical dilatation, premature silent 272
cervical dysplasia, treatment 272
cervical examination, favorability 395, 403
cervical insufficiency 271–7, **277–8**
acute 274–5
adjunctive management 276–7
cerclage 272, 273–4, 275, **278**
complications 276
history-indicated 272, 273, 275–6
ultrasound-indicated 275–6
vaginal pessary comparison 277
chorioamnionitis **277**
diagnosis 272
incidence 272
management 273
postcerclage management 276
PPROM **277–8**
risk factors 272
sonographic diagnosis 275
cervical length
inflammation 340
preterm birth 339–40, 341
preterm delivery risk 354–5
preterm labor 375
transvaginal surveillance 321, **323**
ultrasound measurement 339, 374, 375, 402
cervical ripening, prostaglandin E₂ 190
cervix
changes with preterm birth 339–40
unfavourable 403
cesarean delivery 406–10, **411–12**
abdominal surgical incision 407, 416
vaginal birth after cesarean delivery 416
abdominal wall closure 408
anesthesia 436–7
antibiotic prophylaxis 407
breech presentation 416, 427
cephalopelvic disproportion 416
on demand 406
diabetes mellitus 176
evidence-based operative considerations
406–8
failure to progress in labor 409–10, 416
fetal distress 410
fetal status 436
following failed induction 400
gestational diabetes **172**
HELLP syndrome 284, **285**
HIV transmission prevention 250
hysterotomy
closure 407–8
subsequent to 465

indications 409–10
malpresentation 410
manual removal of placenta 407
maternal cardiac arrest 304–5
maternal morbidity/mortality 304–5, **306**,
406
motor block 436
multifetal pregnancy 13
number of prior 417–18
perimortem 301, 304–5, **306**
perinatal morbidity/mortality 304–5, **306**, 406
peritoneal closure 408
postoperative analgesia 437
PPROM **356**, **371**
preeclampsia 283
prior
labor induction 403–4
placenta accreta risk 387–8
uterine rupture risk 403–4
prolonged pregnancy 392
rate 406, *407*
patient populations 409
repeat 408–9, 410, **411–12**
Robson classification 409
shoulder dystocia 416
thromboprophylaxis 408
transplant patients 165
uterine incision extra-/intra-abdominal
repair 407
vaginal antiseptic prophylaxis 407
vasa previa 387
women with physical disabilities 256
see also vaginal birth after cesarean delivery
cesarean hysterectomy, adherent placenta 294
CFTR gene mutations 44
ΔF508 mutation **46**
CHARGE syndrome, IUGR 66
chelation therapy, lead toxicity 34
chest X-ray
pregnancy **132**
pulmonary embolism 125, 127
Chiari malformation 61
chickenpox (varicella) 227–8
Chlamydia trachomatis 365, 366
chorioamnion, amniotic fluid composition/
volume 329
chorioamnionitis **146**, 348–9
cerclage complication 276
cervical insufficiency **277**
PPROM 366
preterm birth 339, 374
chorionic villus, surface area 6
chorionic villus sampling (CVS) 45, 453, 456–9
array comparative genomic hybridization
459–60
confined placental mosaicism 460–1
congenital malformations 458
cytogenetic diagnosis 459
diagnostic studies 459–61
DNA analysis 461
enzymatic analysis 461
fetal aneuploidy diagnosis 320
genetic counseling 459
limb abnormalities 458
maternal cell contamination 460
miscarriage risk 457–8
patient safety 458–9
septated cystic hygroma 57–8, **61**
sickle cell disease 96
transabdominal 456–7, 459
transcervical 456, 458, 459
chorionicity
ultrasound diagnosis 315–16
see also monochorionicity
chorioretinitis 223
chromosome abnormalities
IUGR 65
multifetal pregnancy 320
spontaneous abortion 261
see also Down syndrome; *trisomy entries*
circle of Willis, Doppler ultrasound 68

clindamycin
　　group B streptococcus infection 234–5, **236**
　　malaria treatment 232
　　resistance 234–5
clonidine 434–5
clotting factors 122, 123
　　amniotic fluid embolism 304
　　disseminated intravascular coagulation
　　　　303
　　pregnancy levels 108, **132**
　　replacement 304
　　thrombosis risk 123
coagulation cascade 122, *305*
　　disseminated intravascular coagulation 302
　　dysregulation biomarkers 353
　　pregnancy 131, **132**
coagulopathy, amniotic fluid embolism 301
cocaine dependence 27
cognitive development, lead level risk 33
cognitive disorders, family history 41
cold-knife cone, cervical dysplasia treatment
　　272
color Doppler imaging
　　DVT 124–5
　　fetal echocardiography 51, Plate 6.2, Plate
　　　　6.3
　　placenta accreta 388
coma, eclampsia 285
combined spinal-epidural (CSE) approach
　　435
　　timing 436
comparative genomic hybridization 459–60
computed tomographic pulmonary
　　　　angiography, spiral (CTPA), pulmonary
　　　　embolism 126–7
condyloma lata 221
confidentiality, HIV infection 251
confined placental mosaicism 65
congenital cytomegalovirus (CMV) 226
congenital diaphragmatic hernia, fetoscopic
　　surgery 469–70
congenital heart block
　　risk **215**
　　systemic lupus erythematosus 212–13
congenital heart disease 133–4, 139–41
　　cardiac anomalies 139–41
　　　　risk 134
　　color Doppler imaging 51, Plate 6.2, Plate
　　　　6.3
　　counseling **53**
　　fetal echocardiography 48–51
　　　　expectations 51–3
　　fetal karyotyping **53**
　　maternal 133–4
　　screening 47–53
　　　　benefits 47
　　　　expectations 51–3
　　　　high-risk populations 48
　　　　low-risk populations 47
　　time of occurrence 52
　　valvular heart disease 134, **135**
congenital malformations
　　alcohol abuse 24
　　antiepileptic drugs 194, 195, **200**
　　asthma in pregnancy 184, 185
　　chorionic villus sampling 458
　　diabetes mellitus 174
　　discordance in multiple gestations 317–18
　　family history 41
　　fetal anticonvulsant syndrome 194, 195
　　monoamnionicity 318
　　oligohydramnios 332, 333
　　organic solvents 36
　　polyhydramnios 331
　　risk 134
　　see also neural tube defects
congenital pulmonary airway malformation
　　468
congenital rubella syndrome 220
congenital syphilis 222
congenital toxoplasmosis 223
congenital varicella 227

conjoined twins 314
connexin 43 351
　　preterm delivery 347
contraception
　　alcohol abuse 30
　　substance abuse 30
　　women on antiepileptic drugs 193, **194**
contraction stress test (CST) 79, 82–3
　　chronic hypertension 207
　　contraindications 82
cord entanglement 314, 316
　　monoamnionicity 318
cord occlusion techniques 317
cordocentesis, fetal thrombocytopenia 105
Cornelia de Lange syndrome **66**
coronary artery arteriosclerosis *166*
corticosteroids 6, 146
　　amniotic fluid embolism 302
　　congenital pulmonary airway malformation
　　　　468
　　fetal maturation 369
　　inhaled in asthma 187–8, 189, **190**
　　PPROM 369, **371**
　　preterm labor prevention 375–6, **380**
　　systemic in asthma 189
　　see also glucocorticoids
corticotrophin-releasing hormone (CRH) 347
cortisol 347
counseling
　　alcohol abuse 24
　　cardiac disease 131–4
　　carrier screening 43–4
　　chorionic villus sampling 459
　　congenital heart disease **53**
　　cytomegalovirus infection 227
　　Down syndrome 58–9
　　fetal aneuploidy 58–9
　　hysterotomy 465
　　multiple gestations 319, 320
　　posttest for HIV seropositive women 244
　　septated cystic hygroma **61**
　　substance abuse 24
　　systemic lupus erythematosus 213
　　toxoplasmosis prevention 223–4
　　transplant recipients 160
　　vaginal birth after cesarean delivery 419–20,
　　　　421
crew resource management, patient safety
　　441
crown-rump length 63
cryoprecipitate 304
Cushing syndrome, chronic hypertension 205
cyclo-oxygenase 2 (COX-2) 351
　　preterm delivery 347
cyclo-oxygenase (COX) inhibitors, preterm
　　　　labor prevention 378–9
cyclophosphamide, contraindication in
　　　　pregnancy 213, **214**
cyclosporine 162
cyclosporine A, tacrolimus 146
cystic fibrosis
　　carrier screening 42–3, 44, **45–6**
　　lung transplant 165
cystic hygroma
　　first trimester 57–8
　　septated 57, **61**, Plate 7.1
　　spontaneous abortion 261
cytogenetic diagnosis 453, 459
cytomegalovirus (CMV) 225–7
　　clinical manifestations 225–6
　　diagnosis 226
　　management 226–7
　　pathogenesis 225, *226*
　　prevention 227
　　transmission 225

D-dimer assays
　　deep vein thrombosis 124
　　pulmonary embolism 126
dacliximab 162
damage-associated molecular pattern
　　　　molecules (DAMPs) 349

decidua basalis 350
decidual-amnion-chorion inflammation,
　　preterm delivery 348–9
decidual hemorrhage, biomarkers 353
decubitus ulcers, women with physical
　　　　disabilities 254, 256
deep vein thrombosis 121
　　clinical presentation 124
　　D-dimer assays 124
　　diagnosis 124–5
　　diagnostic algorithm 125
　　treatment **128**
　　venous imaging 124–5
dehydroepiandrosterone sulfate (DHEAS) 347,
　　　　348
delivery
　　asthma in pregnancy 189–90
　　chronic hypertension 207
　　epilepsy 198–9
　　estimated date 391, *392*
　　five-minute rule *305*
　　gestational diabetes 171
　　HELLP syndrome 284–5
　　HIV infection *251*
　　multiple gestations 322, **323**
　　placenta previa 385
　　preeclampsia 282–3, **287**
　　preterm labor 380
　　seizures during 198
　　sickle cell disease 95
　　timing in prolonged pregnancy 393
　　women with physical disabilities 256, **258**
　　see also breech delivery; cesarean delivery;
　　　　preterm delivery
delta virus infection **239**, 240
dental amalgam, mercury exposure 35
depression
　　postpartum 254, 434
　　preterm delivery 346–7
　　recurrent spontaneous abortion 266
　　women with physical disabilities 254
　　see also postpartum depression
desamino-8-D-arginine vasopressin (DDAVP)
　　151
development, fetal, alcohol/substance abuse
　　effects 26
dexamethasone 181
　　preterm labor prevention 375–6
diabetes mellitus 174–6
　　chronic hypertension 205
　　congenital malformations 174
　　dietary management 169–70, **176**
　　evaluation 174–5
　　glucose control in pregnancy 77
　　management during pregnancy 176
　　maternal glycemia regulation 175
　　multifetal pregnancy 13
　　pancreatic transplant patients 163–4
　　perinatal intervention 387.121
　　perinatal mortality 174
　　polyhydramnios 331
　　screening in pregnancy 168–9
　　treatment 169–70
　　weight gain during pregnancy 8
　　see also gestational diabetes
diabetic nephropathy **158**
diet
　　diabetes mellitus management **176**
　　gestational diabetes management 169–70
dietary recommendations
　　lactation 10, 18–19
　　pregnancy 10, 18–19, **20**
diethylstilbestrol (DES), *in utero* exposure 272
diltiazem, hypertension treatment 155
dioxin toxicity **37**
disseminated intravascular coagulation (DIC)
　　　　122, 301, 302–3
　　blood product replacement 303–4
　　platelet transfusion 304
disulfiram 27
DNA, free fetal 309
DNA analysis 461

DNA sequencing 43
Doppler ultrasound
    clinical application 69–71
    fetal arterial 67–8
    fetal growth restriction 67–71
    fetal venous 68–9, *70*
    see also color Doppler imaging
Doppler velocimetry 79, 83, **86**
    chronic hypertension 207
    middle cerebral circulation 67, 308–9, 310,
        312
    multiple gestations 322
Down syndrome
    cardiac malformations 58
    combined first-trimester serum and
        sonographic screening 57
    contingent screening 60
    counseling 58–9
    detection 320
    first-trimester sonographic screening 55–7
    frontomaxillary facial angle measurement
        56
    hCG screening 57
    integrated screening 59–60
    minor markers 58, **59**
    nasal bone absence/hypoplasia 58
    nuchal fold thickening 58
    nuchal translucency measurement 55–7
    screening 55–60, **61**
        combined first- and second-trimester
            59–60
        multiple gestations 60
        second-trimester serum 59
        second-trimester sonographic 58–9
        sequential 60
    septated cystic hygroma 57
    tricuspid regurgitation 56
    triple screen 59
Dubowitz syndrome, IUGR **66**
Duchenne muscular dystrophy 42
ductal arch, fetal echocardiography Plate 6.1
ductus arteriosus, patent 52
    maternal 139–40
ductus venosus
    Doppler waveform 67
        reverse flow 67, 69, **71**
    flow 56, Plate 7.1, Plate 7.2
Dutch famine, World War II 8
dyspnea of pregnancy 185

Ebstein anomaly, maternal 140
echocardiogram
    pregnancy **132**
    pulmonary embolism 125, 127
    see also fetal echocardiography
eclampsia 285–7
    blood pressure control 286
    coma 285
    definition 285–6
    diagnosis 286
    labor 286
    magnesium sulfate 286, 287
    management 286–7
    seizures 285, 286
    symptoms 286
    transplant patients 165
    uterine activity 286–7
edema, nephrotic syndrome 152–3
Eisenmenger syndrome
    lung transplant 165
    maternal 140
electrocardiogram (ECG)
    pregnancy **132**
    pulmonary embolism 125
emergency care 301–5, **306**
emphysema, lung transplant 165
encephalomalacia, multicystic 317
end-stage renal disease, maternal 154, *155*
endocrinopathies, spontaneous abortion
    262–3
endoglin 281
endomysial antibodies 262

endothelial cell protein C receptor (EPCR)
    123
energy
    requirement in pregnancy 6
    supplementation 14
enoxaparin, factor V Leiden mutation 264
environmental agents 32–6, **37**
    adverse outcome incidence 32
    animal studies 32
    epidemiologic studies 32
    toxicity 32, **33**
        principles 33
environmental factors, systemic lupus
        erythematosus 209
enzymatic analysis 461
epidural analgesia 435, **437**
    patient-controlled 435–6
    vaginal birth after cesarean delivery 419,
        435
epidural anesthesia 436, 437
    asthma 190
    pulmonary hypertension 140
epilepsy, maternal 193–200
    antiepileptic drug management 197–8
    delivery 198–9
    fetal anticonvulsant syndrome 193–5
    labor 198–9
    neurodevelopmental outcome 196
    obstetric complications 198
    postpartum care 199
    prenatal screening 195–6
    seizures during pregnancy 196–7
epinephrine 434–5
Epstein–Barr virus (EBV) 226
ergometrine, uterine atony 290
erythroblastosis fetalis 331
erythromycin
    group B streptococcus infection 234–5, **236**
    resistance 234–5
erythropoiesis, fetal 310
erythropoietin, iron deficiency anemia 100
Escherichia coli 348
    risk with amniocentesis 455
esmolol 181
estimate of date of delivery (EDD) 391, 392
estrogen receptor β (ER-β) 348
ethylenediaminetetraacetic acid (EDTA)
        therapy for lead toxicity 34
evidence-based perinatology 3
exercise, gestational diabetes management
        170
external cephalic version (ECV) 424

factor V Leiden mutation 108
    inherited thrombophilia 109–10, 263–4
factor VIIa, recombinant 304, *305*
factor VIII, activated, postpartum hemorrhage
        295
factor Xa, protein Z-dependent protease
        inhibitor 111
famciclovir, herpes simplex virus 225
familial dysautonomia, carrier screening 44,
        45, **46**
family history, genetic screening 41
Fanconi anemia
    carrier screening 43, 45
    IUGR **66**
    type C 43
3-N fatty acids
    maternal nutrition 17
    preterm birth 339
febrile paroxysms, malaria 231, 232
femur length 63
fetal activity, monitoring in maternal asthma
        187
fetal alcohol syndrome 24
fetal anomalies
    alcohol abuse 24
    polyhydramnios 331
    see also congenital malformations
fetal anticonvulsant syndrome 193–5
fetal condition, comprehensive evaluation 1, 3

fetal demise
    after PPROM 366
    malaria 232
    preeclampsia **450–1**
    twin pregnancy **472**
    see also intrauterine fetal death (IUFD)
fetal distress, cesarean delivery 410
fetal echocardiography
    color Doppler imaging 51, Plate 6.3
    congenital heart disease screening 48
    four-chamber view 48–9, *50*, 51–2,
        Plate 6.3
    technique 48–51
    three-vessel view 53
    two-dimensional cross-sectional imaging 48,
        49, 50–1, Plate 6.1
    ventricular outflow tracts 49–51, 52–3
fetal fibronectin (fFN) 321, 351, 352
    preterm delivery marker 353–5
    preterm labor 375
fetal growth
    curves 5, 64
    discordant 316, 322, **334**
    maternal nutrition 4–7
    monitoring in maternal asthma 187
    multiple gestations 316
    placenta role 5–6
    systemic lupus erythematosus 213
    velocity 5
fetal growth restriction
    multifetal pregnancy 13
    see also intrauterine growth restriction
        (IUGR)
fetal heart rate tracing (FHT) 80
    contraction stress test 82
    evaluation frequency 89
    interpretation 89–91
        guidelines 89
    see also heart rate, fetal
fetal intervention guided by sonography 471,
    472
fetal karyotype 43
    congenital heart disease **53**
    recurrent spontaneous abortion 266
fetal loss
    antiepileptic drug exposure 196
    antiphospholipid antibodies 115
    antiphospholipid antibody syndrome 265
    inherited thrombophilias 113, 116
    multiple gestations 316–17
    twin effect on surviving fetus 317
    see also fetal demise; intrauterine fetal death
        (IUFD); miscarriage
fetal maturation, corticosteroids 369
fetal monitoring
    standardization of electronic monitoring
        441–2
    see also antepartum fetal monitoring
fetal movements 79–80
    assessment in chronic hypertension 207
fetal stress, preterm delivery 346–8
fetal surveillance, antenatal 392–3
fetal weight
    discordant **334**
    estimation 64
    prolonged pregnancy 392
fetomaternal transfusion, amniocentesis 454
fetoscopic surgery 468–71
    congenital diaphragmatic hernia 469–70
    indications 469–71
    percutaneous 469
    twin–twin transfusion syndrome 469, 470
    urinary tract obstruction 470–1
fetus
    alcohol effects 23–4, **25**, 26
    genotype 348
    placenta previa complications 384–5
    substances of abuse effects 23–4, **25**, 26
    surgery 464–71, **472**
    swallowing 329
    teratogenic effects 24, **25**
    see also antepartum fetal monitoring

fibrin plug formation 122
fibrinogen, pregnancy levels 108, **109**, 131
fibrinolysis 123
fibronectin, fetal levels 321, 351, 352
    preterm delivery marker 353–5
    preterm labor 375
fish consumption, mercury exposure 34–5, **37**
fluid administration, postpartum hemorrhage 295, 297, **298**
fluoride toxicity 18
fms-like tyrosine kinase 1, soluble (sFlt-1):placental growth factor (PLGF) ratio 281
foam stability index (FSI) 76
folate
    maternal nutrition 16–17
    recommended dietary allowance 16
folate deficiency 16–17
    macrocytic anemia 99
    meiotic nondisjunction 261
    neural tube defects 16, 17
    risk **20**
folic acid supplementation 16–17
    women with epilepsy 196
    women with spina bifida 257
folinic acid, toxoplasmosis treatment 223
foramen ovale, patent 49, 52
forced expiratory volume in 1 sec (FEV$_1$) 185
forceps delivery 429, 430, 431, **433**
fragile X syndrome, carrier screening 42–3
fresh frozen plasma (FFP)
    amniotic fluid embolism 304
    postpartum hemorrhage 295, **298**
frontomaxillary facial (FMF) angle 56

Gardnerella vaginalis 348, 349
Gaucher disease, carrier screening 45
gender, fetal lung maturity 76
general anesthesia 437
generalized tonic-clonic seizures 197
    during labor 199
genetic disorders, discordance in multiple gestations 317–18
genetic evaluation, sickle cell disease 95–6
genetic factors
    preterm delivery 347
    recurrent spontaneous abortion 260–2, **266**
    systemic lupus erythematosus 209
genetic screening
    carrier screening 42–4
    family history 41
    Mendelian disorders 41–5, **45–6**
    newborn screening 45
    partner testing **45–6**
    preconception/prenatal 42
    prenatal diagnosis 45
genetic syndromes, IUGR 65, **66**
genetics, preimplantation 3
genital herpes, recurrent 224
germline mosaicism 42
gestational age
    adverse perinatal outcomes 66
    chronic hypertension 207
    estimates 8, 63–4
        accuracy 77
    labor induction 400, **401**
    overestimation 63
    prolonged pregnancy 395
gestational diabetes 168–71, **172**
    antenatal testing 170–1
    delivery 171
    dietary management 169–70
    exercise management 170
    familial diabetes **172**
    fetal lung maturity **77**
    high risk women 169
    insulin resistance 170
    macrosomia 171
    multiple gestations **323**
        maternal complications 318, **319**
    obesity 11–12

postpartum management 171
relative insulin deficiency 170
shoulder dystocia 171
treatment 169–70
gestational hypertension 280
    etiology 281
    lead level risk 33
    management 281–2
    maternal complications with multiple gestations 319
    pathophysiology 281
    perinatal outcome 281
    postpartum management 283–4
gestational sac, measurement 63
gestational thrombocytopenia 102, **106**
gestational transient thyrotoxicosis 180
glomerular filtration rate (GFR) 152
    renal transplantation 163
glucocorticoids
    idiopathic thrombocytopenic purpura 103
    systemic lupus erythematosus 213, **214**
    see also corticosteroids
glucose challenge test (GCT) 168, 169, **172**
glucose tolerance, impaired 169, 171, **172**
glucose tolerance testing (GTT)
    gestational diabetes **172**
    pancreatic transplant patients 164
    see also oral glucose tolerance test (OGTT)
glyburide 170
glycemia, maternal regulation 175
glycoprotein (GP) Ib/IX/V receptor 121
glycoprotein (GP) IIb/IIIa 121
glycosuria 151–2
goiter 178
Graves disease 179, 180
    follow-up 181
group B streptococcal (GBS) infection 234–6, 237
    antibiotic prophylaxis 234–5
    bacteriuria 236
    epidemiology 234
    immunization 3
    intrapartum prophylaxis 367
    isolation of bacterium 234
    perinatal 234
    PPROM 235–6, 237
        evaluation 366
        management 369
    prevention 235
    prophylaxis 234–5, 236, 237
        preterm labor 377
growth curves, fetal 5, 64

Hashimoto thyroiditis 178
head circumference 63
head circumference:abdominal circumference ratio 5
hearing loss, sensorineural in infant 310
heart, fetal
    normal anatomy 48
    see also congenital heart disease; heart defects
heart defects
    prenatal diagnosis 47
    screening 47–53
heart failure
    sickle cell disease 95
    thyroid storm 180–1
heart-lung transplantation 165
heart rate, fetal
    accelerations 90
    category I 90, **91**
    category II and III 90–1
    decelerations 90, **91**
    evaluation 89–91
    monitoring 419
    pattern definitions 90–1
    variability 67, 90, **91**
    see also fetal heart rate tracing (FHT)
heart rate, maternal in pregnancy *132*
heart valves, mechanical 137–9

HELLP syndrome 284–5
    cesarean delivery 284, **285**
    delivery 284–5
    liver transplantation 164
    management 284–5
    multiple gestations **323**
        maternal complications 319
    perinatal outcome 284–5
    platelet count 284–5
    platelet transfusion 304
    postpartum management 285
    symptoms 284
    systemic lupus erythematosus differential diagnosis 211
    thrombocytopenia 103
    transplant patients 165
hematocrit, pregnancy *132*
hemoglobin, levels in anemia 98
hemoglobin, maternal glycosylated (HbA$_{1c}$) 174, **175**
hemoglobin C 93
hemoglobin S 93
hemoglobin SC disease 93, 94, **95**
hemoglobin SS disease 93, 94, **95**, **96**
hemoglobinopathies, carrier screening 42–3, 44
hemolysis, elevated liver enzymes, and low platelet count *see* HELLP syndrome
hemolytic disease of the fetus and newborn (HDFN) 307
    end-stage 308
    non-RhD antibodies 310, **311**
    RhD antibodies 307–10
hemophilia 42
    recombinant factor VIIa 304, *305*
hemosiderin, decidual 350
hemostasis
    coagulation cascade 122
    endogenous anticoagulants 122–3
    fibrinolysis 123
    physiology 121–3
    platelet plug formation 121–2
heparin
    antiphospholipid antibody syndrome 108, 116, 215, 265, 266
    disseminated intravascular coagulation 303
    factor V Leiden mutation **116**, 264
    mechanical heart valves 138–9
    peripartum cardiomyopathy 142
hepatic steatosis syndrome 245
hepatitis 238–9, **240**
hepatitis A 238, **239**
hepatitis B 239–40, **241**
    vaccine 240
hepatitis C 239, 240, **241**
    hepatitis B association 239
    liver transplant patients 164
    substance abuse 30
hepatitis D 239, 240, **241**
hepatitis E 238–9
hepatitis G **239**, 240
herbicides, toxicity 35
herpes simplex virus (HSV) 224–5
    neonatal 224
    PPROM 370
herpes zoster infections 227
highly active antiretroviral therapy (HAART) 245, 250, **251**
HIV infection 243–5, **246–9**, 250–1
    breastfeeding recommendations 250
    care of seropositive women 244–5
    confidentiality 251
    delivery **251**
    drug therapy 245, **246–9**
    ethical considerations 250–1
    hepatitis B association 239
    identification of infected patients 243–4
    immunization 3
    labor 250, **251**
    legal considerations 250–1
    membrane rupture 250

mother-to-child transmission prevention 244, 250
  opt-out process for testing 243
  PPROM 370
  rapid tests 244
  resistance testing 244
  responsibility to patient 251
  seropositive women posttest counseling 244
  substance abuse 30
homocysteine 112
hormonal factors, systemic lupus erythematosus 209
HPA-1a antigen 104
HPA-1a gene 104, **106**
human chorionic gonadotrophin (hCG)
  Down syndrome screening 57, 59, 320
  elevated maternal serum **71**
  free β-subunit 57
  maternal screening with renal disease 157
human leukocyte antigens (HLA), recurrent spontaneous abortion 265, 266
human placental lactogen 5, 6
human platelet antigen (HPA) 104
humeral length 63
Huntington procedure 297
Huntington's disease, carrier screening 42–3
hydralazine **181**
  chronic hypertension treatment 206
  preeclampsia **287**
hydration, maternal
  oligohydramnios 334
  preterm labor 377
hydrocephalus 261
hydrops 261
  congenital pulmonary airway malformation 468
  polyhydramnios 331
  RhD alloimmunization outcome 310
15-hydroxy-prostaglandin dehydrogenase (PGDH) 348–9
hydroxychloroquine 213, **214**
1,25-hydroxycholecalciferol 16
17α-hydroxyprogesterone caproate 341, 342, **342**, 365
hyperaldosteronism, chronic hypertension 205
hypercoagulability, pregnancy-associated 123
hyperhomocystinemia 108
  inherited thrombophilias 112
hyperprolactinemia, recurrent spontaneous abortion 262–3
hypertension, maternal
  cardiac transplant patient **166**
  chronic 204–7, **208**
    antepartum fetal evaluation 207
    classification 204
    diagnosis 204
    differential diagnosis 205
    evaluation 205
    indications for delivery 207
    major catastrophic events 207
    postpartum follow-up 207
    preconceptual therapy 204–5
    with renal insufficiency 154–5
    treatment 205–7, **208**
  essential **208**
  fetal monitoring **86**
  hypothyroidism **181**
  obesity 11–12
  paroxysmal 205
  postpartum management **208**
  renal transplantation patients 163
  sickle cell disease 95, **96**
  transplant patients 165
  see also gestational hypertension
hypertensive crises 205
hyperthyroidism, maternal 179–81
  diagnosis 180
  follow-up 181
  management 180–1
  presentation 180
  treatment 180–1
hypocalciuria 15

hyponatremia, labor induction 402
hypophysectomy 178
hypospadias, glandular 195
hypotension, labor induction 402
hypothalamic–pituitary–adrenal (HPA) axis, placental-fetal 347
hypothermia, hypoxic ischemic encephalopathy 450
hypothyroidism, maternal 178–9, **181**
  diagnosis 178–9
  follow-up 179
  management 179
  postpartum thyroiditis 181
  presentation 178
  subclinical 179
  treatment 179
hypoxemia 68–9
  fetal adaptation 70
hypoxia
  amniotic fluid embolism 301
  intrapartum 445–6
hypoxic ischemic encephalopathy 445
  hypothermia 450
  uterine rupture 417
  vaginal birth after cesarean delivery 420
hysterectomy
  adherent placenta 294
  postpartum hemorrhage 292–3
  uterine rupture 417
hysterotomy 464–8
  benefits 464–7
  cesarean section in subsequent pregnancies 465
  closure 466–7
    cesarean delivery 407–8
  congenital pulmonary airway malformation 468
  counseling 465
  indications 467–8
  myelomeningocele 468
  postoperative recovery 467
  risks 464–7
  sacrococcygeal teratoma 468
  technique 465–7

idiopathic thrombocytopenic purpura (ITP) 102–3
  delivery route 104
  splenectomy 103
immunity, adaptive/innate 348
immunoglobulin E (IgE), asthma during pregnancy 184
immunologic disorders
  alloimmune thrombocytopenia 104
  recurrent spontaneous abortion 265–6
  see also autoimmune conditions
immunosuppressive agents 146
  effects on baby 166
  transplant patients 161–2, 164
incontinentia pigmenti 261
indomethacin 190
  cervical insufficiency 277
  polyhydramnios 332
  preterm labor prevention 378–9, **380**
infections
  asthma during pregnancy 184
  intraamniotic 374
  intrauterine subclinical 272, 274
  neonatal 164
  perinatal 218–28
  PPROM risk 365, 370
  preterm birth 339
  preterm delivery 347
  recurrent spontaneous abortion 262
  risk with amniocentesis 455
  see also named conditions and diseases; viral infections
inferior vena cava, Doppler waveform reverse flow 69, *70*
inflammation
  cervical length 340
  decidual-amnion-chorion 348–9

informed consent, vaginal birth after cesarean delivery 420
inhibin-A, Down syndrome screening 59
inotropic agents **145**
Institute of Medicine (IOM) guidelines for weight gain in pregnancy **10**, 12
insulin
  gestational diabetes levels 170
  during labor 176
  management during labor 176
  maternal glycemia regulation 175
  postpartum requirement 175
insulin resistance 168
  gestational diabetes 170
integrase inhibitors 245, **249**
interleukin 8 (IL-8), preterm delivery 347, 349, 350, 351, 352
internal iliac artery embolization in postpartum hemorrhage 293, 295
interpregnancy interval, vaginal birth after cesarean delivery 418
intracranial aneurysm rupture risk 139
intracranial hemorrhage (ICH), fetal thrombocytopenia 104, 105
intracranial translucency (IT) 61
intramembranous (IM) pathway 329
intrauterine fetal death (IUFD) 79, 314
  antepartum testing 79–81
  fetal movement decrease 79–80
  maternal complications with multiple gestations 319
  monoamnionicity 318
  multiple gestations 317
  nonstress test 80
  risk 79
  see also fetal demise
intrauterine growth restriction (IUGR) 64–71
  antiphospholipid antibodies 115
  antiphospholipid antibody syndrome 265
  asthma in pregnancy 186
  asymmetric 65
  definition 64, **65**
  diagnosis 64, **86**
  Doppler ultrasound 67–71
  immunosuppressive agents 166
  inherited thrombophilias 112
  liver transplantation 164
  malaria 232
  management 66–71
  monoamnionicity 318
  multiple gestations 316, 322
  neonatal encephalopathy 447
  oligohydramnios 333
  outcome 65–6
  risk factors 65
  symmetric 65
  systemic lupus erythematosus 212, **215**
  systolic:diastolic ratio 83
  vascular adaptation late-stage changes 69–70
  vascular bed deterioration 70
  women with physical disabilities 256
intrauterine transfusion 1
  RhD alloimmunization 310, **312**
intravascular transfusion (IVT), RBCs 310
intravenous immunoglobulin (IVIG)
  antiphospholipid antibody syndrome 215
  idiopathic thrombocytopenic purpura 103
intraventricular hemorrhage (IVH)
  magnesium sulfate for prevention 448–9
  prevention with corticosteroids 375–6
iodide 180–1
iodine
  endemic deficiency 178
  toxicity 17
iron
  requirements in pregnancy 14
  toxicity 17
iron deficiency anemia 14–15
  blood transfusion 100
  diagnosis 14–15
  erythropoietin 100

iron deficiency anemia (*cont.*)
    microcytic 99
    prevalence 14
    prophylaxis 99
    treatment 99–100
iron supplementation
    dosage 100
    intravenous 100
    maternal nutrition 14–15
    normocytic anemia **100**
    oral preparations 99, **100**

Jarisch-Herxheimer reaction 222
Jewish heritage, Eastern European
    carrier screening 42, **43**, 44–5, **45–6**
    Fanconi anemia type C carrier screening 43
Johanson-Blizzard syndrome **66**

karyotype *see* fetal karyotype
Kell antibodies 310, **311**
ketamine, epidural anesthesia 190
ketorolac, postoperative analgesia 437
kick counts 79–80
kidney, anatomic changes in pregnancy 152
killer cell immunoglobulin-like receptors (KIR) 265–6
Korotkoff sounds 204
kyphoscoliosis, posttraumatic 256

labetalol 181
    hypertension treatment 155, 206
labor
    analgesia 434–6
    asthma in pregnancy 189–90
    augmentation in vaginal birth after cesarean delivery 419
    dystocia 392
    eclampsia 286
    epilepsy 198–9
    failure to progress 409–10
    fetal condition continuous readout 3
    HIV infection 250, **251**
    insulin management in diabetes mellitus 176
    management for breech delivery 426
    polyhydramnios 331
    protracted **297**
        prolonged pregnancy 392
    seizures during 199
    sickle cell disease 95
    women with physical disabilities 256, **258**
    see also preterm labor
labor induction 399–404
    amniotic fluid embolism 403
    cesarean delivery following failed induction 400
    complications 402–3
    contraindications 399, **400**
    elective 399–400
    failed 402–3
    hyponatremia 402
    hypotension 402
    indications 399, **400**
    management 403–4
    maternal risks 400–1
    oxytocin 402
    pediatric issues 400–1
    postterm 395
    preeclampsia **443**
    preinduction assessment 401
    prior cesarean delivery 403–4
    sonographic cervical length measurement 402
    success prediction 401–2
    unfavourable cervix 403
    uterine overactivity 402
    uterine rupture 403
    vaginal birth after cesarean delivery 418–19
lactation
    dietary recommendations **10**, 18–19
    maternal nutrition 18
    multivitamin supplements 11
    see also breastfeeding

lactic acidosis 245
lamellar body count (LBC) 75, 76
lamivudine **246**, 250
lamotrigine 195, 196, 197, **200**
large for gestational age, vaginal birth after cesarean delivery 416
laser cone, cervical dysplasia treatment 272
lead toxicity 33–4
lecithin:sphingomyelin ratio 75
leflunomide 162
left ventricular failure, amniotic fluid embolism 302
left ventricular filling, mitral stenosis 135
lemon sign 61
leukotriene receptor antagonists 188
levothyroxine 179, **181**
limb abnormalities
    amniocentesis 456
    chorionic villus sampling 458
liver transplant patients 164
local anesthetics 434
loop electrosurgical excision procedure (LEEP), cervical dysplasia treatment 272
low birthweight infants, asthma in pregnancy 184
lung transplantation 165
lungs, fetal
    congenital pulmonary airway malformation 468
    fluid 328–9
    hypoplastic 470
    tracheal occlusion 470
lungs, fetal maturity 75–7, 367, 374
    cascade tests 76
    diabetes mellitus 176
    gestational diabetes **77**
    indications for assessment 75
    labor induction 400, **401**
    multiple tests 76
    predictive value of tests 76
    reduction in testing 77
    testing in gestational diabetes 171
lupus anticoagulant 214, 264
lupus flares 210, 211–12
    diagnosis 213
lupus nephritis, maternal 156, **158**
lupus nephropathy 212
lupus syndrome, neonatal 210
    systemic lupus erythematosus impact 212
lymphocytic hypophysitis 178

macrocytic anemia 98–9
    folate deficiency 99
macrosomia
    diabetes mellitus 176
    excessive weight gain in pregnancy 19
    gestational diabetes 171
    labor induction 400
    prolonged pregnancy 392
    vaginal birth after cesarean delivery 416
magnesium
    maternal nutrition 15–16
    toxicity 17, **286**
magnesium sulfate
    cerebral palsy prophylaxis 376, 448–50
    dosage in renal disease 157
    eclampsia 286, 287
    neuroprotection
        preterm birth 449–50
        preterm labor 376
    preeclampsia **287**
    preterm labor 190, 338, 376, 379
    seizure prophylaxis **181**
        eclampsia 286
    tocolysis **342**
magnetic resonance imaging (MRI), placenta accreta 388
magnetic resonance (MR) venography, DVT 124–5
malaria 231–2, **232–3**
    clinical features 231
    complications 232

diagnosis 231–2
    prevention 232
    treatment 232
malpresentation
    cesarean delivery 410
    see also breech delivery
Marfan syndrome, maternal 141
marine oils, maternal nutrition 17
maternal conditions 9–13
maternal mortality 131, **133**
    cesarean delivery 406
    Eisenmenger syndrome 140
maternal serum α-fetoprotein (MSAFP), placenta accreta 388
maternal stress, preterm delivery 346–8
matrix metalloproteinases (MMPs) 351
    decidual 350
    preterm delivery 347
McDonald procedure for cerclage 273–4, **278**
measles, mumps and rubella (MMR) vaccination 221
meconium aspiration syndrome, prolonged pregnancy 392
meiotic errors 460
meiotic nondisjunction, folate deficiency 261
meiotic rescue 461
membrane rupture
    HIV infection 250
    polyhydramnios 331
Mendelian diagnosis 453
Mendelian disorders
    carrier screening 42–4
    genetic screening 41–5, **45–6**
    newborn screening 45
    partner testing **45–6**
    prenatal diagnosis 45
Mendelian inheritance 41–2
meperidine 198
mercury toxicity 34–5, **37**
metformin 170
methacholine challenge test 185
methadone 26, 27
methimazole 180
methotrexate contraindication 213, **214**
α-methyldopa 155
methylergonovine 290
microcephaly, *in utero* antiepileptic drug exposure 196
microcytic anemia 99
micturition, fetal 328
middle cerebral circulation
    Doppler ultrasound 68
    Doppler velocimetry 67, 308–9, 310, **312**
    impedance 67
mineral intake, toxicity 17–18
minimal change disease 153
miscarriage
    amniocentesis-induced 455–6
    chorionic villus sampling 457–8
    lead level risk 33
    malaria 232
    sporadic 260
    see also abortion; fetal loss
misoprostol
    postpartum hemorrhage **298**
    uterine atony 291
    uterine rupture 403
mite allergy **190**
mitotic errors 460–1
mitral stenosis 135–6
mitral valve prolapse 136
mobility, women with physical disabilities 254
molar pregnancy, chronic hypertension 205
molybdenum toxicity 17
monoamnionicity 318
monochorionic diamniotic placentation 315, 316
monochorionicity
    complications 314, 317, 318
    fetal intervention guided by sonography 471
monozygosity, fertility treatment 318
mosaicism, placental confined 460–1

MTHFR A1298C gene, inherited
    thrombophilias 112
MTHFR C677T gene
    cerebral palsy 445
    inherited thrombophilias 112
mucolipidosis type IV, carrier screening 45
multifetal pregnancy reduction (MPR) 317,
    319–20, **323**
    elective first-trimester 315
multiorgan damage, multiple gestations
    317
multiple gestations 314–22, **323**
    amniocentesis 454
    anatomic abnormalities 320–1
    antenatal surveillance 322
    antepartum management 319–20
    back-bleeding of dead fetus 317
    cervical cerclage 321
    chorionicity 315–16
    chromosome abnormalities 320
    delivery 322, **323**
    discordant anatomic abnormalities 317–18
    Doppler velocimetry 322
    Down syndrome screening 60
    embryology 315
    fetal complications 316–18
    fetal loss 316–17
    gestational diabetes 318, **319**, **323**
    HELLP syndrome 319, **323**
    intrapartum period 322
    intrauterine growth restriction 316, 322
    maternal obstetric complications 318–19
    multiorgan damage 317
    neurologic impairment 314–15
    nuchal translucency measurement 60, 320
    nutritional requirements 13
    oligohydramnios 334
    perinatal mortality 395–6
    perinatal outcomes 314–15
    postterm 395–6
    prenatal diagnosis 320–1
    preterm delivery 317
        prevention 321
    preterm labor 317
    ultrasound **322**
    zygosity 315–16
    see also twin pregnancy
multiple sclerosis 253
    women with physical disabilities 256
multivitamin supplements 11
    containing folic acid 17
    maternal nutrition 13–14
muscle cramp **128**
mycophenolate mofetil 146, 162
    embryopathy 162, Plate 19.1
Mycoplasma hominis 348, 349
myelomeningocele, hysterotomy indication
    467–8
myometrium, overstretched in
    polyhydramnios 331

naltrexone 27
nasal bone absence/hypoplasia, Down
    syndrome 58
National Quality Forum (NQF) consensus
    standards 440
natural killer (NK) cells 265–6
necrotizing enterocolitis 376
Neisseria gonorrhoeae 365, 366
neonatal alloimmune thrombocytopenia
    (NAIT) 104–5, **106**
neonatal encephalopathy 445
    antecedents 446
    brain imaging 448
    brain injury patterns 448
    definition 445
    differential diagnosis **446**
    genetic factors 446
    IUGR 447
    preeclampsia and fetal demise **450–1**
    risk factors 446, 447
    task force 447–8

watershed injury pattern 448
    see also hypoxic ischemic encephalopathy
neonatal infections, liver transplantation 164
neonatal lupus syndrome 210
    systemic lupus erythematosus impact 212
neonatal mortality
    breech delivery 425
    prevention with corticosteroids 375–6
    prolonged pregnancy 392, *394*
neonatal outcome 387.121
neonates
    death with preterm birth 337
    herpes simplex virus 224
    vitamin K deficiency 198
    weight in prolonged pregnancy 392
neostigmine 435
nephrotic syndrome, maternal 152–3
    management 153
    thromboembolism risk 157
Neu-Laxova syndrome, IUGR 66
neural tube defects
    antiepileptic drugs 194, 195
    diagnosis 453
    drug-induced 16
    folate deficiency 16, 17, **20**
    intracranial translucency 61
    screening 55, 60–1
        multiple gestations 320
neurologic impairment, multiple gestations
    314–15
nevirapine **247**
    contraindication in pregnancy 245
New York Heart Association classification,
    cardiac disease 131, **132**
Niemann-Pick disease type A, carrier screening
    45
nifedipine
    eclampsia management 287
    hypertension treatment 206
    preterm labor prevention 378
nitric oxide, exhaled (eNO) 185
non-steroidal anti-inflammatory drugs
    (NSAIDs)
    postoperative analgesia 437
    systemic lupus erythematosus 213, **214**
nonnucleoside reverse transcriptase inhibitors
    (NNRTIs) 245, **247**, 250
nonstress test (NST) 79, 80, **86**
    with Amniotic Fluid Index 81
    biophysical profile 81
    diabetes mellitus 176, **176**
    gestational diabetes 171
    nonreactive 80
    prolonged labor prevention 393
    systemic lupus erythematosus 213
nontechnical surgical skills (NOTSS) for
    operative vaginal delivery 431–2
Noonan syndrome, IUGR 66
NPH insulin, maternal glycemia regulation
    175
nuchal fold thickening 58
nuchal translucency (NT)
    cystic hygroma Plate 7.1
    measurement 55–7, **61**
        multifetal pregnancy 60, 320
        septated cystic hygroma 57–8
    nuchal translucency (NT) sonography 55–7
        Down syndrome 57
        with serum assays 59
nucleoside reverse transcriptase inhibitors
    (NRTIs) 245, **246–7**, 250
nutriments, transfer to fetus 5, 6
nutrition, maternal 4–20
    breastfeeding 18
    dietary recommendations for pregnancy/
        lactation **10**, 18–19
    distribution 6
    fetal growth 4–7
    fetal growth curves 5
    maternal conditions 9–13
    multifetal pregnancy 13
    nutritional assessment 9–11

nutritional interventions 13–18
    pregnancy outcome 4
    records of food intake 10–11
nutritional assessment
    24-hour recall method 9–10
    maternal nutrition 9–11
    standardized survey 10
    see also nutrition, maternal
nutritional growth restriction 5
nutritional interventions, maternal nutrition
    13–18

obesity
    gestational diabetes 11–12
    hypertension 11–12
    pregnancy outcome 11–13
    small for gestational age infants 12
    women with physical disabilities 254
    wound infections 12
obstetric hospitalist 441
obstetric patient safety committee 441
oligohydramnios 332–4
    associations 333–4
    clinical significance 332–3
    congenital malformations 332, 333
    definition 332
    diagnosis 332
    fetal urinary system malformation 328
    idiopathic 333
    IUGR 333
    management 334
    multiple gestations 334
    postdate pregnancy 333
    preterm premature rupture of membranes
        333
    scoring system 332
    twin pregnancy 333–4, **334**
    twin-twin transfusion syndrome diagnosis
        470
    umbilical artery end-diastolic flow 68
omega-3 fatty acids 17
    preterm birth 339
opiates
    dependence 26–7
    postoperative analgesia 437
opioids 434
oral glucose tolerance test (OGTT) 169
    diabetes mellitus **176**
    postpartum in gestational diabetes 171
organic solvents, toxicity 36
oxygen, transfer to fetus 5, 6
oxygen supplementation, asthma in pregnancy
    189
oxytocin
    adherent placenta 290
    labor induction 402
    postpartum hemorrhage 290
    uterine atony 290
    uterine rupture 403, 419
oxytocin receptor, preterm delivery 347
oxytocin receptor antagonists 379

P-selectins 122
packed red blood cells (PRBC) 303
    amniotic fluid embolism 304
pain
    unrelieved 434
    see also analgesia, obstetric
pancreatic transplant patients 163–4
paradoxical embolism, maternal 139
parathyroid hormone (PTH) 15
parenting, women with physical disabilities
    255
parvovirus B$_{19}$ 218–20, **228**
    clinical manifestations 218
    diagnosis 218–19
    management 219–20
    transmission 218
pathogen-associated molecular pathogens
    (PAMPs) 348, 349
patient-controlled analgesia, intravenous,
    postoperative analgesia 437

patient-controlled epidural analgesia 435–6
  postoperative analgesia 437
patient education, asthma during pregnancy
    187, **190**
patient safety 439–42, **443**
  Adverse Outcome Index 439–40, 442, *443*
  amniocentesis 454–5
  anonymous event reporting system 441, **443**
  checklists 440–1
  chorionic villus sampling 458–9
  computerized order entry 441
  crew resource management 441
  culture measures 440
  evidence for improvement tools 442
  guidelines 440–1, 442
  induction for preeclampsia **443**
  measurement 439–40
  obstetric hospitalist 441
  obstetric patient safety committee 441
  outcome measures 439–40
  outside expert review 440
  perinatal patient safety nurse 441
  process measures 440
  protocols 440–1, 442
  safety attitude questionnaire 441
  simulation 442
  standardization of fetal monitoring
      assessment 441–2
  team training 441
  tools for improving 440–2
pelvic artery occlusion, placenta accreta/
    percreta 294
pelvic pressure pack 293
  postpartum hemorrhage 295
Pena-Shokier phenotype **66**
penicillin
  allergy 235, **236**
  group B streptococcal infection 234, 235
  syphilis treatment 222
perinatal death
  chronic hypertension 207
  HELLP syndrome 284
  multifetal pregnancy 13
perinatal infections 218–28
perinatal medicine, advances 1, **2**, 3
perinatal mortality
  asthma in pregnancy 184
  cesarean delivery 406
  multiple gestations 395–6
  underweight women 7–8
perinatal patient safety nurse 441
perinatal team 3
perineal lacerations 392
peripartum cardiomyopathy (PPCM) 141–3
  management 142, *143*
  recurrent 142–3
  risk factors 142
peritoneal closure, cesarean delivery 408
pesticides, toxicity 35, **37**
pharmacotherapy, alcohol/substance abuse
    26–7
phenobarbital 194
  alcohol abuse withdrawal 27
  bilirubin conjugation by fetal liver 310, **312**
phenytoin 194–5, 196, **200**
pheochromocytoma, chronic hypertension 205
phosphatidylglycerol (PG) 75–6
phototherapy 310, **312**
physical disabilities, maternal 253–7, **257–8**
  antepartum consultation 254
  autonomic dysreflexia 256, **257–8**
  barriers to care 254–5
  bladder dysfunction 253
  cerebral palsy 257
  delivery 256, **258**
  labor 256, **258**
  medication use 254, **255**
  mobility 254
  multiple sclerosis 256
  parenting 255
  planning for baby care **257**
  pregnancy outcomes 255–7

preterm birth 256
psychosocial risk factors 254
respiratory function 256
rheumatoid arthritis 256–7
skin integrity 254, 256
spinal cord injuries 253, 255–6, **257–8**
urinary tract infection 253, 256, **257**
venous thromboembolism 253
weight gain 253–4
physical violence/abuse, women with physical
    disabilities 254
placenta 5–6
  adherent 289–90, 294, **297–8**
  confined mosaicism 460–1
  manual removal with cesarean delivery 407
  migration 384
  retained 289
  systemic lupus erythematosus 211
  trapped 289
placenta accreta 293–6, 387–8
  clinical presentation 388
  diagnosis 388
  imaging 388
  incidence 387–8
  management 293–6
  pathophysiology 388
  risk after hysterotomy 465
  risk factors 387–8
  unexpected at delivery 296
placenta percreta
  management 293–6
  postpartum hemorrhage 293–6
  unexpected at delivery 296
placenta previa 382–5
  case presentation **388–9**
  classification 382, *383*
  clinical presentation 382
  complications 384–5
  delivery mode/timing 385
  diagnosis 382–4
  incidence 382
  management 384
  placental migration 384
  risk factors 382
  ultrasound 383–4
  uterine incisions 385
placental α-microglobulin 1 (PAMG-1) 365
placental abruption
  antiphospholipid antibody syndrome 265
  chronic hypertension 207
  decidual hemorrhage biomarker 353
  inherited thrombophilias 112–13
  maternal complications with multiple
      gestations 318, **319**
  PPROM 349–50
  preterm delivery 349–50
    decidual hemorrhage biomarker 353
placental hormones 5, 6
placentation, abnormal 318, **319**
plasma osmolality 151
plasma volume in pregnancy 131, *132*
plasminogen activator inhibitor 1 (PAI-1) 123
  inherited thrombophilia 111–12
  levels in pregnancy 108, **109**
plasminogen activator inhibitor 2 (PAI-2) 123
Plasmodium (malaria) 231
platelet α-granules 122
platelets
  activation 121–2
  adhesion 121
  aggregation 122
  count in HELLP syndrome 284–5
  plug formation 121–2
  postpartum hemorrhage 295
  recruitment stimulation 304, *305*
  transfusion 303–4
    idiopathic thrombocytopenic purpura 103
pneumonia
  sickle cell disease 94–5
  varicella 227
polychlorinated biphenyls (PCBs) 35–6, **37**
polycystic ovarian syndrome 262

polyhydramnios 330–2
  anencephaly 329
  associations 331
  complications 331
  congenital malformations 331
  definition 330
  diabetes mellitus 176, 331
  diagnosis 330–1
  erythroblastosis fetalis 331
  fetal anomalies 331
  idiopathic 331
  labor 331
  management 331–2
  postpartum hemorrhage **297–8**
  renal agenesis 328
  sequelae 331
  twin pregnancy **334**
  twin-twin transfusion syndrome diagnosis
    470
ponderal index *see* body-length ratio
postdate pregnancy
  oligohydramnios 333
  see also prolonged pregnancy
postpartum depression 434
  women with physical disabilities 254
postpartum hemorrhage 289–97, **297–8**
  activated factor VIII 295
  adherent placenta 289–90, 294, **297–8**
  aortic clamping 295
  arterial embolization 292, 295
  blood products 295
  conservative management 295–6
  fluid administration 295
  hysterectomy 292–3
  internal iliac artery embolization 293, 295
  magnesium supplementation 15–16
  maternal complications with multiple
      gestations 318, **319**
  mechanical control 291
  pelvic pressure pack 293, 295
  persistent 295
  placenta accreta 293–6
  placenta percreta 293–6
  polyhydramnios **297–8**
  postoperative management 295
  primary 289
  retained placenta 289
  secondary 289
  surgical control 291
  temporizing management 295
  trapped placenta 289
  uncontrolled 295
  uterine atony 290–3
  uterine brace sutures 291
  uterine devascularization 291–2
  uterine inversion 296–7
  uterine tamponade 291
posttraumatic stress disorder (PTSD)
  recurrent spontaneous abortion 266
  unrelieved pain 434
potassium chloride intracardiac injection
    317
Potter syndrome, oligohydramnios 333
prednisone 161
preeclampsia 280–4
  abnormal angiogenesis 281
  antiphospholipid antibodies 115
  antiphospholipid antibody syndrome 265
  asthma in pregnancy 184
  cardiac transplant patient **166**
  chronic hypertension 205, 207, **208**
  definition 280
  delivery 282–3, **287**
  diagnosis 280
  fetal demise **450–1**
  hydralazine **287**
  hypocalciuria 15
  hypothyroidism **181**
  inherited thrombophilias 112
  labor induction **443**
  liver transplantation 164
  lupus flare differential diagnosis 211

magnesium sulfate **287**
management 281–4
maternal complications with multiple
    gestations 318, 319
multifetal pregnancy 13
pathophysiology 281
perinatal outcome 281
plasminogen activator inhibitor 1 levels 112
postpartum management 283–4
prediction 287
prevention 287
proteinuria 153
renal disease **158**
renal transplantation patients 163
severe 280, 281, **287**
    management 282–3
severity 280
sickle cell disease 95, **96**
systemic lupus erythematosus 212, **215**
thrombocytopenia 103
transplant patients 165
weight gain during pregnancy 8
pregnancy (general)
    adverse cardiac events 133
    blood volume 131
    dating 63–4
        first trimester 63
        second/third trimesters 63–4
    dietary recommendations **10**, 18–19, **20**
    energy requirement 6
    hemostatic changes 108, **109**
    high risk **394**
    outcome
        adverse 7–9
        maternal nutrition 4
        obesity 11–13
    physiologic changes 131, **132**
        anesthesia 436–7
    sickle cell disease 93–4
    weight gain 6, 7–9
    see also prolonged pregnancy
pregnancy-associated plasma protein A
    (PAPP-A) 57, **61**
    Down syndrome diagnosis 320
    with NT measurement 59, 320
preimplantation genetic screening (PGS) 261
preimplantation genetics 3
prematurity
    adverse outcomes 321
    multiple gestations 314
prenatal care, comprehensive 27, **28–9**, 30
prenatal diagnosis, indications 453
preterm birth
    abruption-associated 349–50
    acute-phase reactant inflammatory
        biomarkers 353
    amniotic fluid protein biomarkers 353
    antibiotic therapy 339
    asthma in pregnancy 184, 186
    cerebral palsy 337
    cervical cerclage 339–41
    cervical changes 339–40
    cervical length 339–40, 341, 354–5
    chorioamnionitis 339, 374
    consequences 374
    costs 337
    decidual-amnion-chorion inflammation
        348–9
    definition 337, 346
    etiology 346–51
    handicap risk 337
    immunosuppressive agents 166
    incidence 346
    infections 339
    inflammatory biomarkers 352–3
    likelihood ratios 351–2
    liver transplantation 164
    magnesium sulfate neuroprotection 449–50
    markers of final common pathway 353–5
    maternal BMI 8–9
    mechanical stretching of uterus 350–1
    medically indicated 346

monoamnionicity 318
multifetal pregnancy 13
multiple gestations 314, 317
malaria-induced 232
omega-3 fatty acids 339
pathogenesis 346–51
placental abruption 353
PPROM 339, **342**, 346
prediction 351–3
prevention 337–43
progesterone prophylaxis 341–3
prostaglandins 347, 351
proteomics 352–3
racial factors 337, 348
rate 337
retained placenta 289
risk with hysterotomy 465
spontaneous 271, 346
social phenomenon 337–8
systemic lupus erythematosus 212, **215**
tocolytic agents 338
women with physical disabilities 256–7
preterm labor 375
    activity restriction 376–7
    antibiotic prophylaxis 377
    assessment 375
    β-mimetics 377–8
    calcium channel blockers 378
    case presentation **380**
    cervical length 375
    corticosteroids 375–6, **380**
    COX inhibitors 378–9
    delivery mode 380
    diagnosis 375
    evaluation 374, **375**
    fetal fibronectin 375
    group B streptococcal infection prophylaxis
        377
    history taking 374
    hydration 377
    indomethacin 378–9, **380**
    magnesium sulfate 190, 338, 379
    management 374–80
    multiple gestations 317
    neonatal morbidity/mortality prevention
        375–6
    neuroprotection 376
    oxytocin receptor antagonists 379
    physical exam 374
    progesterone use 377
    prophylaxis 375–6
    risk factors 374, **375**
        hysterotomy 465
    screening tests 374
    tocolysis 377–9
    tocolytic agents 338
preterm premature rupture of membranes
    (PPROM) 364–70, **371**
    African-American mothers 348
    antibiotic therapy 339
    cerclage complication 276, 370
    cervical insufficiency **277–8**
    cesarean delivery **371**
    clinical course 365–6
    complications 366
    diagnosis 365
    emergency cesarean delivery **356**
    evaluation 366–7
    fetal demise 366
    fetal membrane resealing 370
    gestational age estimation 369
    group B streptococcal infection 235–6, *237*
    labor induction 369–70
    latency to delivery 365
    liver transplantation 164
    management 367–70, **371**
    maternal complications with multiple
        gestations 318, **319**
    mechanisms 364
    near-term 367
    oligohydramnios 333
    placental abruption 349–50

prediction 364–5
preterm birth 339, **342**
preterm delivery 346
prevention 365
previable 369–70
prostaglandin synthesis 347
remote from term 367–9
resuscitation **356**
risk factors 364–5
    hysterotomy 465
special circumstances 370
systemic lupus erythematosus 212, **215**
tocolytic agents 369
vaginal pool specimens 75
primidone 194
progesterone
    cervical insufficiency 277
    PPROM prevention 365
    preterm birth prevention 341–3
    preterm delivery 346
    preterm labor prevention 377
    recurrent spontaneous abortion 262
    safety 342
progesterone receptors (PR) 346
progestogens, preterm birth prevention 342
prolonged pregnancy 391–3, *394*, 395–6, **396–7**
    antepartum fetal assessment 393, 395
    cervical examination favorability 395
    cesarean delivery 392
    complications 391–2
    definition 391
    delivery timing 393
    etiology 391, **392**
    fetal risk 391–2
    gestational age 395
    intrapartum management 396
    management 392–3, *394*, 395–6
    maternal risk 392
    multiple gestations 395–6
    neonatal mortality 392, *394*
    nutritional growth restriction 5
    oligohydramnios 333
    prevalence 391
    prevention 392–3, *394*, 395–6
    prognosis 396
    stillbirth 392, *394*, 395
propranolol 181
propylthiouracil 180
prostacyclin PGI$_2$ 351
prostacyclin PGI$_2$ synthase 351
prostaglandin(s), preterm delivery 351
prostaglandin E$_2$
    cervical ripening 190
    preterm delivery 347
    uterine atony 290, 291
    uterine rupture 403
prostaglandin F$_{2\alpha}$ 347
    uterine atony 290–1
prostaglandin synthetase inhibitors,
    polyhydramnios 332
protease, preterm delivery 346, 351
protease-activated receptor (PAR) type 1 350
protease inhibitors 245, **247–9**, 250
protein C deficiency 108
    inherited thrombophilia 110–11
protein kinase C (PKC), activation 121
protein S, pregnancy levels 108, **109**
protein S deficiency 108
    inherited thrombophilia 110
protein supplementation, maternal nutrition
    14
protein X deficiency, inherited thrombophilia
    111
protein Z-dependent protease inhibitor (ZPI)
    123
proteinuria
    maternal 152–3
    preeclampsia 153
prothrombin G20210A mutation 108
    inherited thrombophilia 110
psychiatric disorders, alcohol/substance abuse
    26

psychosocial interventions, alcohol/substance
    abuse 26
psychosocial risk factors, women with physical
    disabilities 254
pterygium syndromes, lethal multiple 261
pulmonary arteriography, pulmonary
    embolism 125–6
pulmonary edema, amniotic fluid embolism
    301
pulmonary embolism 121
    clinical presentation 125
    diagnosis 125–7, *128*
    diagnostic algorithm *128*
    maternal complications with multiple
        gestations 318
    spiral computed tomographic pulmonary
        angiography 126–7
    work-up of patients 127
pulmonary hypertension
    epidural anesthesia 140
    lung transplant 165
    maternal 140
    sickle cell disease 95
pulmonary hypoplasia, oligohydramnios 332
pulmonary outflow tract 50
pulmonary valve stenosis 135
pyelonephritis, sickle cell disease 94
pyrimethamine, toxoplasmosis treatment 223

quinine, malaria treatment 232

racial factors
    fetal lung maturity 76
    preterm birth 337, 348
radio-iodine therapy 178
radiofrequency ablation 471, **472**
receptor for advanced glycated end-products
    (RAGE) 349
red blood cells (RBCs)
    hemolysis in sickle cell disease 93
    intravascular transfusion 310
    prophylactic transfusion in sickle cell disease
        95
    volume in pregnancy *132*
red cell alloimmunization 307–10, **311**, **312**
reflux, asthma during pregnancy 187
renal agenesis, polyhydramnios 328
renal artery stenosis, chronic hypertension 205
renal dialysis, maternal 156, **158**
renal disease, maternal 151, 152–7
    chronic hypertension 205
    diabetic nephropathy **158**
    dialysis 156, **158**
    fetal surveillance 157
    lupus nephritis 156, **158**
    management 157
    nephrotic syndrome 152–3, 157
    preeclampsia **158**
    proteinuria 152–3
    renal insufficiency 153–5, **158**
    renal transplantation 156
    renal tubular acidosis **157**
renal function, physiologic changes in
    pregnancy 151–2
renal insufficiency, maternal 153–5
    mild 153, **158**
    moderate/severe 153–4
renal plasma flow (RPF) 152
renal transplantation patients 156, 160–3
    antepartum care 160–1
    glomerular filtration rate 163
    pregnancy 162–3
    rejection 163
    technique *161*
    urinary tract infection 161
    viral infection prophylaxis 161
renal tubular acidosis **157**
respiration, fetal 5
respiratory distress syndrome (RDS)
    gestational diabetes 171
    labor induction 400–1
    lecithin:sphingomyelin ratio 75

prevention with corticosteroids 375–6
    risk 76
    transient tachypnea 400–1
respiratory function, women with physical
    disabilities 256
resuscitation, fetal 91
reticulocyte count, anemia 99, **100**
retrochorionic hematoma 350
RhD alloimmunization 307–10, **312**
    antibody titer 308
    clinical management 309–10
    fetal blood typing 309
    fetomaternal transfusion with amniocentesis
        454
    first sensitized pregnancy 309–10
    intrauterine transfusion 310, **312**
    outcome 310
    phototherapy 310, **312**
    previous severely affected fetus/infant 310
    surveillance 308
    ultrasound 308–9
RhD positivity 103, 307–9, **312**
    idiopathic thrombocytopenic purpura 103
rhesus (Rh) immune prophylaxis 1
rhesus (Rh) immunization 1
rhesus immunoglobulin (RhIg) 307–8
rheumatic heart disease 134
rheumatoid arthritis, women with physical
    disabilities 256–7
ritodrine 377–8
Roberts syndrome, IUGR **66**
root cause analysis (RCA) **443**
rubella, perinatal infection 220–1

sacrococcygeal teratoma, hysterotomy
    indication 468
safety *see* patient safety
Safety Attitude Questionnaire (SAQ) 440, 441
salmeterol 187–8
Seckel syndrome **66**
seizures 193
    amniotic fluid embolism 301
    during delivery 198
    eclampsia 285, 286
    during labor 199
    magnesium sulfate prophylaxis **181**, 286
    perimortem cesarean delivery **306**
    during pregnancy 196–7
    see also epilepsy, maternal
selective termination 315, 317
selenium toxicity 17
serine protease inhibitors (SERPINs) 123
sex steroids 6
shingles 227
Shirodkar cerclage 273
shoulder dystocia 392
    cesarean delivery 416
    gestational diabetes 171
sickle cell disease 93–6
    bacteriuria 94
    carrier screening 44
    crises 95, **96**
    delivery 95
    fetal assessment 95
    genetic evaluation 95–6
    heart failure 95
    hemoglobin SC disease 93, 94, **95**
    hemoglobin SS disease 93, 94, **95**, **96**
    hypertension 95, **96**
    labor 95
    pneumonia 94–5
    preeclampsia 95, **96**
    pregnancy 93–4
    prophylactic RBC transfusions 95
    pulmonary hypertension 95
    pyelonephritis 94
    vasoocclusion 93
Silver-Russell syndrome, IUGR **66**
single deepest pocket (SDP) measurement of
    amniotic fluid 330
single-gene disorders 43
    spontaneous abortion 261–2

sinusitis, asthma during pregnancy 184, 187
sirolimus 162
Sjögren syndrome **157**
skin integrity, women with physical disabilities
    254
sleep apnea syndrome, chronic hypertension
    205
small for gestational age (SGA) infants 64
    excessive weight gain 19
    maternal birthweight 65
    obesity 12
    paternal birthweight 65
    plasminogen activator inhibitor 1 levels 112
    prepregnancy BMI 8, 9
    sirolimus association 162
Smith-Lemli-Opitz syndrome **66**
SMN1 gene mutations 43
smoking
    asthma in pregnancy 187
    education 27
socioeconomic factors, preterm birth 337–8
sodium excretion/reabsorption 151
sonographic dating 63–4
sphingomyelin 75
spina bifida, maternal 253, 257
spinal anesthesia 436, 437
    fetal intervention guided by sonography 471
spinal cord injuries 253, 255–6, **257–8**
spinal muscular atrophy, carrier screening
    42–3
spiral computed tomographic pulmonary
    angiography (CTPA) 126–7
splenectomy, idiopathic thrombocytopenic
    purpura 103
spontaneous preterm birth syndrome 271, 276
status epilepticus 197
stillbirth
    prolonged pregnancy 392, *394*, 395
    systemic lupus erythematosus impact 212
streptococcal infection *see* group B
    streptococcal (GBS) infection
stress
    preterm delivery 346–8
    women with physical disabilities 254
stroke
    prevention 206
    transplant patients 165
stroke volume
    perimortem cesarean delivery 304–5
    pregnancy *132*
stuck twin 316
substance abuse 23–4, **25**, 26–7, **28–9**, 29–30
    breastfeeding 30
    comprehensive prenatal care 27, **28–9**, *29*
    contraception 30
    development effects 26
    fetal effects 23–4, **25**, 26
    follow-up 30
    following childbirth 30
    hepatitis C 30
    HIV infection risk 30
    hospital care 29–30
    pharmacotherapy 26–7
    postpartum care 29–30
    psychiatric disorders 26
    psychosocial interventions 26
    screening for 23, **24**
    therapy during pregnancy 26–7
    women with physical disabilities 254
sulfadoxine-pyrimethamine, malaria
    prevention 232
sulfonamides, toxoplasmosis treatment 223
sulfonylurea drugs 170
surfactant, lamellar body count 76
surfactant:albumin ratio (SAR) 75, 76
surgery *see* cesarean delivery
surgery, fetal 464–71, **472**
    fetoscopic 468–71
    open 464–8
    sonographic guided intervention 471, **472**
    see also hysterotomy
swallowing, fetal 329

syphilis 221–2
systemic bacterial endocarditis (SBE)
    prevention 134
systemic lupus erythematosus (SLE) 209–15
    autoantibodies 209–10
    chronic hypertension 205
    congenital heart block 212–13
    counseling 213
    diagnosis **215**
    differential diagnosis 211
    early pregnancy assessment 213
    environmental factors 209
    epidemiology/etiology 209, **210**
    genetic factors 209
    hormonal factors 209
    lupus flares 210, 211–12
        diagnosis 213
    management during pregnancy 213–15, **215**
    morbidity 211–13
    pathogenesis 209–11
    placenta 211
    postpartum damage 212
    pregnancy
        adverse outcomes 212
        effects on 212–13
        impact of 211–12
    systemic manifestations 209
systolic:diastolic ratio 83

tacrolimus 162
Tay-Sachs disease 42
    carrier screening 44, **45**, **46**
TDx test 76
team training, patient safety 441
teratogens
    fetal effects 24, **25**
    immunosuppressant drugs 162
terbutaline 377–8
tetralogy of Fallot, maternal 141
thalassemias 44
theophylline 188
thioamide drugs 180, 181
thrombin 122, 304, *305*
    activation 123
    decidual hemorrhage biomarker 353
    PPROM 350
thrombin-activatable fibrinolysis inhibitor
        (TAFI) 123
thrombin-antithrombin complex (TAT) 353
thrombocytopenia 102–5, **106**
    alloimmune 104
    autoimmune 102–3, 104
    disseminated intravascular coagulation 302
    fetal 104–5, **106**
        cordocentesis 105
        intracranial hemorrhage 104, 105
        treatment 105
    folate deficiency 99
    gestational 102, **106**
    HELLP syndrome 103
    maternal 102–3, **106**
    platelet transfusion 303–4
    preeclampsia 103
thromboembolic disorders 121–8
    predisposition in pregnancy 131
thromboembolism
    maternal complications with multiple
        gestations 318, **319**
    risk with nephrotic syndrome 157
thrombophilias 108–16, **117**
    acquired 108, 114–15
        screening **116**
    adverse pregnancy outcome prevention
        115–16
    inherited 109–14, 263–4
        pregnancy complications 112–14
        screening **116**
    recurrent spontaneous abortion 263–5
thrombophilic mutations 108
thromboprophylaxis, cesarean delivery 408
thrombosis 122, 123
thromboxane A$_2$ 121

thrombus formation, disseminated
        intravascular coagulation 303
thyroid-stimulating hormone (TSH) 178–9,
        180, **181**
thyroid storm 180–1
thyroidectomy 178
thyroiditis, postpartum 181
thyrotoxicosis 179–81
    transient 181
thyroxine, free (fT$_4$) 178–9
thyroxine replacement 181
tissue factor 122
    decidual 123
    pregnancy levels 108
    thrombin generation 122
tissue factor pathway inhibitor (TFPI) 123
tissue-type plasminogen activator (tPA) 123
tocolysis
    magnesium sulfate **342**
    preterm labor 377–9
        maintenance 379
tocolytic agents 321
    cervical insufficiency 277
    PPROM 369
    preterm birth 338
    preterm labor 338
Toll-like receptors (TLRs) 348, 349
toxoplasmosis, perinatal infection 222–4
transesophageal echocardiogram (TEE),
        pulmonary embolism 125, 127
transplant patients 160–6
    cardiac transplantation 164–5, **166**
        pregnancy after 144, 146
    contraindications to pregnancy 160
    counseling 160
    immunosuppressive agents 161–2
    intrapartum management 165
    life expectancy 160, **166**
    liver transplantation 164
    lung transplantation 165
    obstetric emergencies 165–6
    optimum outcome **161**
    pancreatic transplant patients 163–4
    pregnancy assessment 160
    renal transplantation 156, 160–3
    timing of pregnancy 160
transposition of the great arteries
    fetal **53**
    maternal 141
Treponema pallidum (syphilis) 221
Trichomonas vaginalis, PPROM risk 365
tricuspid lesions 135
tricuspid regurgitation
    Down syndrome 56
    post-cardiac transplant 164
trinucleotide repeats 42
triploidy, IUGR 65
trisomy 13 55
    IUGR 65
trisomy 16 461
trisomy 18 55
    cardiac malformations 58
    IUGR 65
    neural tube defects 61
    septated cystic hygroma 57
trisomy 21 55
    frontomaxillary facial angle measurement 56
trisomy 22 **266**
trisomy rescue 461
trophoblast inclusions **266**
tryptase, amniotic fluid embolism 301
Turner syndrome, septated cystic hygroma 57
twin clinics, specialized 321
twin pregnancy
    acardiac 471, **472**
    amniocentesis 76
    conjoined 314
    fetal demise **472**
    fetal growth 4–5
    oligohydramnios 333–4, **334**
    polyhydramnios **334**
    weight discordancy **334**

twin reverse arterial perfusion (TRAP) 314,
        471, **472**
twin-twin transfusion syndrome 314, 318
    diagnosis 470
    endoscopic laser ablation of
        intercommunicating placental vessels
        334
    fetoscopic surgery 470
        percutaneous 469
    nuchal translucency measurement 320
    oligohydramnios 334, **334**
    polyhydramnios **334**

uE3, Down syndrome screening 59
ultrasound
    amniotic fluid volume assessment 329–30
    cervical insufficiency 275
    cervical length measurement 339, 374, 375,
        402
    chorionicity diagnosis 315–16
    Doppler studies in fetal growth restriction
        67–71
    fetal intervention guided by 471
    maternal renal disease 157
    multiple gestations **322**
    placenta previa 383–4
    pregnancy dating 63–4
        chronic hypertension 207
    preterm labor evaluation 374
    prior to amniocentesis 453–4
    RhD alloimmunization 308–9
    uterine scar evaluation 419
    uterine wall stretch/activation markers
        353
    vasa previa 387
    venous
        DVT 124–5
        lower extremity in pulmonary embolism
            127
    see also color Doppler imaging; Doppler
        ultrasound; Doppler velocimetry
umbilical arterial circulation, Doppler
        ultrasound 67–8
umbilical artery
    Doppler velocimetry 83, **86**
    end-diastolic flow
        reversed 67, 83
        velocity absence 67, **71**
undernourished women, energy/protein
        supplementation 14
underweight women, perinatal mortality
        7–8
uniparental disomy (UPD) 461
upper respiratory tract infections 184
Ureaplasma urealyticum 349
urethral obstruction, fetal 470
urinary tract, anatomic changes in pregnancy
        152
urinary tract infection, maternal
    maternal complications with multiple
        gestations 318, **319**
    renal transplantation patients 161
    women with physical disability 253, 256,
        257
urinary tract obstruction, fetoscopic surgery
        470–1
urine, fetal 328
uterine activity
    cerclage 276
    eclampsia 286–7
    prophylactic bedrest 321
uterine brace sutures, postpartum hemorrhage
        291
uterine closure technique, vaginal birth after
        cesarean delivery 418
uterine contractions, ambulatory home
        monitoring 321
uterine devascularization, postpartum
        hemorrhage 291–2
uterine incisions
    extra-/intra-abdominal repair 407
    placenta previa 385

uterine inversion, postpartum hemorrhage 296–7
uterine overactivity, labor induction 402
uterine-placental dysfunction 65
uterine polyps, recurrent spontaneous abortion 263
uterine relaxation, uterine inversion 297
uterine rupture
  hysterectomy 417
  labor induction 403
  oxytocin 403, 419
  risk factors 417
  risk with prior cesarean delivery 403–4, 416–19
  sequelae 417
  vaginal birth after cesarean delivery 420
uterine scar, sonographic evaluation 419
uterine tamponade, postpartum hemorrhage 291
uterine wall stress 350
uterus
  abnormalities causing recurrent spontaneous abortion 263, 266
  atony and postpartum hemorrhage 290–3
  blood flow 205–6
  involution 305
  mechanical stretching 350–1
    ultrasonographic markers 353
  submucous myoma 263

vacuum extraction 429, 430, 431, **433**
vaginal antiseptic prophylaxis, cesarean delivery 407
vaginal birth after cesarean delivery 406, *407*, 408–9, 414–20, **421**
  birthweight 416
  counseling 419–20, **421**
  epidural analgesia 419, 435
  fetal heart rate monitoring 419
  hypoxic ischemic encephalopathy 420
  informed consent 420
  interpregnancy interval 418
  labor augmentation 419
  labor induction 418–19
  large for gestational age 416
  macrosomia 416
  management 419–20, **421**
  maternal demographics 416
  multiple prior cesarean deliveries 416, **421**
  number of prior cesarean deliveries 417–18
  previous incision type 416
  prior indication for cesarean delivery 416
  prior vaginal delivery 416, 418
  risks 416–19
  trends 414–15
  trial of labor 414–15
    candidates for 415
    risks 420, **421**
    success rates 415–16

uterine closure technique 418
uterine rupture 420
  risk 416–19
uterine scar sonographic evaluation 419
vaginal bleeding, cardiac transplant patient **166**
vaginal delivery
  analgesia 434–6
  breech presentation 424–7
  operative 429–32, **433**
    classification 430
    criteria for forceps delivery **430**
    indications 429
    instrument selection 429–30
    nontechnical surgical skills 431–2
    outcomes 432
    prerequisites 429
    skill 431–2
    training 432
vaginal pessaries, cervical insufficiency 277
vaginal pool specimen collection 75
valaciclovir, herpes simplex virus 225
valproic acid 195, **200**
  neural tube defects 194
    induced 16
  neurodevelopmental outcome 196
valvular heart disease 134, **135**
vancomycin, group B streptococcal infection 235
vanishing twin 317
varicella vaccine 228
varicella zoster virus (VZV) 227–8
vasa previa 385–7
  cesarean delivery 387
  clinical presentation 386, *387*
  diagnosis 386–7
  incidence 386
  management 387
  outcomes 387
  pathophysiology 386
  risk factors 386
vasculopathy, nutritional growth restriction 5
vasoconstrictors **145**
vasodilators **145**
vasoocclusion (VOC) 93, 94, **96**
vasopressin 151
vasopressors 437
venous thromboembolism 121
  acquired thrombophilia 115
  antithrombin deficiency 111
  diagnosis 124–7, *128*
  women with physical disability 253
venous ultrasonography
  DVT 124–5
  lower extremity in pulmonary embolism 127
ventilation/perfusion (V/Q) scans, pulmonary embolism 126–7

ventricular hypoplasia, time of occurrence 52
ventricular outflow tracts, fetal echocardiography 49–51, 52–3
ventricular septal defect (VSD)
  fetal echocardiography Plate 6.3
  maternal 139
ventricular systolic function 49
vibroacoustic stimulation (VAS) 80
video display terminals 36
viral infections
  asthma during pregnancy 184
  liver transplant patients 164
  perinatal 218–21, 224–8
  renal transplantation patients 161
  see also named conditions and diseases
Virchow's triad 123
vitamin(s), toxicity 17–18
vitamin A toxicity 17
vitamin B$_6$ toxicity 17
vitamin B$_{12}$ deficiency 98
vitamin C
  maternal nutrition 17
  PPROM prevention 365
  toxicity 17
vitamin D
  maternal nutrition 16
  supplementation in antiphospholipid antibody syndrome 215
  toxicity 17
vitamin E, maternal nutrition 17
vitamin K
  deficiency in neonates affected by antiepileptic drugs 198
  transport inhibition by antiepileptic drugs 198
von Willebrand factor (vWF)
  platelet adhesion 121
  pregnancy levels 108

Weibel-Palade bodies 121, 122
weight gain
  adverse pregnancy outcome 7–9, 19
  preterm delivery incidence 8–9
  retained postpartum 12–13
  women with physical disabilities 253–4
white blood cells (WBC), maternal count in PPROM 366–7
Williams syndrome **66**
World War II, Dutch famine 8
wound infections, obesity 12

X-linked inheritance 41, 42

zidovudine 245, **246**, 250
  during labor 250, **251**
zinc toxicity 17–18
zygosity, multiple gestations 315–16